Perrino and Reeves' Practical Approach to Transesophageal Echocardiography

Fifth Edition

Perrino and Reeves' Practical Approach to Transesophageal Echocardiography

Fifth Edition

Editors

Albert C. Perrino, Jr, MD
Professor of Anesthesiology
Yale School of Medicine
Chief, Anesthesiology
VA Connecticut Healthcare System
New Haven, Connecticut

Scott T. Reeves, MD, MBA, FACC, FASE
The John E. Mahaffey, MD Professor and Chairman
Senior Associate Dean for Clinical Affairs
Anesthesia & Perioperative Medicine
Medical University of South Carolina
Charleston, South Carolina

Joshua M. Zimmerman, MD, FASE
Professor and Vice Chair
Director, Perioperative Echocardiography
Department of Anesthesiology
University of Utah
Associate Director, Echocardiography
Director, Cardiopulmonary Exercise Testing
George E. Wahlen VA Medical Center
Salt Lake City, Utah

Chirojit Mukherjee, MD, PhD, FASE, MBA
Chief of Anesthesiology
Department of Anesthesia and Intensive Care
Helios Heart Hospital
Karlsruhe, Germany

Wolters Kluwer

Philadelphia • Baltimore • New York • London
Buenos Aires • Hong Kong • Sydney • Tokyo

Acquisitions Editor: Keith Donnellan
Senior Development Editor: Ashley Fischer
Editorial Coordinator: Thirupura Sundari
Marketing Manager: Kirsten Watrud
Production Project Manager: Jennifer L. Harper
Manager, Graphic Arts & Design: Stephen Druding
Manufacturing Coordinator: Lisa Bowling
Prepress Vendor: S4Carlisle Publishing Services

Fifth edition

9 8 7 6 5 4 3 2 1

Printed in Mexico

Library of Congress Cataloging-in-Publication Data

ISBN-13: 978-1-975238-36-0

Library of Congress Control Number: 2025941645

shop.lww.com

QUADM0925

To Anita, Mary, Isabella, and Juliana for sustaining another of my adventures and to Winston Churchill whose keen observation also served as a source of support. "Writing is an adventure. To begin with, it is a toy and an amusement. Then it becomes a mistress, then it becomes a master, then it becomes a tyrant. The last phase is that just as you are about to be reconciled to your servitude, you kill the monster and fling him to the public." —ACP

❖

To my wife, Cathy, who loves and puts up with me. . .
My children, Catherine, Carolyn, Townsend, and
their spouses, Brandon, David, and Megan. . .
And finally, to the next generation of grandchildren,
Fletcher, Jason, David, and Elizabeth who give me great joy. . .
Train up a child in the way he should go; even when old he will not depart from it.
Proverbs 22:6—STR

❖

To my wonderful, thoughtful wife, Susan—thanks for being patient while I worked on the textbook (and while I repeatedly ultrasounded you and the cats).
To my mentor, Dr. Dan Vezina, who taught me that "if you don't look. . . you don't know"—thanks for the years of teaching and support.
To my students of all sorts in Utah and around the world—thanks for your enthusiasm, it keeps me stoked to teach!—JMZ

❖

To my beloved wife, Atashi, and our daughters, Ishikaa and Vedikaa—
Your love, patience, and unwavering support have been the quiet strength behind every page of this work. Thank you for your boundless encouragement, understanding, and the joy you bring into my life.
This book is as much yours as it is mine.
I am deeply grateful to Drs. Albert C. Perrino and Scott T. Reeves for the opportunity to contribute as an editor to this esteemed volume. Their mentorship, trust, and enduring contributions to the field of echocardiography continue to set a high standard for academic excellence and clinical leadership.
As Sir William Osler wisely noted, "The good physician treats the disease; the great physician treats the patient who has the disease."
It is in that spirit of patient-centered care and lifelong learning that I have approached this work, and I am honored to have played a part in advancing this educational mission.—CM

Preface

THE FIFTH EDITION represents a landmark in the publication of *A Practical Approach to Transesophageal Echocardiography*, now titled *Perrino and Reeves' Practical Approach to Transesophageal Echocardiography*. Five editions as editors is a rarity in medical publishing and an achievement beyond our wildest expectations when we began this project in 2001. The longevity serves as a testament to the enduring enthusiasm echocardiography engenders in clinical practice and the intrinsic value this handbook provides. Having witnessed early technology transformations, such as the biplane probe and color Doppler imaging, it is remarkable to witness the advancements imbedded in the current practice of echocardiography covered in this edition. The applications of 3-D imaging, 4-D quantitative analysis, and echocardiography's role expanding from the heart room to critical care and structural heart units are inspiring. For this latest edition to fully capture the state of the art of perioperative echocardiography, we recruited new contributors who are internationally renowned and acknowledged for their independent contributions and teaching ability. They were given the task of presenting a highly readable and clinically relevant survey of the current practice of perioperative echocardiography. Their enthusiasm backed with the strong support of the publisher has produced this volume.

And while perioperative echocardiography endures and expands, we recognize our role as lead editors is term limited. Twenty-five years is a remarkable run and we look forward to the contributions the next generation of editors and writers will bring. To that effect, Joshua M. Zimmerman and Chirojit Mukherjee enthusiastically agreed to come aboard as associate editors for this latest edition and lead the project forward in upcoming editions. Both are uniquely talented echocardiographers and educators that have enriched this edition both as editors and as authors. They have overseen a Fifth Edition that has been extensively updated, with many chapters rewritten with new images, illustrations, multiple-choice chapter-based questions and answers, as well as videos. Examples include echocardiography's evolving role in structural heart interventions and valve surgeries to the growing impact of artificial intelligence on image acquisition and interpretation.

We would especially like to thank the scores of Wolters Kluwer publication team members for their support through these five editions. To the artists, editors, and production team members who took our efforts and visions and embodied them into the finished product you hold today, we truly could not have found better partners for our project.

Lastly, to the readers, this edition further establishes the reputation of *A Practical Approach to Transesophageal Echocardiography* as the practicing clinicians' premier resource to acquire the essential skills of transesophageal (TEE) practice. The presentation, illustrations, and media content create a surprisingly portable and readable text that is conducive to rapid appreciation of the critical elements in the use of TEE for a particular clinical challenge. The associated e-book contains over 400 videos and 300 interactive multiple-choice chapter-based questions and answers to reinforce the reader's knowledge.

It is our hope that this Fifth Edition textbook will become a well-worn and valued asset to your echocardiography practice.

Albert C. Perrino, Jr, MD
Scott T. Reeves, MD, MBA, FACC, FASE

Contents

SECTION I: ESSENTIALS OF TWO-DIMENSIONAL IMAGING

SECTION II: ESSENTIALS OF DOPPLER ECHO

SECTION III: VALVULAR DISEASE

SECTION IV: CLINICAL CHALLENGES

APPENDICES

Contributors

Michael Benson, MD
Assistant Professor of Anesthesiology
Department of Anesthesiology and Perioperative Medicine
Oregon Health and Science University
Portland, Oregon

Mary Beth Brady, MD
Director, Intraoperative and Interventional Echocardiography
Department of Anesthesiology and Critical Care Medicine
The Johns Hopkins University School of Medicine
Baltimore, Maryland

Albert T. Cheung, MD
Professor
Department of Anesthesiology, Perioperative and Pain Medicine
Stanford Medicine
Stanford, California

Ettienne Coetzee, FCA, MBChB, MMed, DA
Specialist Anesthetist
Department of Anesthesia and Perioperative Medicine
University of Cape Town
Western Cape, South Africa

Ira S. Cohen, MD
Emeritus Professor of Medicine, Cardiovascular Disease
Department of Internal Medicine
Thomas Jefferson University, Sidney Kimmel School of Medicine of Free State
Philadelphia, Pennsylvania

Etienne J. Couture, MD
Anesthesiologist and Intensivist
Department of Anaesthesiology
Institut Universitaire De Cardiologie Et De Pneumologie de Québec—Université Laval
Quebec City, Quebec, Canada

Serena Dasani, MD, MBA
Assistant Professor
Department of Anesthesiology, Critical Care and Pain Medicine
The University of Texas Health Science Center at Houston
Houston, Texas

Jennifer Decou, MD
Anesthesiologist
Department of Anesthesiology
University of Utah School of Medicine
Salt Lake City, Utah

André Y. Denault, MD, PhD
Professor of Anesthesiology
Department of Anesthesiology
Montreal Heart Institute
Montreal, Canada

Jörg Ender, MD
Head of the Department of Anesthesiology and Intensive Care Medicine
Herzzentrum Leipzig
Leipzig, Germany

Joachim M. Erb, MD, DEAA
Chair, Cardiothoracic and Vascular Anaesthesia
Clinic for Anaesthesiology, Intermediate Care, Prehospital Emergency Medicine and Pain Therapy
University Hospital Basel
Basel, Switzerland

T. Robert Feng, MD, FASE
Clinical Assistant Professor
Department of Anesthesiology, Perioperative and Pain Medicine
Stanford Medicine
Stanford, California

Anna Flo Forner, MD
Senior Consultant, Anesthesiology
Department of Anesthesiology and Critical Care
Heart Center Leipzig
Leipzig, Germany

Michelle B. Gorgone, MD, MAS
Clinical Assistant Professor
Department of Anesthesia
Warren Alpert Medical School of Brown University
Providence, Rhode Island

Lars Grønlykke, MD, PhD
Anesthesiologist
Department of Cardiothoracic Anesthesia
Copenhagen University Hospital, Rigshospitalet
Copenhagen, Denmark

Fabio Guarracino, MD
Director
Cardiothoracic and Vascular Anesthesia and Intensive Care
Azienda Ospedaliero Universitaria Pisana
Pisa, Italy

Maurice Hogan, MB, BCh, MSc, MBA, FCAI, FASE
Consultant Intensivist
Cardiothoracic and Vascular Intensive Care Unit
Auckland City Hospital
Auckland, New Zealand

Karel Huard, MD
General Internist
Department of Critical Care Medicine
Université de Montréal
Montreal, Canada

Farid Jadbabaie, MD
Director of Echocardiography Laboratory
Department of Cardiology
VA Connecticut Healthcare System
West Haven, Connecticut

Worasak Keeyapaj, MD
Clinical Associate Professor
Department of Anesthesiology, Perioperative and Pain Medicine
Stanford Medicine
Stanford, California

Benjamin Kogelschatz, MD
Resident
Department of Internal Medicine
University of Utah School of Medicine
Salt Lake City, Utah

Megan P. Kostibas, MD
Assistant Professor
Department of Anesthesiology and Critical Care Medicine
The Johns Hopkins University School of Medicine
Baltimore, Maryland

Marc-Antoine Lepage, MD, MSc, FRCPC, RPNI
Internist and Intensivist
Department of Anesthesia and Critical Care
CHU de Quebec-Universite Laval
Quebec City, Quebec, Canada

Dai-Yin Lu, MD, PhD
Physician
Division of Cardiology
University of Utah Health
Salt Lake City, Utah

Nicholas W. Markin, MD
Associate Professor
Department of Anesthesiology
University of Nebraska Medical Center
Omaha, Nebraska

Andrew Maslow, MD
Attending Anesthesiologist
Department of Anesthesiology
Rhode Island Hospital
Providence, Rhode Island

Praveen Mehrotra, MD
Director of Echocardiography
Division of Cardiology
Thomas Jefferson University Hospital
Philadelphia, Pennsylvania

Anand R. Mehta, MD
Staff Anesthesiologist
Department of Cardiothoracic Anesthesia
Cleveland Clinic
Cleveland, Ohio

Massimiliano Meineri, MD
Leitender Oberrartz
Anesthesia dn Critical Care
Herzzentrum Leipzig
Leipzig, Germany

Wanda C. Miller-Hance, MD
Adjunct Professor
Departments of Anesthesiology, Critical Care and Pain Medicine and Pediatrics
Memorial Hermann Hospital
Children's Memorial Hermann Hospital
Houston, Texas

Candice Morrissey, MD, MSPH
Professor
Department of Anesthesiology, Perioperative and Pain Medicine
University of Utah School of Medicine
Salt Lake City, Utah

Pablo Motta, MD
Associate Professor
Department of Anesthesiology, Perioperative and Pain Medicine
Texas Children's Hospital
Baylor College of Medicine
Houston, Texas

Chirojit Mukherjee, MD, PhD, FASE, MBA
Chief of Anesthesiology
Department of Anesthesia and Intensive Care
Helios Heart Hospital
Karlsruhe, Germany

Jacques Neelankavil, MD
Director, Division of Cardiac Anesthesia
Department of Anesthesiology
Ronald Reagan UCLA Medical Center
Los Angeles, California

Charles Nyman, MBBCh
Director of Interventional Cardiac Anesthesiology
Department of Anesthesiology, Perioperative and Pain Medicine
Brigham and Women's Hospital
Boston, Massachusetts

Albert C. Perrino, Jr, MD
Professor of Anesthesiology
Yale School of Medicine
Chief, Anesthesiology
VA Connecticut Healthcare System
New Haven, Connecticut

Sophia P. Poorsattar, MD
Assistant Clinical Professor
Director of Perioperative Echocardiography
Divisions of Cardiothoracic and Liver Transplant Anesthesiology
David Geffen School of Medicine at UCLA
Ronald Reagan UCLA Medical Center
Los Angles, California

Wanda M. Popescu, MD
Professor of Anesthesiology
Department of Anesthesiology
Yale School of Medicine
New Haven, Connecticut

Satvik Ramakrishna, MD
Assistant Professor of Medicine
Division of Cardiology
Department of Medicine
University of Utah School of Medicine
Salt Lake City, Utah

Andrew Roscoe, MBChB
Consultant
Department of Anaesthesiology
Singapore General Hospital
Singapore, Singapore

John Ryan, MD
Cardiologist
Fellowship Program Director
Division of Cardiovascular Medicine
University of Utah Health
Salt Lake City, Utah

Marcus Salvatori, MSc, MBBS, FRCPC
Anesthesiologist
Department of Anesthesiology
Toronto General Hospital
Toronto, Canada

Roman M. Sniecinski, MD, MSc
Professor of Anesthesiology
Department of Anesthesiology
Emory University School of Medicine
Atlanta, Georgia

Michele L. Sumler, MD
Associate Professor
Department of Anesthesiology
Emory University School of Medicine
Atlanta, Georgia

Justiaan Swanevelder, MBChB, DA (SA), FCA (SA), MMed (Anes), FRCA
Emeritus Professor and Specialist Anesthesiologist
UCT Department of Anaesthesia and Perioperative Medicine
University of Cape Town
Cape Town, South Africa

Carolyn Taylor, MD
Professor
Department of Pediatric Cardiology
Medical University of South Carolina
Charleston, South Carolina

Sascha Treskatsch, MD, PhD
Head of Department
Department of Anesthesiology and Intensive Care Medicine, Campus Benjamin Franklin
Charite—Universitätsmedizin Berlin
Berlin, Germany

Ethan Tumarkin, MD, PhD
Assistant Professor of Medicine
Department of Internal Medicine
University of Utah School of Medicine
Salt Lake City, Utah

Edwin Turton, MD
Affiliated Lecturer
Department of Anesthesiology
University of Free State
Bloemfontein, South Africa

Annette Vegas, MD
Staff Anesthesiologist
Anesthesia and Pain Management
Toronto General Hospital
Toronto, Canada

Joshua M. Zimmerman, MD, FASE
Professor and Vice Chair
Director, Perioperative Echocardiography
Department of Anesthesiology
University of Utah
Associate Director, Echocardiography
Director, Cardiopulmonary Exercise Testing
George E. Wahlen VA Medical Center
Salt Lake City, Utah

Essentials of Two-Dimensional Imaging

1 Principles and Technology of Two-Dimensional Echocardiography

Michelle B. Gorgone, Andrew Maslow, and Albert C. Perrino, Jr

Two-dimensional (2D) echocardiography generates dynamic images of the heart from reflections of transmitted ultrasound. The echocardiography system transmits a brief pulse of ultrasound that propagates through, and is subsequently reflected from, the cardiac structures encountered. The sound reflections travel back to the ultrasound transducer, which records the time delay for each returning reflection. As the speed of sound in tissue is constant, the time delay allows for a precise calculation of the location of the cardiac structures from which the echocardiography system can then create an image map of the heart. Not surprisingly, successful cardiac imaging requires a firm understanding of the interactions of sound and tissue. This chapter reviews the basic principles of ultrasound, its propagation through tissues, and the technologies that create moving images of the heart.

PHYSICAL PROPERTIES OF SOUND WAVES

Vibrations

Sound is the vibration of a physical medium. In clinical echocardiography, a mechanical vibrator, known as the *transducer*, is placed in contact with the esophagus (transesophageal echocardiography [TEE]), skin (transthoracic echocardiography), or the heart (epicardial echocardiography) to create tissue vibrations. The resulting tissue vibrations or sound waves consist of areas of *compression* (areas where molecules are tightly packed) and *rarefaction* (areas where molecules are dispersed) resembling a sine wave (Figure 1.1).

Amplitude

The amplitude of a sound wave represents its peak pressure and is appreciated as loudness. The level of sound energy in an area of tissue is referred to as *intensity*. The intensity of the sound signal is proportional to the square of the amplitude and is an important factor regarding the potential for tissue damage with ultrasound. For example, lithotripsy uses high-intensity sound signals to fragment renal stones. In contrast, cardiac ultrasound uses low-intensity signals to image tissue, which produces only limited bioeffects. Since levels of sound pressure vary over a large range, it is convenient to use the logarithmic decibel (dB) scale:

$$\text{Decibel (dB)} = 10 \log_{10} I/I_r = 10 \log_{10} A^2/A_r^2$$
$$= 20 \log_{10} A/A_r$$

where A is the measured sound amplitude of interest and A_r is a standard reference sound level, I is the intensity and I_r is a standard reference intensity.

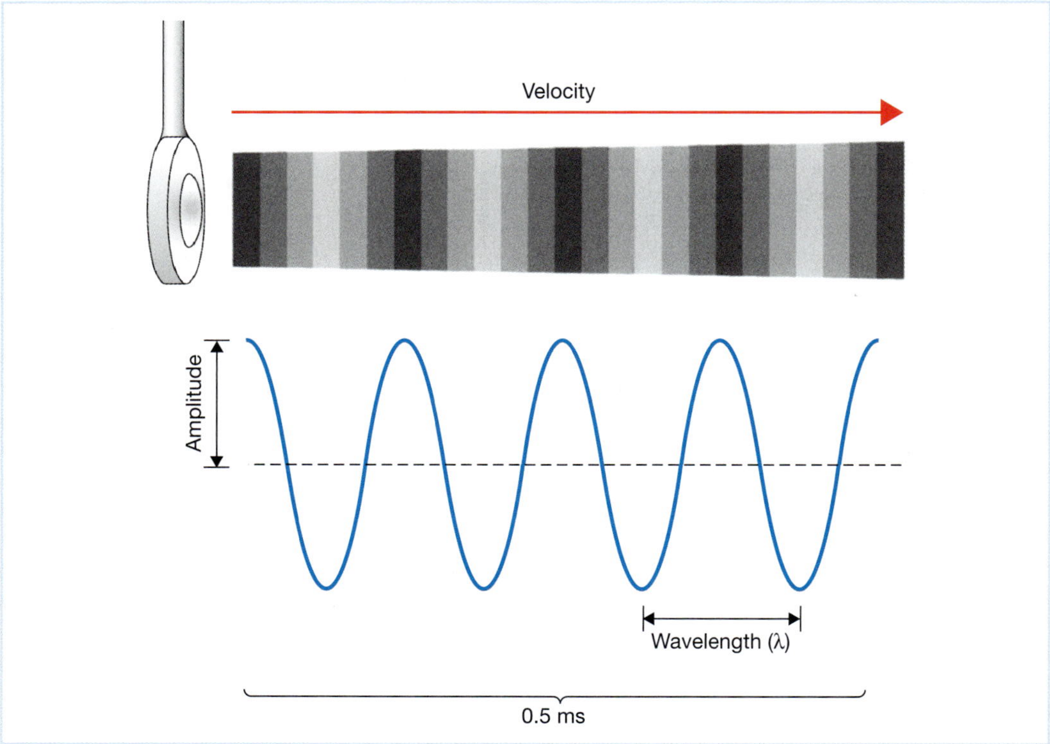

FIGURE 1.1 Sound wave. Vibrations of the ultrasound transducer create cycles of compression and rarefaction in adjacent tissue. The ultrasound energy is characterized by its amplitude, wavelength, frequency, and propagation velocity. In this example, four sound waves are shown in a period of 0.5 μs. The frequency can be calculated as four cycles divided by 0.5 μs and equals 8 MHz.

More simply expressed, each doubling of the sound pressure equals a gain of 6 dB. The U.S. Food and Drug Administration limits the maximum intensity output of cardiac ultrasound systems to be less than 720 W/cm^2 due to concerns with possible tissue and neurologic damage from mechanical injury (resulting from cavitation or microbubbles caused by rarefaction) and thermal effects. The ALARA principle recommends that clinicians limit exposure levels to that which is As Little As Reasonably Achievable to protect patients.

Frequency and Wavelength

Sound waves are also characterized by their *frequency* (f), or pitch, expressed in cycles per second, also known as hertz (Hz), and by their *wavelength* (λ). These attributes have a significant impact on the depth of penetration of a sound wave in tissue and the image resolution of the ultrasound system.

Propagation Velocity

The travel velocity or propagation velocity of sound (v) is determined solely by the medium through which it passes. For example, the speed of sound in soft tissue is approximately 1,540 m/s. Velocity can be calculated as the product of wavelength and frequency: $v = \lambda \times f$

It becomes apparent that the wavelength and frequency are necessarily inversely related:

$$\begin{aligned}\lambda &= v \times 1/f \\ &= 1{,}500 \text{ m/s}/f\end{aligned}$$

Table 1.1 lists the corresponding sound wavelengths and frequencies commonly used in clinical ultrasonography.

WHAT IS SO SPECIAL ABOUT ULTRASOUND?

Several favorable physical properties of ultrasound explain its usefulness in clinical imaging. *Ultrasound* is sound with frequencies above those in the audible range for humans (>20,000 Hz). In clinical echocardiography, frequencies of 2 to 10 MHz are typically used. These high-frequency, short-wavelength ultrasound

TABLE 1.1 Corresponding Frequencies and Wavelengths in Soft Tissue

Frequency (MHz)	Wavelength (mm)
1.25	1.20
2.5	0.60
5	0.30
7.5	0.20
10	0.15

beams can be more easily manipulated, focused, and directed to a specific target. Image resolution also increases when higher-frequency sound waves are used (see later).

INTERACTIONS OF SOUND AND TISSUE

The propagation, or passage, of a sound wave through the body is markedly affected by its interactions with the various tissues encountered. These interactions result in reflection, refraction, scattering, and attenuation of the ultrasound signal. The exact manner in which sound is affected by the various tissues it encounters determines the resulting appearance of the 2D image (Figure 1.2).

$$\text{Energy lost} = 1\ \text{dB/cm/MHz}$$

Reflection

Echocardiographic imaging depends on the transmission and subsequent reflection of ultrasound energy back to the transducer. A sound wave propagates through uniform tissue until it reaches another tissue type with different acoustic properties. At the tissue interface, the ultrasound energy undergoes a dramatic alteration, after which it can be reflected back toward the transducer or transmitted into the next tissue, often in a direction that deviates from the original course. Precisely how the ultrasound beam will be affected is predicted by factoring the acoustic properties of the tissues that create the interface and the angle at which the ultrasound beam strikes this interface.

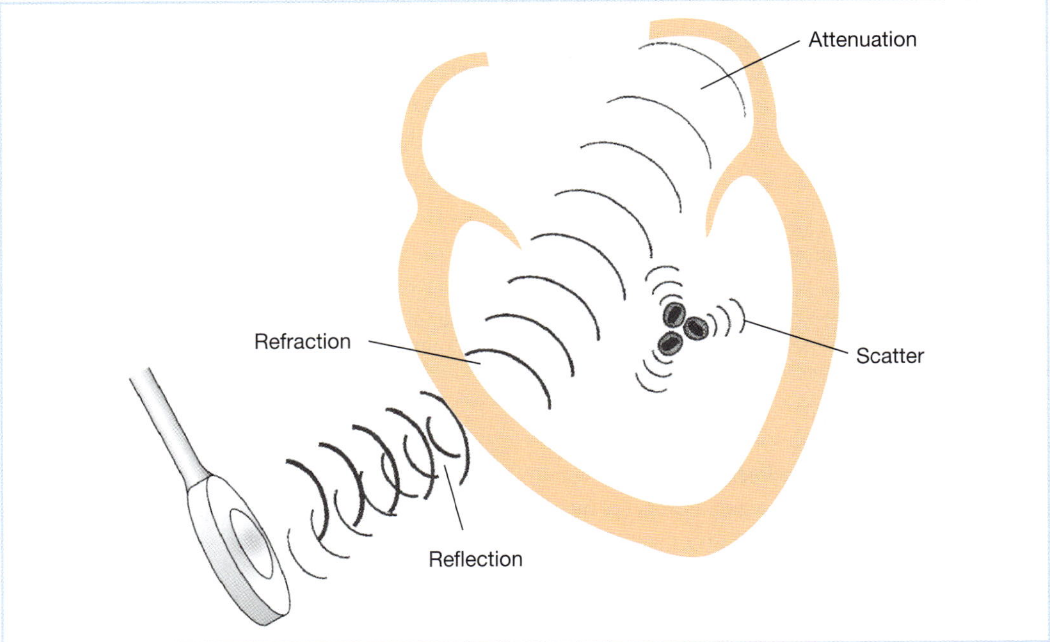

FIGURE 1.2 Interactions of sound and tissue. Traveling through various tissues, sound energy is altered by four major events. Specular *reflection* creates strong echoes directed back toward the transducer. *Refraction* bends the ultrasound beam, directing it in a new path. As the ultrasound beam travels deeper in tissue, *attenuation* occurs as the beam is dispersed, and the sound energy is converted to heat. *Scattering*; reflections from small objects such as red cells disperse the sound energy in all directions.

TABLE 1.2 Characteristics of a Variety of Tissues/Mediums on the Transmission of Sound

Tissue/Medium	Attenuation Coefficient (cm^{-1})	Acoustic Impedance (kg/m^2s)	Speed of Sound (m/s)	Half-Power Distance (2.5-MHz TDR) (cm)
Air		394.4	330	0.08
Lung		0.26×10^6	600	0.05
Fat	0.04–0.09	1.35×10^6	1,460	
Water	0.0003	1.52×10^6	1,480	380.0
Liver	0.07–0.13		1,555	1.0–5.0
Blood	0.02	1.62×10^6	1,560	15.0
Kidney			1,565	
Muscle	0.25–0.35	$1.65–1.74 \times 10^6$	1,600	0.6–1.0
Bone		7.80×10^6	4,080	0.7–0.8

Note: The half-power distances are for a 2.5-MHz transducer (TDR) frequency. Although the impedance of sound through air is low, the speed of sound and the half-power distances are comparatively low, reflecting the effects of dispersion of sound in air. Bone, which also has a relatively low half-power distance, is a highly reflective surface. Air travels farthest through water, which has minimal attenuation and intermediate impedance.

The Tissue Interface: Acoustic Impedance

An important acoustic property of a tissue is its capacity for transmitting sound, known as *acoustic impedance* (Z). This property is largely related to the *density* (ρ) of the material and the speed with which ultrasound travels (v):

$$Z = \rho \times v$$

As seen in Table 1.2, denser materials such as bones and fluids effectively transmit ultrasound, whereas air and lung tissue have a low level of acoustic impedance and are poor transmitters of sound energy. This property explains why whales can hear sound over great expanses of the ocean, yet an amplification system is required to be heard even in a small lecture hall.

When sound reaches an interface of two tissues of similar acoustic impedance, the ultrasound beam travels across the interface largely undisturbed. When the tissues differ in impedance, a percentage of the ultrasound energy is *reflected,* and the remainder is *transmitted. The larger the absolute difference in the levels of acoustic impedance across the interface, the greater the percentage of the ultrasound energy that is reflected.* Reflection can be calculated by using the reflection coefficient (R):

$$\text{Reflection coefficient} = \frac{(Z_2 - Z_1)^2}{(Z_1 + Z_2)^2}$$

The reflective properties of an interface are key factors in the imaged appearance of a structure. When the absolute difference between the levels of acoustic impedance of the two interfacing media is large, as when soft tissue interfaces with air or bone, more energy is reflected back to the transducer. These interfaces are represented by echo-dense or bright signals on the echogram. When the absolute difference is small, as when soft tissue interfaces with soft tissue, the interface will not appear as bright and may even be echolucent or dark.

Specular and Scattering Reflectors

The reflection of sound is also greatly affected by the size and surface of the tissue. Two types of reflection, specular and scattered, are commonly encountered.

Specular reflection occurs when a sound wave encounters a large object with a smooth surface. Such surfaces act like an acoustic mirror, generating strong reflections that travel away from the interface at an angle equal and opposite to that at which the ultrasound beam traveled to the interface. Reflection is maximal when the angle of incidence is 90°—that is, the ultrasound beam and the object are perpendicular to each other. With an angle of incidence other than 90°, less energy is reflected back to the transducer. Because of the important effect of strong specular reflection on image quality, echocardiographers adjust the position of the TEE transducer so that the direction of its beam is near perpendicular to the cardiac structure of interest.

Scattering reflection occurs when an ultrasound beam encounters small or irregularly shaped surfaces. These small objects, such as red blood cells, scatter ultrasound energy in all directions so that far less energy is reflected back to the transducer than in the case of a specular reflector. This type of reflection is the basis of the Doppler analysis of red blood cell movement.

Both types of reflection contribute to the 2D image. Although the strongest signals and best images are obtained from interfaces that are perpendicular to the beam orientation, cardiac tissue is, to a large extent, irregular and nonlinear in shape. Therefore, a significant component of the reflected energy comes from scattering off the smaller irregular components of tissue. An example is imaging of the lateral and septal walls of the left ventricle from esophageal windows. Although the ventricular walls are parallel to the ultrasound beam, they can be imaged as a result of both specular reflection and scattering off the irregular surfaces of the myocardium. However, the total amount of ultrasound returning to the transducer is low, which accounts for the poor quality of images, which often include dark spots called *echo dropout.* Adjusting the transducer angle or using a different echocardiographic window to orient the beam more perpendicularly to the structure of interest will often dramatically improve image quality.

Refraction

The portion of the ultrasound beam that is not reflected propagates through the interface, but its direction is often altered or refracted. Refraction is most pronounced when the difference in sound velocities in the two tissues is large and the angle of incidence is acute. When the angle of incidence is 90°, or when the difference in levels of acoustic impedance is minimal, refraction does not occur because the ultrasound energy is either reflected or continues to travel in the same direction.

Refraction is an important factor in the formation of artifacts. Although the ultrasound beam may proceed in an altered direction, the transducer does not recognize this change.

Consequently, the refracted energy may interact with a cardiac structure outside the *intended* scanning field. The reflected energy from this interaction returns to the transducer, which then incorrectly displays the structure alongside structures detected by the beam along its original course (Figure 1.3). Altering the viewing angle so that the ultrasound energy is perpendicular to the area of interest minimizes refraction and any resultant artifact.

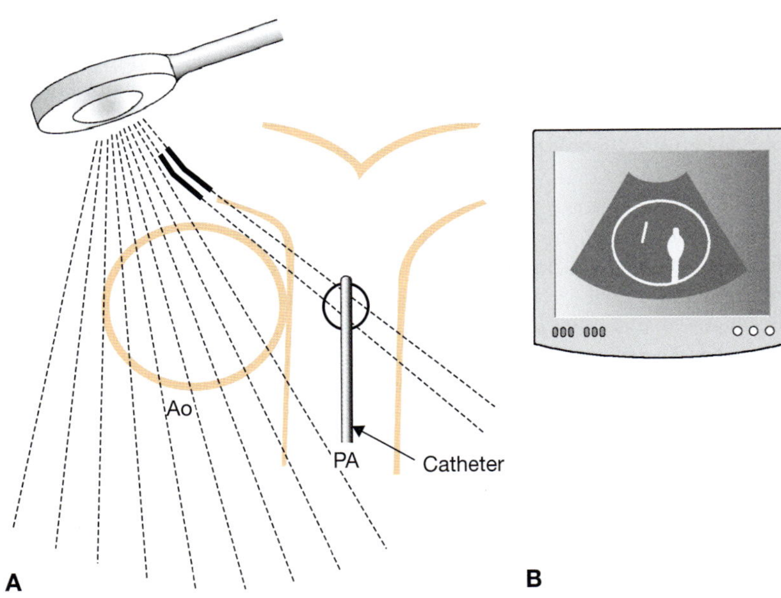

FIGURE 1.3 Refraction artifact. A: Refraction of a portion of the ultrasound beam in the near field (solid line) deflects the beam laterally, where it interacts with a strong reflector, a pulmonary artery (PA) catheter. B: The transducer is unable to recognize that these scan lines have been refracted and incorrectly assumes that the returning reflections have originated from the original course of the beam. Echocardiography display illustrates the resulting artifact as the reflections from the PA catheter are mistakenly positioned within the aorta (Ao).

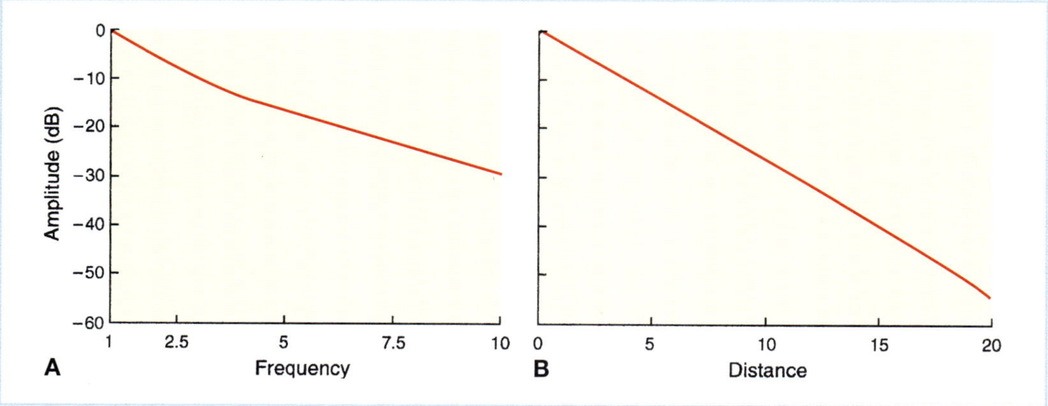

FIGURE 1.4 Attenuation of ultrasound. The effects of transducer frequency and distance on signal strength are plotted in decibels. A: The lower-frequency signals are less attenuated. B: The amplitude of a 1-MHz signal traveling through cardiac tissue is plotted. Signals reaching the far field can be more than 60 dB less than those lying close to the transducer. These effects warrant careful selection of the transducer frequency, imaging view, and gain settings to mitigate attenuation.

Attenuation

In addition to being reflected and refracted from tissue interfaces, the ultrasound signal is altered as it travels through uniform tissue. Most notable is the steady loss (ie, attenuation) in transmitted intensity as a consequence of dispersion and absorption. The attenuation in ultrasound energy caused by dispersion and absorption results in less energy returning to the transducer and subsequently a weaker signal on the display with a poor signal-to-noise ratio.

Dispersion occurs as the ultrasound beam diverges over a greater area in the far field. In addition, since the cellular structure of tissue is irregular, scattering further disperses the ultrasound energy. The amount of scattering varies greatly with tissue type.

Absorption occurs as frictional forces convert ultrasound energy into heat. Since friction is related to the level of tissue movement, it is not surprising that the higher the frequency of the signal and the greater the distance traveled, the greater the absorption (Figure 1.4). The dependence of attenuation on frequency and distance is reflected in the *attenuation coefficient* (dB/cm/MHz), which allows for a comparison of the degree of attenuation between tissue types. The penetration of ultrasound can also be expressed by the *half-power distance* specific for each tissue, which expresses the distance sound will travel until half of its original energy is lost. The acoustic properties of various tissues are summarized in Table 1.3.

As a result of these phenomena, the returning echoes from deeper structures are weakened. To decrease the negative effects of attenuation during an examination, echocardiographers may improve penetration by choosing a lower-frequency signal (eg, a 2.5- instead of a 7.5-MHz transducer frequency) and viewing the structure from a window that is either closer to the structure of interest or avoids a strong near-field reflector (eg, prosthetic valve). In addition, the incoming signal can be enhanced by adjusting the gain controls to amplify the weakened returning signals. These adjustments are discussed in greater detail in Chapter 21: 3D Transesophageal Echocardiography Imaging.

TABLE 1.3 Attenuation or Loss of Energy per Centimeter of Penetration With Different Transducer Frequencies

Transducer Frequency (MHz)	Attenuation (dB/cm)
1	0.5
2	1.0
3	1.5
5	2.5
10	5.0

TRANSDUCER DESIGN AND BEAM FORMATION

Transducer Components

The transducers used in echocardiography systems create a brief pulse of ultrasound that is transmitted into the tissue (Figure 1.5). To achieve this goal, most TEE transducer designs use the following components:

1. A *ceramic piezoelectric crystal,* which acts as an ultrasonic vibrator and receiver
2. *Electrodes,* which both conduct electric energy to stimulate the piezoelectric crystal and record the voltage signal from returning echoes
3. *Backing,* which acts to rapidly dampen the vibrations of the crystal
4. *Insulation,* which prevents unwanted vibration of the transducer from standing waves or extraneous incoming waves
5. *A faceplate,* which optimizes the acoustic contact between the piezoelectric crystal and the esophagus. The faceplate may also include an acoustic lens to focus the beam.

The following sections detail the inner workings of the modern ultrasound transducer and their effects on the transmitted sound beam and the echocardiographic image.

Formation of Ultrasound Waves: The Piezoelectric Crystal

The heart of the transducer consists of a piezoelectric crystal, which contains polarized molecules trapped within a matrix. The formation of the sound wave used in echocardiography is based on the principle of *piezoelectricity.* When stimulated by alternating electric current, polarized particles within the crystal matrix vibrate, generating ultrasound. Conversely, when an ultrasound wave strikes the crystal, the resulting vibrations of the polarized particles generate an alternating electric current. Therefore, a piezoelectric crystal can function as both a transmitter and a receiver of ultrasound. This process is the hallmark of piezoelectricity—that is, the transformation of electric energy into mechanical energy and the reverse transformation of mechanical energy into electric energy.

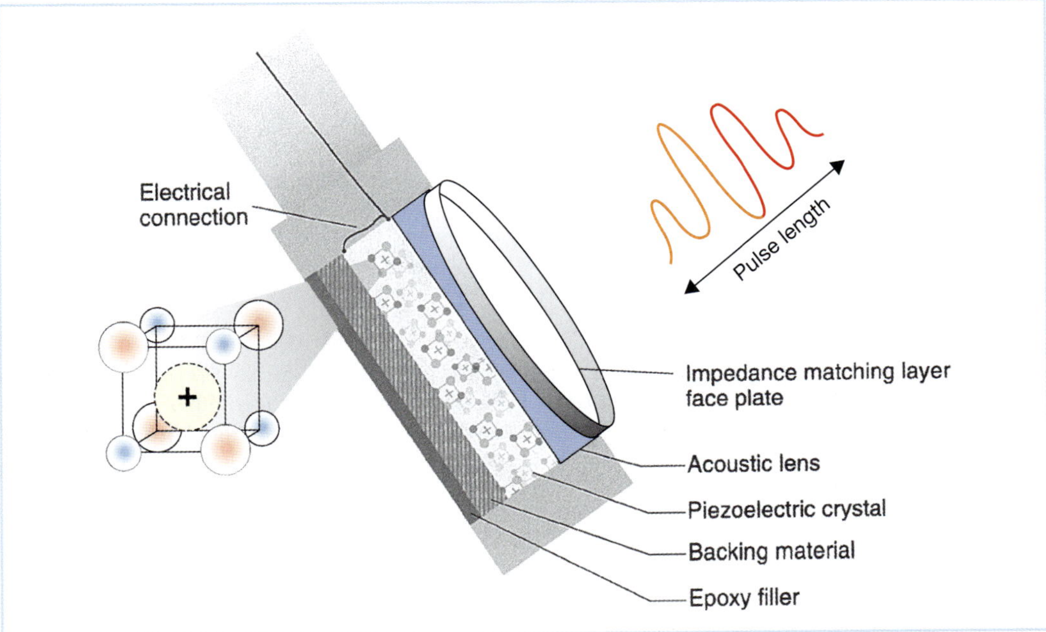

FIGURE 1.5 Transducer components: Creating a sound pulse. A brief transmission of alternating current from the *electric connector* causes charged particles within the matrix of the piezoelectric crystal to vibrate. The *backing material* helps to dampen the crystal vibrations quickly, keeping the pulse length short; in this example, it is four wavelengths. An *acoustic lens* aids in focusing the sound energy. The *faceplate* contains layers of material that match the acoustic impedance of the esophagus, to avoid unwanted reflections and ensure excellent sound transmission. *Epoxy filler* secures the working components to the probe.

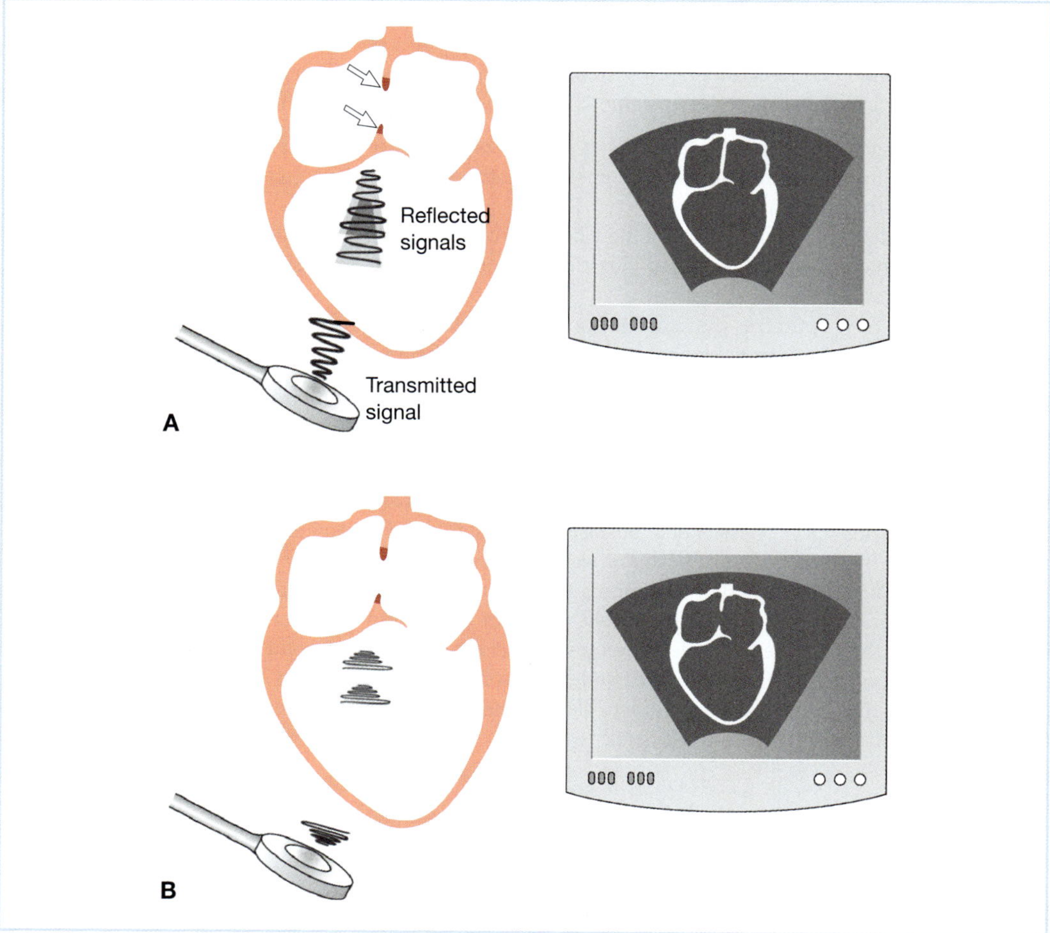

FIGURE 1.6 Effect of pulse length on axial resolution. A: The transducer emits a long sound pulse. Since the length of this pulse is greater than the length of the atrial septal defect (arrows), the reflections from the two tips of atrial septum are smeared, and the defect cannot be resolved. Consequently, the resulting two-dimensional echocardiographic display (right) does not show the abnormality. B: The pulse length has been shortened and is now less than the length of the atrial septal defect. The reflections from each interface are clearly identifiable, and the resulting display (right) shows the defect.

For imaging purposes, the transducer emits a brief burst of ultrasound. Typically, 2D transducers emit a sound pulse of two to four wavelengths. As illustrated in Figure 1.6, the shorter the length of the sound pulse, the better the axial resolution of the system. Therefore, the shorter the wavelength, the shorter the resulting pulse length and the greater the axial resolution.

The Three-Dimensional Ultrasound Beam

Near and Far Fields

The ultrasound transducer emits a three-dimensional (3D) ultrasound beam similar to the beam of a flashlight (Figure 1.7; Video 1.1). The physical dimensions of this beam determine the following:

1. The specific area of the heart examined
2. The intensity distribution of ultrasound energy
3. The lateral (side-to-side) and elevational (top-to-bottom) resolution of the system

Narrower beams are preferred because they improve resolution, increase the intensity of returning echoes, and reduce artifact. Most commonly, ultrasound beams have either a disk or rectangular shape and

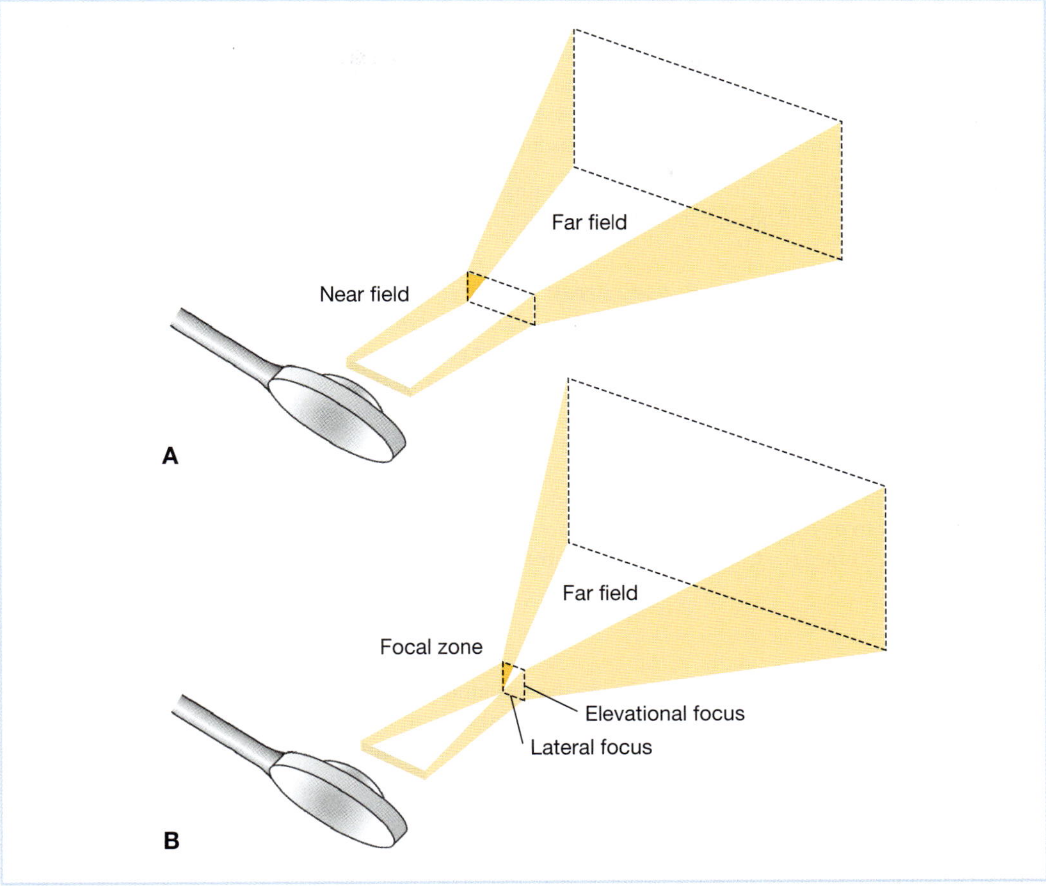

FIGURE 1.7 Three-dimensional (3D) beam. The ultrasound probe projects a 3D beam. The dimensions of this projection have important effects on imaging resolution and artifact. Typically, a narrow profile is preferred. A: Unfocused beam. The beam is narrow in the near field and then diverges in the far field. B: Focused beam. Focusing has resulted in a narrower beam in both the lateral and the elevational planes so that the imaging resolution of structures in the focal zone is improved. Distal to the focal zone, the beam rapidly diverges, and the images of structures in this area will be of lower quality. See Video 1.1.

comprise two main zones: the *near-field (Fresnel)* and *far-field (Fraunhofer) zones.* Beam manipulation and image resolution are greatest within the near field. Also, ultrasound energy is more concentrated within this zone, yielding stronger echoes and better imaging.

In the near-field zone, the ultrasound beam is narrow. The length of the near-field zone is proportional to the diameter (D) of the transducer face and inversely proportional to the wavelength.

$$L_n = D^2/\lambda$$

Distal to the near-field zone, the ultrasound beam diverges, forming the far-field zone. The angle of divergence (θ) is inversely related to the diameter (D) of the transducer face:

$$\sin \theta = 1.22\ \lambda/D$$

Accordingly, larger transducers with high-frequency (small λ) signals produce the most desirable beam profile:

A long, narrow near field and a less divergent far field.

Focusing

Focusing can further narrow the ultrasound beam. This is accomplished in three ways, as follows:

1. By creating a concave shape in the piezoelectric crystal
2. By gluing an acoustic lens to the front of the crystal
3. Electronically with the use of phased array transducers

The narrow beam at the focal zone enhances imaging at this location. However, the beam diverges widely distal to the focal zone, reducing the intensity of the ultrasound energy and impairing imaging of the far field.

Electronic Beam Focusing: The Phased Array

Modern echocardiography systems allow the echocardiographer to adjust the depth of the focal zone selectively to optimize image quality. A single element transducer emits a wave front that diverges in a hemispheric pattern. By aligning several crystals side by side in a *linear array,* the interaction of the individual sound waves emitted by each crystal creates a narrow, forwardly directed wave front (Figure 1.8A; Video 1.1). The beam's shape can be focused further by electrically activating the crystals at the ends of the array before those located at the center. This creates a concave wave front, thereby focusing the beam at a selected distance from the transducer face (Figure 1.8B; Video 1.1).

It is important to be cognizant of both the advantages and the disadvantages of selecting the focus depth of the beam. As discussed next, beam shape is of prime importance in determining the resolution of an imaging system.

Resolution

Three parameters are evaluated when assessing the resolution of an ultrasound system: the resolution of objects lying along the axis of the ultrasound beam (axial resolution), the resolution of objects lying horizontal to the beam's orientation (lateral resolution), and the resolution of objects lying vertical to the beam's orientation (elevational resolution).

Axial Resolution

Axial resolution is the ability of the ultrasound system to identify two separate objects that lie along the path of the ultrasound beam axis. Axial resolution is determined by the *bandwidth* of the ultrasound pulse. The bandwidth is the resonant frequencies that are emitted about the center frequency. *High-bandwidth pulses are best for axial resolution as they are characterized by high-frequency signals of short duration.* As seen in Figure 1.6, short pulses of high-frequency ultrasound offer the greatest axial resolution. A general rule is that the axial resolution of a system is approximately 1.5 times the wavelength of the system. Therefore, for a 7.5-MHz transducer, axial resolution is 0.3 mm. Improved axial resolution does not come without a cost. The shorter the pulse, the lower its energy level, resulting in weaker penetration and returning echoes. Similarly, high-frequency sound is quickly attenuated. Accordingly, the echocardiographer must select these parameters based on the imaging needs.

Lateral (Azimuth) Resolution

Lateral resolution is the ability of the ultrasound system to distinguish between objects that are horizontally aligned and perpendicular to the path of the ultrasound beam. Beam width is a primary determinant of lateral resolution. Wide beams produce a "smeared" image of two such objects, whereas narrow beams can identify each object individually. Signal frequency and transducer size impact lateral resolution, but for typical cardiac ultrasound transducers the beam width is approximated as depth/50, yielding at 10 cm of depth a beam width of approximately 2 mm.

Elevational Resolution

Elevational resolution is the ability of the ultrasound system to distinguish between objects that are vertically aligned and perpendicular to the emitted ultrasound beam. Although 2D images appear to display a thin slice

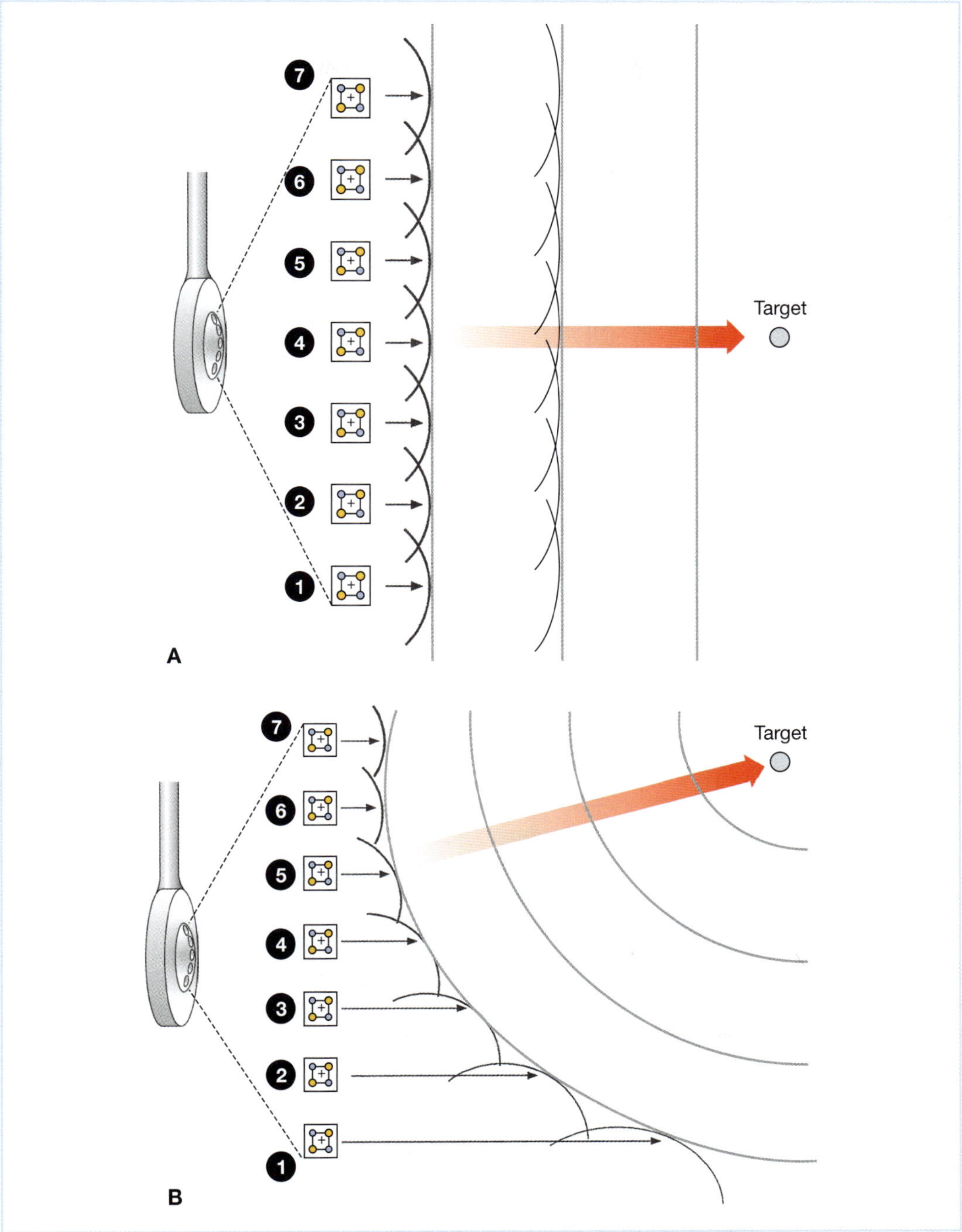

FIGURE 1.8 Phased array transducers. A: This illustration shows seven crystal elements in an array. The interactions of the individual hemispheric wave fronts create a flat, profiled, forwardly directed wave front. B: Phased array transducer. Here, the crystals have been activated sequentially: Crystal 1 first, followed by crystal 2, and so on. This causes the beam to be steered upward toward the target. Note that crystals 6 and 7 have been activated before crystal 5, creating a concave wave front to focus the energy of the beam at the target. The ability to steer electronically and focus the beam is a major advantage of the phased array system. See Video 1.1.

of cardiac anatomy, in actuality the information gathered from the entire thickness of the beam is averaged and displayed. For this reason, the thinner the ultrasound beam, the better the elevational resolution of the system (see Figure 1.7). Signal frequency and transducer size impact elevational resolution, but a typical cardiac ultrasound transducer has a beam height approximated as depth/30. Accordingly, at 10-cm depth the beam height is approximately 3.3 mm. Note that axial resolution offers 50% greater fidelity than that achieved in the lateral and elevational planes.

Optimizing Resolution

The interplay of the transducer size, signal frequency, and focal length and the distance of the structure of interest determine beam width and height. The beam is narrowest in the near-field or focal zone and divergent in the far field. Resolution is therefore better in the near field and decreases in the far field. Factors that lengthen the near field, such as a higher transducer frequency and a larger transducer radius, improve lateral and elevational resolution. Focusing further decreases the width of the ultrasound beam and improves lateral and elevational resolution at the focal point. However, focusing often increases beam divergence distal to the focal zone, with an associated loss of lateral and elevational resolution. These factors explain why it is preferable to position a transducer with a relatively high frequency (smaller wavelength) close to the target of interest to optimize both lateral and elevational resolution. More precise measurements are made along the axial plane due to the superior resolution in this orientation.

Extraneous Sound Beams

Side Lobes

Unfortunately, in addition to the powerful forwardly directed beam of sound energy produced by linear array transducers, additional beams of sound are emitted that travel off-axis to the main beam (Figure 1.9; Video 1.1). These extraneous beams of sound, called side lobes, can significantly affect imaging quality because the transducer incorrectly processes their reflections as reflections of the main beam. Consequently, structures off-axis to the imaging plane appear incorrectly located on the 2D image.

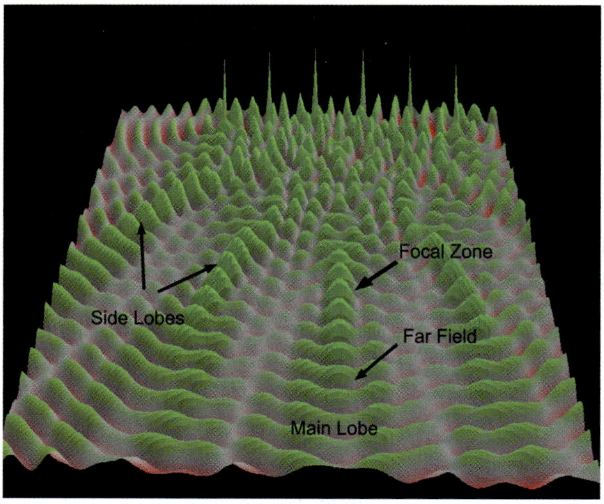

FIGURE 1.9 Ultrasound beam pattern: The spatial distribution of sound energy from a phased array transducer is characterized by focal zone, near and far fields, as well as side lobes. A 6-crystal transducer is shown at the top of the image (sharp peaks), and the emitted waves interact, causing constructive and destructive interference. The resulting pattern includes the forwardly directed, high-intensity main lobe, with its focal zone showing both narrow dimensions and peak intensity. Side lobes are also created, and reflections from these off-axis lobes reduce image quality and are a well-described source of imaging artifact (Video 1.1).

Grating Lobes

Grating lobes are side lobes generated with multielement array transducers. Each crystal of the linear array can be considered a point source of sound emission. When these individual sound waves meet in phase and off-axis to the main beam (constructive interference), a grating lobe is created. The position of a grating lobe is predictable as it is related to the spacing of the crystals and the wavelength of the signal.

Side Lobe Artifacts

Both side and grating lobes contain less energy than the main beam and usually do not significantly affect the echocardiographic image. However, when these lobes of energy contact a highly reflective surface (catheter, prosthesis, calcium), sufficient energy can be reflected back to the transducer to create an artifact. The transducer believes these reflections have arisen from the main forwardly directed field and mistakenly displays them together with those from the main beam. To reduce such artifacts, the echocardiographer should minimize gain settings to decrease the likelihood of strong reflections from the weaker lobes. To further differentiate an artifact from a real structure, the field should be imaged from another window. An artifact is not likely to be reproduced in multiple planes.

SIGNAL RECEPTION AND PROCESSING

The conversion of reflected ultrasound signals into high-fidelity cardiac images is a complex process in which returning ultrasound pulses are received, electronically processed, and displayed. Understanding the basic principles of these steps is essential both to optimize image acquisition and to avoid misdiagnosis caused by artifacts.

Cycling of Transducer Transmit and Receive Modes

The ultrasound transducer acts first as a transmitter and then as a receiver of sound signals. An oscillator signals the discharge of electric current to the piezoelectric crystal, thereby determining the rate of sound pulse transmission. After emitting a short burst of ultrasound, the transducer switches to receive mode to listen for the returning ultrasound reflections from the tissues.

Electrical Processing

Amplification: Gain Controls

The echoes that return to the transducer are converted from sound energy to a radiofrequency electric signal by the piezoelectric crystal. As a large proportion of the sound energy is lost as the ultrasound wave travels, the electric signal must be amplified before it can be further processed. This amplification is controlled by the *system gain* control. Furthermore, since signal attenuation is proportional to distance traveled, signals from distant structures can be 12 to 30 dB weaker than those from closer structures. *Time gain compensation* allows the echocardiographer to selectively amplify signals from structures of varying distances from the transducer. With this feature, signals from distant targets and weaker reflectors are boosted so that their amplitudes more closely match those from nearby structures.

Compression and Display

The amplified and time gain–compensated electric signal must be processed before it can be displayed on a monitor. The radiofrequency signal has a large dynamic range of more than 100 dB, far too large for monitors to display. To reduce the dynamic range, two processes are commonly used. First, *reject* circuits filter out low-amplitude signals, which typically represent background noise or speckle. The remainder of the signal is then *compressed,* so that both low- and high-amplitude components can be displayed. *Digital scan conversion* then converts the electric signal into a standard video format for display.

Preprocessing and Postprocessing

The digital scan converter requires the analog electric signal to be digitized so that it can be processed and then converted to an analog video format. This process offers two important opportunities for the echocardiographer to control the display of the imaging data. By adjusting the *preprocessing settings,* which affect the analog-to-digital conversion, and the *postprocessing settings,* which affect the conversion to analog video format, the echocardiographer can modify the appearance of the displayed image. These adjustments can be used, for example, to emphasize edge detection versus tissue texture or to improve the delineation of weaker reflectors. Again, the choice of these settings is dictated by the examination and the personal preferences of the echocardiographer.

DISPLAY FORMATS

The Golden Rule: Time Is Distance

Ultrasonic imaging is based on the amplitude and time delay of the reflected signals (Figure 1.10). Since the velocity in tissue is relatively constant, only the distance of the structure from the transducer alters the time required for the ultrasound wave to travel to and from the reflected structure:

$$\text{Distance} = \text{velocity} \times \text{time}$$

As sound travels at the rate of 1,540 m/s through soft tissue, the round-trip travel time for each centimeter of separation between transducer and reflector is calculated as:

$$\text{Travel time} = 13\ \mu\text{s/cm}$$

By timing the interval between transmission and return of the reflections, the echocardiography system can precisely calculate the location of a structure.

Amplitude Mode

The original display format is ***amplitude mode*** (A-mode), in which the amplitudes of the returning signals are represented as a series of horizontal spikes along the vertical axis of the display. The horizontal spikes correspond to the distance of the reflecting tissue and the strength of the returning echoes.

Brightness Mode

Current imaging is based on ***brightness-mode*** (B-mode) technology. Instead of horizontal spikes, the amplitudes of the returning echoes are represented as pixels of varying brightness along the vertical axis of the display. The brightness correlates with the strength of the returning signal.

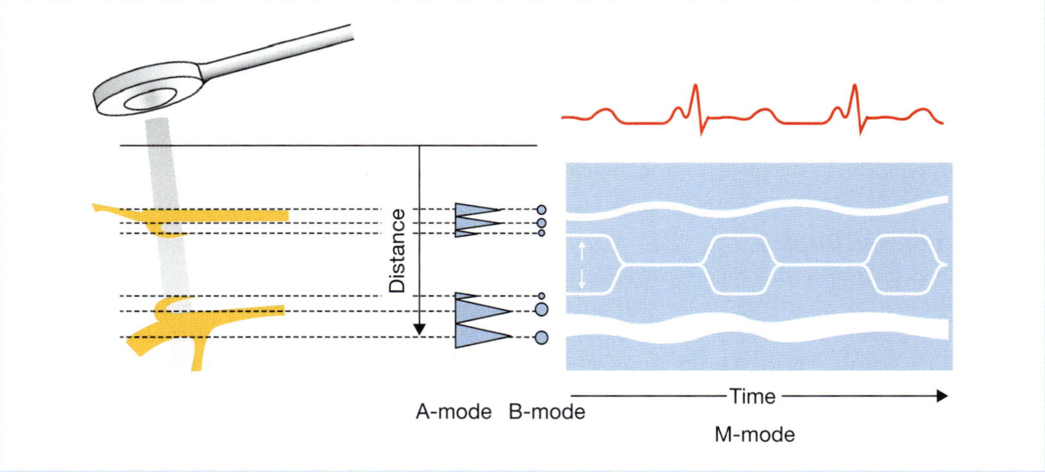

FIGURE 1.10 Display formats. The ultrasound beam is directed through the aortic valve leaflets. Amplitude-mode (A-mode) display shows the resulting reflections as horizontal spikes. In the brightness-mode (B-mode) display, the spikes are replaced with pixels of varying brightness. Motion mode (M-mode) shows sequential B-mode frames to capture cardiac motion. The "boxcar" pattern depicts normal opening and closing of the aortic valve leaflets.

Motion Mode

Motion mode (M-mode) adds temporal information to B-mode by displaying a series of collected B-mode images. M-mode echocardiography provides a one-dimensional, "ice-pick" view through the heart and updates the B-mode images at a very high rate, allowing dynamic real-time imaging. *It is important to realize that before it emits the next pulse of energy, the transducer element must first receive the reflected energy of the previously emitted pulse.* The frequency at which the B-mode images are updated is the *frame rate* and is calculated as 1/round-trip travel time. The frame rate with M-mode imaging is very high (>2,000 frames/s), affording a superior display of dynamic motion in comparison with other techniques. However, M-mode imaging displays only axial motion and provides a limited view of cardiac anatomy. Because of its superior dynamics and axial resolution, M-mode is the best mode for examining the timing of cardiac events when displayed with the electrocardiogram.

Two-Dimensional Echocardiography

2D echocardiography is a modification of B-mode echocardiography and the mainstay of the echocardiographic examination. Instead of repeatedly firing ultrasound pulses in a single direction, the transducer in 2D echocardiography sequentially directs the ultrasound pulses across a sector of the cardiac anatomy. In this way, 2D imaging can display a tomographic section of the cardiac anatomy, and, unlike M-mode, it can show shape and lateral motion (Figure 1.11).

TWO-DIMENSIONAL SCAN SYSTEMS

Both electronic and mechanical systems have been developed to sweep the beam across an area of interest. Most commonly, the transducer consists of multiple crystals (or elements) aligned next to one another in a *linear array.* The individual sound waves from each crystal combine to provide a unified wave front that can be better focused and directed than that of a single crystal. Furthermore, with alterations in the timing of the electric activation of each crystal in the array, hence the term *phased array,* the beam can actually be steered without the transducer itself being moved. The advantages of an electronic system over a mechanical one, including an absence of moving parts and easy manipulation (steering, focusing, narrowing) of the ultrasound beam, have made it the dominant technology in echocardiography scanners. The two commonly used electronic scanning systems in medical ultrasound are the linear scanners and sector scanners.

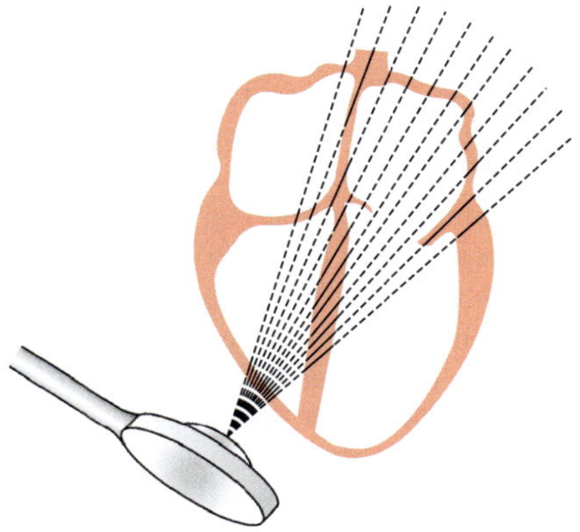

FIGURE 1.11 Scan lines. Illustration of the arced sector from a phased array two-dimensional echocardiogram. Each dotted line represents an individual B-mode (brightness mode) scan line. Any structure that interacts with a scan line will create reflections (dark highlight); however, structures that lie between the scan lines are not interrogated, and the echocardiography system averages the neighboring signals to fill in this defect. Accordingly, the closer the scan lines, the better the image quality. With a phased array scan, the gap between scan lines increases with the distance from the transducer.

Linear Scanners

The linear scanner uses a long transducer composed of several crystals. Groups of crystals are activated sequentially from one end of the transducer to the other. The firing of each group of crystals images the structures directly in front of them. With sequential firing of the groups of crystals, the anatomic features under the entire transducer are imaged. However, the disadvantage of this approach is that the transducer face must be large enough to cover a broad anatomic area effectively. The linear array is commonly used in vascular, obstetric, and regional anesthesia applications.

Sector Scanners

The phased array sector scanner is most commonly used in echocardiography. This is an electronic system that by precisely timing the activation of the individual transducer elements is able to sweep the sound beam in an arc across a predetermined field. With activation of the transducer elements in different sequences, the ultrasound beam in the phased array system can be easily narrowed, steered, and focused (see Figure 1.8). The ability to direct a series of beams electronically over an arced sector also makes it possible to use the smaller transducer face required for TEE and transthoracic echocardiography.

CREATING THE TWO-DIMENSIONAL IMAGE

Imaging a Sector

To construct the 2D image, the echocardiographic system records the B-mode data from the first pulse, redirects the next beam, records the returning signals, and so on until the entire sector has been scanned. Typically, the scanner images a sector of 30° to 90°. The orientation of each B-mode line (also called the *scan line*) is recorded so that the information can be displayed in the correct position on the display screen. The 2D scanner then repeats the entire process to update the image and capture motion. Each image created by a sector scan is a *frame*. 2D imaging typically requires 100 to 200 scan lines per frame, resulting in a *frame rate* of 30 to 60 frames/s. Since this rate is significantly slower than that of M-mode echocardiography, 2D imaging is not as precise for demonstrating dynamic motion or the timing of cardiac events.

Image Quality and Dynamic Motion

2D imaging is characterized by several factors that are operator controlled and that have important (and often opposing) effects on image quality and dynamic motion. The proper settings vary depending on the particular examination at hand.

The *pulse repetition frequency* (PRF) is the rate at which new sound pulses are generated (ie, pulses per second). The greater the PRF, the greater the number of scan lines that are emitted in a given period of time. The PRF is inversely related to the sector depth because a longer period of time is required for the ultrasound to travel increased distances.

The *frame rate* is the frequency at which the sector is rescanned. Each frame consists of one or two scans across the sector of interest. The information from two sweeps can be interlaced to improve image quality. A high frame rate improves the capture of movement. Typically, a frame rate greater than 30/s allows the dynamic representation of some relatively fine movements (eg, intermediate positions of the aortic valve). The frame rate is critically dependent on the sector depth, which determines the time required for each scan line to be received, and sector width, which increases the number of scan lines to be processed. Consequently, increases in the sector size and depth come at the cost of a decreased frame rate.

The scan line density, calculated as the number of lines per degree of the sector, greatly affects the image quality. Line densities should be maintained at 1.5 to 2.2 lines per degree. Doubling the scan line density essentially doubles the lateral resolution. However, the cost is a decrease in the frame rate. The scan line density is calculated by dividing the number of scan lines per sweep by the angle of the sector. The greater the sector angle, the larger the area and the lower the line density. Since phased array transducers produce a fan-shaped sector, scan line density, and hence lateral resolution, is greater closer to the transducer and decreases in direct proportion to distance.

Image Quality Versus Dynamic Motion

It quickly becomes apparent that the echocardiographer must choose between the size of the imaging field and the frame rate. If the frame rate is high (100 frames/s), the number of scan lines per frame is reduced, resulting in a lower line density. Although the dynamics of the image may be excellent, the spatial image quality is decreased. We caution against the practice of assessing several structures in a single large view because it compromises both the dynamics and the quality of the images. We recommend that the clinician focus each part of the examination on a given structure of interest and select the imaging plane that best delineates the structure in the near field. Motion can then be enhanced without costs in lateral resolution by decreasing the sector angle and depth. In situations in which the maximal frame rate is desired, M-mode should be considered. This results in a very dynamic image with a high level of axial resolution. For these reasons, M-mode echocardiography remains an important adjunct to both 2D and color Doppler echocardiography.

ADVANCEMENTS

Recent advancements in echocardiography include harmonic imaging, 3D imaging, tissue Doppler, and strain (and strain rate) analysis. These advancements improve the image quality and the assessment of specific cardiac structures and add to the quantitative assessment of global and regional cardiac function. It should be recognized that these advancements in technology are each guided by the same underlying physical principles and limitations as basic ultrasound.

Harmonic Imaging

Echocardiography involves emission of ultrasound from the transducer into the body, which then, after being reflected at a tissue interface, returns to the transducer after a period of time and of a particular signal strength. The emission of the ultrasound beam causes the tissues to vibrate or resonate, not just at the original or fundamental frequency but also at harmonic frequencies, which are typically multiples of the originally transmitted, or fundamental, frequency. For example, a 5.0-MHz transducer may create harmonics waves with 10- and 15-MHz frequencies. These harmonic echoes are the basis of tissue harmonic imaging. The second harmonic has a frequency twice that of the original fundamental one and can be isolated and recorded by filtering out other frequencies. As these waves originate from the tissue itself (ie, not the transducer), they pass through the tissues once to arrive at the transducer. Accordingly, there is less attenuation, that is, the acoustic signal is stronger and less distorted. This stronger, higher-frequency signal presents itself as a narrower central beam (Figure 1.12). The higher-frequency (therefore smaller wavelength), narrow (focused) ultrasound beam creates an image with higher axial and lateral resolution that has fewer artifacts (eg, side lobes, reverberations), which are typically filtered out.

TISSUE DOPPLER AND SPECKLE TRACKING

Tissue Velocity, Strain, and Strain Rate

Quantitative assessment of regional heart function has been limited by technology. Traditionally, assessment has been largely visual (qualitative) and global, with a greater emphasis on circumferential contraction and thickening. Longitudinal assessment or shortening from apex to base, which is representative of endocardial function, has been absent. However, tissue Doppler imaging (TDI) and speckle tracking analysis allow for quantitative regional assessment (shortening/lengthening), including radial, circumferential, and longitudinal contraction.

Tissue Doppler Imaging (Figure 1.13)

Tissue Doppler uses conventional Doppler principles and techniques to measure the velocity and direction of the contracting myocardium. Compared to Doppler signals from blood cells, which are high velocity and low amplitude, tissue Doppler signals are low velocity and high amplitude. To isolate tissue Doppler signals, the high-velocity signals are filtered out, allowing low-velocity signals to be analyzed. Similarly to Doppler analysis of blood, the velocity and direction of tissue movement is determined by the frequency shift. If the frequency shift is negative, then the myocardial tissue was moving away from the transducer; if positive, then it was moving toward the transducer. Mitral and tricuspid annular (lateral and septal) tissue Doppler velocities are used to estimate ventricular function and chamber pressures.

Doppler signals are optimized by aligning the Doppler ultrasound beam with either blood flow or tissue motion. When applied during four, two, or long axis windows, the longitudinal muscle velocity, or contraction, is measured. Circumferential muscle motion can be assessed from short-axis views of the myocardium.

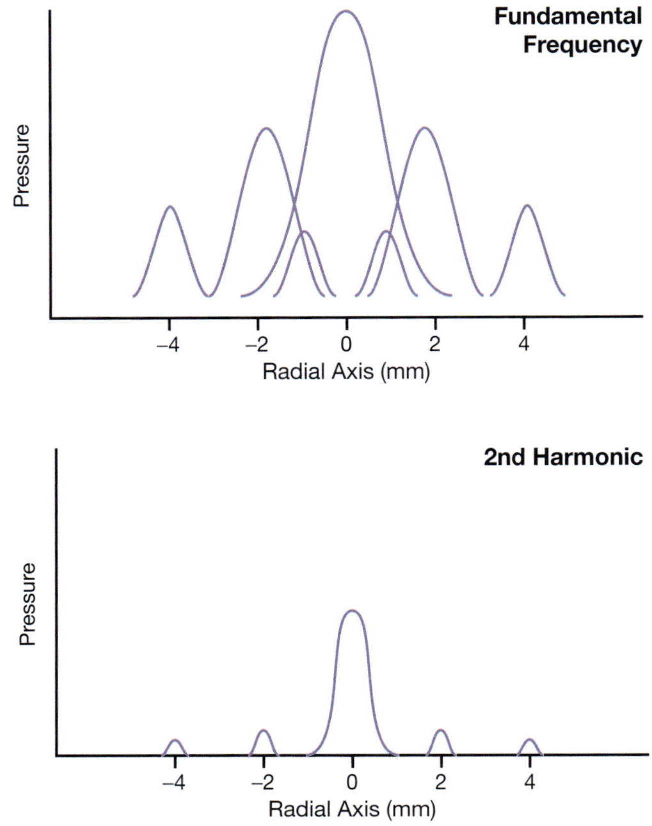

FIGURE 1.12 Harmonic imaging. Schematic describing tissue harmonic imaging compared to conventional imaging.

Pulsed-wave tissue Doppler measures single myocardial segments, while color tissue Doppler interrogates velocities from multiple sites simultaneously. PW TDI can measure higher velocities during specific phases of the cardiac cycle from specific myocardial segments. Color tissue Doppler measures mean peak velocities.

Tissue Doppler is constrained by the same limitations as conventional Doppler, most notably that accurate assessment requires near-parallel alignment between tissue movement and the ultrasound beam. A second limitation is that precise and accurate TDI requires frame rates >100 FPS. Finally, tissue Doppler does not differentiate active contraction from passive motion. Myocardium that has normal intrinsic contraction could have the same velocity as a scarred segment that is tethered to normal functioning myocardium.

Strain, Strain Rate, and Speckle Tracking

Strain and strain rate measure myocardial mechanical function, displacement, or deformation of muscle tissue. Strain is a dimensionless number expressed as an object's percentage change (shortening or lengthening) from its initial position. Strain rate is the change over time. When the ventricle contracts, strain and strain rate are positive in the radial dimension and negative in the longitudinal and circumferential dimensions.

These techniques are rarely used in intraoperative examinations due to angle dependence and the limitations in the beam orientation afforded with TEE as well as the low accuracy of strain technique overall.

Speckle tracking is an extension of B-mode ultrasound technology that relies on the detection of myocardial speckles, or reflectors, to assess contraction- and relaxation-related motion of the myocardium to calculate myocardial strain throughout the cardiac cycle (Figure 1.13). Its speed of change and direction form a vector that is independent of the angle of the ultrasound beam. By tracking myocardial speckle patterns,

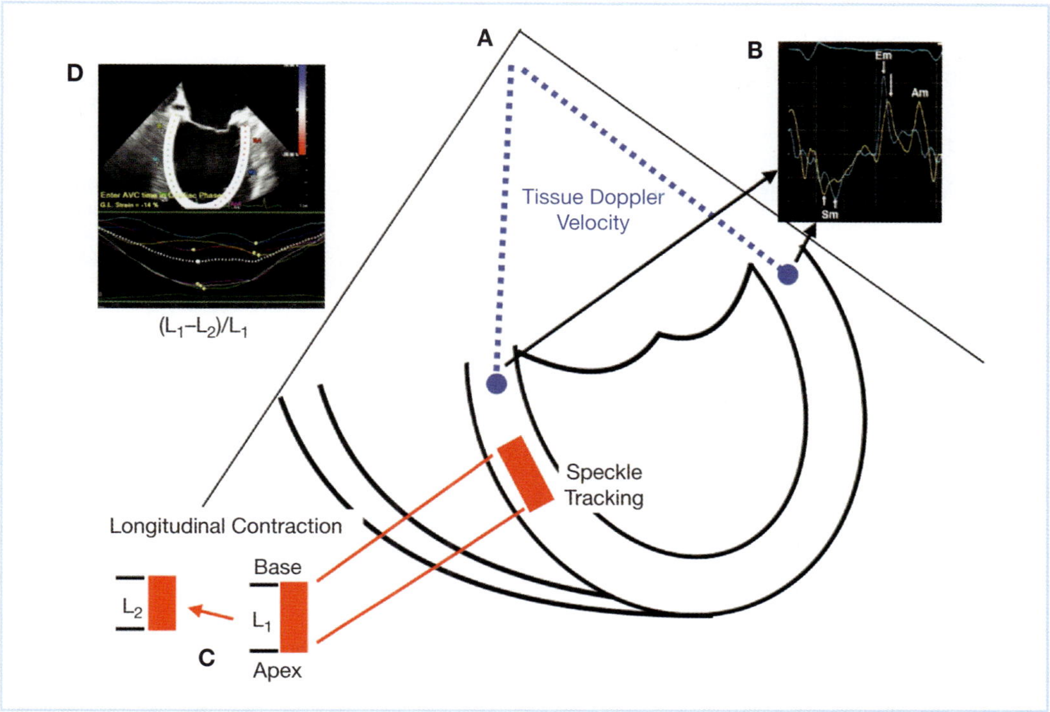

FIGURE 1.13 Tissue Doppler and speckle tracking. The central schematic (A) is used to highlight tissue Doppler imaging of the mitral annulus (black arrows) shown in B. The *blue dashed ultrasound beams* are targeting the annular sites, and the tissue velocities are displayed in B. From these, strain patterns can be assessed. The red box seen in the ventricular septum represents tissue speckle which deforms from L1 to L2 as seen with the red arrow in C, which is converted (double red line) to strain assessment as seen in D.

the displacement is measured over time to yield a strain value. Speckle tracking assesses myocardial motion or deformation over a larger user-defined region compared to TDI.

3D speckle tracking is available, and full-volume data sets are obtained for analysis, permitting assessment of a cardiac segment in the three imaging planes, improving the quantitative assessment of regional and global ventricular function. 3D speckle analysis yields information regarding myocardial torsion and twisting.

Temporal resolution is a limiting variable, and assessment relies on a high-resolution B-mode image. Similarly to other B-mode imaging, narrowing of the sector beam will increase both temporal resolution (frame rate) and image resolution (higher scan line density) and improve speckle tracking.

Although these newer applications of ultrasound enhance the assessment of cardiac function, they are based on the same underlying principles of B-mode and Doppler ultrasound, and, therefore, image quality will be improved and hindered in a similar fashion.

SUMMARY

Echocardiography is based on the interaction of ultrasound and the patient. Between the generation of the ultrasound pulse and its subsequent reflection, reception, and display, a complex series of events takes place. Echocardiographers who ignore the physical realities of the imaging process will suffer from poor image resolution and interference from artifacts. However, by applying an understanding of the principles and selecting the most appropriate views and machine settings, the echocardiographer can reliably optimize the imaging of a particular structure of interest. No patient or echocardiographic system is ideal. Rather, echocardiographers must compromise between conflicting imaging needs, such as between dynamic motion and the visual quality of an image, based on the primary diagnostic goal. Although advancements in technology might offer greater automaticity, understanding the basic principles is key to performing a qualitative and quantitative examination of the heart. We expand on the important relationship between the echocardiographer and the echocardiography machine in Chapter 23: Techniques and Tricks for Optimizing Transesophageal Images.

SUGGESTED READINGS

Blessberger I, Binder T. Two dimensional speckle tracking echocardiography: basic principles. *Heart.* 2010;96:2032-2040.

Fischer GW, Salgo IS, Adams DH. Real-time three-dimensional transesophageal echocardiography: the matrix revolution. *J Cardiothorac Vasc Anesth.* 2008;22:904-912.

Geiser EA. Echocardiography: physics and instrumentation. In: Marcus ML, Skorton DJ, Schelbert AR, et al, eds. *Cardiac Imaging.* 2nd ed. WB Saunders; 1991.

Geyer H, Caracciolo G, Abe H, et al. Assessment of myocardial mechanics using speckle tracking echocardiography: fundamentals and clinical applications. *J Am Soc Echocardiogr.* 2010;23:343-458.

Hoit BD. Strain and strain rate echocardiography and coronary artery disease. *Circ Cardiovasc Imaging.* 2011;4:179-190.

Hung J, Lang R, Flachskampf F, et al. 3D echocardiography: a review of the current status and future directions. *J Am Soc Echocardiogr.* 2007;20:213-233.

Kadappu KK, Thomas L. Tissue Doppler imaging in echocardiography: value and limitations. *Heart Lung Circ.* 2015;24:224-233.

Lang RM, Badano L, Tsang W, et al. EAE/ASE recommendations for image acquisition and display using three-dimensional echocardiography. *Eur Heart J Cardiovasc Imaging.* 2012;13:1-46.

Thomas JD, Rubin DN. Tissue harmonic imaging: why does it work? *J Am Soc Echocardiogr.* 1998;11:803-808.

Uppal T. Tissue harmonic imaging. *Australas J Ultrasound Med.* 2010;13:29-31.

Weyman A, ed. *Principles and Practice of Echocardiography.* 2nd ed. Lea & Febiger; 1994:3-55.

QUESTIONS

1. Which of the following affects a sound wave's propagation velocity?
A. Signal frequency
B. Signal amplitude
C. Tissue density
D. Transducer size

2. Sound waves propagate in all of the following except:
A. Vacuum
B. Blood
C. Bone
D. St. Jude mitral valve

3. The speed of sound in soft tissue is approximately:
A. 1,500 cm/s
B. 1,500 m/s
C. 1,500 km/h
D. 1,500 mph

4. High-frequency sound waves are advantageous in cardiac imaging because they provide:
A. Better penetration through fatty tissue
B. Better amplitude in the far field
C. Smaller transducer face
D. Better focus

5. The signal amplitude is related to the:
A. Square root of the intensity
B. Intensity squared
C. Intensity divided by sector width
D. Intensity times sector width

6. The sharply demarcated border between the ascending aortic walls and aortic blood in the ME AV LAX view:
A. Results from specular reflections
B. Results from scattering reflections
C. Depends on the Nyquist limit
D. Is not affected by reflection coefficient

7. Factors in loss of ultrasound signal amplitude include:
A. Dispersion and reflection coefficient
B. Absorption and sector width
C. Frequency and PRF
D. Distance and gain settings

8. Which of the following is false regarding piezoelectric crystals?
A. They transmit ultrasound
B. They convert an AC electrical signal to ultrasound
C. They receive the reflected sound signals
D. They are controlled by gain settings

9. The length of the near field is:
A. Increased with large transducers and large wavelength
B. Increased with large transducers and high frequency
C. Increased with small transducers and large wavelength
D. Increased with small transducers and low frequency

10. Side lobe artifacts:
A. Can be mitigated by increasing gain settings
B. Can be mitigated by increasing transducer output
C. Are reduced in the near field
D. Are lower with a larger wavelengths

11. The transducer is most commonly operating in transmit mode.
A. True
B. False

12. Reject circuits are best employed to:
A. Reduce white out
B. Reduce background speckle
C. Protect against electrical injury
D. Reduce side lobe artifacts

13. Round-trip travel time (time from emission to return of reflected signals) in a TEE cardiac examination:
A. Varies significantly based on tissues encountered
B. Is impacted by sector width
C. Equals 13 μs/cm
D. Is highest with high-frequency signals

14. The round-trip travel time for a 10-MHz signal reflected from a target 20 cm from the transducer is:
A. 3,080 μs
B. 3,080 ms
C. 260 μs
D. 2,600 ms

15. M-mode has higher temporal resolution than 2D ultrasound because:
A. M-mode employs higher-frequency signals
B. 2D employs sector display
C. Effective depth of M-mode is one-half that of 2D
D. 2D employs B-mode

16. Phased array:
A. Is a passing fad
B. Is critical to M-mode display
C. Is an advancement over B-mode
D. Features electronic control over the activation of individual transducer elements

17. Frame rate is related to the PRF.
A. True
B. False

18. A freeze frame's image quality is directly impacted by all of the following ***except*****:**
A. Pulse length
B. Scan line density
C. Frame rate
D. Amplitude of returning signals

19. Dynamic motion appearance will be negatively impacted by:
A. Increase in sector width
B. Decrease in signal frequency
C. Decrease in depth setting
D. Decrease in scan line density

20. All are true regarding sound except:
A. Ultrasound obeys the same principles as sound.
B. Wavelength and frequency are inversely related.
C. The velocity of sound in soft tissue is relatively constant at 1,540 m/s.
D. Higher sound frequencies result in less absorption.
E. Sound is a vibration in a physical medium.

21. True statements regarding reflection of ultrasound are:
A. Two-dimensional echocardiographic imaging consists of both specular and scattering reflections.
B. Scattered reflections come from larger regular surfaces.
C. Specular reflections are greatest when the ultrasound beam and tissue interface are perpendicular (90°).
D. A and C

22. The following are true regarding reflection of the ultrasound beam except:
A. Reflection occurs at a tissue interface or area of acoustic mismatch.
B. Reflection is directly related to the absolute difference of the acoustic impedances between two tissues.
C. The ultrasound beam is reflected at an angle equal and opposite of that of the incident beam.
D. All of the above

23. Attenuation is least with:
A. Specular reflection of ultrasound with a 90° angle of incidence
B. Scattered reflection
C. Dispersion
D. Divergence of the ultrasound beam

24. All of the following are true regarding wavelength and frequency except:
A. Resolution is improved with higher-frequency sounds.
B. Resolution is improved with higher wavelength.
C. Lower-frequency sound waves have less absorption than higher-frequency sound waves.
D. Axial resolution is approximately 2 times the wavelength.

25. The ultrasound beam:
A. Is a two-dimensional beam, which results in a two-dimensional image
B. Is more concentrated in the near field and produces stronger signals
C. Width determines the lateral and elevational resolution
D. B and C

26. Resolution of a two-dimensional object:
A. Is improved with focusing
B. Is better with high-frequency/low-wavelength sound
C. Is better in the near-field imaging
D. All of the above

27. True statements regarding image resolution include all except:
A. Narrow ultrasound beams improve lateral resolution.
B. Higher frequencies increase resolution *and* imaging of deeper structures.
C. Focusing improves resolution in the near field but creates a more divergent beam thereafter.
D. Beam width is related to the frequency of the sound wave.

28. The following statements regarding echocardiographic displays are true except:
A. A-mode imaging used horizontal spikes along a vertical axis to represent tissue character and axial position.
B. M-mode imaging is characterized by high-resolution axial imaging with superdynamic display of cardiac motion.
C. M-mode imaging not only shows axial (vertical) motion but also displays lateral relations.
D. Two-dimensional imaging displays lateral and axial relations.

29. The following are false with respect to scan systems except:
A. An array consists of a single transducer element that is mechanically moved across the field of interest.
B. A linear scan emits a narrow beam from a small transducer face, making this ideal for imaging through small apertures (echocardiographic windows).
C. A phased array scan emits sweeps the ultrasound beam across a sector characterized by a narrow near field and diverging far field.
D. Neither phased array nor linear array scans are subject to side or grating lobes.

30. The process that is responsible for steering and focusing the transmitted and received scan lines is called:
A. Harmonics
B. Beamforming
C. Attenuation
D. Acquisition

31. What patient would provide the most optimal 3D, 4-beat full-volume data set?
A. Lightly sedated and in normal sinus rhythm (NSR)
B. Intubated and paralyzed and in atrial fibrillation
C. Lightly sedated and in atrial fibrillation
D. Intubated and paralyzed, and in NSR

32. How is strain usually expressed?
A. As a percentage change from its initial position
B. In centimeters per second
C. In hertz
D. In cm^3

33. Speckle tracking uses which mode of scanning?
A. M-mode
B. B-mode
C. A-mode
D. CWD
E. PWD

34. Tissue Doppler signals are:
A. High amplitude and high velocity
B. High amplitude and low velocity
C. Low amplitude and high velocity
D. Low amplitude and low velocity

35. Which statement is True.

A. Strain and speckle tracking are both dependent on the angle of the ultrasound beam to the direction of tissue movement.

B. Strain is angle independent, whereas speckle tracking is dependent on the angle of the ultrasound beam to the direction of tissue movement.

C. Strain and speckle tracking are both independent of the angle of the ultrasound beam to the direction of tissue movement.

D. Strain is dependent, whereas speckle tracking is independent of the angle of the ultrasound beam to the direction of tissue movement.

ANSWERS

1. Answer is C.
Rationale: The ultrasound energy is characterized by its amplitude, wavelength, frequency, and propagation velocity. The speed of ultrasound is determined solely by the medium through which it passes. $\lambda = v \times 1/f$

2. Answer is A.
Rationale: Ultrasound is a mechanical wave and needs particles to vibrate and transfer energy. A vacuum has no particles. Ultrasound is known to propagate through the other choices but at different speeds, which are dependent on the medium.

3. Answer is B.
Rationale: The speed of ultrasound through blood is approximately 1,500 m/s. By contrast, the speed of ultrasound through air and through lung is 330 and 600 m/s, respectively. While the ultrasound image appears echolucent through blood, it appears echo bright through air.

4. Answer is D.
Rationale: Frequency and wavelength are inversely related. Higher frequency sound waves are associated with smaller wavelengths. This results in smaller wavelengths, longer, narrower near field beams which have better focus and resolution. $\lambda = v \times 1/f$

5. Answer is A.
Rationale: Intensity (I) is ≅ Amplitude A^2. Amplitude is a measure of particle displacement.

6. Answer is A.
Rationale: B-mode imaging is *optimal* when the ultrasound beam is perpendicular to the flat tissue surface, that is, specular reflections. However, clinically since tissue surfaces are irregular, the returning or reflected ultrasound is a combination of specular and scatter reflections, with the former providing the strongest reflections.

7. Answer is A.
Rationale: Dispersion and the reflection coefficient are both correct. Although a higher frequency transducer loses more energy, the pulse repetition frequency is not a factor. The signal energy is lost with greater distance and absorption. PRF is the rate at which pulse signals are transmitted and would determine the maximal detectable velocity or Nyquist limit. The further away the area of interrogation the longer it takes to transmit and receive, the lower the PRF, and the smaller the maximal detectable velocity (Nyquist limit).

8. Answer is D.
Rationale: Piezoelectric crystals convert and generate ultrasound signals from electricity and then vice versa, the latter allowing them to be displayed on a monitor. While the transmission and conversion are independent, because the signals may be weak, amplification may be necessary by adjusting gain settings.

9. Answer is B.
Rationale: The length of the near field is increased with a larger transducer face and a higher frequency, permitting greater resolution of the near field. While focusing might improve imaging and resolution at a desired point, the field then disperses widely thereafter, resulting in a weaker signal beyond the focal point. Frequency and wavelength are inversely related.

10. Answer is C:
Rationale: Side lobes can be reduced by reducing gain and output to make the signal weaker. Side lobes are reduced with higher frequency and near field imaging. A larger wavelength is associated with smaller frequencies.

11. Answer is B:
Rationale: **False.** The ultrasound transducer is in receiver mode nearly 99% of the time. After it sends out a short pulse, it waits until the reflected wave returns.

12. Answer is B.
Rationale: Reject circuits filter out low-amplitude signals or background noise or speckle to allow concentration on the lower and higher amplitude signals.

13. Answer is C.
Rationale: Ultrasonic imaging is based on the amplitude and time delay of the reflected signals. Since the velocity in tissue is relatively constant, only the distance of the structure from the transducer alters the time required for the ultrasound wave to travel to and from the reflected structure. In other words, travel time = distance of the object from the transducer.

Distance = velocity × time

The round-trip travel time for each centimeter of separation between transducer and reflector is calculated as: Travel time for transesophageal exams is generally 13 μs/cm.

14. Answer is C.
Rationale: Travel time for transesophageal exams is generally 13 μs/cm. For a target 20 cm away, the travel time would be 20 × 13 μs = 260 μs.

15. Answer is B.
Rationale: M-mode is a unidimensional technique that provides an ice-pick view through the heart. Based on the size of the region that is interrogated, the frame rate is very high, approximately 100 times that of two-dimensional sector scanning. Although M-mode imaging does not display lateral resolutions, its ability to align motion with time and a very high axial resolution make M-mode unique.

16. Answer is D.
Rationale: As above, M-mode is a single dimension imaging mode while sector scanning is two or three dimensional. Phased array is an electronic process that allows control over individual transducer activation that permits narrowing of the sector width and/or focusing.

17. Answer is A.
Rationale: PRF and frame rate are related but distinct concepts. PRF is the rate at which pulses of ultrasound are emitted by the transducer, while frame rate is the rate at which complete images (frames) are displayed. A higher PRF can allow for a higher frame rate, but the two are not directly equivalent.

18. Answer is C.
Rationale: The image quality includes lateral, axial, and elevational resolutions as well as temporal resolution, the latter in regard to viewing the moving cardiac structures. Pulse length and scan line density impact on resolution and information and amplitude affects the appearance of structures. Since the question is asking about a "freeze frame," then temporal resolution or frame rate does not apply.

19. Answer is A.
Rationale: The dynamic resolution is the temporal resolution and is reflected by the frame rate. Anything that increases the amount of information that the system is asked to do will decrease the frame rate. Increasing the sector scan, the depth, and scan line density will increase the amount of information.

20. Answer is D.
Rationale: Absorption of the ultrasound energy is increased with increasing depth and frequency. The attenuation coefficient = db/cm/MHz.

21. Answer is D.
Rationale: Scattered reflections come from irregular and smaller surfaces. Specular reflections, which result in greater reflection, come from larger, flatter surfaces that are perpendicular to the desired object being imaged.

22. Answer is D.
Rationale: All are true: Acoustic impedance $z = \rho \times v$.

Reflection coefficient = Between two mediums Z_1 and Z_2

$$\frac{(Z_2 - Z_1)^2}{(Z_1 + Z_2)^2}$$

23. Answer is A.
Rationale: Loss of ultrasound energy is least with a 90° angle of incidence or a perpendicular path between the ultrasound beam and a flat regular surface.

24. Answer is B.
Rationale: Higher frequency sounds have a better axial and lateral resolution. Frequency and wavelength are inversely related, so higher frequencies have smaller wavelengths and are able to distinguish between smaller spaced objects. However, higher frequency sounds lose energy faster and do not penetrate as well as lower frequency sounds.

25. Answer is D (B and C).
Rationale: The ultrasound beam is a three-dimensional structure, but the display is two dimensional. The near field is a narrower width and has better resolution than the far field. Since the ultrasound beam diverges in the far field, the ultrasound tends to disperse, and returning signals are weaker when compared to the near field.

26. Answer is D (All of the above).
Rationale: All of the options are consistent with improved image resolution. Focusing narrows the field to improve both imaging and resolution. The near field is narrower, includes better image strength, and able to better distinguish between objects closer together.

27. Answer is B.
Rationale: While higher frequencies have a favorable beam width and longer near field and improve resolution, more energy is used and does not image deeper structures with the same signal strength. The attenuation coefficient = db/cm/MHz.

28. Answer is C.
Rationale: M-mode imaging only shows axial relations and not lateral ones. M-mode imaging is a unidimensional imaging tool, while 2D imaging displays both axial and lateral relations. Display formats. The ultrasound beam is directed through the aortic valve leaflets. Amplitude-mode (A-mode) display shows the resulting reflections as horizontal spikes. In the brightness-mode (B-mode) display, the pikes are replaced with pixels of varying brightness. Motion mode (M-mode) shows sequential B-mode frames to capture cardiac motion.

29. Answer is C.
Rationale: A single element (crystal) emits a wave front that diverges. Aligning multiple crystals in an array allows interaction between multiple wave fronts that creates a forward narrower wave front with a stronger signal. Furthermore, the crystals of the array can be electrically activated to steer and focus. However, the stronger the signal (higher intensity main lobe) the greater the chance for energy away from the main energy beam (lobe), increasing the chance for artifacts called side lobes.

30. Answer is B.
Rationale: Beamformer is a unit that shapes the ultrasound beam, including focusing. Harmonics is a process in which the object acts as a reflecting or emitting source of ultrasound to increase the image resolution. Attenuation is the loss of the ultrasound energy.

31. Answer is D.
Rationale: Three-dimensional imaging is a summation of multiple two-dimensional slices that are captured and processed to build a comprehensive image of the cardiac tissues. Current technology includes processors that are fast for single-beat three-dimensional imaging; however, depending on the size of the sector scanned, these result in a lower frame rate and miss important information combined with a lower temporal resolution. If multi-beat acquisition were desired to increase both frame rate and line density, then patients would optimally be completely still and in sinus rhythm. Any other condition increases the risk of stitch artifacts.

32. Answer is A.
Rationale: Strain and strain rate measure myocardial mechanical function, displacement, or deformation of muscle tissue. Strain is a dimensionless number expressed as an object's percentage change (shortening or lengthening) from its initial position. When the ventricle contracts, strain and strain rate are positive in the radial dimension and negative in the longitudinal and circumferential dimensions.

33. Answer is B.
Rationale: Speckle tracking assesses myocardial motion or deformation over a larger user-defined region compared to TDI, an extension of B-mode ultrasound technology that relies on the detection of myocardial speckles, or reflectors, to assess contraction- and relaxation-related motion of the myocardium to calculate myocardial strain throughout the cardiac cycle.

34. Answer is B.
Rationale: Based on conventional Doppler, tissue Doppler measures the lower velocity movements of the myocardium. These signals are lower velocity but of higher amplitude. The processing filters out higher velocities to allow analysis of the lower tissue velocity. Tissue Doppler is constrained by the same limitations as conventional Doppler, most notably that accurate assessment requires near-parallel alignment between tissue movement and the ultrasound beam. A second limitation is that precise and accurate TDI requires frame rates greater than 100 FPS. Finally, tissue Doppler does not differentiate active contraction from passive motion. Myocardium that has normal intrinsic contraction could have the same velocity as a scarred segment that is tethered to normal functioning myocardium.

35. Answer is D.
Rationale: Strain and strain rate measure myocardial mechanical function, displacement, or deformation of muscle tissue. Strain, which is tissue Doppler based, is a dimensionless number expressed as an object's percentage change (shortening or lengthening) from its initial position. As it is a Doppler-based technology, it is angle-dependent with parallel alignment yielding more accurate data. Speckle tracking is an extension of B-mode ultrasound technology that relies on the detection of myocardial speckles, or reflectors, to assess contraction- and relaxation-related motion of the myocardium to calculate myocardial strain throughout the cardiac cycle. Its speed of change and direction form a vector that is independent of the angle of the ultrasound beam.

2 Two-Dimensional Examination

Michael Benson and Candice Morrissey

Two-dimensional (2D) transesophageal echocardiography (TEE) is an indispensable tool in modern medicine. It allows for the real-time assessment of the heart and surrounding structures, assessment of volume status and hemodynamics, and intraoperative and periprocedural guidance. Despite the advancements in complex three-dimensional (3D) and strain imaging, the 2D TEE exam remains a mainstay of cardiac imaging because of its speed, reproducibility, and ease of real-time application. In experienced hands, it can optimize patient safety and improve outcomes (1). It is important to note, however, that 2D TEE is challenging and takes time to master. Misinterpretation of critical information in a clinical setting can be as harmful as a lack of information. As such, minimum standards for independent practice in echocardiography have been created (2).

The 2013 American Society of Echocardiography Guidelines for Performing a Comprehensive TEE Examination and 2022 ASE Guidelines for Transesophageal Screening for Structural Heart Intervention describe essentially all the TEE views available to the echocardiographer (3,4) and will be referenced throughout this chapter. In practice, it is rare that every view described in these guidelines is needed because of time constraints and limited value added to the exam. The purpose of this chapter is to describe the *practical* application of the 2D TEE exam. A standardized and disciplined approach to the exam is strongly recommended and will be described along with practical tips for image optimization.

PROBE INSERTION

The beginning of every TEE exam is the insertion of the probe, a medical procedure that is not without risks. Potential complications range from the more common and less severe, such as transient hoarseness and difficulty swallowing, to the less common and more severe, such as major bleeding, esophageal perforation, and death (5).

Contraindications to TEE, both absolute and relative, must be appreciated. Absolute contraindications include: perforated viscus, esophageal stricture, esophageal tumor, esophageal perforation/laceration, esophageal diverticulum, and active upper gastrointestinal (GI) bleed. Relative contraindications include a history of neck or mediastinal radiation, a history of GI surgery, recent upper GI bleed, Barrett esophagus, history of dysphagia, restriction of neck mobility, symptomatic hiatal hernia, esophageal varices, coagulopathy, active esophagitis, and active peptic ulcer diseases (6). While these contraindications are uncommon, it is important to consider them and to weigh the risks and benefits of TEE placement in each case.

In anesthetized patients, the probe will typically be inserted with the patient in the supine position. Supporting or suspending the probe handle allows the use of both hands for probe placement, with the left hand providing tongue and jaw lift and the right gently inserting the ultrasound probe. Placement of a TEE probe should never require more pressure than can be delivered with a gentle two-finger grip, and a closed-fist "hammer grip" should never be employed. While slight anteflexion may help guide the probe around the tongue, it's important that the probe be in a neutral or retroflexed position in the posterior oropharynx. Constant gentle pressure directed in the orientation of the esophagus, toward the patient's feet, typically allows for easy passage of probe. If passage remains difficult, either direct or video laryngoscopy can serve to expand the posterior oropharynx as well as visualize passage of the probe into the esophagus.

PROBE MANIPULATION

Subtle probe manipulations are critical to creating and optimizing each view, and employing a standard language to describe these motions is helpful when communicating with colleagues and trainees. The probe can be advanced and withdrawn, turned to the patient's left (counterclockwise) and the patient's right (clockwise), flexed to the left and the right, or anteflexed and retroflexed (4) (Figure 2.1).

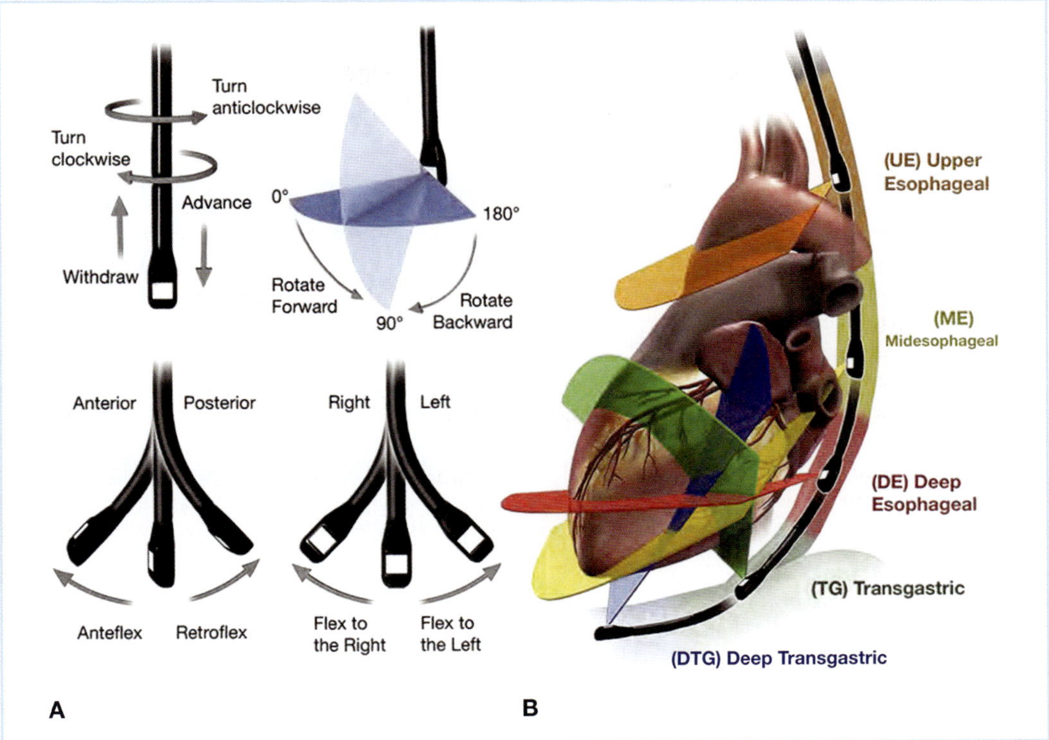

FIGURE 2.1 Probe manipulation and levels of imaging. The terminology for probe manipulation (A) is as follows: (1) advancing or withdrawing the probe within the esophagus, (2) rotating the probe clockwise (toward the right chest) or counterclockwise (toward the left chest), (3) axial flexion of the probe (anteflexion and retroflexion), (4) lateral flexion of the probe (right flexion and left flexion), and (5) mechanical rotation (forward rotating by increasing the degrees of rotation and backward rotating by decreasing the degrees of rotation). The five levels of imaging (B) are UE, ME, DE, TG, and DT or DTG. (From Hahn RT, Saric M, Faletra F, et al Recommended standards for the performance of transesophageal echocardiographic screening for structural heart intervention: from the American Society of Echocardiography. *J Am Soc Echocardiogr*. 2022;35(1):1-76, Figure 1 with permission.)

Probe positions or "windows" are described starting proximally in the upper esophageal (UE) window. Advancing the probe brings it to the midesophageal (ME), deep esophageal (DE), transgastric (TG), and finally deep transgastric (DTG) windows. Each of the windows can be recognized by the structures nearest the TEE probe. In the UE window, the great vessels are closest to the TEE probe. In the ME window, the left atrium (LA) is closest to the TEE probe. In the DE window, the coronary sinus (CS) is closest to the TEE probe. In the TG window, the left or right ventricle (RV) is closest to the TEE probe. In the DTG window, the cardiac apex is closest to the TEE probe (4).

Turning of the probe has been described as toward the patient's left or counterclockwise versus toward the patient's right or clockwise. These terms may be used interchangeably. The probe is turned to the patient's left to optimize left-sided cardiac structures and to the patient's right to optimize right-sided cardiac structures. When turning the probe, it is important to turn from the probe handle while supporting the probe shaft near the mouth so as not to torque the shaft.

Finally, while there may be variation among vendors, the probe handle typically has two control wheels or knobs. The larger wheel will retroflex or anteflex the probe and imaging plane. The smaller wheel will flex the probe and imaging plane to the patient's left or right (3).

IMAGING PLANE ANGLE

Modern TEE probes have improved significantly from the early generations that employed only M-mode or single-plane 2D imaging. Today's probes have matrix array ultrasound transducers allowing for multiplane

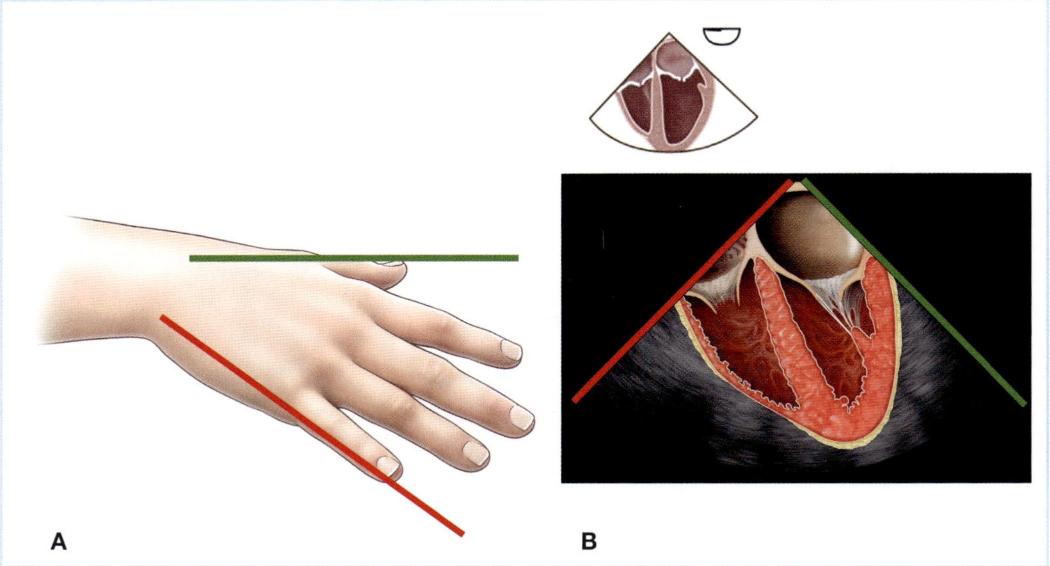

FIGURE 2.2 A: Orientation of a 0° imaging plane. Imagine that "you are the probe" and your right hand held horizontally is the ultrasound plane. Your **L**ittle finger will be shown on the **L**eft side of the screen. The red and green lines correspond with those shown in image B. B: A schematic representation of the imaging plane (above) and the cardiac anatomy (below) for a midesophageal (ME) four-chamber view. The TEE probe lies in the esophagus behind the left atrium with the imaging plane projecting like a wedge anteriorly through the heart. On the monitor, the "red edge," corresponding to your little finger, will be shown on the left of the screen.

imaging angles from 0° to 180°. These probes can perform simultaneous multiplane imaging, strain analysis, and real-time 3D imaging (3).

The creation of successful 2D images requires an understanding of the relationship between the ultrasound beam and the cardiac anatomy of interest. The ultrasound beam originates from the probe and projects perpendicularly away from the transducer. The structures closest to the transducer are displayed at the pointy "top" of the ultrasound image (the near field) and will typically be anatomically posterior. Structures at the arc of the imaging sector (the far field) are farther from the transducer and are typically anatomically anterior cardiac structures (3).

Another important principle to appreciate in 2D TEE is that the left-right orientation of the image depends on the rotation of the multiplane angle. The rotation of the multiplane angle is analogous to the physical clockwise and counterclockwise rotation of a probe when performing surface ultrasound. The degree of rotation is manipulated in 1° increments using the up and down buttons on the probe handle.

The image starts at a baseline of 0°. At this multiplane angle, the sector orientation can be understood by placing your right hand in front of you with your palm facing downward. Your thumb points to the left and your little finger points toward the right. With this orientation, structures on the left side of the heart will be displayed on the right of the image, and structures on the right side of the heart will be displayed on the left side of the image (Figure 2.2).

You can remember that the **L**eft side of the image shows what's by your **L**ittle finger. By increasing the multiplane, the imaging plane angle moves in a clockwise manner. The movement of this plane is simulated by rotating your right hand clockwise. At 90°, this would be analogous to the palm of your right hand facing to your left and your thumb pointing upward (anterior) and little finger pointing downward (inferior) (Figure 2.3).

As mentioned previously, simultaneous biplane imaging is a capability of most modern TEE probes. To accomplish this, the initial image is created, and the "biplane" function on the machine is enabled. A cursor line is placed through the area of interest and both orthogonal views are displayed side by side. This allows for a more efficient and more comprehensive examination of the heart. An important point to remember is that if the initial image has an angle of rotation greater than 90°, the orthogonal image will be right-left inverted. Most machines have a "right-left invert" function that will allow a more traditional view to be displayed.

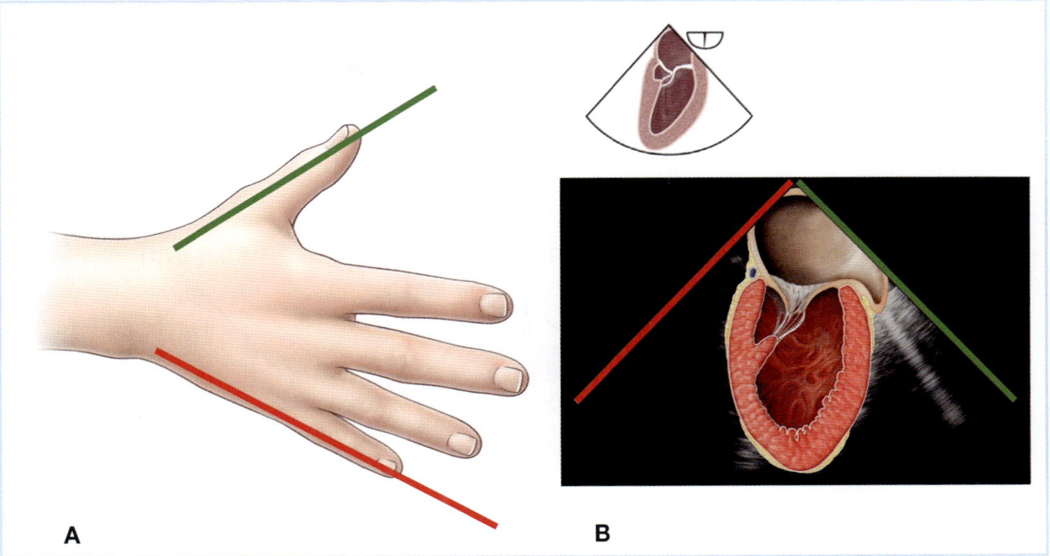

FIGURE 2.3 A: Orientation of a 90° imaging plane. Imagine that "you are the probe" and your right hand held vertically is the ultrasound plane. Your Little finger will be shown on the Left side of the screen. The red and green lines correspond with those shown in image B. B: A schematic representation of the imaging plane (above) and the cardiac anatomy (below) for a midesophageal (ME) two-chamber view. Now, the red plane (little finger, left side of the screen) is inferior, and the green plane (thumb, right side of the screen) is anterior.

By combining probe manipulation with the adjustment of the multiplane angle, essentially all cardiac structures can be well visualized with TEE. As we describe the views, recall that the orientation of the heart and its relationship to the TEE transducer vary from patient to patient, and structures may be relatively displaced secondary to differences in anatomy and pathology. As such, the positions and angles described will serve as general guidelines rather than rigid protocols.

A STANDARDIZED APPROACH TO THE TRANSESOPHAGEAL ECHOCARDIOGRAPHY EXAM

The 2013 ASE Guidelines for Performing a Comprehensive TEE Examination and the 2022 ASE Guidelines for Transesophageal Screening for Structural Heart Intervention outline all the described views for the 2D TEE exam. Practical constraints limit the need for obtaining every view in every exam. For example, while it may not be imperative to identify all four pulmonary veins on every TEE exam, there are images that should be obtained almost without exception. We will call this standard collection of essential images a "Basic TEE exam" (Figure 2.4). In this section, we advocate for maintaining a consistent and standardized approach to the TEE exam and ask the reader to consider developing a core set of images used in every exam—both for individuals and within groups.

While TEE is typically utilized to address specific clinical questions, unexpected abnormalities are commonly encountered and must be identified. Failing to systematically explore all the major structures of the heart can lead to avoidable errors. This risk is exacerbated by production pressure and the urgent nature of perioperative imaging. Perioperative TEE is one of the only times in medicine in which a single provider must simultaneously perform a complex diagnostic procedure, interpret the findings in real time, integrate those findings into a challenging clinical scenario, act on the findings, then observe and repeat. This high cognitive load creates a setup for errors and cognitive biases (7). Some of these cognitive biases include but are not limited to: search satisfaction (failing to search for additional abnormalities after identifying the initial one), anchoring bias (influence of one's initial impression), and confirmation bias (favoring findings that confirm one's initial beliefs) (8). While error and cognitive bias can never be eliminated, they can be mitigated by employing cognitive forcing strategies and consistent search patterns (8). The disciplined and systematic performance and interpretation of perioperative TEE represent such an approach.

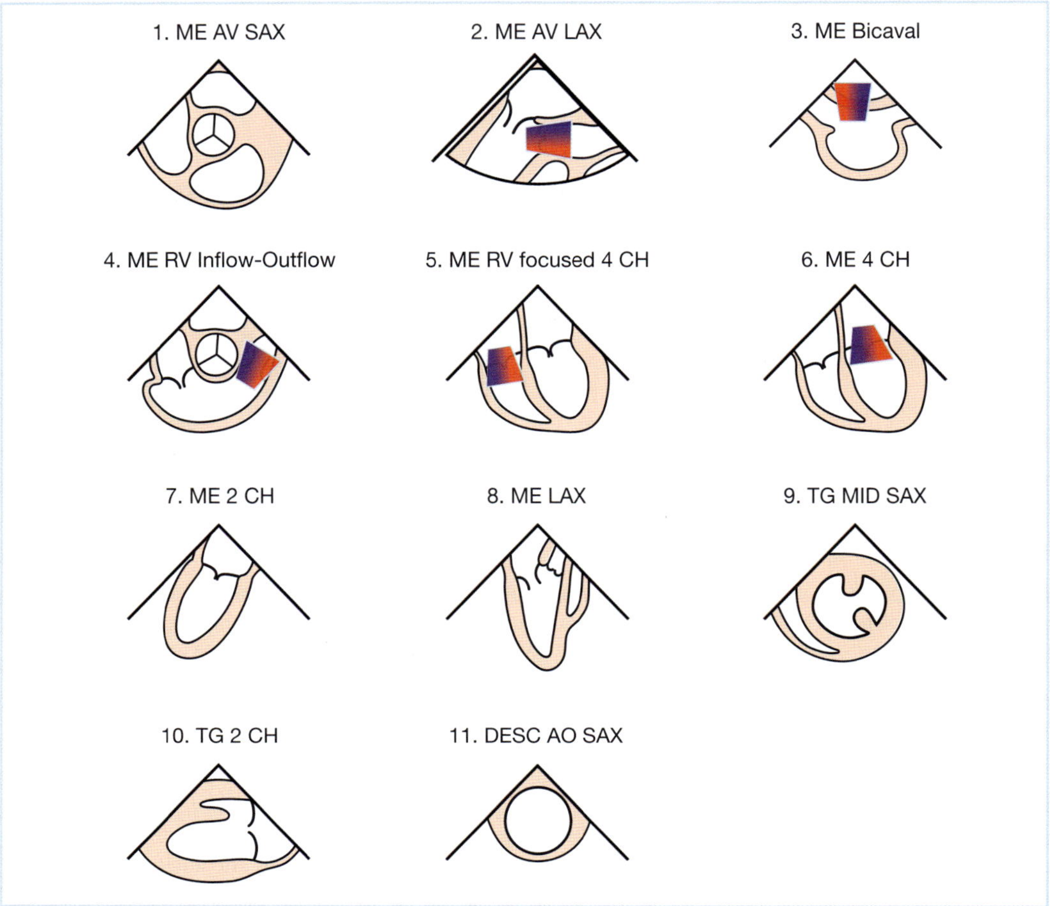

FIGURE 2.4 The authors' recommended Basic Exam sequence. Color flow Doppler should be used for each valve in one view (the aortic valve in long axis, the pulmonic valve in the RV I-O, and the tricuspid and mitral valves in the corresponding four-chamber views). The interatrial septum should be assessed with color flow Doppler in the bicaval view. Finally, in order to visualize both the complete right and left heart, the four chamber should be seen as two views -- an RV focused, where the complete RA and RV are demonstrated, and an LV focused, where the left ventricle is directly under the transducer. 2 CH, two chamber; 4 CH, four chamber; AO, aorta; AV, aortic valve; DESC, descending; LAX, long axis; ME, midesophageal; RV, right ventricular; SAX, short axis; TG, transgastric; CFD, color flow doppler; MID, mid-papillary. (Adapted from Hahn RT, Abraham T, Adams MS, et al. Guidelines for performing a comprehensive transesophageal echocardiographic examination: recommendations from the American Society of Echocardiography and the Society of Cardiovascular Anesthesiologists. *J Am Soc Echocardiogr*. 2013;26:921-964, with permission.)

THE "BASIC EXAM" (FIGURE 2.4)

The "Basic Exam" described here represents our approach for evaluating the heart using a limited number of views. This represents an evolution of the exam created by Drs Michael Cahalan (often described as the father of perioperative echocardiography) and Dan Vezina at the University of California, San Francisco then perfected at the University of Utah (9,10). While we may call it the "Basic Exam," it is by no means basic in practice. The aim of this exam is to efficiently visualize all major cardiac structures at least once with 2D and color flow Doppler. It is the authors' experience that the described exam can be performed and interpreted within 3 to 5 minutes. This exam entails assessing all left ventricular (LV) segments, the RV, the interatrial and interventricular septa, all cardiac valves, and the thoracic aorta.

This Basic Exam minimizes probe manipulation by starting in the midesophagus, progressing into the stomach, and returning to the midesophagus for completion. Any identified pathology should prompt further investigation after completion of this initial evaluation. While this approach may not be universally applicable to all clinical scenarios, it provides an efficient, thorough, and consistent starting point for most clinical situations.

Midesophageal Aortic Valve Short-Axis View (Figure 2.5; Video 2.1)

The ME aortic valve (AV) short-axis view is the starting point for our Basic Exam. After insertion of the TEE probe into the esophagus, the probe is advanced until the ascending aorta is seen, then advanced until the AV is visualized. The imaging plane is rotated to approximately 45° to visualize the AV in short axis at the center of the image. For this and every subsequent view, it should be noted that a suggested multiplane angle will be given as a general guide with the understanding that significant patient-to-patient variability exists. In practice, the multiplane angle that creates the optimal view should be used, and the depth should be set to include only the structures of interest and nothing more.

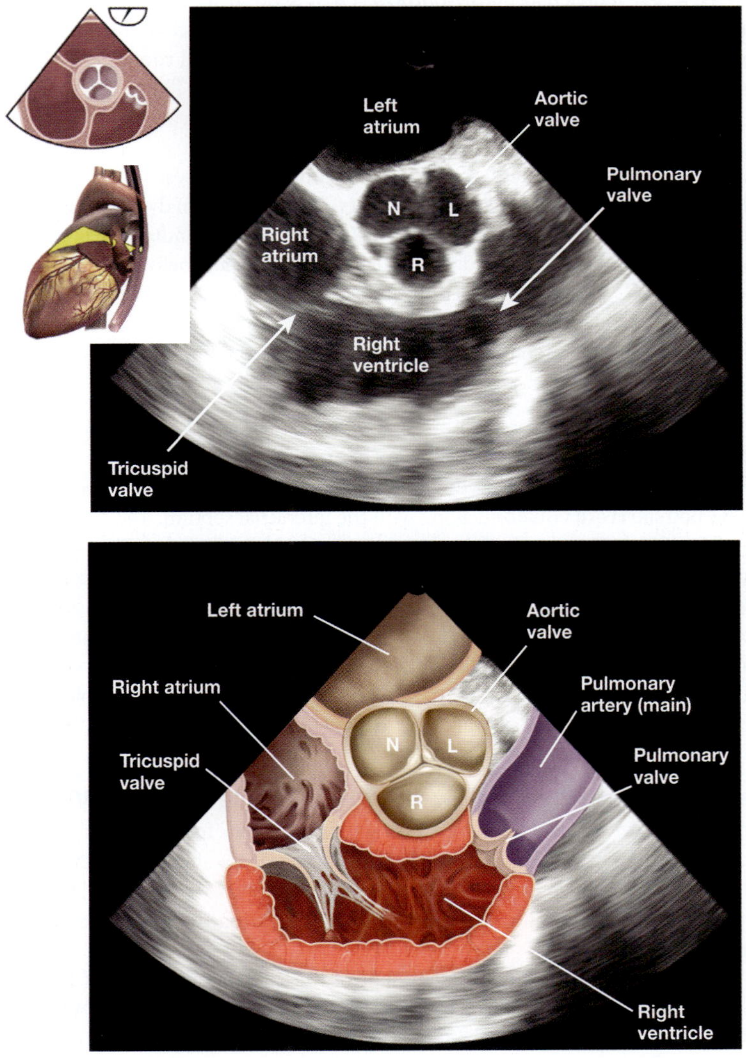

FIGURE 2.5 Midesophageal aortic valve short-axis view (above). Anatomic representation (below). Inset: anatomic representation with approximate imaging plane. L, left coronary aortic valve cusp; N, noncoronary aortic valve cusp; R, right coronary aortic valve cusp.

As with all ME windows, the LA is seen in the near field of the image closest to the TEE probe. The AV in short axis is below the LA. This has been described as the "Mercedes Benz" view of the AV, with the non-coronary cusp on the left (always associated with the interatrial septum), the right coronary cusp (RCC) on the bottom (associated with the RV), and the left coronary cusp on the right. The origins of the right coronary artery and the left main coronary artery may be visualized from their respective coronary cusps. While other structures such as the atria, interatrial septum, and RV are often visualized in this view, the primary focus of this view is on the AV.

The purpose of this view is to compare the relative size of the AV to the atria, identify the morphology of AV, and assess overall valvular function by gauging the degree of the calcification of the leaflets, the mobility of the leaflets, and identifying coaptation defects. The interatrial septum is well visualized in this view as well and is evaluated during structural heart procedures requiring crossing of the interatrial septum.

Midesophageal Aortic Valve Long-Axis View (Figure 2.6; Video 2.2)

The ME AV long-axis view is obtained by increasing the image plane to approximately 120° to 140°. This view should be considered a "left ventricular inflow-outflow" cross-section and should be created to optimize both features. This can be done by rotating the probe to optimize the appearance of the mitral valve (inflow) while increasing the multiplane angle to optimize the appearance of the AV and root (outflow).

In the ME AV long-axis view, the left ventricular outflow tract (LVOT), the AV, and the aortic root are all visualized in a long-axis orientation. The RCC of the AV is the cusp nearest the RV in this view, with the remaining cusp most commonly being the left coronary cusp.

The purpose of this view is to evaluate overall valvular function by assessing leaflet calcification, the mobility of the leaflets, and any significant coaptation defects. The presence of dynamic LVOT obstruction from systolic anterior motion of the mitral leaflets should be sought. The ascending aorta should be assessed for significant pathology such as dilation, atheroma, or dissection especially before and after aortic cannulation. Measurements of the LVOT, sinotubular junction, sinuses of Valsalva, and proximal ascending aorta can be done in this view. After the 2D examination, the AV should be evaluated with color flow Doppler to screen for aortic insufficiency as well as to identify flow acceleration or turbulence that point toward either valvular or LVOT obstruction.

Midesophageal Bicaval View (Figure 2.7; Video 2.3)

The ME bicaval view is obtained by rotating the probe to the patient's right and decreasing the imaging plane to 100°. In this view, both atria are visualized along with the interatrial septum. The superior vena cava (SVC) is seen entering the right atrium (RA) on the right side of the image while the inferior vena cava (IVC) may be seen on the left. Often, both structures are not perfectly aligned in the same plane, and it is common to only visualize the SVC. Slightly modifying depth and imaging plane angle can help to visualize the CS just proximal to the IVC.

One of the primary purposes of the bicaval view is to assess the interatrial septum. Continuous bowing of the interatrial septum to the left or right can indicate relatively elevated pressures on one side of the heart. This view can also be used to identify wires or cannulas placed on the right side. Color flow Doppler can be used to assess for the presence of atrial septal defect or large patent foramen ovale.

Midesophageal Right Ventricular Inflow-Outflow View (Figure 2.8; Video 2.4)

The ME RV inflow-outflow view is obtained by rotating the probe back to the patient's left and decreasing the imaging plane to approximately 60°. This view is similar to the ME AV short-axis view; however, rather than focusing on the AV, the goal is to optimize the atria, interatrial septum, tricuspid valve, RV, right ventricular outflow, pulmonic valve, and main pulmonary artery (PA). Increasing the imaging depth is often needed to optimize this view.

The ME RV inflow-outflow view allows assessment of the 2D characteristics of the tricuspid valve, the pulmonic valve with and without color flow Doppler, and RV systolic function. It will often be difficult to determine which leaflets of the tricuspid valve are visualized in this view; however, the anterior leaflet of the pulmonic valve is typically the most anterior (furthest from the AV) at 4 o'clock position.

This image may provide good alignment for spectral Doppler interrogation of the tricuspid valve. Right ventricular outflow tract diameter can be measured in this view to calculate right-sided cardiac output. This view is also helpful for PA catheter insertion and confirmation of placement in the main PA.

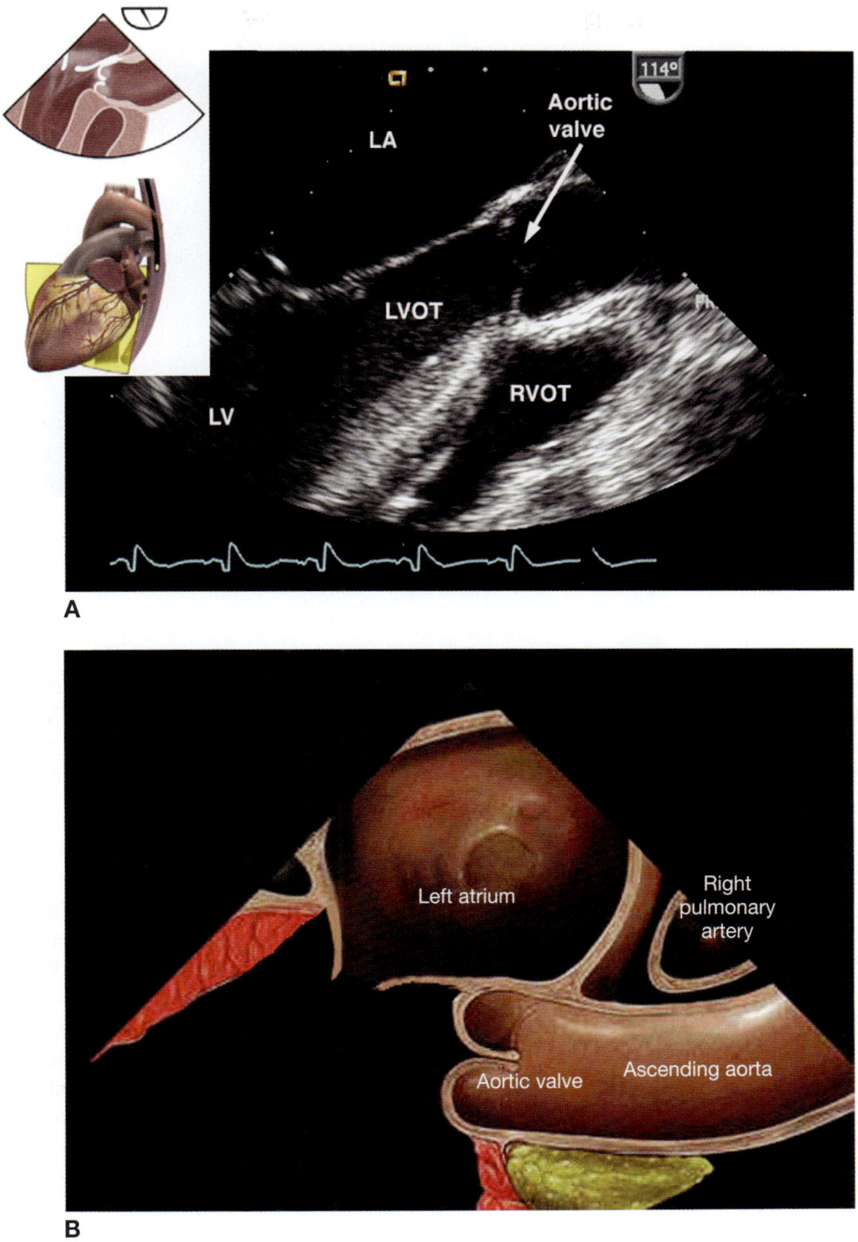

FIGURE 2.6 A: Midesophageal (ME) aortic valve long-axis view. B: Anatomic representation of the ME aortic valve long-axis view. Inset: anatomic representation with approximate imaging plane. LA, left atrium; LV, left ventricle; LVOT, left ventricular outflow tract; RVOT, right ventricular outflow tract. (B from Patrick J. Lynch, illustrator; C. Carl Jaffe, MD, cardiologist, Yale University Center for Advanced Instructional Media; Medical illustrations by Patrick Lynch, generated for multimedia teaching projects by the Yale University School of Medicine, Center for Advanced Instructional Media, 1987-2000. Patrick J. Lynch, http://patricklynch.net. Creative Commons Attribution 2.5 License 2006; no usage restrictions except please preserve our creative credits: Patrick J. Lynch, medical illustrator; C. Carl Jaffe, MD, cardiologist. http://creativecommons.org/licenses/by/2.5/.)

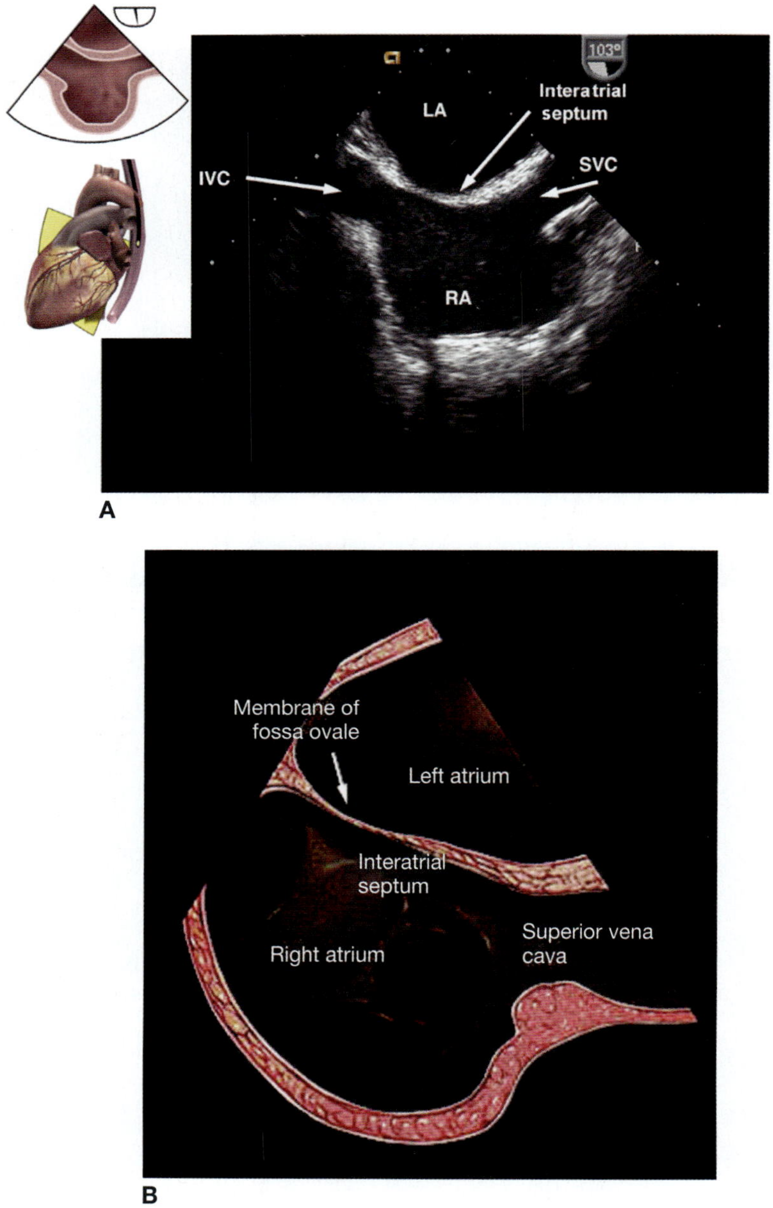

FIGURE 2.7 A: Midesophageal (ME) bicaval view. B: Anatomic representation of the ME bicaval view. Inset: anatomic representation with approximate imaging plane. IVC, inferior vena cava; LA, left atrium; RA, right atrium; SVC, superior vena cava. (B from Patrick J. Lynch, illustrator; C. Carl Jaffe, MD, cardiologist, Yale University Center for Advanced Instructional Media; Medical illustrations by Patrick Lynch, generated for multimedia teaching projects by the Yale University School of Medicine, Center for Advanced Instructional Media, 1987-2000. Patrick J. Lynch, http://patricklynch.net. Creative Commons Attribution 2.5 License 2006; no usage restrictions except please preserve our creative credits: Patrick J. Lynch, medical illustrator; C. Carl Jaffe, MD, cardiologist. http://creativecommons.org/licenses/by/2.5/.)

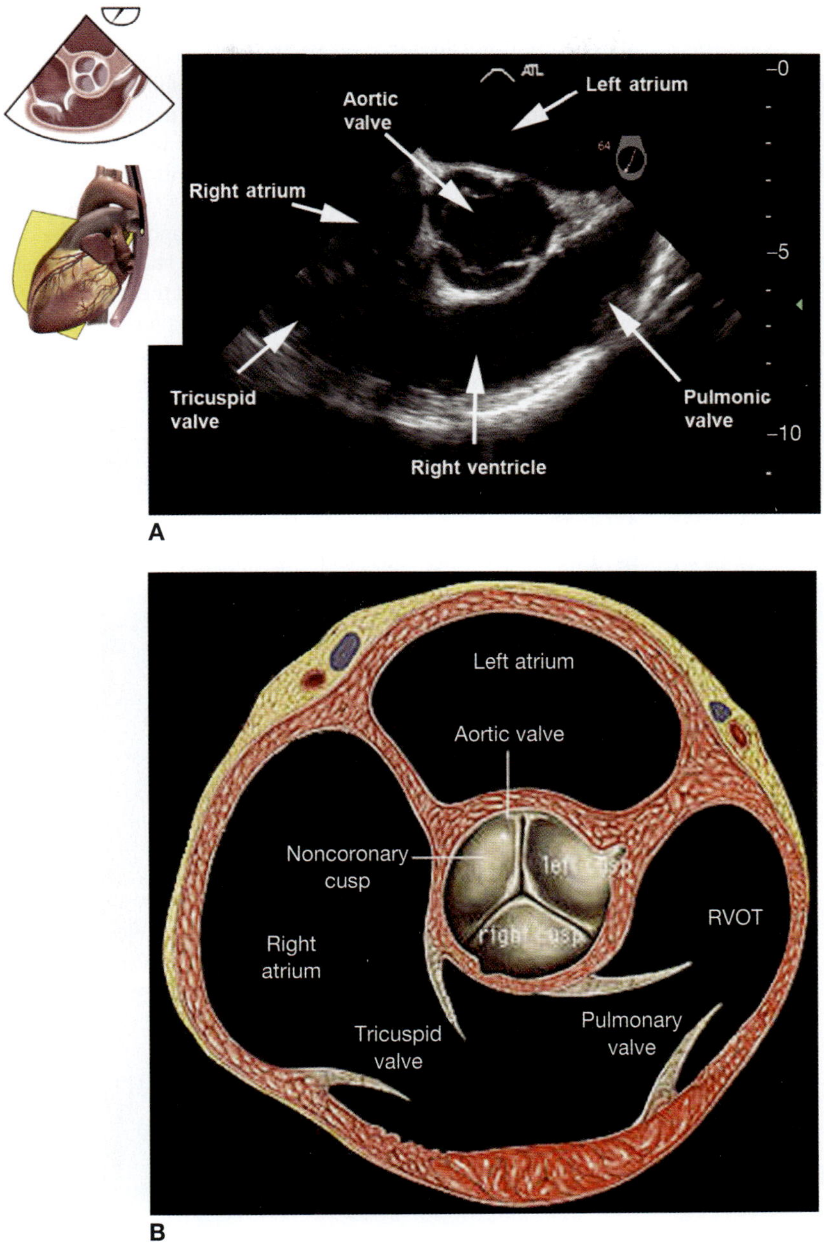

FIGURE 2.8 A: Midesophageal (ME) right ventricular inflow outflow. B: Anatomic representation of the ME right ventricular inflow-outflow view. The reader should compare this image to the adjacent echocardiographic image for a better understanding of cardiac anatomy. Inset: anatomic representation with approximate imaging plane. RVOT, right ventricular outflow tract. (From Patrick J. Lynch, illustrator, C. Carl Jaffe; MD, cardiologist Yale University Center for Advanced Instructional Media; Medical illustrations by Patrick Lynch, generated for multimedia teaching projects by the Yale University School of Medicine, Center for Advanced Instructional Media, 1987-2000. Patrick J. Lynch, http://patricklynch.net. Creative Commons Attribution 2.5 License 2006; no usage restrictions except please preserve our creative credits: Patrick J. Lynch, medical illustrator; C. Carl Jaffe, MD, cardiologist. http://creativecommons.org/licenses/by/2.5/.)

Midesophageal Four-Chamber View (Figure 2.9; Video 2.5)

The ME four-chamber view is obtained by slightly advancing the probe and decreasing the imaging plane to approximately 0°. Rotation to the patient's left is often required to center the LA and help to fix the LV apex in the center of the far field. Retroflexion is often necessary to prevent foreshortening of the LV. In some cases, the AV and LVOT are initially visualized. These are anterior structures in the heart; therefore, further advancement or retroflexion of the probe can help to remove these from view and optimize the image. If the probe is advanced or retroflexed, the CS will be visualized communicating with the RA from the right side of the screen.

The classic four-chamber view of the heart includes the LA, mitral valve, and LV on the right side of the image and the RA, tricuspid valve, and RV on the left side of the image. Depth should be adjusted, so the image just includes the LV apex. The apex should remain thin and in the center of the image during contraction. If the apex appears to move toward the mitral valve with contraction, there is foreshortening of the image, which can cause overestimation of LV ejection fraction. It should be noted that, while this view is called a "four chamber," it is uncommon to adequately visualize all four chambers in a single image. A separate view

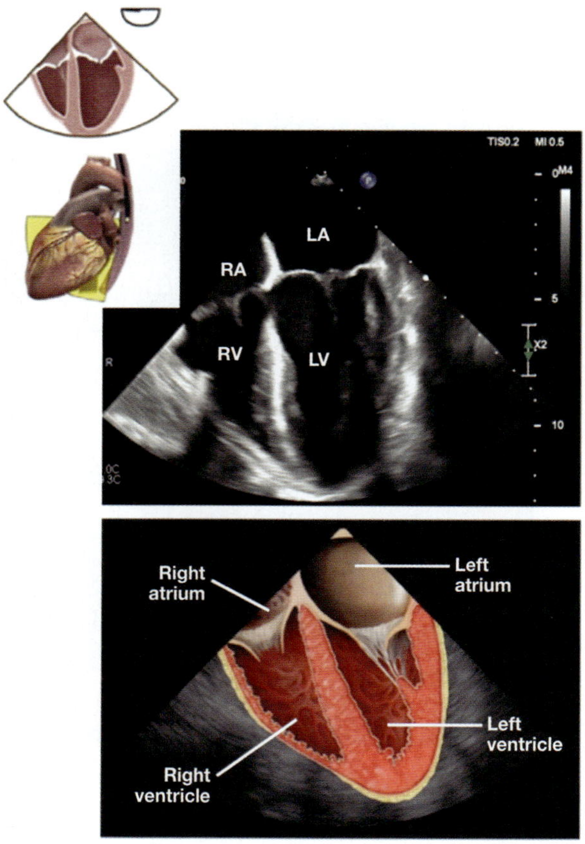

FIGURE 2.9 Midesophageal four-chamber view (above). Anatomic representation (below). Note that the authors suggest creating both right ventricular–focused and left ventricular–focused views (as shown in Video 2.5) to ensure the entire heart is visualized. Inset: anatomic representation with approximate imaging plane. LA, left atrium; LV, left ventricle; RA, right atrium; RV, right ventricle. (From Patrick J. Lynch, illustrator, C. Carl Jaffe; MD, cardiologist Yale University Center for Advanced Instructional Media; Medical illustrations by Patrick Lynch, generated for multimedia teaching projects by the Yale University School of Medicine, Center for Advanced Instructional Media, 1987-2000. Patrick J. Lynch, http://patricklynch.net. Creative Commons Attribution 2.5 License 2006; no usage restrictions except please preserve our creative credits: Patrick J. Lynch, medical illustrator; C. Carl Jaffe, MD, cardiologist. http://creativecommons.org/licenses/by/2.5/.)

that focuses on the right heart (an "RV-focused four chamber") created by rightward probe rotation from the classic "LV-focused" four chamber will be necessary in most cases.

The ME four-chamber view has a high diagnostic yield for global assessment of cardiac structure and function. One should compare the relative sizes of the atria and ventricles, assess global biventricular systolic function, evaluate segmental wall motion, and assess the mitral and tricuspid valves in 2D and with color flow Doppler. In this image, the anterolateral and inferoseptal walls of the LV are visualized. The anterior leaflet of the mitral valve is seen on the left and posterior on the right. For the tricuspid valve, the septal leaflet is typically seen closest to the interventricular septum and the long anterior leaflet is visualized laterally.

The ME four-chamber view can be used to measure the annulus of the tricuspid valve and can also be helpful in observing intraventricular air following cardiopulmonary bypass (CPB), which is seen as echodense bubbles often present at the apex and along the interventricular septum.

Midesophageal Two-Chamber View (Figure 2.10; Video 2.6)

This ME two-chamber view is obtained by ensuring the LV is centered in the previous view and increasing the imaging plane to approximately 90°. This view shows the LA, mitral valve, and LV. The image is optimized

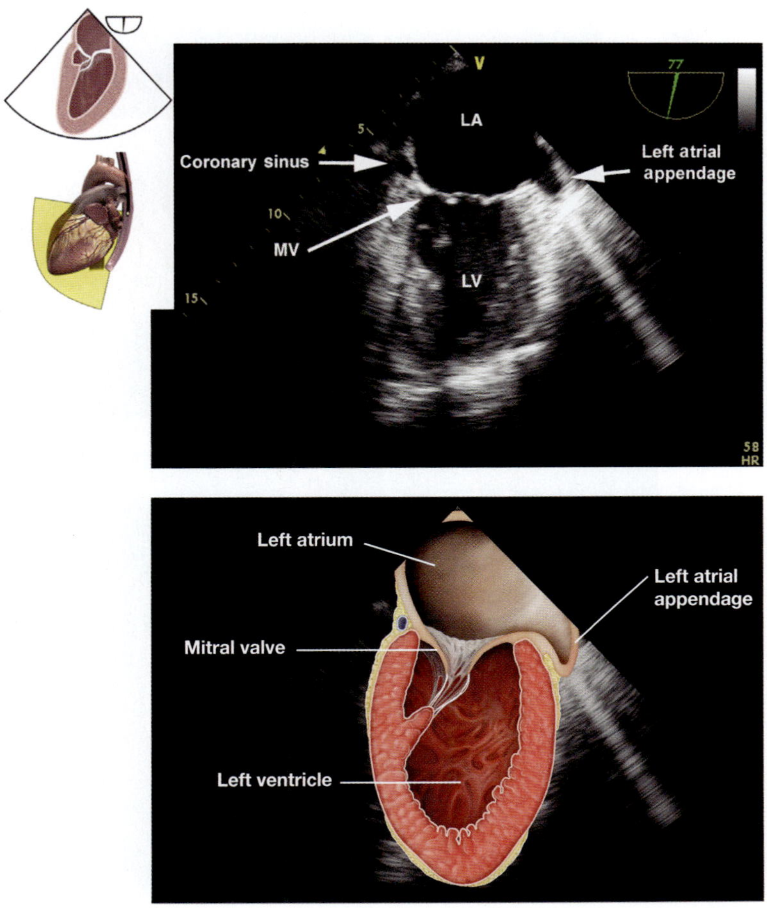

FIGURE 2.10 Midesophageal two-chamber view (above). Anatomic representation (below). Inset: anatomic representation with approximate imaging plane. (From Patrick J. Lynch, illustrator, C. Carl Jaffe; MD, cardiologist Yale University Center for Advanced Instructional Media; Medical illustrations by Patrick Lynch, generated for multimedia teaching projects by the Yale University School of Medicine, Center for Advanced Instructional Media, 1987-2000. Patrick J. Lynch, http://patricklynch.net. Creative Commons Attribution 2.5 License 2006; no usage restrictions except please preserve our creative credits: Patrick J. Lynch, medical illustrator; C. Carl Jaffe, MD, cardiologist. http://creativecommons.org/licenses/by/2.5/.)

when the left atrial appendage is visualized communicating with LA on the right side of the image, the CS is seen in the atrioventricular groove on the left side of the image, and the characteristic appearance of the long anterior mitral leaflet is seen near the appendage. This ensures visualization of the anterior wall of the LV on the right side of the image and the inferior wall on the left side of the image.

The utility of this image includes evaluation of the mitral valve, further assessment of global LV systolic function, and assessing for anterior and inferior segmental wall motion abnormalities (SWMAs). The CS can be visualized for confirmation of a retrograde cardioplegia catheter. The left atrial appendage can be evaluated for the presence of thrombus; however, a complete assessment of the left atrial appendage requires additional imaging.

Midesophageal Long-Axis View (Figure 2.11; Video 2.7)

The ME long-axis view is obtained by increasing the imaging plane to approximately 120° to 140°. An optimized ME long axis allows for visualization of the mitral valve, the LV cavity, the LVOT, the AV, and

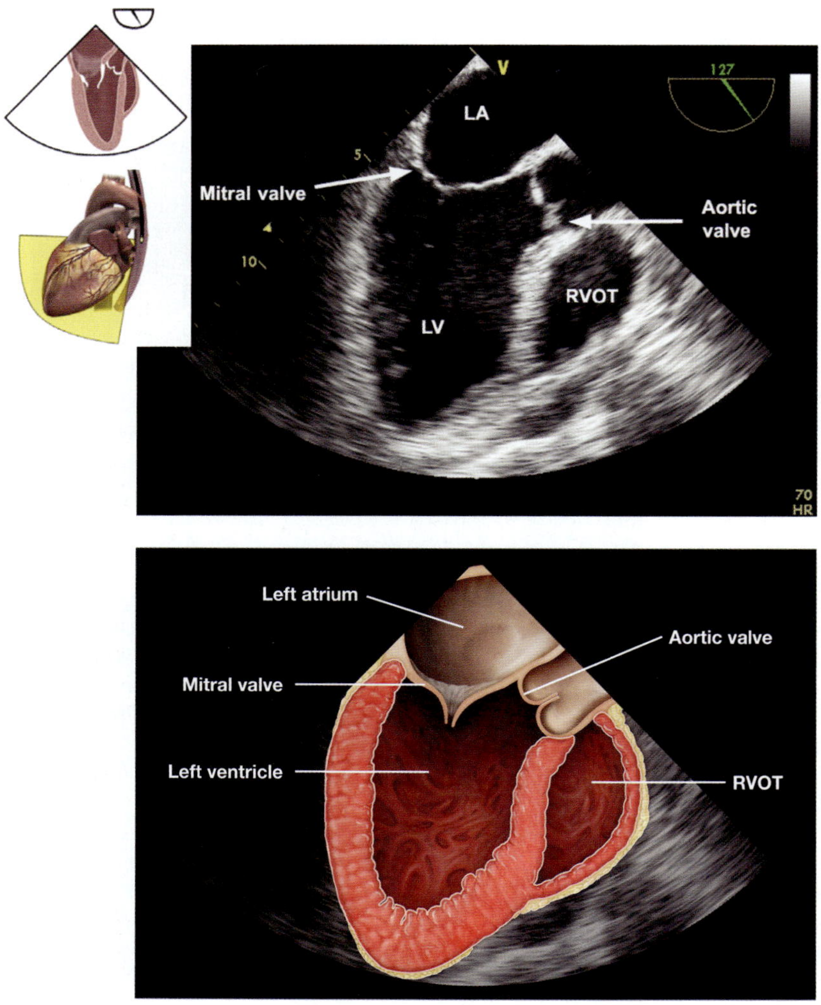

FIGURE 2.11 Midesophageal long-axis view (above). Anatomic representation (below). Inset: anatomic representation with approximate imaging plane. LA, left atrium; LV, left ventricle; RVOT, right ventricular outflow tract. (From Patrick J. Lynch, illustrator, C. Carl Jaffe; MD, cardiologist Yale University Center for Advanced Instructional Media; Medical illustrations by Patrick Lynch, generated for multimedia teaching projects by the Yale University School of Medicine, Center for Advanced Instructional Media, 1987-2000. Patrick J. Lynch, http://patricklynch.net. Creative Commons Attribution 2.5 License 2006; no usage restrictions except please preserve our creative credits: Patrick J. Lynch, medical illustrator; C. Carl Jaffe, MD, cardiologist. http://creativecommons.org/licenses/by/2.5/.)

the ascending aorta in a continuous long-axis orientation. The walls of the LV seen in this view are the anteroseptal wall, between the LV and RV, and the inferolateral wall visualized on the left side of the image. If the ultrasound beam is centered through the LVOT, there will typically be no large papillary muscles visualized, and the A2 segment of the anterior leaflet of the mitral valve is seen closest to the AV with the P2 segment of the posterior leaflet on the left side of the image. Rightward rotation will show the medial aspect of the mitral valve (A3 and P3), and leftward rotation will show the lateral aspect of the mitral valve (A1 and P1).

The combination of the ME four-chamber, ME two-chamber, and ME long-axis views provides visualization of all 16 segments of the LV for complete assessment of segmental wall motion. In addition, this view is excellent for assessing dynamic LVOT obstruction from systolic anterior motion of the mitral valve.

Transgastric Midpapillary Short-Axis View (Figure 2.12; Video 2.8)

The TG midpapillary short-axis view is obtained by decreasing the imaging plane back to 0°, centering the LV, then advancing the probe into the stomach. Before passing into the stomach, it's worth double checking that the probe is in a neutral position, neither locked nor flexed. Contact is often lost between the probe and the stomach, and slight anteflexion is required to begin to bring the ventricle into view. The probe should be advanced or withdrawn to physically place the probe at the level of the posteromedial papillary muscle, with adjustment of the degree of anteflexion to optimize the short axis. If the mitral valve or chordae are visible, the probe is likely too basal and needs to be advanced. If no papillary muscles are visible, the probe is likely too apical and needs to be withdrawn.

The TG midpapillary short-axis view shows all the coronary perfusion territories of the LV. The posteromedial and anterolateral papillary muscles are also visualized. The posteromedial papillary muscle is most proximal to the probe. A small cross-section of the RV is also visualized at the left side of the image.

This view is used to characterize LV systolic function, LV volume status, and to assess for SWMAs. Though no single view is adequate to evaluate global or regional function, this image shows all three coronary territories, so it can be helpful in identifying which coronary artery is responsible for SWMAs. Another benefit of this view is to assess relative chamber pressures between the LV and RV. Relative sizes of the RV and LV can be compared, and flattening of the interventricular septum can be observed in this view. Flattening of the intraventricular septum in systole is consistent with RV pressure overload, whereas flattening during diastole is more consistent with RV volume overload.

Transgastric Two-Chamber View (Figure 2.13; Video 2.9)

The TG two-chamber view is obtained by increasing the imaging plane to approximately 90°. This view will show the LA on the right side of the image with the left atrial appendage often visualized in the far field and the LV on the left side of the image. The TG two-chamber view is excellent for evaluating the anterior and inferior walls of the LV and is among the best views for evaluating the mitral valve subvalvular apparatus because the angle of insonation of the ultrasound beam is perpendicular to the structures of interest. Finally, the TG two chamber is a recommended view for measuring chamber size and wall thickness with TEE.

Descending Aorta Short-Axis View (Figure 2.14; Video 2.10)

The descending aorta short-axis view is obtained by decreasing the imaging plane to 0° and rotating the probe to the patient's left. Often a slight withdrawal is necessary to bring a transverse view of the aorta into the image. The aorta is relatively small and, therefore, the image may require a reduction in depth to adequately visualize the aorta. It is necessary to include enough depth, however, to adequately assess the left pleural space. The aorta should be examined along its entire course by withdrawing the probe until the level of the arch is reached.

This image is useful for evaluating a dissection both before and after procedures requiring CPB and to assess the degree of atherosclerotic disease. This view can also be useful in helping to position an intraaortic balloon pump. A left-sided pleural effusion can be visualized in the far field as an echolucency often described as "tiger claw appearance" (11).

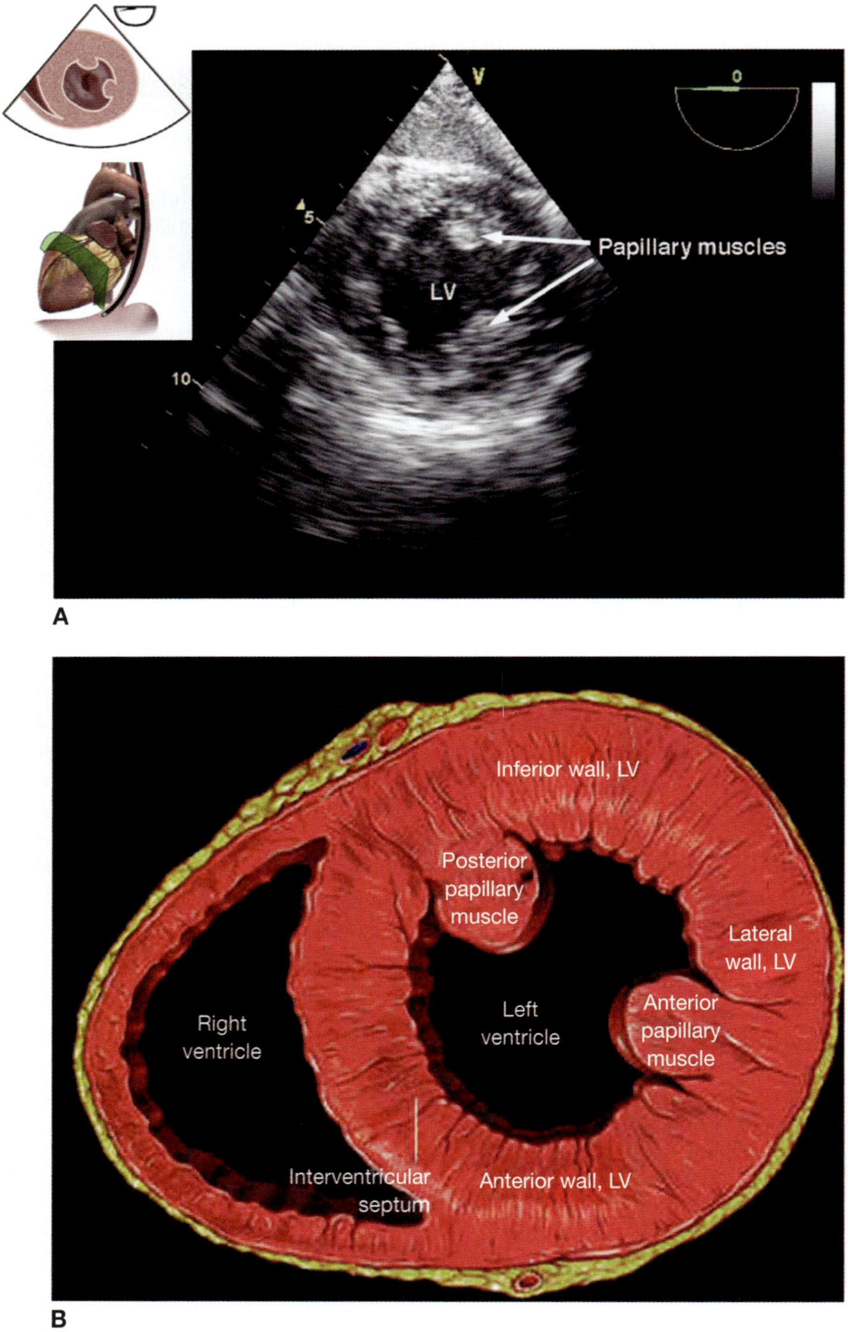

FIGURE 2.12 A: Transgastric (TG) midpapillary short-axis view. B: Anatomic representation of a TG midpapillary short-axis view. Inset: anatomic representation with approximate imaging plane. LV, left ventricle. (B from Patrick J. Lynch, illustrator; C. Carl Jaffe, MD, cardiologist Yale University Center for Advanced Instructional Media; Medical Illustrations by Patrick Lynch, generated for multimedia teaching projects by the Yale University School of Medicine, Center for Advanced Instructional Media, 1987-2000. Patrick J. Lynch, http://patricklynch.net. Creative Commons Attribution 2.5 License 2006; no usage restrictions except please preserve our creative credits: Patrick J. Lynch, medical illustrator; C. Carl Jaffe, MD, cardiologist. http://creativecommons.org/licenses/by/2.5/.)

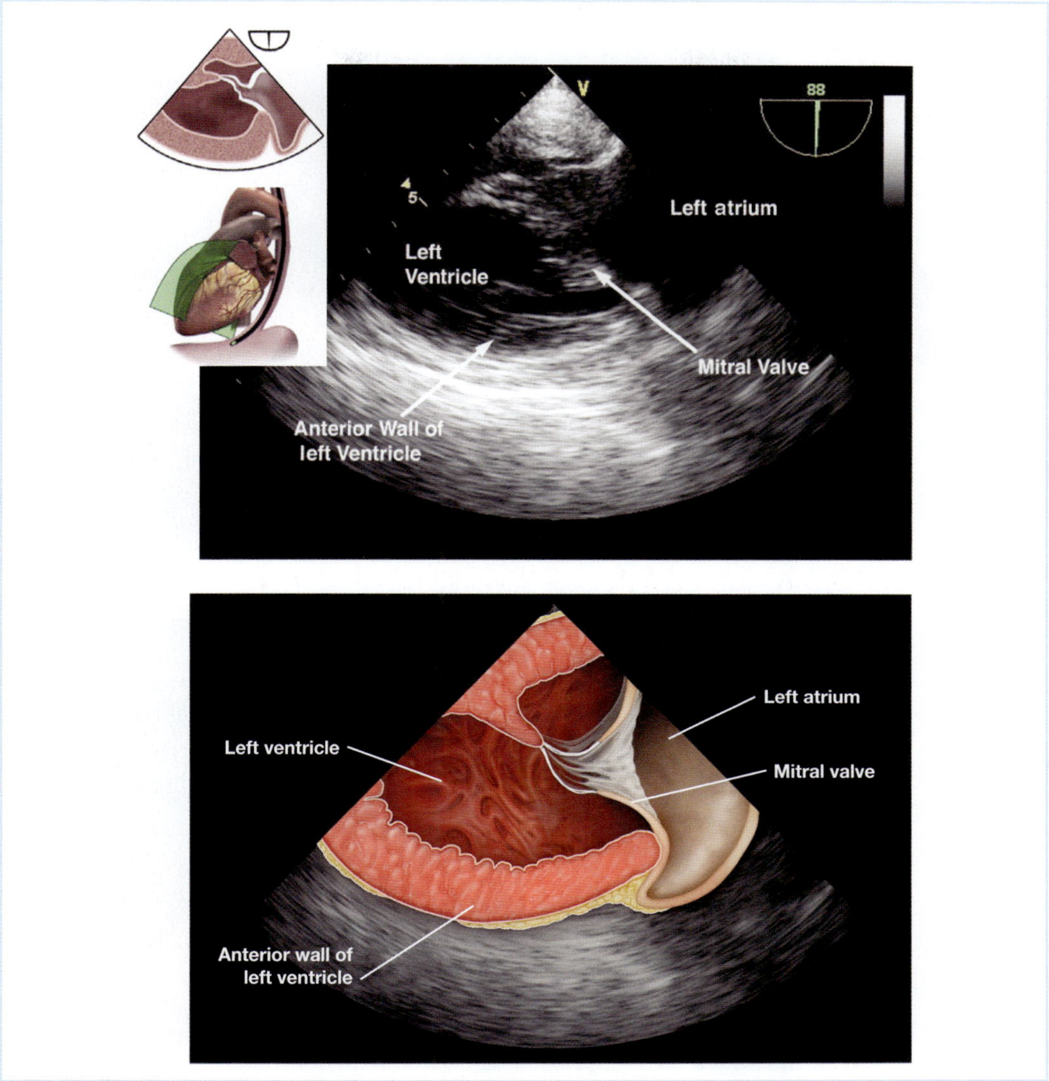

FIGURE 2.13 Transgastric two-chamber view (above). Anatomic representation (below). Inset: anatomic representation with approximate imaging plane. (From Patrick J. Lynch, illustrator, C. Carl Jaffe; MD, cardiologist Yale University Center for Advanced Instructional Media; Medical illustrations by Patrick Lynch, generated for multimedia teaching projects by the Yale University School of Medicine, Center for Advanced Instructional Media, 1987-2000. Patrick J. Lynch, http://patricklynch.net. Creative Commons Attribution 2.5 License 2006; no usage restrictions except please preserve our creative credits: Patrick J. Lynch, medical illustrator; C. Carl Jaffe, MD, cardiologist. http://creativecommons.org/licenses/by/2.5/.)

ADDITIONAL VIEWS

The "Basic Exam" is concluded with the evaluation of the descending thoracic aorta. At this point in the study, additional views can be added for further investigation based upon the clinical scenario and the findings of the initial TEE survey. In the following section, the additional views will be described as presented in the ASE (American Society of Echocardiography) comprehensive exam guideline, although they will often be obtained in a different sequence (3).

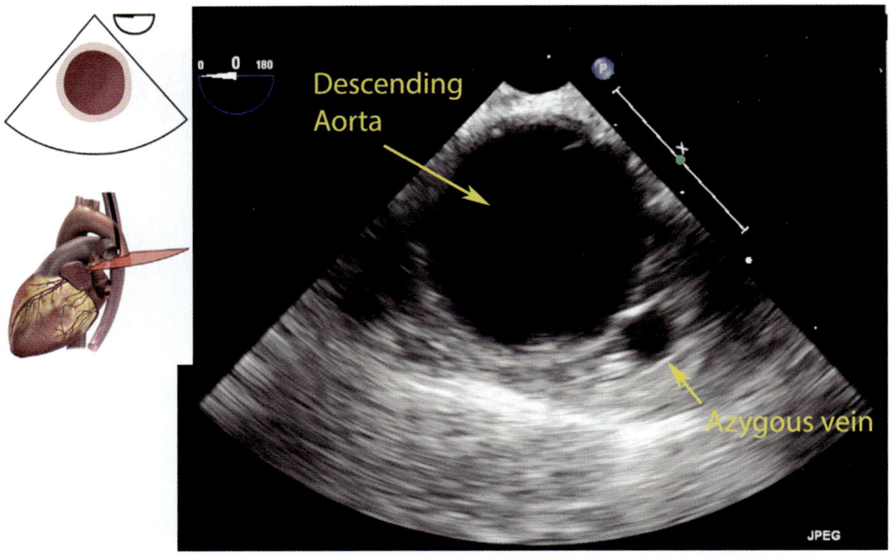

A

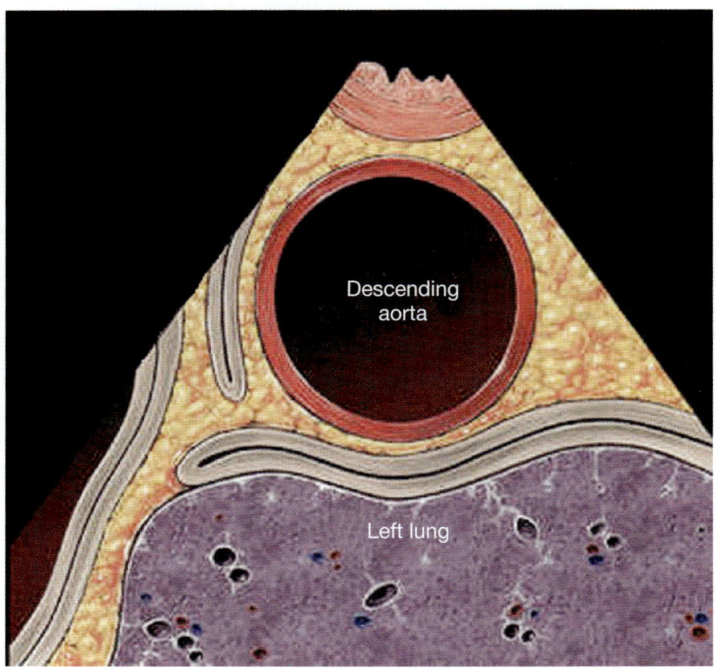

B

FIGURE 2.14 A: Descending aorta short-axis view. B: Anatomic representation. Inset: anatomic representation with approximate imaging plane. (From Patrick J. Lynch, illustrator, C. Carl Jaffe; MD, cardiologist Yale University Center for Advanced Instructional Media; Medical illustrations by Patrick Lynch, generated for multimedia teaching projects by the Yale University School of Medicine, Center for Advanced Instructional Media, 1987-2000. Patrick J. Lynch, http://patricklynch.net. Creative Commons Attribution 2.5 License 2006; no usage restrictions except please preserve our creative credits: Patrick J. Lynch, medical illustrator; C. Carl Jaffe, MD, cardiologist. http://creativecommons.org/licenses/by/2.5/.)

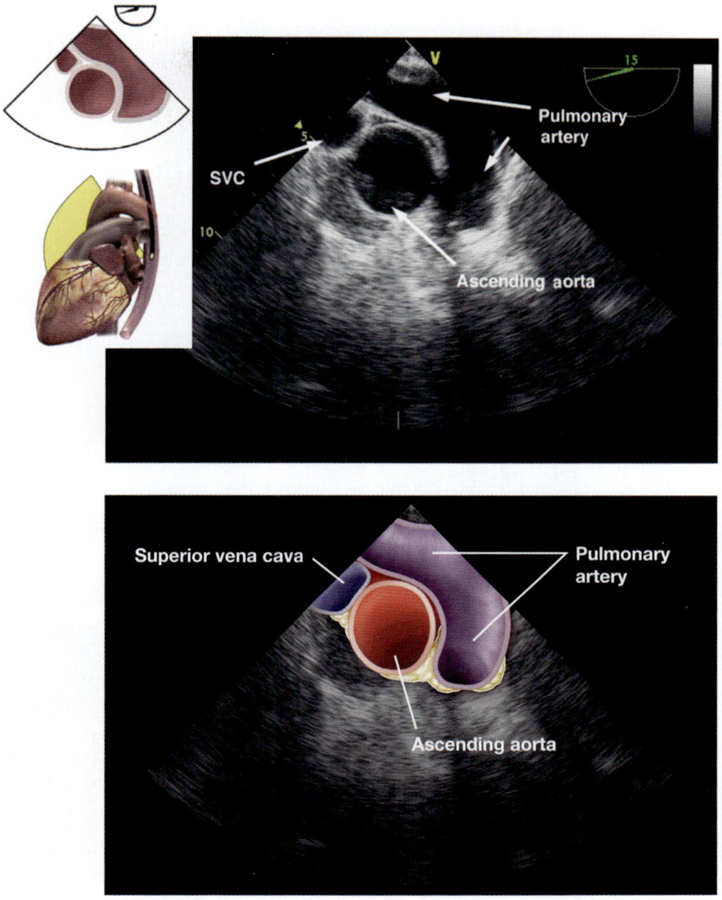

FIGURE 2.15 Midesophageal ascending aortic short-axis view with still image above and anatomic representation below. Inset: anatomic representation with approximate imaging plane. SVC, superior vena cava.

Midesophageal Ascending Aorta Short-Axis View (Figure 2.15; Video 2.11)

The ME ascending aorta short-axis view can be visualized from high in the esophagus above the level of the heart. Adjusting the imaging plane in the range of 0° to 30° will optimize the view to show a short-axis view of the ascending aorta. This view can also reliably be obtained from the short axis of the AV from which the ultrasound probe is withdrawn, multiplane decreased, and the probe anteflexed to bring in the short axis of the ascending aorta.

This view shows a short-axis view of the ascending aorta in the center of the image. The main PA is seen bifurcating with the right PA posterior to the ascending aorta. The SVC is seen in short axis to the left of the ascending aorta, and in a portion of cases, the right upper pulmonary vein can be visualized next to the SVC. This view allows assessment of the ascending aorta for abnormalities as well as confirm PA catheter location. It may also identify saddle pulmonary thromboembolism.

Midesophageal Right Pulmonary Vein View (Figure 2.16; Video 2.12)

From the ME ascending aorta short-axis view, the probe is rotated to the patient's right. Often small changes in depth and/or imaging angle are needed to optimize the image.

This view shows the right pulmonary veins entering the LA on the left side of the image. Typically, the right lower pulmonary vein is oriented perpendicular to the beam while the right upper pulmonary vein is more parallel allowing for more accurate spectral Doppler interrogation. The SVC may be visualized in the

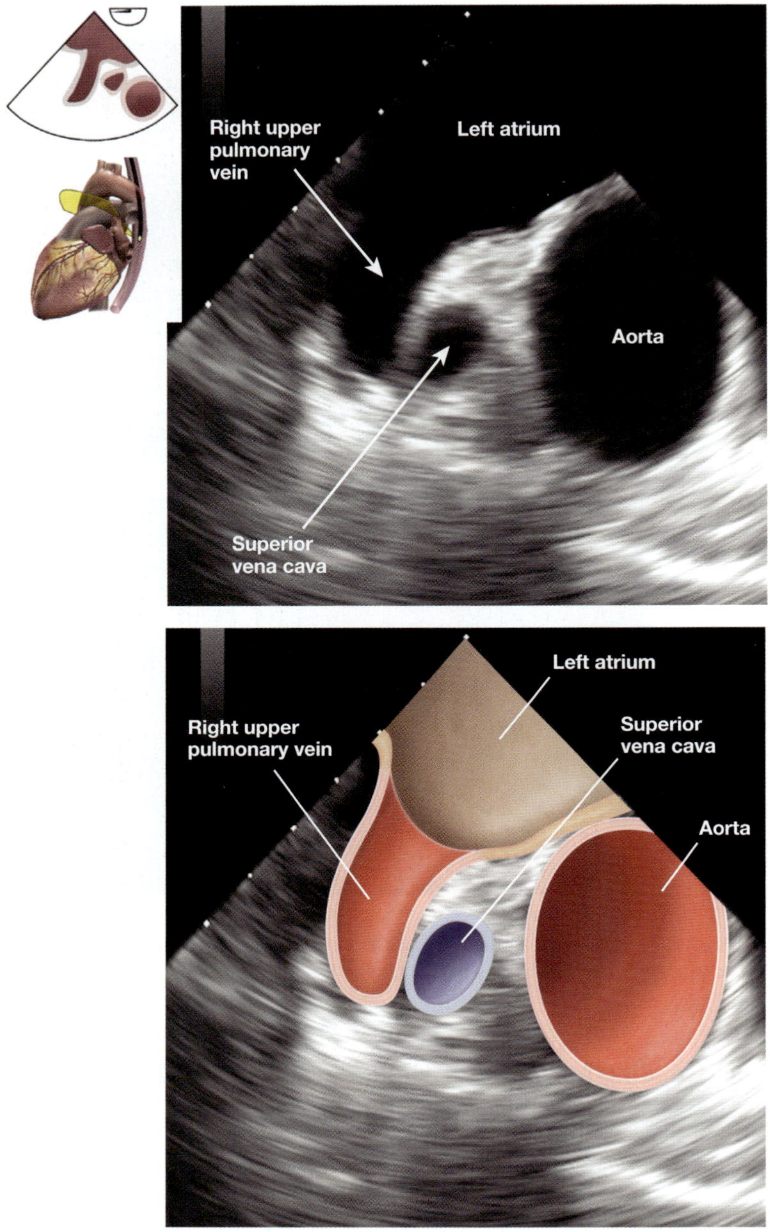

FIGURE 2.16 Midesophageal right pulmonary vein view with still image above and anatomic representation below. Inset: anatomic representation with approximate imaging plane.

short-axis orientation to the right of the right upper pulmonary vein. The utility of this view is to assess for abnormalities in the pulmonary veins, particularly after lung transplant surgery.

Midesophageal Ascending Aortic Long-Axis View (Figure 2.17; Video 2.13)

From the ME right pulmonary vein view, the probe is rotated back toward the patient's left to obtain the ME ascending aorta short-axis view. Increasing the imaging plane to approximately 90° to 120° will often show a true long-axis view of the ascending aorta. The short axis of the right PA is visualized at the apex of

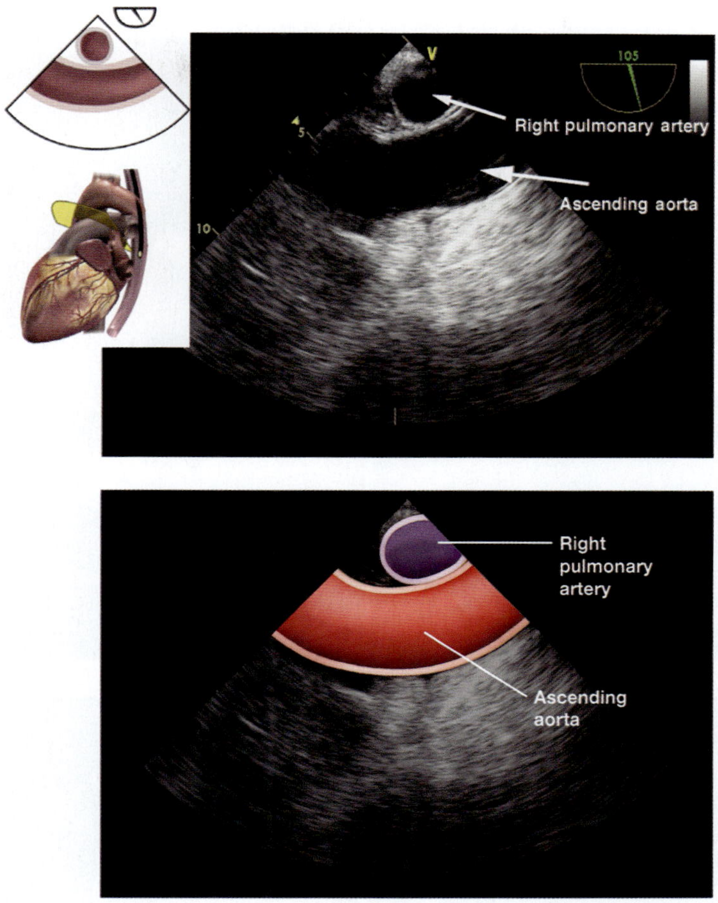

FIGURE 2.17 Midesophageal ascending aortic long-axis view with still image above and anatomic representation below. Inset: anatomic representation with approximate imaging plane.

the image coursing behind the ascending aorta in long axis. This view is good for assessing the ascending aorta for dissection or atheroma as well as for attempting to evaluate aortic and left ventricular assist device outflow cannulas.

Midesophageal Modified Bicaval Tricuspid Valve View (Figure 2.18; Video 2.14)

From the ME bicaval view, the probe is rotated slightly to the left or the imaging plane increased and the probe anteflexed. The tricuspid valve is visualized in the far field beyond the RA. The anterior leaflet of the tricuspid valve is typically seen on the right side of the image, while the left-sided leaflet is either the septal or posterior leaflet. This image may provide good Doppler alignment for assessment of tricuspid regurgitation. It can also be helpful in PA catheter insertion.

Midesophageal Five-Chamber View (Figure 2.19; Video 2.15)

From the ME four-chamber view, the probe is withdrawn and retroflexed to visualize the LVOT and AV in the center of the screen while ideally still visualizing the LV apex. This view shows the four traditional cardiac chambers in addition to the LVOT, which is considered the "fifth chamber." In the setting of aortic root aneurysm, the "fifth chamber" can be prominent. The ME five-chamber view can be used for a global assessment of cardiac structure and function specifically related to the outflow of the heart as well as for assessment of the anterior aspect of the mitral valve.

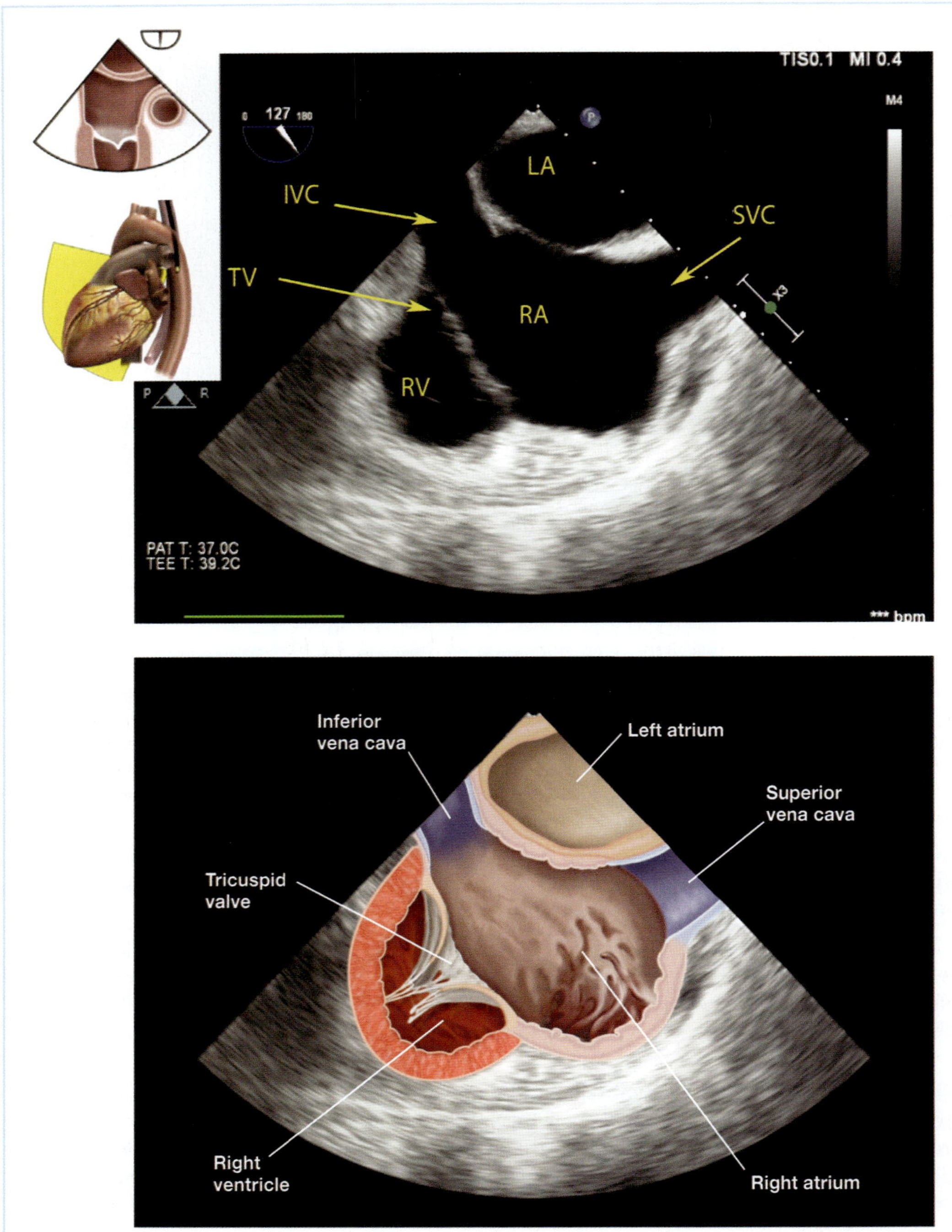

FIGURE 2.18 Midesophageal modified bicaval tricuspid valve view with still image above and anatomic representation below. Inset: anatomic representation with approximate imaging plane. IVC, inferior vena cava; LA, left atrium; RA, right atrium; RV, right ventricle; SVC, superior vena cava; TV, tricuspid valve.

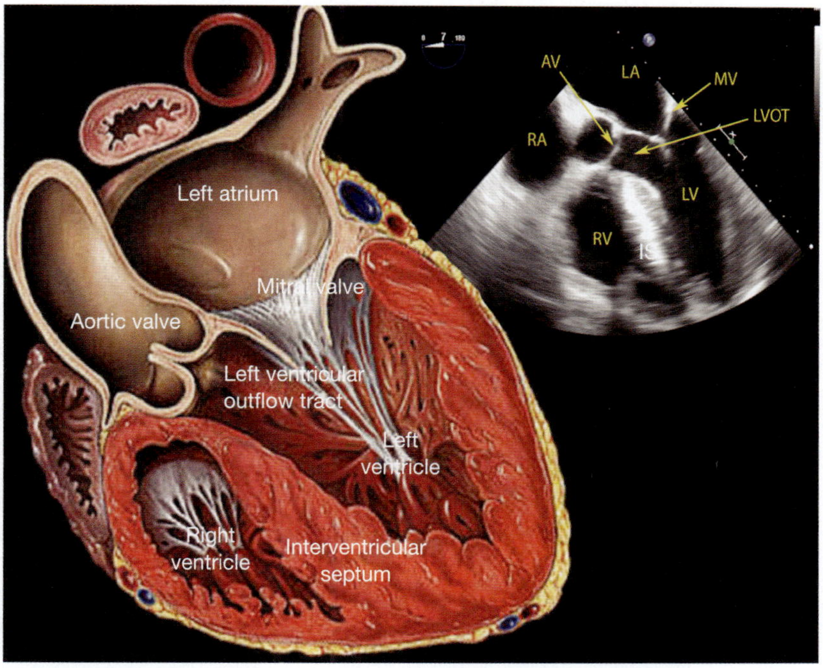

FIGURE 2.19 Midesophageal five-chamber view. Anatomic representation (inset). AV, aortic valve; LA, left atrium; LV, left ventricle; LVOT, left ventricular outflow tract; MV, mitral valve; RA, right atrium; RV, right ventricle. (From Patrick J. Lynch, illustrator; C. Carl Jaffe, MD, cardiologist, Yale University Center for Advanced Instructional Media; Medical illustrations by Patrick Lynch, generated for multimedia teaching projects by the Yale University School of Medicine, Center for Advanced Instructional Media, 1987-2000. Patrick J. Lynch, http://patricklynch.net. Creative Commons Attribution 2.5 License 2006; no usage restrictions except please preserve our creative credits: Patrick J. Lynch, medical illustrator; C. Carl Jaffe, MD, cardiologist. http://creativecommons.org/licenses/by/2.5/.)

Midesophageal Mitral Commissural View (Figure 2.20; Video 2.16)

From the ME four-chamber view, the imaging plane is increased to approximately 60°. This view shows the LA and LV with the classic P3-A2-P1 segments of the mitral valve from left to right. The posteromedial and anterolateral papillary muscles can typically be visualized in this view as well. The view is useful to aid localization of mitral valve pathology and in percutaneous mitral valve interventions.

Midesophageal Left Atrial Appendage View (Figure 2.21; Video 2.17)

From the ME two-chamber view, depth is reduced to focus on the left atrial appendage, which is visualized on the right side of the image. Small changes in rotation and/or angle are used to maximize the appearance of the opening of the appendage into the LA. The left atrial appendage is a complex structure, and this view alone will not provide complete visualization of the appendage. This view shows the left circumflex coronary artery, which is visualized in short axis between the mitral valve and left atrial appendage. This view is used to assess for thrombus of the left atrial appendage and to assist in left atrial appendage closure procedures.

Midesophageal Left Pulmonary Vein View (Figure 2.22; Video 2.18)

From the ME left atrial appendage view, the probe is withdrawn slightly to visualize the left upper pulmonary vein entering the LA above the "coumadin ridge." Small changes in rotation and/or angle are needed to optimize the view.

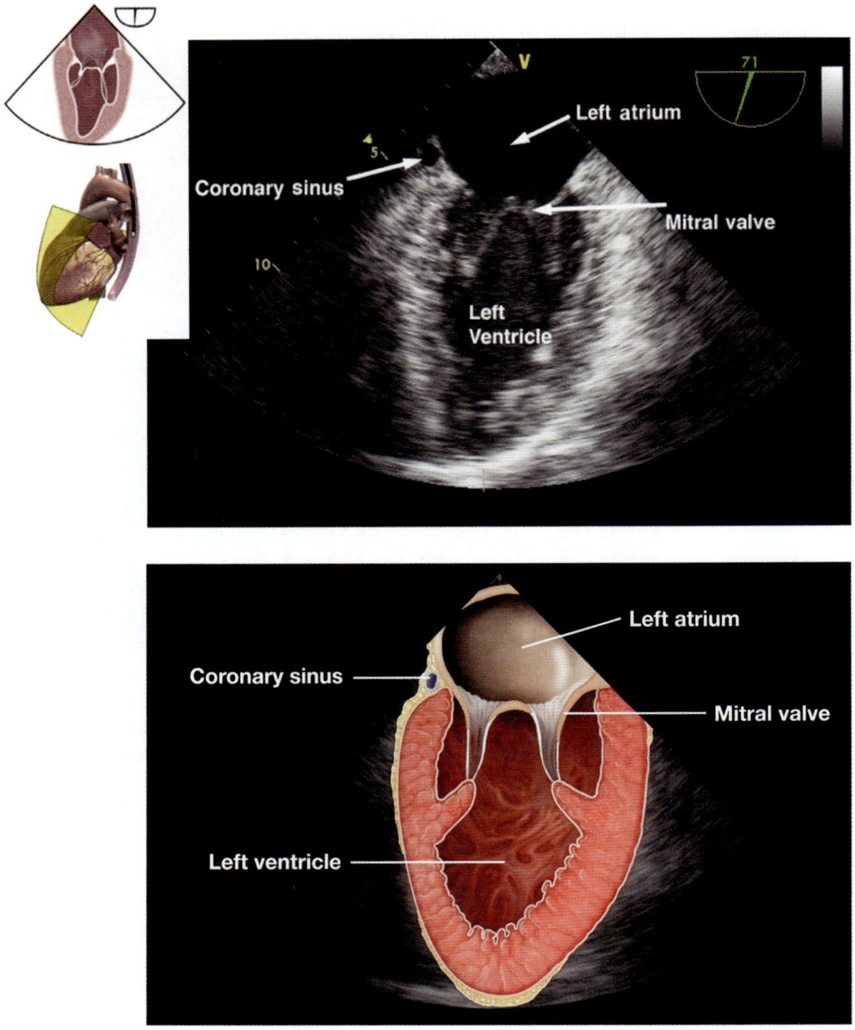

FIGURE 2.20 Midesophageal mitral commissural view (above). Anatomic representation (below). Inset: anatomic representation with approximate imaging plane. (From Patrick J. Lynch, illustrator, C. Carl Jaffe; MD, cardiologist Yale University Center for Advanced Instructional Media; Medical illustrations by Patrick Lynch, generated for multimedia teaching projects by the Yale University School of Medicine, Center for Advanced Instructional Media, 1987-2000. Patrick J. Lynch, http://patricklynch.net. Creative Commons Attribution 2.5 License 2006; no usage restrictions except please preserve our creative credits: Patrick J. Lynch, medical illustrator; C. Carl Jaffe, MD, cardiologist. http://creativecommons.org/licenses/by/2.5/.)

This view can show both the left upper and left lower pulmonary veins. Typically, the left lower pulmonary vein is seen in a slightly more transverse orientation, and the left upper pulmonary vein is seen entering more parallel to the beam. Manipulation of the probe by advancing and withdrawing is often required to differentiate the left upper from the left lower pulmonary vein, the upper being visualized when the probe is withdrawn and the lower when the probe is advanced. The view allows assessment of abnormalities in the pulmonary veins, including after lung transplantation.

Transgastric Basal Short-Axis View (Figure 2.23; Video 2.19)

From the TG short-axis view, the probe is withdrawn to visualize more basal structures of the heart. Often, small changes in rotation and/or flexion of the probe are necessary to optimize this image. This view shows

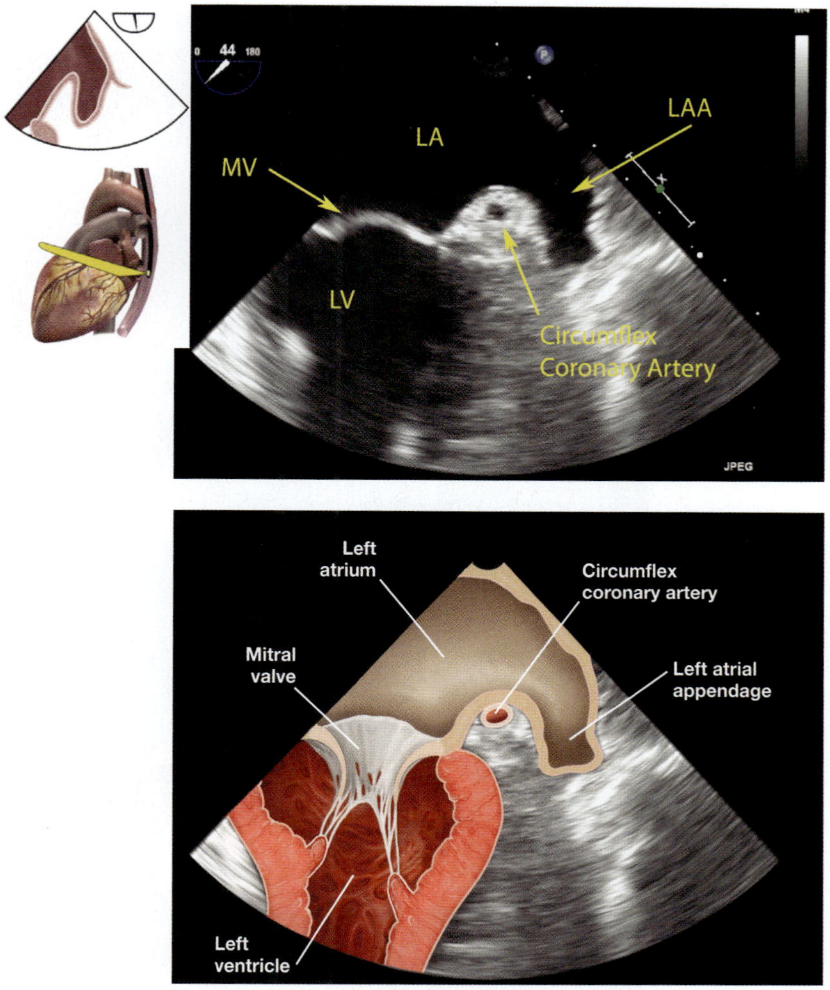

FIGURE 2.21 Midesophageal left atrial appendage view with still image above and anatomic representation below. Inset: anatomic representation with approximate imaging plane. LA, left atrium; LAA, left atrial appendage; LV, left ventricle; MV, mitral valve.

the traditional "fish-mouth" appearance of the mitral valve allowing one to visualize all segments of the mitral simultaneously. The view can aid in localization of mitral valve pathology, as well as to assess basal SWMAs of the LV.

Transgastric Apical Short-Axis View (Figure 2.24; Video 2.20)

From the TG short-axis view, the probe is advanced to visualize more apical structures of the heart. This view shows the anterior, lateral, inferior, and septal apical wall segments of the LV and allows assessment of SWMAs in the apical segments of the LV.

Transgastric Long-Axis View (Figure 2.25; Video 2.21)

From the TG two-chamber view, the imaging plane is increased to approximately 120°. Anteflexion is sometimes required to bring the LVOT into view. The LVOT and AV should be visualized on the right side of the image, in the far field. The LA will be on the right side of the image and LV on the left. This view provides good spectral Doppler alignment for interrogation of the AV and LVOT.

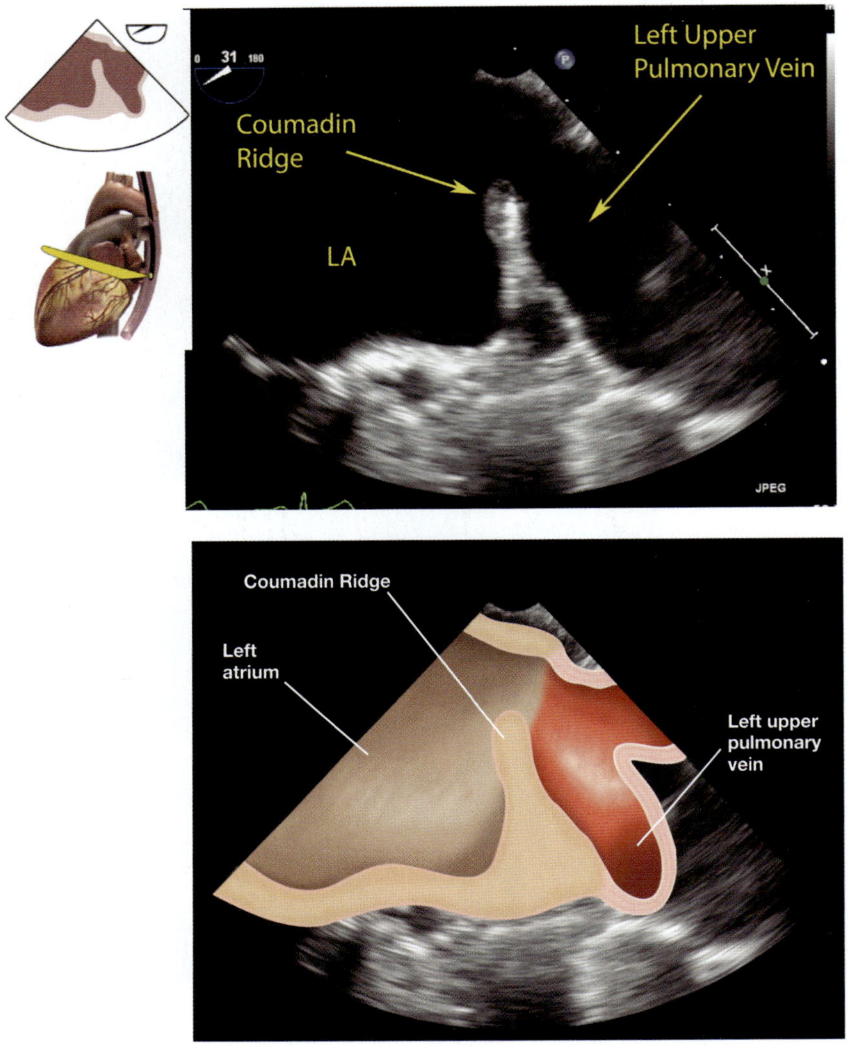

FIGURE 2.22 Midesophageal left pulmonary vein view with still image above and anatomic representation below. Inset: anatomic representation with approximate imaging plane. LA, left atrium.

Transgastric Right Ventricular Inflow View (Figure 2.26; Video 2.22)

From the TG two-chamber view, the probe is rotated to the patient's right, until the RA, tricuspid valve, and RV are visualized. This image is the right-sided analog to the TG two-chamber view. This view shows the RA on the right side of the image and the RV on the left side of the image. The tricuspid valve is visualized between the two chambers. This view allows additional assessment of right ventricular systolic function and wall thickening, as well as tricuspid leaflet morphology.

Deep Transgastric Five-Chamber View (Figure 2.27; Video 2.23)

From the TG short-axis view, the probe is advanced past the LV apex, then maximally anteflexed and gently withdrawn to obtain this view. Slight rotation and left flexion are needed to optimize this image. This view shows the apex of the LV in the near field with the LA, mitral valve, and LV on the right side of the image. The RA, tricuspid valve, and RV are on the left of the image. The LVOT and AV are visualized in the far field, and

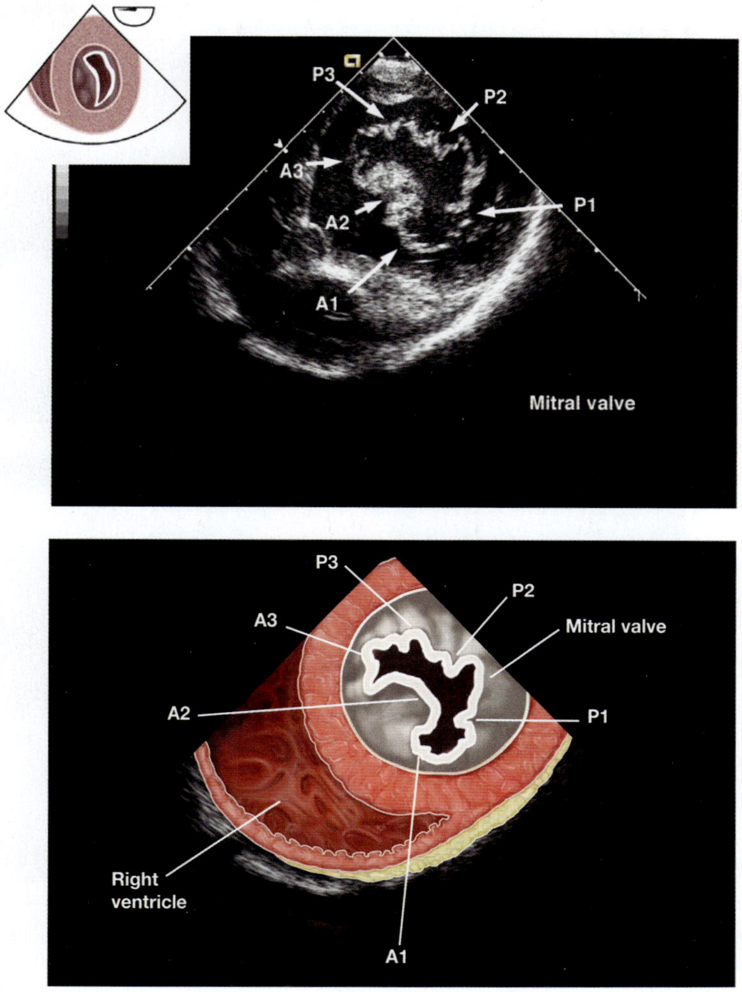

FIGURE 2.23 Transgastric basal short-axis view with still image above and anatomic representation below. Inset: anatomic representation with approximate imaging plane. A1, A2, A3, P1, P2, P3.

the ascending aorta and arch can often be visualized as well. Along with the TG long axis, this is a valuable view for Doppler alignment and interrogation of the LVOT and AV.

Transgastric Right Ventricular Basal View (Figure 2.28; Video 2.24)

From the deep TG five-chamber view, the probe is anteflexed, withdrawn, and rotated to the patient's right. Small changes in flexion, rotation, and/or imaging angle are needed to optimize this image. This view shows the tricuspid valve in short axis in the near field with the right ventricular outflow tract and pulmonic valve in the far field. Traditionally, all three leaflets of the tricuspid valve can be visualized in this image with the septal leaflet on the right closest to the LV, the posterior leaflet in the left near field, and the anterior leaflet in the right far field. This view can aid in localization of tricuspid valve pathology.

Transgastric Right Ventricular Inflow-Outflow View (Figure 2.29; Video 2.25)

From the TG RV basal view, the probe is right flexed, anteflexed, and rotated to the right. This view shows the same structures visualized in the traditional ME RV inflow-outflow view but rotated approximately 90°

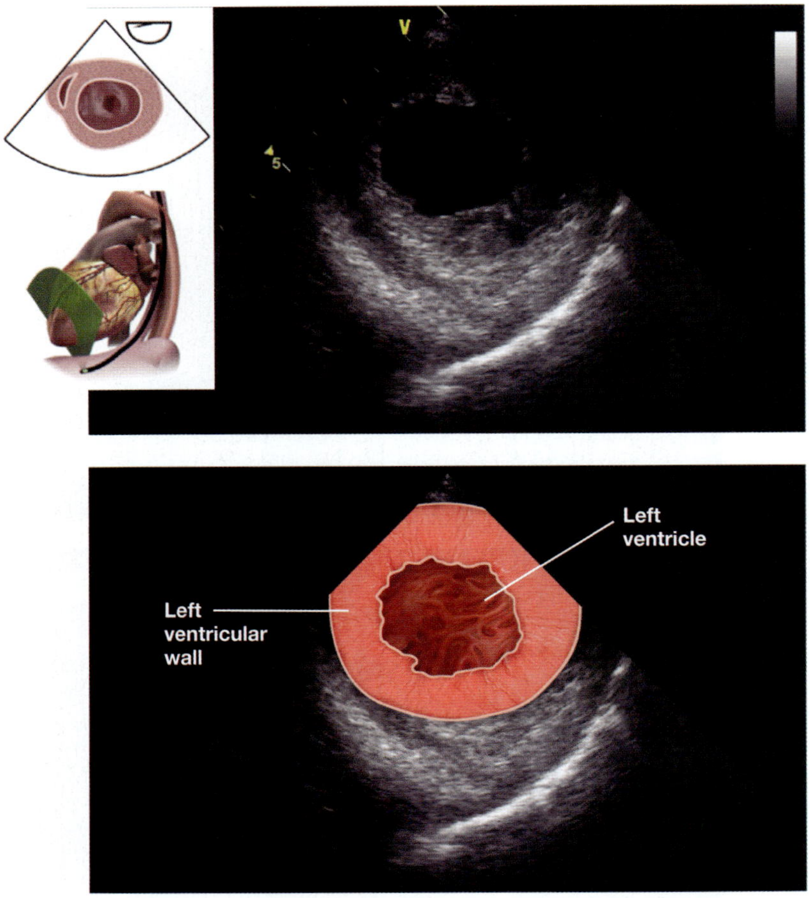

FIGURE 2.24 Transgastric apical short-axis view with still image above and anatomic representation below. Inset: anatomic representation with approximate imaging plane.

clockwise. The value of this view is for general assessment of the tricuspid and pulmonic valves as well as assessment of global RV systolic function.

Descending Aorta Long-Axis View (Figure 2.30; Video 2.26)

From the descending aorta short-axis view, the imaging plane is rotated 90° to visualize the descending aorta in long axis. This view shows the proximal descending aorta on the right side of the image and distal on the left. The left chest cavity can be visualized in the far field with appropriate imaging depth. The view provides good visualization of the aorta for evaluation of dissection, both before and after procedures requiring CPB, and to assess the burden of atherosclerotic disease. This view can also be useful in helping to position an intraaortic balloon pump. Again, with appropriate depth of the image, a left-sided pleural effusion can be visualized in the far field as an echolucency around the aorta.

Upper Esophageal Aortic Arch Long-Axis View (Figure 2.31; Video 2.27)

From the descending aorta short-axis view at the level of the arch, the probe is rotated to the patient's right (passing the left subclavian artery) to visualize the distal aortic arch. In some cases, the left innominate vein can be seen just distal to the aorta. The view can be used to assess the aortic arch and provides an angle of insonation that allows Doppler interrogation of aortic flow.

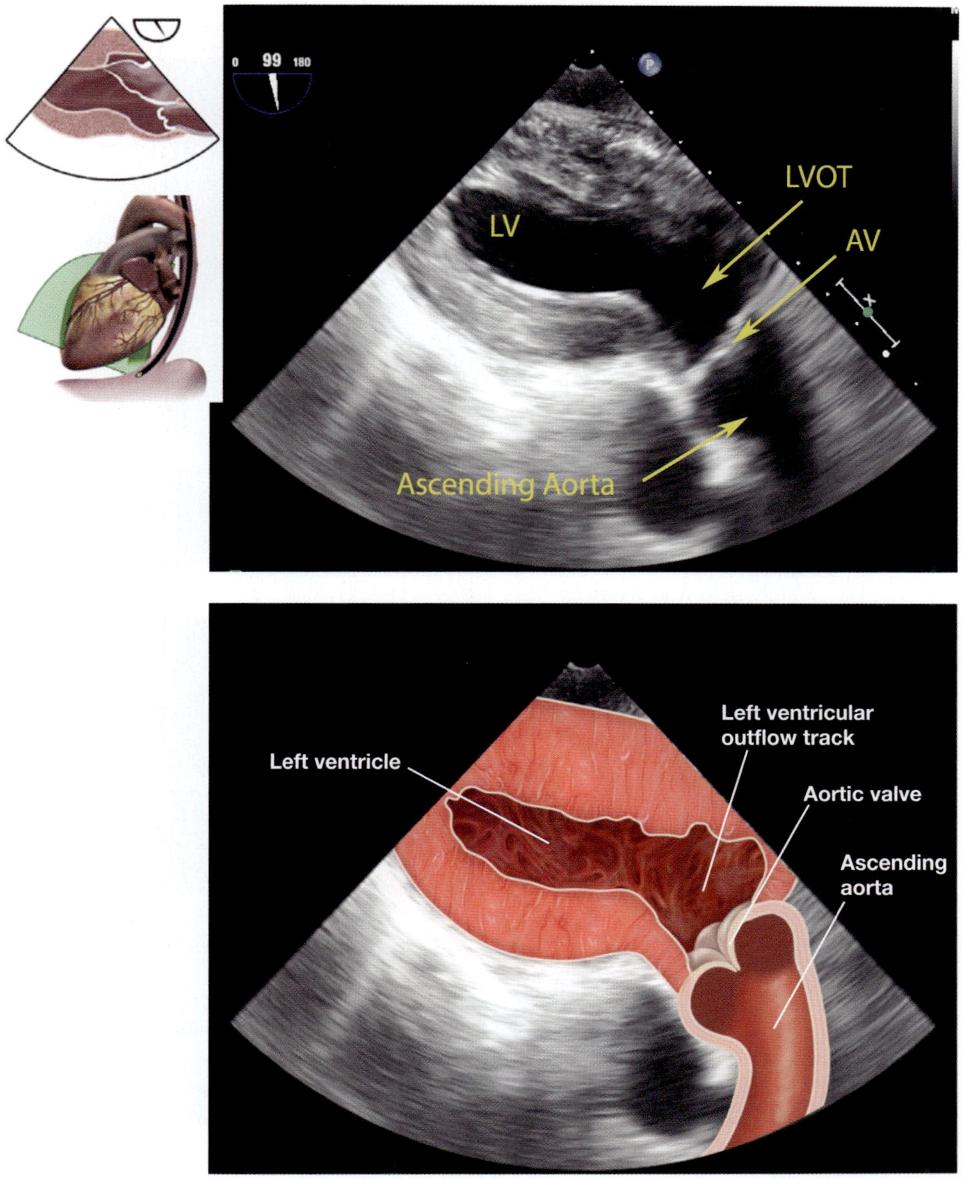

FIGURE 2.25 Transgastric long-axis view with still image above and anatomic representation below. Inset: anatomic representation with approximate imaging plane. AV, aortic valve; LV, left ventricle; LVOT, left ventricular outflow tract.

Upper Esophageal Aortic Arch Short-Axis View (Figure 2.32; Video 2.28)

From the UE aortic arch long-axis view, the imaging plane is increased to 70° to 90° to show the aortic arch in short-axis view. Often, the main PA in long axis and pulmonic valve are visualized in the left side. Small changes in flexion, rotation, and/or imaging angle can allow for visualization of the origin of the left subclavian artery in this image. The greatest utility of this view is for good Doppler interrogation of the pulmonic valve and PA.

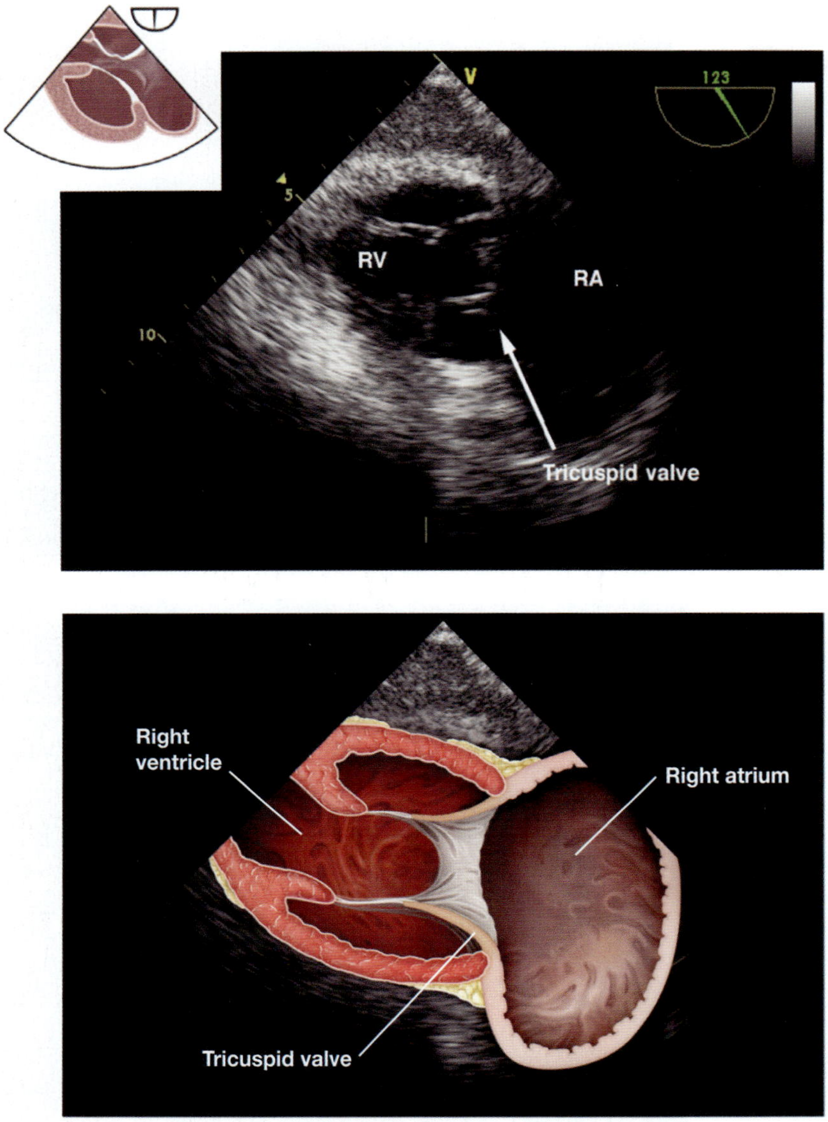

FIGURE 2.26 Transgastric right ventricular inflow view (above). Anatomic representation (below). Inset: anatomic representation with approximate imaging plane. RA, right atrium; RV, right ventricle. (From Patrick J. Lynch, illustrator, C. Carl Jaffe; MD, cardiologist Yale University Center for Advanced Instructional Media; Medical illustrations by Patrick Lynch, generated for multimedia teaching projects by the Yale University School of Medicine, Center for Advanced Instructional Media, 1987-2000. Patrick J. Lynch, http://patricklynch.net. Creative Commons Attribution 2.5 License 2006; no usage restrictions except please preserve our creative credits: Patrick J. Lynch, medical illustrator; C. Carl Jaffe, MD, cardiologist. http://creativecommons.org/licenses/by/2.5/.)

Deep Esophageal Right Ventricular Two-Chamber View (Figure 2.33; Video 2.29)

From the ME four-chamber view, the probe is advanced into the distal esophagus. This brings the probe closer to the tricuspid annulus. This view typically does not show the LA, rather the CS is visualized in the near field communicating with the RA. The tricuspid valve and RV are also visualized. The posterior leaflet of the tricuspid valve is typically visualized near the CS with the anterior leaflet opposite (4). This view allows imaging of the tricuspid valve without shadowing from the adjacent mitral valve and, as such, shows

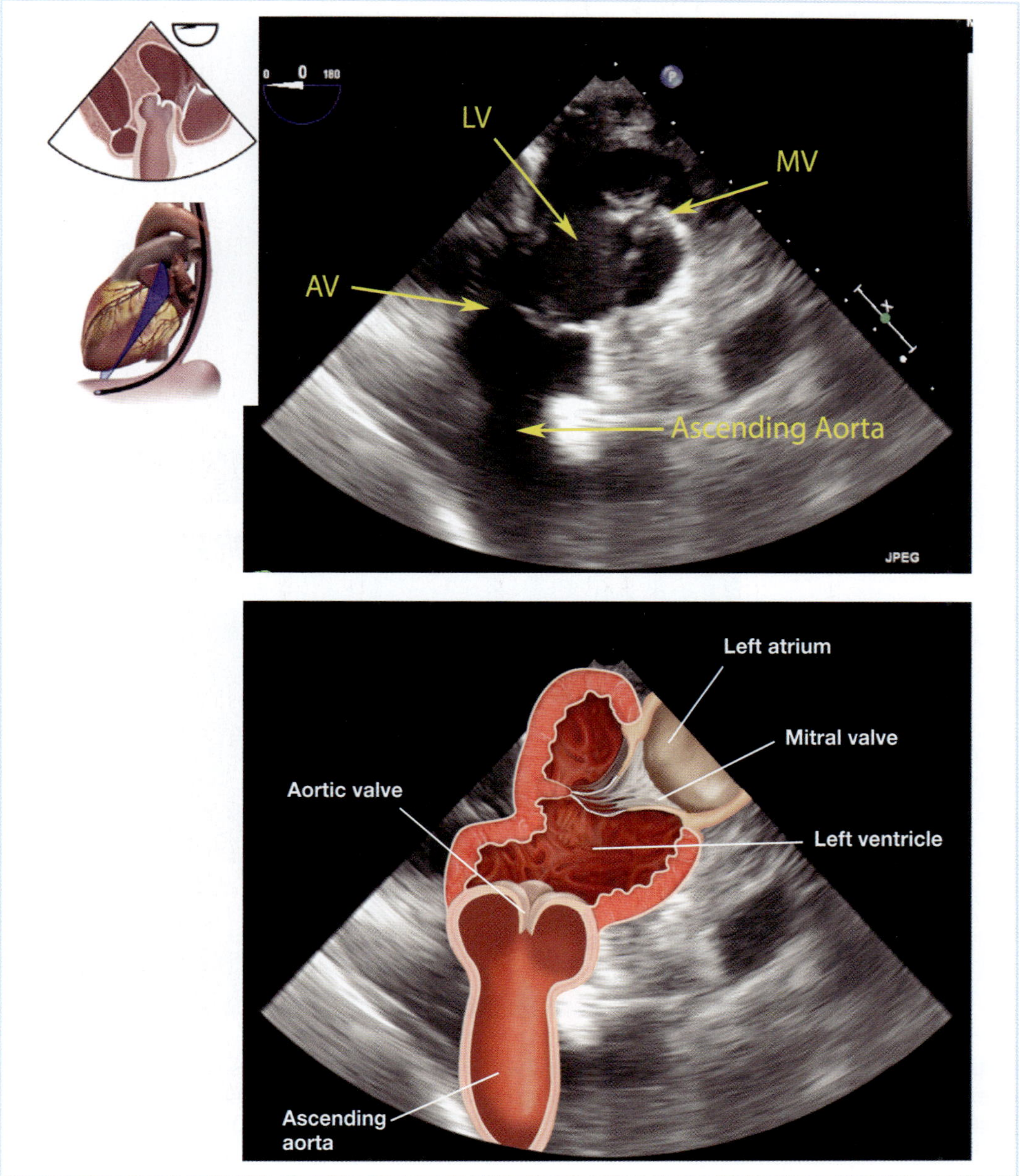

FIGURE 2.27 Deep transgastric five-chamber view (above). Anatomic representation (below). Inset: anatomic representation with approximate imaging plane. AV, aortic valve; LV, left ventricle; MV, mitral valve.

particular value in 3D tricuspid imaging and in structural heart interventions. The CS is well visualized for confirmation of a retrograde cardioplegia catheter.

Deep Esophageal Right Ventricular Inflow Outflow (Video 2.30)

From the DE right ventricular two-chamber view, the imaging plane is increased to 70° to 90°. This view is similar to the ME inflow-outflow view. While this view is called the "inflow-outflow" view, it is primarily utilized to focus on the tricuspid valve. Typically, a small portion of the LA is visualized near field. The RA,

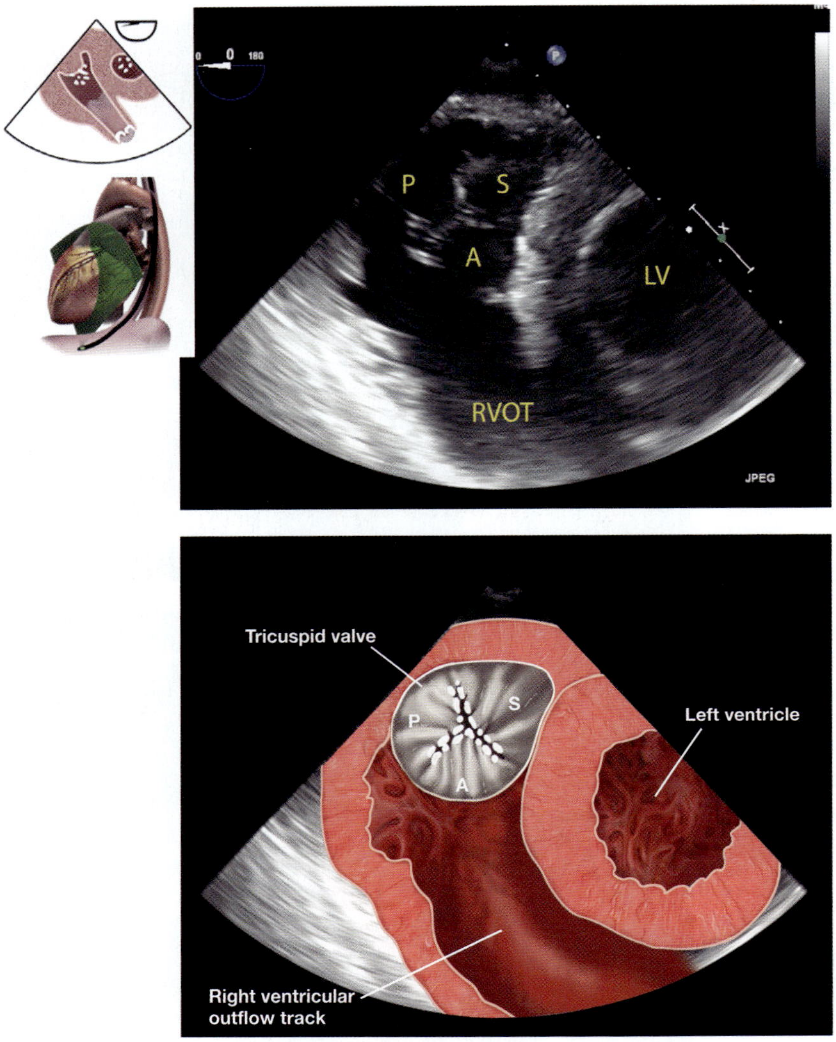

FIGURE 2.28 Transgastric right ventricular basal view with still image above and anatomic representation below. Inset: anatomic representation with approximate imaging plane. A, anterior leaflet of tricuspid valve; LV, left ventricle; P, posterior leaflet of tricuspid valve; RVOT, right ventricular outflow tract; S, septal leaflet of tricuspid valve.

tricuspid valve, and RV are visualized in the far field. The anterior leaflet of the tricuspid valve is typically the leaflet on the right and the posterior leaflet is typically opposite (4).

Although this is referred to as the "inflow-outflow" view, the tricuspid valve is the primary focus of this view, as this orientation often removes shadowing from the mitral valve, allows for optimal Doppler alignment, and by using biplane imaging, can allow for imaging of all leaflets of the tricuspid valve simultaneously. Portions of the pulmonic valve can be visualized on the right side of the image around 3 o'clock position.

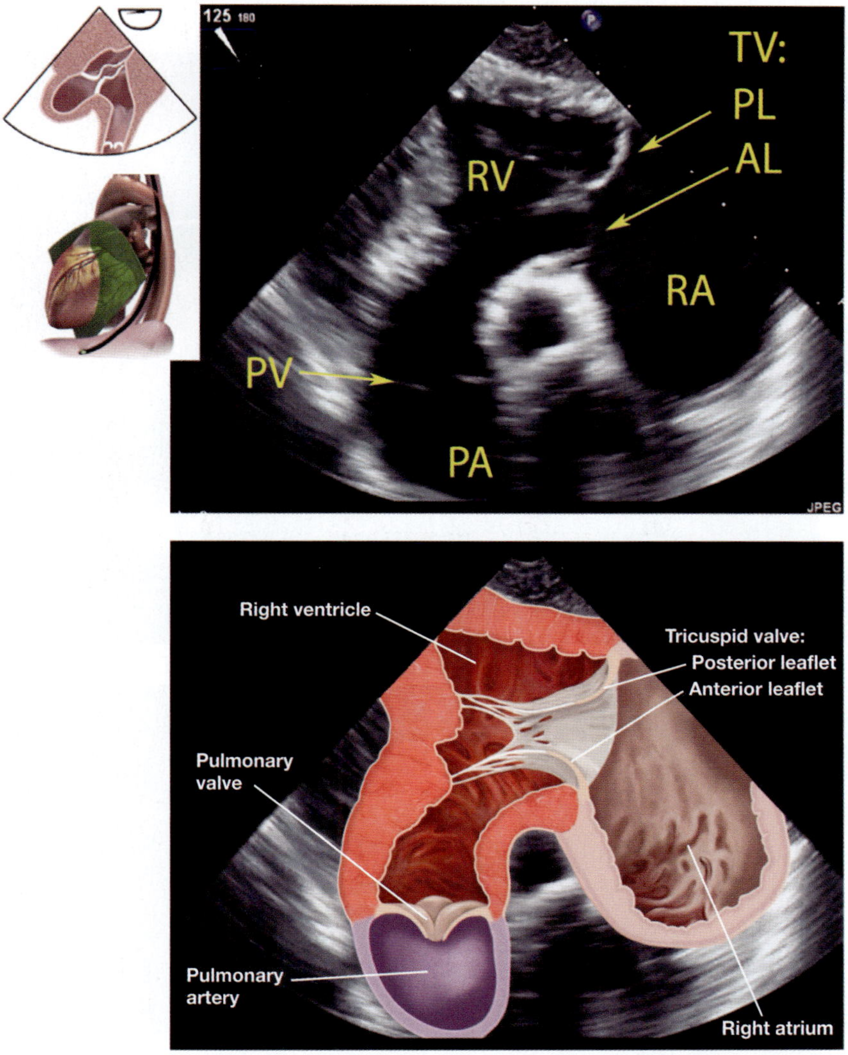

FIGURE 2.29 Transgastric right ventricular inflow-outflow view with still image above and anatomic representation below. Inset: anatomic representation with approximate imaging plane. AL, anterior leaflet; PA, pulmonary artery; PL, posterior leaflet; PV, pulmonic valve; RA, right atrium; RV, right ventricle; TV, tricuspid valve.

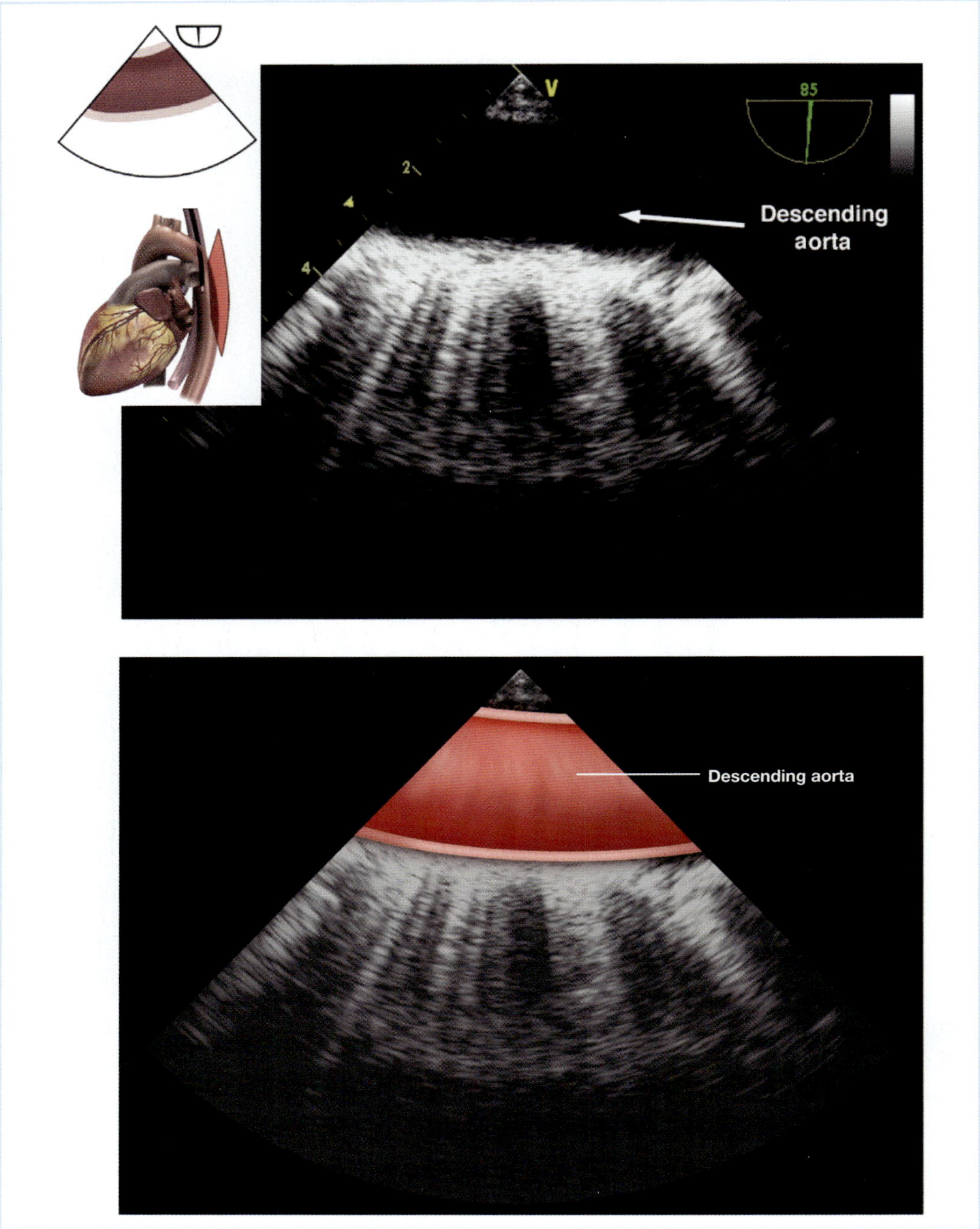

FIGURE 2.30 Descending aorta long-axis view with still image above and anatomic representation below. Inset: anatomic representation with approximate imaging plane.

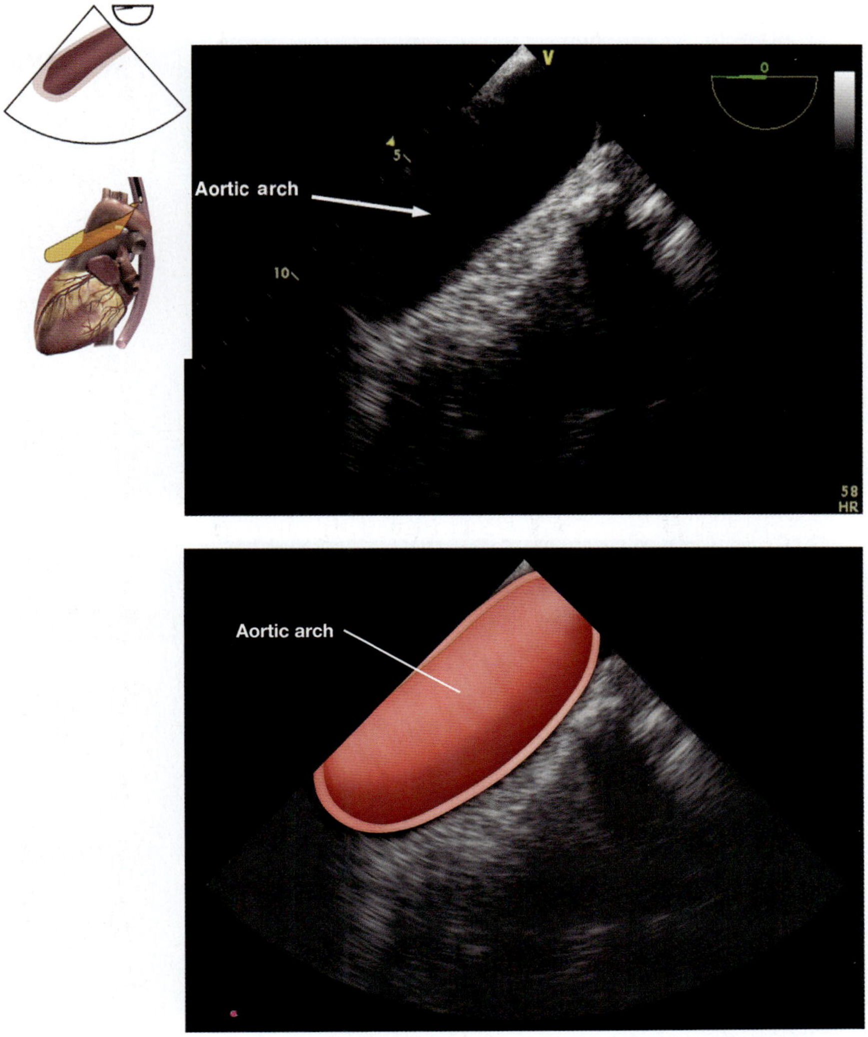

FIGURE 2.31 Upper esophageal aortic arch long-axis view with still image above and anatomic representation below. Inset: anatomic representation with approximate imaging plane.

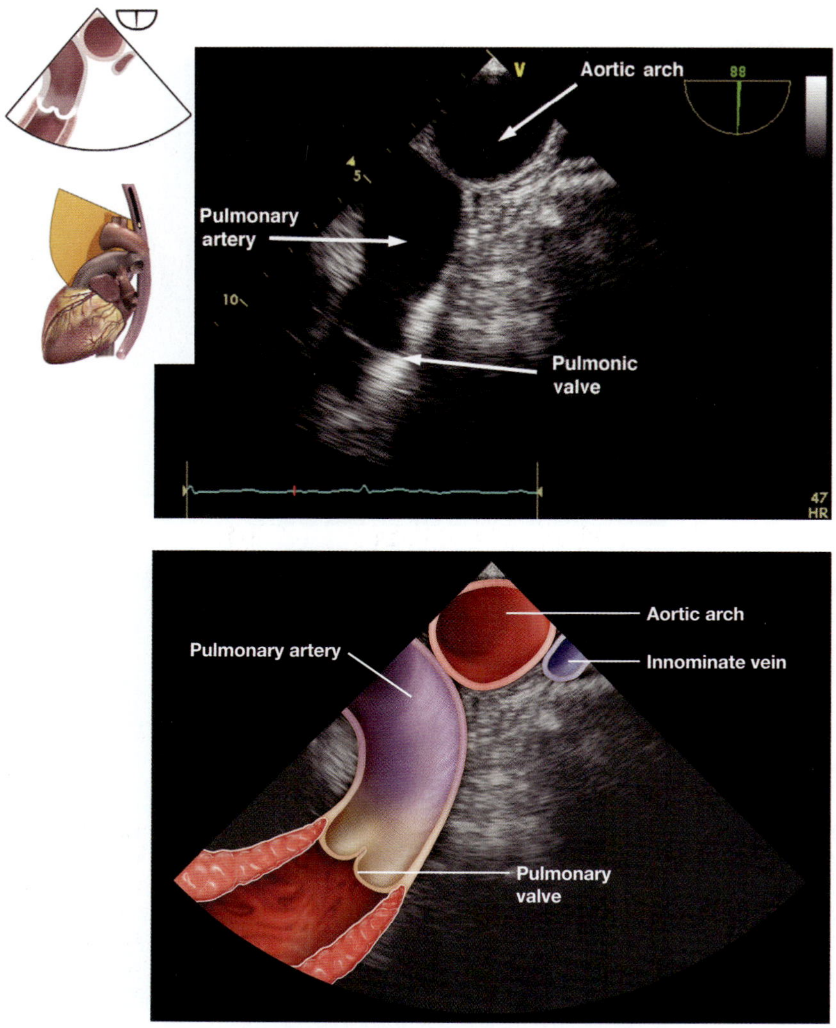

FIGURE 2.32 Upper esophageal aortic arch short-axis view with still image above and anatomic representation below. Inset: anatomic representation with approximate imaging plane.

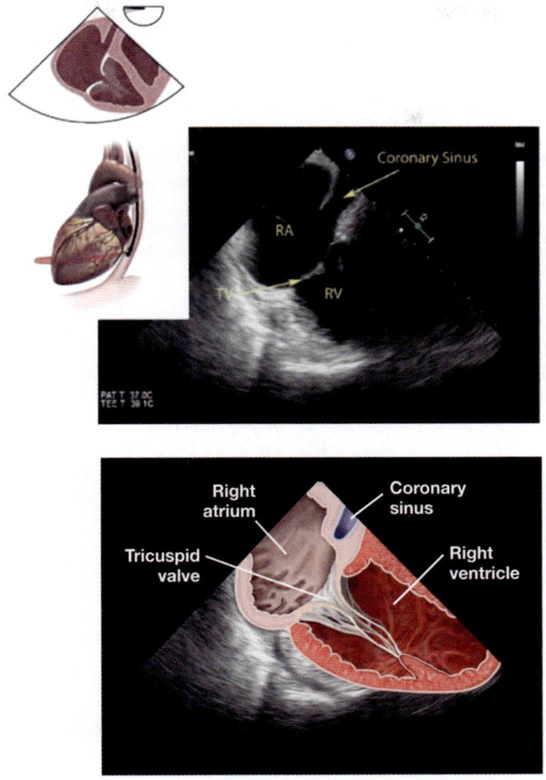

FIGURE 2.33 Deep esophageal right ventricular two-chamber view (above). Anatomic representation of the DE RV two-chamber view (below). Inset: anatomic representation with approximate imaging plane. RA, right atrium; RV, right ventricle; TV, tricuspid valve. (From Patrick J. Lynch, illustrator, C. Carl Jaffe; MD, cardiologist Yale University Center for Advanced Instructional Media; Medical illustrations by Patrick Lynch, generated for multimedia teaching projects by the Yale University School of Medicine, Center for Advanced Instructional Media, 1987-2000. Patrick J. Lynch, http://patricklynch.net. Creative Commons Attribution 2.5 License 2006; no usage restrictions except please preserve our creative credits: Patrick J. Lynch, medical illustrator; C. Carl Jaffe, MD, cardiologist. http://creativecommons.org/licenses/by/2.5/.)

CONCLUSION

The 2D TEE exam is a complex procedure that benefits from a comprehensive understanding of anatomy, physiology, and pathology as well as the spatial relationship of structures in different imaging planes. Developing the knowledge and experience to master this exam not only requires a significant investment of time and effort but also pays significant dividends.

We have described our stepwise approach to the 2D exam. There are potential variations depending on preferences and local demands. Whatever exam sequence is chosen, it is imperative that a standardized and consistent approach to performance and interpretation of images is implemented to limit errors of omission and minimize cognitive bias.

ACKNOWLEDGMENTS

We gratefully acknowledge the contributions of the previous edition author, Joseph P. Miller, as portions of those chapters have been retained in this revision.

REFERENCES

1. MacKay EJ, Neuman MD, Fleisher LA, et al. Transesophageal echocardiography, mortality, and length of hospitalization after cardiac valve surgery. *J Am Soc Echocardiogr*. 2020;33(6):756-762.e1.
2. Reeves ST, Finley AC, Skubas NJ, et al. Basic perioperative transesophageal echocardiography examination: a consensus statement of the American Society of Echocardiography and the Society of Cardiovascular Anesthesiologists. *J Am Soc Echocardiogr*. 2013;26(5):443-456.
3. Hahn RT, Abraham T, Adams MS, et al. Guidelines for performing a comprehensive transesophageal echocardiographic examination: recommendations from the American Society of Echocardiography and the Society of Cardiovascular Anesthesiologists. *J Am Soc Echocardiogr*. 2013;26(9):921-964.
4. Hahn RT, Saric M, Faletra FF, et al. Recommended standards for the performance of transesophageal echocardiographic screening for structural heart intervention: from the American Society of Echocardiography. *J Am Soc Echocardiogr*. 2022;35(1):1-76.
5. Kallmeyer IJ, Collard CD, Fox JA, Body SC, Shernan SK. The safety of intraoperative transesophageal echocardiography: a case series of 7200 cardiac surgical patients. *Anesth Analg*. 2001;92(5):1126-1130.
6. Hilberath JN, Oakes DA, Shernan SK, Bulwer BE, D'Ambra MN, Eltzschig HK. Safety of transesophageal echocardiography. *J Am Soc Echocardiogr*. 2010;23(11):1115-1127; quiz 1220-1221.
7. Webster CS, Taylor S, Weller JM. Cognitive biases in diagnosis and decision making during anaesthesia and intensive care. *BJA Educ*. 2021;21(11):420-425.
8. Busby LP, Courtier JL, Glastonbury CM. Bias in radiology: the how and why of misses and misinterpretations. *Radiographics*. 2018;38(1):236-247.
9. University of Utah Department of Anesthesiology Perioperative Echocardiography Website. Basic TEE exam lectures. Accessed June 17, 2024. https://echo.anesthesia.med.utah.edu/tee/basic-tee-exam-lecture/
10. Zimmerman J. A recipe for success in echocardiography training: the University of Utah experience. *J Cardiothorac Vasc Anesth*. 2018;32(6):2607-2613.
11. Capper SJ, Ross JJ, Sandström E, Braidley PC, Morgan-Hughes NJ. Transoesophageal echocardiography for the detection and quantification of pleural fluid in cardiac surgical patients. *Br J Anaesth*. 2007;98(4):442-446.

QUESTIONS

1. Which of the following will optimize imaging of right-sided cardiac structures?
A. Anteflexion
B. Retroflexion
C. Rotation to patient right
D. Rotation to patient left

2. Which view allows for optimal imaging of the tricuspid valve?
A. ME two chamber
B. TG midpapillary short axis
C. DE RV two chamber
D. ME long axis

3. Which view is necessary to identify all cusps of the AV?
A. ME AV short axis
B. ME AV long axis
C. ME ascending aortic short axis
D. ME ascending aortic long axis

4. Which view is most helpful in placing and determining the position of a PA catheter?
A. ME four chamber
B. ME RV inflow outflow
C. ME two chamber
D. ME five chamber

5. All segments of the mitral valve are visualized simultaneously in which TEE view?
A. TG basal short axis
B. ME two chamber
C. ME four chamber
D. ME five chamber

6. **Which of the following views may be useful for confirmation of placement of femoral cannula for CPB?**
   A. ME bicaval
   B. ME four chamber
   C. ME four chamber
   D. TG midpapillary short axis

7. **In which view can a left-sided pleural effusion be visualized?**
   A. ME four chamber
   B. TG midpapillary short axis
   C. Descending aorta short axis
   D. All of the above

8. **The left atrial appendage is best evaluated in which view?**
   A. ME bicaval
   B. ME two chamber
   C. ME four chamber
   D. All of the above

9. **Which of the following views is most useful for spectral Doppler interrogation of the AV?**
   A. ME AV long axis
   B. TG two chamber
   C. Deep TG five chamber
   D. None of the above

10. **In which view is the interventricular septum best evaluated for relative pressure differences between the LV and RV?**
   A. TG midpapillary short axis
   B. TG two chamber
   C. ME long axis
   D. All of the above

11. **Which cusp of the AV is indicated by the arrow in this ME AV short-axis view (QVideo 2.1)?**
   A. Right coronary cusp
   B. Left coronary cusp
   C. Noncoronary cusp
   D. None of the above

12. **Which leaflet of the mitral valve is indicated by the arrow in this ME AV long-axis view (QVideo 2.2)?**
   A. Anterior leaflet
   B. Posterior leaflet
   C. Septal leaflet
   D. None of the above

13. **What is the arrow indicating in this ME bicaval view (QVideo 2.3)?**
   A. Superior vena cava
   B. Inferior vena cava
   C. Left atrium
   D. Coronary sinus

ANSWERS

1. **Correct Answer: C.**
Rationale: Anatomic relationships of cardiac structures are the same for the patient and the echocardiographer. To view right-sided structures, rotate to the patient's right. To view left-sided structures, rotate to the patient's left. To view posterior structures, retroflex. To view anterior structures, anteflex.

2. **Correct Answer: C.**
Rationale: Of the listed views, only the DE RV two-chamber view allows for visualization of the tricuspid valve. It provides the added benefit of optimal viewing of the tricuspid valve without shadowing from the adjacent mitral valve.

3. **Correct Answer: A.**
Rationale: The ME AV short-axis view is the only view that allows visualization of all cusps of the AV simultaneously.

4. **Correct Answer: B.**
Rationale: Of the listed views, the ME RV inflow-outflow view shows the RA, RV, and main PA, allowing for visualization of the path of a PA catheter. The ME-modified bicaval view can also assist in crossing the tricuspid valve, but this was not listed as an option.

5. **Correct Answer: A.**
Rationale: While all views show some segments of the mitral valve, only the TG basal short-axis view allows for visualization of all segments of the mitral valve at once.

6. **Correct Answer: A.**
Rationale: Of the listed views, only the ME bicaval view shows the IVC that is needed to confirm wire placement for the placement of a femoral cannula for CPB.

7. **Correct Answer: C.**
Rationale: In the descending aorta short-axis view, with appropriate depth of the image, a left-sided pleural effusion can be visualized in the far field as an echolucency often described as "tiger claw appearance."

8. **Correct Answer: B.**
Rationale: The left atrial appendage is visualized in the ME two-chamber view and not in the other listed views.

9. **Correct Answer: C.**
Rationale: While the AV is also visualized in the ME AV long-axis view, Doppler interrogation is best achieved when blood flow is most parallel to the ultrasound beam. This is best achieved for the AV in the deep TG five-chamber view.

10. **Correct Answer: A.**
Rationale: The TG midpapillary short-axis view allows the assessment relative chamber pressures between the LV and RV. Flattening of the interventricular septum can be observed in this view. This finding can be consistent with right-sided pressure or volume overload, seen in significant pulmonary hypertension and/or right-sided valvular regurgitation.

11. **Correct Answer: C.**
Rationale: The noncoronary cusp is always associated with the interatrial septum.

12. **Correct Answer: A.**
Rationale: The right of this image is more anterior based on the imaging plane. Additionally, the anterior leaflet is associated with the other anterior structure in this view, the AV.

13. **Correct Answer: A.**
Rationale: The right of this image is more superior based on the imaging plane. In this view, the SVC is always on the right and IVC on the left.

3 Left Ventricular Systolic Performance and Pathology

Serena Dasani and Charles Nyman

Transesophageal echocardiography (TEE) has been a valuable way to evaluate left ventricular (LV) systolic function and LV pathologies since 1976 when an M-mode transducer was combined with a steerable catheter. Over the past several decades, medical device innovation has advanced such that function may be assessed via integration of numerous parameters including color flow and pulsed-wave Doppler; biplane, multiplane, and three-dimensional (3D) imaging, with higher frequency and matrix array probes (1). Accordingly, the American Society of Echocardiography and European Association of Cardiovascular Imaging have provided formal recommendations on how echocardiographers should best quantify LV systolic function through specific measurements and techniques. Updates were made in 2015 to the societal guidelines given the generation of newer techniques (3D TEE), establishment of partition values, and expanded awareness of gender differences when quantifying cardiac chambers (2).

LEFT VENTRICULAR MEASUREMENTS

To comprehensively quantify the LV, echocardiographers should measure diameter, volume, mass, and wall thickness. Cardiac chamber measurements should be obtained on more than one cardiac cycle to avoid discrepancies in quantification due to interbeat variability. For patients in normal sinus rhythm, measurements should be averaged over three beats and for patients with atrial fibrillation over five beats. End-diastolic measurements should be made in the first frame after mitral valve closure, or the frame of largest ventricular size if the mitral valve is not visualized. End-systolic measurements should be made in the first frame after aortic valve closure, or the frame with the smallest chamber size if the aortic valve is not visualized.

It should be noted that, while some cardiac structures may be better visualized with TEE in comparison to transthoracic echocardiography (TTE), there may be differences in chamber dimension and thickness measurements when comparing the two modalities. Large studies of normative data for TEE are not currently available, and, as such, it is recommended that the same normal values be utilized for both TEE and TTE (2).

Chamber Size (Left Ventricular Diameter)

Linear measurements of both LV diameter and wall thickness should be obtained perpendicular to the long axis of the ventricle with measurements obtained just below the mitral leaflets. The recommended view is the transgastric two chamber, though the transgastric LV long-axis or mid-papillary short-axis views may be considered if necessary. Measurements are performed at end diastole and end systole and can be further indexed to a patient's body surface area (BSA; Figure 3.1) (3,4).

Normal values for LV dimension in the minor axis (LVID) during diastole are 50.2 ± 4.1 mm for men and 45.0 ± 3.6 mm for women. Normal values for LVID during systole are 32.4 ± 3.7 mm for men and 28.2 ± 3.3 mm for women. A minor-axis diameter during diastole of greater than 59 mm for men and greater than 53 mm for women is considered abnormal. A minor-axis diameter during systole of greater than 41 mm for men and greater than 36 mm for women is considered abnormal (2).

Chamber Size (Left Ventricular Volume)

The biplane method of disks (MOD, also called the Simpson method) is the recommended approach for the calculation of LV volumes using 2D echocardiography (Figure 3.2). The views required for this calculation are the midesophageal two-chamber view and the midesophageal four-chamber view, which will allow the LV cavity to be imaged from the base of the heart to the apex in two orthogonal planes. The LV chamber is traced at the interface between the LV cavity and the compacted myocardium, excluding the papillary muscles, and connecting the mitral valve annulus with a straight line. The software then divides the LV into a series of 20 disks along its length. The volume of each disk is calculated by multiplying the area of the disk by the height of the disk and the volumes are added to provide a total LV volume. The MOD can underestimate LV volume

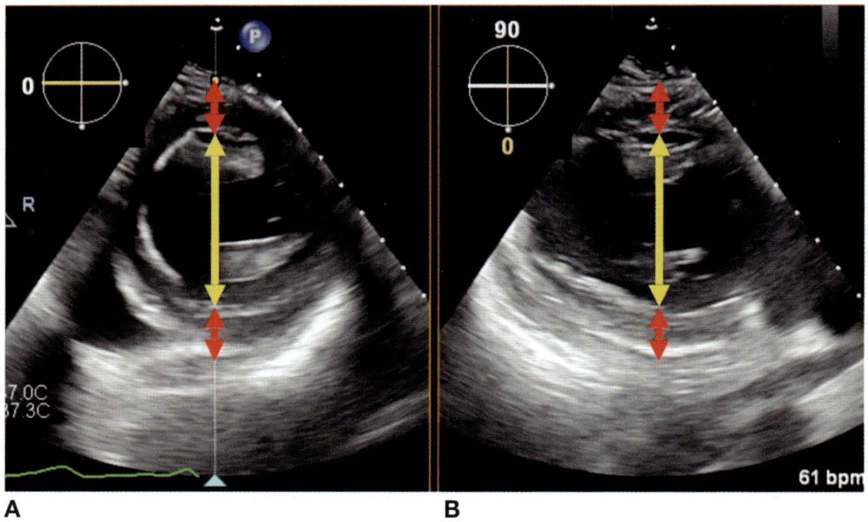

FIGURE 3.1 Recommended method for measuring LV diameter (yellow double arrow) and wall thickness (red double arrows) from (A) TG LV mid-papillary short axis and (B) TG LV two-chamber views. The green line at the bottom of the figure shows the EKG tracing for the patient. LV, left ventricle; TG, transgastric.

when apical foreshortening is present or there is endocardial dropout. In addition, as this approach only visualizes the LV in two planes, distortions to the LV that are not present in either plane may be missed (2,5).

Normal LV diastolic volumes (and indexed volumes) are 106 ± 22 mL (54 ± 10 mL/m^2) for men and 76 ± 15 mL (45 ± 8 mL/m^2) for women. Normal LV systolic volumes utilizing biplane MOD are 41 ± 10 mL (21 ± 5 mL/m^2) for men and 28 ± 7 mL (16 ± 4 mL/m^2) for women.

The use of 3D echocardiography data sets to calculate LV volume overcomes the limitations of foreshortening found with 2D imaging as LV volumes are calculated without geometrical assumptions (Figure 3.3; Video 3.1). Thus, 3D echocardiography can be helpful in assessing LV volumes in patients with pathology that has affected the shape of their LV such as cardiomyopathy, aneurysm, and myocardial infarction. LV volumes obtained by 3D echocardiography have been demonstrated to correlate better to cardiac magnetic resonance imaging (MRI) than 2D measurements. Although 3D echocardiography measures larger LV volumes in comparison to 2D echocardiography (6), the larger values are not typically significant enough to change the LV size classification. 3D echocardiography is also limited by lower temporal resolution compared with 2D echocardiography (2).

Left Ventricular Wall Thickness and Relative Wall Thickness

LV wall thickness is assessed in the transgastric mid-papillary short axis and/or transgastric two-chamber views with 2D imaging and excluding the papillary muscles (Figure 3.1). In these views, the anterior and inferior walls are measured at end diastole. Normal wall thickness is 0.6 to 1.0 cm in men and 0.6 to 0.9 cm in women (3). It should be noted that different walls are measured with TEE (anterior and inferior) than TTE (anteroseptal and inferolateral). This is true both for wall thickness and chamber size, and reflects the fact that different views create the most perpendicular alignment with the endocardium in the two modalities.

Relative wall thickness (RWT) is calculated to identify the presence of LV hypertrophy. The formula for RWT is RWT = IWTd/LVIDd, where IWTd = inferior wall thickness in diastole and LVIDd = LV internal diameter in diastole. This formula represents an adaptation of that used in TTE, recognizing that different walls are measured best with the two modalities. Normal RWT is 0.24 to 0.42 in men and 0.22 to 0.42 in women. Increased RWT (>0.42) can be used to classify patients as having either concentric LV hypertrophy (if patient also has increased LV mass, see later) or concentric LV modeling (if patient also has normal LV mass) (2).

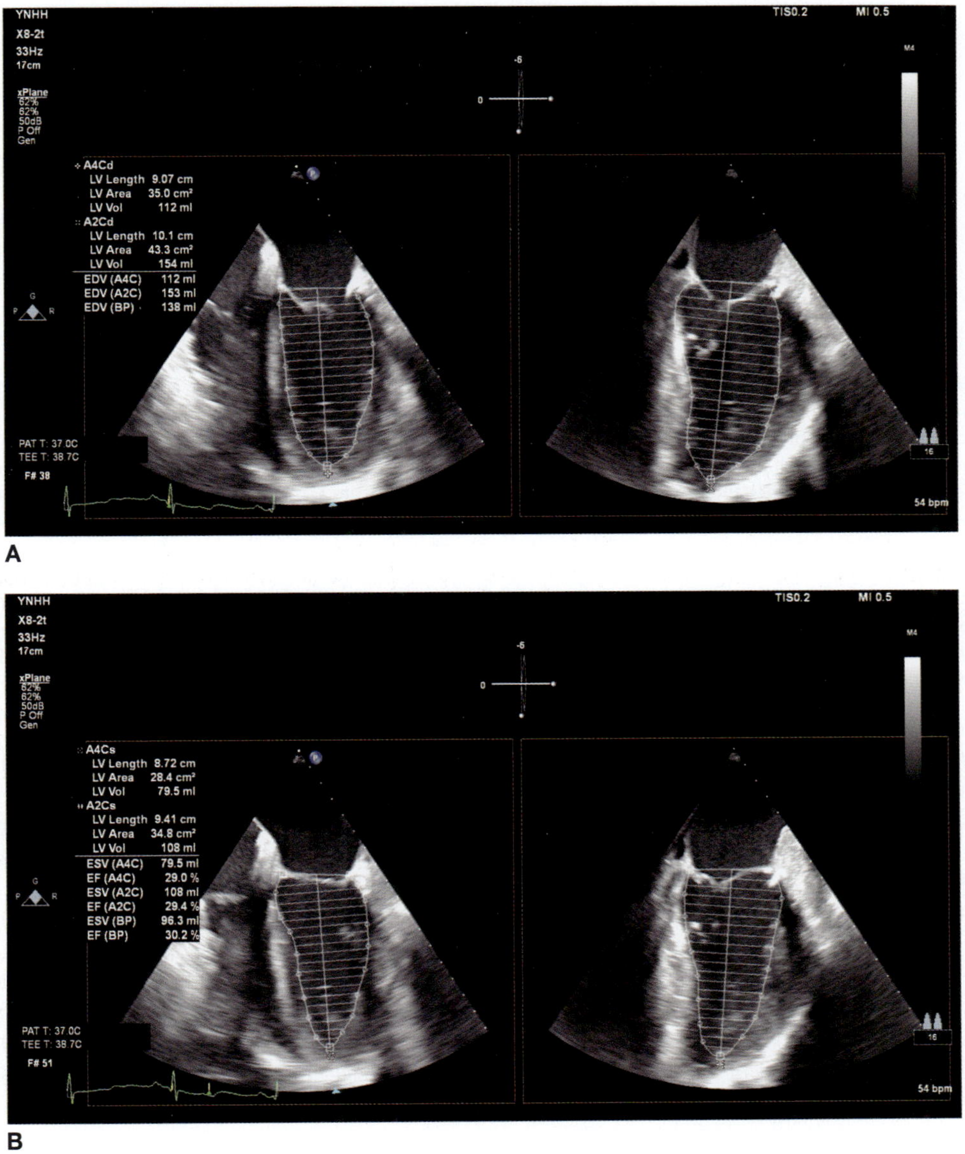

FIGURE 3.2 Example of the 2D measurements required for the biplane method of disks calculation of LV volumes and LVEF. A: ME four-chamber and ME two-chamber views at end diastole; the endocardium (border of the compacted myocardium) is manually traced by the user and the software calculates the long-axis diameter and divides the LV cavity into 20 disks. B: ME four-chamber and ME two-chamber views at end systole; the same measurements are made as in part A. To minimize the impact of foreshortening, there should be less than a 10% difference between the lengths of the four-chamber and two-chamber views in systole as well as in diastole. 2C(d), two chamber (in diastole); 4C(d), four chamber (in diastole); BP, biplane; EDV, end-diastolic volume; EF, ejection fraction; ESV, end-systolic volume; LV, left ventricle; LVEF, left ventricular ejection fraction; ME, midesophageal; vol, volume. Note that the vendor identifies the image by the equivalent transthoracic view in spite of it being a transesophageal image (eg, A4C is the apical four-chamber view, which is equivalent to the midesophageal four-chamber view).

Left Ventricular Mass

LV mass is a strong predictor of cardiovascular events and is typically calculated with 2D echocardiography using measurements performed at end diastole. LV mass increases as body size increases and thus is corrected for BSA. Mass measurements conceptually reflect subtraction of the LV cavity volume from the LV

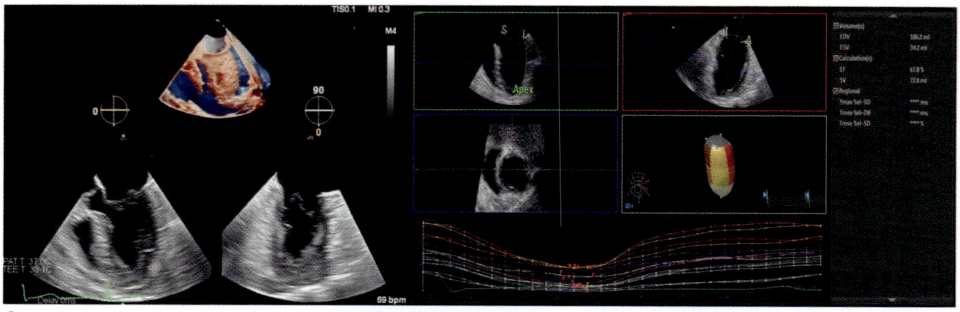

A B

FIGURE 3.3 LV volumes and LVEF calculated using 3D echocardiography. A: The left ventricle is acquired as a pyramidal volume and displayed utilizing automated border detection and cropped to show a 3D rendering of the left ventricular (LV) cavity. The midesophageal (ME) four-chamber and two-chamber views are displayed below. B: LV volume from a 3D echocardiography full-volume data set. Top panels: The multiplanar reconstruction allows for generation of midesophageal ME four- and ME two-chamber views on which reference points at the septal, lateral, inferior, and anterior mitral annulus and the LV apex in end diastole and end systole are placed (similar to biplane Simpson method of disks), automated border detection then generates a 3D-derived LV volume, stroke volume, and ejection fraction. Middle panels: Transgastric short-axis view and AHA/ASE 17-segment volumetric model. Bottom panel: Individual-segment contribution to overall left ventricular volume throughout the cardiac cycle. Colored lines on the graph of volume against time represent the same-colored segment of the volumetric model. AHA/ASE, American Heart Association/American Society of Echocardiography; EDV, end-diastolic volume; EF, ejection fraction; ESV, end-systolic volume; LV, left ventricle; LVEF, left ventricular ejection fraction; SV, stroke volume.

epicardial volume to obtain the LV muscle or shell volume. This volume is converted to mass by multiplying by myocardial density.

There are several approaches that can be taken to calculate LV mass using M-mode, 2D, or 3D imaging, each using a different mathematical model. We suggest the simplest approach with the most robust prognostic value, which uses the cube formula and linear measurements. The cube formula (modified for a TEE approach) is:

$$\text{LV mass (g)} = 0.8 \times 1.04 \times [(\text{AWT} + \text{LVIDd} + \text{IWT})^3 - \text{LVIDd}^3] + 0.6\ \text{g}$$

where AWT, is the anterior wall thickness; LVIDd, the LV internal diameter in diastole; and IWT, the inferior wall thickness. Because numbers in this equation are cubed, small measurement errors are exacerbated thereby limiting the utility of this equation in patient with poor image quality. This approach is also increasingly inaccurate in diseased ventricles including those that are dilated, asymmetrically hypertrophied, or suffer from regional wall motion abnormalities.

While the 2D-based formulas to calculate LV mass, called the truncated ellipsoid and area-length methods, are less dependent on geometrical assumptions and partially correct for shape distortions in comparison to the cube formula, those formulas have cumbersome methodology, higher measurement variability, and fewer studies published on normative data. 3D echocardiography can also be utilized to assess LV mass by subtracting the LV cavity volume from the LV volume encompassed by the epicardium. These volumes are calculated utilizing the 3D MOD also known as the modified Simpson rule. While 3D echocardiography is helpful in that it directly measures LV volumes without geometrical assumptions, there are few studies that assess its value and generalizability to entire patient populations; thus, the ASE guidelines do not provide normal reference values for 3D-derived LV mass (2).

Normal values for LV mass indexed to BSA (g/m^2) are 43 to 95 for women and 49 to 115 for men. LV mass index thresholds for hypertrophy are greater than 115 g/m^2 for men and greater than 95 g/m^2 for women. LV remodeling patterns include normal geometry, concentric remodeling, eccentric hypertrophy, and concentric hypertrophy. Normal geometry is indicated by a normal RWT (<0.42) and normal LV mass index. Concentric remodeling is typically seen earlier in pressure overload states and is indicated by increased RWT of greater than 0.42 and an LV mass index within the normal range. Concentric hypertrophy, which carries a

TABLE 3.1 Normal Values for **LV** Mass Indices (2)

Parameter	ASE Range	
	Women	Men
Linear method	67-162	88-224
LV mass (g)	43-95	49-115
LV mass/BSA (g/m²)	0.22-0.42	0.24-0.42
Septal thickness (cm)	0.6-0.9	0.6-1.0
Posterior wall thickness (cm)	0.6-0.9	0.6-1.0
2D method		
LV mass (g)	66-150	96-200
LV mass/BSA (g/m²)	44-88	50-102

ASE, American Society of Echocardiography; BSA, body surface area; LV, left ventricle.
Reprinted from Lang RM, Badano LP, Mor-Avi V, et al. Recommendations for cardiac chamber quantification by echocardiography in adults: an update from the American Society of Echocardiography and the European Association of Cardiovascular Imaging. *J Am Soc Echocardiogr*. 2015;28[1]:1-39.e14. With permission from Elsevier.

worse prognosis and is often seen later in pressure overload pathology, is indicated by both increased RWT and increased LV mass. Finally, eccentric hypertrophy (LV dilation) is typically from volume overload and is demonstrated by a normal RWT with an increased LV mass index (2) (Table 3.1).

QUANTITATIVE MEASURES OF LEFT VENTRICULAR SYSTOLIC PERFORMANCE

Systolic function of the LV can be measured in numerous ways via qualitative visual assessment, M-mode echocardiography, 2D echocardiography, and 3D echocardiography. While visual estimation of LV systolic performance is quick and improves with experience, it has not been found to be universally accurate (7) and should be supported by quantitative assessment whenever possible.

Common Measures of Left Ventricular Systolic Function

Fractional Shortening

Fractional shortening can be calculated using either M-mode or, preferably, linear measurements from 2D images of the transgastric mid-papillary LV short-axis view. The diameter of the LV is measured at end diastole (LVIDd) and at end systole (LVIDs) with exclusion of the papillary muscles (Figure 3.4). The fractional shortening equation is ([LVIDd − LVIDs]/LVIDd) × 100 and is reported as a percentage. A fractional shortening value of more than 25% is considered normal (2). Notably, this methodology measures function in one plane and only observes two of the four LV walls: the inferior and anterior walls. Additionally, measurements are load dependent and cannot capture any concurrent regional wall motion abnormalities (5).

Fractional Area Change

Fractional area change is an area measurement of LV function, and measurements are also performed in the transgastric mid-papillary LV short-axis view (Figure 3.5). The area of the LV cavity is traced at the border of the compacted myocardium at end diastole (LVEDA) and at end systole (LVEDS) with exclusion of the papillary muscles. The fractional area change equation is ([LVEDA − LVEDS]/LVEDA) × 100 and is presented as a percentage; a fractional area change value of more than 35% is considered normal (2). Like fractional shortening, this measurement is load dependent and assessed in one plane of the LV and may miss regional wall motion abnormality in other planes (5).

Left Ventricular Ejection Fraction

Left ventricular ejection fraction (LVEF) is the most used and reported measure of global LV systolic function. It is fundamental to the evaluation and management of heart failure and has been correlated with clinical outcome in countless studies (8,9). To patients' detriment, however, the LVEF is sometimes the only "takeaway" from the detailed reports of comprehensive echocardiograms, and the limitations of LVEF must be recognized. The ejection fraction is a load-dependent measure of ventricular ejection (not contractility, which is much harder to assess) and is subject to significant variability—intraobserver,

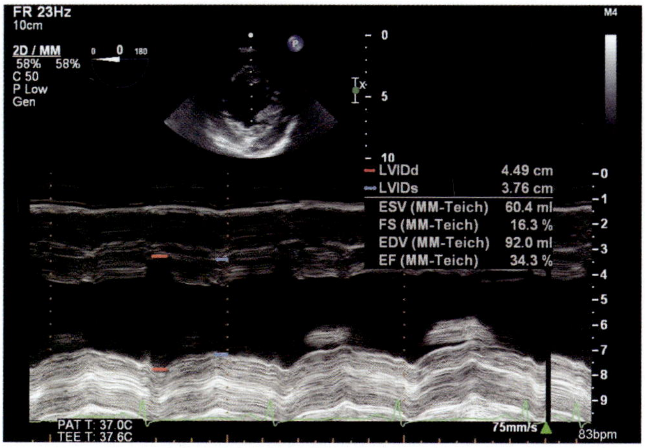

FIGURE 3.4 Fractional shortening (FS) calculated from an M-mode of the transgastric short axis. Calipers are placed on the endocardium at end diastole (largest internal diameter) and at the end systole (smallest internal diameter). FS = (LVIDd − LVIDs)/LVIDd expressed as a percentage. Note that the posteromedial papillary muscle is not included in the measurement. While the machine displays "volumes" using the Teicholz method, it should be noted that neither ventricular volume nor LVEF should be extrapolated from the FS measurements. EDV, end-diastolic volume; EF, ejection fraction; ESV, end-systolic volume; LVEF, left ventricular ejection fraction; LVIDd, left ventricular internal diameter in diastole; LVIDs, left ventricular internal diameter in systole; MM, M-mode.

interobserver, and across modalities (10). As LVEF represents the proportion of diastolic blood that is ejected, it correlates poorly with stroke volume with either low or high ventricular volumes. Patients with hypovolemia with high LVEF still have low stroke volume, and the stroke volume of patients with dilated cardiomyopathy (DCM) can sometimes be surprisingly near normal. That being said, LVEF assessment is a critical component of every comprehensive echocardiogram, and the measurements should be made with care and attention.

To calculate LVEF, LV volumes must be obtained either via the biplane MOD with 2D echocardiography (as described earlier) or with 3D echocardiography. The ejection fraction formula is LVEF = ([LVEDV − LVESV]/LVEDV) × 100, where LVEDV is the end-diastolic volume and LVESV, the end-systolic volume. Ejection fraction is presented as a percentage. Normal LVEF by biplane MOD for men is 62 ± 5% and for women is 64 ± 5% (2) (Figures 3.2 and 3.3).

dP/dt

While most measures of global LV systolic function provide information on contraction or ejection, it is much harder to assess contractility or the inherent contractile state of the myocardium. LV contractility is best assessed with echocardiography by observing the rate of LV pressure rise during isovolumetric contraction, referred to as dP/dt. This is achieved by interrogating a mitral regurgitation jet with continuous wave Doppler, which reflects the pressure difference between the LV and the left atrium during ventricular systole. To perform this calculation, the time at two velocities, 1 and 3 m/s of the mitral regurgitation jet, is measured. The modified Bernoulli equation is applied to calculate the pressure differential (dP) $= 4(3^2) - 4(1^2) = 32$ mm Hg (Figure 3.6). This pressure difference is then divided by the time interval (dt) of the continuous wave Doppler–derived mitral regurgitant jet between 1 and 3 m/s. In an LV with normal contractility, the dP/dt should be greater than 1,200 mm Hg/s. Although this measurement is independent of loading conditions, it is angle dependent due to the reliance on continuous wave Doppler. Additionally, this measurement becomes less accurate in cases of acute mitral regurgitation where elevated left atrial pressures alter the expected pressure gradient (5).

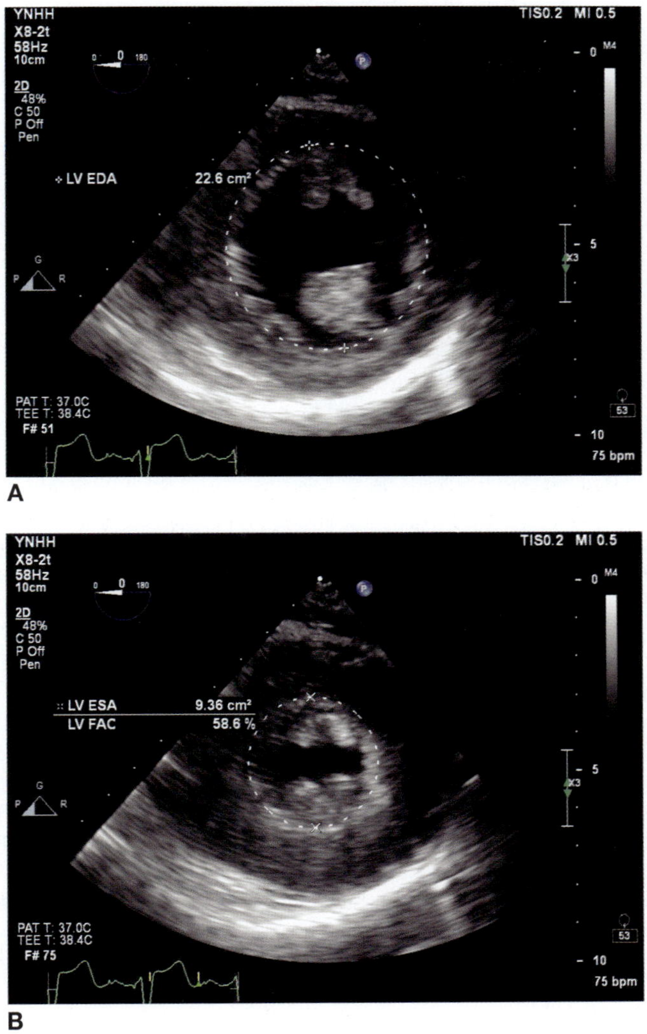

FIGURE 3.5 Fractional area change. A: Transgastric short-axis view at end diastole. B: Transgastric short-axis view at end systole. The area of the LV cavity is measured at end diastole and at end systole, excluding the papillary muscles; FAC = (LVAd − LVAs)/LVAd expressed as a percentage. LVAd, left ventricular area in diastole; LVAs, left ventricular area in systole; LV EDA, left ventricular end-diastolic area; LV ESA, left ventricular end-systolic area.

Other Measures of Global Left Ventricular Systolic Function

Tissue Doppler–Derived Left Ventricular Systolic Function (s′)

Tissue Doppler–derived LV systolic function (*s*′) utilizes tissue Doppler imaging to quantify systolic LV function. It is of increased utility when image quality is poor, and thus, more robust 2D and 3D quantifications of LV function are limited. The *s*′ velocity averages four basal segments and measures longitudinal LV contraction, which then serves as a proxy for overall LV systolic function. The *s*′ velocities are measured by placing the sample volume at the mitral annular level at the septal annulus and at the lateral annulus (11) (Figure 3.7). The normal reference ranges of *s*′ tissue Doppler imaging (TDI) values in healthy adults are 8.1 ± 1.5 cm/s (septal velocity), 10.2 ± 2.4 cm/s (lateral velocity), and 9.2 ± 1.7 cm/s (average of septal and lateral velocities) (11).

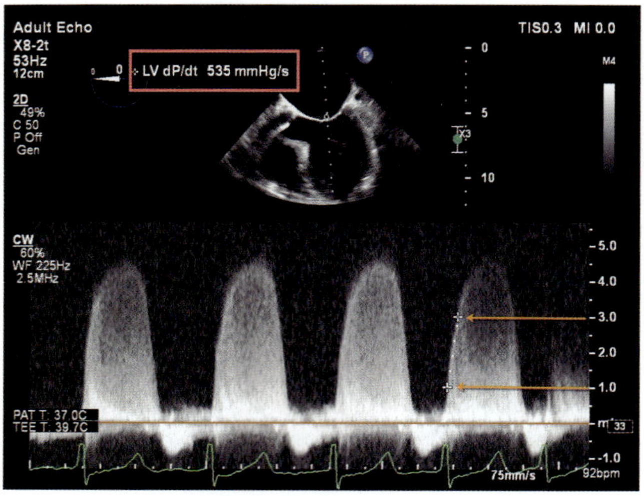

FIGURE 3.6 Calculation of dP/dT using a continuous wave Doppler sampling of a jet of mitral regurgitation. The caliper is placed on the jet envelope at 1 m/s and again at 3 m/s to measure the time for the pressure gradient between the left ventricle (LV) and left atrium (LA) to rise from 4 to 36 mm Hg.

2D Speckle-Tracking Echocardiography

Speckle-tracking echocardiography (STE) observes how ultrasound interacts with the myocardium to produce "speckles," which are then tracked over time (Figures 3.8 and 3.9).

The tracking of speckle displacements allows for calculation of tissue velocities, strain, and strain rates of specific segments of the heart (12). Global longitudinal strain (GLS) obtained by 2D STE allows for accurate and reproducible quantification of LV systolic function (Video 3.2). Of note, global circumferential and global radial strains are less reliable and are thus not utilized clinically for evaluation of LV systolic function (13). GLS is defined as the myocardial length change between end diastole and end systole: GLS (%) = (myocardial length at end systole − myocardial length at end diastole)/myocardial length at end diastole.

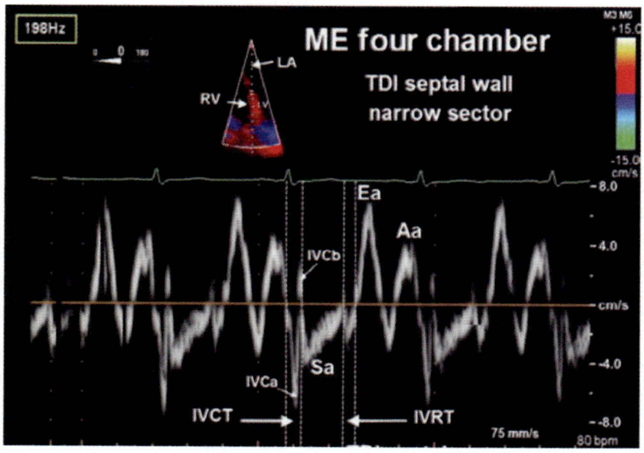

FIGURE 3.7 Typical left ventricle mitral annulus tissue Doppler imaging (TDI). Aa, atrial contraction (late diastolic) tissue velocity; Ea, early diastolic peak tissue velocity; IVC, isovolumic contraction; IVCT, isovolumic contraction time; IVRT, isovolumic relaxation time; LA, left atrium; LV, left ventricle; RV, right ventricle; Sa, mitral annular systolic tissue velocity.

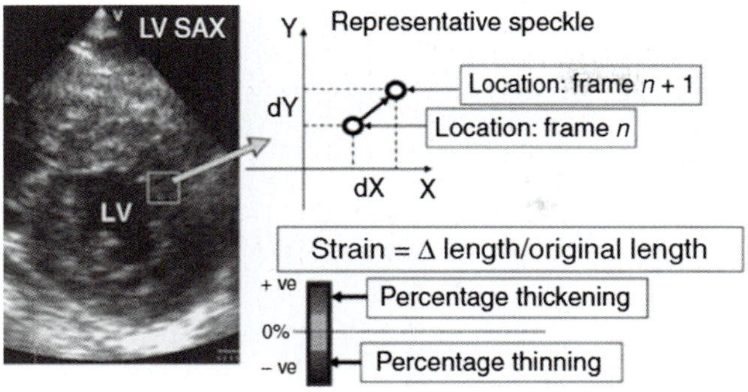

FIGURE 3.8 Speckle tracking. Localized region of the myocardium is marked by the box; speckles are identified in frame (*n*) and tracked over time to frame (*n* + 1); velocity vector is calculated and used to derive strain. LV, left ventricle; SAX, short axis. (From Suffoletto MS, Dohi K, Cannesson M, et al. Novel speckle-tracking radial strain from routine black-and-white echocardiographic images to quantify dyssynchrony and predict response to cardiac resynchronization therapy. *Circulation*. 2006;113[7]:960-968.)

The specific methodology to obtain GLS by speckle tracking varies by vendor, but GLS is measured in previously acquired midesophageal four-chamber, midesophageal two-chamber, and midesophageal long-axis views. The automated software will define the myocardial borders, with the ability for manual correction in each view at end diastole and end systole; subsequently, the software will track the change over the cardiac cycle to generate a GLS. An average GLS is reported, and a peak GLS of −18% is considered normal (14). The value is negative given that myocardial length at end systole is smaller than myocardial length at end diastole. Abnormal strain is defined when the absolute GLS number is greater than 18 and as the absolute number of GLS decreases, the LV strain worsens (2). Bull's eye blots can be generated by strain analysis programs using 2D STE data; blue represents positive strain, and red represents negative strain. This allows for visualization of all 17 segments of the LV and for specific localization of abnormal strain (12).

Mitral Annular Plane Systolic Excursion and Mitral Tissue Motion Annular Displacement

Mitral annular plane systole excursion (MAPSE) measures the movement of the annulus of the mitral valve toward the apex of the heart to quantify LV systolic function with M-mode echocardiography. This can be achieved by placing the M-mode cursor on the medial and lateral annulus of the mitral valve in the apical four-chamber view of TTE, where it has been validated. It can also be obtained in the midesophageal four-chamber view of TEE; however, this has not been validated. A normal MAPSE range is 12 to 15 mm, and a MAPSE of less than 8 mm is associated with an LVEF of less than 50% (15). MAPSE is angle dependent, given it utilizes M-mode echocardiography.

Contrast Echocardiography for Left Ventricular Function Assessment

Intravenous echocardiography contrast (called in the literature an "ultrasound-enhancing agent" or UEA) consists of microbubbles of a high-molecular-weight gas with high persistence due to a low solubility and diffusivity. The bubbles are of a size that easily passes through the pulmonary circulation (unlike agitated saline) and opacifies the blood when viewed with ultrasound. This improves the visualization of blood-tissue boundaries, which can be helpful in the assessment of global and regional biventricular systolic function as well as in the evaluation of masses and thrombi. As an adjunct to 2D echocardiography, UEAs improve both the manual and automatic border detection for the evaluation of LV volumes as well as global and regional systolic function (16) (Figure 3.10). There are various contrast agents that can be administered as either bolus injections or infusions. Additionally, as ultrasound machine vendors have their own unique imaging presets available for contrast echocardiography, echocardiographers should educate themselves on platform settings to optimize contrast imaging (17,18).

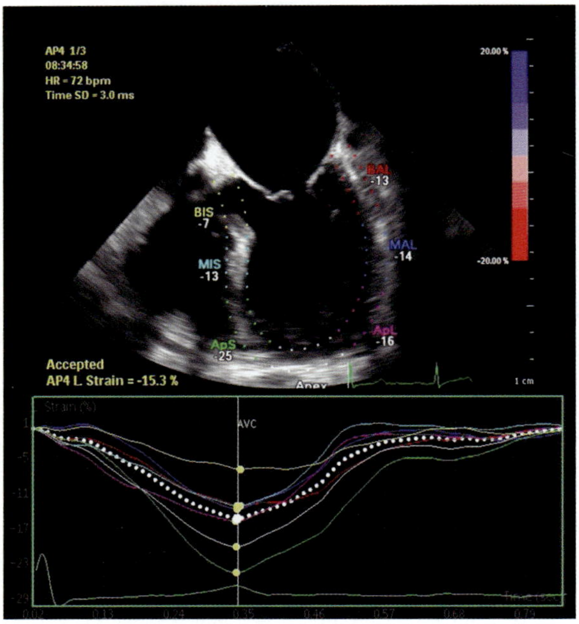

A

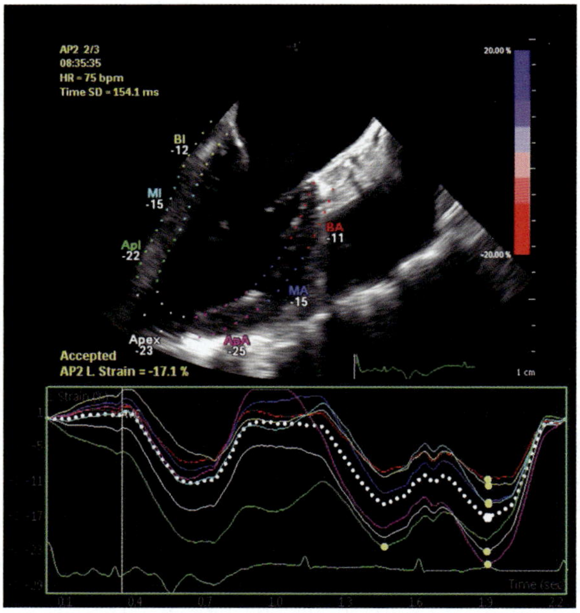

B

FIGURE 3.9 Global longitudinal strain (GLS). Speckle-tracking echocardiography (STE) is performed on the entirety of the LV myocardium in the midesophageal (ME) four-chamber, two-chamber, and long-axis views. Speckles are sampled in each segment, and strain is calculated from the change in length then displayed graphically. An average or global strain is calculated for each view. A: STE and calculated strain in the ME four-chamber view. Upper panel: The left ventricle is divided into segments, and the average strain is calculated for each. Lower panel: Longitudinal strain for each segment plotted against time (cardiac cycle). Dotted line represents the average longitudinal strain. Panels B and C show similar displays for the ME two-chamber and ME long-axis views. D: Global longitudinal strain. Longitudinal strain data from an ME four chamber, ME two chamber and LV long axis are displayed as the 17-segment "bull's eye" and an average global longitudinal strain (GLS) reported. Note the "bull's eye" is oriented as in a transthoracic view. AP2, apical ME two chamber; AP3, apical ME LV long axis; AP4, apical ME four chamber; Avg, average; HR, heart rate; L, longitudinal; LV, left ventricle; SD, standard deviation.

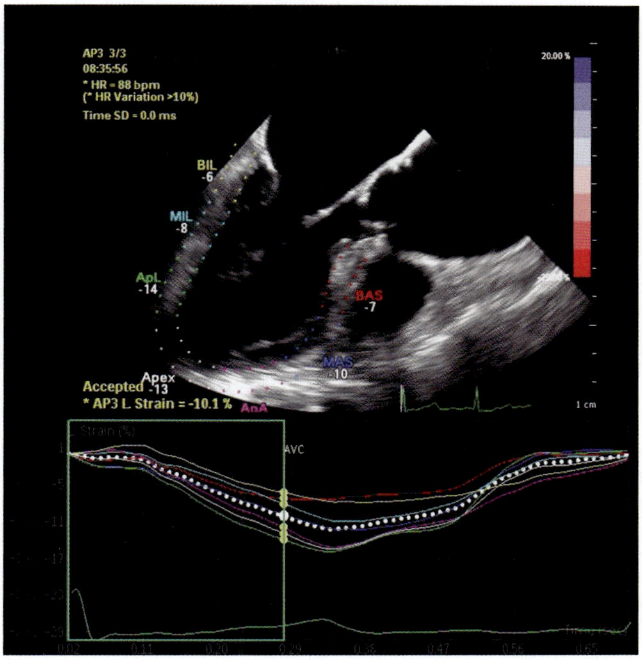

C

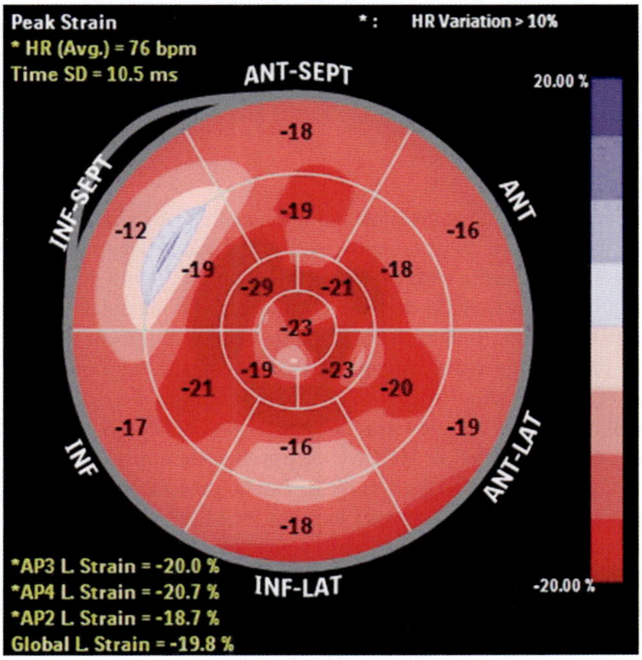

D

FIGURE 3.9 *(continued)*

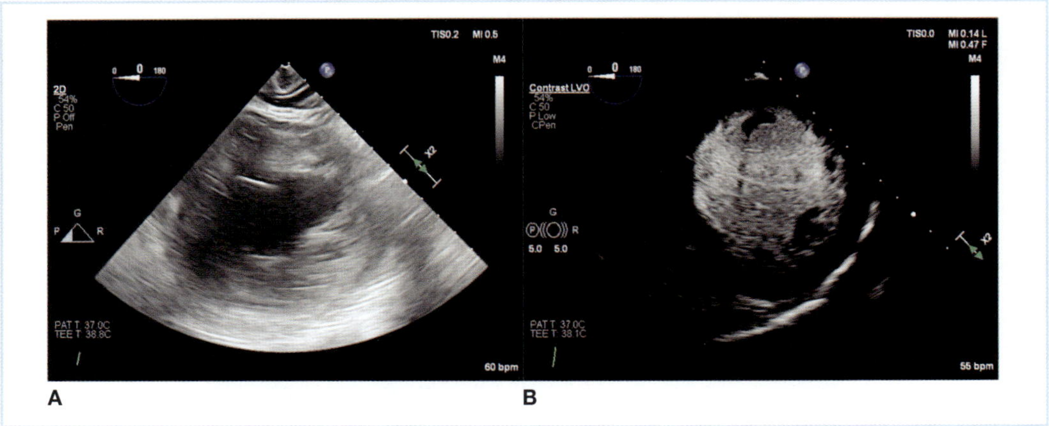

FIGURE 3.10 Transgastric short-axis still images without (A) and after administration (B) of an ultrasound-enhancing agent (UEA). Notice that in image A, the endocardial border is difficult to distinguish while in B, it is easily identifiable. The use of UEA is recommended when two or more LV segments are not well visualized.

VENTRICULAR PATHOLOGY

Cardiomyopathies

Cardiomyopathy is best (though variably) defined as a disorder of the myocardium in which the heart muscle is abnormal both in structure and function and that is not due to other etiologies, including coronary artery disease, valvulopathies, congenital heart disease, or hypertension. More recently, given the complexity of the disease spectrum of cardiomyopathies, the 2023 European Society of Cardiology created a task force to create a new categorization system of cardiomyopathies by phenotype (19,20). Cardiomyopathies will be described by phenotype outlined in Figure 3.11.

Hypertrophic Cardiomyopathy

Hypertrophic cardiomyopathy (HCM) is the most common genetic abnormality of the myocardium and is an autosomal dominant disease with variable expressivity and variable penetrance. While global LV systolic function is typically preserved, patients with HCM commonly present with diastolic dysfunction. Echocardiographic findings in patients with HCM include: (a) unexplained maximal wall thickness of more than 15 mm in any myocardial segment, (b) anteroseptal/inferolateral wall thickness ratio of greater than 1.3 in normotensive patients, or (c) anteroseptal/inferolateral wall thickness ratio of greater than 1.5 in patients with hypertension (21) (Video 3.3).

While HCM with left ventricular outflow tract obstruction (LVOTO) is commonly referred to as "hypertrophic obstructive cardiomyopathy" or HOCM, the appropriate nomenclature is now considered to be "HCM with obstruction." This acknowledges that HCM can be present with or without obstruction, and it should be noted that LVOTO can also be present without HCM. HCM with obstruction presents unique physiologic challenges that are distinct from nonobstructive HCM. Echocardiographic features are crucial for diagnosing and differentiating HCM with obstruction from other pathologies. Systolic anterior motion (SAM) of the mitral valve leaflets is a hallmark feature of obstruction and is best seen in the midesophageal long-axis view. SAM occurs when mitral leaflet tissue, typically the anterior mitral leaflet, is displaced into the LVOT during systole causing obstruction (Figure 3.12).

Additionally, hypertrophy of the interventricular septum is an important risk factor for SAM that can be seen with TEE. In the midesophageal long-axis view, SAM *may* be associated with coarse fluttering of the aortic valve leaflets and early closure of the aortic valve in mid-systole, which can be seen on 2D or M-mode (Video 3.4). Color flow Doppler in the subaortic region will demonstrate flow acceleration due to turbulent flow in the LVOT, suggestive of dynamic obstruction. Color flow Doppler can also help distinguish mitral regurgitation secondary to SAM, which often causes posteriorly directed mitral regurgitation, from intrinsic mitral valve pathology that would more likely result in a central or anteriorly directed jet. Continuous wave

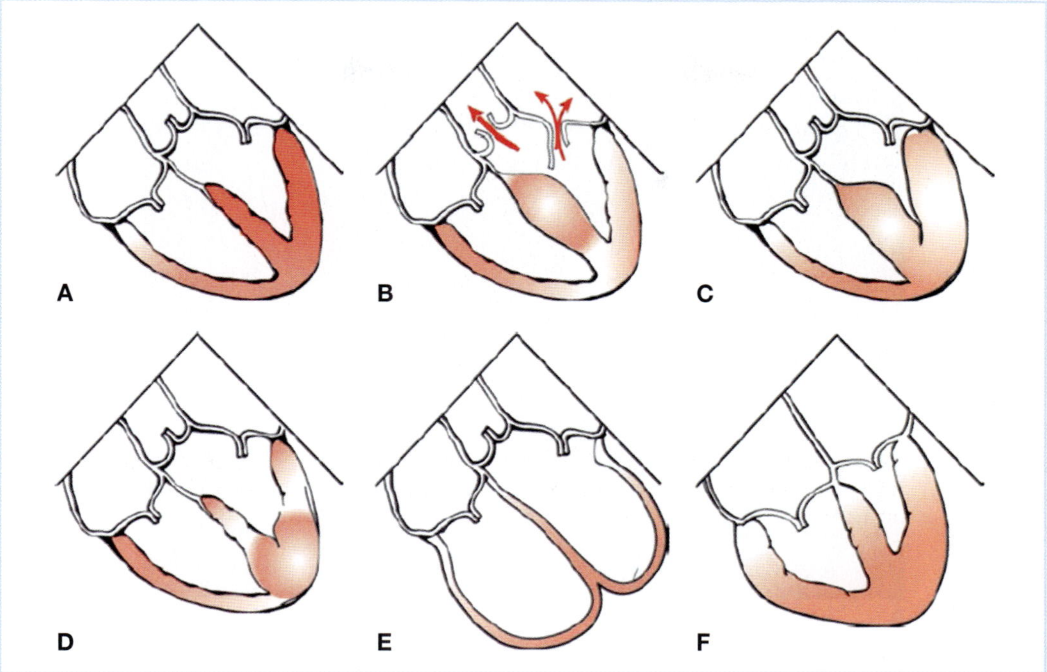

FIGURE 3.11 Cardiomyopathy variants. A: Normal. B: Hypertrophic cardiomyopathy (HCM) with anteroseptal hypertrophy. Note systolic anterior motion of the mitral leaflets with left ventricular outflow tract obstruction and mitral regurgitation. **C:** Concentric HCM. The basal inferolateral segment is frequently spared. D: Apical HCM. E: Dilated cardiomyopathy; dilation may be confined to the left ventricle or biventricular with or without atrial involvement. F: Restrictive cardiomyopathy. Note thick ventricles with small intraventricular cavities and biatrial enlargement.

Doppler of the LVOT, typically from the deep transgastric five-chamber or transgastric long-axis views, will show a late-peaking, dagger-shaped velocity curve (22) (Figure 3.13). A peak instantaneous LVOT gradient of more than 30 mm Hg defines LVOT obstruction. An LVOT gradient of more than 50 mm Hg is considered hemodynamically significant. It is recommended that septal myectomy be considered to reduce LVOT obstruction in patients who have an LVOT gradient of 50 mm Hg or more, moderate-to-severe symptoms (eg, New York Heart Association functional Class III-IV), or recurrent exertional syncope despite drug therapy (23) (Figure 3.14).

There are other pathologies that may mimic HOCM such as fixed subvalvular obstruction, valvular aortic stenosis, and supravalvular stenosis. Echocardiography can help distinguish these pathologies from HCM. LVOT obstruction can be differentiated from fixed subvalvular, valvular, or supravalvular stenosis because the continuous wave Doppler envelope in fixed obstruction will not be late peaking (21). Moreover, valvular aortic stenosis can be distinguished by thickening and calcification of the aortic valve leaflets. Supravalvular stenosis will demonstrate a narrowed aortic root or ascending aorta on 2D imaging and turbulence localized above the valve on color flow Doppler versus in the subaortic region as observed in dynamic LVOT obstruction.

Dilated Cardiomyopathy

The DCM phenotype is defined by the combination of LV dilation and systolic dysfunction. Patients with DCM will have enlarged ventricles with an LV end-diastolic diameter (LVEDd) or volume more than 2 *z*-scores above the expected mean value. For men, this corresponds to an LVEDd of greater than 58 mm and for women, greater than 52 mm. LV systolic dysfunction is defined by an ejection fraction of less than 50%. These patients commonly have right ventricular (RV) dilation and dysfunction, biatrial enlargement, as well as mitral and tricuspid regurgitation, though these findings are not required for the diagnosis. While there is a degree of mitral annular dilation in DCM, it is the increased tethering from tension on the mitral

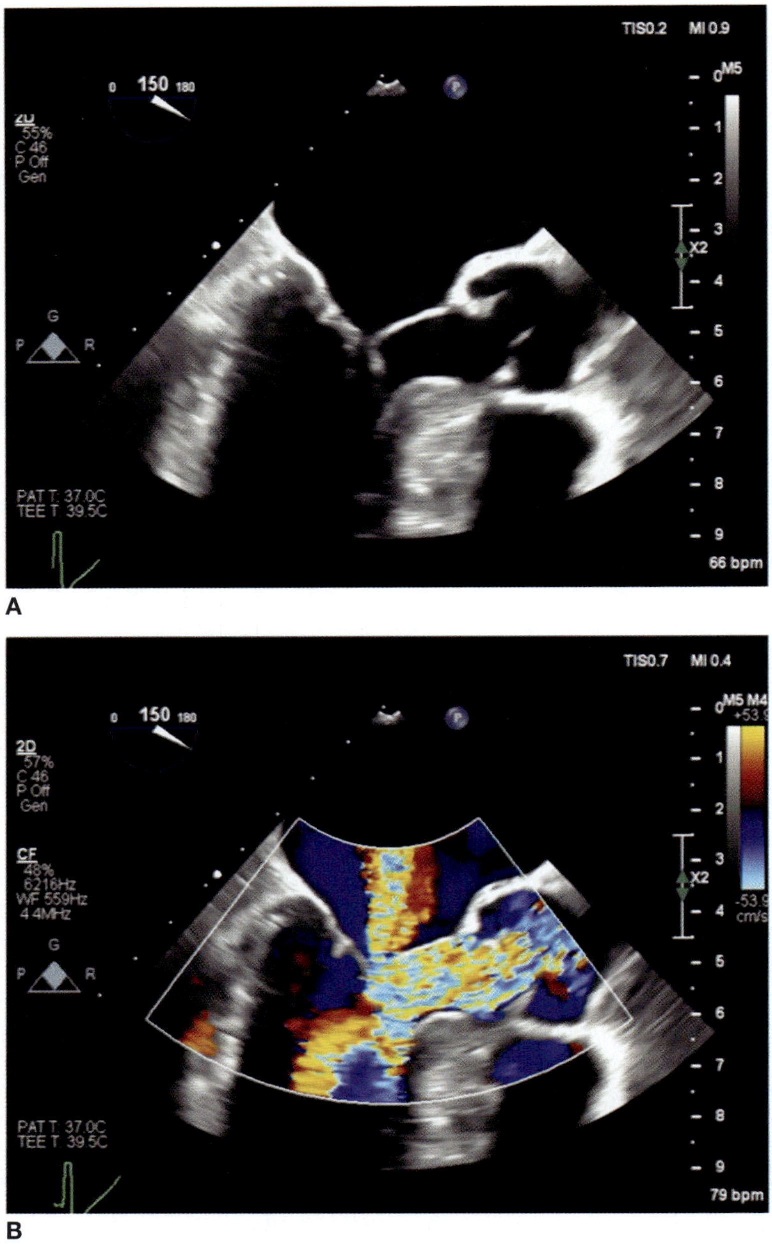

FIGURE 3.12 Hypertrophic cardiomyopathy with systolic anterior motion (SAM) of the mitral valve. A: Midesophageal left ventricle long-axis (ME LV LAX) view. Note that the anterior leaflet of the mitral valve abuts the septum during systole. It is also apparent from the coaptation defect that significant mitral regurgitation can be expected. B: Color flow Doppler findings in SAM with left ventricular outflow tract (LVOT) obstruction. There is evidence of flow acceleration in the LV approaching the obstruction. There is then turbulent flow in the LVOT as well as mitral regurgitation. This pattern has been called by one of our editors (JZ) the "Y" sign. While this finding should alert the echocardiographer to the presence of LVOT obstruction, its absence does not preclude it.

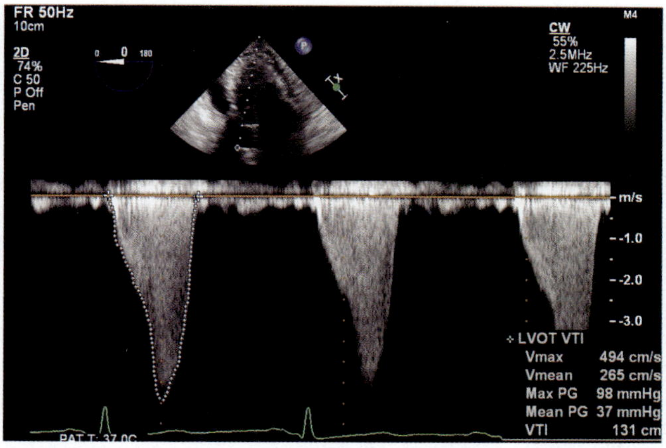

FIGURE 3.13 Left ventricular outflow tract (LVOT) obstruction demonstrating typical late systolic peaking ("dagger-shaped") gradient across the LVOT as the cross-sectional area becomes progressively smaller during systole. Note the high gradients generated.

subvalvular apparatus that is the greatest contributor to the functional mitral regurgitation in these cases (Figure 3.15; Video 3.5). The combination of ventricular dilation and dysfunction seen in DCM also creates the substrate for LV apical thrombus, which should be sought in every echo for a patient with DCM.

DCM is the third most common cause of heart failure with 20% to 35% of cases having a heritable component and the remainder being nongenetic. Potential nongenetic etiologies include toxins such as alcohol or doxorubicin, thiamine deficiency, infections such as Chagas disease or viral infections, and idiopathic. Of note, patients who have DCM secondary to Chagas disease experience focal disease. These individuals have an LV apical aneurysm and their interventricular septum is typically spared (24).

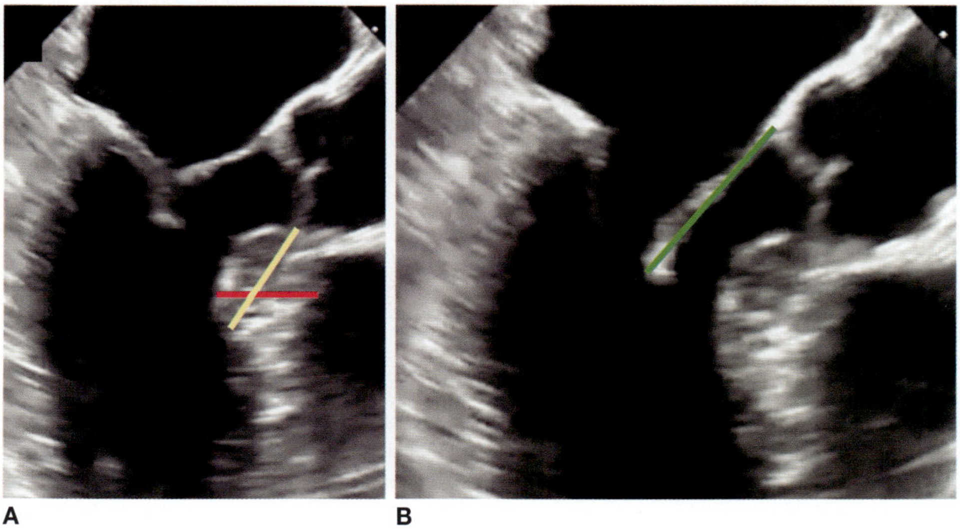

FIGURE 3.14 Example of common measurements made to guide the surgical approach to septal myectomy. A: End-diastolic maximal basal anteroseptal thickness (red) and the distance from right coronary cusp insertion to the "end of the bulge" if present (yellow). B: Anterior mitral leaflet length in diastole, measured from the tip to the insertion of the noncoronary cusp (green). Long anterior mitral leaflets may benefit from plication. Additional measures may be helpful or requested in some cases.

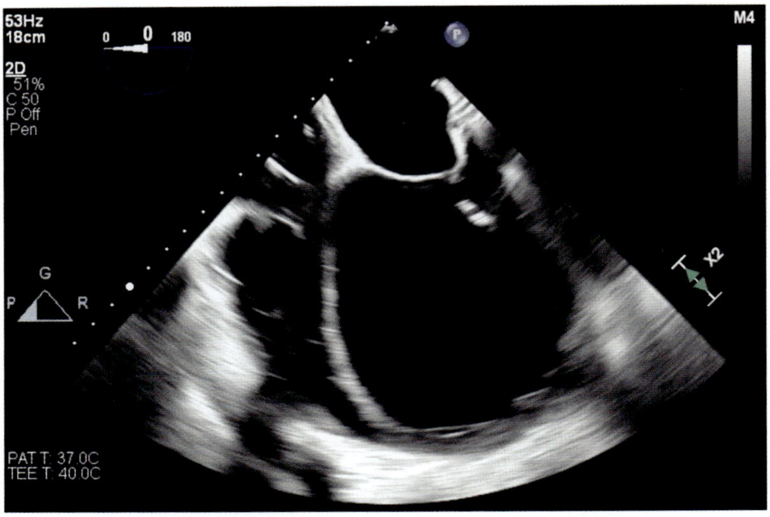

FIGURE 3.15 Midesophageal four chamber demonstrating the 2D findings of dilated cardiomyopathy (DCM). The left ventricle is dilated with an appearance of increased sphericity. This results from a disproportional increase in the diameter of the mid-portion of the left ventricle (LV). There is also evidence of increased tethering of the mitral leaflets, displacing them toward the LV apex and reducing their coaptation length. In this example, the right ventricle is not (yet) dilated. LV, left ventricle.

Non-Dilated Left Ventricular Cardiomyopathy

Non-dilated LV cardiomyopathy is defined by nonischemic LV scarring with impaired global LV systolic function (LVEF <50%) in the absence of significant LV dilation (19).

Arrhythmogenic Cardiomyopathy

Arrhythmogenic cardiomyopathy is a genetic disorder that leads to progressive replacement of the myocardium with fibrofatty tissue that leads to arrhythmias. The classification has expanded to include not only the classic arrhythmogenic RV cardiomyopathy phenotype, but also disease that affects the LV as well. Thus, the phenotypic variants of arrhythmogenic cardiomyopathy include (a) right-dominant variant (eg, classic arrhythmogenic RV cardiomyopathy phenotype characterized by RV involvement with no LV abnormalities) and (b) left-dominant variant characterized by LV involvement with no RV abnormalities, and biventricular disease variant that affects both ventricles (25). Echocardiographic features of the right-dominant variant include RV dilation and reduced RV function, often with RV wall motion abnormalities (Video 3.6).

Restrictive Cardiomyopathy

Restrictive cardiomyopathy represents a heterogenous group of diseases characterized by increased LV stiffness and with low compliance. There is a normal or decreased volume of both ventricles with biatrial enlargement and diastolic dysfunction (24,26). Echocardiography should be used to distinguish restrictive cardiomyopathy from constrictive pericarditis. In restrictive cardiomyopathy, patients have restrictive diastolic filling profiles on pulse wave Doppler whereas in constrictive pericarditis, patients have normal diastolic function or grade 1 diastolic dysfunction. Patients with constrictive pericarditis will have respirophasic septal shift and septal bounce due to enhanced ventricular interdependence. This is due to the early diastolic biventricular filling present in constrictive pericarditis. Further characteristics differentiating restrictive cardiomyopathy and constrictive pericarditis are elaborated on in Table 3.2 (27).

Amyloidosis is the most common cause of restrictive cardiomyopathy and occurs due to deposition of amyloid fibrils in the myocardium. Echocardiographic features of amyloidosis include: increased LV and RV wall thickening, biatrial enlargement, diastolic dysfunction, severely reduced mitral annular tissue Doppler

TABLE 3.2 Two-Dimensional and Doppler Characteristics of Constrictive Pericarditis and Restrictive Cardiomyopathy

	Constrictive Pericarditis	Restrictive Cardiomyopathy
2D echocardiography or M-mode		
Thickened pericardium	+++	±
Biatrial enlargement	±	+++
LV chamber size	±	Small
Wall thickness	±	++
Myocardium	Normal	Sparkling, granular
Systolic function	Intact	Reduced
Septal movement	Septal "bounce" = rapid anterior movement during early diastole; ventricular interdependence	No ventricular interdependence
IVC and hepatic veins	Enlarged	Enlarged
Mitral regurgitation	±	Usually present
Tricuspid regurgitation	±	Usually present
Doppler findings		
E/A ratio	May be normal or <1	>2.2
MV inflow deceleration time (ms)	Low normal	Shortened (<150)
Mitral E wave changes during respiration	>25% reduction in inspiration and increase in expiration[a]	Normal (~5%)
IVRT during inspiration	++	No variation
Pulmonary vein flow (left-sided filling pattern)	Inspiration *S* approximately = *D*, expiration produces increased D waves	*S* < *D*, *S/D* ratio <0.5 deep and wide A wave; no respiratory variation
Hepatic vein flow (right-sided filling pattern)	W waveform (prominent A wave) with respiratory variations (decrease in diastolic flow during expiration)	Blunted systolic flow, deep atrial reversal, may be reversed during systole (secondary to significant TR)

A, late diastolic filling; E, early diastolic filling; IVC, inferior vena cava; IVRT, isovolumetric relaxation time; LV, left ventricle; MV, mitral valve; TR, tricuspid regurgitation; TV, tricuspid valve; W waveform, reversal of flow in late systole and late diastole.
[a]This pattern occurs in spontaneously breathing patients; in those receiving positive pressure ventilation, the pattern is reversed.

velocities, reduced GLS with apical sparing, paradoxical low-flow low-gradient aortic stenosis, pericardial effusion, increased atrial septal thickness, diffuse valve thickening, and preserved ejection fraction with low stroke volume index (28) (Video 3.7; Figures 3.16 and 3.17).

Left Ventricular Hypertrabeculation

LV hypertrabeculation (frequently called LV noncompaction in the past) is characterized by the presence of an increase in the proportion of noncompacted to compacted LV myocardium with associated increased trabeculation and associated intertrabecular recesses. While there is debate about whether this represents a true cardiomyopathy (the current ESC guidelines do not consider it a cardiomyopathy), it has been included for the sake of completeness.

The Jenni criteria are often used to evaluate the presence of LV noncompaction and include a bilayered myocardium, a noncompacted to compacted ratio of more than 2:1, communication with the intertrabecular space demonstrated by Doppler, absence of coexisting cardiac abnormalities, and the presence of multiple prominent trabeculations in end systole (29). LV hypertrabeculation has historically been attributed to abnormal myocardial embryogenesis in utero; however, a different LV noncompaction cardiomyopathy that is reversible has been described in patients who have an increase in cardiac output and stroke volume such as pregnant patients or athletes. This increase in cardiac output leads to the de novo formation of trabeculations that then regress when physiology normalizes (30) (Video 3.8).

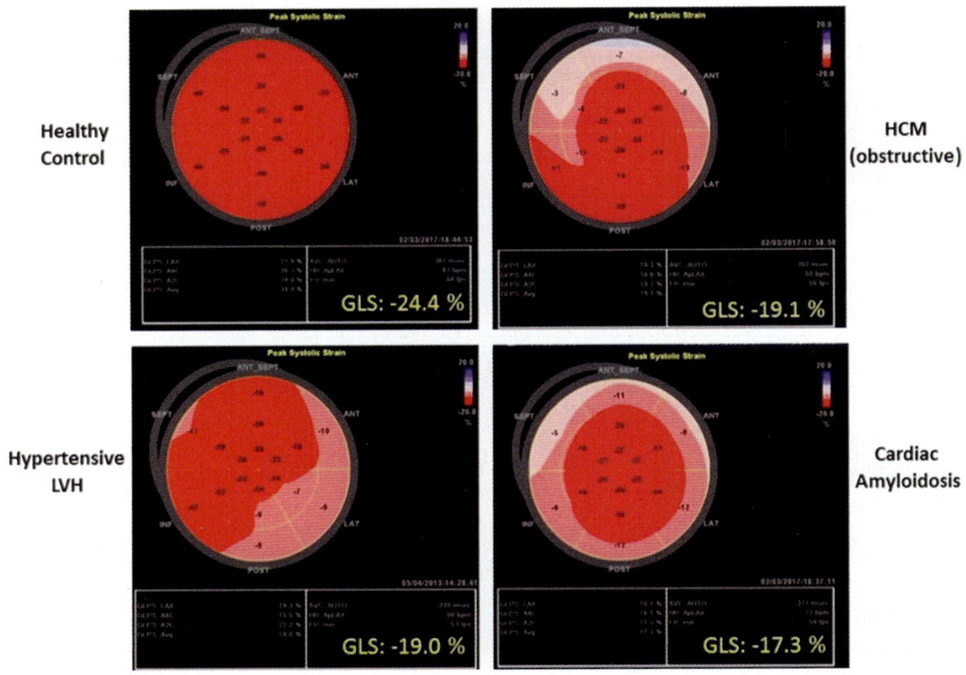

FIGURE 3.16 Strain in cardiomyopathy. Strain patterns from speckle-tracking echocardiography. Red denotes normal strain, lighter shades of pink denote lower strain values. Healthy control—normal strain throughout myocardium; hypertrophic obstructive cardiomyopathy—lower strain values in anterior, septal, and anteroseptal segments; hypertensive hypertrophy—lower strain values in a large area of the myocardium; cardiac amyloidosis—apical sparing. GLS, global longitudinal strain; HCM, hypertrophic cardiomyopathy; LVH, left ventricular hypertrophy. (From Inciardi RM, Galderisi M, Nistri S, et al. Echocardiographic advances in hypertrophic cardiomyopathy: three-dimensional and strain imaging echocardiography. *Echocardiography*. 2018;35[4]:1-11.)

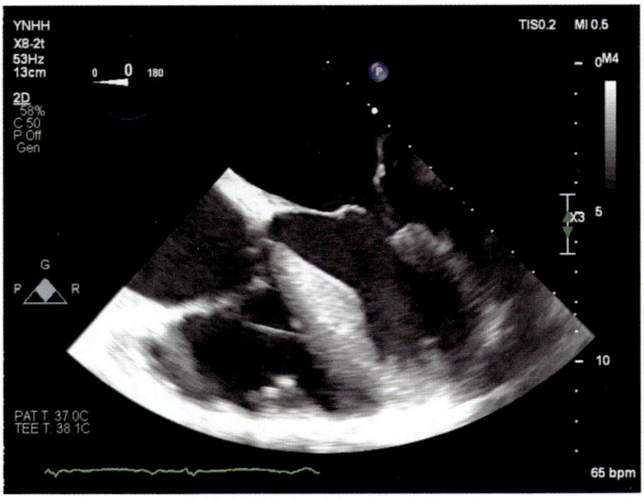

FIGURE 3.17 Amyloid restrictive cardiomyopathy. Midesophageal four-chamber view. Note "sparkling" granularity of myocardium especially in the septum.

Takotsubo Syndrome

Stress-induced "cardiomyopathy" is described as an acute and transient LV systolic dysfunction in the setting of emotional or physiologic stress and is not explained by the presence of obstructive coronary disease. The apex and mid-portion of the heart is stunned, which causes characteristic "apical ballooning" of the akinetic or dyskinetic apex combined with a hypercontractile basal LV during systole (19,20,24). The RV may or may not be involved, and this syndrome is seen most commonly in postmenopausal women. This constellation is called takotsubo syndrome or transient LV apical ballooning syndrome and is not currently considered a true cardiomyopathy (Video 3.9).

Peripartum or Postpartum Cardiomyopathy

Peripartum or postpartum cardiomyopathy is a DCM that presents in a patient's third trimester through first 5 months postpartum. While 50% of cases either completely or nearly recover by 6 months, a subset of patients who suffer from peripartum cardiomyopathy have significant clinical deterioration (24).

Left Ventricular Hypertrophy

LV hypertrophy occurs when LV mass increases, which can be due to (a) increase in ventricular wall thickness, (b) LV cavity enlargement, or (c) both. Wall thickening typically occurs due to pressure overload whereas ventricular cavity enlargement usually occurs due to volume overload. Several circumstances can lead to LV hypertrophy and include hypertension; athletic heart with physiologic LV hypertrophy; aortic pathologies such as aortic stenosis, coarctation of the aorta, or aortic regurgitation; and infiltrative cardiac disease such as amyloidosis. The most common causes of LV hypertrophy are hypertension and aortic valve stenosis, where the heart must contract against a high afterload.

RWT and LV mass index are two echocardiographic parameters that can categorize four different states of the LV: normal geometry, concentric remodeling, concentric hypertrophy, and eccentric hypertrophy (Figure 3.18). Patients with normal LV geometry will have a normal RWT and a normal LV mass index.

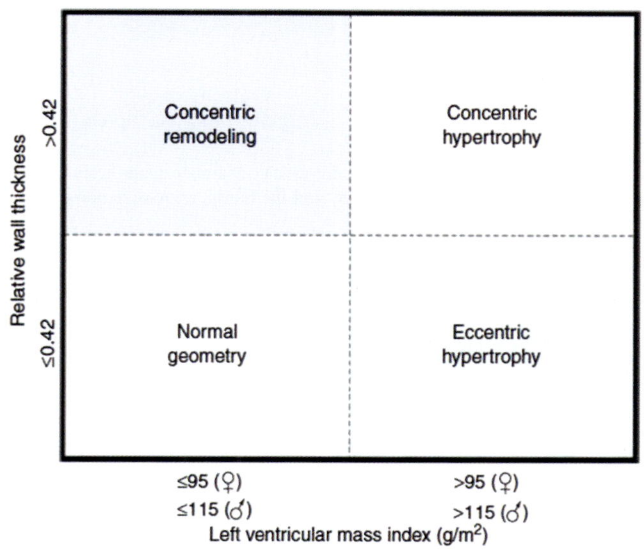

FIGURE 3.18 Left ventricular mass may be combined with relative wall thickness to categorize patients into various classes of left ventricle (LV) hypertrophy. (From Lang RM, Bierig M, Devereux RB, et al; Chamber Quantification Writing Group; American Society of Echocardiography's Guidelines and Standards Committee; European Association of Echocardiography. Recommendations for chamber quantification: a report from the American Society of Echocardiography's Guidelines and Standards Committee and the Chamber Quantification Writing Group, developed in conjunction with the European Association of Echocardiography, a branch of the European Society of Cardiology. *J Am Soc Echocardiogr*. 2005;18[12]:1440-1463.)

Patients with increased RWT will either have concentric remodeling or concentric hypertrophy. Concentric remodeling patients will have a normal LV mass index, and patients with concentric hypertrophy will have an increased LV mass index. Concentric LV hypertrophy occurs when the LV sees an increased afterload leading to pressure overload. Both chronic hypertension and aortic stenosis cause concentric LV hypertrophy. Eccentric hypertrophy occurs when the RWT is normal, but the LV mass index is elevated. This occurs when there is volumetric or diastolic LV overload such as in the setting of regurgitant lesions.

Patients with LV hypertrophy develop myocardial fibrosis that initially causes diastolic dysfunction. As the LV hypertrophy and subsequent myocardial fibrosis progress systolic dysfunction may follow (31).

Left Ventricular Hypertrophy Versus "Athlete's Heart"

Physical exercise leads to an increase in one's heart rate and blood pressure and may cause the heart to adapt in the setting of an increased observed workload. One of the adaptations is LV hypertrophy and, in these individuals, it is commonly referred to as "athlete's heart." Echocardiography may show an increased LV wall thickness, increased LV diastolic and systolic dimensions, increased stroke volume, preserved fractional shortening, no diastolic dysfunction, and no abnormalities on LV strain imaging (32).

It is important to note that although both athletes and patients with hypertension may develop LV hypertrophy, their echocardiographic features are distinct. While hypertrophy from both an athlete's heart and hypertension will demonstrate an increase in LV wall thickness and LV mass, athlete's heart does not show diastolic dysfunction and abnormal LV strain (33). In addition, the athlete's heart is less likely to have mitral annular and aortic valve calcification compared with the hypertensive heart.

CONCLUSION

Advances in echocardiographic technology and imaging techniques have allowed for increasingly precise quantification of LV systolic function and LV pathologies. As such, echocardiographers should be familiar with the various ways to quantify LV systolic function and the benefits and limitations of each modality. Innovations in TDI, strain assessments, and 3D echocardiography have contributed to the evolving approach to assessing LV function. It is additionally of significant importance to understand the various disease processes of the LV and how echocardiography can be applied to distinguish these pathologies from one another.

REFERENCES

1. Skiles JA, Griffin BP. Transesophageal echocardiographic (TEE) evaluation of ventricular function. *Cardiol Clin.* 2000;18(4):681-697.
2. Lang RM, Badano LP, Mor-Avi V, et al. Recommendations for cardiac chamber quantification by echocardiography in adults: an update from the American Society of Echocardiography and the European Association of Cardiovascular Imaging. *J Am Soc Echocardiogr.* 2015;28(1):1-39.e14.
3. Lang RM, Bierig M, Devereux RB, et al. Recommendations for chamber quantification: a report from the American Society of Echocardiography's Guidelines and Standards Committee and the Chamber Quantification Writing Group, developed in conjunction with the European Association of Echocardiography, a branch of the European Society of Cardiology. *J Am Soc Echocardiogr.* 2005;18(12):1440-1463.
4. Hahn RT, Abraham T, Adams MS, et al. Guidelines for performing a comprehensive transesophageal echocardiographic examination: recommendations from the American Society of Echocardiography and the Society of Cardiovascular Anesthesiologists. *J Am Soc Echocardiogr.* 2013;26(9):921-964.
5. Chengode S. Left ventricular global systolic function assessment by echocardiography. *Ann Card Anaesth.* 2016;19(suppl 1):S26-S34.
6. Rong LQ. An update on intraoperative three-dimensional transesophageal echocardiography. *J Thorac Dis.* 2017;9(suppl 4):S271-S282.
7. Berdnikov A, Roifman I, Tang E, Muhtaseb O, Chenkin J. Structured cardiac assessment outperforms visual estimation in novice ultrasound users: a randomized controlled trial. *J Emerg Med.* 2023;65(6):e563-e567.
8. Angaran P, Dorian P, Ha ACT, et al. Association of left ventricular ejection fraction with mortality and hospitalizations. *J Am Soc Echocardiogr.* 2020;33:802-811.e6.
9. Writing Committee Members; ACC/AHA Joint Committee Members. 2022 AHA/ACC/HFSA guideline for the management of heart failure. *J Card Fail.* 2022;28:e1-e167.
10. Pellikka PA, She L, Holly TA, et al. Variability in ejection fraction measured by echocardiography, gated single-photon emission computed tomography, and cardiac magnetic resonance in patients with coronary artery disease and left ventricular dysfunction. *JAMA Netw Open.* 2018;1(4):e181456.

11. Kadappu KK, Thomas L. Tissue Doppler imaging in echocardiography: value and limitations. *Heart Lung Circ.* 2015;24(3):224-233.
12. Abraham TP, Dimaano VL, Liang HY. Role of tissue Doppler and strain echocardiography in current clinical practice. *Circulation.* 2007;116(22):2597-2609.
13. Reant P, Barbot L, Touche C, et al. Evaluation of global left ventricular systolic function using three-dimensional echocardiography speckle-tracking strain parameters. *J Am Soc Echocardiogr.* 2012;25(1):68-79.
14. Haji K, Marwick TH. Clinical utility of echocardiographic strain and strain rate measurements. *Curr Cardiol Rep.* 2021;23(3):18.
15. Schick AL, Kaine JC, Al-Sadhan NA, et al. Focused cardiac ultrasound with mitral annular plane systolic excursion (MAPSE) detection of left ventricular dysfunction. *Am J Emerg Med.* 2023;68:52-58.
16. Timperley J, Mitchell ARJ, Becher H. Contrast echocardiography for left ventricular opacification. *Heart.* 2003;89(12):1394-1397.
17. Hampson R, Senior R, Ring L, et al. Contrast echocardiography: a practical guideline from the British Society of Echocardiography. *Echo Res Pract.* 2023;10(1):23.
18. Porter TR, Mulvagh SL, Abdelmoneim SS, et al. Clinical applications of ultrasonic enhancing agents in echocardiography: 2018 American Society of Echocardiography guidelines update. *J Am Soc Echocardiogr.* 2018;31(3):241-274.
19. Arbelo E, Protonotarios A, Gimeno JR, et al. 2023 ESC guidelines for the management of cardiomyopathies. *Eur Heart J.* 2023;44(37):3503-3626.
20. McKenna WJ, Maron BJ, Thiene G. Classification, epidemiology, and global burden of cardiomyopathies. *Circ Res.* 2017;121(7):722-730.
21. Mitevksa IP. Focus on echocardiography in hypertrophic cardiomyopathy—fourth in series. *e-J Cardiol Pract.* 2015;13(20). Accessed November 27, 2024. https://www.escardio.org/Journals/E-Journal-of-Cardiology-Practice/Volume-13/Focus-on-echocardiography-in-hypertrophic-cardiomyopathy-third-in-series
22. Nagueh SF, Phelan D, Abraham T, et al. Recommendations for multimodality cardiovascular imaging of patients with hypertrophic cardiomyopathy: an update from the American Society of Echocardiography, in collaboration with the American Society of Nuclear Cardiology, the Society for Cardiovascular Magnetic Resonance, and the Society of Cardiovascular Computed Tomography. *J Am Soc Echocardiogr.* 2022;35(6):533-569.
23. Authors/Task Force members; Elliott PM, Anastasakis A, et al. 2014 ESC guidelines on diagnosis and management of hypertrophic cardiomyopathy: the Task Force for the Diagnosis and Management of Hypertrophic Cardiomyopathy of the European Society of Cardiology (ESC). *Eur Heart J.* 2014;35(39):2733-2779.
24. Maron BJ, Towbin JA, Thiene G, et al. Contemporary definitions and classification of the cardiomyopathies. *Circulation.* 2006;113(14):1807-1816.
25. Corrado D, Zorzi A, Cipriani A, et al. Evolving diagnostic criteria for arrhythmogenic cardiomyopathy. *J Am Heart Assoc.* 2021;10(18):e021987.
26. Rapezzi C, Aimo A, Barison A, et al. Restrictive cardiomyopathy: definition and diagnosis. *Eur Heart J.* 2022;43:4679-4693.
27. Lloyd JW, Anavekar NS, Oh JK, Miranda WR. Multimodality imaging in differentiating constrictive pericarditis from restrictive cardiomyopathy: a comprehensive overview for clinicians and imagers. *J Am Soc Echocardiogr.* 2023;36(12):1254-1265.
28. Cuddy SAM, Chetrit M, Jankowski M, et al. Practical points for echocardiography in cardiac amyloidosis. *J Am Soc Echocardiogr.* 2022;35(9):A31-A40.
29. Jenni R, Oechslin E, Schneider J, et al. Echocardiographic and pathoanatomical characteristics of isolated left ventricular noncompaction: a step towards classification as a distinct cardiomyopathy. *Heart.* 2001;86:666-671.
30. Kawtar M, Zineb G, Eddine LA, Nawal D, Mohamed C. Reversible left ventricular noncompaction after pregnancy: a physiological cardiomyopathy. *Int J Adv Res.* 2018;6(9):975-978.
31. Bornstein AB, Rao SS, Marwaha K. Left ventricular hypertrophy. In: *StatPearls.* StatPearls Publishing; 2024. Accessed July 19, 2024. http://www.ncbi.nlm.nih.gov/books/NBK557534/
32. Lovic D, Narayan P, Pittaras A, Faselis C, Doumas M, Kokkinos P. Left ventricular hypertrophy in athletes and hypertensive patients. *J Clin Hypertens (Greenwich).* 2017;19(4):413-417.
33. D'Ascenzi F, Fiorentini C, Anselmi F, Mondillo S. Left ventricular hypertrophy in athletes: how to differentiate between hypertensive heart disease and athlete's heart. *Eur J Prev Cardiol.* 2021;28(10):1125-1133.

QUESTIONS

1. Which is an expected finding of cardiac amyloidosis?
   A. Normal left ventricular diastolic function
   B. A normal pattern of LV strain imaging
   C. Asymmetric septal hypertrophy
   D. Significantly reduced tissue Doppler velocities of the left ventricle

2. Which of the following is required to diagnose the DCM phenotype?
   A. Increased LV wall thickness
   B. RV dilation
   C. Increased LV chamber size
   D. Presence of mitral regurgitation

3. **What is a limitation of 3D STE?**
   A. Worse assessment of GLS
   B. Less accurate in patients with regional wall motional abnormalities
   C. Less accurate when beat-to-beat variability is present.
   D. Less accurate in individuals with valvular pathologies

4. **What parameter would help differentiate LV hypertrophy secondary to hypertension from that seen in athlete's heart?**
   A. Impaired diastolic function
   B. Increased LV diastolic dimension
   C. Increased LV systolic dimension
   D. Increased LV wall thickness

5. **What parameters are required for calculation of RWT?**
   A. Anterior wall thickness and LV internal diameter
   B. Inferior wall thickness and LV internal diameter
   C. Posterior wall thickness and LV external diameter
   D. Septal wall thickness and LV external diameter

6. **What angle of incidence should not be exceeded to ensure TDI does not underestimate myocardial velocities?**
   A. 5°
   B. 15°
   C. 30°
   D. 45°

7. **What is the gold standard for measurement of LV volume?**
   A. 3D volume assessment using Simpson method
   B. 3D speckle-tracking echocardiography
   C. Cardiovascular MRI
   D. Strain-volume loops

8. **What is the most frequent pathology that leads to patients being listed for heart transplantation?**
   A. Restrictive cardiomyopathy
   B. Noncompaction of the left ventricle
   C. Hypertrophic cardiomyopathy
   D. Dilated cardiomyopathy

9. **What portion of the heart *most commonly* experiences myocardial stunning in Takotsubo cardiomyopathy?**
   A. Lateral wall
   B. Anterior wall
   C. Basal segments
   D. Apical segments

10. **What would be seen in a patient with concentric remodeling?**
   A. Normal RWT and normal LV mass index
   B. Normal RWT and increased LV mass index
   C. Increased RWT and normal LV mass index
   D. Increased RWT and increased LV mass index

ANSWERS

1. **Correct Answer: D.**
Rationale: Cardiac amyloidosis is an example of a restrictive cardiomyopathy. There is significant diastolic dysfunction with abnormal strain and a diffuse pattern of ventricular hypertrophy (with a sparkly appearance).

2. **Correct Answer: C.**
Rationale: While the RV may be involved and regurgitation of the atrioventricular valves may be present, neither is required to diagnose DCM. LV dilation and systolic dysfunction, however, are required.

3. **Correct Answer: C.**
Rationale: 3D GLS is a good predictor of adverse remodeling of the left ventricle. It is useful in assessing LV function in patients with ischemic heart disease, LV hypertrophy, valvular heart disease, and cardiac resynchronization therapy. Beat-to-beat variability, however, interferes with accurate 3D STE.

4. **Correct Answer: A.**
Rationale: In both patients with LV hypertrophy secondary to athlete's heart and hypertension, echocardiography will show increased LV wall thickness. Individuals with athlete's heart will have increased LV diastolic and systolic dimensions whereas those with hypertension may have decreased, preserved, or increased LV diastolic and systolic dimensions. Diastolic dysfunction will likely be present in individuals with hypertension but will not be seen in those with athlete's heart.

5. **Correct Answer: B.**
Rationale: RWT is measured in the transgastric short-axis view. The RWT equation adapted for TEE is RWT $= 2 \times$ (inferior wall thickness distance)/LV internal diameter in diastole.

6. **Correct Answer: B.**
Rationale: TDI is a Doppler technique and thus subject to underestimation of velocities with increasing angles of insonation. As such, the pulsed-wave sampling volume should be positioned parallel to the motion being examined. A good rule of thumb is to attempt to achieve no more than a 15° angle between the beam and the tissue motion.

7. **Correct Answer: C.**
Rationale: While transesophageal echocardiography has multiple ways to assess LV areas, volumes, and ejection fractions, cardiovascular MRI is the gold standard for acquiring these measurements.

8. **Correct Answer: D.**
Rationale: DCM is a common cause of heart failure and is the most common reason why patients are listed for heart transplants. HCM is the most common familial heart disease. Noncompaction of the left ventricle is an uncommon cardiac disease.

9. **Correct Answer: D.**
Rationale: Takotsubo cardiomyopathy is also known as apical ballooning cardiomyopathy. Though other patterns may be observed, the mid and apical segments of the heart most commonly become akinetic or dyskinetic while the basal segments are hyperdynamic.

10. **Correct Answer: C.**
Rationale: Concentric remodeling is associated with increased RWT and normal left ventricular mass index and is often seen earlier in pathologies that create LV pressure overload, prior to the development of concentric hypertrophy. Patients with normal geometry will have normal RWT and normal LV mass index. Patients with eccentric hypertrophy will have normal RWT and increased LV mass index. Patients with concentric hypertrophy will have increased RWT and increased LV mass index.

4 Diagnosis of Myocardial Ischemia

Joachim M. Erb and Sascha Treskatsch

ANATOMY AND PATHOPHYSIOLOGY OF THE MYOCARDIAL BLOOD SUPPLY

Coronary Anatomy

The myocardium has its own independent blood supply and drainage (Figure 4.1). Two coronary arteries originate from the aortic root: the left main coronary artery (LCA) from the left coronary sinus (CS) and the right coronary artery (RCA) from the right CS, both adjacent to the respective left or right cusp of the aortic valve.

The LCA bifurcates at around 10 mm from its origin into the left anterior descending (LAD) and the left circumflex (LCX) coronary arteries. The LAD runs along the anterior interventricular sulcus passing the ventricular apex to reach the posterior interventricular sulcus. On its way to the apex, it gives rise to the diagonal branches and septal arteries. It thereby supplies the left ventricular (LV) anterior wall, the apex, and the anterior part of the interventricular septum. The LCX runs along the left atrioventricular sulcus and gives rise to mostly one large marginal branch and the posterolateral branches supplying the lateral wall.

The RCA runs along the right atrioventricular sulcus, where its middle section gives off the right ventricular (RV) marginal branches. These marginal branches supply the RV free wall and the conduction system including the sinus and atrioventricular node. The RCA bifurcates into the posterior descending artery and the right posterolateral branch. Their supply territory is the inferolateral RV wall, the inferior part of the interventricular septum, and the inferior wall of the LV.

Variations in Coronary Anatomy and Main Distribution Types

Many segments have a consistent coronary artery perfusion; however, there are three major variations of coronary distribution. These distribution types affect the posterior descending artery and posterolateral branch, which supply the inferior septum and inferior wall of the LV (Figures 4.1-4.5). The right-dominant coronary distribution type is the most common (80%-85%), where the supply originates from the RCA. In patients with left-dominant coronary distribution, the distal LCX extends as a posterolateral branch within the posterior intraventricular sulcus to supply part of the inferior LV wall. A balanced or codominant type is present in approximately 5% of individuals, where the posterior descending artery and the posterolateral branch receive supply from both the RCA and the LCX. Imaging studies, however, have altered traditional concepts of coronary perfusion zones as well as revealed the significant individual variation in coronary supply to the myocardial segments. For example, the apical segments are now understood in the majority of cases to be supplied by the LAD with the LCX and RCA seen in a minority of individuals. The greatest overlap in coronary artery distribution occurs in the inferolateral region corresponding either to RCA or LCX territories, as well as the inferoseptal region that may be supplied by the LAD, RCA, or even a left-dominant LCX artery. Figures 4.2 to 4.5 incorporate these findings and emphasize the large amount of myocardium supplied by the LAD artery and the potential for substantial infarct size with LAD occlusion (1,2).

In segments with physiologic variability in coronary supply, the culprit coronary artery of myocardial ischemia can often be identified by examining neighboring segments whose coronary supply is known. For example, the combination of ischemia in the anterolateral and inferolateral walls is consistent with a left-dominant or codominant LCX occlusive disease while the presence of anterolateral ischemia without inferolateral wall ischemia is specific for a nondominant LCX occlusion.

The coronary anatomy can be defined by cardiac catheterization and/or coronary computed tomography/angiography (CTA), and this information is valuable when communicating regional wall motion abnormalities (RWMAs) to the surgeon.

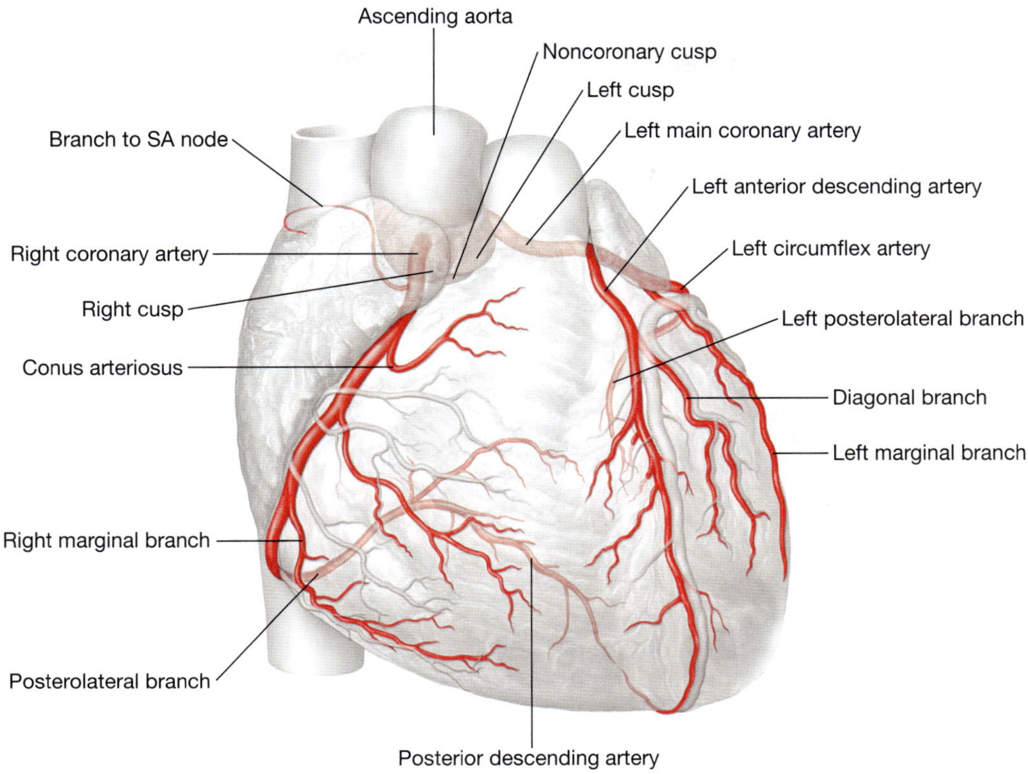

FIGURE 4.1 Anatomy of the coronary arteries of the heart.

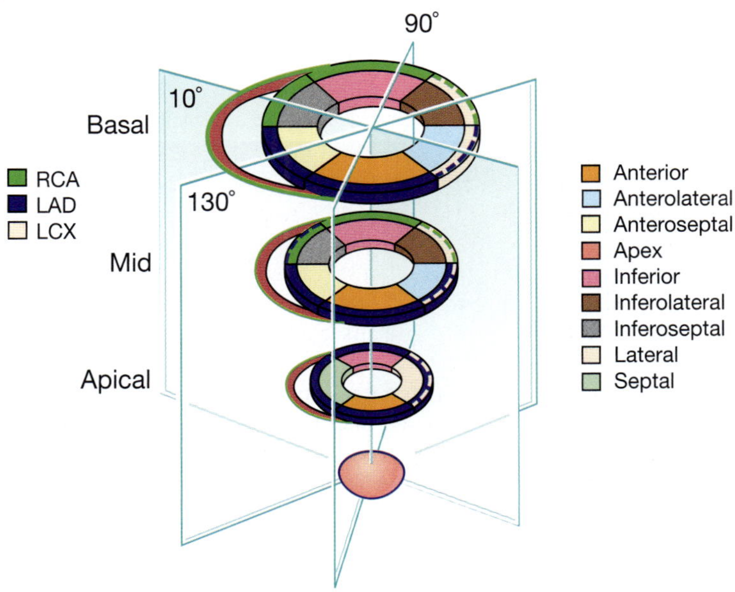

FIGURE 4.2 The 17-segment model of the left ventricle (inner ring) as demonstrated in the transgastric short-axis views. The outer ring shows the common (solid line) and variant (dashed line) coronary artery distributions. LAD, left anterior descending artery; LCX, left circumflex artery; RCA, right coronary artery.

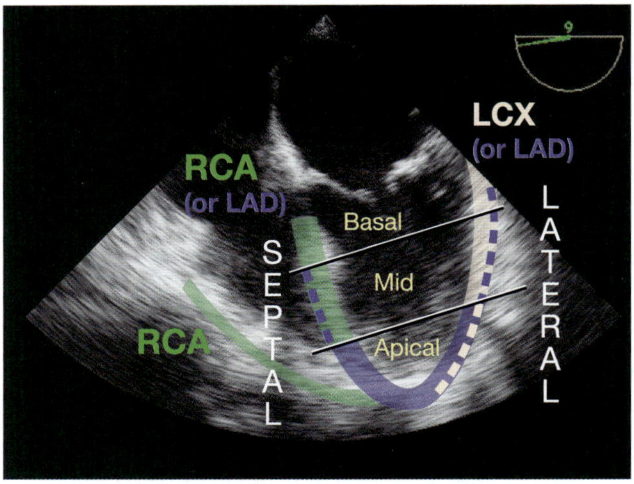

FIGURE 4.3 Segmental anatomy of the left ventricle in the midesophageal four-chamber view and corresponding coronary perfusion (common solid color, variant dashed color). LAD, left anterior descending; LCX, left circumflex; RCA, right coronary arteries.

Echocardiographic Assessment of Coronary Arteries

Two-Dimensional Visualization of Coronary Artery Anatomy

Coronary ostia: From the midesophageal aortic valve short-axis (ME AV SAX) view, the coronary ostia can be visualized by a small degree of anteflexion or withdrawal of the probe (Figure 4.6; Video 4.1A,B) (3). The left coronary ostium and the full length of the LCA to its bifurcation into the LAD and LCX are visible in the middle of the left coronary cusp at the 1 to 2 o'clock positions (Video 4.2). The right coronary ostium is visible in the middle of the right coronary cusp at the 6 to 7 o'clock positions.

Left coronary artery: The LAD is visualized by further rotation to approximately 120° to 130° and a slight turn of the probe to the left (Video 4.3). To follow the LCX from the left main bifurcation in ME AV SAX view, the probe is turned leftward and advanced slightly while following the LCX on its way around the atrioventricular groove (Figure 4.7; Video 4.4) (4). Within this groove, the LCX is close to the CS, with

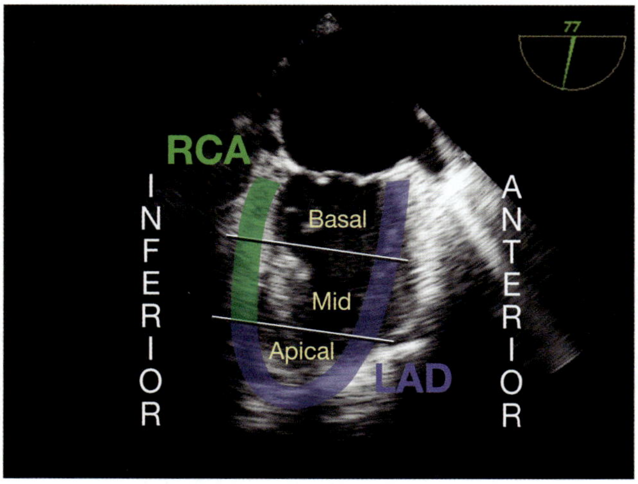

FIGURE 4.4 Segmental anatomy of the left ventricle in the midesophageal two-chamber view and corresponding coronary perfusion. LAD, left anterior descending; RCA, right coronary arteries.

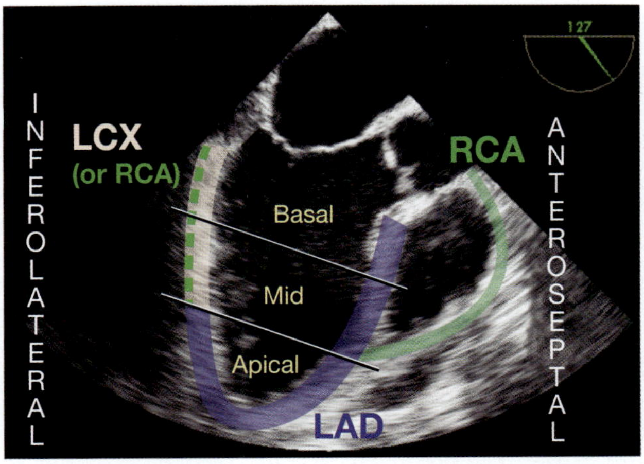

FIGURE 4.5 Segmental anatomy of the left ventricle in the midesophageal long-axis view and corresponding coronary perfusion (common solid color, variant dashed color). LAD, left anterior descending; LCX, left circumflex; RCA, right coronary arteries.

which it must not be confused. As a rule of thumb, it may be helpful that while the LCX diminishes in its distal diameter, the CS will enlarge.

Right coronary artery: The proximal RCA can also be imaged from the ME AV SAX view supported by slight anteflexion (Figure 4.6; Video 4.1A,B). In addition, the ostium and proximal parts of the RCA can be imaged in a modified midesophageal aortic valve long-axis (ME AV LAX) view at 120° to 160° (Figure 4.8; Video 4.5). In the older adult patients, RCA visualization may be quite more challenging if aortic cusp calcification is present.

Visualization of the coronary ostia in (transesophageal) three-dimensional (3D) echocardiography is possible, but requires extensive postprocessing efforts in cropping the data sets appropriately (5). Furthermore, the lower resolution compared to two-dimensional (2D) echocardiography prevents gathering superior information, which is also true for the 3D color flow mode. Therefore, 3D echocardiography is not routinely used in the operating room for assessment of the coronary arteries.

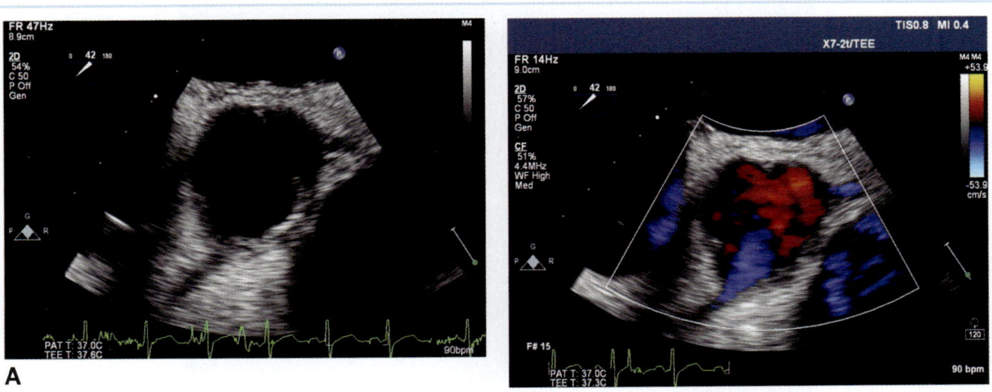

FIGURE 4.6 The left and the right coronary ostia in the two-dimensional aortic short-axis view (A) and with added color flow Doppler (B). The left coronary ostium is visible in the middle of the left coronary cusp at the 1 to 2 o'clock positions. The right coronary ostium is visible in the middle of the right coronary cusp at the 6 o'clock position (see Video 4.1A, B).

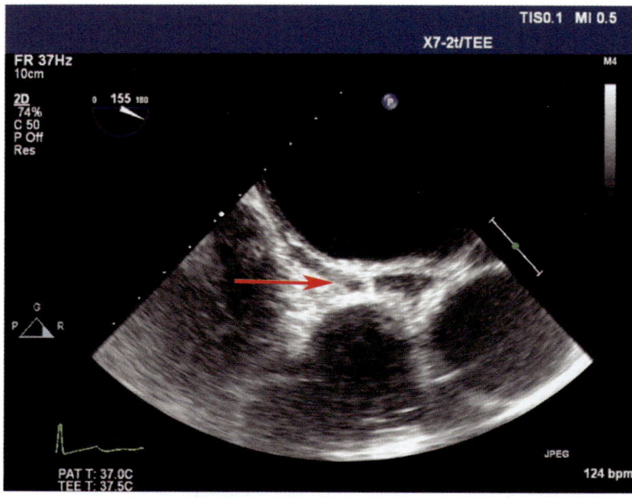

FIGURE 4.7 The left circumflex coronary artery (arrow) in long axis (see Video 4.4).

Doppler Evaluation of Coronary Artery Blood Flow

For qualitative color flow Doppler assessment of coronary blood flow, it is recommended to initially set the Nyquist limit to 50 cm/s for examination of the left coronary artery and to 20 cm/s for the RCA (6). However, further reduction in the Nyquist limit is often required to obtain adequate signals. The angle of incidence has to be taken into account when interpreting the results, as the angle may continuously change for neighboring sections of the same vessel due to the curved course of the coronary arteries. Normal coronary arterial blood flow shows a biphasic, laminar pattern with a short systolic wave of slower velocity and a longer diastolic wave of higher velocity with a deceleration slope. This can be quantitatively measured using pulse-wave (PW) Doppler (Figure 4.9). Reported normal mean peak coronary flow velocities are in the range of 30 to 35 cm/s during systole and 70 to 75 cm/s during diastole for the LCA, and approximately 25 cm/s during systole and 40 cm/s during diastole for the RCA (7). *Visualization of the coronary ostia and arteries and of intracoronary flow may be of importance in situations with acute new segmental wall motion abnormalities,*

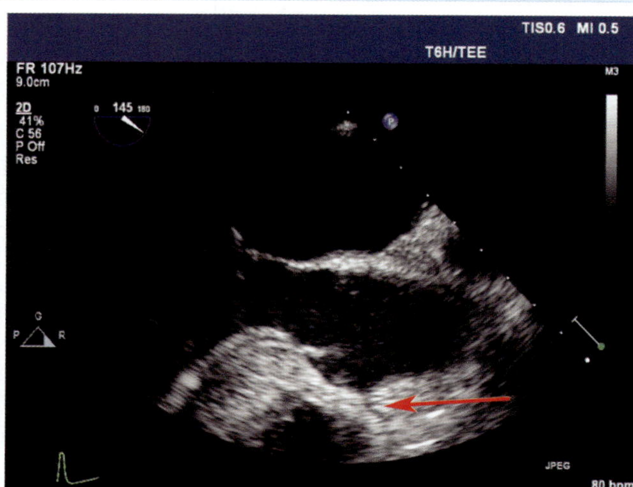

FIGURE 4.8 The right coronary ostium and proximal RCA (arrow) in a modified ME AV LAX view (see Video 4.5). ME AV LAX, midesophageal aortic valve long axis; RCA, right coronary arteries.

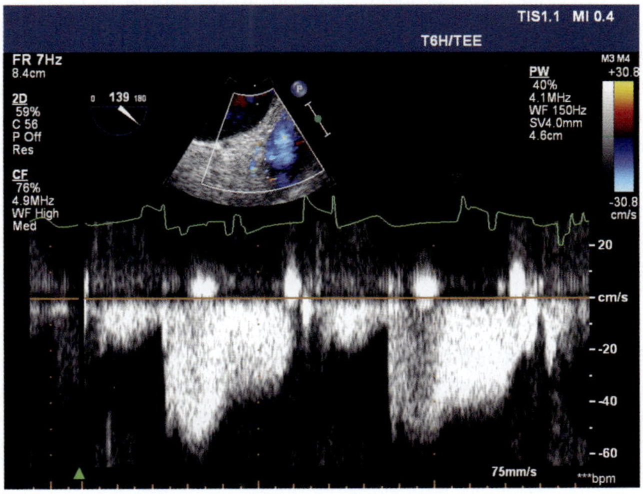

FIGURE 4.9 Pulsed wave Doppler recording of coronary flow. Normal coronary arterial blood flow shows a biphasic, laminar pattern with a short systolic wave of slower velocity and a longer diastolic wave of higher velocity.

for example, during separation from cardiopulmonary bypass (CPB) after mitral valve surgery (8), in patients with aortic dissection (9), during transcatheter aortic valve implantation (10), or transcatheter mitral valve reconstruction (11).

Detection of Coronary Artery Pathology

Although echocardiographic diagnosis of coronary artery stenosis and myocardial viability is not a daily practice in perioperative medicine, it can be clinically valuable for assessing proximal vessel disease when coronary angiography is not practical (ie, during emergent cardiac surgery and/or hemodynamic instability in noncardiac surgery) (12). Indicators are increased echo density, suggesting calcification of the vascular intima and velocity acceleration with turbulent color flow Doppler signals. The following velocities have been published as the threshold for hemodynamically relevant stenosis (>50%): LCA greater than 140 cm/s, LAD greater than 90 cm/s, LCX greater than 110 cm/s (13). The percentage reduction in vessel diameter or increase in diastolic velocity-time integral at the site of stenosis compared to the normal segment proximal to the stenosis correlates well with the degree of stenosis diagnosed by coronary angiography (14,15).

PHYSIOLOGIC BASIS FOR THE DETECTION OF ISCHEMIA

Segmental endocardial motion and myocardial thickening in systole are the foundations for echocardiographic detection of myocardial ischemia. As first observed by Tennant and Wiggers in 1935, occlusion of a coronary artery results in severe RWMA in the corresponding myocardium (16). Decades later, Pandian et al established the value of echocardiography for detecting ischemic RWMAs (17,18). Since then, multiple human studies have shown that RWMAs (ie, reductions in systolic wall motion and/or thickening) detected by echocardiography are an earlier and more sensitive indicator of ischemia than electrocardiography (ECG) (14,15,19-21).

The progression in wall dysfunction from hypokinesia to dyskinesia correlates to the progression in degree of perfusion abnormalities, which has been established in dog studies. Reductions in systolic wall thickening reflect subendocardial ischemia, while akinesia reflects ischemia sparing the subepicardial myocardial layer only, and dyskinesia plus acute wall thinning are seen in the setting of transmural ischemia (22). An echocardiographic dog study has found that segmental contraction abnormalities are induced only when myocardial perfusion is less than 25% of control (18). Although human data on the possible quantitative relationship between myocardial perfusion and segmental wall contraction are missing, from a clinical point of view, acute changes in segmental function are highly indicative of acute ischemia.

Prolonged reduction or cessation of coronary flow leads to infarction. By echocardiography, an acutely infarcted myocardium may look similar to an acutely ischemic myocardium. In contrast, scar tissue presents echocardiographically as a thin, dense, and permanently akinetic or dyskinetic wall.

Although reduced or absent wall thickening may be the most sensitive indicator of ischemia, reduced endocardial motion may be the more conspicuous echocardiographic sign of severe ischemia. However, adjacent nonischemic regions may pull the endocardium of an ischemic area inward; this points out the importance of also considering wall thickening that will still indicate ischemia. Quite typically, unaffected, nonischemic regions develop exaggerated inward movement (termed *compensatory hyperkinesis*) that partially offsets the adverse effects of akinesis or dyskinesis in other regions on cardiac stroke volume. This is the principal reason why hemodynamic instability is a late and ominous sign of ischemia and usually only occurs with very severe regional or global ischemia.

Clinical Syndromes of Myocardial Ischemia

The echocardiographer must be aware of the various presentations of ischemic tissue, including myocardial stunning and hibernation (Table 4.1), which complicate the echocardiographic assessment of myocardial viability (23). *Acute ischemia* results from severe reductions in coronary blood flow and is associated with reductions in wall thickening and endocardial inward motion. *Stunned myocardium* occurs following an acute episode of ischemia when a potentially reversible RWMA transiently persists despite full restoration of blood flow. *Hibernation* is a chronic ischemic condition where RWMAs persist in viable myocardium with marginal resting blood flow. LV function may improve markedly, and mortality may be reduced

TABLE 4.1 Characteristics, Echocardiographic Findings, and Clinical Implications of Myocardial Ischemia

Condition	Acute Ischemia	Stunned Myocardium	Hibernating Myocardium	Infarction
Definition	Reversible hypoperfusion	Postreperfusion contractile dysfunction	Chronic, ischemic dysfunction	Permanent ischemia with myocyte damage
Histomorphology	Normal	Normal, intra- and extracellular edema	Cardiomyocyte dedifferentiation, reduced myofibrils	Contraction band necrosis, destruction of membranes and mitochondria
Metabolism	ATP deficiency	Reduced Ca sensitivity	Altered	Destructed, inflammatory infiltration
Resting coronary flow	Reduced	Normal	Reduced	Severely reduced/ absent
Regional wall motion	Hypokinesia	Hypokinesia	Hypokinesia	Akinesia-dyskinesia
Response to inotropes	Worsens	Sustained improvement in wall motion	Biphasic: low dose improves kinesis, deterioration with higher doses, hypokinetic with high dose.	No change
Contractile recovery after revascularization	Full	Full to partial	Full to partial	None
Perioperative implications	Urgent pharmacologic or interventional treatment indicated, infarction if ongoing	Common following CPB	Revascularization superior to medical management may show immediate improvement after CPB.	Revascularization not indicated

CPB, cardiopulmonary bypass (23,53,54).
From Almeida AG, Carpenter JP, Cameli M, et al. Multimodality imaging of myocardial viability: an expert consensus document from the European Association of Cardiovascular Imaging (EACVI). *Eur Heart J Cardiovasc Imaging*. 2021;22(8):e97-e125.
From Opie LH. The multifarious spectrum of ischemic left ventricular dysfunction: relevance of new ischemic syndromes. *J. Mol. Cell. Cardiol*. 1996;28(12):2403-2414.
From Nihoyannopoulos P, Vanoverschelde JL. Myocardial ischaemia and viability: the pivotal role of echocardiography. *Eur. Heart J*. 2011;32(7):810-819.

spontaneously (stunning) or following successful coronary revascularization (hibernation). The time course of recovery is variable (days to months). Dobutamine stress echocardiography is still frequently used for the detection of significant coronary artery disease (CAD) as well as viable hibernating myocardium. In contrast to stress-induced RWMAs in patients with CAD, viable myocardium shows improved regional contractile function (inotropic reserve) in response to low-dose dobutamine administration. For patients with ischemic heart disease, dobutamine stress echocardiography predicts the likelihood of LV functional recovery following revascularization. In addition, in patients with LV dysfunction caused by myocardial infarction, dobutamine stress echocardiography is useful for evaluating the presence of hibernating myocardium due to a residual stenosis that warrants intervention. Patients with LV dysfunction who demonstrate myocardial viability with dobutamine stress echocardiography have better survival with revascularization than with medical therapy (24). *A key message is that an RWMA is not always caused by acute ischemia but may reflect stunning, hibernation, or nonviable infarcted tissue.*

ECHOCARDIOGRAPHIC ASSESSMENT OF ISCHEMIA

Anatomic Localization of Ischemia: The 17-Segment Model

The 17-segment model of LV topographical anatomy (Figure 4.2) provides a common nomenclature across imaging specialties to define the LV segmental anatomy (25). Using the 17-segment model, perioperative transesophageal echocardiography (TEE) has the advantage of applying the same topographical concept for describing the regional function of the LV as in transthoracic echocardiography (TTE), cardiovascular magnetic resonance imaging (MRI), nuclear cardiology (positron emission tomography/single-photon emission computed tomography [PET/SPECT]), and cardiac computed tomography (CTA). It also serves as the basis for correlating the location of RWMAs with coronary perfusion.

Echocardiographic Imaging of the 17 Myocardial Segments

The 17-segment model divides the LV along its longitudinal axis into three levels plus the apical cap (Figure 4.2). The basal and mid (midpapillary) levels are subdivided into six segments: the anteroseptal, anterior, anterolateral, inferolateral (formerly "posterior"), inferior, and inferoseptal segments. The apical level is subdivided into anterior, lateral, inferior, and septal segments as well as the apical cap (apex).

The three standard ME views (ME four-chamber, ME two-chamber, and ME long axis) (Figures 4.3-4.5) together allow visualization of all 17 segments (26). Although all the three views theoretically visualize the distant apical slice (segment 17), often the echo imaging plane transects the ventricle above the true apex and the TEE image is "foreshortened." Bi-/multiplane or 3D full-volume mode may be useful for detecting foreshortening. To obtain the correct alignment of the imaging plane along the long axis of the LV, the echocardiographer should focus on obtaining the maximum long-axis dimension in each view. A reliable indicator of a "true" long axis is the lack of movement of the apical epicardium toward the TEE probe during systole as well as displacement or wandering of the LV during rotation. The reason is that the entire LV moves into an apical direction during systole with little displacement of the apex (27). Favorable settings include the use of low ultrasound frequency (usually no higher than 6 MHz) because the apex is in the far field of the TEE image; a focal zone placed in the area of the apex; and optimized gain settings in that field. Foreshortening may be ruled out if the long axis in two ME views of the LV (eg, four- and two-chamber view; biplane views helpful) is no more different than 10% in its length.

The *transgastric (TG) short-axis (SAX) views* (basal, mid, and apical) allow the visualization of 16 segments excluding the apical cap. The TG basal and midpapillary short-axis views each show the entire radius of six segments and are unique in that myocardial territories perfused by all the three main coronary arteries are visualized (Figure 4.2). *Although ischemia monitoring in TG midpapillary short-axis view is popular, using this view alone is inadequate because ischemia caused by stenosis in an artery more distal to this plane will be missed.* Repeated assessment of multiple views is essential as limiting the examination to the TG midpapillary SAX view alone will miss the majority of RWMAs (28). Comprehensive monitoring of all 17 segments for ischemia utilizing both ME and TG imaging planes is advised.

Assessment and Grading of Regional Wall Motion Abnormalities

To grade the severity of ischemia, it is important to analyze both systolic myocardial thickening and endocardial inward motion ("radial shortening") (Table 4.2). The American Society of Echocardiography/Society of Cardiovascular Anesthesiologists (ASE/SCA) guidelines for TEE examination classify systolic ventricular

TABLE 4.2 Five-Grade Scale of Segmental Wall Contraction Abnormalities

		Radial Shortening	Myocardial Thickening
Grade 1	Normal contractility	>30%	+++ (30%-50%)
Grade 2	Mild hypokinesis	10%-30%	++
Grade 3	Severe hypokinesis	<10%	+
Grade 4	Akinesis	0	0
Grade 5	Dyskinesis	Lengthening	Thinning

Diagnostic of ischemia when contractility worsens by two grades (14,29).
From Wang J, Filipovic M, Rudzitis A, et al. Transesophageal echocardiography for monitoring segmental wall motion during off-pump coronary artery bypass surgery. *Anesth Analg*. 2004;99(4):965-73.
From Shanewise JS, Cheung AT, Aronson S, Stewart WJ, Weiss RL, Mark JB, et al. ASE/SCA guidelines for performing a comprehensive intraoperative multiplane transesophageal echocardiography examination: recommendations of the American Society of Echocardiography Council for Intraoperative Echocardiography and the Society of Cardiovascular Anesthesiologists Task Force for Certification in Perioperative Transesophageal Echocardiography. *Anesth Analg*. 1999;89(4):870-84.

contraction in five grades: normal wall motion/contractility (normokinesis), mild hypokinesis, severe hypokinesis, akinesis, and dyskinesis (Table 4.2) (29). For systolic myocardial thickening, a 50% increase is regarded as normal, but given substantial intersegment and intersubject variability, a value of 30% thickening has been defined as the lower normal limit. Similarly, systolic radial shortening has been defined as normal if it exceeds 30%.

In clinical practice, 2D visual assessment of systolic regional contraction is most commonly used as it provides a quick, qualitative monitor for ischemia. Motion mode (M-mode) imaging provides a quantitative assessment of systolic myocardial thickening and radial shortening (Figure 4.10). The high temporal resolution and better delineation of endocardial and epicardial borders are advantages of M-mode. However, with TEE, the ability to place the ultrasound beam perpendicular to the myocardial wall is limited to the inferior and anterior walls. One alternative is provided by the free (anatomic) M-mode, where a virtual ultrasound beam can be placed anywhere in the imaging sector. A limitation of this technique is that the free M-mode image is calculated from the 2D image and, thus, lacks the high temporal and spatial resolution of the real M-mode. As a result, quantitative assessments are limited in clinical practice and the visual assessment of regional myocardial contraction remains the method generally used in the operating room.

Wall motion abnormalities can reflect acute or chronic ischemic conditions or nonischemic pathologies (ie, viral cardiomyopathy). *Only (acute) regional systolic contraction deterioration by two grades (ie, from normal contraction to severe hypokinesia) confirms the diagnosis of new-onset myocardial ischemia (14).* Side-by-side comparison of corresponding digital cine loops acquired at different periods of the intraoperative

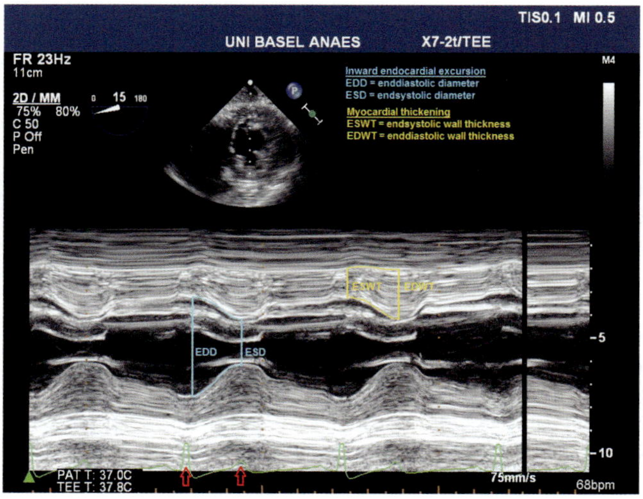

FIGURE 4.10 Normal LV M-mode (motion mode) reading. Normal inward endocardial excursion and wall thickening are illustrated on an M-mode image through the inferior (top) and anterior (bottom) walls in the transgastric short-axis view (***top inset***). Systole starts at the onset of the QRS complex and ends near the end of the T wave (arrows). M-mode echocardiographic imaging coupled with the electrocardiogram can on occasion provide helpful information regarding the timing of wall motion. LV, left ventricular; M-mode, motion mode.

course greatly aids the comparative analysis of regional contraction. The defined requirement of a temporal deterioration in regional systolic contraction implies that myocardial ischemia cannot be diagnosed by a single echocardiographic examination alone.

Important Methodologic Aspects of Wall Motion Analysis and Potential Pitfalls

Considering endocardial motion alone may result in incorrect segmental grading in situations with the rotational or translational movement of the heart (Figure 4.11; Video 4.6), with bundle branch block or ventricular pacing (Video 4.7A,B), or in ischemic segments where the endocardium is pulled inward by adjacent, normally contracting myocardium ("tethering"). *Wall contraction analysis must also consider that the basal septum is mainly membranous and physiologically does not thicken as much as its more muscular brethren.* This segment is well known to be read as falsely positive for RWMAs by inexperienced echocardiographers.

Systolic translation and rotation of the heart (Figure 4.11; Video 4.6) may complicate segmental wall contraction analysis (30). Translational and rotational movements are minimal at the midpapillary SAX levels (31). During cardiac surgery, translational and rotational movements frequently increase after separation from CPB and complicate the analysis of segmental wall contraction (32). Application of fixed reference systems after CPB (Figure 4.11A) can result in the false-positive diagnoses of septal akinesis or dyskinesis and lateral hyperkinesis. In contrast, the application of a floating reference system (Figure 4.11B), which compensates for heart movements, reduces the alleged septal RWMAs that occur post-CPB. *To minimize diagnostic errors in ischemia, detection analysis of both wall motion and myocardial thickening and the choosing of a floating reference system in cardiac surgical patients with significant translational cardiac motion are recommended.*

An endocardial inward motion may markedly overestimate the area of hypoperfused ischemic myocardium (33). One cause for this observation is the *tethering* effect of the hypokinetic segment on an adjacent nonischemic myocardium. In clinical practice, this potential overestimation of the ischemic area by impaired endocardial motion may facilitate echocardiographic detection of ischemia, and the skillful echocardiographer will estimate the true extent of the ischemic area more reliably by assessing myocardial thickening.

Correct alignment of the imaging plane with the long axis of the ventricle is another important prerequisite for obtaining correct echocardiographic information. Incorrect alignment in the long-axis views results in *foreshortening*. Foreshortening is particularly problematic in the ME TEE views as the true apex is easily missed (Figure 4.12; Video 4.8A-C). Incorrect alignment also results in a nonperpendicular intersection of walls and consequently overestimation of diastolic wall thickness and pseudothickening during systole (Figure 4.13A-D). Pseudothickening may mimic normal wall contraction in segments with severe wall

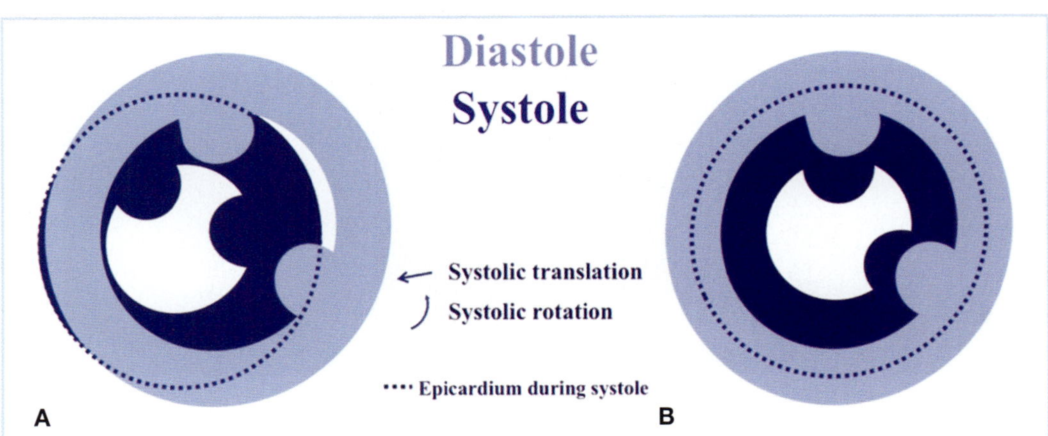

FIGURE 4.11 Effects of translational and rotational movements of the heart on analysis of segmental contraction. A: With a fixed reference system not compensating for translation and rotation, segmental contraction looks severely impaired in the anteroseptal segment and hyperkinetic in the inferolateral segment. B: With a floating reference system compensating for translation and rotation, segmental contraction is correctly diagnosed as normal in all segments (see Video 4.6).

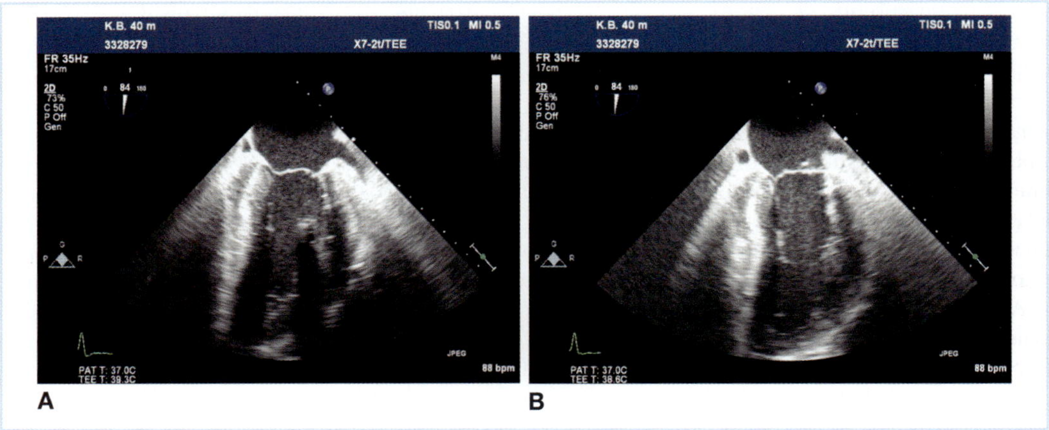

FIGURE 4.12 End-systolic frames illustrating that foreshortening may mimic normal contraction in pathologic segments. A: Foreshortening mimicking normal contraction of the anteroapical segment. B: After correct alignment, it becomes clear that inward motion and thickening of the akinetic anteroapical segment were mimicked by foreshortening (see Video 4.8A-C).

contraction abnormalities, as illustrated in Figure 4.12 (Video 4.8A,B). As noted before, the biplane mode may be very helpful for detecting foreshortening. Pseudothickening with associated incorrect imaging of wall contraction similarly occurs when the systolic translation of the heart (Figure 4.11; Video 4.6) displaces the imaging plane away from the axis of the ventricle.

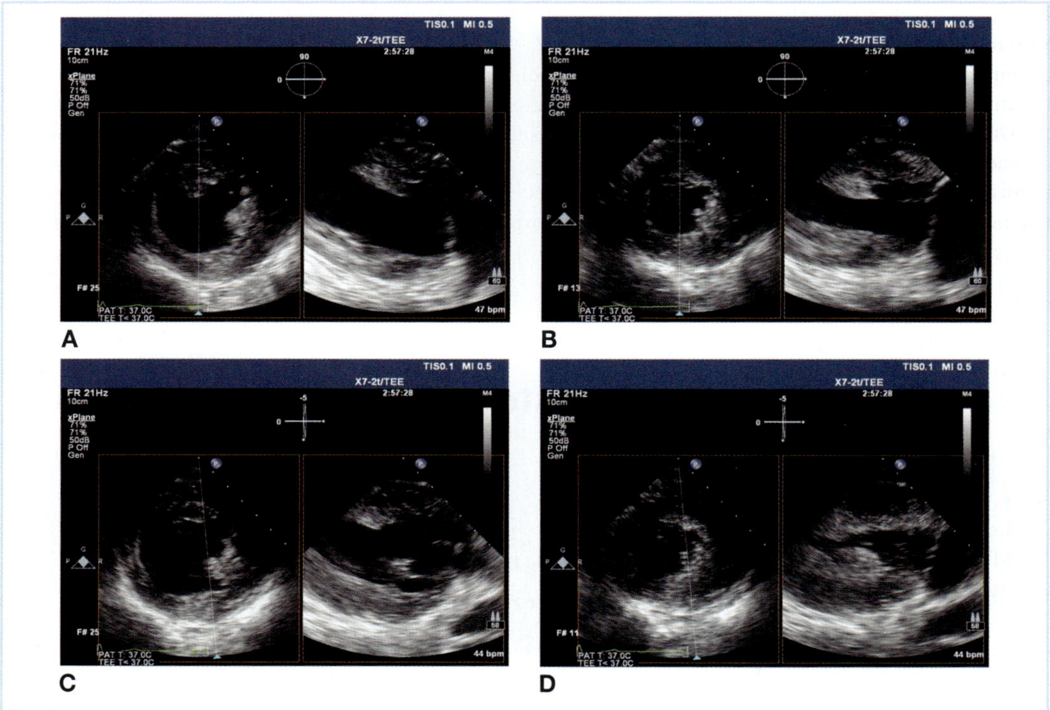

FIGURE 4.13 X-plane transgastric short-axis and corresponding long-axis views illustrating correctly centered (A, B) and foreshortened long-axis views (C, D), each during diastole (A, C) and systole (B, D). Foreshortening mimics inadequate wall thickness in diastole (C), excessive endocardial inward motion and myocardial thickening in systole (D), and decreased diastolic and systolic diameters of the left ventricle (C, D).

Limitations of Echocardiographic Detection of Myocardial Ischemia

Even if the echocardiographer copes well with all potential pitfalls, some methodologic limitations remain and must be taken into account. The fact that a single echocardiographic examination alone cannot provide definite evidence of myocardial ischemia is one limitation of echocardiography. Echocardiography is more sensitive and specific for diagnosing ischemia than ECG when acute deterioration of regional systolic function is observed. However, if an RWMA is detected during an initial echocardiographic examination, causes other than acute ischemia must also be taken into consideration. These causes include stunning, hibernation, previous myocardial infarction, or nonischemic pathology such as myocarditis or cardiomyopathy (Table 4.1). "New" (perioperative) echocardiographic findings, thus, must always be interpreted in the context of previous echocardiographic results and within the clinical context.

A major limitation of the above-described visual regional wall motion analysis is that it is not based on quantitative measurements but relies on qualitative ("semiquantitative" at best) assessment. The qualitative character implies a degree of subjective bias that may impair the reliability of wall contraction readings. Automated, quantitative analysis of regional and global LV function is offered by color kinesis based on real-time, spatiotemporal analysis of endocardial motion (34). Despite its advantages, color kinesis has not become widely adopted in the perioperative setting because it is time consuming, and neither considers myocardial thickening nor corrects for translational or rotational movement. In addition, color kinesis is limited by the requirement of a clearly delineated endocardial border throughout the cardiac cycle.

In clinical practice, endocardial and epicardial borders are rarely perfectly delineated in each frame of the cardiac cycle. Accordingly, a practical approach has been adopted in which a segment is only graded as normal if at least 50% of endocardial and epicardial borders are visible and contracting normally. In contrast, a segment with a clearly detectable RWMA is graded as pathologic even if less than 50% of endocardial and epicardial borders are visible.

Echo contrast agents in combination with default echocardiographic machine settings improve the delineation of endocardial borders in patients with suboptimal image quality but do not improve the assessment of myocardial thickening. During stress echocardiography, they have been found to improve the detection of RWMAs even in patients with apparently adequate grayscale image quality (35). In the perioperative setting, contrast-enhanced echocardiography is rarely used, and studies suggesting beneficial indications for their intraoperative use are still missing. In addition, contrast agents have been associated with rare acute, life-threatening anaphylactoid events, which have been the reason for a black box warning from the U.S. Food and Drug Administration.

Another limitation is that echocardiographic monitoring for ischemia is time consuming. It cannot be performed in an automated fashion like electrocardiographic ST-segment analysis but requires repeated imaging and analysis of multiple long- and short-axis views. Monitoring restricted to a single cross-sectional view ignores major parts of the LV wall and results in missing a majority of RWMAs, even if the view visualizes myocardium supplied by each of the three main coronary arteries, like the TG SAX views. The time needed for repeatedly analyzing multiple views may also explain the observation that echocardiographic real-time detection of ischemia by busy anesthesiologists in the operating room was slightly less reliable than offline detection by examiners who had no other concomitant duties (36). Finally, acute changes in LV loading conditions have important impacts on regional LV contraction. Acute decreases in preload can cause a new RWMA in the absence of ischemia, and acute increases in afterload mimic RWMAs in postischemic myocardium (37).

Alternative Echocardiographic Methods for Detection of Myocardial Ischemia

Doppler indicators: Diastolic function is impaired at an early stage of ischemia, and Doppler indices of diastolic function can be monitored quickly and quantitatively. Studies in awake patients have revealed that changes in transmitral inflow patterns are diagnostic of myocardial ischemia. In anesthetized patients, however, the E/A ratio of diastolic transmitral flow failed to reliably indicate ischemia induced by dobutamine stress testing or transient coronary occlusion during off-pump CPB surgery (38). Explanations for the failure of the diastolic E/A ratio to detect myocardial ischemia in anesthetized surgical patients include the confounding effects of general anesthesia and the frequent changes in preload seen intraoperatively.

3D echocardiography: Using semiautomated endocardial border detection software, 3D TEE allows quantification of end-diastolic and end-systolic volumes, stroke volume, and ejection fraction. It also allows for quantitative analysis of the endocardial motion of the 17 LV segments. Recently, 3D measurements do not have to be performed only offline requiring a time-consuming manual definition of key points of the endocardial border at end diastole and end systole. New software applications have been developed, encouraging detailed full-volume analysis within a short time period directly on the machine in the operating room. Fully automated 3D quantification should be a major advance by saving time and increasing the reproducibility of 3D measurements but is at an early stage of scientific evaluation (39). Nevertheless, it must be noted that the lower frame rate with 3D echocardiography may limit image quality and that the diagnostic accuracy of 3D measurements has to be confirmed in the perioperative setting. The accuracy of this approach is also limited, as myocardial thickening is not considered. This limitation becomes particularly important in cardiac surgical patients after CPB where confounding factors such as translational and rotational movements and ventricular pacing occur more frequently.

Tissue Doppler imaging: Tissue Doppler imaging (TDI) of the mitral annulus and analysis of strain and strain rate are additional, potentially useful techniques for quantitative assessment of regional ventricular systolic and diastolic function (40). Strain and strain rate (deformation) imaging is less influenced by tethering effects than visual regional wall motion analysis. It might enable a more precise assessment of the extent of ischemia (41), but still is not implemented for routine use in the perioperative setting. Reasons include that it is unknown which of the various strain parameters provide(s) the most reliable and robust information on regional dysfunction and that there is a marked variability of regional strain parameters between vendor-specific software (42). Lastly, all TDI measurements as in all Doppler techniques are dependent on the correct alignment of the intercept angle.

Speckle tracking: Another novel and promising method for quantitative analysis of segmental myocardial function is called speckle tracking. 2D Speckle tracking has become available for TEE, but to date, the more promising 3D speckle tracking technology has only been released for transthoracic use. However, all these quantitative methods also have substantial limitations, and recent studies have questioned whether their diagnostic value for detecting ischemia is superior to qualitative wall motion reading. For example, a multiparametric mathematical model based on quantitative deformation markers has failed to provide incremental value to visual assessment of wall motion during stress echocardiography (43). Possible reasons are technical limitations of quantitative imaging, including inadequate spatial and temporal resolution, noise, and artifacts (44). In addition, inter- and intragrader variability, which is a well-known limitation of wall motion reading, is not eliminated by speckle tracking (45). Nevertheless, transthoracic assessment of the LV global longitudinal strain (GLS) at rest has been shown to be superior to visual wall motion analysis in acute coronary syndromes (ACS) (46). Therefore, the recent recommendations on noninvasive imaging in coronary syndromes state that speckle tracking is the method of choice for the assessment of LV strain and is particularly useful in the acute setting when left ventricular ejection fraction (LVEF) is normal or RWMA is not visible (47).

Right Ventricular Ischemia

The RV plays an important role in morbidity and mortality after cardiac surgery, and TEE is a crucial tool for assessing its function. This fact has resulted in the scientific evaluation of a variety of cross-sectional views for the assessment of the right heart, and the inclusion of additional views focused on the RV in the updated guidelines for performing a comprehensive TEE examination (26). The anterior location of the RV in the chest and its thin walls make the RV more susceptible than the LV to incomplete myocardial preservation from cardioplegia during cardiac surgery. As the RCA originates more anterior from the aorta in the supine patient, it is also at a higher risk of acute air lock than the LCA in situations with incomplete de-airing after open-heart surgery or air entrainment from an assist device cannula. For these reasons, assessment of the RV according to current guidelines should not be neglected (26,48,49). Interestingly, most vendors have now implemented specific RV assessment tools in their machines, for example, 3D RVEF and RV strain.

Coronary perfusion of most RV walls originates from the RCA. Nevertheless, a more sophisticated appreciation of RV coronary perfusion is clinically important. For example, the RV anteroseptal wall and minor parts of the anterior wall receive blood supply from the LAD coronary artery, from which also the moderator band artery has its source. The latter may provide collateral blood supply in case of occlusion of the RCA and, thus, influence the extent of RV infarction. In addition, a separate ostial origin of the conal artery, which is found in 30% of subjects, may explain the preserved myocardial function of the RV outflow tract despite proximal occlusion of the RCA.

There are no established rules for detailed analysis of regional contraction of the RV similar to those for the LV, or criteria for diagnosis of acute RV ischemia. Most of the knowledge on RV function is based on studies performed by TTE in awake patients. Acute ischemia will result in acute diastolic and systolic dysfunction with akinesis and, because RV walls are thin, in marked RV distension (Video 4.10). Marked distension of the RV in the absence of a markedly elevated pulmonary artery pressure is a strong indicator of RV ischemia.

COMPLICATIONS OF MYOCARDIAL ISCHEMIA

The immediate and obvious consequence of myocardial ischemia is the impairment of diastolic and systolic myocardial function and consequently systemic hemodynamics (Table 4.3). Ischemic mitral or tricuspid regurgitation, as discussed before, may further increase hemodynamic instability (50,51).

When ischemia progresses to infarction, more disastrous sequelae must be considered. Local inflammation can lead to pericarditis and subsequent pericardial effusion (Video 4.11), hindering ventricular filling and performance. The infarcted, akinetic region of the myocardium is a trigger for thrombus formation (Video 4.12). If the infarcted area dilates during fibrous transformation, an aneurysm (Video 4.13) may develop, further reducing cardiac performance and increasing the risk for thrombus formation. Recognition of thrombi is important because intraoperative surgical manipulation of the heart can dislodge the thrombus,

TABLE 4.3 Complications of Myocardial Infarction

Ischemic mitral or tricuspid regurgitation 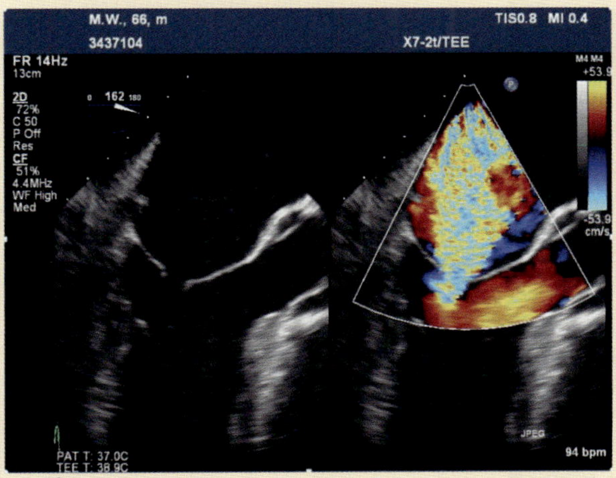 (see Video 4.9A,B)	Ischemia causes diastolic stiffness and reduced systolic ventricular contraction and may result in ventricular dilatation. Changes in ventricular geometry lead to changes in chord tension and direction, called "tethering." Annular dilatation will cause valvular insufficiency as well. Additional papillary muscle dysfunction will aggravate the pathology. Echo findings: Central insufficiency jet and vena contracta as direct measurement for the grade of severity are most helpful. Annular dilatation, reduced area of coaptation, and increased tethering distance and tethering area are predictors.
Pericardial effusion-pericardial tamponade 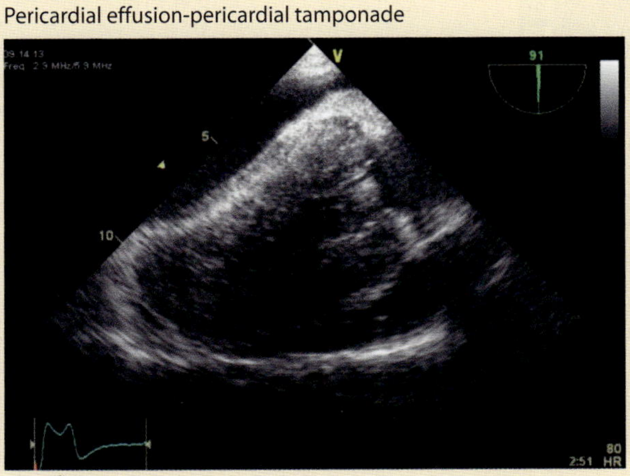 (see Videos 4.11 and 4.14)	Pericardial effusion of serous fluid in pericarditis or blood originating from postoperative bleeding or myocardial rupture presents as black, echo-free space in the pericardium. With clot formation, echo density similar to thrombus develops. Signs of ventricular compression start with impaired diastolic expansion, followed by paradoxical septal motion. Reduced systolic contraction (beyond the initial impairment caused by the infarction itself) may follow. Because of low pericardial compliance, even small amounts of fluid (<2 cm in diameter) can be clinically significant. Cave: Tamponade is a clinical diagnosis.

(continued)

TABLE 4.3 Complications of Myocardial Infarction (*continued*)

LV thrombus 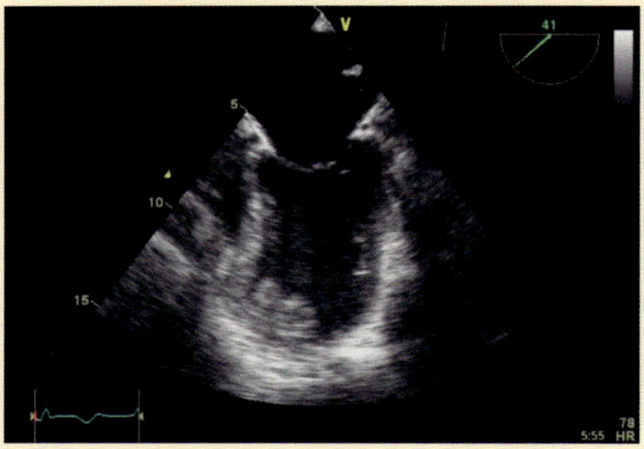 (see Video 4.12)	Blood stasis in the trabecular wall with RWMA favors thrombus formation. No thrombus formation without adjacent RWMA. TEE has a high sensitivity and specificity for detecting thrombi, but special attention to a possible apical thrombus is needed. Use deep transgastric views. Echo findings: Acute thrombi look similar to myocardium; old thrombi may be more echo dense. Shape of thrombi is variable, more frequently sessile and laminated than pedunculated and mobile. Cave: Differentiation from artifact. A thrombus should be visible in ≥2 planes in an area with severe RWMA.
LV aneurysm 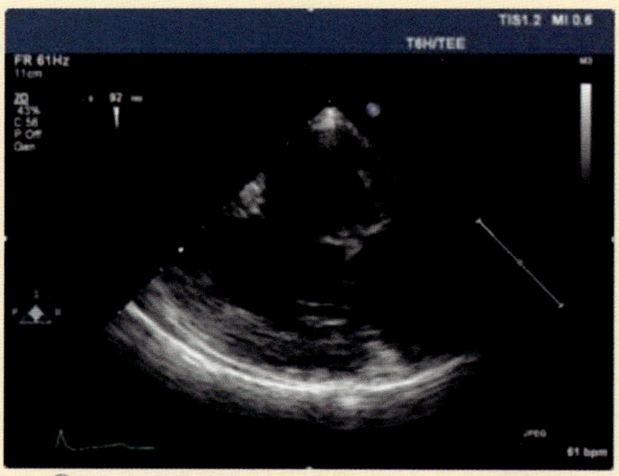 (see Video 4.13)	LV aneurysm develops after transmural infarction. Wall stress increases with LV dilatation and thinning of the infarct zone, causing stretching of the fibrous scar. It is more common after infarction in the supply area of the LAD (anterior wall). Most common locations are the LV apex (90%) or the basal inferior or inferolateral wall. Echo features: Thin wall without systolic thickening and dyskinetic motion, wide neck. Frequently with thrombus formation Cave: If akinetic or dyskinetic wall is not thin: Suspect thrombus.
Postinfarction VSD 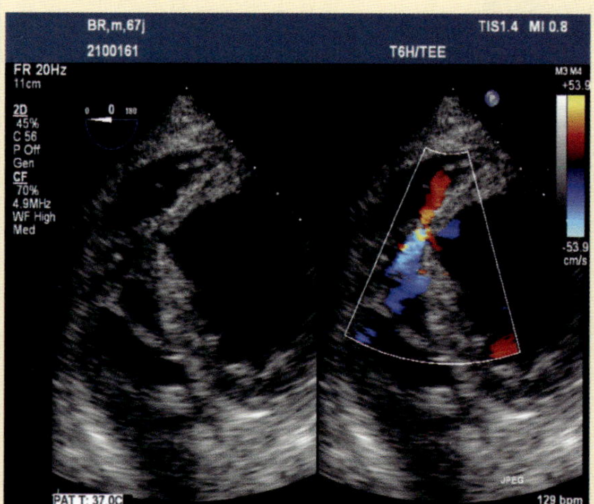 (see Video 4.15)	Usually develops 3-6 d post myocardial infarction, with single or multiple defects. Left-to-right shunt causes RV dilatation and decrease in function. The LV seems hypercontractile through acute LV afterload reduction by VSD. The VSD is often difficult to locate. Use color flow Doppler for locating; transgastric views are preferable due to angle dependency in Doppler studies. Use pulse-wave Doppler or continuous-wave Doppler to measure pressure gradients between LV and RV; beware of angle mismatch. Interpretation: Larger defect → lower gradient → lower velocities measured (volume transfer increases RV pressure and lowers LV pressure).

TABLE 4.3 Complications of Myocardial Infarction (*continued*)

Papillary muscle rupture 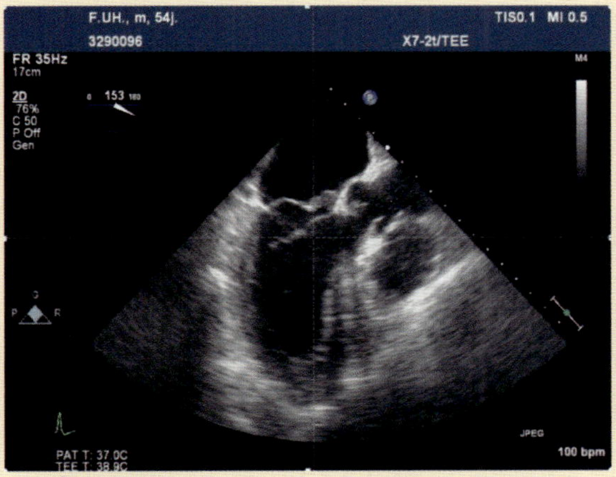 (see Video 4.16)	Rupture is more likely in posteromedial than anterolateral papillary muscle (single vs dual artery supply). • Complete rupture: Both leaflets involved, flail leaflets and chords, often with attached piece of the papillary muscle. Grade 3 insufficiency with usually central jet, vena contracta >6 mm, large PISA, pulmonary venous S inversion. • Incomplete rupture: Prolapse or partial flail of one or both leaflets. Grade of insufficiency varies, often asymmetric jet. Other findings: RWMA in wall segments adjacent to papillary muscle, but globally hyperdynamic LV with acute mitral regurgitation and retrograde LV "unloading."
Pseudoaneurysm 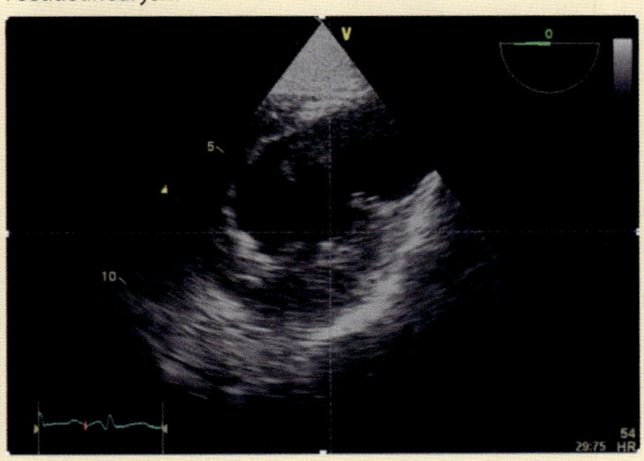 (see Video 4.17)	Pseudoaneurysm has the same pathology as VSD. Most frequently in the inferior wall, small free rupture contained by pericardium. The size of the tear in the myocardium determines the flow of blood into the pericardial space and, together with the speed of coagulation, the amount and extent of pericardial blood and pericardial tamponade. Echo signs: Small neck, variable amount of pericardial fluid and/or thrombus, varying signs of tamponade.

LAD, left anterior descending; LV, left ventricular; PISA, proximal isovelocity surface area; RWMA, regional wall motion abnormality; VSD, ventricular septal defect.

with potentially fatal embolic consequences. Differentiation of intracardiac thrombus from artifacts (caused by near-field echoes, reverberations, marked trabeculation in hypertrophic LV, tendons, false chordae, etc) may be difficult (52). True thrombi are located in areas with severe RWMA and should be diagnosed using multiple views.

The most catastrophic complication of myocardial infarction is myocardial rupture. A rupture in the cardiac free wall leads to massive pericardial tamponade (Video 4.14) and is usually a lethal complication. A rupture isolated to the interventricular septum causes a ventricular septal defect (VSD) with a left-to-right shunt (Video 4.15) and ultimately, if untreated, cardiac failure. Acute ischemic papillary muscle rupture results in severe mitral regurgitation and requires immediate surgical treatment (Video 4.16). A small, incomplete myocardial rupture can be contained, leading to a pseudoaneurysm that usually shows thrombus formation (Video 4.17).

Acute ischemia frequently causes new or worsening (acute) mitral regurgitation. Ischemic mitral regurgitation occurs due to impaired contraction of the left ventricle, or ischemic dysfunction of one or both papillary muscles resulting in restricted leaflet motion, or by acute annular enlargement (Figure 4.14; Video 4.9A, B). Progressive mitral regurgitation is a marker for the clinical severity of LV myocardial ischemia and, if it resolves, an indicator for effective therapy (see Chapter 8: Mitral Regurgitation).

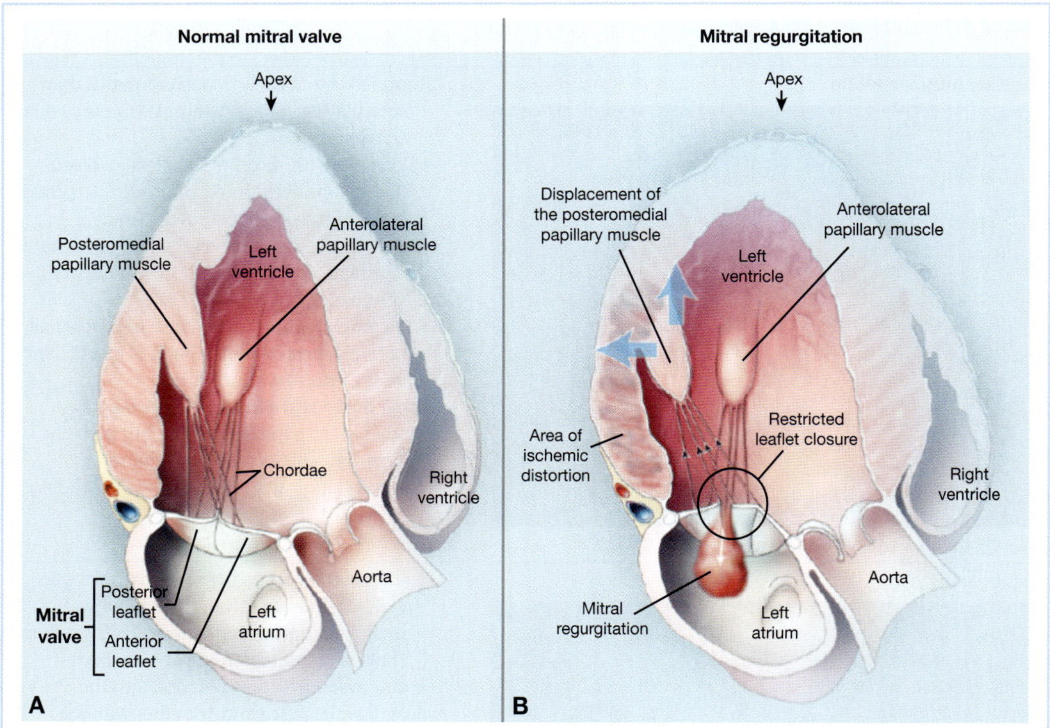

FIGURE 4.14 Ischemic mitral regurgitation. A normal mitral valve is shown in (A). Ischemic mitral regurgitation, in which the leaflets cannot close effectively, is shown in (B). The orientation of the illustration is typical of transthoracic echocardiographic imaging (see Video 4.9).

SUMMARY

Detecting ischemia, grading its severity, and recognizing its complications are important priorities for the intraoperative echocardiographer. Monitoring for ischemia is based on analysis of regional endocardial motion and wall thickening according to established concepts and criteria (ie, on the 17-segment model and the five-grade scale of regional systolic contraction). In addition, the clinician needs to be aware of the limitations and potential pitfalls of regional wall contraction analysis in order to avoid misdiagnosis.

ACKNOWLEDGMENTS

We gratefully acknowledge the contributions of the previous edition author, Manfred D. Seeberger, as portions of those chapters have been retained in this revision.

REFERENCES

1. Ortiz-Pérez JT, Rodríguez J, Meyers SN, Lee DC, Davidson C, Wu E. Correspondence between the 17-segment model and coronary arterial anatomy using contrast-enhanced cardiac magnetic resonance imaging. *JACC Cardiovasc Imaging.* 2008;1(3):282-293.
2. Edvardsen T, Asch FM, Davidson B, et al. Non-invasive imaging in coronary syndromes: recommendations of the European Association of Cardiovascular Imaging and the American Society of Echocardiography, in collaboration with the American Society of Nuclear Cardiology, Society of Cardiovascular Computed Tomography, and Society for Cardiovascular Magnetic Resonance. *Eur Heart J Cardiovasc Imaging.* 2022;23(2):e6-e33.
3. Salerno P, Jackson A, Shaw M, Spratt P, Jansz P. Transesophageal echocardiographic imaging of the branches of the aorta: a guide to obtaining these images and their clinical utility. *J Cardiothorac Vasc Anesth.* 2009;23(5):694-701.
4. Ender J, Singh R, Nakahira J, Subramanian S, Thiele H, Mukherjee C. Echo didactic: visualization of the circumflex artery in the perioperative setting with transesophageal echocardiography. *Anesth Analg.* 2012;115(1):22-26.

5. Faletra FF, Agricola E, Flachskampf FA, et al. Three-dimensional transoesophageal echocardiography: how to use and when to use—a clinical consensus statement from the European Association of Cardiovascular Imaging of the European Society of Cardiology. *Eur Heart J Cardiovasc Imaging.* 2023;24(8):e119-e197.
6. Theunissen T, Coddens J, Foubert L, Cammu G, Degrieck I, Deloof T. Intraoperative severity assessment of coronary artery stenosis in patients at risk: the role of transesophageal echocardiography. *Anesth Analg.* 2006;102(2):366-368.
7. Kasprzak JD, Drozdz J, Peruga JZ, Rafalska K, Krzemińska-Pakuła M. Definition of flow parameters in proximal nonstenotic coronary arteries using transesophageal Doppler echocardiography. *Echocardiography.* 2000;17(2):141-150.
8. Ender J, Gummert J, Fassl J, Krohmer E, Bossert T, Mohr FW. Ligation or distortion of the right circumflex artery during minimal invasive mitral valve repair detected by transesophageal echocardiography. *J Am Soc Echocardiogr.* 2008;21(4):408.e4-408.e5.
9. Kyo S, Takamoto S, Omoto R, et al. Intraoperative echocardiography for diagnosis and treatment of aortic dissection. Utility of color flow mapping for surgical decision making in acute stage. *Herz.* 1992;17(6):377-389.
10. Gurvitch R, Tay EL, Wijesinghe N, et al. Transcatheter aortic valve implantation: lessons from the learning curve of the first 270 high-risk patients. *Catheter Cardiovasc Interv.* 2011;78(7):977-984.
11. Anker SD, Friede T, von Bardeleben RS, et al. Transcatheter valve repair in heart failure with moderate to severe mitral regurgitation. *N Engl J Med.* 2024;391(19):1799-1809.
12. Ahmari SA, Idris A, Amri HA, Habbab M. Failure of multiple coronary angiographies to identify left main coronary artery disease in a patient diagnosed by transesophageal echocardiography. *Eur J Echocardiogr.* 2005;6(4):308-310.
13. Vrublevsky AV, Boshchenko AA, Karpov RS. Diagnostics of main coronary artery stenoses and occlusions: multiplane transoesophageal Doppler echocardiographic assessment. *Eur J Echocardiogr.* 2001;2(3):170-177.
14. Wang J, Filipovic M, Rudzitis A, et al. Transesophageal echocardiography for monitoring segmental wall motion during off-pump coronary artery bypass surgery. *Anesth Analg.* 2004;99(4):965-973.
15. Seeberger MD, Skarvan K, Buser P, et al. Dobutamine stress echocardiography to detect inducible demand ischemia in anesthetized patients with coronary artery disease. *Anesthesiology.* 1998;88(5):1233-1239.
16. Tennant R, Wiggers C. The effect of coronary occlusion on myocardial contraction. *Am J Physiol.* 1935;112:351-361.
17. Pandian NG, Kerber RE. Two-dimensional echocardiography in experimental coronary stenosis. I. Sensitivity and specificity in detecting transient myocardial dyskinesis: comparison with sonomicrometers. *Circulation.* 1982;66(3):597-602.
18. Pandian NG, Kieso RA, Kerber RE. Two-dimensional echocardiography in experimental coronary stenosis. II. Relationship between systolic wall thinning and regional myocardial perfusion in severe coronary stenosis. *Circulation.* 1982;66(3):603-611.
19. Wohlgelernter D, Cleman M, Highman HA, et al. Regional myocardial dysfunction during coronary angioplasty: evaluation by two-dimensional echocardiography and 12 lead electrocardiography. *J Am Coll Cardiol.* 1986;7(6):1245-1254.
20. Lambertz H, Kreis A, Trümper H, Hanrath P. Simultaneous transesophageal atrial pacing and transesophageal two-dimensional echocardiography: a new method of stress echocardiography. *J Am Coll Cardiol.* 1990;16(5):1143-1153.
21. Agati L, Renzi M, Sciomer S, et al. Transesophageal dipyridamole echocardiography for diagnosis of coronary artery disease. *J Am Coll Cardiol.* 1992;19(4):765-770.
22. Gallagher KP, Kumada T, Koziol JA, McKown MD, Kemper WS, Ross J Jr. Significance of regional wall thickening abnormalities relative to transmural myocardial perfusion in anesthetized dogs. *Circulation.* 1980;62(6):1266-1274.
23. Almeida AG, Carpenter JP, Cameli M, et al. Multimodality imaging of myocardial viability: an expert consensus document from the European Association of Cardiovascular Imaging (EACVI). *Eur Heart J Cardiovasc Imaging.* 2021;22(8):e97-e125.
24. Colucci WS. Dobutamine stress echocardiography in the evaluation of hibernating myocardium. *UpToDate.* Published 2012. Accessed February 6, 2013. http://www.uptodate.com/contents/dobutamine-stress-echocardiography-in-the-evaluation-of-hibernating-myocardium?source=search_result&search=Dobutamine+stress+echocardiography%2C+Colucci&selectedTitle=1~71
25. Cerqueira MD, Weissman NJ, Dilsizian V, et al. Standardized myocardial segmentation and nomenclature for tomographic imaging of the heart. A statement for healthcare professionals from the Cardiac Imaging Committee of the Council on Clinical Cardiology of the American Heart Association. *Circulation.* 2002;105(4):539-542.
26. Hahn RT, Abraham T, Adams MS, et al. Guidelines for performing a comprehensive transesophageal echocardiographic examination: recommendations from the American Society of Echocardiography and the Society of Cardiovascular Anesthesiologists. *Anesth Analg.* 2014;118(1):21-68.
27. Codreanu I, Robson MD, Golding SJ, Jung BA, Clarke K, Holloway CJ. Longitudinally and circumferentially directed movements of the left ventricle studied by cardiovascular magnetic resonance phase contrast velocity mapping. *J Cardiovasc Magn Reson.* 2010;12(1):48.
28. Rouine-Rapp K, Ionescu P, Balea M, Foster E, Cahalan MK. Detection of intraoperative segmental wall-motion abnormalities by transesophageal echocardiography: the incremental value of additional cross sections in the transverse and longitudinal planes. *Anesth Analg.* 1996;83(6):1141-1148.
29. Shanewise JS, Cheung AT, Aronson S, et al. ASE/SCA guidelines for performing a comprehensive intraoperative multiplane transesophageal echocardiography examination: recommendations of the American Society of Echocardiography Council for Intraoperative Echocardiography and the Society of Cardiovascular Anesthesiologists Task Force for Certification in Perioperative Transesophageal Echocardiography. *Anesth Analg.* 1999;89(4):870-884.
30. Sengupta PP, Tajik AJ, Chandrasekaran K, Khandheria BK. Twist mechanics of the left ventricle: principles and application. *JACC Cardiovasc Imaging.* 2008;1(3):366-376.
31. Schnittger I, Fitzgerald PJ, Gordon EP, Alderman EL, Popp RL. Computerized quantitative analysis of left ventricular wall motion by two-dimensional echocardiography. *Circulation.* 1984;70(2):242-254.
32. Lehmann KG, Lee FA, McKenzie WB, et al. Onset of altered interventricular septal motion during cardiac surgery. Assessment by continuous intraoperative transesophageal echocardiography. *Circulation.* 1990;82(4):1325-1334.

33. Buda AJ, Zotz RJ, Pace DP, Krause LC. Comparison of two-dimensional echocardiographic wall motion and wall thickening abnormalities in relation to the myocardium at risk. *Am Heart J.* 1986;111(3):587-592.
34. Mor-Avi V, Vignon P, Koch R, et al. Segmental analysis of color kinesis images: new method for quantification of the magnitude and timing of endocardial motion during left ventricular systole and diastole. *Circulation.* 1997;95(8):2082-2097.
35. Larsson MK, Da Silva C, Gunyeli E, et al. The potential clinical value of contrast-enhanced echocardiography beyond current recommendations. *Cardiovasc Ultrasound.* 2016;14:2.
36. Bergquist BD, Leung JM, Bellows WH. Transesophageal echocardiography in myocardial revascularization: I. Accuracy of intraoperative real-time interpretation. *Anesth Analg.* 1996;82(6):1132-1138.
37. Buffington CW, Coyle RJ. Altered load dependence of postischemic myocardium. *Anesthesiology.* 1991;75(3):464-474.
38. Filipovic M, Seeberger MD, Rohlfs R, et al. Doppler indices of diastolic transmitral flow velocity are invalid indicators of myocardial ischaemia during high-dose dobutamine infusion in anaesthetized patients. *Eur J Anaesthesiol.* 2002;19(11): 789-795.
39. Sun L, Feng H, Ni L, Wang H, Gao D. Realization of fully automated quantification of left ventricular volumes and systolic function using transthoracic 3D echocardiography. *Cardiovasc Ultrasound.* 2018;16(1):2.
40. Liel-Cohen N, Tsadok Y, Beeri R, et al. A new tool for automatic assessment of segmental wall motion based on longitudinal 2D strain: a multicenter study by the Israeli Echocardiography Research Group. *Circ Cardiovasc Imaging.* 2010;3(1):47-53.
41. Takagi Y, Hozumi T, Takemoto Y, et al. Detection of prolonged regional myocardial systolic dysfunction after exercise-induced myocardial ischemia by strain echocardiography with high frame rate tissue Doppler echocardiography. *J Echocardiogr.* 2011;9(3):90-96.
42. Mirea O, Pagourelias ED, Duchenne J, et al. Intervendor differences in the accuracy of detecting regional functional abnormalities: a report from the EACVI-ASE Strain Standardization Task Force. *JACC Cardiovasc Imaging.* 2018;11(1):25-34.
43. Čelutkienė J, Burneikaitė G, Petkevičius L, Balkevičienė L, Laucevičius A. Combination of single quantitative parameters into multiparametric model for ischemia detection is not superior to visual assessment during dobutamine stress echocardiography. *Cardiovasc Ultrasound.* 2016;14:13.
44. Argyle RA, Ray SG. Stress and strain: double trouble or useful tool? *Eur J Echocardiogr.* 2009;10(6):716-722.
45. Tschöpe C, Kasner M. Can speckle-tracking imaging improve the reliability of echocardiographic parameters for outcome evaluation in clinical trials? *Eur Heart J.* 2014;35(10):605-607.
46. Grenne B, Eek C, Sjøli B, et al. Acute coronary occlusion in non-ST-elevation acute coronary syndrome: outcome and early identification by strain echocardiography. *Heart.* 2010;96(19):1550-1556.
47. Stanton T, Leano R, Marwick TH. Prediction of all-cause mortality from global longitudinal speckle strain: comparison with ejection fraction and wall motion scoring. *Circ Cardiovasc Imaging.* 2009;2(5):356-364.
48. Rudski LG, Lai WW, Afilalo J, et al. Guidelines for the echocardiographic assessment of the right heart in adults: a report from the American Society of Echocardiography endorsed by the European Association of Echocardiography, a registered branch of the European Society of Cardiology, and the Canadian Society of Echocardiography. *J Am Soc Echocardiogr.* 2010;23(7): 685-713; quiz 86-88.
49. Surkova E, Cosyns B, Gerber B, Gimelli A, La Gerche A, Ajmone Marsan N. The dysfunctional right ventricle: the importance of multi-modality imaging. *Eur Heart J Cardiovasc Imaging.* 2022;23(7):885-897.
50. Kono T, Sabbah HN, Rosman H, et al. Mechanism of functional mitral regurgitation during acute myocardial ischemia. *J Am Coll Cardiol.* 1992;19(5):1101-1105.
51. Glasson JR, Komeda M, Daughters GT, et al. Early systolic mitral leaflet "loitering" during acute ischemic mitral regurgitation. *J Thorac Cardiovasc Surg.* 1998;116(2):193-205.
52. Stratton JR, Lighty GW Jr, Pearlman AS, Ritchie JL. Detection of left ventricular thrombus by two-dimensional echocardiography: sensitivity, specificity, and causes of uncertainty. *Circulation.* 1982;66(1):156-166.
53. Opie LH. The multifarious spectrum of ischemic left ventricular dysfunction: relevance of new ischemic syndromes. *J Mol Cell Cardiol.* 1996;28(12):2403-2414.
54. Nihoyannopoulos P, Vanoverschelde JL. Myocardial ischaemia and viability: the pivotal role of echocardiography. *Eur Heart J.* 2011;32(7):810-819.

QUESTIONS

1. **Which statement regarding coronary artery anatomy is true?**
   A. The LCA bifurcates into the LAD and the RCA.
   B. The LAD gives rise to the marginal branches.
   C. The acute marginal branches supplying the conduction system run off the RCA.
   D. The LCX gives rise to septal arteries.

2. **Which statement regarding coronary blood distribution type is true?**
   A. The supply of the inferior wall and inferior septum determines the coronary distribution type.
   B. The right-dominant coronary distribution type is rarely present.
   C. The left-dominant coronary distribution type is the most frequent one.
   D. The balanced distribution type is found in about 30% of individuals.

3. **Acute occlusion of the RCA will not cause:**
   A. Inferior wall motion abnormalities of the LV
   B. Anterolateral wall motion abnormalities of the LV
   C. RV wall motion abnormalities
   D. Dysfunctions of the conduction system

4. **Doppler evaluation of coronary artery blood flow:**
   A. Is usually performed using continuous-wave Doppler
   B. Shows highest blood flow velocity during diastole for the LCA
   C. Shows highest blood flow velocity during systole for the RCA
   D. Should be performed by setting the highest possible Nyquist limit for color flow Doppler

5. **Echocardiographic detection of hypokinesis/akinesis indicating myocardial ischemia may be complicated by all the following factors** *except:*
   A. Translational and rotational movements of the heart
   B. Ventricular pacing
   C. Incorrect alignment of the imaging plane with the axis of the ventricle
   D. The use of 3D or X-plane modes in echocardiography

6. **Which statement is correct regarding echocardiographic findings during acute ischemia?**
   A. Wall thinning is not an indicator of acute ischemia.
   B. The degree of ischemic mitral regurgitation is typically independent of changes in preload and afterload.
   C. Coronary air embolism directly after open-heart surgery most frequently causes systolic wall contraction abnormalities of the anterior wall.
   D. Acute akinesia indicates myocardial ischemia, acute dyskinesia myocardial infarction.

7. **Which of the following statements regarding complications of ischemia is true?**
   A. Acute myocardial ischemia and acute myocardial infarction cannot be differentiated by echocardiography.
   B. Ischemic rupture in the septum causes a VSD with an interventricular left-to-right shunt.
   C. A pseudoaneurysm has the same pathology as a VSD.
   D. All of the above apply.

8. **Which of the following is not a complication of myocardial infarction?**
   A. Pericardial tamponade
   B. Papillary muscle rupture
   C. Membranous VSD
   D. Ventricular thrombus

9. **All 17 segments of the LV model adopted by the ASE/SCA can be visualized by the combination of:**
   A. The ME four-chamber and LAX views and the TG mid-SAX view
   B. The TG mid-SAX, two-chamber, and LAX views
   C. The ME four-chamber, two-chamber, and LAX views
   D. The TG basal SAX, mid-SAX, and apical SAX views

10. **Which of the following is not a mechanism for chronic ischemic mitral regurgitation?**
    A. Ventricular dilatation with incomplete leaflet coaptation
    B. Papillary muscle rupture
    C. Ischemic dysfunction of one or both papillary muscles
    D. Hypokinesis of the ventricular segment underlying a normal papillary muscle

ANSWERS

1. **Correct Answer: C.**
Rationale: The LCA bifurcates into the LAD (giving offspring to diagonal branches and septal arteries) and the LCX giving offspring to the marginal branches. The RCA gives off the RV acute marginal branches which supply the conduction system.

2. **Correct Answer: A.**
Rationale: The supply of the inferior wall and septum is the indicator for the coronary blood distribution type. This is by the RCA in the right-dominant type (80%-85%), by the LCX in the left-dominant type, and only in 5% by both the RCA and the LCX, which defines the balanced distribution type.

3. **Correct Answer: B.**
Rationale: The RCA supplies the right ventricle including the conduction system and, in most individuals (80%-85% right-dominant type), the inferior wall of the LV. The anterolateral wall of the LV is only supplied by the LCA.

4. **Correct Answer: B.**
Rationale: For Doppler evaluation of the coronary blood flow, PW Doppler using a reduced Nyquist limit due to low flow velocities is required. Blood flow occurs predominantly and with the highest velocities in diastole in all coronary arteries.

5. **Correct Answer: D.**
Rationale: Translational and rotational movements as well as incorrect alignment of the imaging plane (foreshortening) can lead to improper cross-sectional views of the ventricular walls, impairing the assessment of wall thickness and its changes. The use of 3D or X-plane modes in echocardiography thus may help to overcome these limitations. Ventricular pacing can lead to dyssynchrony of wall contractions mimicking dyskinesis.

6. **Correct Answer: A.**
Rationale: As air bubbles in blood by gravidity float upward, they are much more likely to enter the anteriorly placed RCA ostium in a patient lying supine. Akinesia and dyskinesia depend on the extent of the ischemia in the layers of the myocardial wall and not on the reversibility, with myocardial infarction being irreversible. Ischemic mitral regurgitation worsens with increases in pre- and afterload. Wall thinning occurs after an infarction due to the replacement of myocyte by fibrotic tissue.

7. **Correct Answer: D.**
Rationale: Both acute ischemia and infarction echocardiographically will show hypokinesis or akinesis. A pseudoaneurysm will develop after a transmural infarction when the myocardium ruptures, and the rupture remains contained by the epicardial and pericardial layers, which adhere due to the inflammatory process involved.

8. **Correct Answer: C.**
Rationale: A muscular, but not a membranous, VSD would be a complication of myocardial infarction as well as a papillary muscle rupture or a pericardial tamponade in case of ventricular rupture. Thrombus formation is likely at chronic severely hypokinetic or akinetic wall segments.

9. **Correct Answer: C.**
Rationale: Only the combination of the three standard ME views (four-chamber, two-chamber, and long axis or a 3D data set) guarantees to visualize all segments. In the TG SAX views, the apical cap cannot be visualized, and the apical and basal views are often cut obliquely.

10. **Correct Answer: B.**
Rationale: Papillary muscle rupture leads to acute ischemic mitral regurgitation.

II Essentials of Doppler Echo

5 Doppler Technology and Technique

Albert C. Perrino, Jr and Jennifer Decou

Two-dimensional echocardiography provides remarkable high-resolution, full-motion display of cardiac structures. Yet despite the ability to reveal the most intricate anatomic detail, two-dimensional imaging is unable to visualize blood flow. Blood flow in cardiac chambers and the great vessels is simply presented in black on the two-dimensional display. Since the movement of blood is the raison d'être of the cardiovascular system, this limitation presents a serious challenge to the diagnostic capability of echocardiography. Doppler ultrasonography overcomes this limitation in the assessment of blood flow. Its color flow display affords the echocardiographer dramatic views of blood flow. In addition, spectral Doppler provides the tools to quantify the magnitude and direction of flow. Since Doppler evaluation is quantitative, it provides a means of grading the severity of disease in many cases in which two-dimensional echocardiography merely demonstrates the presence of an abnormality. As such, mastery of Doppler examinations is a critical element in the training of a perioperative echocardiographer.

DOPPLER FREQUENCY SHIFT

Doppler examinations are based on principles fundamentally different from those underlying two-dimensional imaging. As is addressed in the following sections, these differences necessitate altered approaches and techniques when Doppler examinations are performed. Many times, the required view and imaging frequencies are contrary to those selected for two-dimensional imaging of the same anatomic region. To obtain an optimal assessment of both the form and function of the desired cardiac structure, it is essential to remain cognizant of the underlying physical principles of the two approaches and how they differ.

The Doppler Effect

As explained in Chapter 1: Principles and Technology of Two-Dimensional Echocardiography, two-dimensional imaging is based on the intensity and time delay of reflected ultrasound. To determine the velocity of blood flow, Doppler systems examine the change in frequency of the ultrasound reflected from red blood cells. Our ability to use the movement of red blood cells to gauge blood flow velocity dates back to the experiments of the Austrian physicist Christian Doppler. Trumpeters on a high-speed locomotive played a tone at a specific pitch so that the effects of motion on sound frequency could be examined. A second group of musicians stationed on a loading dock played the same tone as the train passed by. As Doppler had predicted, the two tones were audibly different. The change in pitch, known as the Doppler effect, occurs because the motion of an object causes the sound wave to be compressed in the direction of the motion and expanded in the direction opposite to the motion.

Signal Frequency and Blood Flow

Red blood cells reflect ultrasound as they travel through the bloodstream. By directing an ultrasound signal at flowing blood and listening for the change in frequency produced by the red cell reflections, Doppler echocardiography can assess the direction and speed of blood flow.

Figure 5.1 illustrates the principle of the Doppler effect for cardiac applications. When ultrasound is transmitted to blood, it is scattered by the multitude of red blood cells, and a small portion of this scattering is reflected back toward the transducer. The strength of the echoes returning to the transducer is related to the number of particles reflecting the ultrasound. If the hematocrit is increased, more interfaces are available for reflection and the ultrasound signal is stronger. However, this effect is self-limited because, at a hematocrit exceeding 30%, the reflected signal strength is weakened by destructive interference. Modern echocardiography systems are designed to detect Doppler signals over a wide range of hematocrit values.

If the red cells are stationary, the signal is reflected at the same frequency as the transmitted signal. Since no Doppler frequency shift occurs, the situation is similar to that of two-dimensional echocardiography. When blood flows toward the ultrasound transducer, the reflected signal is compressed by the motion of the red cells, and its frequency is higher than that of the transmitted signal. Conversely, when blood flows away from the ultrasound transducer, the frequency of the reflected signal received by the transducer is lower than that of the transmitted signal. The technical term for the alterations in the frequency of the ultrasound signals caused by the Doppler effect is *modulation*. Through analysis of the modulated signal, both the direction and speed of the red blood cells can be determined.

DOPPLER ANALYSIS

The Doppler Equation: Linking the Frequency Shift to Velocity

The *Doppler equation* describes the relationship between the alteration in ultrasound frequency and blood flow velocity (Figure 5.2):

$$\Delta f = v \times \cos\theta \times 2f_t/c,$$

where Δf is the difference between transmitted frequency (f_t) and received frequency, v is blood velocity, c is the speed of sound in the blood (1,540 m/s), and θ is the angle of incidence between the ultrasound beam and blood flow.

Conceptually, the equation can be simplified based on the observation that the change in ultrasound frequency is directly related to just two variables: blood velocity and cos θ. The remaining factors in the

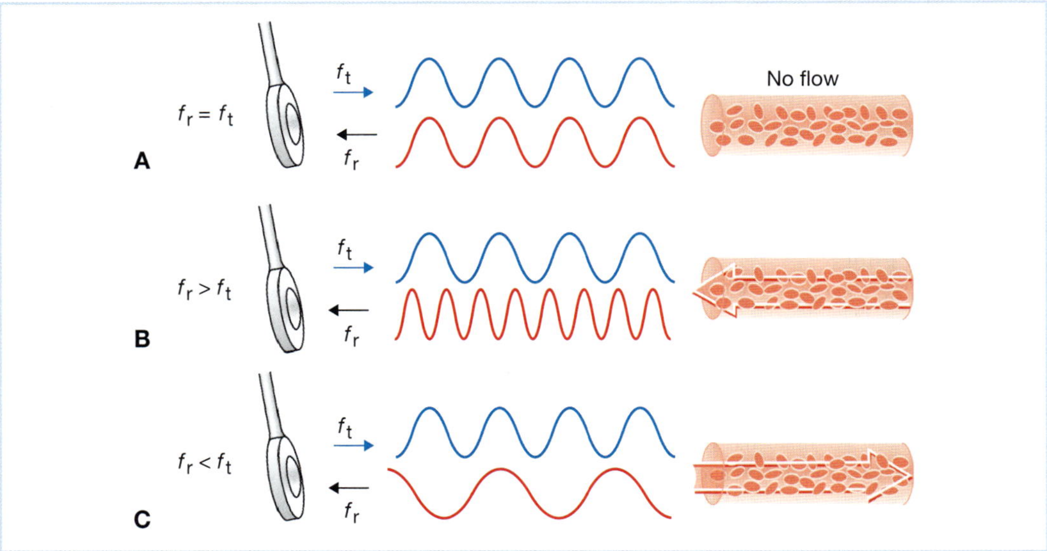

FIGURE 5.1 Detecting blood flow: Effects of red cell motion on ultrasound frequency. The motion of an object alters the frequency of a reflected ultrasound signal. A: The reflected echoes from a stationary target are of the same frequency as the transmitted signal. B: Objects such as red blood cells moving toward the transducer compress the sound signal, and the reflected frequency is increased. C: When red cells travel away from the transducer, the frequency of the reflected echoes is decreased. These modulations in the frequency of the reflected ultrasound are used to detect blood flow. f_t, transmitted signal frequency; f_r, reflected signal frequency.

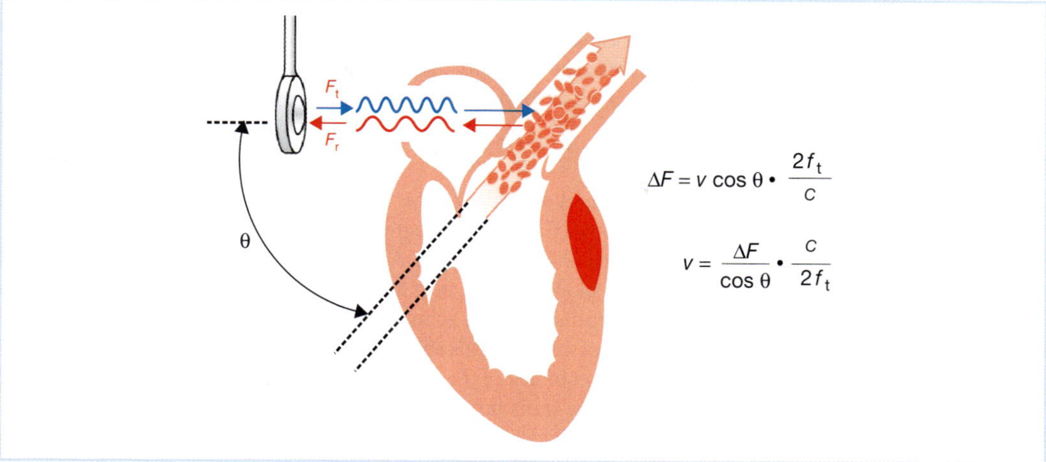

FIGURE 5.2 Calculating blood flow velocity: The Doppler equation. The Doppler equation calculates blood flow velocity based on two variables: the Doppler frequency shift (ΔF) and the cosine of the angle of incidence between the ultrasound beam and the blood flow. The Doppler frequency shift is measured by the echocardiographic system, but cos θ is unknown, and manual entry by the echocardiographer is required for its estimation. v, blood flow velocity; f_t, transmitted signal frequency; f_r, reflected signal frequency; ΔF, difference between f_r and f_t; c, speed of sound in tissue; θ, angle of incidence between the orientation of the ultrasound beam and that of the blood flow.

equation, the speed of sound in the blood (c) and the transmitted frequency (f_t), are constants. The Doppler signal is shifted only by the component of the blood velocity that is in the direction of the beam path (ie, $v \cos \theta$). For example, when the direction of the ultrasound beam is parallel to the blood flow, the observed Δf fully reflects total blood velocity ($\cos\theta = 1$). With nonparallel orientation of the ultrasound beam to blood flow, Δf is reduced by the factor cos θ. As illustrated in Figure 5.3, when the beam angle divergence is small, the effects on Δf are limited. However, *with angles greater than 30°, the value of cos θ decreases rapidly*. When the direction of the beam is perpendicular to the blood flow (90°, cos 90 = 0), the movement of blood is no longer appreciated by the Doppler system ($\Delta f = 0$).

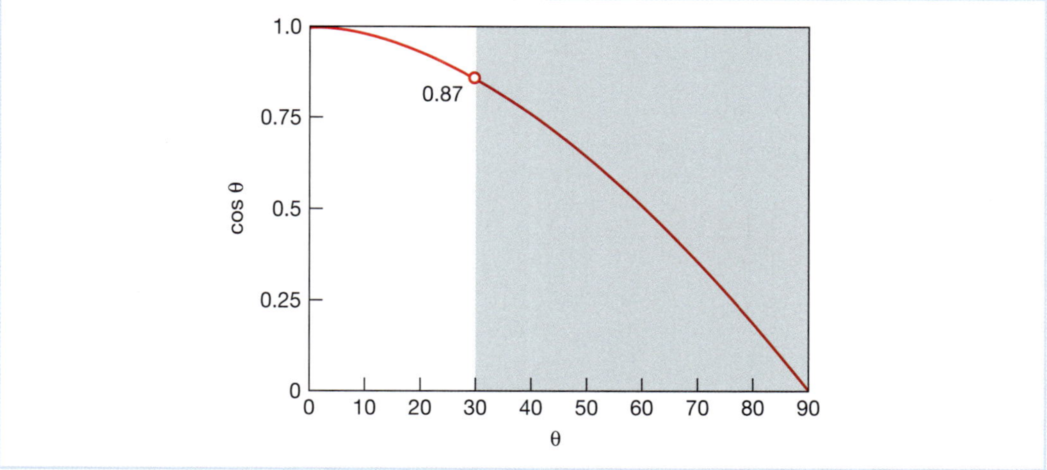

FIGURE 5.3 Cosine relationship. Most devices default to a simplified Doppler equation in which cos θ is ignored, with the assumption that the Doppler beam is nearly parallel to the blood flow so that the cos θ factor is negligible. However, at angles between beam and blood flow greater than 30°, a precipitous drop in the cosine curve results in a substantial underestimation of blood flow velocity. θ, angle of incidence between the orientation of the ultrasound beam and that of the blood flow.

Implications of Beam Orientation

The effect of the beam angle on Doppler measurements has important clinical implications. In clinical practice, the ultrasound system measures the frequency shift to calculate velocity. By rearranging the Doppler equation, the calculated blood velocity is derived as follows:

$$v = \Delta f/\cos\theta \times c/2f_t.$$

The angle of incidence between the beam and the blood flow is not easily determined. Although a two-dimensional image of the blood vessel allows the echocardiographer to estimate the angle in the x- and y-planes, the orientation in the z-plane remains indeterminate. Assessment of the interrogation angle is further complicated by eccentrically directed blood flow, as in mitral regurgitation. Most Doppler systems default to a value of cos θ of 1, with the assumption that the echocardiographer has directed the ultrasound beam to be nearly parallel with the blood flow of interest. This approach has the advantages of stronger Doppler signals and a lower rate of errors as a consequence of the plateau shape of the cosine curve at angles of low incidence. Therefore, in clinical practice, the transducer should be positioned such that the beam and blood flow are nearly parallel for accurate velocity calculations. Figure 5.3 illustrates the basis for the clinical practice of requiring the beam angle to be within 30° of the direction of blood flow, so that the rate of angle-related errors remains less than 15%. The assumption that the orientation of the ultrasound beam is parallel to the blood flow leads to a common error in Doppler velocity calculations. *Because of the shape of the cosine curve, when the incident angle between the beam and the blood flow is greater than 30, the blood flow is markedly underestimated* (Figure 5.4). However, even the 30° standard may not be acceptable in certain conditions. For example, when very high velocities are interrogated, as in aortic stenosis, even a 15% underestimation will correspond to a large difference in velocity and may result in an underestimation of the severity of aortic stenosis.

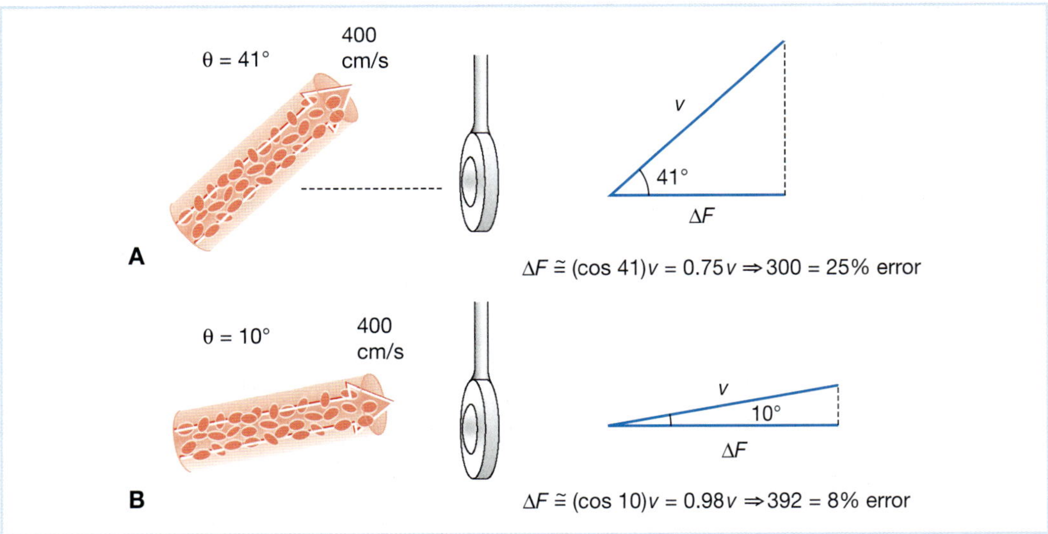

FIGURE 5.4 Underestimation of blood flow velocity with nonparallel beam orientation. A: With an angle of 41°, the vector component of blood flow velocity in the direction of the ultrasound beam is only 75% of the total. Therefore, a velocity estimation based on ΔF alone will lead to a clinically unacceptable underestimation of the true blood flow velocity of 25%. B: With an angle of 10°, the vector component of blood flow velocity in the direction of the ultrasound beam is 92%, and the practice of ignoring the cos θ leads to a clinically acceptable 8% underestimation of velocity. ΔF, difference between f_r and f_t; v, blood flow velocity; θ, angle of incidence between the orientation of the ultrasound beam and that of the blood flow.

Clinical Caveats in Transesophageal Echocardiographic Doppler Examinations

1. Positioning the transesophageal echocardiography (TEE) probe so that the orientation of the Doppler beam is parallel to the blood flow is often a significant challenge. Unlike the position of a transthoracic probe, which can be moved freely about the chest wall to achieve proper orientation, the position of the TEE probe is limited to the confines of the esophagus and stomach.
2. The standard views used for two-dimensional imaging are often inadequate for Doppler assessments. Optimal two-dimensional images are obtained by directing the beam perpendicular to the structure of interest to obtain strong, mirror-like reflections. Paradoxically, Doppler measurements are best obtained when the beam is parallel to the blood flow to avoid underestimates of blood flow velocity. The view that provides the best two-dimensional image of a structure typically provides only limited flow information and can result in a failure to detect abnormal flow. Figure 5.5 illustrates the application of this principle in examining the aortic valve.

Isolating the Doppler Frequency Shift

For the Doppler system to determine the frequency shift caused by red blood cells, it must first distinguish red cell–modulated echoes from all the other nonfrequency-shifted echoes created by reflections from tissue (Figure 5.6). This *demodulation process* is often accomplished by comparing the returning echoes with internal reference signals that are in phase and 90° out of phase with the transmitted signal, a process known as *quadrature demodulation.* Once the Doppler signal has been isolated, its frequency content can then be determined by means of the *fast Fourier transform (FFT)* technique. This approach transforms the demodulated Doppler signal into its individual frequency components. The process is analogous to identifying the

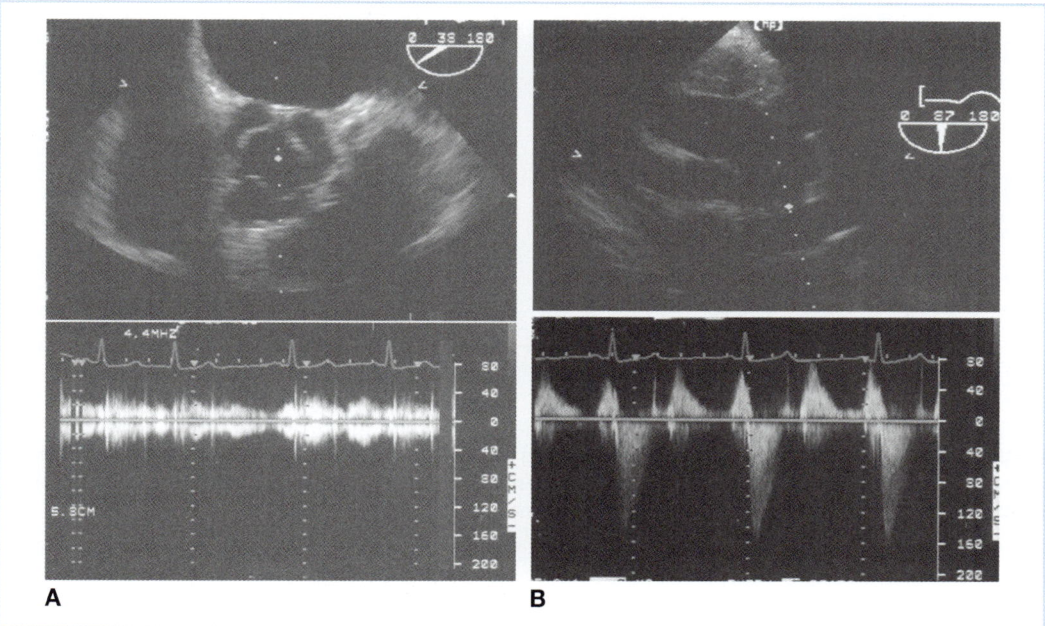

FIGURE 5.5 Comparison of views selected for two-dimensional imaging versus Doppler flow measurement. A: Two-dimensional echocardiography from the midesophageal aortic valve short-axis view (top) provides high-fidelity images of the valve leaflets and their excursion. Since the direction of blood flow is orthogonal to the ultrasound beam in this view, the CW Doppler measurement of blood flow velocity (bottom) will substantially underestimate blood flow velocity. B: After repositioning the probe to obtain the transgastric long-axis view (top), the direction of the ultrasound beam is parallel to the left ventricular outflow tract and ascending aorta, providing excellent CW measurements of blood flow velocity (bottom).

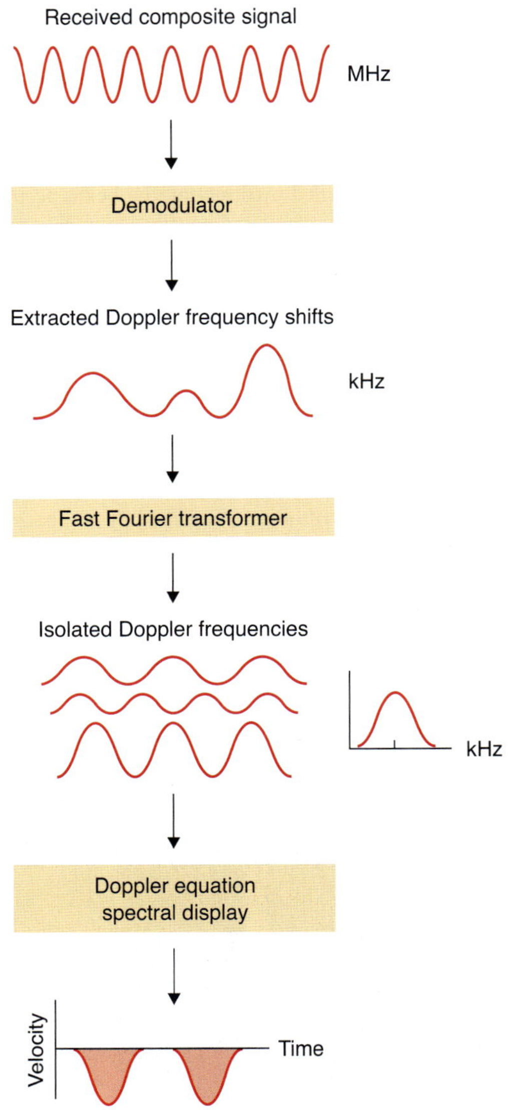

FIGURE 5.6 Looking for a needle in a haystack. Extracting the low-frequency, low-amplitude Doppler signal from the received composite signal is a technical challenge requiring several procedures, including demodulation and fast Fourier transform. Once isolated, the Doppler frequencies can be analyzed and displayed.

individual harmonics that comprise a musical chord. At each time point, the analysis provides the range of frequencies (ie, velocities) detected and their magnitude (ie, the number of red cells moving at this speed).

PRESENTATION OF DOPPLER DATA

Audible Broadcast

Blood flow in the heart and great vessels creates a Doppler frequency shift in the kilohertz (kHz) range, with a high-velocity aortic stenotic jet generating a Doppler frequency shift in the order of 20 kHz. Since these frequencies are within the audible range, most echocardiography machines provide a sound system that amplifies and broadcasts the signal to the operator. *By listening to the loudness and pitch of the broadcast Doppler frequencies, the echocardiographer can precisely position the Doppler beam to interrogate the desired flow signal.* Typically, the ideal location is identified when the signal reaches its highest frequency and greatest loudness. Soft, low-decibel signals indicate that the Doppler beam is misdirected and is only glancing at a small part of the blood flow. In addition, the texture and pitch of the Doppler signal are useful in diagnosis. For example, when transvalvular flow across the aortic valve is examined, a coarse, high-pitched signal is diagnostic of a high-velocity, turbulent jet caused by aortic stenosis and contrasts markedly with the smooth-sounding, low-pitched signals generated by the laminar flow in a normal aortic valve. The ability to use the audible Doppler signal to guide beam positioning is a favored technique of experienced echocardiographers, and the development of this skill remains a goal for all trainees.

Spectral Display

Presenting Doppler data as a time-velocity plot is known as a *spectral display* (Figure 5.7). At each point in time, the spectrum of velocities detected by the Fourier transformation is displayed. For blood flow measurements, the low-velocity signals emanating from myocardial motion are filtered and not displayed (the use of these "tissue Doppler" signals is presented in Chapters 3: Left Ventricular Systolic Performance and Pathology and 7: Echocardiographic Evaluation of Ventricular Diastolic Function). Frequencies with greater amplitude (loudness) are marked with brighter pixels. The excellent temporal resolution of the spectral display allows beat-to-beat assessment of blood flow and is the basis for the quantitative calculations of cardiovascular hemodynamics. Measurements of peak velocity, acceleration ($\Delta v/\Delta t$), and the velocity-time integral (represented by the area under the velocity-time plot from a single cardiac cycle) are examples of the many important measurements that are easily obtained from the spectral display (see Chapter 6: Quantitative Doppler and Hemodynamics for a detailed examination of the use of these measurements in clinical echocardiography).

Despite the ease with which velocity measurements are made from the spectral display, vigilance is required on the part of the echocardiographer. The measurements will be accurate only when the underlying principles of good Doppler technique have been followed. First, the Doppler beam must be properly positioned to interrogate the targeted blood flow. For example, small alterations in beam position determine whether the displayed spectral velocities represent a targeted high-frequency jet of mitral stenosis or the lower blood flow velocities found along its perimeter. Second, the direction of the Doppler beam must be

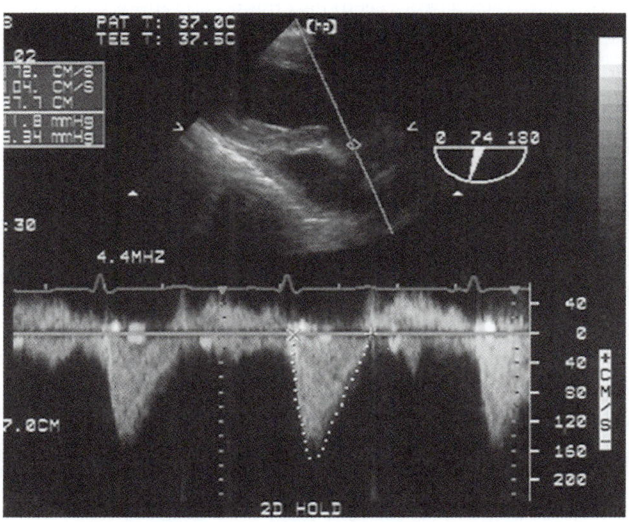

FIGURE 5.7 Doppler spectral display. Blood flow through the left ventricular outflow tract and aorta is captured using continuous-wave Doppler directed from the transgastric long-axis view. This time-velocity display shows the Doppler-calculated velocities on the *x*-axis, with flow toward the transducer as positive deflections and flow away from the transducer as negative deflections. Planimetry of the velocity waveform has been performed by the operator, and the machine's analysis package calculates the velocity-time integral and the mean and peak flow velocities.

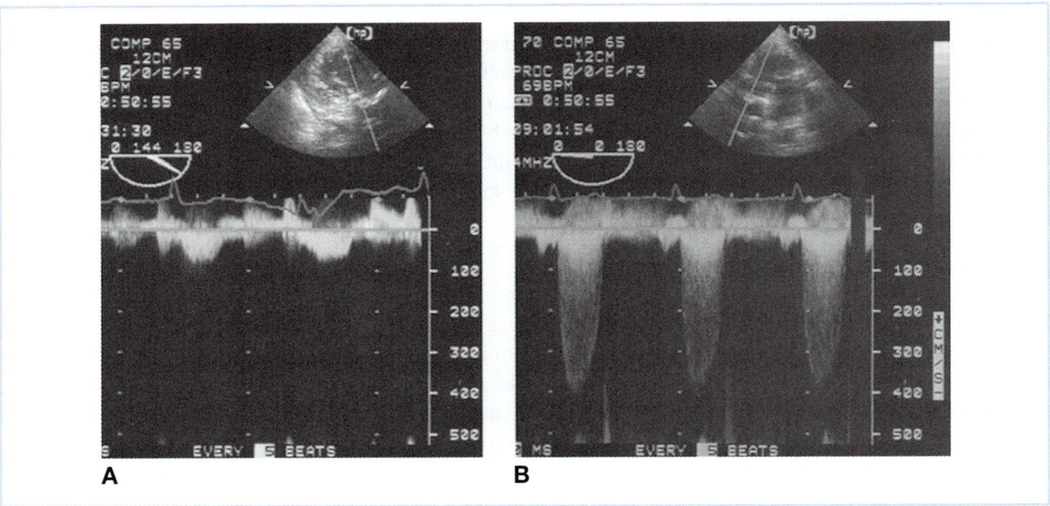

FIGURE 5.8 Hunting for the jet core. A: Despite high-quality two-dimensional imaging of the transgastric long-axis view, Doppler interrogation of the transvalvular flow fails to detect the high-velocity flow of aortic stenosis. The wispy signal waveform provides no clear definition of peak velocities. B: After adjustment of the probe position to obtain the deep transgastric long-axis view, the resulting Doppler interrogation detects a 400-cm/s high-velocity jet, revealing aortic stenosis. Note the potential for misdiagnosis if the echocardiographer bases the diagnosis on the initial signal obtained in (A).

parallel to the path of the targeted blood flow. Errors in diagnosis are often related to failure to meet these essential requirements.

Poor ultrasound technique can often be detected by an examination of the spectral display. High-quality signals result in a pattern commonly referred to as a *clean envelope*, denoted by a sharply demarcated border, bright pixels, and clear peaks. When these features are lacking, the echocardiographer should be reluctant to accept the data from the spectral display and improve the Doppler signal through alterations in probe position or imaging view (Figure 5.8). Inexplicably, seemingly minor alterations can resolve difficulties in obtaining a flow signal. In this regard, there is no substitute for perseverance and experience.

DOPPLER TECHNIQUES

Two Doppler techniques, *pulsed wave* and *continuous wave*, are commonly used to evaluate blood flow. A thorough understanding of the advantages and disadvantages of each technique is critical in selecting the one most appropriate for the clinical setting at hand.

In clinical practice, pulsed-wave (PW) and continuous-wave (CW) Doppler are frequently used in conjunction with two-dimensional imaging. The two-dimensional image is used to identify the area of interest and guide the echocardiographer in precisely localizing the sampling volume in a PW study or in directing the beam in a CW study.

Pulsed-Wave Doppler

The PW transducer uses a single crystal as both the emitter and the receiver of ultrasound waves. Like the pulsed-echo system described for two-dimensional imaging, the PW Doppler system transmits a short burst of ultrasound toward the target and then switches to receive mode to interpret the returning echoes. Since the speed of sound (c) in tissue is constant, the time delay for a signal to reach its target and return to the transducer depends solely on the distance (d) to the target:

$$\text{Time delay} = 2d/c.$$

Consequently, reflected signals from locations more distant from the transducer return after a greater time interval. The electronic circuitry of the PW transducer interprets returning echoes only after a predetermined time period has elapsed following the transmission of an ultrasound pulse. In this way, only those signals associated with a specific depth or location are selected for evaluation, a process known as *time gating.* It is important to remember that the transducer transmits a three-dimensional beam. Therefore, the small portion of reflected sound accepted by the time-gating process corresponds to a volume of blood at a specific location, called the *sample volume.* The pulse length, which equals the product of the wavelength and the number of cycles contained in each sound pulse, determines the length of the sample volume. The width and height of the sample volume are related to the transducer size, signal frequency, and beam focus.

Clinical Caveats for Pulsed-Wave Doppler

Since red cells scatter the ultrasound signal, the reflected Doppler signal returning to the transducer represents only a fraction of the transmitted signal. Therefore, the returning signal is much weaker than the strong specular reflections from tissue interfaces. Accordingly, the clinician faces a trade-off between good range resolution (ie, a small sample length) and an accurate determination of velocity. *In contrast to the preferred settings in two-dimensional echocardiography, in which axial resolution is a priority and the pulse length is kept very short, large Doppler sample volumes (length >10 mm) are preferred by most echocardiographers to improve the accuracy of the velocity measurement because they provide more wavelength for demodulation.* A more powerful Doppler signal is produced because the signal-to-noise ratio is increased.

In summary, PW Doppler allows the echocardiographer to select both the location and dimensions of the sample volume to determine blood flow velocity at a discrete location. The ability to select a sample volume from which to record blood velocities was a major advancement in the diagnostic capability of echocardiography.

Pulsed-Wave Doppler System Processing

The pulsed Doppler system uses a repeating pattern of ultrasound transmission and reception. After producing a short burst of ultrasound, it waits for a period of time, proportional to the selected distance, to receive the signal from the sample volume. The transducer then sends another burst of ultrasound, waits and receives, and so on. The rate at which the device repeatedly generates sound bursts is known as the *pulse repetition frequency (PRF).* The longer the PW system waits for the returning echoes, the lower the PRF. Since the speed of sound through tissue is a constant, the PRF is directly related to the depth of the sample volume. The PRF is analogous to the frame rate of a movie camera. Like the multiple frames on a roll of movie film, each ultrasound pulse interacts with the blood flow for a brief period of time, and just as a series of movie frames display motion, a series of pulsed cycles are consecutively analyzed to determine the blood flow. The demodulation process examines the returning echoes from a series of pulses to determine the Doppler frequency shift and calculate blood flow velocity.

Limitations of Pulsed-Wave Doppler

Since these Doppler data are collected intermittently, the maximal frequency and blood flow velocity that can be accurately measured by PW Doppler are limited. The maximal frequency, which equals one-half the PRF, is known as the *Nyquist limit.* Figure 5.9 illustrates the principle of the Nyquist limit with the example of an orbiting comet. A similar effect is seen in movie animation, in which a rapidly spinning wheel appears to spin backward because of the slow frame rate. At Doppler shifts above the Nyquist limit, analysis of the returning signal becomes ambiguous, so that the velocity is indeterminate. This ambiguous signal for frequencies above the Nyquist limit, known as *aliasing,* appears on the spectral display as a signal on the other side of the baseline, often referred to as *wraparound* (Figure 5.10). The intermittent sampling of the pulsed system can resolve only frequencies that are less than half the pulse repetition rate.

Maximizing Pulsed-Wave Velocity Measurements

The echocardiographer has several techniques available to maximize the velocity performance of a PW system:

1. The first clinical principle is to select the view that places the transducer closest to the sample volume. Lessening the target distance increases the PRF, thereby increasing the velocity that can be assessed.

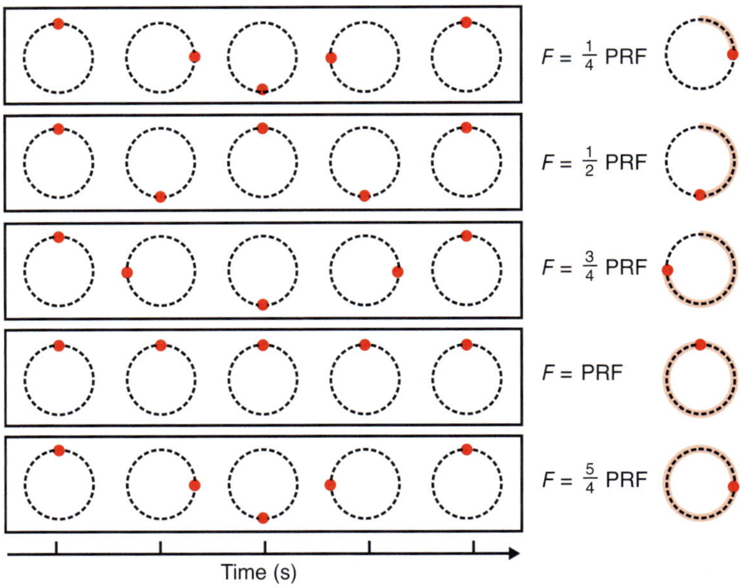

FIGURE 5.9 Nyquist illusions. The Nyquist limit of one-half the pulse repetition frequency (PRF) applies to any system based on intermittent observation. In this illustration, the position of the orbiting comet at each observation point is displayed. The orbiting velocity of the comet is progressively increased from the *top* to the *bottom* rows. At the low orbiting velocity of one-fourth PRF, the serial observations properly portray the comet as moving in a clockwise direction. As the speed of the comet is increased so that its orbiting velocity is three-fourth the PRF, it appears to be traveling counterclockwise. It appears to be moving not at all when its orbiting velocity equals the PRF. At five-fourth the PRF, it appears to be orbiting at the same speed as when it was traveling at the much slower speed of one-fourth the PRF.

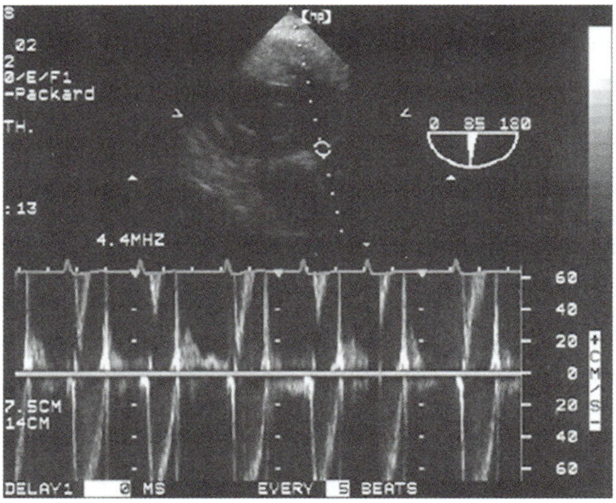

FIGURE 5.10 Alias artifact. Alias artifact appears once velocities exceed the Nyquist limit. In this example, the pulsed-wave Doppler sample volume is located in the left ventricular outflow tract, and when the peak velocities of the spectral signal exceed 70 cm/s, aliasing occurs and they appear on the opposite side of the baseline, a condition known as *wraparound*.

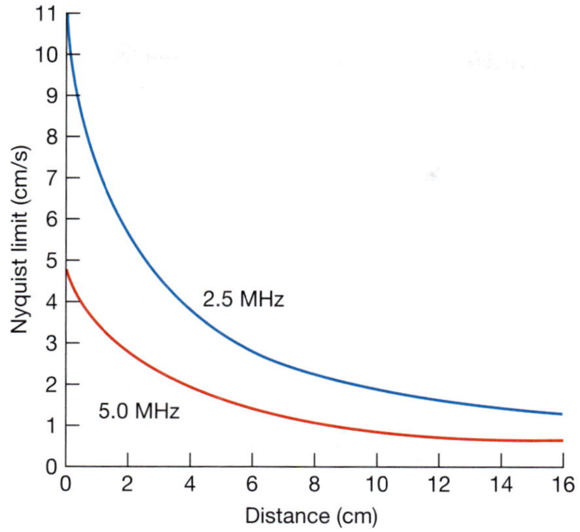

FIGURE 5.11 Effect of distance and frequency on the Nyquist limit. Two important variables under the echocardiographer's control that can be used to minimize the potential for aliasing in Doppler signals are target distance and transmitted frequency. As the transducer is moved closer to the target or the transmitted frequency is lowered, the pulsed-wave Nyquist limit rises substantially, allowing higher-velocity signals to be measured accurately.

2. The second clinical principle is to select a low-transmitted frequency. The lower-transmitted frequency has two major advantages:
   a. The modulated echo (f_r) will be of a lower frequency for any given blood velocity because $f_r = f_t + \Delta f$. Therefore, increased velocities can be measured without the aliasing that would be caused by a Doppler signal with a higher-transmitted frequency.
   b. Lower frequencies provide a stronger signal because they are less attenuated by tissue. This is important because Doppler signals are much weaker than those used for imaging. Figure 5.11 illustrates the importance of target distance and transmitted frequency to the velocity performance of a Doppler system.
3. The third clinical principle is to set the baseline of the spectral display to provide the greatest range of velocities in the direction of interest. Figure 5.12 illustrates the practical implications of baseline adjustment.

Echocardiography technology has also tried to address the velocity limitation of PW Doppler systems with the development of *high-frequency-pulsed Doppler*. This approach sacrifices some of the spatial resolution of the PW system in exchange for the ability to measure significantly faster flows. The principle of high-frequency-pulsed Doppler is to emit a second or third pulse signal before the first signal has returned. In this way, the PRF is doubled or tripled, and it becomes possible to calculate a greater maximal velocity. However, with high-frequency-pulsed Doppler, the operator cannot be sure that the reflected echoes have come from the intended target rather than from other targets located more proximally.

Despite technologic advancements, the Nyquist limit remains a major impediment to the measurement of high-velocity blood flows, such as those across stenotic valves and in congenital cardiac lesions, with PW Doppler. This limitation has led to an alternative approach for the Doppler assessment of high-velocity blood flows, which is CW Doppler.

Continuous-Wave Doppler

The CW Doppler technique avoids the maximal velocity limitation of PW systems. The transducer of a CW system is composed of two crystals, one continuously transmitting and the other continuously receiving the reflected ultrasound signal. With continuous reception of the Doppler signal, the Nyquist limit is not applicable, and blood flows with very high velocities can be recorded accurately. A CW transducer can measure velocities in excess of 7 m/s and is therefore useful in measuring the high-velocity flows associated

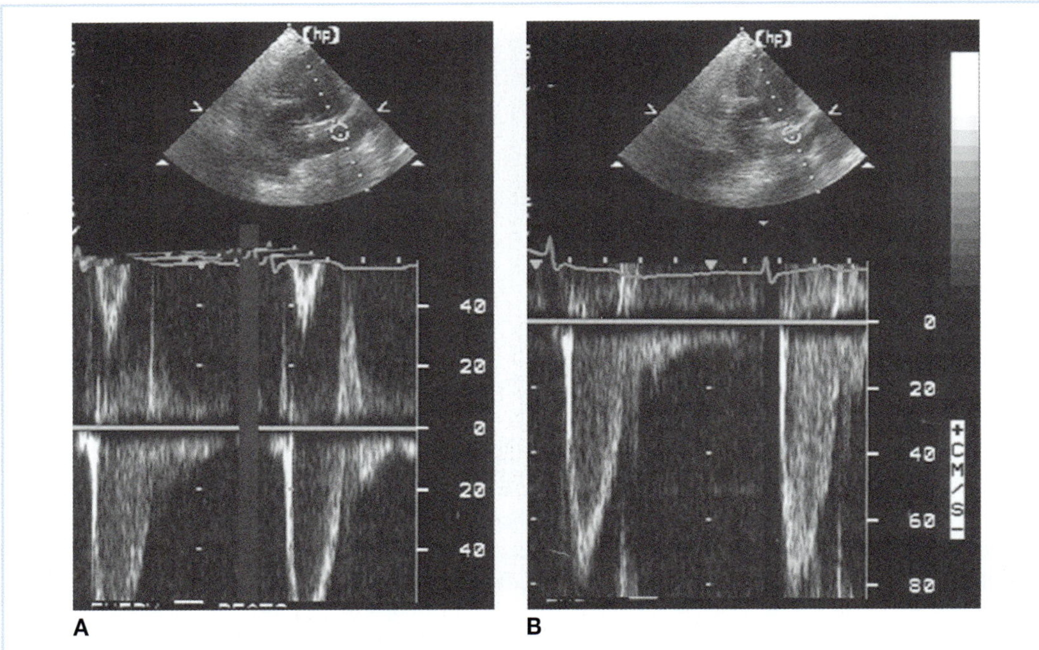

FIGURE 5.12 Effect of baseline setting on pulsed-wave Doppler aliasing. A: With the velocity baseline set in the mid-portion of the display, the signal aliases at 50 cm/s. B: The baseline has been adjusted to the upper portion of the display, which increases the Nyquist limit to more than 80 cm/s for flow away from the transducer and captures the spectral signal without aliasing.

with stenotic valvular disease. Other differences between the PW and CW techniques are important. Since the CW signal is not time-gated like the PW technique, the CW mode receives reflected signals from blood flow throughout its beam path. Unlike the clean envelope achieved with PW Doppler, the spectral display of CW Doppler is typically shaded with the multitude of velocities recorded along the beam path (Figure 5.13). Consequently, the use of CW Doppler is limited primarily to detecting the highest velocities along the beam path, represented by the edge of the spectral envelope.

Color Flow Mapping

Color flow mapping provides a dramatic display of both blood flow and cardiac anatomy. To achieve these remarkable images, the technique combines two-dimensional ultrasonic imaging and PW Doppler methods. The PW Doppler used for color flow mapping differs from that previously discussed in two important ways. First, instead of recording from a single, operator-selected sample volume, color flow mapping performs multiple PW sample determinations of velocity along the depth of each scan line. Multiple sample volume recordings are obtained along each scan line as the beam is swept through the sector. This approach provides flow data matched with the structural data obtained by two-dimensional imaging. The second difference is that the Doppler velocity data from each sample volume are color-coded and superimposed on top of the grayscale two-dimensional image. *In the most widely accepted color code, red indicates flow toward the transducer and blue indicates flow away from the transducer.* In addition to flow direction, flow velocity alters the color map. Increasing flow velocities are displayed in various hues; high-velocity flow toward the transducer is displayed as yellow, and high-velocity flow away from the transducer is displayed as cyan. Flow with directional variance, as in areas of turbulence, is displayed as green.

The ability to provide a real-time, integrated display of flow and structural information makes color flow Doppler useful for assessing valvular function, aortic dissection, and congenital heart abnormalities. However, several important caveats to its use in the clinical setting must be noted. Since it relies on PW Doppler measurements, color flow mapping is susceptible to alias artifacts. In fact, *color flow will alias at a lower*

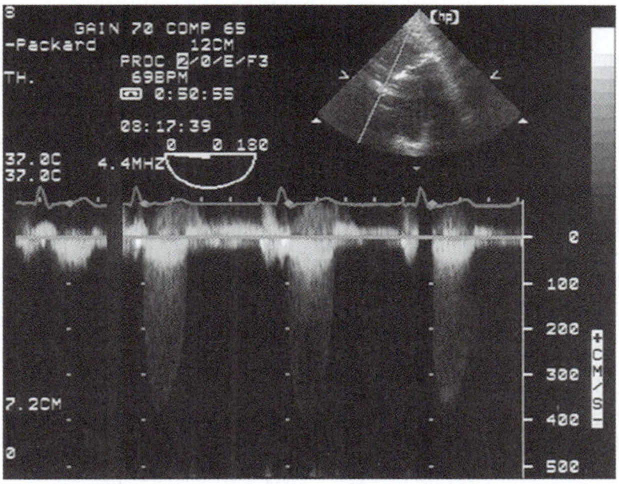

FIGURE 5.13 Continuous-wave spectral signal. Whereas pulsed-wave Doppler obtains targeted sample volume recordings, the continuous-wave system detects blood flow along the entire beam path. Top: In this example, the Doppler beam was positioned from the deep transgastric long-axis view. Bottom: The resulting spectral signal shows two distinct peaks, a pattern often referred to as a *double envelope*. The major peak at 400 cm/s is the high-velocity jet caused by aortic stenosis recorded from that portion of the beam in the aorta. The minor peak of 100 cm/s represents the blood velocity in the left ventricular outflow tract.

velocity than a conventional PW device because a part of the signal must be used for image generation, and this effectively decreases the PRF. Aliasing in the color flow map is illustrated in Figure 5.14. At the extreme of accurate velocity measurement (eg, bright yellow for flow toward the transducer), progressively increasing flow rates appear cyan, then dark blue, and then dark red. In a high-velocity jet, several cycles of color aliases can occur, which appear as a tiger stripe pattern in hues of red and blue. Because of the complex acquisition of multiple Doppler samples and the sharing of acquisition time with the imaging processor, the velocities

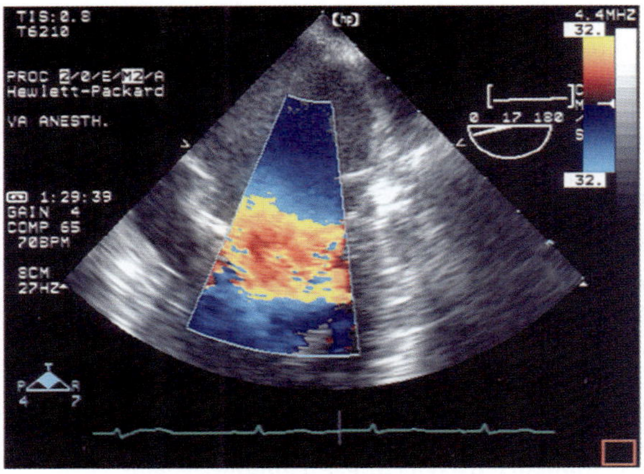

FIGURE 5.14 Aliasing of color display. Blood flow through the mitral valve (midesophageal four-chamber view) during early diastole results in aliasing in the color flow mapper. Flow velocity accelerates in the left atrium as blood is funneled to the mitral valve orifice, shown as the color code of dark blue transitioning to light blue, and reaches 32 cm/s (the Nyquist limit), as seen on the color bar. As a result, aliasing signals are coded bright yellow, then red, as the velocity reaches a maximum at the level of the leaflet tips. Once in the left ventricle, the blood flow decelerates to fall below the Nyquist limit and is again appropriately coded blue by the echocardiographic system.

displayed by the color flow mapper lack the fidelity of a conventional PW device. Color flow mapping neither measures blood flow velocity nor tracks alterations in velocity through the cardiac cycle with the precision of a conventional Doppler device. *Because of these limitations, the color flow mapper is often used to identify a flow abnormality that is subsequently characterized by a conventional Doppler approach.*

SUMMARY

Doppler echocardiography has greatly expanded the diagnostic capabilities of clinical echocardiography. Quantitative measurements of blood velocity derived from the spectral display of PW and CW Doppler signals are widely used to characterize systolic and diastolic cardiac performance and valve function. Color flow mapping allows the visualization of cardiac blood flow. The broad clinical applications of Doppler echocardiography are described in detail in the next chapters. The clinician must remain mindful of the underlying principles of good technique to obtain optimal Doppler signals and avoid incorrect diagnoses related to erroneous measurements.

SUGGESTED READINGS

Hatle L, Angelsen B. *Doppler Ultrasound in Cardiology*. Lea & Febiger; 1985.

Nishimura RA, Miller FA, Callahan MJ, et al. Doppler echocardiography: theory, instrumentation, technique, and application. *Mayo Clin Proc.* 1985;60:321-343.

Quinones MA, Otto CM, Stoddard M, et al. Recommendations for quantification of Doppler echocardiography: a report from the Doppler quantification task force of the nomenclature and standards committee of the American Society of Echocardiography. *J Am Soc Echocardiogr.* 2002;15:167-184.

Weyman A. *Principles and Practice of Echocardiography*. Lea & Febiger; 1994.

QUESTIONS

1. Which of the following statements about Doppler echocardiography is true?
A. The received Doppler signal is stronger than the two-dimensional signal.
B. Christian Doppler was a Swedish echocardiographer.
C. Doppler velocity measurements are based on the change in the signal's frequency.
D. Doppler velocity measurements are based on reflections from plasma.

2. In clinical practice, the Doppler frequency shift is:
A. Typically 2.5 to 7.5 MHz
B. Less than 1 MHz
C. Not relevant to the Nyquist limit
D. Negative for flow directed perpendicular to the ultrasound beam

3. The Doppler frequency shift is affected by all of the following *except*:
A. Transmitted frequency
B. Blood velocity
C. Incident angle of the ultrasound beam
D. Distance of the target from the transducer

4. Fast Fourier analysis is applied to:
A. PW but not CW Doppler signals
B. Identify the Doppler frequency shift.
C. Identify the component frequencies of the Doppler frequency shift.
D. Extract noise from weaker Doppler signals.

5. All of the following statements are true of PW Doppler *except*:
A. Requires two separate crystals
B. Is useful to identify blood flow in a particular area
C. Has a limited maximum velocity that can be measured
D. Is the basis for color flow Doppler

6. Techniques useful to correct an alias signal include all the following *except*:
A. Adjust baseline.
B. Position transducer closer to target.
C. Increase transmitted frequency.
D. Use high-frequency-pulsed Doppler.

7. The Nyquist limit is directly related to:
A. Blood flow velocity
B. Pressure gradient
C. PRF
D. Red cell mass

8. Which of the following statements about color flow Doppler is true?
A. It is susceptible to aliasing.
B. It is a good choice for measuring high blood velocities.
C. It is based on CW technology.
D. It provides nonquantitative information.

9. Demodulation:
A. Filters out noise in the Doppler signal
B. Identifies the Doppler shift
C. Is not necessary for color flow Doppler
D. Is not necessary for CW Doppler

10. A spectral display with sharp, dense edges:
A. Is diagnostic of stenotic lesions
B. Suggests echoes from a strong reflector such as a nearby calcified valve
C. Assures that the beam is parallel to blood flow
D. Suggests proper interrogation of blood flow

11. Increasing distance will increase the Nyquist limit.
A. True
B. False

12. Which of the following is likely in the case of a double envelope spectral signal obtained from the transgastric long-axis (TG LAX) view with peak velocities of 115 cm/s?
A. Severe aortic stenosis is present.
B. Fractional area change of 55%
C. Bicuspid aortic valvular disease is present.
D. Subaortic stenosis is present.

13. Which of the following increases accuracy in velocity measurements of subpulmonic artery blood flow in a patient with pulmonic stenosis from the upper esophageal (UE) aortic arch short-axis view (SAX) view?
A. The selected sample volume should have a length greater than 10 mm.
B. Range resolution should be adjusted to high.
C. CW Doppler should be employed.
D. The imaging array should be adjusted to 0° to obtain the UE aortic arch LAX view.

14. In obtaining blood velocity measurements of the right ventricular outflow tract using PW Doppler, the angle of incidence is 70°. The resulting measurement:
A. Will display blood flow in the opposite direction of true blood flow
B. Will underestimate blood flow by approximately 70%
C. Will underestimate blood flow by approximately 30%
D. Will be more accurate using the color flow Doppler setting

15. All the following are true concerning color flow Doppler *except*:
A. High-velocity flow away from the transducer can appear dark red.
B. Color flow Doppler displays B-mode acquired images.
C. Color flow Doppler uses pulse-wave technology.
D. Turbulent flow is displayed as bands of red, yellow, and blue.

16. As per the Doppler equation, the difference between the reflected and received frequency is inversely related to the cosine of the angle of incidence between the ultrasound beam and blood flow.
A. True
B. False

17. Time gating:
A. Filters out low-frequency signals
B. Filters out high-frequency signals
C. Requires a fixed speed of sound
D. Selects a defined distance from the transducer face

18. Compared to PW Doppler, CW Doppler can more accurately measure high blood flow velocities because:
A. It uses two transducers rather than one.
B. It uses M-mode technology.
C. It time gates the signal.
D. It uses high-frequency signal.

19. The color flow map is set at +32 cm/s. Blood flow traveling away from the transducer at 77 cm/s will appear:
A. Green
B. Blue
C. Red
D. As banded colors

20. The color flow map is set at +32 cm/s. Blood traveling perpendicular to the probe at 77 cm/s will appear as:
A. Green
B. Blue
C. Red
D. Black

21. CW Doppler interrogation of ascending aortic blood flow from the TG LAX view in a patient with known history of high gradient aortic stenosis shows a peak velocity of 80 cm/s. This finding most likely represents:
A. Wraparound
B. Nyquist limit error
C. Left ventricular outflow tract (LVOT) blood flow
D. Mitral inflow

22. Modulation describes:
A. Alterations in the frequency of ultrasound signals
B. Process to determine the frequency shift of reflected ultrasound
C. The breakdown of a complex waveform into coherent components
D. The velocity-time integral

23. Nyquist limit increases with:
A. High-frequency, near-field imaging
B. Low-frequency, near-field imaging
C. High-frequency, far-field imaging
D. Low-frequency, far-field imaging

24. Doppler frequency shift decreases with:
A. CW Doppler
B. Lower-frequency signals
C. Imaging in air-filled medium versus blood
D. Increasing gain

25. A beam orientation of 40° off parallel from blood flow will result in:
A. Approximately 25% velocity underestimation compared to parallel
B. Approximately 50% velocity underestimation compared to parallel
C. Approximately 80% velocity underestimation compared to parallel
D. Approximately 100% velocity underestimation compared to parallel

26. Characteristics of an optimized CW Doppler signal necessarily include all of the following *except*:
A. Sharply demarcated border
B. Bright pixels
C. Clear peaks
D. Clear inner envelope

27. Imaging from the midesophageal aortic valve short-axis (ME AV SAX) view shows leaflet pathology consistent with aortic stenosis. Which of the following is the best choice to measure associated blood flow velocities:
A. Color flow Doppler from ME AV SAX
B. Rotate imaging array 90° to obtain the ME LAX view.
C. Apply PW Doppler from the deep TG LAX view.
D. Obtain the TG LAX view.

28. In typical practice, Doppler sample volumes:
A. Equal 1/2 of transmitted wavelength
B. Are minimized to reduce aliasing
C. Exceed the two-dimensional pulse length
D. Equal color flow Doppler window

29. High-frequency-pulsed Doppler:
A. Improves spatial resolution
B. Utilizes higher-transmitted frequencies
C. Interrogates velocities proximal to the target sample volume
D. Has a PRF similar to CW Doppler

30. With color flow imaging, blood flow of the carotid artery:
A. Appears red
B. Appears blue
C. Appears black
D. Varies with probe angulation

ANSWERS

1. **Correct Answer: C.**
Rationale: Doppler echocardiography measures blood flow velocity by detecting changes in the frequency of the reflected ultrasound waves. When blood cells move toward or away from the transducer, the frequency of the returning signal shifts. The Doppler equation uses this frequency shift to calculate the blood flow velocity. Option A is incorrect because Doppler signals are generally weaker than two-dimensional signals. Doppler signals rely on reflections from small moving particles like red blood cells, which produce lower amplitude signals. Option B is incorrect because Christian Doppler was an Austrian physicist, not an echocardiographer. He first described the Doppler effect in 1842. Option D is incorrect because Doppler measurements are based on reflections from red blood cells, not plasma, as plasma itself is generally nonreflective to ultrasound waves.

2. **Correct Answer: B.**
Rationale: The Doppler frequency shift refers to the change in frequency between the transmitted and the reflected ultrasound waves. Ultrasound systems used in echocardiography operate at a much higher frequency, typically 2.5 to 7.5 MHz for the transmitted signal. However, the actual frequency shift due to blood flow is much smaller, generally in the range of a few kilohertz to less than 1 MHz. The Doppler frequency shift is highly relevant to the Nyquist limit, which determines the maximum detectable velocity before aliasing occurs. When blood flow is perpendicular to the ultrasound beam, there is no Doppler shift detected by the transducer (zero frequency shift), not a negative frequency shift. The Doppler effect is most accurate when the beam is parallel to flow.

3. **Correct Answer: D.**
Rationale: Options A, B, and C are all components of the Doppler equation. The Doppler shift primarily depends on motion (such as blood flow) and the angle of insonation, not the distance between the red blood cells and the transducer. While the strength of the reflected signal decreases with distance, the frequency shift itself remains unaffected by how far away the moving target is.

4. **Correct Answer: C.**
Rationale: FFT is a mathematical technique used in Doppler ultrasound to break down complex signals into their individual frequency components. Doppler ultrasound measures blood flow velocity by detecting frequency shifts in reflected sound waves. However, because blood flow is not uniform, different regions move at varying speeds, creating a range of frequency shifts. FFT processes the Doppler signal to separate and display these individual frequency components, producing a spectral Doppler waveform that provides detailed information about blood flow patterns, turbulence, and velocity distribution. FFT can be used in both PW and CW Doppler to analyze frequency shifts. Option B is partially correct but too broad. FFT doesn't just identify the shift; it decomposes it into its component frequencies, allowing for precise spectral Doppler analysis. Option D is incorrect. While FFT helps distinguish different frequency components, its primary function is not noise reduction but frequency analysis.

5. **Correct Answer: A.**
Rationale: PW Doppler uses a single crystal that alternates between sending and receiving ultrasound signals. PW Doppler is designed to measure blood flow velocity at a specific location by sending short bursts (pulses) of ultrasound and then waiting for the reflected signal to return. Since it uses only one transducer element (or crystal) for both transmission and reception, it can precisely sample blood flow at a chosen depth. PW Doppler is subject to the Nyquist limit, which restricts the highest velocity it can measure before aliasing occurs. Color Doppler imaging is essentially an extension of PW Doppler, using multiple sample volumes to create a color-coded map of blood flow direction and velocity.

6. **Correct Answer: C.**
Rationale: Aliasing in Doppler ultrasound occurs when the Doppler frequency shift exceeds half the PRF, known as the Nyquist limit, causing the displayed velocities to "wrap around" and appear incorrectly. To correct aliasing, an echocardiographer aims either to reduce the magnitude of the Doppler

shift or to increase the Nyquist limit. For example, adjusting the baseline shifts the zero-velocity line on the Doppler display, effectively expanding the range available for displaying velocities before aliasing occurs and making high-velocity flows easier to interpret. Similarly, positioning the transducer closer to the target reduces the travel distance for the ultrasound pulse, which allows the system to use a higher PRF; this increased PRF raises the Nyquist limit and enables the accurate measurement of larger Doppler shifts. Using high-frequency pulsed Doppler also supports a higher PRF, thereby increasing the Nyquist limit and further reducing the likelihood of aliasing. In contrast, increasing the transmitted frequency would directly raise the Doppler shift (since the shift is proportional to the transmitted frequency), making aliasing more likely rather than correcting it.

7. **Correct Answer: C.**
Rationale: The Nyquist limit represents the maximum Doppler frequency that can be accurately measured without aliasing, and it is defined as half of the PRF. Although blood flow velocity (Option A) influences the Doppler frequency shift observed in ultrasound, it does not determine the Nyquist limit. Similarly, while pressure gradient (Option B) can be estimated from blood flow velocity through the Bernoulli equation, it does not directly impact the Nyquist limit. Furthermore, red cell mass (Option D) may affect the strength or quality of the Doppler signal but has no bearing on the maximum measurable frequency shift.

8. **Correct Answer: A.**
Rationale: Color flow Doppler is known to be susceptible to aliasing. This susceptibility arises because color flow Doppler is based on PW technology, where the Doppler shift is measured relative to the PRF, limiting the measurable velocity range. Option B is incorrect because color flow Doppler is not ideal for measuring high blood velocities; its PW nature makes it prone to aliasing when the velocity exceeds the Nyquist limit. Option C is also incorrect since color flow Doppler relies on PW rather than CW technology—the latter is more suitable for high velocities but lacks range resolution. Finally, Option D is not true because, although color flow Doppler primarily provides qualitative data in the form of a color-coded visual display, it is not devoid of quantitative information. In practice, clinicians can extract numerical data, such as estimated velocity values, from color flow images.

9. **Correct Answer: B**
Rationale: Demodulation is the process of extracting the Doppler frequency shift from the high-frequency ultrasound signal and converting it into a lower-frequency signal that can be easily analyzed and displayed. It does this by comparing the returning echoes with internal reference signals that are in phase and 90° out of phase with the transmitted signal. The primary role of demodulation is to identify the Doppler shift (Option B), which indicates the movement of blood cells. While demodulation may incidentally reduce some noise, its main function is not noise filtering (Option A). In addition, demodulation is essential for both color flow Doppler and CW Doppler techniques, meaning it is necessary for each (making Options C and D incorrect).

10. **Correct Answer: D.**
Rationale: A clear and well-defined display shows that the ultrasound system's settings—such as gain, sample volume placement, and PRF—are optimized to capture the full range of blood velocities accurately. Option A is incorrect because while stenotic lesions can alter the spectral waveform, a sharp spectral display by itself is not diagnostic of stenosis. Option B is not accurate since echoes from strong reflectors, such as a calcified valve, typically produce artifacts rather than the well-defined spectral edges associated with optimal blood flow interrogation. Option C is also incorrect; although aligning the beam parallel to blood flow can improve the quality of the spectral display, the presence of sharp, dense edges does not necessarily ensure proper beam alignment.

11. **Correct Answer: B.**
Rationale: The Nyquist limit in Doppler ultrasound is defined as one-half of the PRF, which is the rate at which ultrasound pulses are emitted. The PRF is determined by the depth of the target; as the distance increases, the ultrasound system must wait longer for echoes to return before sending the next pulse, thereby lowering the PRF. A lower PRF means that the Nyquist limit is also reduced, not increased.

12. **Correct Answer: B.**
In the TG LAX view, a double envelope spectral display typically shows two distinct signals: one envelope represents the blood flow velocity in the LVOT and the other represents the peak velocity through the narrowest portion, along the axis of the aortic valve. In this case, the peak velocity is 115 cm/s, which is relatively low and indicates that there is no significant obstruction at the aortic valve. This finding is consistent with normal blood flow, which is further supported by a fractional area change of 55% (Option B), suggesting preserved left ventricular systolic function. Option A, indicating severe aortic stenosis, is unlikely because severe stenosis would produce much higher velocities. Option C, relating to bicuspid aortic valvular disease, is not confirmed or excluded solely by this velocity measurement. Option D, suggesting subaortic stenosis, would also typically result in elevated velocities. Therefore, the data best support Option B.

13. **Correct Answer: A.**
Rationale: Using a sample volume longer than 10 mm captures a broader section of the blood flow, which helps average out the variability caused by turbulent flow in pulmonic stenosis. Option B—adjusting the range resolution to high—mainly improves spatial detail rather than directly enhancing the accuracy of velocity measurements. Option C, employing CW Doppler, is not appropriate here because it does not allow for precise localization of the sample volume (range resolution). Option D, which involves adjusting the imaging array to 0° to obtain the UE aortic arch long-axis (LAX) view, is incorrect because it changes the imaging plane entirely; the goal is to optimize the measurement from the UE aortic arch SAX view, not to switch to LAX.

14. **Correct Answer: B.**
Rationale: When using PW Doppler to measure blood velocity in the right ventricular outflow tract at an angle of incidence of 70°, the Doppler equation—which relies on the cosine of the angle between the ultrasound beam and the direction of blood flow—becomes critical. At 70°, the cosine value is approximately 0.34, meaning that only about 34% of the true velocity is detected; in other words, the measurement underestimates the true velocity by roughly 70%. Option A is incorrect because although a very high angle can sometimes reverse the sign (indicating flow direction), a 70° angle still yields a positive cosine. Option D is not valid because using the color flow Doppler setting does not correct for the error introduced by the steep angle of incidence; the fundamental cosine dependence remains the same regardless of the Doppler modality.

15. **Correct Answer: D.**
Rationale: Color flow Doppler is a technique that overlays color-coded blood flow information on B-mode images using pulse-wave technology. In Option A, it is true that high-velocity flow away from the transducer can appear as dark red, depending on the system's color scale. However, in the most widely accepted color code, red indicates flow toward the transducer and blue indicates flow away. Option B is also correct because color flow Doppler is superimposed on the B-mode images, providing anatomic context alongside flow data. Option C is accurate since the technology relies on pulse-wave sampling to generate the color map of blood flow. Option D is false: turbulent flow is usually depicted as a chaotic mosaic of colors resulting from aliasing, where the mix of colors reflects the complexity and variability of the flow.

16. **Correct Answer: B.**
Rationale: The Doppler equation states that the frequency shift (the difference between the reflected and transmitted frequencies) is directly proportional to the cosine of the angle of incidence between the ultrasound beam and the blood flow.

17. **Correct Answer: D.**
Rationale: Time gating is a technique that isolates echoes from a specific depth by selecting a defined time interval after the transmitted pulse. Since the time it takes for an echo to return is directly related to the distance from the transducer (given a known speed of sound in tissue, 1,540 m/s), time gating effectively selects a defined distance from the transducer face (Option D). Option A is incorrect because time gating does not filter out low-frequency signals, and Option B is not correct because it does not filter out high-frequency signals either. While Option C mentions a fixed speed of sound, this

assumption is simply used to calculate distance from the time delay and is not a defining requirement of time gating.

18. Correct Answer: A.
Rationale: CW Doppler can more accurately measure high blood flow velocities compared to PW Doppler because it uses two transducers—one for transmitting and one for receiving ultrasound signals (Option A). This dual-transducer setup allows CW Doppler to continuously capture the Doppler frequency shift without interruption. This avoids the aliasing issues that arise in PW Doppler due to its inherent PRF limitations. In PW Doppler, time gating restricts the measurement to a specific depth and creates a maximum limit, the Nyquist limit, beyond which high velocities cannot be accurately recorded. Option B is incorrect because the use of M-mode technology is not related to measuring high blood flow velocities in this context. Option C is also incorrect, as time gating is a characteristic of PW Doppler, not CW Doppler, and it actually limits its ability to accurately measure high velocities. Option D is not accurate because the key factor is the continuous, ungated nature of its signal acquisition and not the frequency of the signal.

19. Correct Answer: B.
Rationale: In color flow Doppler imaging, the baseline velocity setting of ±32 cm/s determines the range within which velocities are mapped according to standard color conventions—typically, red indicates flow toward the transducer and blue indicates flow away. Even though the measured blood flow velocity of 77 cm/s exceeds the baseline threshold, the color assignment is still based on the *direction* of flow. Since the flow is moving away from the transducer, it will be displayed as blue, making Option B the correct answer. Options A and C are incorrect because green generally indicates turbulence and red is reserved for flow toward the transducer. Option D (banded colors) refers to the discrete bands or stripes of alternating colors that are seen in aliasing, which is not applicable in this case.

20. Correct Answer: D.
Rationale: In color flow Doppler, the color displayed is determined by the Doppler frequency shift, which is calculated using the cosine of the angle between the ultrasound beam and the blood flow. When blood flow is perpendicular to the probe, the angle is 90° and the cosine of 90° is zero. This means no Doppler shift is detected, regardless of the actual velocity—in this case, 77 cm/s. Since no shift is detected, the system does not assign any color, and the area appears black.

21. Correct Answer: C.
Rationale: CW Doppler interrogation from the TG LAX view in a patient with severe aortic stenosis should typically show a high-velocity jet through the stenotic valve. A measured peak velocity of only 80 cm/s is much too low for such a jet, which should be several meters per second. This suggests that the Doppler beam is instead capturing the slower blood flow in the LVOT. Wraparound (Option A) refers to aliasing artifacts seen with PW Doppler, and Nyquist limit error (Option B) is not an issue with CW Doppler. Mitral inflow (Option D) would have a distinct pattern with E and A waves.

22. Correct Answer: A.
Rationale: Modulation in ultrasound refers to the alterations in the frequency of the ultrasound signals caused by the Doppler effect. Option B describes the process of determining the frequency shift from reflected ultrasound, which is more accurately called demodulation. Option C refers to the breakdown of a complex waveform into its component frequencies—a process typically performed by the FFT rather than modulation. Option D, the velocity-time integral, is a measurement that reflects the distance blood travels during a cardiac cycle and is unrelated to the concept of modulation.

23. Correct Answer: B.
Rationale: The Nyquist limit—the maximum velocity measurable without aliasing—is half the PRF. In near-field imaging, the imaging depth is shallow, so echoes return quickly, allowing the system to use a higher PRF and thereby increasing the Nyquist limit. Additionally, the Doppler shift for a given blood flow velocity is directly proportional to the transmitted frequency; using a low-frequency transducer produces a smaller Doppler shift compared to a high-frequency one. This means that for the same PRF, a lower-frequency setting allows a higher

measurable velocity before aliasing occurs. Combining these factors, low-frequency, near-field imaging (Option B) results in a higher Nyquist limit.

24. Correct Answer: B.
Rationale: The Doppler frequency shift is given by the equation:

$\Delta f = v \times \cos\theta \times 2 f_t / c.$

This equation shows that the Doppler frequency shift is directly proportional to the transmitted frequency. Therefore, when lower-frequency signals are used, the resulting Doppler shift is smaller for a given blood flow velocity. Option A refers to the type of Doppler used (CW Doppler) which does not inherently alter the frequency shift. Option C refers to imaging in different media (air-filled vs blood) which affects sound propagation but not directly the proportionality of the Doppler shift to the transmitted frequency. Option D (increasing gain) only amplifies the signal without altering its frequency content.

25. Correct Answer: A.
Rationale: In Doppler ultrasound, the measured velocity is proportional to the cosine of the angle between the ultrasound beam and the blood flow direction. When the beam is perfectly parallel to the flow (0°), the cosine is 1, and the true velocity is accurately measured. However, if the beam is 40° off parallel, the cosine of 40° is approximately 0.77, meaning that only about 77% of the true velocity is recorded. This results in an underestimation of roughly 23%—which is approximately a 25% underestimation compared to a parallel alignment.

26. Correct Answer: D.
Rationale: An optimized CW Doppler signal is characterized by a well-defined outer border, bright pixels, and clear peaks that depict the maximum velocities. The sharply demarcated border (Option A) defines the flow envelope, bright pixels (Option B) ensure the signal is easily distinguished, and clear peaks (Option C) indicate the highest velocities. An inner envelope (Option D), which can be part of a double envelope signal, is not a required characteristic because it may represent lower-velocity components and is not always present.

27. Correct Answer: D.
Rationale: To accurately measure blood flow velocities associated with aortic stenosis, the Doppler beam must be as parallel as possible to blood flow. The ME AV SAX view is useful for assessing leaflet pathology but does not provide the proper alignment for velocity measurements. Color Doppler in this view (Option A) can show turbulence but is not suitable for precise velocity assessment. Rotating to the ME LAX view (Option B) improves alignment slightly but is still suboptimal for parallel alignment to blood flow. Using PW Doppler from the deep TG LAX view (Option C) is not ideal because PW Doppler cannot measure the high velocities seen in stenosis. The TG LAX view (Option D) is the best choice because it aligns the ultrasound beam more parallel to the stenotic jet, allowing for accurate velocity measurement using CW Doppler.

28. Correct Answer: C.
Rationale: In Doppler ultrasound, the sample volume refers to the specific region from which returning echoes are analyzed to measure blood flow velocity. The sample volume needs to be larger than just a single ultrasound pulse to collect enough data for accurate velocity measurements. Option A is incorrect because the sample volume is not directly related to the wavelength. The wavelength affects Doppler frequency shifts but does not define the physical size of the sample volume. Option B is incorrect because aliasing in Doppler ultrasound is primarily controlled by adjusting the PRF and the Doppler shift frequency, not necessarily by minimizing the sample volume. Option D is also incorrect because the sample volume in spectral Doppler is independent of the color flow Doppler window, which is a broader region used for qualitative flow assessment rather than precise velocity measurements.

29. Correct Answer: C.
Rationale: Pulsed Doppler has aliasing limitations due to its dependence on the PRF, which determines how frequently pulses are sent and received. To avoid this, a high-frequency pulsed Doppler system often detects velocities that are closer (proximal) to the target sample volume, making Option C correct. This means that the actual measured

velocities may come from areas just before the intended sample region due to range ambiguity and potential signal overlap.
Option A is incorrect because while higher frequencies can improve spatial resolution in imaging, high-frequency pulsed Doppler refers to PRF, not the transmitted frequency. Option B is also incorrect because "high frequency" in this context refers to PRF, not the actual transmitted frequency of the ultrasound waves. Option D is incorrect because pulsed Doppler uses discrete pulses, while CW Doppler has an infinitely high PRF.

30. Correct Answer: D.
Rationale: Color Doppler imaging assigns colors based on blood flow direction relative to the transducer. Typically, flow toward the probe appears red, while flow away appears blue, but this depends on the probe's angle. If the angle changes, the perceived color may shift. When the beam is perpendicular to the vessel, or 90°, no Doppler shift is detected and blood may appear black. Since the displayed color is not fixed and varies with angulation, D is the most accurate answer.

6 Quantitative Doppler and Hemodynamics

Benjamin Kogelschatz, Dai-Yin Lu, Ethan Tumarkin, John Ryan, and Satvik Ramakrishna

Doppler ultrasound, through its determination of blood flow velocities, has proven an immensely valuable tool to obtain quantitative hemodynamic assessments. Cardiac output, flows within the great vessels, the extent of valvular disease, intracardiac pressures and shunts, and systolic and diastolic dysfunction are just a sampling of the assessments available with Doppler techniques. Transesophageal echocardiography (TEE) provides access to a range of imaging windows, which in some cases, enables more precise measurements than transthoracic echocardiography, while in other cases provides a useful adjunct to surface imaging. The objective of this chapter is to survey the multiples uses of Doppler ultrasound in TEE for the quantitative assessment of hemodynamics.

VOLUMETRIC FLOW CALCULATIONS

Stroke Volume and Cardiac Output

Doppler Ultrasound Concepts and Volumetric Flow

Clinically, two of the most valuable hemodynamic markers are stroke volume (SV) and cardiac output (CO). When compared to thermodilution, numerous studies have shown that echocardiography can provide accurate estimates of both SV and CO (1-4). The calculation of SV relies on the principle that the volumetric flow rate (Q) at any instant is equal to the velocity of blood (v) multiplied by the cross-sectional area (CSA) through which that blood flows:

$$Q = v \times \text{CSA (cm}^3\text{/s)}$$

In a pulsatile system like the heart, the velocity of blood flow varies dynamically during each ejection period. To accurately calculate the volume of blood ejected during a systolic cycle, a single velocity measurement is therefore not reliable, and the instantaneous velocities throughout systole must be calculated. In a spectral Doppler display, the individual velocities are displayed graphically as a spectrum (hence the term spectral Doppler), with the x-axis representing time and the y-axis the number of red blood cells moving at each velocity. When a spectral Doppler curve is traced, the individual instantaneous velocities (cm/s) are integrated with respect to time (sec). The resulting velocity-time integral (VTI) (cm) represents the distance that the red blood cells have traveled in one systolic beat, sometimes referred to as the "stroke distance." The stroke distance (cm) is multiplied by the CSA (cm^2) of the conduit through which the blood traveled to calculate the SV (cm^3) (Figure 6.1):

$$\text{SV} = \text{CSA} \times \text{VTI cm}^3 \text{ (or mL)}$$

CO, which represents the volume of blood pumped by the heart per unit of time (typically expressed in ml/min), is simply calculated as the product of the SV and the heart rate.

$$\text{CO} = \text{SV} \times \text{HR mL/min}$$

LVOT Stroke Volume

The most common location used to calculate SV with TEE is the left ventricular outflow tract (LVOT). Flow at the LVOT is more likely to be laminar with a spatially flat profile, meaning that the velocities at the center and at the periphery are nearly equal. The LVOT is also relatively circular in shape, with less change in size during the cardiac cycle than the pulmonary artery or ascending aorta. The LVOT can become more elliptic in the setting of aortic stenosis or hypertrophic cardiomyopathy, however, possibly leading to underestimation of the CSA and, subsequently, the SV (5). It should also be recognized that LVOT SV will be larger than the right ventricular outflow tract (RVOT) or thermodilution-derived SV in the setting of aortic regurgitation as it is augmented by the ejected regurgitant volume.

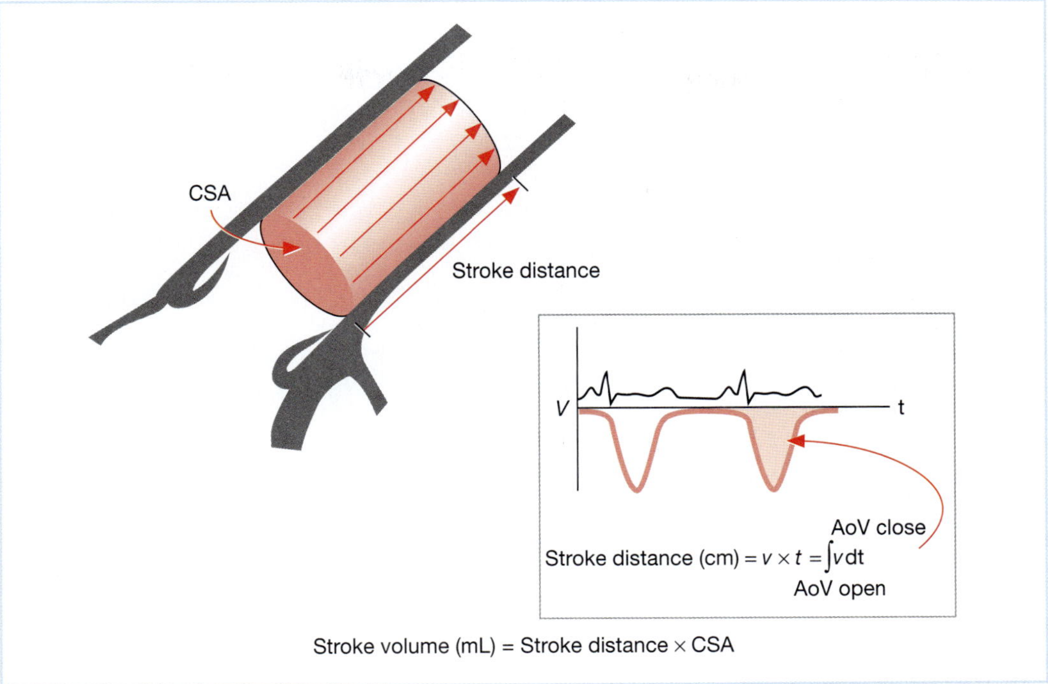

FIGURE 6.1 Calculation of stroke volume. The volume, here shown in the ascending aorta, can be thought of as a cylinder of blood with a CSA and a length. The CSA is typically calculated from a 2D diameter. The length (stroke distance) is calculated by tracing the spectral Doppler signal of flow measured with pulsed-wave Doppler. The instantaneous velocities are integrated over time to calculate the velocity-time integral, or stroke distance. CSA, cross-sectional area.

Calculation of the Left Ventricular Outflow Tract Stroke Volume

1. 2D measurements of the LVOT diameter should be made from the midesophageal aortic valve long axis view in midsystole using an inner edge-to-inner edge technique. While some suggest that the LVOT be measured at 0.5 to 1.0 cm proximal to the aortic valve annulus, we recommend that this measurement be made at the level of the aortic valve annulus for the best accuracy and reproducibility (reference (6), figure 2). If possible, multiplanar reconstruction of the aortic annulus can provide a more accurate SV calculation as it does not make assumptions about the shape of the structure. Caution should be taken applying a 3D SV to the assessment of aortic stenosis, however, as discussed in Chapter 12: Aortic Stenosis.
2. The LVOT VTI is then obtained with pulsed-wave Doppler (PWD) from the deep transgastric five-chamber and the transgastric long axis views. We recommend obtaining both signals and using that with the best alignment and therefore the highest velocity. In patients without aortic stenosis, the PWD gate should be placed just at the level of the aortic valve annulus. This signal should demonstrate a valve closing click as well as a narrow range of velocities and a well-defined peak. Every SV measurement should strive to measure the Doppler flow and CSA in the same location for best accuracy.
3. Having obtained this data, the calculation of the LVOT CSA is as follows:

$$CSA_{LVOT} = \pi(\text{diameter}/2)^2$$

The SV and CO is then calculated using as (Figure 6.2):

$$SV_{LVOT} = VTI_{LVOT} \times CSA_{LVOT}$$

$$CO_{LVOT} = SV_{LVOT} \times HR$$

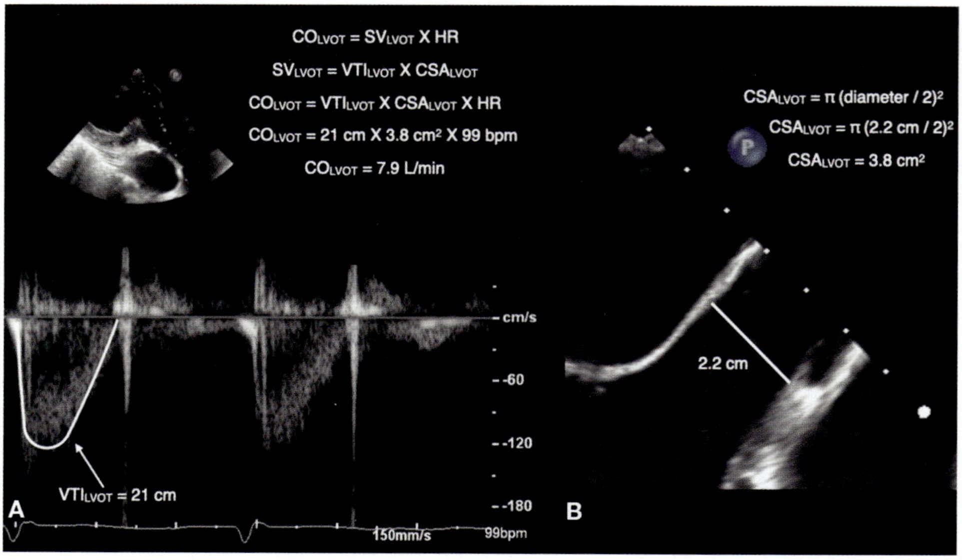

FIGURE 6.2 CO calculated at the LVOT. A: A pulsed-wave Doppler sample is made at the level of the aortic annulus in the transgastric long axis view. The signal shows a narrow range of velocities with a clear closing click. Tracing this allows the system to calculate the VTI. B: The diameter of the LVOT is measured in the midesophageal long axis view at the level of the annulus from the base of the right coronary cusp to the interleaflet trigone between the left and noncoronary cusps. The CSA_{LVOT} is determined by the equation $(D_{LVOT}/2)^2$. These measurements are then used to calculate stroke volume and CO. CO, cardiac output; CSA, cross-sectional area; D, diameter; HR, heart rate; LVOT, left ventricular outflow tract; SV, stroke volume; VTI, time-velocity integral or "stroke distance."

Right Heart Stroke Volume

SV of the right heart can be calculated from either the RVOT or the main pulmonary artery. Although this approach is less common due to challenging acoustic windows, it may provide value in cases of aortic regurgitation or in the assessment of intracardiac shunts.

1. RVOT diameter is measured in the midesophageal right ventricular (RV) inflow-outflow view at the level of the pulmonic valve annulus in midsystole.
2. RVOT VTI is determined from a PWD measurement made at the level of the pulmonic valve annulus, typically in the transgastric RV basal, transgastric RV inflow-outflow, or the upper esophageal aortic arch short axis views.
3. The ascending aorta short axis view can be used as an alternative, as shown in Figure 6.3, with diameter measurements of the main pulmonary artery and PWD signals sampled at the same location.

Intracardiac Shunts

The ratio of total pulmonary blood flow (Q_p) to total systemic blood flow (Q_s), the Q_p/Q_s ratio, is a useful tool for quantifying intracardiac shunts (7). Q_p and Q_s are calculated from the respective SVs of each ventricle (assuming that there is no significant regurgitation of either pulmonic or aortic valves) and the ratio calculated as:

$$Q_p/Q_s = \text{RVOT SV}/\text{LVOT SV}$$

A normal Q_p/Q_s ratio is 1:1 as the blood volume flowing through the pulmonary circulation should be equivalent to the volume flowing through the systemic circulation in the absence of a shunt. A Q_p/Q_s ratio of >1:1 indicates that pulmonary flow exceeds systemic flow and defines a net left-to-right shunt. Conversely, a Q_p/Q_s ratio of <1:1 indicates a net right-to-left shunt.

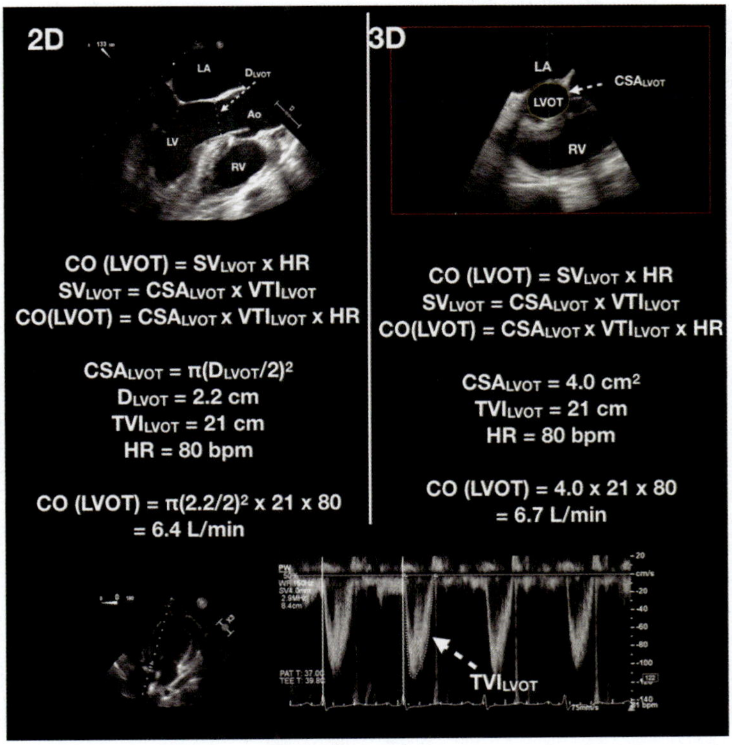

FIGURE 6.3 Calculation of cardiac output from the MPA can be performed from the ascending aorta short axis view. The MPA diameter is measured, in this case 2.8 cm. The cross-sectional area of the pulmonary artery ($\pi(D_{MPA}/2)^2$) is then calculated to be 6.2 cm^2. The PW Doppler signal is aligned with blood flow in the pulmonary artery (at the site where the MPA diameter is measured), the signal is traced, and the VTI is calculated, in this case 10.5 cm. When multiplied by the cross-sectional area, the stroke volume is calculated to be 64.6 mL, and when multiplied by the heart rate, the CO is calculated to be 5.3 L/min. Ao, ascending aorta; CO, cardiac output; CSA, cross-sectional area; D, diameter; HR, heart rate; MPA, main pulmonary artery; SV, stroke volume; VTI, velocity-time integral.

Regurgitant Volume

Regurgitant volume is defined as the quantity of blood that flows backward through a cardiac valve during a single cardiac cycle. It is a useful measure of the severity of valvular heart disease, and the calculation can be accomplished by two different methods: the volumetric method (described further on) and the proximal isovelocity surface area method (further described in Chapter 8: Mitral Regurgitation).

The volumetric method uses the principle that the forward flow across a regurgitant valve is equal to the sum of the systemic SV and the regurgitant volume. The regurgitant volume is therefore calculated as the difference between the total SV across the regurgitant valve and the total SV across a normal reference valve.

$$\text{Regurgitant volume} = \text{forward flow through regurgitant valve} - \text{forward flow through reference valve}$$

$$\text{Regurgitant fraction (\%)} = (\text{regurgitant volume/forward flow through regurgitant valve}) \times 100$$

Using mitral regurgitation as an example, the regurgitant volume is estimated by measuring the mitral inflow volume (regurgitant valve) and subtracting the SV across the AoV (reference valve):

$$\text{Regurgitant volume}_{MV} = \text{forward flow through MV} - \text{forward flow through AoV} = SV_{MV} - SV_{AoV}$$

Valve Area: The Continuity Equation

The continuity equation is a fundamental principle of fluid dynamics as well as echocardiography and is based on the concept of conservation of mass. The equation is used to calculate the area of a stenotic or regurgitant valve as the volume entering a valve (eg, LVOT flow) is equal to the volume exiting the valve (eg, flow across a stenotic aortic valve) (Figure 6.4). As valve stenosis severity progresses and its CSA decreases, the velocity of the blood flow across the valve must increase to preserve the continuity of flow. This is applied clinically using the principle of volumetric flow, as discussed previously:

$$\text{Volumetric flow}_1 = \text{Volumetric flow}_2$$

$$\text{CSA}_1 \times \text{VTI}_1 = \text{CSA}_2 \times \text{VTI}_2$$

$$\text{CSA}_1 = \text{CSA}_2 \times \text{VTI}_2/\text{VTI}_1$$

Figure 6.4B illustrates the use of the continuity equation to calculate the area of a stenotic aortic valve. Note that the SV across the LVOT must equal the SV across the stenotic aortic valve. Because of the high velocities across the stenotic valve, continuous wave Doppler (CWD) is employed in this region (described in more detail in Chapter 12: Aortic Stenosis) to calculate the aortic valve area.

$$\text{Area}_{\text{AV}} = \text{Area}_{\text{LVOT}} \times (\text{VTI}_{\text{LVOT}}/\text{VTI}_{\text{AV}})$$

$$\text{Area}_{\text{AV}} = \pi(\text{diameter}_{\text{LVOT}}/2)^2 \times (\text{VTI}_{\text{LVOT}}/\text{VTI}_{\text{AV}})$$

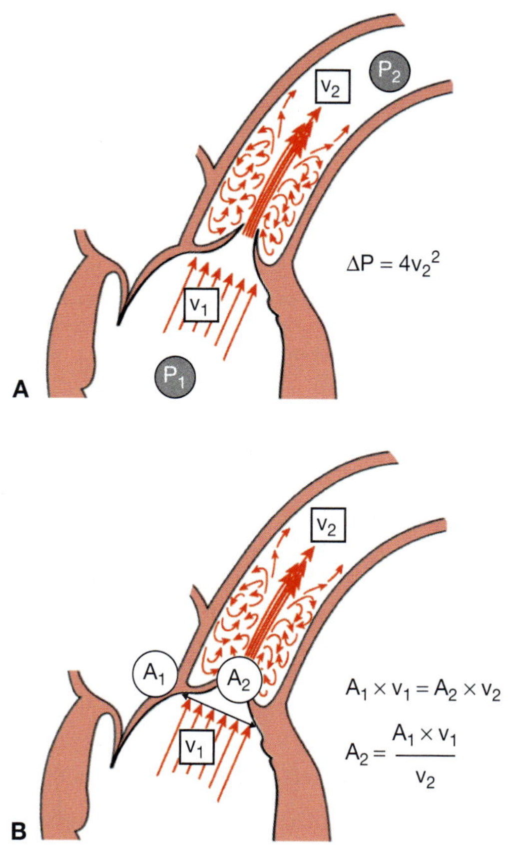

FIGURE 6.4 Calculation of the pressure gradient and valve area. A: The simplified Bernoulli equation states that the pressure difference across a stenotic valve is equal to 4 times the square of the velocity of the high-velocity jet through the valve. B: The continuity equation describes conservation of flow, meaning that flow proximal to a valve should equal flow exiting the valve. A_1, cross-sectional area proximal to the valve; A_2, cross-sectional area through the valve; P_1, pressure proximal to the valve; P_2, pressure distal to the valve; v_1, flow velocity proximal to the valve; v_2, flow velocity through the valve.

INTRACARDIAC PRESSURES AND PRESSURE GRADIENTS: THE BERNOULLI EQUATION

The Bernoulli equation is used to estimate the pressure gradients to assess the severity of valvular disease (eg, aortic stenosis), intracardiac pressures, outflow tract abnormalities (eg, LVOT obstruction), and shunts. The equation employs a key concept in fluid dynamics that relates the pressure difference between two points to the velocity difference between those points. For example, when blood flows across a stenotic valve, the velocity will increase to a value that is directly proportional to the degree of narrowing. The relationship between pressure and velocity is described by the Bernoulli equation as:

$$P_1 - P_2 = 1/2\rho\,(v_2^2 - v_1^2) + \rho\,(dv/dt)dx + R(v)$$

Convective acceleration + Flow acceleration + Viscous friction

where P is the pressure in the areas of interest (mm Hg), ρ is the density of blood (1.06×103 kg/m^3), v_1 is the peak velocity of blood flow proximal to the area of interest (m/s), and v_2 is the peak velocity of blood flow across the area of interest (m/s).

In clinical practice, the Bernoulli equation is simplified by ignoring the effects of flow acceleration, viscous friction, and the velocity proximal to the area of interest (v_1) because:

1. Peak flows are of interest in clinical measurements. During peak flow, the flow acceleration is virtually nonexistent and can thus be ignored.
2. Viscous friction contributes significantly only in discrete orifices with an area of less than 0.25 cm^2. Blood flow is thought to be constant for orifices with an area greater than this, so viscous friction is also eliminated in the Bernoulli calculation.
3. For clinically significant lesions, v_2 is substantially greater than v_1, such that $v_2^2 - v_1^2$ is approximated by just v_2^2.

The elimination of these factors yields the simplified Bernoulli equation:

$$\text{Simplified Bernoulli equation: } \Delta P = 4v_2^2$$

Therefore, a pressure gradient is obtained in clinical echocardiography by the straightforward process of measuring the peak velocity of blood flow across the lesion of interest (**Figure 4A**). *However,* when v^1 is greater than 1.4 m/s, then the ***Modified Bernoulli equation*** is considered to account for the higher proximal velocity:

$$\text{Modified Bernoulli equation: } \Delta P = 4v_2^2 - 4v_1^2 \text{ or } 4\,(v_2^2 - v_1^2)$$

To calculate the pressure gradient, the PWD sample volume or CWD beam is directed across the region of interest. The measured peak velocity is then entered into the simplified Bernoulli equation ($\Delta P = 4v_2^2$) to estimate the pressure gradient. When blood flow velocities are high (≥1.4 m/s), CWD is preferred to avoid the aliasing that may occur with PWD. It is imperative that the Doppler beam be so positioned that it interrogates the jet with the highest velocity; otherwise, the pressure gradient will be significantly underestimated (8). To obtain the highest velocity flow, interrogation from multiple windows is preferred. Also, accuracy is improved by assessing multiple flow profiles (3-5 for a regular rhythm and 10 for an irregular rhythm) at end-expiration. *The simplified Bernoulli equation is the basis for most pressure gradient calculations in clinical echocardiography.*

Assessment of Valvular Disease

The most common clinical use of the Bernoulli equation is to determine the pressure gradient across a stenotic valve. Utilizing the peak Doppler velocity yields the instantaneous, maximal pressure gradient. The average of the pressure gradients over the ejection period estimates the mean gradient. This is accomplished by tracing the velocity signal and utilizing built-in software, which then automatically calculates the mean gradient from the obtained velocities through the narrowed valve (9).

In addition to the pressure gradient itself, the rate of decline in the gradient is an important parameter in evaluating the severity of valvular disease, particularly in the context of mitral stenosis and aortic regurgitation. *Pressure half-time* (PHT) describes the time interval for the peak pressure gradient to decrease by 50% and is inversely proportional to valve area. As such, a shorter PHT is indicative of more rapid equilibration between the two chambers of interest. In the context of aortic regurgitation, a short PHT corresponds to severe regurgitation due to the rapid increase in LV diastolic pressure and decrease in aortic pressure. In evaluating mitral stenosis, a longer PHT suggests a highly stenotic MV due to the slower rate of pressure decay during diastole through a smaller orifice (10,11).

Measurement of Intracavitary Pressures

As mentioned previously, the Bernoulli equation relates a velocity across a valve to the pressure difference between the chambers on either side of the valve. Intracavitary and pulmonary arterial pressures can be measured by combining a Doppler-derived pressure gradient from a regurgitant jet and a known (or estimated) pressure either proximal or distal to the chamber of interest (**Appendix C**).

Right Ventricular and Pulmonary Artery Systolic Pressures

The peak velocity of the tricuspid regurgitation jet enables calculation with the Bernoulli equation of the pressure gradient between the right atrium (RA) and the RV (12) (Figure 6.5). This measurement is performed by aligning a CWD beam with a jet of tricuspid regurgitation. The optimal views for this measurement will be the midesophageal 4-chamber, inflow-outflow, or modified bicaval. To this gradient is added either a known or estimated right atrial pressure or central venous pressure (CVP) to calculate the right ventricular systolic pressure (RVSP). For patients without RVOT obstruction or pulmonic stenosis, the RVSP will be similar to the pulmonary artery systolic pressure (PASP).

$$\text{RVSP or PASP (mm Hg)} = 4(v_{TR})2 + \text{CVP (mm Hg)}$$

Pulmonary Artery Mean and Diastolic Pressures

As pulmonic valve regurgitation occurs during diastole, the velocity of the regurgitant jet can be used to calculate the diastolic pressure gradient between the PA and the RV (13,14). These measurements are best made with CWD from either the upper esophageal short axis or the transgastric RV basal views. The PA diastolic pressure (PADP) is calculated using a measurement of the end diastolic velocity of a jet of pulmonic regurgitation and an estimate of the right atrial pressure or CVP (Figure 6.6).

$$\text{PADP} = 4(v_{\text{late}}\ \text{PI})^2 + \text{CVP}$$

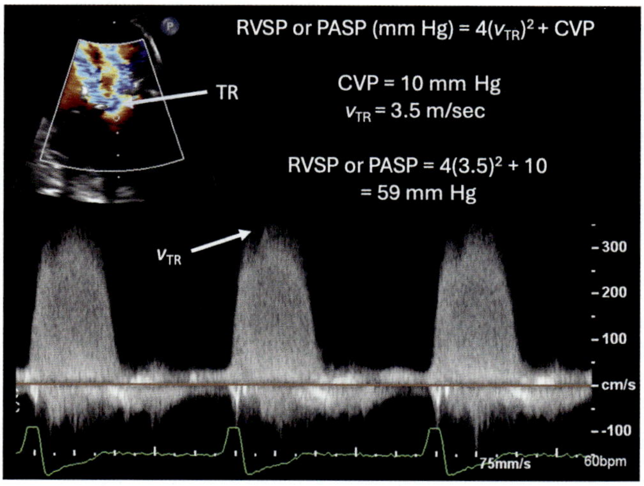

FIGURE 6.5 Calculation of PASP or RVSP. Using the simplified Bernoulli equation, the peak velocity of the tricuspid regurgitant velocity profile (v_{TR}) is utilized to determine the pressure gradient across the tricuspid valve. The product is added to a known right atrial or central venous pressure to yield the PASP or the RVSP. CVP, central venous pressure; PASP, pulmonary artery systolic pressure; RVSP, right ventricular systolic pressure; v_{TR}, tricuspid regurgitant velocity profile.

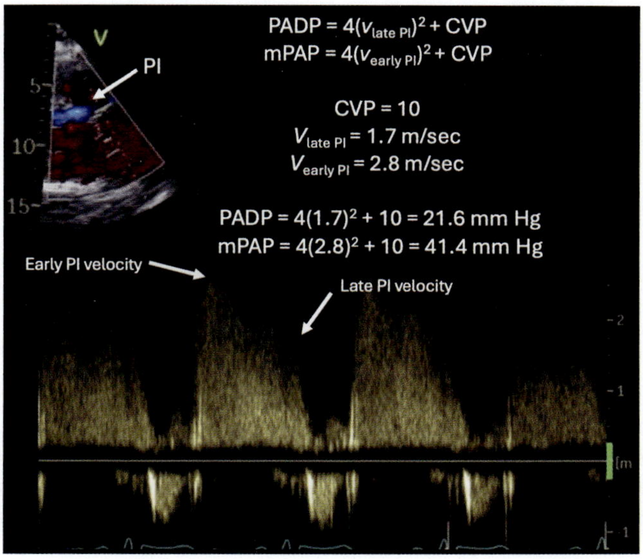

FIGURE 6.6 Calculation of pulmonary artery mean and diastolic pressures. The mean pulmonary artery pressure can be estimated from the early pulmonary insufficiency velocity, and the diastolic pressure is approximated from the late pulmonary insufficiency velocity. The arrows demonstrate the early and late velocities. The pressure gradient across the pulmonic valve is obtained using the simplified Bernoulli equation ($v_{early\ PI}$, $v_{late\ PI}$). The early and late pulmonary insufficiency gradients are added to the central venous pressure to produce the mPAP and PADP. CVP, central venous pressure; mPAP, mean pulmonary artery pressure; PADP, pulmonary artery diastolic pressure; PI, pulmonary insufficiency; *v*, velocity.

To calculate the mean PA pressure (mPAP), the early diastolic velocity of pulmonic regurgitation is measured instead:

$$\text{mPAP} = 4(v_{\text{early}}\ \text{PI})^2 + \text{CVP}$$

Pulmonary Vascular Resistance

Elevated mPAP, as described in the previous section, is suggestive of pulmonary hypertension, which can be further characterized by assessment of the pulmonary vascular resistance (PVR). While the standard technique for measurement remains invasive right heart catheterization, Doppler echocardiography can provide an estimate using the ratio of the peak velocity of the TR jet and the RVOT VTI (15,16). As described in the previous section, the RVOT VTI should be measured at the pulmonic annulus in the transgastric RV basal, transgastric RV inflow-outflow, or the upper esophageal aortic arch short axis views

$$\text{PVR (in Woods units)} = (V_{\text{TR}}/\text{VTI}_{\text{RVOT}} \times 10) + 0.16$$

Pulmonary arterial compliance (PAC) has been suggested as a sensitive marker for pulmonary hypertension severity as well as an independent predictor of functional capacity. Echocardiography can estimate the PAC using the ratio of the RVOT VTI and estimated PASP (17).

$$\text{PAC} = \text{VTI}_{\text{RVOT}}/\text{PASP}$$

Left Atrial Pressure

On the left side of the heart, blood flow through the mitral valve can help estimate the left atrial (LA) pressure in a similar fashion (18,19). The velocity of mitral regurgitation (MR) represents the systolic pressure gradient between the LV and the LA. This velocity is sampled with CWD in the midesophageal view that creates the best alignment with the regurgitant flow. In the absence of AoV disease or LV outflow tract obstruction, it is assumed that the LV systolic pressure is equivalent to the systolic blood pressure (SBP), and thus, the LA pressure can be calculated (although best considered an "estimate") using the following equation (Figure 6.7).

$$\text{LAP} = \text{SBP} - 4(V_{\text{MR}})^2$$

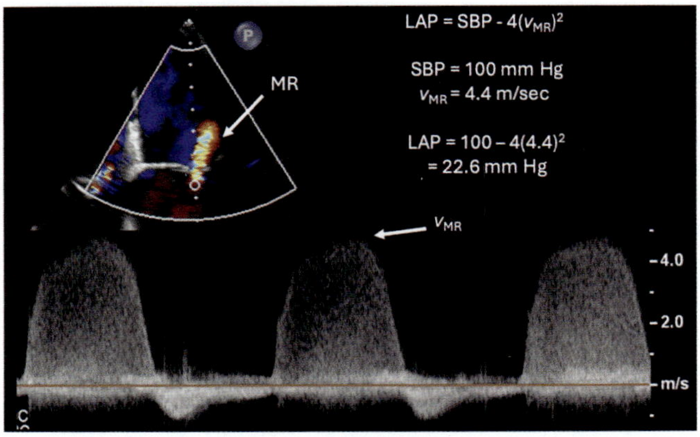

FIGURE 6.7 Calculation of left atrial pressure. The peak MR velocity is utilized to estimate the pressure gradient between the left ventricle and the left atrium using the simplified Bernoulli equation. This is subtracted from the systolic blood pressure to equal the left atrial pressure. LAP, left atrial pressure; MR, mitral regurgitation; SBP, systolic blood pressure; v, velocity.

LV End Diastolic Pressure

The LV end diastolic pressure (LVEDP) is estimated by utilizing the aortic regurgitation (AI) end diastolic jet velocity, typically sampled with CWD from the transgastric long axis or deep transgastric five-chamber views (20). The pressure gradient between the LV and the aorta is calculated from the peak velocity of this signal, then subtracted from the systemic diastolic blood pressure (DBP) (Figure 6.8).

$$\text{LVEDP} = \text{DBP} - 4(V_{\text{AI end}})^2$$

Of note, the LVEDP and LA pressures are commonly estimated using mitral inflow, tissue Doppler, and pulmonary vein velocity patterns, as described in Chapter 7: Echocardiographic Evaluation of Ventricular Diastolic Function (9,21-23).

Intracardiac Shunts

In an atrial septal defect (ASD), a hemodynamically significant left-to-right shunt is defined as a pulmonary to systemic flow ratio (Q_p/Q_s) ≥1.5:1, often associated with RA and/or RV enlargement (24). Using the simplified Bernoulli equation, the maximum velocity of flow across the ASD can be translated into the pressure gradient between the right and the left atria and used to calculate the LA pressure (Figure 6.9).

$$\text{LAP} = 4(v_{\text{ASD}})^2 + \text{CVP}$$

In a ventricular septal defect (VSD), a hemodynamically significant shunt is similarly defined as Q_p:Q_s ≥1.5:1, often associated with LV dilation (24). The maximal velocity of flow across the VSD can be translated into the pressure gradient between the left and the right ventricles. The RV and PA systolic pressure can be estimated by subtracting LV-to-RV pressure gradients from the SBP (Figure 6.10).

$$\text{RVSP or PASP (mm Hg)} = \text{SBP} - 4(v_{\text{ASD}})^2$$

Vascular Resistance

The resistance that the LV or RV must overcome to eject blood during systole, or afterload, is critical to understanding hemodynamics and is commonly used to guide clinical management. Since Ohm's Law states that resistance equals change in pressure divided by flow, echocardiographic calculations are based on the ratio between a valvular regurgitant jet velocity (for pressure gradient) and the respective ventricular outflow tract VTI (reflecting forward flow).

Systemic vascular resistance (SVR, in Wood units) is proportional to the ratio of the peak MR velocity to the LVOT VTI.

$$\text{SVR} \propto V_{\text{MR}}/\text{VTI}_{\text{LVOT}}$$

One study observed that this equation correlates with the following specific SVR values (25):

$$V_{\text{MR}}/\text{VTI}_{\text{LVOT}} > 0.27 = \text{SVR} > 14 \text{ Wood units (WU) (70\% sensitivity, 77\% specificity)}$$

$$V_{\text{MR}}/\text{VTI}_{\text{LVOT}} < 0.20 = \text{SVR} < 10 \text{ WU (92\% sensitivity, 88\% specificity)}$$

Assessment of Cardiac Rhythm

Assessment of mitral inflow performed with PWD at the tips of the leaflets (described further in Chapter 7: Echocardiographic Evaluation of Ventricular Diastolic Function) provides valuable insights to cardiac rhythm as well as diastolic function. A normal mitral inflow pattern demonstrates an E wave, representing early ventricular filling, and a subsequent A wave due to atrial contraction. The presence of both waves indicates a sinus rhythm. In atrial fibrillation, the disorganized electrical activity prevents atrial contraction resulting in the absence of a clear A wave. Atrial flutter or other atrial tachycardias, however, may demonstrate a series of flutter waves.

In a sinus rhythm, PWD in the LA appendage typically demonstrates a single deflection above and below the baseline during each cardiac cycle (once for filling and once for ejection from the appendage). Deviations from this pattern, specifically multiple deflections during each cardiac cycle, can indicate atrial dysrhythmia such as fibrillation. Pulmonary venous flow assessed using PW Doppler technology will also demonstrate abnormalities from atrial fibrillation, including loss of reverse flow during atrial contraction, greater diastolic than systolic flow, and an early systolic reversal of flow (26).

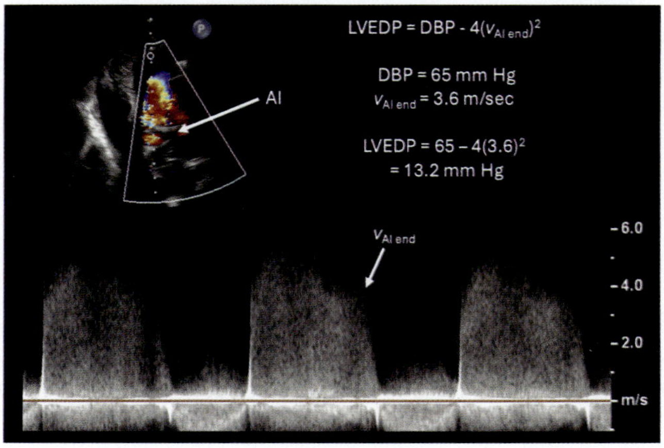

FIGURE 6.8 Calculation of the left ventricular end diastolic pressure. The LVEDP can be estimated using the end velocity of the aortic valve regurgitant flow, as marked by the arrow. Using this velocity, the simplified Bernoulli equation calculates the gradient between the left ventricle and aorta. The pressure gradient is subtracted from the diastolic blood pressure to yield the LVEDP. AI, aortic insufficiency; DBP, diastolic blood pressure; LVEDP, left ventricular end diastolic pressure; v, velocity.

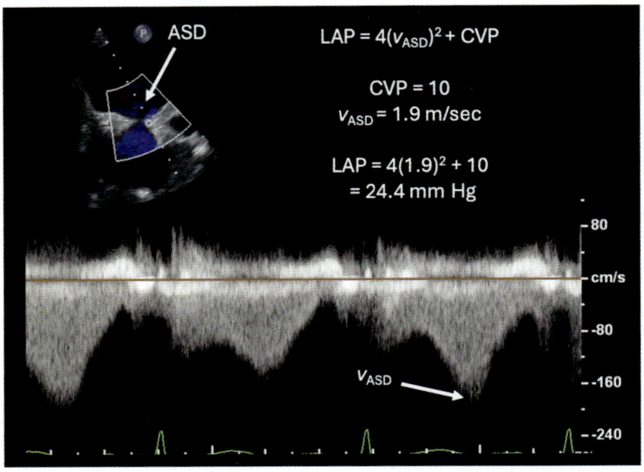

FIGURE 6.9 Calculation of the left atrial pressure using the pressure gradient across an atrial septal defect. The peak velocity across an ASD can be utilized to calculate the pressure gradient between the left and the right atria via the simplified Bernoulli equation. This value is added to the central venous pressure to obtain an estimation of the left atrial pressure. ASD, atrial septal defect; CVP, central venous pressure; LAP, left atrial pressure; *v*, velocity.

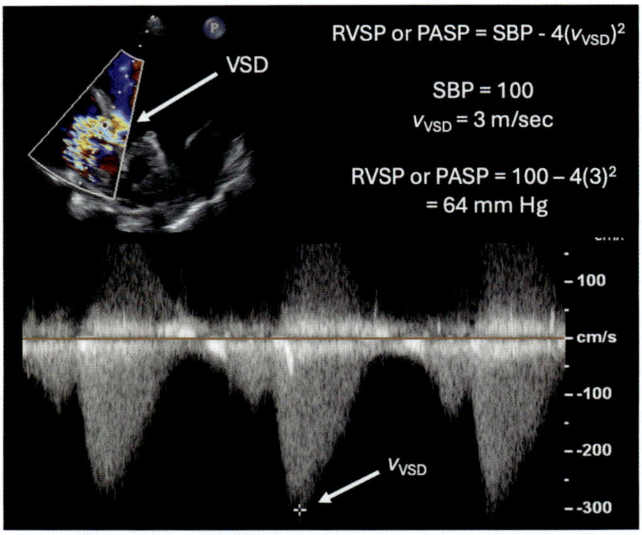

FIGURE 6.10 Calculation of the PASP or the RVSP using a ventricular septal defect. The pressure gradient between the left and the right ventricles can be determined using the peak velocity flow through a VSD. This value is subtracted from the systolic blood pressure to estimate the PASP or the RVSP. PASP, pulmonary artery systolic pressure; RVSP, right ventricular systolic pressure; SBP, systolic blood pressure; *v*, velocity; VSD, ventricular septal defect.

SUMMARY

Doppler echocardiography is an indispensable tool in the assessment of hemodynamics for both diagnosis and management of cardiac disease. By providing accurate, quantitative measurement of the speed and direction of blood flow, it allows for evaluation of valve area and function, pressure gradients, chamber pressures, and shunts. It is a safe, readily available, and cost-effective technique to observe cardiac function and can provide estimates of many hemodynamic measurements that must otherwise be acquired utilizing invasive techniques.

ACKNOWLEDGMENTS

We gratefully acknowledge the contributions of the previous edition authors, Tzong Huei Chen, Andrew Maslow, and Albert C. Perrino, Jr, as portions of those chapters have been retained in this revision.

REFERENCES

1. Zhang Y, Wang Y, Shi J, Hua Z, Xu J. Cardiac output measurements via echocardiography versus thermodilution: a systematic review and meta-analysis. *PLoS One*. 2019;14(10):e0222105.
2. Rong LQ, Kaushal M, Mauer E, et al. Two- or 3-dimensional echocardiography-derived cardiac output cannot replace the pulmonary artery catheter in cardiac surgery. *J Cardiothorac Vasc Anesth*. 2020;34(10):2691-2697.
3. Olivieri PP, Patel R, Kolb S, et al. Echo is a good, not perfect, measure of cardiac output in critically ill surgical patients. *J Trauma Acute Care Surg*. 2019;87(2):379-385.
4. Mercado P, Maizel J, Beyls C, et al. Transthoracic echocardiography: an accurate and precise method for estimating cardiac output in the critically ill patient. *Crit Care*. 2017;21(1):136.
5. Lavine SJ, Obeng GB. The relation of left ventricular geometry to left ventricular outflow tract shape and stroke volume index calculations. *Echocardiography*. 2019;36(5):905-915.
6. Hahn RT, Saric M, Faletra F, Garg R, et al. Recommended standards for the performance of transesophageal echocardiographic screening for structural heart intervention. *J Am Soc Echocardiogr*. 2022;35:1-76.
7. Valdes-Cruz LM, Horowitz S, Mesel E, Sahn DJ, Fisher DC, Larson D. A pulsed Doppler echocardiographic method for calculating pulmonary and systemic blood flow in atrial level shunts: validation studies in animals and initial human experience. *Circulation*. 1984;69:80-86.
8. Mitchell C, Rahko PS, Blauwet LA, et al. Guidelines for performing a comprehensive transthoracic echocardiographic examination in adults: recommendations from the American Society of Echocardiography. *J Am Soc Echocardiogr*. 2019;32(1):1-64.
9. Anavekar NS, Oh JK. Doppler echocardiography: a contemporary review. *J Cardiol*. 2009;54(3):347-358.
10. Nakatani S, Masuyama T, Kodama K, Kitabatake A, Fujii K, Kamada T. Value and limitations of Doppler echocardiography in the quantification of stenotic mitral valve area: comparison of the pressure half-time and the continuity equation methods. *Circulation*. 1988;77(1):78-85.
11. Teague SM, Heinsimer JA, Anderson JL, et al. Quantification of aortic regurgitation utilizing continuous wave Doppler ultrasound. *J Am Coll Cardiol*. 1986;8(3):592-599.
12. Yock PG, Popp RL. Noninvasive estimation of right ventricular systolic pressure by Doppler ultrasound in patients with tricuspid regurgitation. *Circulation*. 1984;70(4):657-662.
13. Ge Z, Zhang Y, Ji X, Fan D, Duran CM. Pulmonary artery diastolic pressure: a simultaneous Doppler echocardiography and catheterization study. *Clin Cardiol*. 1992;15(11):818-824.
14. Lee RT, Lord CP, Plappert T, Sutton MS. Prospective Doppler echocardiographic evaluation of pulmonary artery diastolic pressure in the medical intensive care unit. *Am J Cardiol*. 1989;64(19):1366-1370.
15. Abbas AE, Fortuin FD, Schiller NB, Appleton CP, Moreno CA, Lester SJ. A simple method for noninvasive estimation of pulmonary vascular resistance. *J Am Coll Cardiol*. 2003;41(6):1021-7.
16. Roule V, Labombarda F, Pellissier A, et al. Echocardiographic assessment of pulmonary vascular resistance in pulmonary arterial hypertension. *Cardiovasc Ultrasound*. 2010;8:21.
17. Bhattacharya PT, Troutman GS, Mao F, et al. Right ventricular outflow tract velocity time integral-to-pulmonary artery systolic pressure ratio: a non-invasive metric of pulmonary arterial compliance differs across the spectrum of pulmonary hypertension. *Pulm Circ*. 2019;9(2):2045894019841978.
18. Pressman GS, Ranjan R, Olex S. A simple technique for bedside estimation of left atrial pressure. *Echocardiography*. 2019;36(11):1972-1978.
19. Gorcsan J 3rd, Snow FR, Paulsen W, Nixon JV. Noninvasive estimation of left atrial pressure in patients with congestive heart failure and mitral regurgitation by Doppler echocardiography. *Am Heart J*. 1991;121(3 pt 1):858-863.
20. Nishimura RA, Tajik AJ. Determination of left-sided pressure gradients by utilizing Doppler aortic and mitral regurgitant signals: validation by simultaneous dual catheter and Doppler studies. *J Am Coll Cardiol*. 1988;11(2):317-321.
21. Oh JK, Appleton CP, Hatle LK, Nishimura RA, Seward JB, Tajik AJ. The noninvasive assessment of left ventricular diastolic function with two-dimensional and Doppler echocardiography. *J Am Soc Echocardiogr*. 1997;10(3):246-270.
22. Nagueh SF, Kopelen HA, Quiñones MA. Assessment of left ventricular filling pressures by Doppler in the presence of atrial fibrillation. *Circulation*. 1996;94(9):2138-2145.
23. Nishimura RA, Abel MD, Hatle LK, Tajik AJ. Assessment of diastolic function of the heart: background and current applications of Doppler echocardiography. Part II. Clinical studies. *Mayo Clin Proc*. 1989;64(2):181-204.
24. Abbas AE, Fortuin FD, Patel B, Moreno CA, Schiller NB, Lester SJ. Noninvasive measurement of systemic vascular resistance using Doppler echocardiography. *J Am Soc Echocardiogr*. 2004;17(8):834-838.
25. Bollmann A. Pulmonary venous flow assessed by Doppler echocardiography in the management of atrial fibrillation. *Echocardiography*. 2007;24(4):430-435.
26. Quiñones MA, Otto CM, Stoddard M, Waggoner A, Zoghbi WA; Doppler Quantification Task Force of the Nomenclature and Standards Committee of the American Society of Echocardiography. Recommendations for quantification of Doppler echocardiography: a report from the Doppler Quantification Task Force of the Nomenclature and Standards Committee of the American Society of Echocardiography. *J Am Soc Echocardiogr*. 2002;15(2):167-184.

QUESTIONS

CASE 6.1

A 35-year-old woman with a history of undifferentiated connective tissue disorder is admitted to the hospital with worsening respiratory distress and intubated for hypoxemic respiratory failure. Emergent TEE demonstrates the following:

Vital Signs:

• Heart rate:	120 bpm
• Systemic BP:	100/60 mm Hg
• CVP:	10 mm Hg

TEE Data:

• TR peak velocity:	4.0 m/s
• PI jet early diastolic velocity:	3.0 m/s
• PI jet end diastolic velocity:	2.5 m/s
• TVI_{RVOT}:	8 cm

There is no significant pulmonary stenosis or RVOT obstruction identified.

1. Based on Case 6.1 the estimated PA systolic pressure (mm Hg) is:
A. 64 mm Hg
B. 36 mm Hg
C. 25 mm Hg
D. 74 mm Hg

2. Based on Case 6.1, the estimated PADP (mm Hg) is:
A. 36 mm Hg
B. 35 mm Hg
C. 46 mm Hg
D. 64 mm Hg

3. Based on Case 6.1, the estimated PA mean pressure (mm Hg) is:
A. 36 mm Hg
B. 35 mm Hg
C. 46 mm Hg
D. 64 mm Hg

4. Based on Case 6.1, the estimated PVR (in WU) is:
A. 8
B. 20
C. 5
D. <2

CASE 6.2

A 65-year-old man is undergoing surgery for coronary artery bypass grafting. On the intraoperative transesophageal echo, his aortic valve appears calcified with restricted leaflet mobility. The following measurements are made:

Vital Signs:

• Heart rate:	80 bpm
• Systemic BP:	140/90 mm Hg
• Mean arterial BP:	105 mm Hg
• CVP:	10 mm Hg
• Pulmonary capillary wedge pressure:	15 mm Hg

TEE Data:

• Mitral valve peak velocity:	7.0 m/s
• LVOT diameter:	2.0 cm
• TVI_{LVOT}:	20 cm

Assume that the pulmonary capillary wedge pressure (PCWP) approximates the left atrial pressure (LAP).

5. Based on Case 6.2, the peak aortic valve gradient is approximately:
A. 90 mm Hg
B. 35 mm Hg
C. 70 mm Hg
D. 45 mm Hg

6. Based on Case 6.2, the severity of aortic stenosis is:
A. Mild
B. Moderate
C. Severe
D. There is no significant aortic stenosis

7. Based on Case 6.2, the calculated CO (L/min) is:
A. 3.0
B. 4.0
C. 5.0
D. 6.0

CASE 6.3

A 55-year-old man is undergoing surgery for coronary artery bypass grafting. On the intraoperative transesophageal echo, he is identified to have MR. There is no significant aortic regurgitation. The following measurements are made:

Vital Signs:

• Heart rate:	80 bpm
• Systemic BP:	120/80 mm Hg
• CVP:	10 mm Hg

TEE Data:

• LVOT diameter:	2.0 cm
• TVI_{LVOT}:	18 cm
• Left ventricular end diastolic volume:	180 mL
• Left ventricular end systolic volume:	60 mL
• TVI_{MR}:	140 cm

8. Based on Case 6.3, the severity of MR is:
A. Mild
B. Mild to moderate
C. Moderate
D. Severe

9. Based on Case 6.3, the estimated regurgitant volume of MR (in mL) is:
A. 120 mL
B. 56 mL
C. 64 mL
D. 124 mL

10. The estimated effective regurgitant orifice area (EROA) of MR in cm^2 is:
A. 0.86
B. 0.40
C. 0.46
D. 0.89

ANSWERS

1. **Correct Answer: D.**
Rationale: The TR peak velocity obtained on TEE is 4.0 m/s. With the simplified Bernoulli equation of $4v^2$, the pressure gradient between the right ventricle (RV) and the RA can be identified as 64 mm Hg. By adding the known CVP of 10 mm Hg to the RV-RA pressure gradient, the RVSP is estimated as 74 mm Hg. In the absence of significant pulmonary stenosis or RVOT obstruction, the RVSP and PASP are similar. Answer choice (B) utilizes the simplified Bernoulli equation on the PI jet early diastolic velocity of 3.0 m/s, which yields 36 mm Hg, and can approximate the pulmonary artery mean pressure as 46 mm Hg with the addition of the CVP. Answer choice (C) utilizes the simplified Bernoulli equation on the PI jet end diastolic velocity of 2.5 m/s, which yields 25 mm Hg, and can approximate the pulmonary artery diastolic pressure as 35 mm Hg with the addition of the CVP.

2. **Correct Answer: B.**
Rationale: The PI jet end diastolic velocity obtained on TEE is 2.5 m/s. With the simplified Bernoulli equation of $4v^2$, the pressure gradient between the PA and the RV in end diastole can be identified as 25 mm Hg. By adding the known CVP of 10 mm Hg to the PA-RV end diastolic pressure gradient, the PADP is estimated as 35 mm Hg. Answer choice (A) utilizes the simplified Bernoulli equation on the PI jet early diastolic velocity of 3.0 m/s, which yields 36 mm Hg, and can approximate the pulmonary artery mean pressure as 46 mm Hg with the addition of the CVP. Answer choice (C) is the estimated PA mean pressure. Answer choice (D) is the pressure gradient between the RV and the RA using the simplified Bernoulli equation on the TR peak velocity.

3. **Correct Answer: C.**
Rationale: The PI jet early diastolic velocity obtained on TEE is 3.0 m/s. Utilizing this velocity with the simplified Bernoulli equation of $4v^2$, the pulmonary artery mean pressure (mPA pressure) can be estimated as 36 mm Hg plus the addition of the CVP, which yields 46 mm Hg. Alternatively, the mPA pressure can be approximated as 1/3 (PASP) + 2/3 (PADP). By using the previously calculated PASP of 74 mm Hg and PADP of 35 mm Hg, this yields an estimated mPA pressure of ~48 mm Hg, which is similar. Answer choice (A) fails to add the CVP to the pressure gradient obtained from the PI jet early diastolic velocity. Answer choice (B) is the estimated PADP as obtained from the addition of the CVP to the pressure gradient obtained from the PI jet late diastolic velocity. Answer choice (D) is the pressure gradient between the RV and the RA using the simplified Bernoulli equation on the TR peak velocity.

4. **Correct Answer: C.**
Rationale: PVR can be approximated on echocardiography through the following formula: PVR = $V_{TR}/TVI_{RVOT} \times 10 + 0.16$. Based on a V_{TR} of 4 m/s and a TVI_{RVOT} of 8 cm, the estimated PVR = $(4/8) \times 10 + 0.16 \approx$ 5 WU. Answer choice (B) incorrectly takes the ratio of the TVI_{RVOT}/V_{TR} (which is 2) $\times$ 10.

5. **Correct Answer: C.**
Rationale: The MR peak velocity obtained on TEE is 7.0 m/s. With the simplified Bernoulli equation of $4v^2$, the systolic pressure gradient between the left ventricle and the left atrium can be identified as 196 mm Hg. By adding the LAP of 15 mm Hg (which the PCWP approximates) to the LV-LA systolic pressure gradient, the left ventricular systolic pressure is estimated as 211 mm Hg. Because the SBP is 140 mm Hg, there is a gradient of ~70 mm Hg across the aortic valve, which is the peak aortic valve gradient. Answer choice (A) is the difference between the LV-LA systolic pressure gradient of 196 mm Hg and the mean arterial blood pressure (MAP) of 105 mm Hg, which is incorrect. Answer choice (B) is the difference between the SBP and the MAP. Answer choice (D) is the difference between the SBP + CVP and the MAP, which is incorrect.

6. **Correct Answer: C.**
Rationale: The peak aortic valve gradient is 70 mm Hg. The mean aortic valve gradient can be approximated as 2/3 of the peak aortic valve gradient, which is ~45 mm Hg and consistent with severe aortic stenosis. The echocardiographic images obtained demonstrating a calcified and restricted aortic valve.

7. Correct Answer: C.
Rationale: The volume of flow passing through the LVOT (SV) is calculated as the product of the TVI and the CSA of the LVOT. $CSA_{LVOT} = \pi(\text{diameter}/2)^2 = 3.14\ cm^2$, using an LVOT diameter of 2.0 cm. When multiplied by the TVI_{LVOT} of 20 cm, the estimated stroke volume across the LVOT (SV_{LVOT}) is 63 cm^3 or mL. The CO can be estimated by multiplying the SV_{LVOT} by the heart rate of 80 bpm = 5.0 L/min.

8. Correct Answer: C.
Rationale: The regurgitant volume of MR is 64 mL (see explanation in answers that follow), which corresponds with severe MR.

9. Correct Answer: C.
Rationale: The total SV of the left ventricle is the left ventricular end diastolic volume (LVEDV) − left ventricular end systolic volume (LVESV) = 180 mL − 60 mL = 120 mL. The forward SV of flow passing through the LVOT is calculated as the product of the TVI and the CSA of the LVOT. $CSA_{LVOT} = \pi(\text{diameter}/2)^2 = 3.14\ cm^2$ using an LVOT diameter of 2.0 cm. When multiplied by the TVI_{LVOT} of 18 cm, the estimated forward SV across the LVOT (SV_{LVOT}) is 56 cm^3 or mL. The regurgitant volume of the MR is equivalent to the total left ventricular SV − the forward SV → 120 mL − 56 mL = 64 mL.

10. Correct Answer: C.
Rationale: The regurgitant volume of MR is typically calculated by multiplying the EROA by the TVI of the regurgitant jet. The EROA can therefore be calculated by dividing the regurgitant volume by the TVI_{MR}. Dividing 64 mL (cm^3) by 140 cm yields an estimated EROA of 0.46 cm^2.

7 Echocardiographic Evaluation of Ventricular Diastolic Function

Anand R. Mehta and Wanda M. Popescu

The diastolic phase of the cardiac cycle is recognized as an important, independent component of cardiac performance. Quantification of diastolic function and filling pressures was initially performed via cardiac catheterization. The introduction of two-dimensional (2D) and pulsed-wave Doppler (PWD) echocardiography, and later of tissue Doppler imaging (TDI), has revolutionized the assessment and understanding of diastolic function. Being less invasive, portable, and safer, echocardiography has emerged as the modality of choice for the clinical evaluation of diastolic function and filling pressures.

Over the past several decades, echocardiography has highlighted diastolic dysfunction as a major pathophysiologic component of several cardiac disorders, including acute and chronic heart failure (HF) (1). In the perioperative arena, several studies have identified an association between preoperative left ventricular (LV) diastolic dysfunction, even without the presence of symptoms, and increased short- and long-term morbidity and mortality (2-4). Other echocardiographic studies have suggested that diastolic dysfunction contributes to hemodynamic instability and adverse outcomes following cardiac surgery (5,6). This chapter presents a practical approach to understanding the importance and utility of echocardiography in assessing ventricular filling and diastolic function.

BASICS OF LEFT VENTRICULAR DIASTOLIC PHYSIOLOGY

Diastolic filling is not passive but rather represents a complex, energy-dependent process involving an intricate interplay of several dynamic phenomena (7). Left atrial (LA) contraction, mitral valve (MV) geometry, ventricular myocardial relaxation, viscoelastic properties of the myocardium, pericardial restraint, ventricular interaction, and restoring forces generated by the LV impact ventricular filling (8). In addition, many factors that can vary widely in the perioperative period, such as fluid status, positioning, ventilation, hemodynamics, including heart rate and rhythm, also impact diastolic function and the echocardiographic indices used to assess it. Therefore, diastolic function in the perioperative arena should be regarded as a dynamic process, and the echocardiographer must carefully consider both cardiac and noncardiac factors, which impact their assessments.

Clinically, the diastolic phase of the cardiac cycle is defined as the period from aortic valve closure (AVC) to mitral valve closure (MVC) (Figure 7.1), which comprises an initial isovolumic relaxation period, followed by early LV inflow, diastasis, and, finally, atrial contraction (9). *Isovolumic relaxation* begins with the closure of the aortic valve (AV). Due to ventricular relaxation, the pressure in the LV declines rapidly to levels below left atrial pressure (LAP), thus promoting the opening of the MV and rapid filling. The *early filling phase* is typically responsible for 70% to 80% of diastolic filling. Due to continuing myocardial relaxation as well as the elastic recoil of the myocardium during this phase, the LV pressure (LVP) continues to drop despite the LV volume increase. This continued suction effect supports blood flow from the pulmonary veins (PVs) to the LA and into the LV. *Diastasis* is characterized by the equilibration of LAP and LVP. At this time point, filling is minimal and is based on the passive compliance of the LV. *Atrial contraction* results in an increase in LAP, which again promotes forward flow into the LV and also retrograde flow into the PVs. The contribution of this phase to the total stroke volume (usually 20%-25%) varies depending upon ventricular compliance and atrial contractility. Unlike the early LV filling phase, at this point, any LV volume increase is coupled with an LVP increase. The increasing LVP, along with falling atrial pressures due to atrial relaxation, eventually drives closure of the MV.

Physiologically, diastole is characterized by a relaxation and a diastolic filling phase. The *physiologic relaxation phase* comprises the second half of ejection, isovolumic relaxation, and, last, the early filling phase. Relaxation commences immediately after maximal ejection is reached, while the LV is still in the clinical systolic phase (Figure 7.1). At this point, calcium from the cytosol is resequestrated into the sarcoplasmic reticulum via a complex energy-dependent process. Consequently, the contractile elements are deactivated, and the myofibrils return to their original, precontraction length and force (10). The *physiologic diastolic*

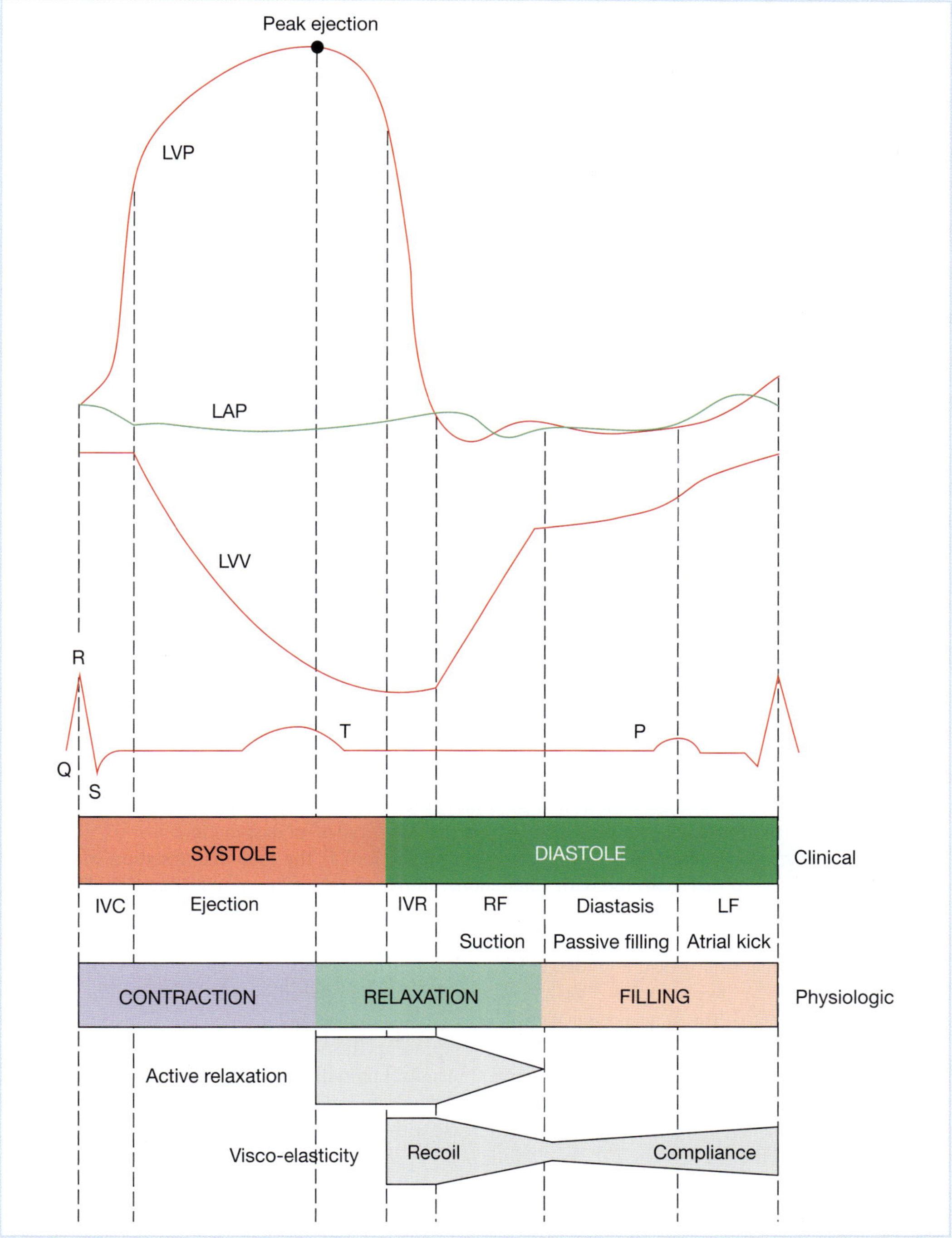

FIGURE 7.1 Division of the cardiac cycle from a clinical and physiologic point of view. After mitral valve closure (MVC), isovolumic contraction (IVC) leads to a significant increase in left ventricular (LV) pressure while the LV volume remains fairly constant. Eventually, the LV pressure increases above the aortic pressure and promotes the aortic valve opening (AVO). With the continuation of LV contraction, LV pressure continues to increase and blood is ejected in the aorta, leading to an LV volume decrease. At the point of maximal ejection, the LV begins to relax, which, coupled with the continued ejection of blood, leads to LV pressure decrease and aortic valve closure. During isovolumic relaxation (IVR) (*1*), LV pressure falls rapidly. When LV pressure decreases below left atrial (LA) pressure, the mitral valve opens (MVO), initiating early, rapid LV filling (*RF*) (*2*). Equilibration of LV and LA pressures results in diminished transmitral flow during diastasis (*3*) until atrial contraction (AC) (*4*), which normally contributes <20% of the total LV end-diastolic volume. Diastole terminates with MVC prior to isovolumic contraction and the AVO, which permits LV ejection.

filling phase comprises, sequentially, the last part of early filling, diastasis, and atrial systole. The interdependency of systole and diastole is underscored by this physiologic process.

Intrinsic Myocardial Factors Affecting Diastolic Performance

Diastolic function is dependent on both intrinsic and extrinsic factors. The intrinsic myocardial factors are ventricular relaxation (dependent upon calcium resequestration) and chamber compliance (related to extracellular matrix and cytoskeleton). *Ventricular relaxation* is gauged by the rate and duration of LVP decline. The traditional method of LV relaxation assessment consists of measuring the LVP rate of decay during isovolumic relaxation. This assessment is performed using high-fidelity, intraventricular, micromanometer catheters, which measure diastolic parameters such as peak instantaneous rate of LVP decline ($-dP/dt$) and the time constant on LV relaxation (tau) (11). Measuring tau is a clinically and experimentally acceptable technique for assessing isovolumic relaxation, although limitations have been described (10). A prolongation of tau is usually consistent with impaired relaxation. *LV chamber compliance* is dependent upon the passive properties of the ventricle (11) and determined by the exponential relationship between the change in volume and the change in pressure during end diastole (dV/dP). The *stiffness modulus*, which can be measured during cardiac catheterization but not with echocardiography, is an index of LV compliance.

Extrinsic Factors Affecting Diastolic Performance

Extrinsic, nonventricular factors significantly impact diastolic function. Tamponade, pleural effusions, mediastinal masses, and pericardial diseases may directly compress the LV and affect filling. Hemodynamic alterations such as tachycardia, rhythm disturbances, and acute hypotension and hypertension all impact filling of the LV. Right ventricular (RV) enlargement may lead to a leftward septal shift, thereby increasing LVP and impeding LV filling. Preload and LA contributions to LV end-diastolic volume are also important determinants of ventricular filling.

PATHOPHYSIOLOGY OF DIASTOLIC DYSFUNCTION AND PROGRESSION OF DISEASE

An impaired capacity of a ventricle to fill at low pressure related to an abnormality in ventricular relaxation and/or chamber compliance is the hallmark of diastolic dysfunction. Diastolic dysfunction is a progressive disorder characterized by the following stages, also described as "grades" of dysfunction:

Impaired ventricular relaxation (grade I diastolic dysfunction) is the first manifestation of diastolic dysfunction unrelated to that expected with aging alone. Impaired relaxation implies that the LV requires a longer time to fully relax. Therefore, the isovolumic relaxation time (IVRT, the time from cessation of systolic ventricular outflow to the onset of LV inflow) is prolonged, and the pressure gradient between the LA and the LV (transmitral pressure gradient) is decreased. It usually occurs in the setting of myocardial ischemia/infarction, LV hypertrophy (LVH), hypertrophic cardiomyopathy, and in the early stages of infiltrative disorders (12). This stage is typically still associated with normal LV filling pressures.

Pseudonormal filling (grade II diastolic dysfunction) represents the next stage of pathophysiology as compensatory mechanisms, aimed at restoring a normal transmitral pressure gradient and promoting LV filling through increases in LAP. With the progression of diastolic dysfunction, compliance decreases, increased stiffness of the LV ensues, and LV filling pressures increase with a further reduction in the pressure gradient between the LA and the LV.

Restrictive filling (grade III diastolic dysfunction) is the ultimate progression of disease as the LV becomes extremely stiff, leading to a markedly decreased compliance and a significantly increased LVP and LAP. In these advanced stages of diastolic dysfunction, compensatory mechanisms are inadequate and little forward flow occurs.

ECHOCARDIOGRAPHIC EVALUATION OF LEFT VENTRICULAR DIASTOLIC FUNCTION

While echocardiography is unable to directly approximate catheter-derived diastolic function parameters, it offers a more practical method for the evaluation of LV diastolic function in clinical practice. However, the perioperative echocardiographer assessing diastolic function must understand that most diastolic indices have been validated in studies with patients breathing spontaneously, undergoing transthoracic echocardiography (TTE), in the left lateral decubitus position, and *not* under general anesthesia. The extrapolation of these results to intubated patients undergoing transesophageal echocardiography (TEE) in the operating room may lead to errors (13,14). PWD indices are particularly impacted by positive pressure ventilation (PPV), preoperative fasting, and intraoperative positioning (15). Whenever possible, the assessment of diastolic function should begin with a clear understanding of preoperative imaging (TTE) and pressure measurements obtained during cardiac catheterization, both of which can help establish a patient's baseline. The perioperative echocardiographer must be cognizant, however, of altered hemodynamic loading conditions, common in the perioperative setting, which have an impact on a patient's diastolic function and filling pressures. An accurate assessment of intraoperative diastolic function should, therefore, include multiple modalities, with an emphasis on those indices that are less load dependent. The evaluation of diastolic function at several time points and under various loading conditions may create a more robust understanding of the patient's diastolic pathology. For instance, a patient who demonstrated significant changes in estimated filling pressures with small changes in volume status might be expected to have poor ventricular compliance. This information can then be utilized to devise a targeted hemodynamic strategy tailored to the patient's physiology.

Two-Dimensional Echocardiography

Indirect evidence of potential diastolic dysfunction can be obtained by 2D echocardiography through evaluations of LV wall thickness and chamber size, global LV systolic function, LA size, and MV structure and function, as these are often impacted by chronic diastolic dysfunction.

Assessment of the Left Ventricle

LVH often indicates a chronic state of elevated LV filling pressures. In addition, in a symptomatic patient, the presence of LVH without LV dilatation and with normal systolic function indicates the presence of diastolic HF.

Assessment of the Left Atrium

The LA serves as a blood reservoir during systole, as a conduit during early LV filling and as a blood pump during atrial systole (16). The LA contribution to LV diastolic filling is usually less than 25% in young healthy patients, yet it may approach 50% in patients with early diastolic dysfunction. The increased LAP, which is the result of chronically elevated LVP, leads to LA remodeling and an increase in size. LA volume has been described as the "HbA1c of left heart disease" as it reflects both the severity and chronicity of elevated LAPs (17). To account for variations in LA size with respect to race and gender, the left atrial volume index (LAVI) can be utilized. This index represents the LA volume normalized for body surface area. An LAVI of greater than 34 mL/m^2 in the absence of significant MV disease is an important indicator of diastolic dysfunction (13). However, due to the close proximity of the LA to the esophagus, the entire LA is difficult to enclose in a single imaging plane when using TEE (18). As such, the LA volume obtained by TEE often underestimates the corresponding volume measured by TTE. Therefore, an LA linear dimension of greater than 4 cm is used as a rough equivalent for dysfunction with TEE (19).

Assessment of Mitral Valve Structure and Function

Mitral regurgitation (MR) and/or stenosis can lead to an increase in LA size in the absence of diastolic dysfunction. Similarly, these pathologies also affect transmitral and PV flow velocities, making the assessment of diastolic function challenging. Mitral annular calcification (MAC) can complicate measurement of mitral annular tissue velocities. The evaluation of diastolic function in these scenarios is discussed in a later section.

Doppler Echocardiographic Evaluation of Left Ventricular Filling

Mitral Valve Inflow Velocities

The utilization of Doppler echocardiography to measure transmitral flow velocities provides valuable information in the assessment of diastolic function. The PWD recording of mitral valve inflow (MVI) velocities is obtained by placing the sample volume at the MV leaflet tips in the midesophageal (ME) four-chamber view (Figure 7.2).

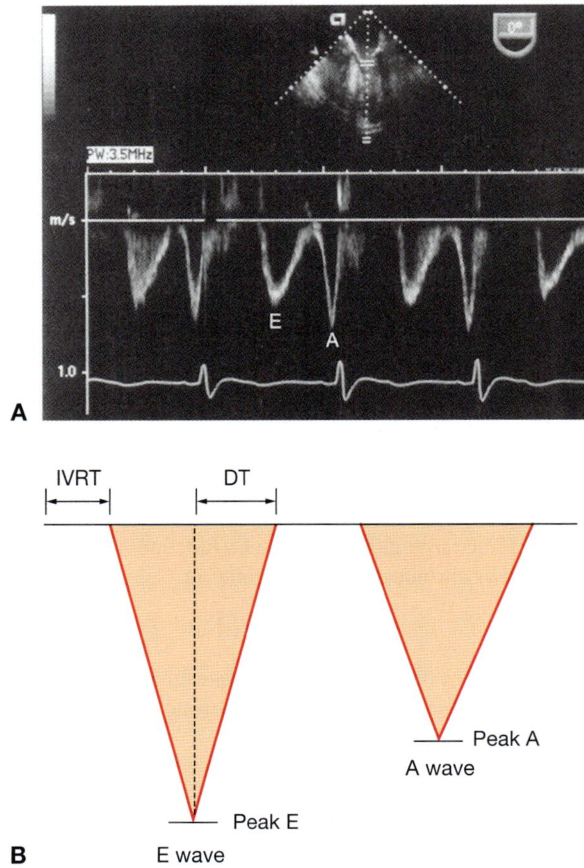

FIGURE 7.2 A: Mitral valve inflow (MVI) velocity profile using transesophageal echocardiography. The MVI profile is obtained by placing a pulsed-wave Doppler sample volume (1-2 mm) at the tips of the mitral leaflets. The initial phase of early left ventricular (LV) filling (E) is followed by a variable period of minimal flow (diastasis) and finally late diastolic filling during atrial contraction (A). B: Schematic of MVI profile depicting relevant indices of diastolic function. Several indices of LV diastolic function can be obtained from this signal including the E- and A-wave peak velocities and ratio, the E-wave deceleration time (DT, the time interval from the peak E-wave velocity to the zero baseline), and the isovolumic relaxation time (IVRT, the time from cessation of systolic ventricular outflow to the onset of transmitral LV inflow).

It is important to ensure that the ultrasound beam is parallel to the direction of transmitral flow. In cases where this is not feasible, an ME long-axis view can be utilized to align the Doppler probe parallel to the transmitral flow.

A typical MVI profile has a biphasic pattern. An initial peak velocity (E wave) occurs during early diastolic filling, and a later velocity (A wave) occurs during atrial contraction. Blood flow during the interposed period of diastasis is usually minimal. Although diastasis is associated with minimal flow, the appearance of a triphasic transmitral inflow pattern occurs occasionally with the presence of an "L wave" during mid-diastole. Mid-diastolic events (L events) can be seen as mitral inflow velocities (L wave), mitral annular tissue velocities (L′ wave), and as MV motion (L motion). The presence of an L wave on MVI, particularly with a velocity greater than 20 cm/s, suggests advanced diastolic dysfunction and is associated with poor outcomes. (13, 20) (Table 7.1; Figures 7.3 and 7.4)

Other than the peak velocities (E and A waves), several additional indices of diastolic function have been derived from mitral inflow signals (Table 7.2) (10,21). A shortening of the deceleration time (DT, the interval from the peak E-wave velocity to the baseline) generally reflects elevation in mean LAP and poor LV compliance (22). The lengthening in the IVRT reflects impaired LV relaxation unless compensatory increases in LAP are present.

TABLE 7.1 Diastolic Events (L Events)

Event	Characteristic	Method
L wave: mitral inflow	Distinguishable forward flow velocity after E wave with a peak velocity >20 cm/s	Pulsed-wave Doppler with sample volume at mitral valve leaflets
L′ wave: mitral annular TDI	Distinguishable basilar-apical tissue velocity after E′	TDI with volume sample at mitral annulus
L motion: mitral valve motion	Opening and closing motion of the mitral valve	M-mode of mitral valve

TDI, tissue Doppler imaging.

MVI velocities reflect the transmitral pressure gradient, which is dependent upon several variables including heart rate and rhythm, LAP and contractility, MV disease, ventricular septal interactions, the intrinsic lusitropic state of the LV, and ventricular compliance (23). An efficient LV relaxation and elastic recoil (restoring forces) observed in young adults is associated with predominant early LV filling corresponding with a greater initial pressure gradient, a large E wave, and a smaller contribution (10%-15%) from atrial contraction.

LV relaxation is delayed with aging, resulting in a lower initial gradient and proportionally less early filling (lower peak E-wave velocity with a longer DT) and a greater, compensatory late filling (higher peak A-wave velocity) accounting for 35% to 40% of LV diastolic inflow.

1. **MVI in diastolic dysfunction**: Changes in LV relaxation and compliance contribute to the spectrum of Doppler LV filling patterns that are observed with worsening diastolic function.
2. **Impaired relaxation (grade I diastolic dysfunction):** Impaired relaxation results in a reduced early MVI velocity characterized by a decreased peak E-wave velocity relative to the peak A-wave velocity (E/A <0.8) and a prolonged IVRT (>110 milliseconds) (26). In addition, as the LAP-LVP gradient takes longer to equilibrate, DT (>220 milliseconds) is prolonged (8). There is a subsequent, compensatory flow increase during atrial contraction accounting for the increased peak A-wave velocity. Due to the relatively

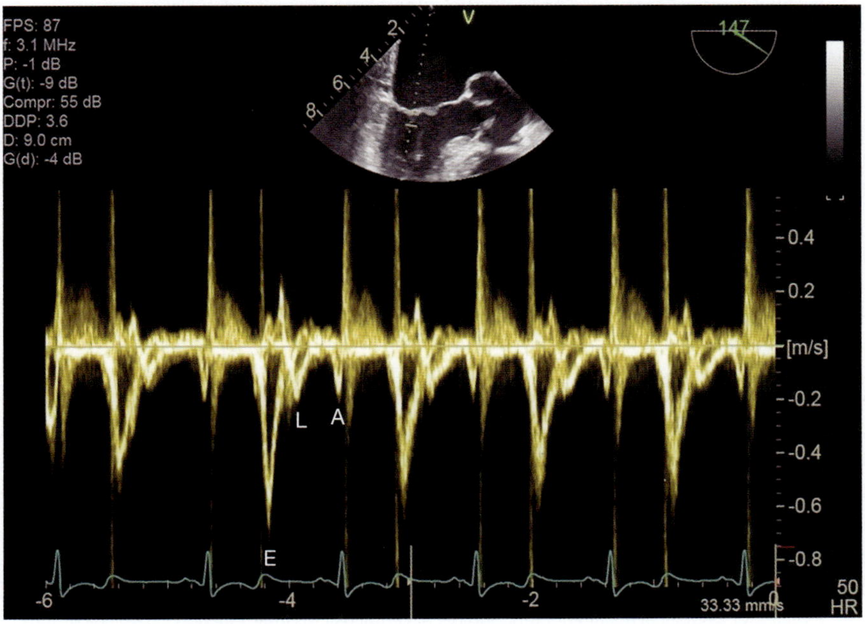

FIGURE 7.3 Transmitral pulsed-wave Doppler demonstrating a mid-diastolic "L" wave.

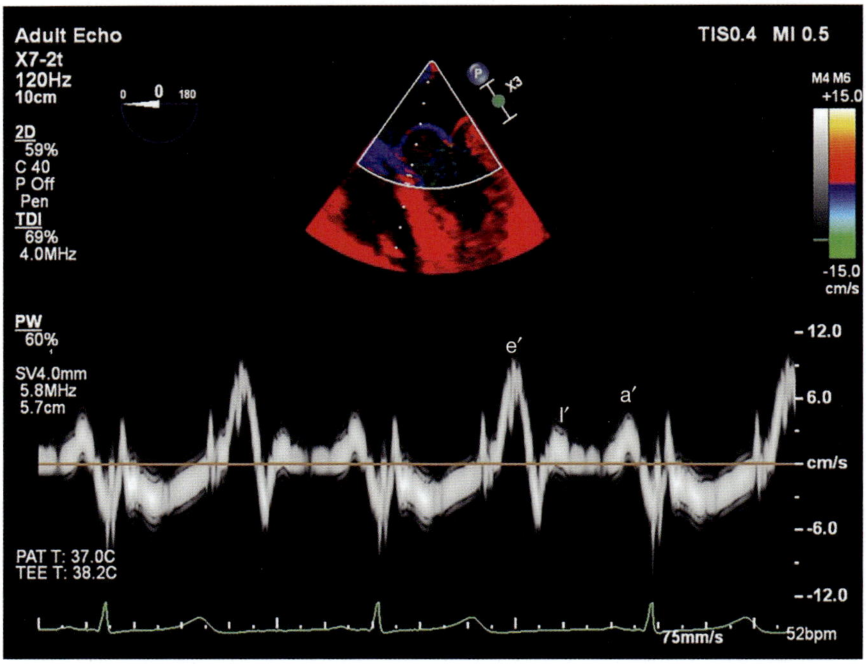

FIGURE 7.4 Tissue Doppler of the mitral annulus demonstrating l′ wave.

TABLE 7.2 Left and Right Ventricular Echocardiographic Indices of Diastolic Function in Normal Subjects

	Age 21-49 y	Age ≥50 y
Left ventricular inflow		
Peak *E* (cm/s)	72 (44-100)	62 (34-90)
Peak *A* (cm/s)	40 (20-60)	59 (31-87)
E/A ratio	1.9 (0.7-3.1)	1.1 (0.5-1.7)
DT (ms)	179 (139-219)	210 (138-282)
IVRT (ms)	76 (54-98)	90 (56-124)
Pulmonary vein		
Peak *S* (cm/s)	48 (30-66)	71 (53-89)
Peak *D* (cm/s)	50 (30-70)	38 (20-56)
S/D ratio	1 (0.5-1.5)	1.7 (0.8-2.6)
Peak *A* (cm/s)	19 (11-27)	23 (–5-51)
Right ventricular inflow		
Peak *E* (cm/s)	51 (37-65)	41 (25-57)
Peak *A* (cm/s)	27 (11-43)	33 (17-49)
E/A	2 (1-3)	1.3 (0.5-2.1)
DT (cm/s)	188 (144-232)	198 (152-244)
Superior vena cava		
Peak *S* (cm/s)	41 (23-59)	42 (18-66)
Peak *D* (cm/s)	22 (12-32)	22 (12-32)
Peak *A* (cm/s)	13 (7-19)	16 (10-22)

Normal reference values for Doppler echocardiographic indices of ventricular diastolic function in two age groups of normal subjects. Data presented are mean values (confidence interval).
A, late diastolic atrial flow velocity associated with atrial contraction; *D*, diastolic flow velocity; DT, deceleration time; *E*, early diastolic flow velocity; IVRT, isovolumic relaxation time; *S*, systolic flow velocity.
Reproduced with permission from Cohen GI, Pietrolungo JF, Thomas JD, et al. A practical guide to assessment of ventricular diastolic function using Doppler echocardiography. *J Am Coll Cardiol*. 1996;27:1753-1760.

high atrial preload, the A-wave duration is prolonged. By convention, the A-wave duration is measured by placing the Doppler sample volume at the level of the MV annulus (as opposed to the MV leaflet tips used for MVI) (13). In summary, the MVI signal of impaired relaxation is characterized by "*E*/*A* reversal" (*E*/*A* <0.8), prolonged IVRT, and prolonged DT.

3. **Pseudonormal filling (grade II diastolic dysfunction):** During the progression from impaired relaxation to restrictive filling, the MVI profile may assume an intermediate *pseudonormalized* pattern that resembles normal LV filling (24). The pseudonormalized pattern represents a moderate stage of diastolic dysfunction where a "normal" early transmitral pressure gradient is generated as gradually increasing LAP from decreased LV compliance balances the lower early mitral inflow velocities from compromised LV relaxation. In summary, the pseudonormalized stage of diastolic dysfunction is thereby characterized by normal values for peak E- and A-wave velocities, IVRT, and DT. Provocative maneuvers can be used to differentiate a patient with normal versus pseudonormal patterns. Reducing preload by utilizing reverse Trendelenburg positioning, partial cardiopulmonary bypass, a Valsalva maneuver (25), or by administering nitroglycerin in a patient with a pseudonormalized transmitral inflow may reveal the underlying impaired LV relaxation (26). In contrast, normal individuals usually respond to preload reduction with a proportional decrease in both E- and A-wave velocities (12). Similarly, preload reduction in patients with a restrictive diastolic dysfunction may result in a pseudonormal pattern on the MVI (9).
4. **Restrictive filling (grade III diastolic dysfunction):** Diastolic dysfunction associated with markedly decreased LV compliance and severely increased LAP is often described as a "restrictive" LV filling pattern (12) and is characterized by an elevated peak E-wave velocity relative to the A-wave velocity due to the elevated LAP (24). Even though impaired relaxation coexists with decreased compliance when diastolic dysfunction has progressed, the substantial increase in LV end-diastolic pressure (LVEDP) results in a markedly elevated LAP and an elevated peak E-wave velocity, consistent with very rapid filling during early diastole. The IVRT is shortened (<60 milliseconds) as the MV opens prematurely due to the elevated LAP. The DT is also abnormally short (<140 milliseconds), as early transmitral flow into the poorly compliant LV results in rapid equilibration of LAP and LVP. This phenomenon may also be associated with diastolic MR (12). Finally, the peak A-wave velocity and duration tend to be compromised by poor atrial contractility and the rapid increase in LVP, which can prematurely terminate late mitral inflow. In summary, a restrictive MVI signal is characterized by an elevated peak E-wave velocity, decreased peak A-wave velocity (*E*/*A* ratio >2), and a shortened IVRT and DT.

In summary, *E*/*A* velocity ratios observed in the progression of diastolic dysfunction begin with high ratios seen with a vigorous LV relaxation pattern of young adults, evolving to a reduction of the ratio with early disease, and terminating with even higher *E*/*A* ratios consistent with the restrictive pattern of severe diastolic dysfunction.

Pulmonary Venous Flow

The evaluation of LA filling can provide important insight into LV diastolic function, especially when combined with data obtained from the MVI signal. A typical pulmonary venous Doppler flow (PVDF) profile consists of an antegrade systolic velocity, which may appear monophasic, or biphasic especially in the presence of low LAP probably owing to temporal dissociation of atrial relaxation and mitral annular motion (Figure 7.5) (27). The first systolic component, PV_{S1}, is dependent upon LA relaxation and the subsequent decrease in pressure. The later peaking PV_{S2} reflects the LA compliance, the effects of early ventricular systole on LAP, any concomitant MR, and the RV stroke volume. An additional, large antegrade velocity occurs during diastole (PV_D) following early transmitral inflow as the LA serves as an open conduit between the PVs and the LV. The late diastolic retrograde velocity, also known as pulmonary venous atrial flow reversal (PV_{AR}), occurs during LA systole and is dependent upon LA contractility, heart rate, and compliance of the LA, PV, and LV (23).

Normally, the PV systolic peak velocity is equal to or slightly greater than the PV_D velocity (Table 7.2) (21). In addition, the normal PV_{AR} duration (≈90-115 milliseconds) is the same or less than the transmitral A-wave duration (≈120-140 milliseconds) (22). In a normally compliant LV, LA contraction should result in a greater net forward blood flow compared with retrograde flow in the PV. A PV_{AR} velocity that exceeds the mitral

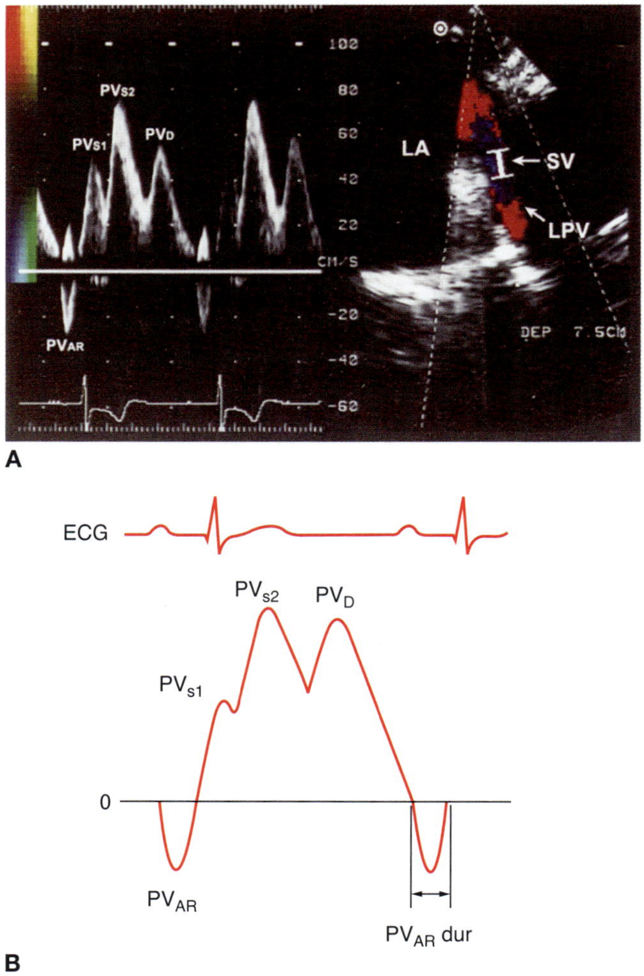

FIGURE 7.5 A: Pulmonary venous flow velocity (PVF) profile. Left atrial (LA) filling can be assessed by placing a PWD sample volume (2-4 mm) ~1 cm into a pulmonary vein (PV) orifice where it joins the LA. B: Schematic of PVF profile depicting relevant indices of diastolic function. Indices of left ventricular (LV) diastolic function obtained from the PVF include the peak *S/D* velocity ratio, as well as the peak A-wave reversal velocity and duration. PV_{AR}, late diastolic retrograde velocity; PV_{AR} dur, PV_{AR} wave duration; PV_{S1}, first systolic component; PV_{S2}, second systolic component; PV_D, diastolic component; SV, sample volume; LPV, left pulmonary vein. ECG, electrocardiogram.

A-wave duration by greater than 35 cm/s or PV_{AR} duration longer than the transmitral A-wave duration by 30 milliseconds usually indicates diastolic dysfunction with increased LVEDP (28).

The analysis of pulmonary vein flow (PVF) compliments the assessment of mitral inflow in the evaluation of diastolic dysfunction.

1. **PVF with impaired relaxation:** The PVF profile consistent with impaired LV relaxation is characterized by a reduced PV_D velocity that parallels the mitral E-wave velocity, and a compensatory increase in the PV_S velocity, resulting in a pattern of *systolic predominance* (PV_S significantly greater than PV_D).
2. **PVF in pseudonormal filling:** The PVF pattern may be helpful in distinguishing a pathologic pseudonormal MVI profile from a normal MVI profile. In such cases, the PV flow profile is often characterized by a pattern of relative systolic blunting and an increased PV_{AR} duration and velocity. It must be emphasized,

however, that in normal young adults and athletes, who do not rely on a significant LA contribution for LV filling, the LA behaves more like a "passive conduit," and PV_s blunting may be observed (29).

3. **PVF with restrictive filling:** Conversely, when the LV filling is restrictive, due to the elevated LAP and decreased LV compliance, the systolic antegrade velocity is reduced and a greater proportion of antegrade flow occurs during diastole, resulting in a pattern of *systolic blunting* (PV_S lower than PV_D). In addition, the PV_{AR} velocity and duration may be increased in the presence of restrictive pathophysiology. However, in patients with severe restrictive filling, the PV_{AR} velocity may be diminished due to atrial mechanical failure (29).

Influence of Physiologic Variables on Doppler Flow Profiles

The utility of MVI and PVF profiles for evaluating LV diastolic function parameters throughout the perioperative period is hindered by frequent changes in preload, afterload, heart rate, and rhythm on peak velocities and proportions of early and late filling (30). *Increases in preload* will often be associated with a more proportionate increase in the transmitral peak E-wave velocity, a shortened IVRT, and steeper DT. *Decreases in preload* will result in opposite changes. *MR* may produce an MVI profile with an increased E-wave velocity due to the elevated LAP and increased volume flow rate across the MV. *Tachycardia* causes fusion of the transmitral E- and A-wave velocities and a pseudo-increase in the A-wave velocity and duration (23). *Dysrhythmias and pacing* may also be associated with alterations in the MVI and PVF profiles. For example, atrial flutter may present with "flutter waves" in the MVI. *Isolated LV systolic dysfunction* may also be associated with an increased transmitral peak E-wave velocity and reduced A wave since diastolic filling occurs at a steeper portion of the LV pressure-volume curve (31).

Mitral Annular Motion Assessed With Tissue Doppler Imaging

As both MV and PVFs are sensitive to alterations in loading conditions, other echocardiographic methods that are less vulnerable to these effects have been sought out, specifically the measurement of mitral annular motion using TDI. This technique utilizes the low-velocity, high-amplitude signal from tissue motion. TDI uses a low-pass frequency filter that eliminates the high velocities associated with blood flow and provides a signal with high temporal and velocity range resolution (32). With TEE, the ME four-chamber view is used with a PWD sample volume placed preferably at the lateral mitral annulus and the PWD beam as parallel as possible to the longitudinal motion of the LV (Figure 7.6). While the septal mitral annulus can be evaluated as

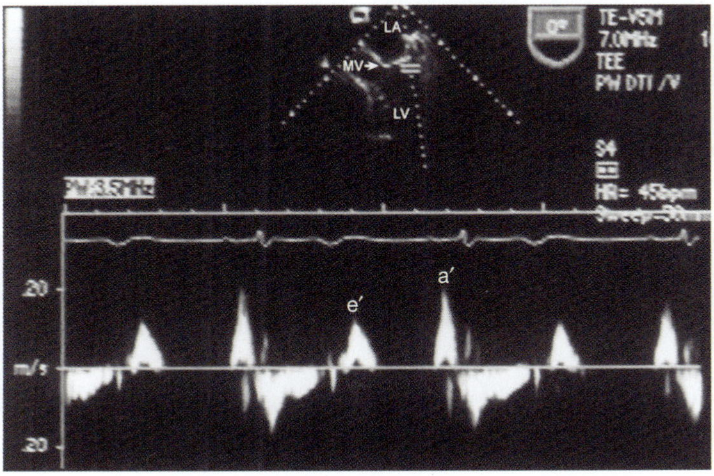

FIGURE 7.6 Mitral annular motion assessed with tissue Doppler imaging (TDI). The PWD sample volume is positioned at the level of the lateral mitral valve (MV) annulus to obtain the TDI profile. A biphasic diastolic component is seen, including an initial early (*e′*) and a later (*a′*) diastolic tissue velocity. LA, left atrium; LV, left ventricle.

well, the alignment between probe and the tissue motion is often poor, resulting in significant underestimation of the tissue velocity. The lowest wall filter and minimal optimal gain should be used to eliminate blood flow velocity signals produced by transmitral flow. Finally, the Nyquist limit, sweep speed, and size of the Doppler profile should be adjusted for optimal visualization.

The mitral annular TDI profile has a systolic component, which has been shown to correlate with ejection fraction (33), and a biphasic diastolic component that mirrors the MVI signal, except that the tissue velocities are much lower (8-15 cm/s). The initial early diastolic tissue velocity (*e′*) begins slightly before mitral inflow, peaks prior to the peak transmitral E-wave velocity, and ends before LV inflow termination (34). In the absence of gross geometric distortion and severe regional wall motion abnormalities, *e′* reflects tissue velocities associated with changes in LV volume and is primarily influenced by the rate of myocardial relaxation and elastic recoil. In the normal patient, the peak *e′* velocity is greater than the later diastolic tissue velocity (*a′*), which tends to reflect LA systolic function (35).

Values of *e′* lower than 8 cm/s are considered a hallmark of diastolic dysfunction. TDI *e′* has been demonstrated to correlate with tau, supporting its value as an index of LV relaxation (36). Due to the relative preload independence of *e′*, these velocities remain depressed in patients with pseudonormal MVI patterns and/or restrictive disease, in contrast to MVI E-wave velocities, which increase along with rising LAP (Figure 7.7). *e′* has been shown to be the best discriminator between normal and pseudonormal patients (31). The *E*/*e′* ratio offers a rough estimate of the LVEDP. A normal value for the *E*/*e′* ratio is less than 8, with a ratio greater than 14 is suggestive of elevated LV filling pressures. An *E*/*e′* ratio between 9 and 13 is considered a "gray zone," in which the filling pressures are indeterminate (13). Similar to transmitral inflow velocities, *e′* and *e′*/*a′* have also been shown to decline with age (33,37). Furthermore, neither peak *e′* velocity nor *e′*/*a′* velocity ratio changes significantly after preload alteration by saline infusion or nitroglycerin (35). This *relative preload insensitivity of e′ makes it particularly useful in the perioperative period when loading conditions can vary considerably.*

Color M-Mode Transmitral Propagation Velocity

The onset of active LV relaxation begins in apical myocardial segments, which creates an intraventricular pressure gradient responsible for accelerating flow and promoting sequential filling toward the apex (36).

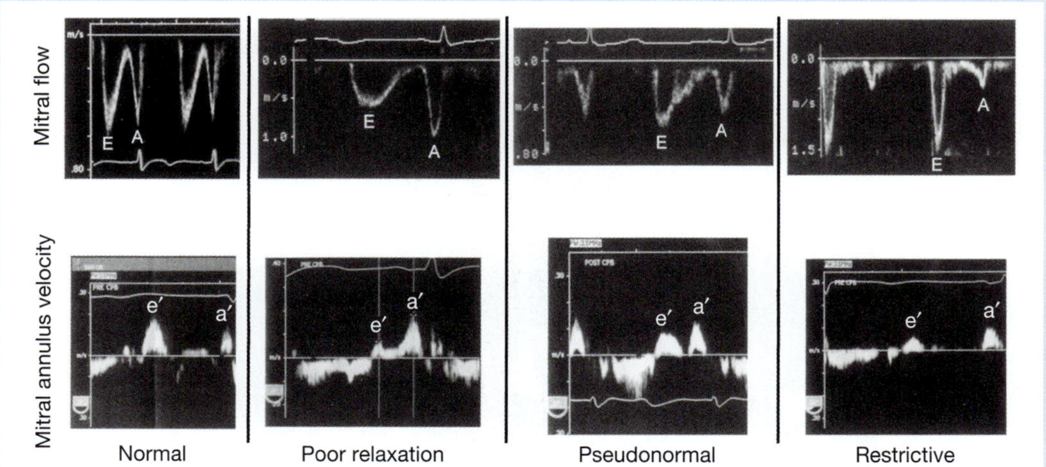

FIGURE 7.7 Patterns of mitral inflow (*E*, *A*) and mitral annular velocities (*e′*, *a′*) associated with progressive left ventricular (LV) diastolic dysfunction. Although both *E*/*A* and *e′*/*a′* decrease with impaired relaxation, that concordance is disrupted with progressive patterns of diastolic dysfunction. Importantly, *e′*/*a′* remains reduced with pseudonormal and restrictive patterns supporting the utility of *e′* as a measure of LV relaxation, and its relative insensitivity to preload compensation.

The propagation rate of LV peak inflow velocity can be evaluated using color M-mode Doppler echocardiography. While standard PWD permits only a temporal distribution of blood flow velocities in a single spatial location, color M-mode Doppler echocardiography provides a spatiotemporal distribution of these velocities, which can be used to delineate the slope of the propagating wavefront (*V*p) from the mitral orifice toward the LV apex (37). The velocity at which flow propagates within the ventricle (*V*p) can be determined from the slope of the color wavefront (Figure 7.8). A significant negative correlation between *V*p and tau has been demonstrated and suggests that rapid LV relaxation (short tau) promotes faster propagation of LV filling from the base to the apex (38).

The technique for obtaining color M-mode Doppler images of LV filling is often described using transthoracic, apical long-axis acoustic windows. An ME four-chamber TEE view also permits visualization of *V*p when an M-mode Doppler beam is aligned parallel to the color-flow Doppler display of transmitral inflow (Figure 7.8). Measurement of *V*p is obtained from the slope of the first aliasing velocity beginning at the mitral annulus and ideally extending 4 cm into the LV toward the apex (37). Visualization of the color wavefront is optimized by shifting the baseline toward the direction of flow, maximizing sweep speed, and adjusting the depth.

In healthy individuals, color M-mode *V*p is between 55 and 100 cm/s (38). Impaired LV relaxation results in a diminished ventricular minimal pressure, thereby compromising the propagation of early filling. In contrast to standard Doppler filling indices, *V*p is relatively independent of preload, yet responds to changes in lusitropic conditions (39,40,41,42) and systolic performance (43). Consequently, *V*p remains reduced through

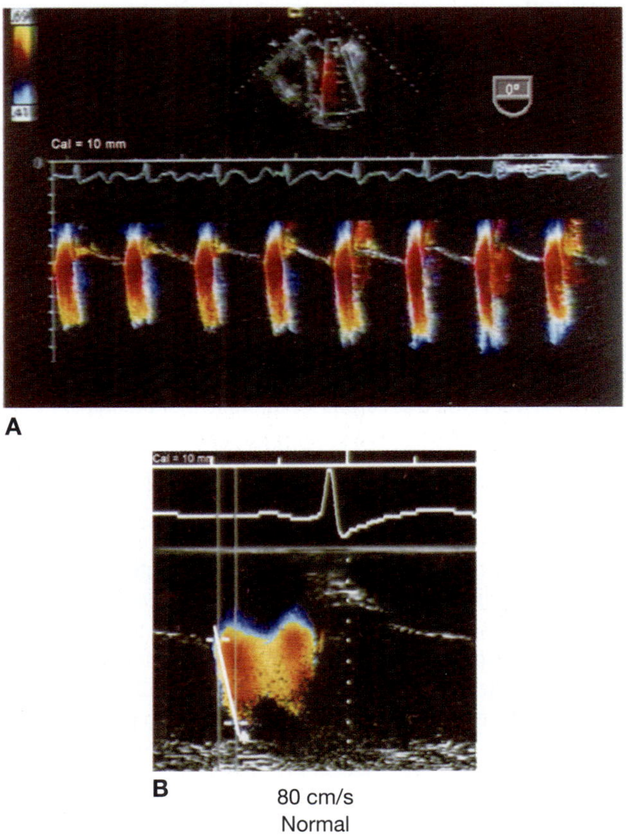

FIGURE 7.8 A: Transmitral color M-mode Doppler flow propagation velocity (*V*p) is obtained by placing the M-mode cursor through the center of the mitral inflow region in a transesophageal midesophageal four-chamber view. B: *V*p is then obtained by measuring the slope of the first aliasing velocity 4 cm into the left ventricular cavity.

all grades of diastolic dysfunction. Interestingly, the ratio of peak E-wave velocity to propagation velocity (*E*/*Vp*) may be useful to predict LAP (43) and also relates directly to LV filling pressures in patients with atrial fibrillation (AF) (44). However, the technique is highly operator dependent and suffers from lower reproducibility and feasibility in the busy perioperative setting. In addition, in patients with normal LVEF but elevated LV filling pressures, *Vp* can be misleadingly normal (13). Finally, improper alignment between the Doppler beam and mitral inflow can lead to erroneous results. Therefore, we advise caution in the use of *Vp* for diastolic function assessment in the perioperative setting.

Assessment of Diastolic Function in Special Clinical Scenarios

Atrial Fibrillation

Determination of diastolic dysfunction and filling pressures in patients with AF can be challenging due to the beat-to-beat variability in LV filling. For measurement of *E* and *e′* velocities, it is recommended to average measurements from 10 consecutive cycles. Since this can be quite cumbersome, velocities averaged from three nonconsecutive beats with cycle lengths within 10% to 20% of the average heart rate may be utilized (44). In patients with AF, the transmitral A waves and PV_{AR} waves are absent, and the E-wave peak velocity and DT vary with the length of the cardiac cycle. AF may also be associated with a loss of PV_{S1} and a decreased PV_{S2} relative to the dominant PV_D (45). Shortening of the transmitral E-wave DT may still correlate with increased LV filling pressure in the presence of AF (45). Several other cutoffs for diastolic dysfunction have been described in patients with AF, such as *E*/mitral V_p 1.4 or greater, IVRT 65 milliseconds or less, and *E*/septal *e′* 11 or greater, and have been suggested, though not validated, in TEE (13,44,46,47).

Mitral Annular Calcification

Severe MAC may result in increases in *E* velocities from mitral stenosis (MS). Moderate-to-severe MAC may also decrease *e′* velocities by restricting annular wall motion. Thus, the measured *E*/*e′* may be disproportionately elevated in such patients. Not surprisingly, in patients with MAC, the *E*/*e′* has been shown ***not*** to correlate well with LV filling pressures (48). *E*/*A* and IVRT have been shown to correlate better with LV filling pressures in this patient population.

Mitral Stenosis

Patients with MS have valve-related elevations of LAP and LA enlargement. Consequently, utilization of *E*/*e′* ratio, PVF Doppler measurements, and LAVI are unreliable metrics for diastolic function assessment in this patient population as the valve lesion's impact on LAP is independent of ventricular diastolic properties. As patients with MS with LV diastolic dysfunction will have delayed onset of *e′* velocity and premature opening of the MV, the time interval from onset of *E* to *e′* ($T_{E\text{-}e'}$) is elevated. An IVRT less than 60 milliseconds and an IVRT/$T_{E\text{-}e'}$ less than 4.2 have been suggested as cutoffs for diastolic dysfunction in this patient population (13). Obtaining a reliable measurement of these parameters is quite difficult, limiting its practical utility in the busy intraoperative environment.

Mitral Regurgitation

Increase in LAP and volume seen with chronic MR often leads to alterations in PVF velocities and LV filling patterns and is often accompanied by AF. Patients with MR often have elevated mitral *E* velocities and a decrease in PV_S due to elevated LAP. Consequently, the measured *E*/*e′* is elevated and *S*/*D* ratio is reduced, resembling diastolic dysfunction. A notable distinction between patients with MR and those with diastolic dysfunction, however, is that the difference in duration of PV_{AR} wave and mitral A wave is normal. Similar to MS, IVRT/$T_{E\text{-}e'}$ is also useful for the estimation of LV filling pressures in patients with MR.

In patients with reduced systolic function, elevated filling pressures often precede the development of MR. Not surprisingly, unlike in patients with primary MR, an increased *E*/*e′* in this patient population has been shown to be a marker for poor outcomes (49).

Right Ventricular Diastolic Function

Indirect evidence of RV diastolic function can first be sought out by examining RV mass or volume. Second, Doppler echocardiographic evaluation of tricuspid valve inflow (TVI) and tricuspid annular velocities is performed to provide more specific information (Figure 7.9A) as RV diastolic dysfunction manifests with the same relative changes in TVI peak E- and A-wave velocities, E/A-wave ratios, and DT that occur with MVI profiles (50,51). TVI velocities mimic those of the MV, though the TVI signals are of lower velocity due to the larger tricuspid valve (TV) annular size. Direct comparisons of RV and LV inflow velocities also reveal differences in timing and reciprocal respiratory variation. During spontaneous inspiration, negative intrapleural pressure results in an increase in right atrial (RA) volume and subsequent greater RV diastolic filling velocities up to 20% compared to end-expiratory values (31). In contrast, LA and LV filling is reduced during spontaneous inspiration relative to end expiration.

RA inflow velocities, including the IVC, hepatic veins (HVs), and superior vena cava (SVC), provide additional echocardiographic evaluation of RV diastolic function. The HVs join the intrahepatic inferior vena cava (IVC) tangentially and can be visualized by advancing and turning the TEE probe rightward

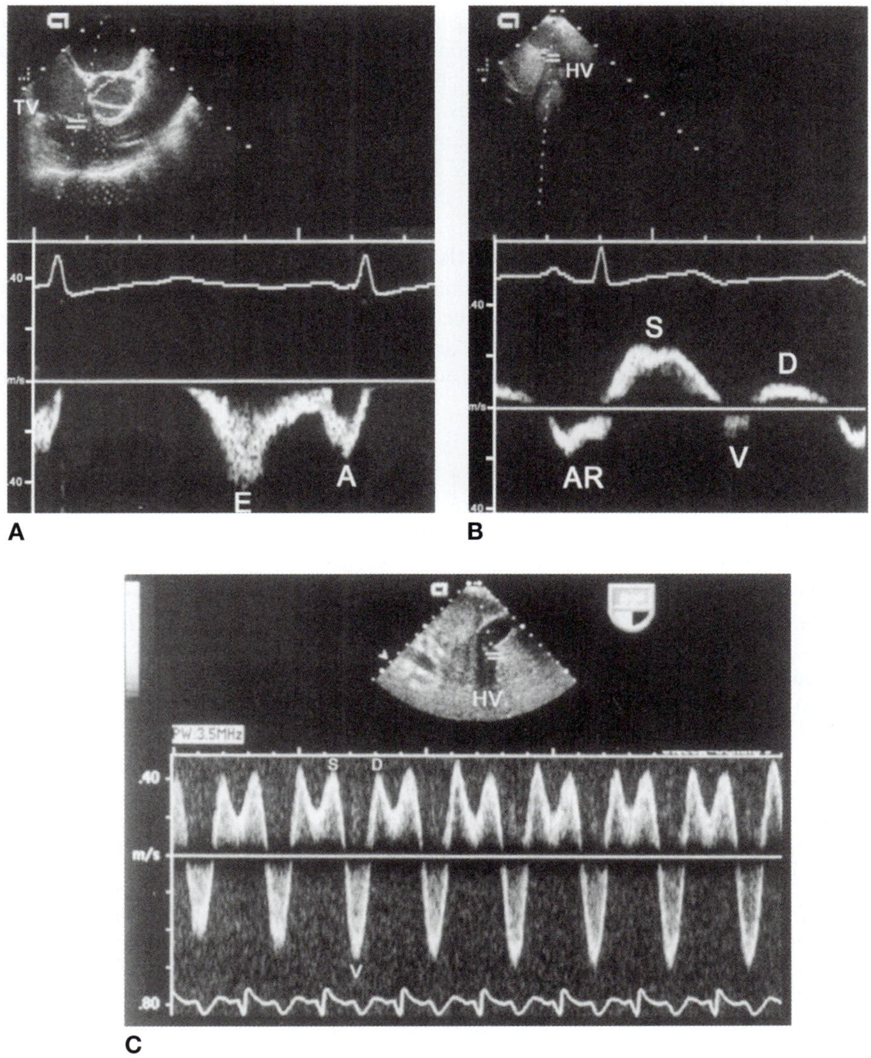

FIGURE 7.9 A: Normal transtricuspid Doppler flow profile. B: Normal hepatic venous Doppler flow velocity profiles. C: Prominent hepatic flow reversal at end systole (*V*) in a patient with decreased right ventricular compliance. *A*, late diastolic velocity; AR, atrial contraction flow reversal; *D*, antegrade flow during right ventricular filling; *E*, early diastolic velocity; HV, hepatic vein; *S*, antegrade early systolic flow; TV, tricuspid valve.

from the ME bicaval view. The normal HV Doppler profile (Figure 7.9B) is characterized by (a) a small reversal of flow following atrial contraction (*AR wave*), (b) an antegrade systolic phase during atrial filling from the SVC and IVC (*S wave*) that is influenced by TV annular motion, RA relaxation, and tricuspid regurgitation (TR), (c) a second small flow reversal at end systole (*V wave*) that is influenced by RV and RA compliance, and (d) a second antegrade filling phase while the RA acts as a passive conduit during RV filling (*D wave*) (31).

The ratio of the total hepatic reverse flow to total forward flow increases with either RV diastolic dysfunction or significant TR but appears to be more affected by the former (52). In addition, a marked shortening of the TVI DT and diastolic predominance of HV flow with prominent V- and A-wave reversals during spontaneous inspiration indicates significant decreases in RV compliance and increased diastolic filling pressures (Figure 7.9C) (23). Diastolic RV dysfunction (lower TV peak E-wave velocity, lower *E*/*A* ratios, and prolonged RV IVRT) has also been demonstrated in patients with pulmonary hypertension (PHT). Symptomatic HF, even in the absence of PHT, presents a similar finding, suggesting a potential role for ventricular interdependence in impaired RV filling (45).

RV diastolic dysfunction is considered when the *E*/*A* ratio is less than 0.8 or greater than 2.1, an *E/E′* ratio is greater than 6, and a DT is less than 120 milliseconds. An impaired relaxation of the RV is defined by an *E*/*A* ratio less than 0.8. Pseudonormal filling is highlighted by an *E*/*A* ratio 0.8 to 2.1 with an *E*/*e′* greater than 6 or a diastolic flow predominance (*D*) of the HV. Restrictive filling is defined by an *E*/*A* greater than 2.1 with an associated DT less than 120 milliseconds. (53) However, more research is required to validate the values of various RV diastolic indices and the grading of RV diastolic dysfunction.

Pericardial Diseases: Constrictive Pericarditis and Cardiac Tamponade

Pericardial diseases may have profound hemodynamic effects, and therefore, promptly establishing the diagnosis and severity of pericardial pathologies is crucial in the perioperative setting. Both constrictive pericarditis (CP) and cardiac tamponade impair diastolic filling and result in chest pain, shortness of breath, tachycardia, and hypotension. Echocardiography may be the only feasible imaging modality in an emergent perioperative setting.

Constrictive Pericarditis

CP is defined as chronic fibrous thickening or calcification of the pericardial sac, which reduces its compliance (54). As the heart functions within a fixed nonelastic casing, the total cardiac volume is severely limited. As such, the constrictive pericardium leads to elevated intracardiac pressures and exaggerated ventricular interdependence. Due to elevated intra-atrial pressures, ventricular filling occurs earlier than usual and results in a steep rise in intraventricular pressures that impedes further filling later in diastole. This process explains the rapid "y" descent on the atrial pressure waveform and "square root" sign on the ventricular pressure tracings (55).

2D echocardiographic hallmarks of CP include thickened pericardium (>4 mm), rapid diastolic biventricular filling with an abrupt halt referred to as "diastolic checking," abnormal septal motion ("septal bounce") due to ventricular interdependence, and biatrial enlargement (56). On TDI, as the pericardium prevents the tethered lateral mitral annulus from moving freely, the *e′* lateral is lower than the *e′* medial. This finding, referred to as "annulus reversus," is often utilized to differentiate between CP and restrictive cardiomyopathy (57). Unlike in restrictive cardiomyopathy, where the *e′* values are reduced, *e′* septal is preserved and may even be increased in patients with CP (58,59). On Doppler examination of the ventricular inflow velocities, patients with CP have a distinct respiratory variation that is discussed in the following sections.

Cardiac Tamponade

Cardiac tamponade is a life-threatening condition. Rapid accumulation of intrapericardial fluid leads to a rise in intrapericardial pressure, impeding diastolic filling of the ventricles. To compensate for the increase in intrapericardial pressure and to maintain cardiac output, the intracavitary filling pressures rise, resulting in an "equalization of pressures" in all cardiac chambers.

TABLE 7.3 Respirophasic Variation in Ventricular Inflow Velocities in Pericardial Diseases

	Tricuspid Valve *E* Peak Velocity		Mitral Valve *E* Peak Velocity	
Ventilation	SV	PPV	SV	PPV
Normal	Insp > Exp $\Delta_{20\%}$	Insp < Exp	Insp < Exp $\Delta_{5\%-10\%}$	Insp > Exp
Cardiac tamponade	Insp > Exp $\Delta_{60\%}$	Insp = Exp	Insp < Exp $\Delta_{30\%}$	Insp = Exp
Constrictive pericarditis	Insp > Exp $\Delta_{40\%}$	Insp < Exp	Insp < Exp $\Delta_{25\%}$	Insp > Exp $\Delta_{20\%}$

Respiratory variation of peak inflow velocity (*E*) in normal state, cardiac tamponade, and constrictive pericarditis under spontaneous or positive pressure ventilation.
By convention, percentage respiratory variation of the mitral and tricuspid inflow is calculated as (Exp – Insp)/Exp. It should be noted that, in some instances, the value may be negative.
Δ, respiratory variation; Exp, peak expiratory inflow velocity; Insp, peak inspiratory inflow velocity; PPV, positive pressure ventilation; SV, spontaneous ventilation.

Although tamponade is a clinical diagnosis, several characteristic echocardiographic features can establish the severity of the disease. Common echocardiographic findings include the presence of a large pericardial effusion persisting throughout the cardiac cycle, a characteristic "swinging motion" of the heart, reduced LV systolic and diastolic dimensions due to reduced filling, and a resulting decreased stroke volume (56). Due to increased systemic venous pressures, the IVC is distended, plethoric (>2 cm), and has minimal respiratory variation. In addition, RA collapse starting early in ventricular systole and lasting more than one-third of the cardiac cycle is a highly sensitive (100%) and specific (94%) sign of cardiac tamponade (60). With a further rise in intrapericardial pressures, RV diastolic collapse occurs. The duration of RV collapse is directly proportional to the severity of tamponade (61). RV diastolic collapse is also a highly sensitive (93%) and specific (100%) finding for tamponade. The duration of collapse can be assessed using M-mode across the RA or RV, respectively, in an ME four-chamber view and correlating it with the electrocardiographic tracing. Like CP, patients with tamponade also have a distinct respiratory variation in ventricular inflow velocities (Table 7.3).

Respirophasic Variation in Ventricular Inflow Velocities in Pericardial Diseases

Under normal conditions, the elastic pericardium transmits intrathoracic pressures to the cardiac chambers, causing the pulmonary capillary-LV diastolic pressure gradient to remain fairly constant during the respiratory cycle. In a healthy spontaneously breathing individual, the decrease in intrathoracic pressure with inspiration augments venous return to the right-sided cardiac chambers, with TVI velocities increasing by 20% compared to expiration (Table 7.3). Conversely, transmitral inflow velocities are lower during spontaneous inspiration as blood is sequestered in the pulmonary capillaries, decreasing LV preload. During spontaneous expiration, blood is squeezed out of the pulmonary vasculature, leading to increased transmitral inflow velocities and a minimal respiratory variation of 5% to 10% (inspiration <expiration) (Table 7.3) (58). Under PPV, the respirophasic transvalvular flow pattern is typically reversed in normovolemic, healthy individuals. Due to positive intrathoracic pressure during inspiration, RV filling is decreased, while during expiration, it increases. Conversely, the transmitral inflow velocity is augmented during inspiration, due to the squeezing of the pulmonary vasculature resulting from the positive intrathoracic pressure, and decreases with expiration. It is important to recognize that the respirophasic flow pattern during PPV is impacted by the tidal volumes administered and the resulting amount of pressure applied to the lung.

In patients with CP, respirophasic variations are impacted by two factors. First, the thickened pericardium impedes the transmission of intrathoracic pressures to the heart, leading to a dissociation between the intracardiac and intrathoracic pressures during respiration. Second, the pericardial pathology impairs expansion of the cardiac chambers, resulting in exaggerated ventricular interdependence. Thus, during spontaneous inspiration, the pressure in the PVs decreases while the LVP remains unchanged. Therefore, the pressure gradient between the PVs and the LV cavity is reduced, leading to markedly decreased peak mitral inflow velocities. During spontaneous expiration, similar to healthy patients, the blood is squeezed out of the pulmonary circulation into the LV, leading to increased velocities in expiration. The typical pattern of right-sided intracardiac flows ($I > E$), which are reciprocal to the left heart, is more pronounced in patients with CP, mainly due to the influence of ventricular interdependence. In total, the transmitral and transtricuspid respiratory inflow velocity variations are exaggerated in patients with CP, exceeding 25% for mitral and 40% for tricuspid inflow (56). Similar to healthy patients, PPV reverses the respiratory variation pattern of ventricular inflow velocities.

As opposed to CP, in patients with tamponade, the pericardial sac filled with fluid easily transmits intrathoracic pressures to the heart chambers. However, due to limited pericardial expansion allowed by tamponade, exaggerated ventricular interdependence is present. Therefore, during spontaneous inspiration, similar to healthy patients, the negative intrathoracic pressure is transmitted to the right side of the heart, which fills preferentially at the expense of the LV. The ventricular septum is pushed toward the LV, further impeding its filling. In expiration, the process is reversed, whereby LV expansion impedes RV filling. Ventricular inflow respiratory variation is more pronounced in patients with tamponade compared to CP, exceeding 30% for mitral and 60% for tricuspid velocities (56). Although mechanical ventilation typically reverses the respiratory variation pattern of ventricular inflow velocities seen during spontaneous breathing, in patients with tamponade, at the edge of their physiologic reserve and with limited circulating volume, this tenet may not hold. Such little blood is squeezed out of the pulmonary vasculature during inspiration in these patients that any LV preload enhancement is limited and ventricular inflow respiratory variation may not be present during PPV (62) (Table 7.3).

A PRACTICAL APPROACH TO DIASTOLIC FUNCTION ASSESSMENT IN THE PERIOPERATIVE PERIOD

We advocate the following approach to the intraoperative assessment of diastolic function, preferably performed during periods of hemodynamic stability, at end expiration, and prior to pericardiotomy. Measurements during periods of tachycardia, pacing, Valsalva maneuvers, or surgical manipulation of the heart/great vessels should be avoided.

1. 2D assessment of cardiac chambers and valves: Evidence of valvular abnormalities, MAC, LVH, and marked LA enlargement should be sought.
2. Doppler interrogation:
    a. TDI of the lateral mitral annulus is performed and the e' velocity measured.
    b. MVI velocities are measured next, maintaining a parallel alignment with transmitral blood flow with the PWD gate at the tips of the mitral leaflets in diastole.
    c. An E/e' velocity is then calculated and the grade of diastolic dysfunction assessed (Figure 7.10). Optimal MVI and TDI waveforms should not display spikes, feathering, or ghosting.
3. PVF: Measurement of PVF velocities and calculation of the S/D ratio can be employed to assess diastolic function. This is particularly helpful in patients with MAC and in patients where 2D visualization of the lateral mitral wall annulus is difficult.

Thus, the evaluation and incorporation of all the parameters with consideration of the pitfalls of each is of paramount importance. *It must also be emphasized that diastolic dysfunction is a continuum and that the grade may vary during the intraoperative period as a result of changing loading conditions and rhythm.* In some instances, diastolic parameters do not converge to a particular grade of diastolic dysfunction. In such situations, the most recent American Society of Echocardiography guidelines recommend grading diastolic dysfunction as "indeterminate" (13). However, due to the paucity of studies validating the correlation between the results of the preoperative TTE with those of the intraoperative TEE examination, further studies are required to "fine-tune" intraoperative TEE evaluation of diastolic function.

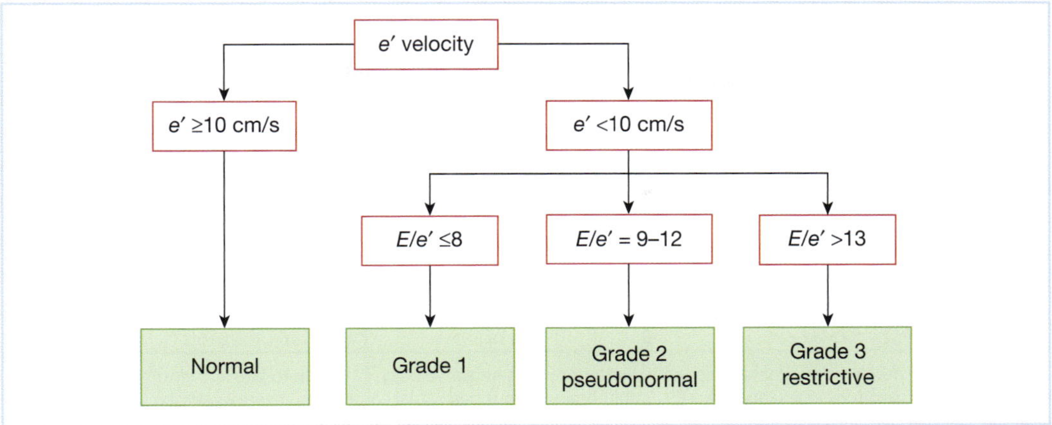

FIGURE 7.10 A simplified algorithm for intraoperative grading of diastolic dysfunction using mitral inflow peak *E* velocity and lateral mitral annulus peak *e′* velocity. EF, ejection fraction; LA, left atrium; LAP, left atrial pressure; LV, left ventricle; TR, tricuspid regurgitation. (Derived from Swaminathan M, Nicoara A, Phillips-Bute BG, et al. Utility of a simple algorithm to grade diastolic dysfunction and predict outcome after coronary artery bypass graft surgery. *Ann Thorac Surg*. 2011;91:1844-1850.)

SUMMARY

The assessment of diastolic function provides vital therapeutic and prognostic information and should be an integral part of every intraoperative TEE. Echocardiography provides an effective, noninvasive means for diagnosing the presence, extent, and etiology of diastolic dysfunction (Figure 7.11; Table 7.4) (63). Doppler echocardiographic measurements of atrial and ventricular inflow velocities remain an important component

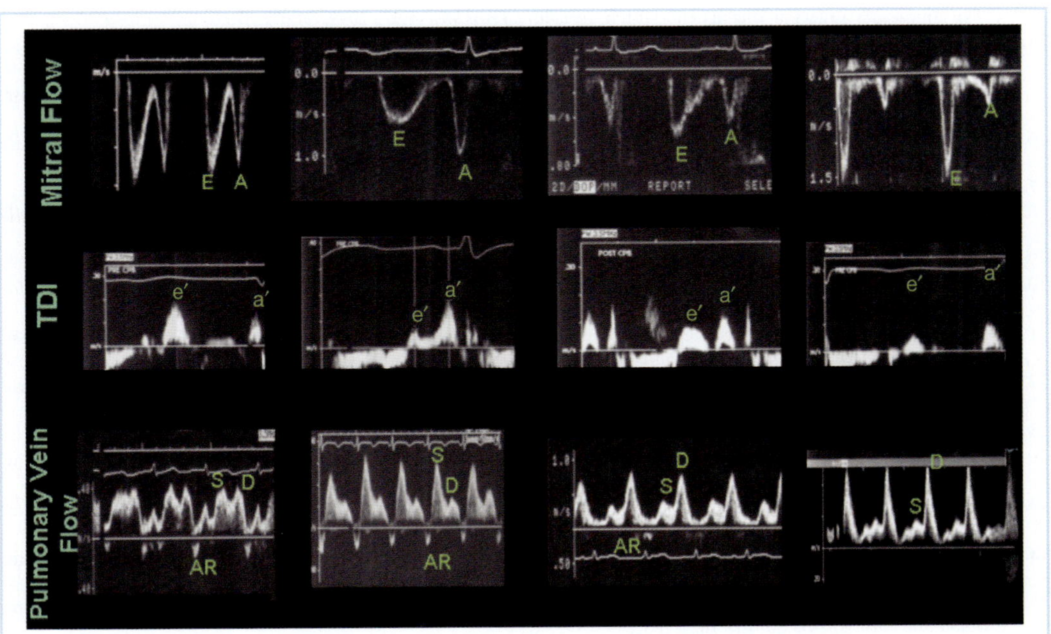

FIGURE 7.11 Doppler echocardiographic measures of diastolic function. *A*, peak late transmitral Doppler flow velocity; *a′*, late diastolic mitral annular tissue velocity; AR, pulmonary venous atrial flow reversal; *D*, diastolic pulmonary venous Doppler flow velocity; *E*, peak early transmitral Doppler flow velocity; *e′*, early diastolic mitral annular tissue velocity; *S*, systolic pulmonary venous Doppler flow velocity.

TABLE 7.4 Doppler Echocardiographic Values of Left Ventricular Diastolic Dysfunction

	Normal (Young)	Normal (Adult)	Impaired Relaxation	Pseudonormal Filling	Restrictive Filling
E/A (cm/s)	>1	>1	<1	1-2	>2
DT (ms)	<220	<220	>220	150-200	<150
IVRT (ms)	<100	<100	>100	60-100	<60
S/D	<1	≥1	≥1	<1	<1
PV_{AR} (cm/s)	<35	<35	<35	≥35[a]	≥25[a]
Vp (cm/s)	>55	>45	<45	<45	<45
e′ (cm/s)	>10	>8	<8	<8	<8

DT, early LV filling deceleration time; e′, peak early diastolic mitral annular velocity; *E/A*, early-to-late left ventricular (LV) filling ratio; IVRT, isovolumic relaxation time; PV_{AR}, pulmonary venous peak atrial contraction reversal velocity; *S/D*, systolic-to-diastolic pulmonary venous flow ratio; *Vp*, transmitral color M-mode propagation velocity.
[a]Unless atrial mechanical failure is present.
Reproduced with permission from Garcia MJ, Thomas JD, Klein AL. New Doppler echocardiographic applications for the study of diastolic function. *J Am Coll Cardiol*. 1998;32:865-875.

of a thorough examination along with mitral annular TDI, which is less sensitive to changes in loading conditions. In the future, the availability of more sensitive echocardiographic techniques for diagnosing diastolic dysfunction will hopefully facilitate both the perioperative evaluation and the development of therapeutic plans to manage this complex and important physiology.

REFERENCES

1. Grossman W. Diastolic dysfunction in congestive heart failure. *N Engl J Med.* 1991;325:1557-1564.
2. Flu WJ, van Kuijk JP, Hoeks SE, et al. Prognostic implications of asymptomatic left ventricular dysfunction in patients undergoing vascular surgery. *Anesthesiology.* 2010;112:1316-1324.
3. Lerman BJ, Popat RA, Assimes TL, et al. Association of left ventricular ejection fraction and symptoms with mortality after elective noncardiac surgery among patients with heart failure. *J Am Med Assoc.* 2019;321:572-579.
4. Fayad A, Ansari MT, Yang H, et al. Perioperative diastolic dysfunction in patients undergoing noncardiac surgery is an independent risk factor for cardiovascular events: a systematic review and meta-analysis. *Anesthesiology.* 2016;125:72-91.
5. Bernard F, Denault A, Babin D, et al. Diastolic dysfunction is predictive of difficult weaning from cardiopulmonary bypass. *Anesth Analg.* 2001;92:291-298.
6. Swaminathan M, Nicoara A, Phillips-Bute BG, et al. Utility of a simple algorithm to grade diastolic dysfunction and predict outcome after coronary artery bypass graft surgery. *Ann Thorac Surg.* 2011;91:1844-1850.
7. Morrissey C. Echo for diastology. *Ann Card Anaesth.* 2016;19:S12-S18.
8. Nishimura RA, Tajik AJ. Evaluation of diastolic filling of left ventricle in health and disease: Doppler echocardiography is the clinician's Rosetta Stone. *J Am Coll Cardiol.* 1997;30:8-18.
9. Plotnick GD. Changes in diastolic function–difficult to measure, harder to interpret. *Am Heart J.* 1989;118:637-641.
10. Pagel PS, Grossman W, Haering JM, et al. Left ventricular diastolic function in the normal and diseased heart. Perspectives for the anesthesiologist (1). *Anesthesiology.* 1993;79:836-854.
11. Zile M, Smith V. Relaxation and diastolic properties of the heart. In: Fozzard H, Haber E, Jennings R, et al, eds. *The Heart and Cardiovascular System: Scientific Foundations*. 2nd ed. Raven; 1991:1353-1367.
12. Oh JK, Appleton CP, Hatle LK, et al. The noninvasive assessment of left ventricular diastolic function with two-dimensional and Doppler echocardiography. *J Am Soc Echocardiogr.* 1997;10:246-270.
13. Nagueh SF, Smiseth OA, Appleton CP, et al. Recommendations for the evaluation of left ventricular diastolic function by echocardiography: an update from the American Society of Echocardiography and the European Association of Cardiovascular Imaging. *J Am Soc Echocardiogr.* 2016;29:277-314.
14. McIlroy DR, Wettig P, Burton J, et al. Poor agreement between preoperative transthoracic echocardiography and intraoperative transesophageal echocardiography for grading diastolic dysfunction. *Anesth Analg.* 2024;138:123-133.
15. Juhl-Olsen P, Hermansen JF, Frederiksen CA, et al. Positive end-expiratory pressure influences echocardiographic measures of diastolic function: a randomized, crossover study in cardiac surgery patients. *Anesthesiology.* 2013;119:1078-1086.
16. Bardia A, Montealegre-Gallegos M, Mahmood F, et al. Left atrial size: an underappreciated perioperative cardiac risk factor. *J Cardiothorac Vasc Anesth.* 2014;28:1624-1632.
17. Teo SG, Yang H, Chai P, et al. Impact of left ventricular diastolic dysfunction on left atrial volume and function: a volumetric analysis. *Eur J Echocardiogr.* 2010;11:38-43.
18. Hahn RT, Abraham T, Adams MS, et al. Guidelines for performing a comprehensive transesophageal echocardiographic examination: recommendations from the American Society of Echocardiography and the Society of Cardiovascular Anesthesiologists. *J Am Soc Echocardiogr.* 2013;26:921-964.

19. Appleton CP, Galloway JM, Gonzalez MS, et al. Estimation of left ventricular filling pressures using two-dimensional and Doppler echocardiography in adult patients with cardiac disease. Additional value of analyzing left atrial size, left atrial ejection fraction and the difference in duration of pulmonary venous and mitral flow velocity at atrial contraction. *J Am Coll Cardiol.* 1993;22:1972-1982.
20. Di Virgilio E, Montillo F Santoro D et al. Mid-diastolic events (L Events): a critical review. *J Clin Med.* 2021;10:1-17.
21. Cohen GI, Pietrolungo JF, Thomas JD, et al. A practical guide to assessment of ventricular diastolic function using Doppler echocardiography. *J Am Coll Cardiol.* 1996;27:1753-1760.
22. Little WC, Ohno M, Kitzman DW, et al. Determination of left ventricular chamber stiffness from the time for deceleration of early left ventricular filling. *Circulation.* 1995;92:1933-1939.
23. Appleton CP, Firstenberg MS, Garcia MJ, et al. The echo-Doppler evaluation of left ventricular diastolic function. A current perspective. *Cardiol Clin.* 2000;18:513-546, ix.
24. Appleton C, Hatle L. The natural history of left ventricular filling abnormalities: assessment by two-dimensional and Doppler echocardiography. *Echocardiography.* 1992;9:437-457.
25. Dumesnil JG, Gaudreault G, Honos GN, et al Use of Valsalva maneuver to unmask left ventricular diastolic function abnormalities by Doppler echocardiography in patients with coronary artery disease or systemic hypertension. *Am J Cardiol.* 1991;68:515-519.
26. Hurrell DG, Nishimura RA, Ilstrup DM, et al. Utility of preload alteration in assessment of left ventricular filling pressure by Doppler echocardiography: a simultaneous catheterization and Doppler echocardiographic study. *J Am Coll Cardiol.* 1997;30:459-467.
27. Nishimura RA, Abel MD, Hatle LK, et al. Relation of pulmonary vein to mitral flow velocities by transesophageal Doppler echocardiography. Effect of different loading conditions. *Circulation.* 1990;81:1488-1497.
28. Yamamoto K, Nishimura RA, Burnett JC Jr, et al. Assessment of left ventricular end-diastolic pressure by Doppler echocardiography: contribution of duration of pulmonary venous versus mitral flow velocity curves at atrial contraction. *J Am Soc Echocardiogr.* 1997;10:52-59.
29. Appleton CP, Hatle LK, Popp RL. Relation of transmitral flow velocity patterns to left ventricular diastolic function: new insights from a combined hemodynamic and Doppler echocardiographic study. *J Am Coll Cardiol.* 1988;12:426-440.
30. Nishimura RA, Abel MD, Hatle LK, et al. Assessment of diastolic function of the heart: background and current applications of Doppler echocardiography. Part II. Clinical studies. *Mayo Clin Proc.* 1989;64:181-204.
31. Otto CM. Ventricular Diastolic Filling and Function. In: Otto CM, ed. *Textbook of Clinical Echocardiography.* 7th ed. Philadelphia, PA: Elsevier; 2023:190-220.
32. Farias CA, Rodriguez L, Garcia MJ, et al. Assessment of diastolic function by tissue Doppler echocardiography: comparison with standard transmitral and pulmonary venous flow. *J Am Soc Echocardiogr.* 1999;12:609-617.
33. Nagueh SF, Middleton KJ, Kopelen HA, et al. Doppler tissue imaging: a noninvasive technique for evaluation of left ventricular relaxation and estimation of filling pressures. *J Am Coll Cardiol.* 1997;30:1527-1533.
34. Garcia MJ, Rodriguez L, Ares M, et al. Differentiation of constrictive pericarditis from restrictive cardiomyopathy: assessment of left ventricular diastolic velocities in longitudinal axis by Doppler tissue imaging. *J Am Coll Cardiol.* 1996;27:108-114.
35. Sohn DW, Chai IH, Lee DJ, et al. Assessment of mitral annulus velocity by Doppler tissue imaging in the evaluation of left ventricular diastolic function. *J Am Coll Cardiol.* 1997;30:474-480.
36. Takatsuji H, Mikami T, Urasawa K, et al. A new approach for evaluation of left ventricular diastolic function: spatial and temporal analysis of left ventricular filling flow propagation by color M-mode Doppler echocardiography. *J Am Coll Cardiol.* 1996;27:365-371.
37. Garcia MJ, Thomas JD, Klein AL. New Doppler echocardiographic applications for the study of diastolic function. *J Am Coll Cardiol.* 1998;32:865-875.
38. Brun P, Tribouilloy C, Duval AM, et al. Left ventricular flow propagation during early filling is related to wall relaxation: a color M-mode Doppler analysis. *J Am Coll Cardiol.* 1992;20:420-432.
39. Garcia MJ, Smedira NG, Greenberg NL, et al. Color M-mode Doppler flow propagation velocity is a preload insensitive index of left ventricular relaxation: animal and human validation. *J Am Coll Cardiol.* 2000;35:201-208.
40. Garcia MJ, Palac RT, Malenka DJ, et al. Color M-mode Doppler flow propagation velocity is a relatively preload-independent index of left ventricular filling. *J Am Soc Echocardiogr.* 1999;12:129-137.
41. Moller JE, Poulsen SH, Sondergaard E, et al. Preload dependence of color M-mode Doppler flow propagation velocity in controls and in patients with left ventricular dysfunction. *J Am Soc Echocardiogr.* 2000;13:902-909.
42. Djaiani GN, McCreath BJ, Ti LK, et al. Mitral flow propagation velocity identifies patients with abnormal diastolic function during coronary artery bypass graft surgery. *Anesth Analg.* 2002;95:524-530.
43. Garcia MJ, Ares MA, Asher C, et al. An index of early left ventricular filling that combined with pulsed Doppler peak E velocity may estimate capillary wedge pressure. *J Am Coll Cardiol.* 1997;29:448-454.
44. Nagueh SF, Kopelen HA, Quinones MA. Assessment of left ventricular filling pressures by Doppler in the presence of atrial fibrillation. *Circulation.* 1996;94:2138-2145.
45. Oh J. Assessment of diastolic function. In: Oh J, ed. *The Echo Manual.* 2nd ed. Lippincott Williams & Wilkins; 1999:45-57.
46. Chirillo F, Brunazzi MC, Barbiero M, et al. Estimating mean pulmonary wedge pressure in patients with chronic atrial fibrillation from transthoracic Doppler indexes of mitral and pulmonary venous flow velocity. *J Am Coll Cardiol.* 1997;30:19-26.
47. Temporelli PL, Scapellato F, Corra U, et al. Estimation of pulmonary wedge pressure by transmitral Doppler in patients with chronic heart failure and atrial fibrillation. *Am J Cardiol.* 1999;83:724-727.
48. Abudiab MM, Chebrolu LH, Schutt RC, et al. Doppler echocardiography for the estimation of LV filling pressure in patients with mitral annular calcification. *JACC Cardiovasc Imaging.* 2017;10:1411-1420.

49. Burch JA, Soares-Weiser K, St John DJ, et al. Diagnostic accuracy of faecal occult blood tests used in screening for colorectal cancer: a systematic review. *J Med Screen.* 2007;14:132-137.
50. Klein AL, Hatle LK, Burstow DJ, et al. Comprehensive Doppler assessment of right ventricular diastolic function in cardiac amyloidosis. *J Am Coll Cardiol.* 1990;15:99-108.
51. Spencer KT, Weinert L, Lang RM. Effect of age, heart rate and tricuspid regurgitation on the Doppler echocardiographic evaluation of right ventricular diastolic function. *Cardiology.* 1999;92:59-64.
52. Nomura T, Lebowitz L, Koide Y, et al. Evaluation of hepatic venous flow using transesophageal echocardiography in coronary artery bypass surgery: an index of right ventricular function. *J Cardiothorac Vasc Anesth.* 1995;9:9-17.
53. Rudski LG, Lai WW, Afilalo J et al. Guidelines for the echocardiographic assessment of the right heart in adults: a report from the American Society of Echocardiography. *J Am Soc Echocardiogr.* 2010;23:685-713.
54. Troughton RW, Asher CR, Klein AL. Pericarditis. *Lancet.* 2004;363:717-727.
55. Geske JB, Anavekar NS, Nishimura RA, et al. Differentiation of constriction and restriction: complex cardiovascular hemodynamics. *J Am Coll Cardiol.* 2016;68:2329-2347.
56. Klein AL, Abbara S, Agler DA, et al. American Society of Echocardiography clinical recommendations for multimodality cardiovascular imaging of patients with pericardial disease: endorsed by the Society for Cardiovascular Magnetic Resonance and Society of Cardiovascular Computed Tomography. *J Am Soc Echocardiogr.* 2013;26:965-1012.e15.
57. Reuss CS, Wilansky SM, Lester SJ, et al. Using mitral 'annulus reversus' to diagnose constrictive pericarditis. *Eur J Echocardiogr.* 2009;10:372-375.
58. Ha JW, Oh JK, Ling LH, et al. Annulus paradoxus: transmitral flow velocity to mitral annular velocity ratio is inversely proportional to pulmonary capillary wedge pressure in patients with constrictive pericarditis. *Circulation.* 2001;104:976-978.
59. Ha JW, Ommen SR, Tajik AJ, et al. Differentiation of constrictive pericarditis from restrictive cardiomyopathy using mitral annular velocity by tissue Doppler echocardiography. *Am J Cardiol.* 2004;94:316-319.
60. Gillam LD, Guyer DE, Gibson TC, et al. Hydrodynamic compression of the right atrium: a new echocardiographic sign of cardiac tamponade. *Circulation.* 1983;68:294-301.
61. Singh S, Wann LS, Klopfenstein HS, et al. Usefulness of right ventricular diastolic collapse in diagnosing cardiac tamponade and comparison to pulsus paradoxus. *Am J Cardiol.* 1986;57:652-656.
62. Faehnrich JA, Noone RB Jr, White WD, et al. Effects of positive-pressure ventilation, pericardial effusion, and cardiac tamponade on respiratory variation in transmitral flow velocities. *J Cardiothorac Vasc Anesth.* 2003;17:45-50.
63. Nagueh SF, Appleton CP, Gillebert TC, et al. Recommendations for the evaluation of left ventricular diastolic function by echocardiography. *J Am Soc Echocardiogr.* 2009;22:107-133.

QUESTIONS

1. Which of the following cardiac cycle phases is depicted by the arrow in Q-Figure 7.1?

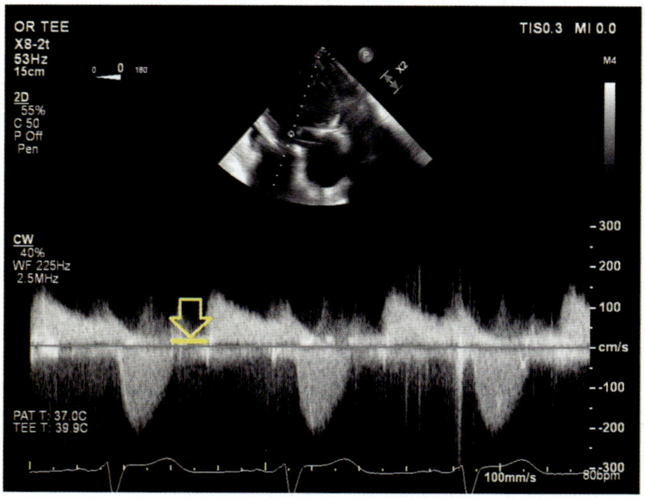

A. Isovolumic relaxation phase
B. Early diastolic filling
C. Diastasis
D. Late diastolic filling

2. **Based on the Doppler images shown in Q-Figure 7.2 the LV filling pressures are:**

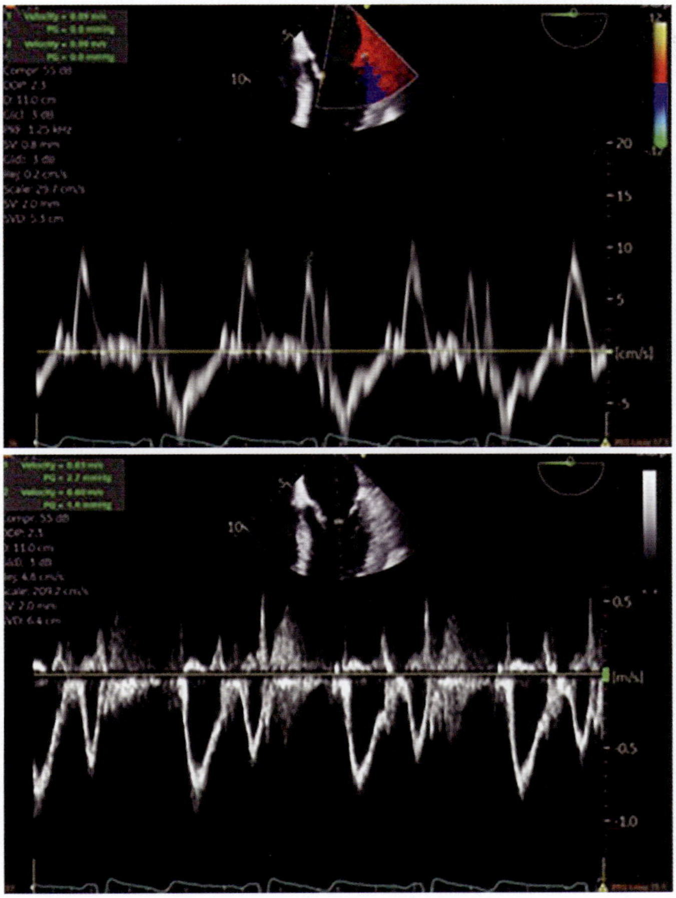

A. Normal
B. Increased
C. Decreased
D. Indeterminate.

3. **Which of the following pathologies is best depicted by the Doppler tracings in Q-Figures 7.3-7.5?**

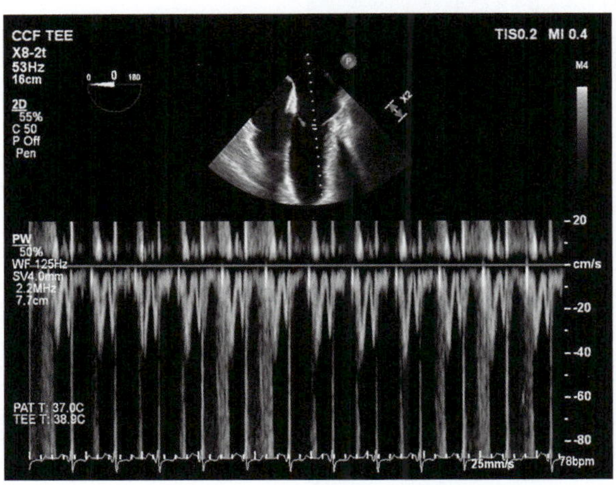

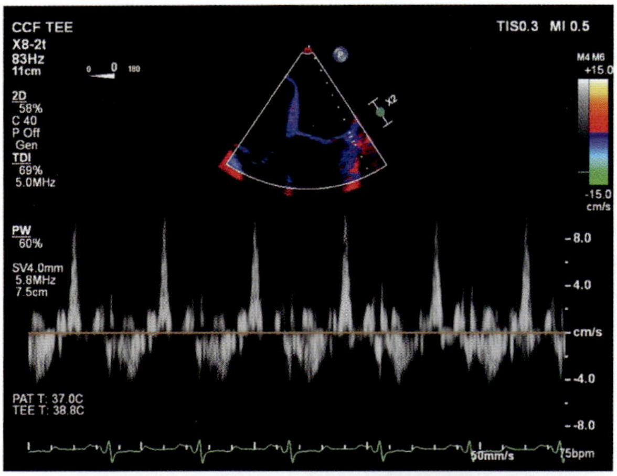

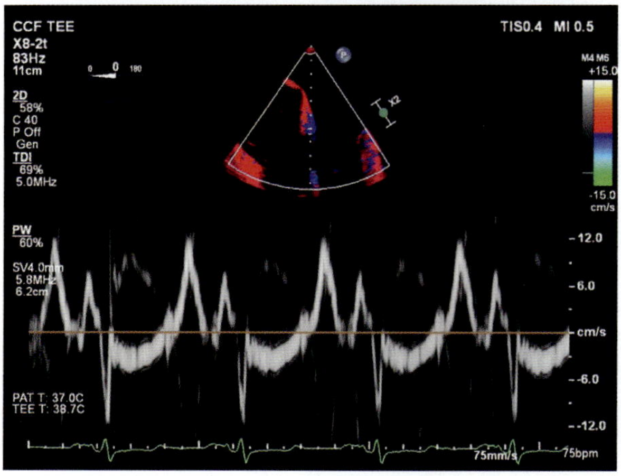

A. Restrictive pericarditis
B. CP
C. Pericardial tamponade
D. Acute pericarditis

4. **In the spectral display shown in Q-Figure 7.6, the arrow depicts which phase of the cardiac cycle?**

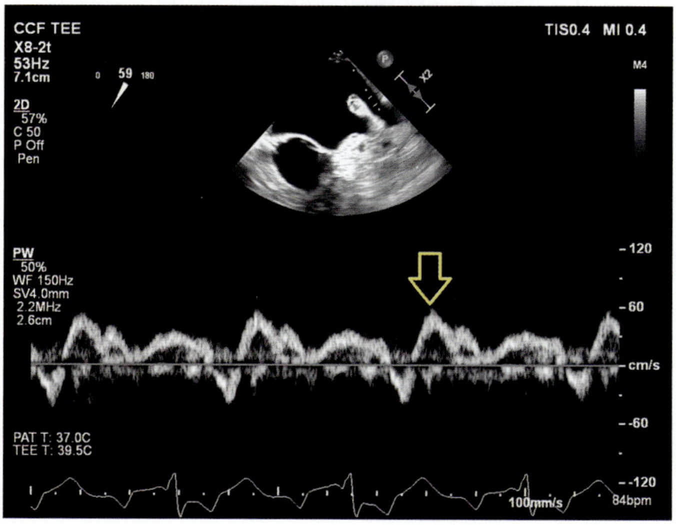

A. Atrial contraction
B. Atrial relaxation
C. Ventricular contraction
D. Ventricular relaxation

5. Which of the following best describes the diastolic function in the patient shown in Q-Figure 7.7?

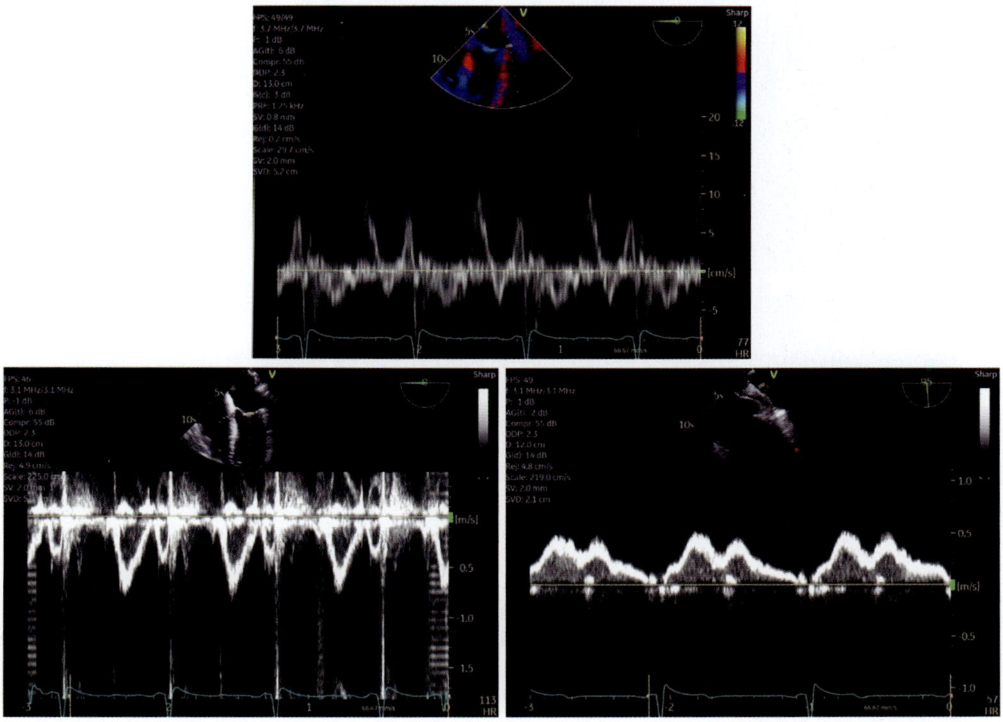

A. Normal
B. Impaired relaxation
C. Pseudonormal
D. Restrictive

6. On the MVI Doppler profile, during which diastolic phase does the L wave occur?
A. Early filling
B. Diastasis
C. Rapid filling
D. Atrial contraction

7. On PVDF, which of the following events represents the PV_{S2} wave?
A. Descent of the base of the heart
B. RA compliance
C. LA contraction
D. Early transmitral inflow

8. In a patient with AF, which of the following diastolic parameters are indicative of a worse prognosis?
A. E/e' less than 8
B. E/A greater than 2
C. DT less than 160 milliseconds
D. PV_{AR} greater than 35 cm/s

9. Based on the Q-Figure 7.8, which of the following is most consistent with the patient's LV filling pattern?

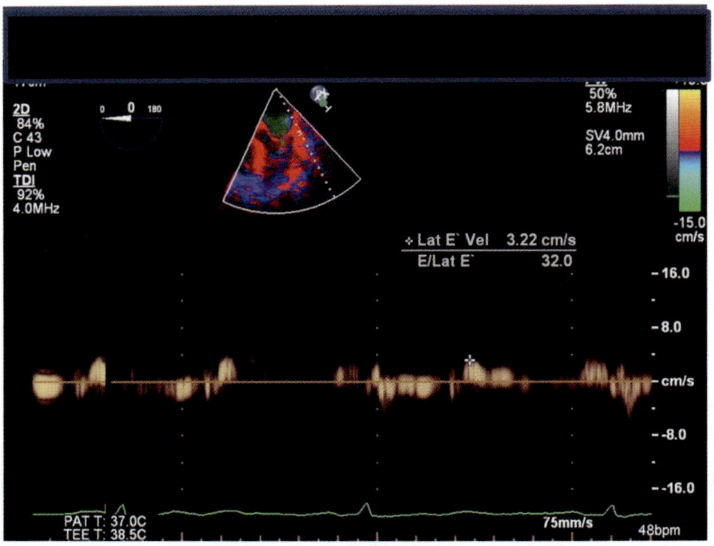

A. Normal
B. Pseudonormal
C. Impaired relaxation
D. Restrictive

10. In a spontaneously breathing patient with pericardial tamponade, the respiratory variation of the early filling velocity across the tricuspid (E_T) and the mitral (E_M) valve can be represented by which of the following equations?

A. Inspiration $E_T >$ Expiration E_T
B. Inspiration $E_T =$ Expiration E_T
C. Inspiration $E_M >$ Expiration E_M
D. Inspiration $E_M =$ Expiration E_M

ANSWERS

1. Correct Answer: A.
Rationale: Q-Figure 7.1 is a spectral display obtained using continuous-wave Doppler from the deep transgastric view. The phase of the cardiac cycle marked by the arrow begins at end systole after closure of the AV and ends with opening of the MV. This phase is the isovolumic relaxation phase, which precedes the early rapid filling of the LV. The yellow line on the x-axis depicts the IVRT.

2. Correct Answer: A.
Rationale: The E/e' ratio for the Doppler image shown in Q-Figure 7.2 is 0.83/0.09, which is 9.2. Values greater than 15 are associated with increased LV filling pressures, whereas values less than 15 are associated with normal LV filling pressures.

3. Correct Answer: B.
Rationale: The PWD of the MVI demonstrates respirophasic variation in the inflow velocities, and the TDI of the mitral annulus shows annulus inversus; that is, the medial annular velocity is higher than the lateral.

4. Correct Answer: B.
Rationale: The arrow in Q-Figure 7.6 depicts the first systolic component of the pulmonary tracing (PV_{S1}), which is due to LA relaxation.

5. Correct Answer: A.
Rationale: Q-Figure 7.7 demonstrates an MVI pattern with the E wave greater than A wave, which can be seen in both normal and pseudonormal filling patterns. However, on the TDI of the lateral mitral annulus, the e' is

greater than 10 cm/s, which is consistent with a normal velocity, suggestive of normal diastolic function. Further confirmation is obtained from the PVDF, which is also normal, displaying $PV_S > PV_D$. An impaired relaxation filling pattern would display E < A on the MVI. A restrictive filling pattern would display E >> A on the MVI, while the TDI of the lateral mitral annulus would show *e′* greater than 8 cm/s and the PVDF would show $PV_S < PV_D$.

6. Correct Answer: B.
Rationale: The L wave occurs in severe forms of diastolic dysfunction and takes place during diastasis. It is caused by the increased atrial pressures. The early filling and rapid filling phases are the same thing and are represented by the E wave on MVI. The atrial contraction phase is represented by the A wave on MVI.

7. Correct Answer: A.
Rationale: The PV_{S2} wave occurs during LV systole. During this time, the base of the heart moves downward, creating a suction effect in the LA and allowing more blood to flow from the PVs. Other determinants of the PV_{S2} wave are LA compliance (not RA compliance), concomitant MR, and RV stroke volume. LA contraction is represented by the retrograde PV_{AR} wave on the PVDF. During early transmitral inflow, the LA serves as a conduit as the blood flows from the PV through the atrium into the LV. The early transmitral inflow is represented by the PV_D wave on the PVDF.

8. Correct Answer: C.
Rationale: In patients with AF, measurement of diastolic indices is difficult. The *E* and *e′* values should be an average measured over 10 consecutive cycles or over 3 nonconsecutive cycles. A DT less than 160 milliseconds is predictive of increased diastolic pressures and worse clinical outcomes. Due to the fact that in AF, there is no meaningful atrial contraction, the A wave on MVI and the PV_{AR} on PVDF are absent. Therefore, *E*/*A* and PV_{AR} cannot be measured. An *E*/*e′* greater than 11 is considered suggestive of increased filling pressures in patients with AF, while an *E*/*e′* less than 8 is suggestive of normal filling pressures.

9. Correct answer: D.
Rationale: The image (Q-Figure 7.8) displays TDI at the lateral mitral annulus. The *e′* velocity is severely decreased, measuring 3.22 cm/s, and the calculated *E*/*e′* is 32, consistent with restrictive filling pressures. An *E*/*e′* less than 8 is found in patients with normal diastolic function as well as in those with impaired relaxation. The distinguishing factor between these two categories is the value of *e′*, which would be greater than 10 cm/s in patients with normal diastolic function and less than 8 cm/s in those with impaired relaxation. In patients with pseudonormal filling pressures, while the *e′* is less than 8 cm/s, the *E*/*e′* would most likely be between 9 and 13.

10. Correct answer: A.
Rationale: There is always a normal degree of respiratory variation of the mitral and tricuspid inflows (~20%). In patients with pericardial tamponade spontaneously breathing, this respiratory variation is further augmented. During inspiration, the negative intrathoracic pressure is transmitted to the right side of the heart, which fills preferentially at the expense of the LV. The ventricular septum is pushed toward the LV, further impeding its filling. In expiration the process is reversed, whereby LV expansion impedes RV filling. Ventricular inflow respiratory variation is more pronounced in patients with tamponade compared to CP, exceeding 30% for mitral and 60% for tricuspid velocities.

III Valvular Disease

8 Mitral Regurgitation

Nicholas W. Markin and Joshua M. Zimmerman

The orientation of the mitral valve with respect to the esophagus permits imaging in an unparalleled fashion (pun intended, as the valve is perpendicular to the ultrasound beam). From the introduction of transesophageal echocardiography (TEE) to the current era of high frame rate three-dimensional (3D) imaging, the ability to elucidate the underlying cause of mitral valve dysfunction continues to showcase the role of TEE in guiding surgical management. TEE permits the qualitative and quantitative evaluation of the etiology, mechanism, and severity of mitral valve disease as well as the adequacy of repair or replacement in the postbypass period.

ANATOMY

Embryology

Cardiac structures form beginning in the third week and are relatively completed by the seventh week of gestation with the mitral valve resulting from an ingrowth of the endocardial cushions. The origin of the valve from the superior and inferior endocardial cushions and its proximity to the septum primum explain the association between anterior leaflet cleft and primum atrial septal defects (ASDs) (1). The valve forms with two leaflets, one anterior leaflet that comprises two-third of the area of the valve opening and one-third of the annulus and the posterior leaflet that represents the other one-third of the valve area and accounts for two-third of the annular perimeter, as shown in Figure 8.1. Together, the leaflets and mitral valve apparatus resist the systemic pressures of the left ventricle (LV) and permit one-way flow of blood between the atrium and ventricle without restricting flow during diastole. The components that comprise the mitral valve apparatus can be further divided into three parts, and understanding each part is crucial in the evaluation of the dysfunctional valve.

Leaflets

The anterior leaflet is the larger and more dynamic of the two with its annulus adjacent to the aortic valve and root, an area commonly referred to as the aortomitral curtain. The posterior leaflet spans most of the mitral annulus with the leaflet itself having a crescentic shape and typically being made up of three scallops or sections. The typical naming convention for the mitral leaflets is that described by Dr Alain Carpentier, the father of modern mitral valve reconstructive surgery, in 1983 (2). As shown in Figure 8.1, the anatomically distinct scallops of the posterior leaflet are called P1, P2, and P3 from anterolateral (near the left atrial [LA] appendage) to posteromedial (near the coronary sinus). While the anterior leaflet does not have anatomically distinct segments, the leaflet is divided into three sections called A1, A3, and A3 based on the anterior leaflet's coaptation with the numbered scallops of the posterior leaflet. It should be noted that, while the leaflets are called "anterior" and "posterior," the anterior leaflet is also relatively medial while the posterior leaflet is lateral.

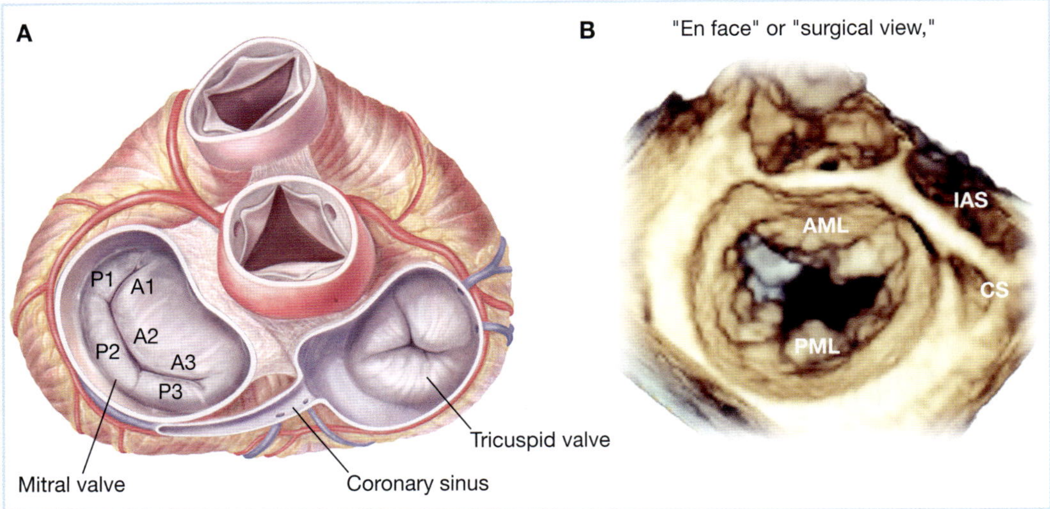

FIGURE 8.1 A: Mitral valve anatomy from the anatomic perspective, which is how the TEE probe "sees the valve." Note that the anterior leaflet is anterior and medial, and the posterior leaflet is posterior and lateral. B: 3D en face view of mitral valve from the "surgeon's view" with anatomic landmarks. Ant, anterior mitral leaflet; IAS, interatrial septum; LAA, left atrial appendage; LCC, left coronary cusp; NCC, noncoronary cusp; Post, posterior mitral leaflet; RCC, right coronary cusp; TEE, transesophageal echocardiography.

The transition between the two leaflets occurs in a region referred to as the commissures, which include an anterolateral commissure adjacent to the LA appendage and fully supported by the anterolateral papillary muscle and a posteromedial commissure near the septum, which is supported by the posteromedial papillary muscle. These commissures are small, complex structures that comprise tiny commissural leaflets, each with its own miniature fan of chordae. Both leaflets have a coaptation zone where they contact each other during closure in systole to prevent regurgitation. This coaptation zone along the entire valve is more textured when compared to the otherwise smooth surface of the mitral valve leaflets. The normal coaptation zone is 8 to 12 mm in length, though this length may be difficult to appreciate in some TEE views (3).

Annulus

The annulus of the mitral valve is a discontinuous band of fibrous tissue from which the leaflets hinge. The thickest portion of the annulus is the trigones, which are located near the commissures, with the annular tissue becoming less prominent as it progresses toward the middle of the posterior leaflet. This lack of support along the posterior annulus permits dilation in response to abnormal hemodynamic states (4). Anteriorly, the annulus is contiguous with the aortomitral curtain (also called the intervalvular fibrosa).

The mitral annulus is a saddle-shaped structure in which the aortic annulus creates a concavity in an otherwise oval-shaped structure, making it kidney-shaped, as seen in Figure 8.2. The annulus is nonplanar, with the most ventricular aspect of the annulus corresponding to its widest dimension and seen echocardiographically in the midesophageal commissural view. The most atrial aspect of the annulus corresponds to the minor dimension and is seen in the midesophageal aortic valve long-axis view. Given the lack of fibrous support in the posterior aspect of the annulus, dilation of the annulus predominately elongates the minor dimension rather than the major (4).

Subvalvular Apparatus

The mitral subvalvular apparatus comprises papillary muscles and chordal attachments. The papillary muscles arise from the LV myocardium and are vascularized in the same way as their adjacent segments. The anterolateral papillary muscle is near the transition between the anterior and anterolateral wall of the LV and is commonly perfused by branches of both the left anterior descending and the left circumflex coronary arteries. The posteromedial papillary muscle arises from the region around the inferoseptal and inferior walls of the LV and therefore is perfused by branches of the posterior descending coronary artery. The papillary

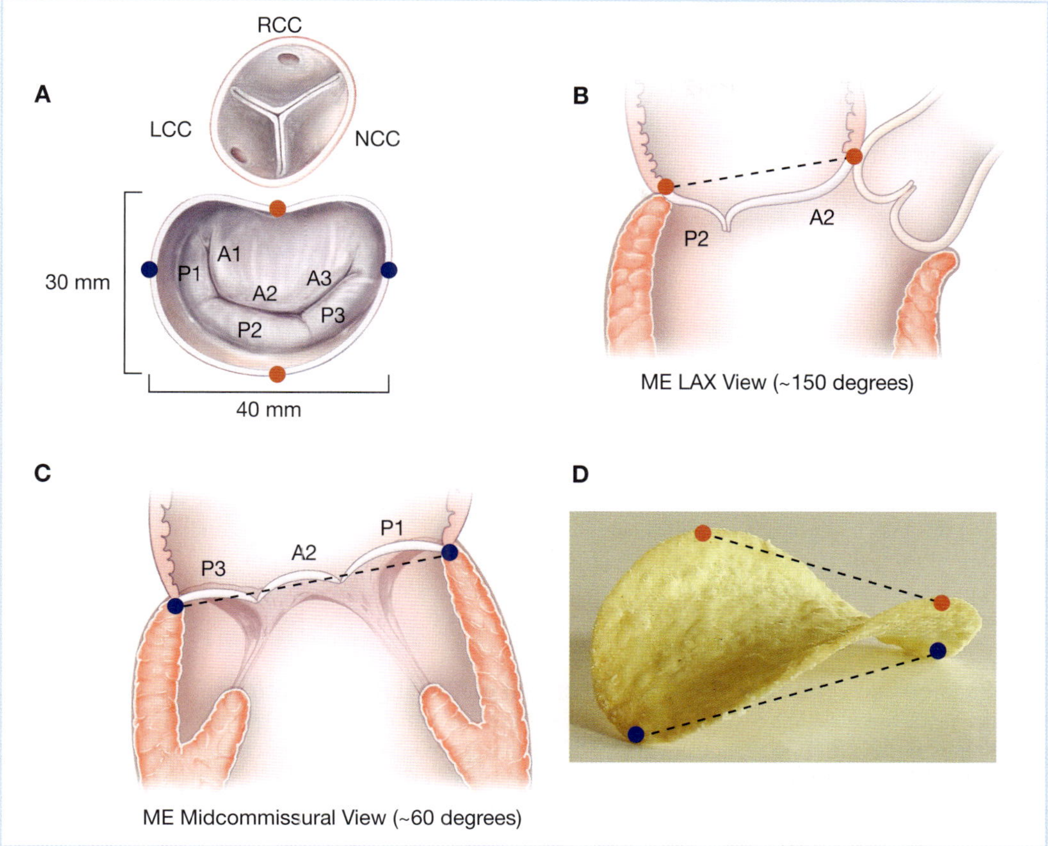

FIGURE 8.2 Overview of mitral valve anatomy. A: Mitral valve from the left atrial perspective in the "surgeon's view." B: Midesophageal long-axis view, showing the A2 and P2 segments. This view demonstrates the most atrial extent of the annulus (red dots) and, as such, is where prolapse is most appropriately identified. C: Midesophageal commissural view, showing the P3, A2, and P1 segments. The most ventricular aspect of the annulus is seen in this view and is denoted by the blue dots. D: While the mitral valve has sometimes been likened to a "saddle shape," our editor (JZ) finds it more helpful to consider the valve like a Pringles potato chip. It has a wide and narrow, and high and low aspect. The wide, or major, dimension is typically less than 40 mm, is more ventricular, and is seen in the commissural cross section. The narrow, or minor, dimension is typically less than 30 mm, is more atrial, and is seen in the long-axis cross section.

muscles have three types of chordal attachments to the mitral valve based on the insertion point. They are primary, secondary, and tertiary chordae (5). The primary chordae are thin and provide fine-tuning of valve closure as they insert into the very edges of the coaptation line. The secondary chordae are thicker and are most critical in establishing leaflet height, in which rupture commonly leads to the "flail" of the associated leaflet. The tertiary chordae attach near or at the annulus, and their presence during systole helps maintain the geometry of the LV. Each papillary muscle contributes chordae to its half of each leaflet, with chordae not crossing an imaginary line through the middle of the A2/P2 coaptation zone.

APPROACH TO THE PATIENT WITH MITRAL REGURGITATION

It is incumbent upon the perioperative echocardiographer not to focus solely on the severity of any valvular lesion but rather to describe the breadth of the complex pathology. While severity is a critical component of the description of a lesion and will be reviewed in detail later, the severity is not the target of the surgical intervention. As one of the authors (JZ) says "Remember that your surgeon operates ***on*** the valvular lesion, ***because of*** the severity and consequences." Dr. Carpentier famously described mitral valve pathology in terms of a "pathophysiologic triad" that included the etiology, lesion, and dysfunction (6). To this surgical perspective, the echocardiographer would add a description of severity and consequences.

TABLE 8.1 Common Etiologies of Mitral Regurgitation

Primary Valvular Diseases (Structural)	Secondary Valvular Diseases (Functional)
Degenerative diseases	Atrial fibrillation
Barlow disease	Dilated cardiomyopathy
Fibroelastic deficiency	Myocardial infarction
Marfan disease	
Ehlers-Danlos	
Calcific degeneration	
Rheumatic valvular disease	
Endocarditis	
Congenital	
Toxins	

Etiology

The etiology is the disease that causes the valvular abnormality (Table 8.1) (7-10). Etiologies are commonly, if imperfectly, divided into primary and secondary causes. Primary, or structural, mitral regurgitation (MR) is caused by abnormalities of the leaflets, annulus, or subvalvular apparatus. In secondary, or "functional," MR, the mitral leaflets are normal with regurgitation caused by dysfunction of the LA and/or LV. The importance of this distinction cannot be overstated, as it helps determine both the medical and surgical management of MR.

Valve Lesions and the Functional Classification of Mitral Regurgitation

Having considered the etiology (cause) of valvular disease, we then describe the specific valvular lesions and the resultant dysfunction. The spectrum of valvular lesions is broad, affecting any combination of the leaflets, annulus, or subvalvular apparatus. Some examples are provided in Table 8.2, along with the resultant valvular dysfunction. The functional classification of MR describes dysfunction in terms of leaflet motion—either normal, excessive, or restricted, respectively (2) (Figure 8.3).

In Type I dysfunction, the leaflets are moving normally and the subvalvular apparatus is intact (Video 8.1). This may occur from annular dilation, commonly from chronic atrial fibrillation or other causes of persistently elevated LA pressure, resulting in insufficient leaflet coaptation and a flat-appearing mitral valve. Alternately, Type I valve disease may be seen in the setting of endocarditis with malcoaptation or leaflet perforation (Video 8.2).

Type II dysfunction is defined by excessive systolic leaflet motion (prolapse) above the mitral annulus (Video 8.3). Echocardiographically, this is best defined in the midesophageal aortic valve long-axis view as it is the most atrial portion of the annulus. Type II dysfunction is often caused by chordal elongation or rupture and less frequently by rupture of a portion of a papillary muscle (Video 8.4). It is common to hear various terms used to describe Type II leaflet motion such as flail, prolapse, and chordal rupture; all of these

TABLE 8.2 Classification of Valve Dysfunction Using the Carpentier Approach Describing Leaflet Motion, Along With Common Lesions Associated With Each Type of Leaflet Motion

Functional Classification	Lesion
Type I (normal motion)	Annular dilation Leaflet perforation (often from endocarditis)
Type II (excessive motion)	Chordal rupture Chordal elongation Papillary muscle rupture
Type III (restricted motion)	Chordal thickening/fusion Leaflet thickening or calcification Commissural fusion Ventricular dilation or aneurysm

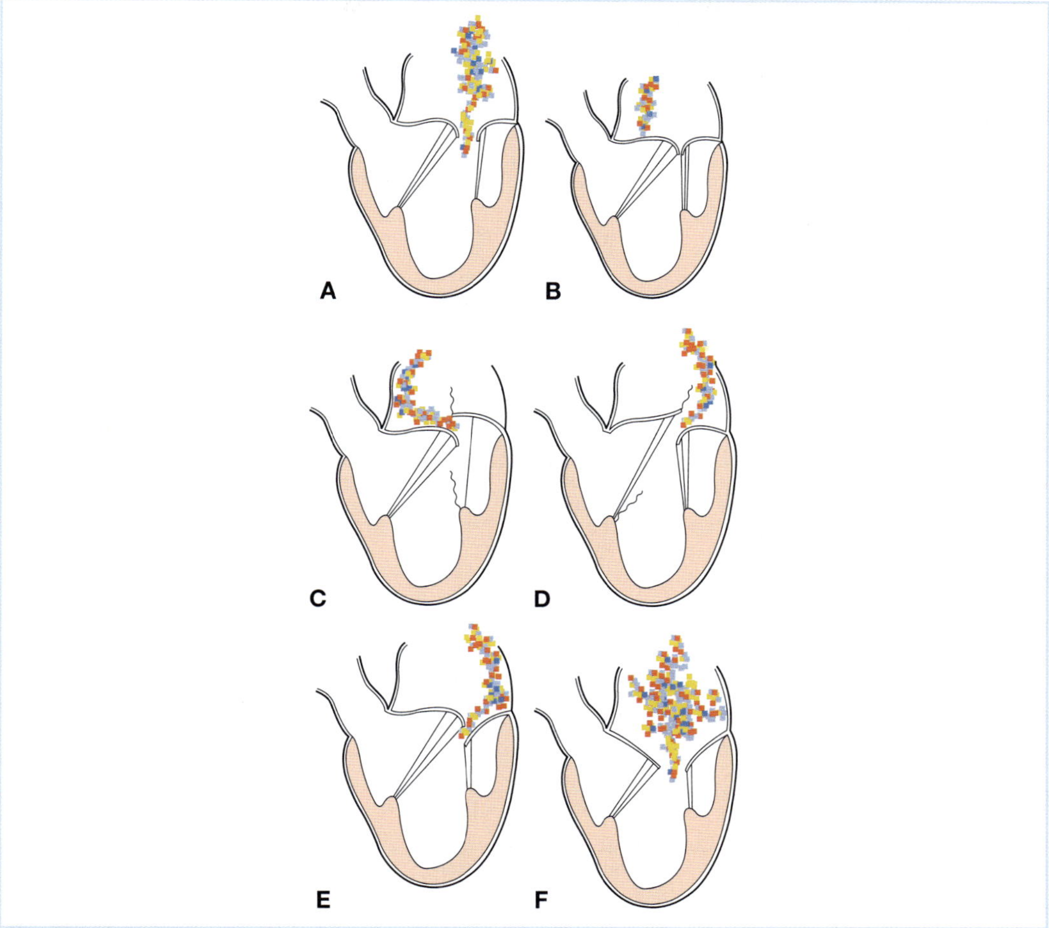

FIGURE 8.3 Carpentier classification of mitral regurgitation (MR) based on leaflet motion. A, B: In Type I regurgitation, the leaflet motion is normal, and the MR jet tends to be central from annular dilation (A) or variable from leaflet perforation (B). C, D: In Type II disease, there is excessive leaflet motion, and the MR jet is typically directed away from the diseased leaflet. E, F: In Type III disease, leaflet motion is restricted. This is further subdivided into Type IIIa (restriction in systole and diastole) and Type IIIb (restriction primarily in systole). In Type III lesions, the regurgitant jet may be directed away from the diseased leaflet if only one leaflet is affected, or it may be central if both mitral leaflets are equally affected. (Courtesy Dr Gregory M. Hirsch.)

are subjective terms that describe excessive leaflet motion. It is suggested that the echocardiographer is best served by simplifying this to excessive motion or Type II motion to communicate with others.

Type III dysfunction results from restricted leaflet motion, which may exist in systole and/or diastole. Restriction that is seen in both systole and diastole is classified as Type IIIa. Type IIIa dysfunction is commonly described in rheumatic mitral valve disease, often with combined stenosis and regurgitation (Video 8.5). Type IIIb dysfunction describes restricted leaflet motion only in systole, which is typically found in LV dilation (Video 8.6 and Video 8.7).

SEVERITY OF MITRAL REGURGITATION—QUALITATIVE AND SEMIQUANTITATIVE (TABLE 8.3)

While the severity of any valvular lesion is only a piece of the understanding necessary for the perioperative echocardiographer and at times will not be the most important piece described intraoperatively, it is nonetheless a critical component of a comprehensive mitral valve assessment. In this section, we will discuss an approach to both image acquisition and interpretation with each of the different echocardiographic

TABLE 8.3 Summary of Assessment Methods to Grade Severity of Mitral Regurgitation

Modality	Method	Type of Assessment	Severity: Mild	Moderate	Severe
2D	Leaflet motion	Qualitative	Normal or abnormal		Flail or restricted
	Leaflet morphology	Qualitative	Normal or abnormal		Typically abnormal leaflets
	Coaptation defect	Qualitative	Absent		Presence of coaptation defect
	Mobile echodensity	Qualitative	Important but not associated directly with severity		
	LA size	Qualitative	Normal	Normal/enlarged	Enlarged
Color flow Doppler	Vena contracta width	Semiquantitative	<3 mm	3-6 mm	≥7 mm (or >8 for biplane)
	Flow convergence zone	Qualitative	None or small	Intermediate	Large
	Flow convergence radius	Quantitative (used for PISA)	(Adjust Nyquist in direction of jet, measure parallel to ultrasound beam)		
	Color flow jet size/shape	Qualitative	Small and central	Intermediate	Very large or eccentric with Coanda effect
Continuous wave Doppler	MR jet density	Qualitative	Faint	Dense	
	MR jet profile	Qualitative	Parabolic		Triangular
	Peak velocity	Quantitative	(Measurement used for PISA calculation)		
Pulse wave Doppler	MV inflow pattern	Semiquantitative	E < A	E > A	E ≫ A
	MV inflow peak velocity	Semiquantitative	<1 m/s	Variable	≥1.2 m/s
	Pulmonary vein flow	Semiquantitative	Systolic dominant	Systolic blunting	Systolic flow reversal
	VTI_{mitral}/VTI_{LVOT}	Semiquantitative	<1	1-1.4	>1.4
3D	Annulus size	Semiquantitative	Annulus should have 4:3 ratio and is dilated when approaching 1:1 ratio.		
3D CFD	Vena contracta area	Quantitative	>0.2 cm^2	0.2-0.4 cm^2	≥0.4 cm^2
Multimodality	PISA $PISA = (2 \times \pi \times r^2 \times V_{alias})/V_{max}$	Quantitative	>0.2 cm^2	0.2-0.4 cm^2	≥0.4 cm^2
	Regurgitant volume[b]	Quantitative	<30 mL	30-44 mL[a] 44-59 mL[a]	≥60 mL
	Regurgitant fraction[b]	Quantitative	<30%	30-39 mL[a] 40-49 mL[a]	≥50%

CFD, color flow Doppler; LA, left arium; MR, mitral regurgitation; MV, mitral volume; PISA, proximal isovelocity surface area; VTI, velocity time integral.

[a]Guidelines subcategorize moderate MR into mild-to-moderate MR and moderate-to-severe MR based on the subgrouping indicated, respectively.

[b]This could be performed using 3D volumetric analysis to determine the total volume change and subtract forward flow via left ventricular outflow tract stroke volume (LVOT SA) to determine regurgitant volume and fraction, or the EROA combined with MR VTI (CWD) can be used to determine MR flow and then compared to 3D volumes or LVOT SV calculation to determine regurgitant volume and fraction.

modalities, as well as the data that will be used, particularly in the qualitative and semiquantitative assessment of MR severity. As described in the ASE guidelines (7), many patients will have findings of either mild or severe regurgitation that are highly specific. In those cases, a more detailed quantitative assessment is unnecessary. For patients lacking these specific findings, however, more quantitative assessment will be necessary and will be described by the modality used to perform these qualitative and semiquantitative methods in the section that follows.

TWO-DIMENSIONAL ECHOCARDIOGRAPHY

The evaluation of MR begins with rigorous two-dimensional (2D) imaging. It should be the goal of every perioperative echocardiographer not to be surprised by either Doppler or 3D findings but rather to anticipate those findings based on a thorough 2D evaluation. This should be the case in general and is particularly true when it comes to the mitral valve. In each view, the echocardiographer is evaluating leaflet thickness, motion, and coaptation. The mitral annulus is being assessed for calcification or annular disjunction. A flail leaflet or clear 2D coaptation defect will have a high specificity for severe MR (Video 8.8). We recommend the following approach for 2D imaging of the mitral valve (Figure 8.4).

- Begin the exam in the midesophageal four chamber (at 0°) with the mitral valve centered in the screen. The LV outflow tract should not be visualized. The anterior mitral leaflet will be medial (by the interatrial septum) while the posterior leaflet will be lateral. This cross section most likely demonstrates the A2/P2 segments of the valve. With retroflexion or advancement of the probe, just before visualizing the coronary

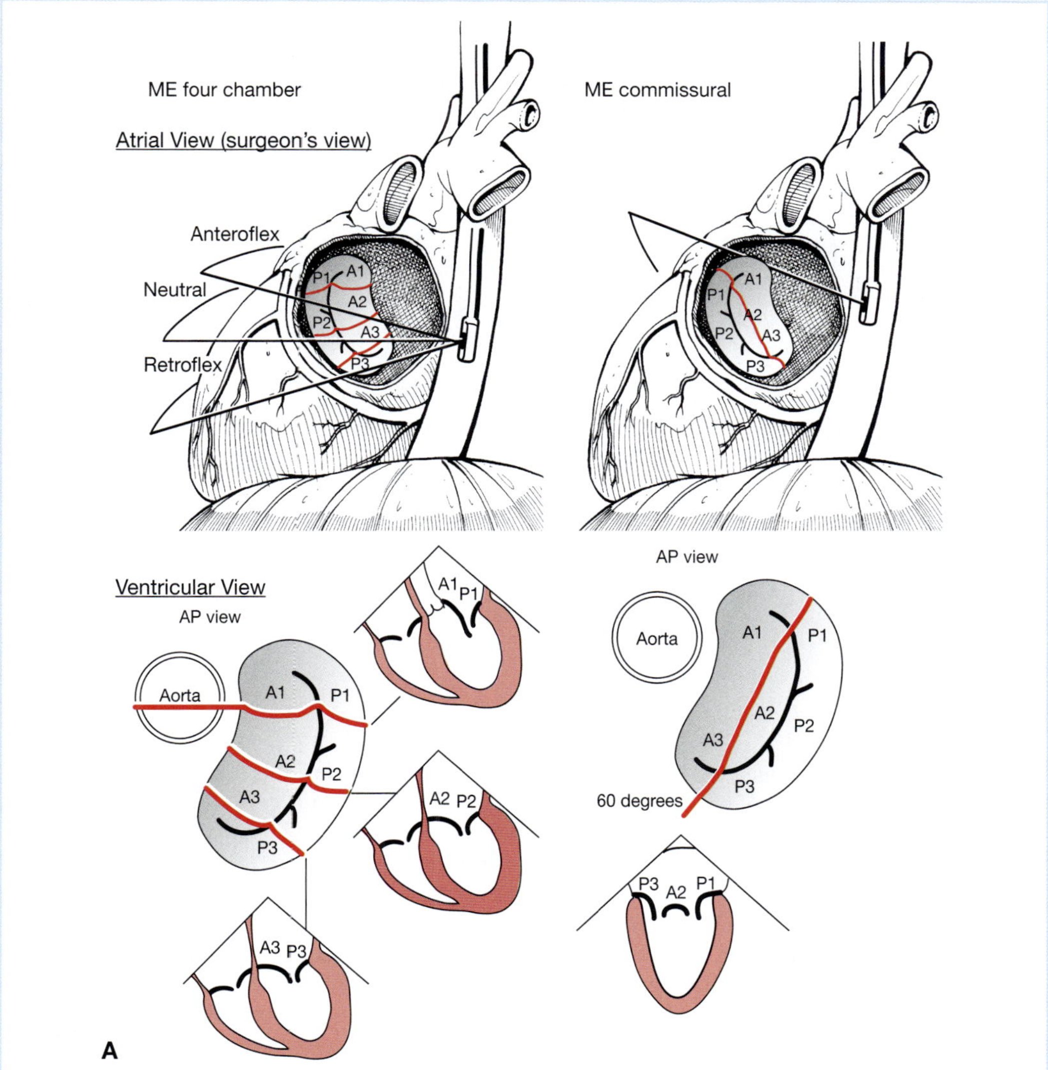

FIGURE 8.4 Systematic 2D examination of the mitral valve. The anatomic view is shown above with the plane of the ultrasound beam. Below, the surgeon's view is shown with lines reflecting the ultrasound beam along with line drawings of the segments of mitral leaflet demonstrated with different probe manipulations. (A) Examination of the midesophageal four chamber (0 degrees) and commissural (60 degrees) cross-sections. (B) Examination of the two chamber (90 degrees) and long-axis (135 degrees) cross sections.

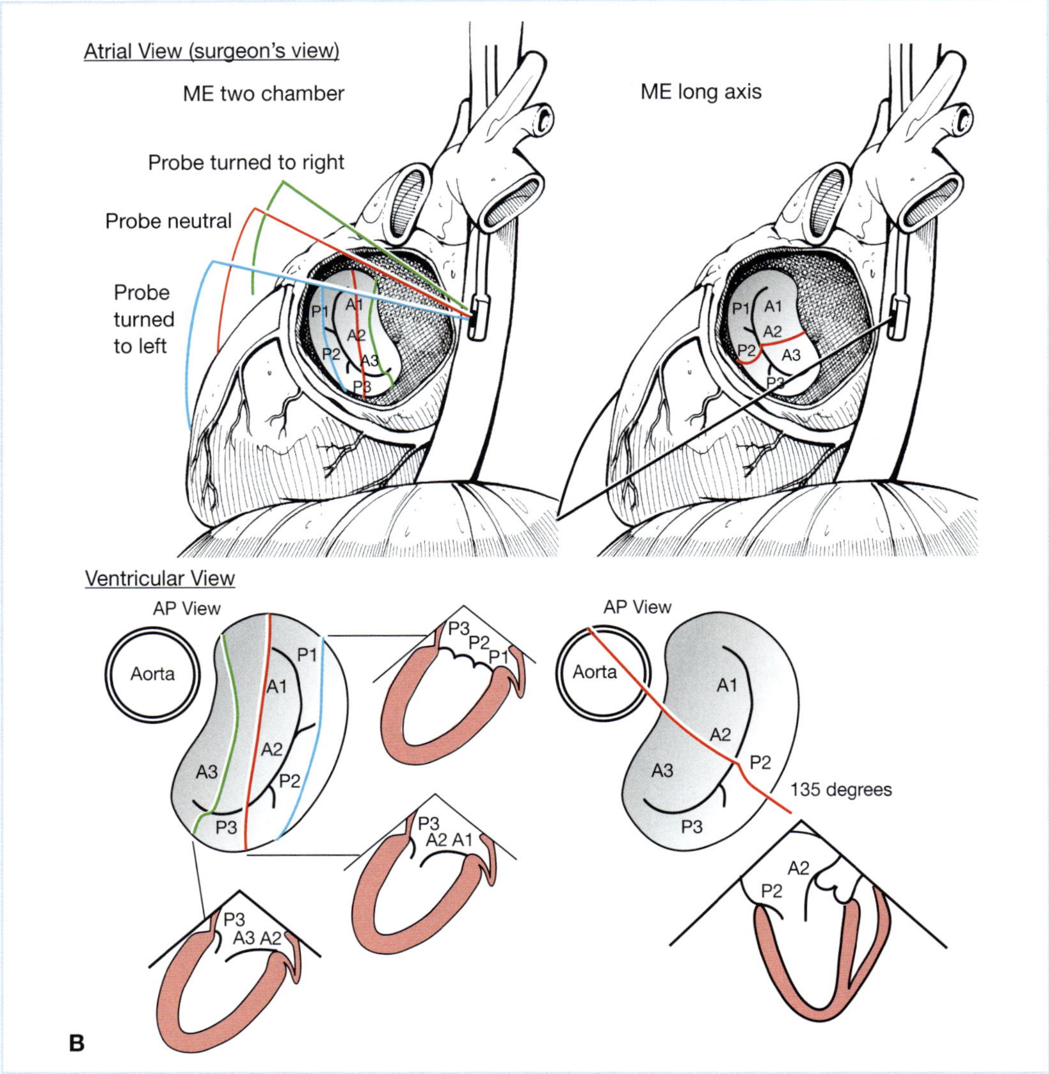

FIGURE 8.4 *(continued)*

sinus, the A3/P3 segments and ultimately the posteromedial commissure will be visualized. With withdrawal or anteflexion of the probe, the left ventricular outflow tract (LVOT) will come into view as will the A1//P1 segments of the valve and ultimately the anterolateral commissure (Figure 8.4).

- With an increase in multiplane angle to approximately 60°, the midesophageal commissural cross section will be created. This view shows a typical "trap door" or "seagull" appearance with P1 anteriorly (near the LA appendage, if it is visualized) and P3 posteriorly (near the coronary sinus). There will be a variable portion of the anterior leaflet, including at least the A2 segment, visualized between the portions of the posterior leaflet. From this view, a slight advancement with rightward rotation will show more of the anterior leaflet, while a slight withdrawal and leftward rotation will show more of the posterior leaflet. This cross section will also be useful for measuring the major axis of the mitral annulus (Figure 8.4).
- The midesophageal two-chamber view is created next with a further increase in the multiplane angle (90°-100°). This view should demonstrate the length of the anterior mitral leaflet from near the appendage (A1), through the body of the leaflet, to the coaptation at A3/P3 (Figure 8.4).
- The final midesophageal view of the mitral valve will be the long axis at a multiplane angle of 120° to 140°. This view theoretically cuts directly through the middle of the mitral valve and the aortic valve at the

A2/P2 level. As such, this view should not visualize either papillary muscle. This is the minor dimension as well as the most atrial aspect of the mitral annulus. With advancement/retroflexion and a slight rightward rotation, the A3/P3 segments and posteromedial papillary muscle can be visualized. With slight withdrawal/anteflexion and a slight leftward rotation, the A1/P1 segments and anterolateral papillary muscle may be seen (Figure 8.4).

- The probe is then advanced into the stomach and anteflexed to create a transgastric basal short axis of the mitral valve. This view serves as a useful adjunct and can be particularly helpful in identifying leaflet clefts.
- Finally, with an increase in multiplane angle to 90°, the transgastric two-chamber view is created. While this view adds less to the evaluation of the valve itself, it is an excellent view to interrogate the subvalvular apparatus and the papillary muscles.

The importance of a thorough 2D exam extends beyond the mitral valve itself, of course, and the LA and LV size can be an indicator of both the severity and chronicity of MR (11). It is unlikely that a patient with chronic, severe MR will have normal LA and LV size (though it is possible in acute severe regurgitation). Through this systematic evaluation process, the echocardiographer begins to build a model in their mind as to what the valve "looks like" and where the identifiable 2D abnormalities occur.

COLOR FLOW DOPPLER

Having established a solid understanding of both the structure and function of the mitral valve apparatus with 2D imaging, the next step is to apply color flow Doppler (CFD). A detailed CFD examination of the mitral valve supplements the understanding of valve structural pathology and adds to the ability to quantify MR severity (Table 8.3; Figure 8.5).

Jet Direction

The orientation of the regurgitant jet can aid in determining the mechanism of regurgitation. Jets that are centrally directed typically result from pathology that is balanced or symmetrical between the two leaflets. This can be annular dilation, bileaflet prolapse, or bileaflet restriction. Jets that are eccentric typically result from "unbalanced" pathology or abnormalities that affect one leaflet more than the other. In prolapse or flail (Type II motion), there will typically be an eccentric jet directed away from the abnormal leaflet. With a single restricted leaflet (Type IIIb motion), the jet typically flows toward the diseased segment.

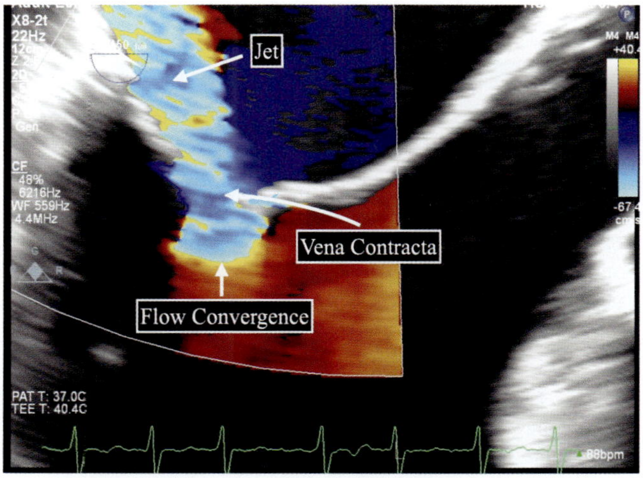

FIGURE 8.5 Demonstration of the three components of a regurgitant jet seen with color flow Doppler. As flow approaches the regurgitant orifice, it accelerates and converges. At or just past the orifice, the narrowest portion of the regurgitant flow is called the vena contracta. Past the vena contracta is the body of the jet itself.

Of critical importance to the intraoperative echocardiographer is the notion that "multiple jets mean multiple lesions." When performing a thorough mitral valve examination, the echocardiographer should not only pay attention to the first or primary regurgitant jet but should also recognize additional jets that may indicate a second pathology. It is only with a clear understanding of all the valvular abnormalities that an effective intervention can be planned.

Jet Area

While cutoffs have been described for the size (area) of jets of MR, we would recommend against quantifying MR based on these measurements. That is not to say that the jet area isn't a valuable piece of the picture. When screening the mitral valve with CFD to decide whether further quantification of MR is necessary, the jet area plays a role. A small, narrow, central jet of MR is almost always mild and does not typically warrant further quantification. Large central jets that appear to take up more than half of the LA, on the other hand, are likely to be severe. The jet area is a result of the mass of blood passing through the regurgitant orifice, and larger volumes of blood will result in greater CFD signals seen further into the LA as it takes longer for a large volume of blood to slow.

Vena Contracta

The vena contracta (VC) is the narrowest area of flow through a regurgitant orifice, is typically located just past the orifice, and is slightly smaller than the anatomic regurgitant orifice. This occurs as the result of the high-pressure low-velocity blood (in the LV) converting to a jet of high-velocity low-pressure blood at the regurgitant orifice. This low-pressure blood, moving at a high velocity, is constrained by the blood in the LA, narrowing the jet briefly until the velocity decreases and the energy is transformed back into pressure with some energy lost as heat.

Measurement of the VC is a commonly used semiquantitative method of describing the severity of regurgitant lesions with CFD (Figures 8.5 and 8.6). The measurement of a single-plane VC should be performed in the midesophageal long axis with the CFD scale set between 50 and 70 cm/s and with the image zoomed in to maximize the size of the measurement. The single-plane VC works well for circular orifices, and it applies to both central and eccentric jets. A large VC measurement (>0.7 cm) is highly specific for severe MR, but the sensitivity suffers particularly in the setting of functional MR where the orifice is likely to be more elliptical. In those situations, a biplane approach averaging the long axis and commissural measurements of VC will better reflect the true regurgitant orifice (>0.8 cm being severe) (12,13).

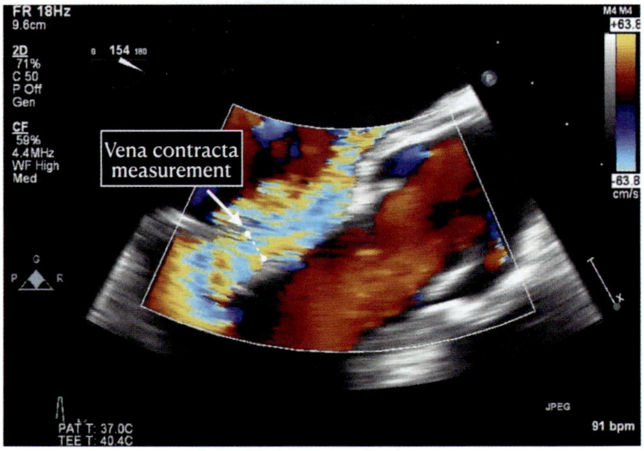

FIGURE 8.6 A midesophageal long-axis view with color flow Doppler during systole demonstrating a mitral regurgitant jet and the measurement of the vena contracta shortly after the jet passes the coaptation defect.

Flow Convergence

Flow convergence is the appearance of a hemispheric CFD pattern on the LV side of the mitral valve adjacent to the regurgitant orifice. This occurs as a result of blood accelerating toward the orifice as it is converted from a high-pressure low-velocity to a high-velocity low-pressure state. The incorporation of the measurements obtained from the area of flow convergence into a detailed quantitative assessment is described later, but there is valuable information in this portion of the regurgitant signal even without complex quantification. Fundamentally, the more the regurgitant flow, the more prominent the area of flow convergence will appear. In severe MR, there is typically a prominent appearance of flow convergence throughout systole. If the radius, measured parallel to the ultrasound beam, of the flow convergence (the PISA radius for proximal isovelocity surface area) is greater than 1 cm at a velocity of 30 to 40 cm, it strongly suggests severe MR. The measurement of PISA radius is typically performed in the four-chamber or long-axis views, with the CFD scale baseline shifted in the direction of flow so that the velocity where the scale aliases is around 40 cm/s (switches color from reds to blues) and with the image zoomed in to maximize the measurement (Figure 8.7). These measurements are most valid when the flow convergence is hemispheric, which is less likely in eccentric jets or when flow acceleration is constrained by the LV wall.

SPECTRAL DOPPLER MODALITIES

Spectral Doppler, which includes both pulsed-wave Doppler (PWD) and continuous wave Doppler, comes into play with the quantitative techniques described later in the chapter, but there is valuable qualitative and semiquantitative data as well.

PULSED-WAVE DOPPLER

The characteristic of PWD that provides utility in assessing MR is the ability to determine the direction and velocity of blood within a specific region of interest. As described in Chapter 5: Doppler Technology and Technique, PWD imaging measures velocities in a specified location though there are limits to the speed that can be sampled.

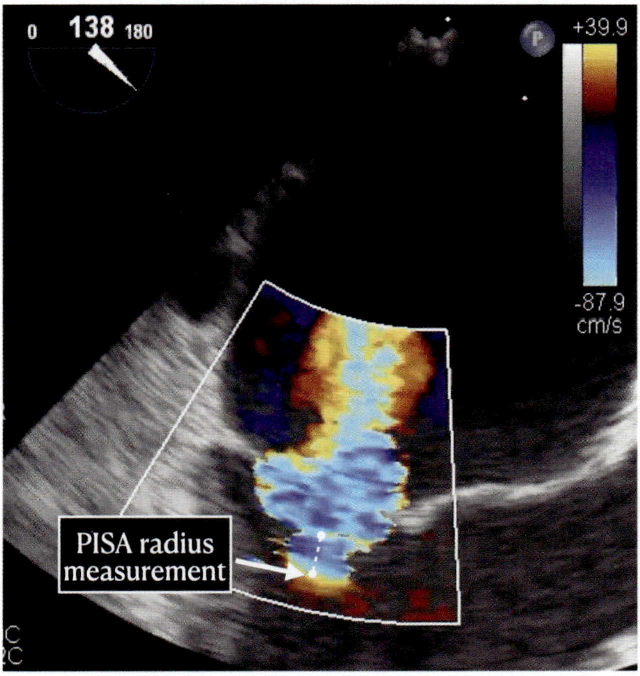

FIGURE 8.7 Measurement of flow convergence (PISA) in a midesophageal long axis. The Nyquist limit baseline is shifted in the direction of flow and is between 30 and 40 cm/s. This radius is less than 1 cm, and the MR was determined to be in the moderate range. MR, mitral regurgitation.

Mitral Inflow Velocity and Velocity Time Integral

In the absence of mitral stenosis or low-flow states, increases in MR will create increased flow across the valve in diastole. This necessarily results in higher velocities of mitral inflow, sampled with PWD at the tips of the mitral leaflets and measured at the peak of the E-wave in early diastole. A peak velocity of 1.2 m/s or more is suggestive of severe MR, while the A-wave dominant pattern of impaired relaxation essentially excludes severe MR.

MR can also be assessed by comparing the velocity time integral (VTI) of mitral inflow in diastole with that of LVOT outflow in systole. The mitral valve signal is sampled at the leaflet tips, and the LVOT sample is placed just at the annulus of the aortic valve where a closing click can be seen. As the volume of MR increases, there will be an increase in the mitral to LVOT VTI ratio. While this approach creates only a rough approximation of regurgitant fraction (RF) and assumes a normal ratio in the size of the mitral and aortic annulus, it is nonetheless a useful adjunct in the assessment of MR (8). A mitral to LVOT VTI ratio of greater than 1.4 is considered specific for severe MR, though some studies have identified a lower cutoff, and a value below 1.4 does not exclude severe MR.

Pulmonary Vein Flow

While pulmonary vein flow should be investigated even in routine TEE studies, it is particularly valuable in cases of MR. Each of the pulmonary veins should be sampled with PWD, placing the sample gate approximately 1 cm inside the vein. A normal pattern would have more flow in systole than diastole, referred to as systolic dominant. With either increasing MR or elevated LA pressure from diastolic dysfunction, a pattern of systolic blunting can be seen where there is less forward flow in systole than diastole. The pattern of systolic reversal, however, where flow is seen back into a pulmonary vein during systole, is a specific finding, suggesting severe MR. These patterns are demonstrated in Figure 8.8.

CONTINUOUS WAVE DOPPLER

Continuous wave Doppler (CWD) allows the echocardiographer to sample velocities all along the scan line. While there is no limit to the velocities measured, the echocardiographer will not be able to discern where along that line the velocities arise (range ambiguity). In addition to being used in the quantitative methods described later, there are characteristics of the CWD signal that can provide more qualitative information as well.

Density

The density or the "brightness" of the CWD signal is related to the amplitude of the returned signal. The larger the volume of blood sampled, the brighter the signal will be as there are more red blood cells moving at that velocity. Faint or incomplete envelopes of CWD are likely associated with trivial or mild regurgitation, while dense signals are more likely to be seen in moderate and severe MR.

Shape

The shape of the CWD signal can clarify the impact of MR on LA pressures and give clues to severity as well. A mild or moderate MR jet, regardless of the CWD density, should have a spectral Doppler profile that is parabolic with a high velocity (4-6 m/s). This means that throughout systole there is a significant pressure gradient between the LV and the LA. The gradient exists because the regurgitant orifice is too small to result in acutely elevated LA pressure toward the end of the systole. This is contrasted with the most severe MR in which the regurgitant volume is so high that the LA pressure increases acutely. In effect, the mitral valve is unable to protect the LA from the LV chamber pressure in systole, and the pressures begin to equalize. An example of a triangular, early peaking CWD signal in severe MR is shown in Video 8.4.

THREE-DIMENSIONAL ECHOCARDIOGRAPHY

3D echocardiography is ideal for evaluating the mitral valve. As the mitral annulus and leaflets are virtually perpendicular to the ultrasound beam in the midesophageal window, very high-resolution images can be obtained. The advent of the matrix array probe and recent improvements in image processing now allow one to obtain real-time 3D images of the mitral valve with a high frame rate and no stitching artifacts.

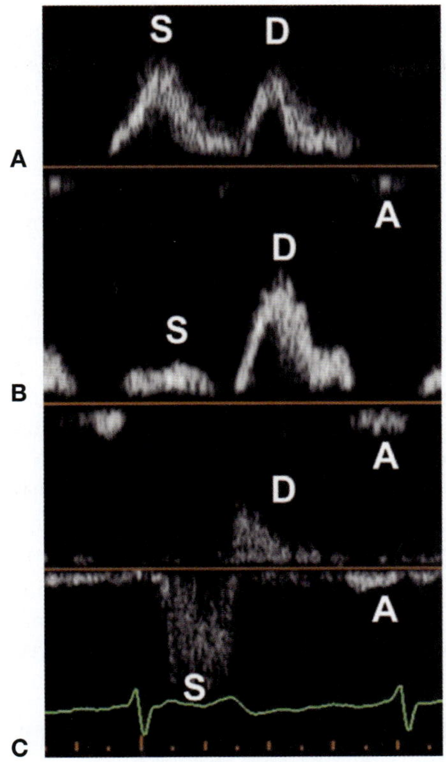

FIGURE 8.8 Pulsed-wave Doppler of pulmonary venous flow. A: An example of a normal pattern, with systolic dominant flow (more forward flow in systole than diastole). B: Systolic blunting, with a diastolic dominant pattern that can be seen either in mitral regurgitation or in diastolic dysfunction and is therefore nonspecific. C: Systolic reversal of flow suggesting severe mitral regurgitation. Flow is away from the transducer, into the pulmonary vein, throughout systole. Note also that the reversed S wave has non-laminar flow caused by the mitral regurgitation.

While 3D echocardiography is revolutionizing the intraoperative assessment of the mitral valve and creates images that add substantially to our understanding of both mechanism and severity, we would caution the enthusiastic new echocardiographer to take time with each of the modalities described in this chapter as they provide complementary information.

Jet Location

With optimal imaging, the locations of lesion(s) causing MR are often immediately apparent on 3D imaging. The standard display of the mitral valve with 3D imaging is from the "surgeon's view," with the mitral valve shown from the LA perspective and the aortic valve in the 12 o'clock position (14). This orientation places the LA appendage orifice and the anterolateral commissure on the left toward the 9 o'clock position and the posteromedial commissure around 3 o'clock position. While the temporal resolution is improved by minimizing the size of the 3D sector scanned, it is helpful to include enough surrounding anatomy to provide a clear orientation of the mitral valve. In particular, the aortic valve and LA appendage orifice should be included whenever possible.

In addition, while the surgeon's view is a helpful way to display the mitral valve, particularly in conversations with our surgeons, the authors find it necessary but not sufficient for turning a 3D data set into a thorough understanding of the mitral valve. We would suggest the routine addition of the views shown in Video 8.9. These views, in addition to other postprocessing options may demonstrate the lesion and associated dysfunction better than a single view.

Mitral Annular Sizing

The use of multiplanar reconstruction (MPR) of 3D data sets expands the value beyond that of qualitative assessment and allows for detailed and directed measurements to be made. As seen in Figure 8.9, one such application is the use of MPR to obtain measurements of mitral annular size.

Three-Dimensional Ejection Fraction

3D echocardiography provides value beyond descriptions of mitral valve anatomy as it can be used to measure LV size and global systolic function. 3D volumes that include the entire LV can determine the largest ventricular volume, LV end-diastolic volume, and the smallest ventricular volume, LV end-systolic volume. Mathematically, the difference between the two is considered the stroke volume and is used to determine Left ventricular ejection fraction (LVEF; as described in Chapter 3: Left Ventricular Systolic Performance and Pathology). In the setting of MR, the volume change represents a combination of regurgitant volume and forward flow through the LVOT. This volume (the forward stroke volume plus regurgitant volume) is the same as the volume crossing the mitral valve in diastole (assuming no aortic insufficiency). These volumes will be used both to describe systolic function and also in the quantification of severity described in the next section. With severe, chronic MR, a normally functioning LV will have hyperdynamic systolic function, and an LVEF below 60% is suggestive of early dysfunction that may warrant intervention (10).

THREE-DIMENSIONAL COLOR FLOW DOPPLER

The addition of color to the 3D assessment of the mitral valve can help in the localization of regurgitant jets as well as in the description of the number and direction of jets. Remember, multiple jets mean multiple lesions. With MPR, the echocardiographer can directly assess the size of regurgitant orifices.

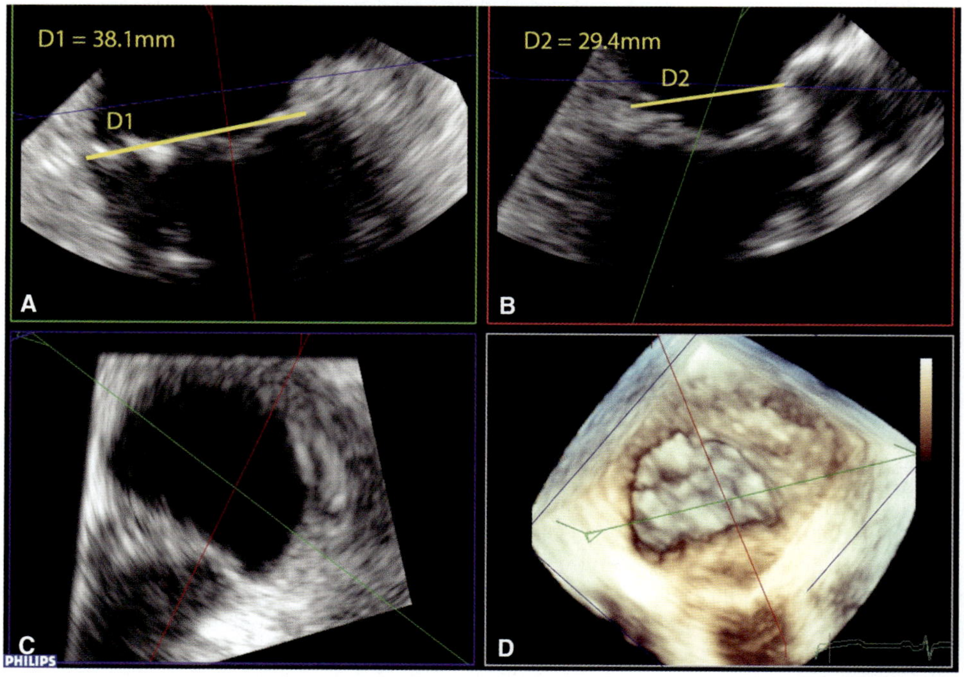

FIGURE 8.9 A still image of a 3D mitral valve data set being measured with multiplanar reconstruction (MPR). In panel A, the lateral plane is seen within the green box and the major dimension of the mitral annulus (at the midcommissural line) is measured. In panel B, the elevational plane demonstrates the minor dimension (at the long-axis view) and the annulus is measured. Note how the two lines are at different levels when referenced to the blue line in each panel. Panel C is the short-axis view and measurements should not be taken in this view as the two measurements of interest are not both within the plane. Panel D is a 3D volume of the mitral valve looking down upon the valve during systole.

Three-Dimensional Vena Contracta Area

The VC, as described earlier, is the narrowest area of the regurgitant jet just on the LA side of the orifice. When measuring the VC in 2D with CFD, it can be difficult to accurately describe a complex regurgitant orifice even with biplane imaging, particularly when the orifice is noncircular (15). This limitation is removed with 3D imaging by using MPR to identify the narrowest area perpendicular to the direction of the jet. Figure 8.10 demonstrates this process of identifying and measuring the VC area with MPR. The authors' approach is:

- Align two of the planes 90° to each other and parallel to the long axis of the jet. This should be done for each jet if there is more than one.
- Once these two planes are aligned, the third plane is oriented so that it is perpendicular to the long axis of the jet. This creates the "short axis of the jet," which is then moved to scan parallel to the jet to identify the narrowest section, often just on the atrial side of the leaflets.
- This cross section can then be traced, and the result is the effective regurgitant orifice area (EROA) in cm (2,16,17). As with EROA calculated by the PISA method (below), a cutoff of VC area of 0.4 cm^2 suggests severe MR.

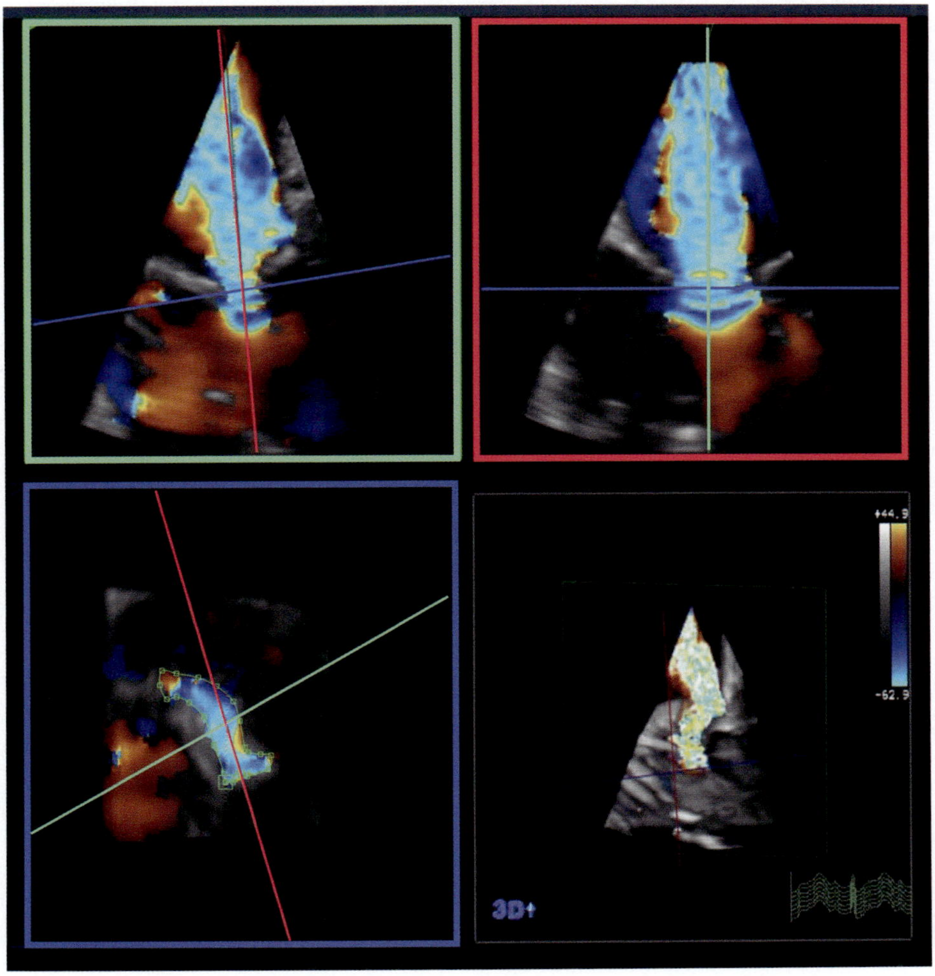

FIGURE 8.10 Still of a 3D color flow Doppler loop in mid-systole with multiplanar reconstruction to measure vena contracta area. The planes are adjusted such that the lateral and elevational planes (in this case red and green) traverse the long axis of the jet with the blue plane placed at the level of the vena contracta. The vena contracta is then measured in the blue plane.

SEVERITY OF MITRAL REGURGITATION—QUANTITATIVE METHODS

While the severity of MR can often be appropriately described after identifying several specific findings of either mild or severe disease, there will remain a proportion of patients for whom a more quantitative approach will be necessary. This includes patients with non-holosystolic MR as well as those whose findings cross categories and allows echocardiographers to avoid the overused catch-all "moderate-to-severe" regurgitation. The quantitative assessment of MR includes the calculation of the EROA, the regurgitant volume (R_{vol}) per beat, and the RF, which represents the ratio of regurgitant volume to forward stroke volume. These concepts are described in more detail in Chapter 6: Quantitative Doppler and Hemodynamics.

Effective Regurgitant Orifice Area

The EROA is a fundamental measure of severity and a strong predictor of clinical outcomes. It can be measured with 3D CFD techniques as described earlier and can also be calculated using the PISA method. The PISA method (also referred to as the "flow convergence" method) of calculating EROA involves an application of the continuity equation using both color flow and CWD data.

To create an optimal measurement, a midesophageal view that best demonstrates flow acceleration proximal to the regurgitant orifice should be chosen, and the image should be zoomed to maximize the size of the PISA shell being measured. The CFD baseline should be shifted in the direction of flow such that aliasing occurs between 30 and 40 cm/s. The PISA radius should be measured parallel to the ultrasound beam from the color change to the LV side of the mitral valve as demonstrated in Figure 8.11. The velocity that was selected by changing the baseline should be used as the aliasing velocity. Switching the modality to CWD will allow the determination of the highest velocity through the valve.

$$\text{EROA (in cm}^2) = (2\pi r^2 \times V_{alias})/V_{max}$$

where $2 \times \pi \times r^2$ is the equation for the surface area of a hemisphere, V_{alias} in cm/s is the shifted aliasing velocity, and V_{max} in cm/s is the peak velocity of MR obtained with CWD.

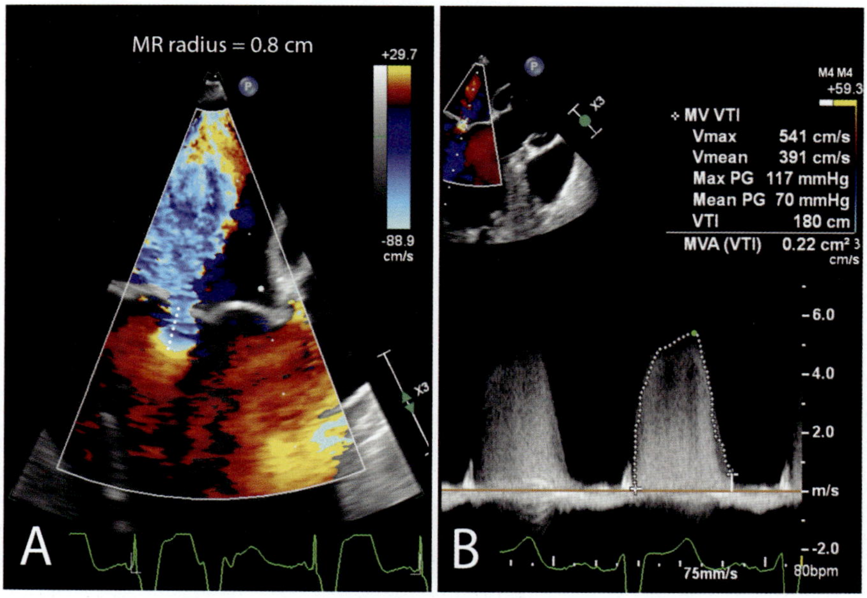

FIGURE 8.11 Example of PISA measurement. Panel A shows a color flow Doppler image of the jet with the baseline shifted to provide a more pronounced hemisphere shape. While the color section looks spherical, the flows on each side are perpendicular to the flow and are not as well visualized, which is why the radius is measured parallel to the ultrasound beam. The radius measures 8 mm in this example. Panel B shows a continuous wave Doppler envelope of the blood as it moves toward the ultrasound probe during systole. From this image, the peak velocity is used to measure the EROA by PISA. When the MR VTI is measured, both the EROA and the regurgitant flow can be estimated. EROA, effective regurgitant orifice area; MR, mitral regurgitation; PISA, proximal isovelocity surface area; VTI, velocity time integral.

Regurgitant Volume (R_{vol})

Regurgitant volumes can be calculated using flow convergence, PWD, or the volumetric method. The volumetric and PWD methods compare a measure of "total volume change" to one of forward stroke volume. The volumetric method uses LV sizes measured with 2D or 3D techniques to calculate total volume change (representing the combination of forward flow and regurgitant flow). From this is subtracted the forward stroke volume measured at a non-regurgitant valve (typically the aortic valve measured at the LVOT).

$$R_{vol} = (\text{LVEDV} - \text{LVESV}) - \text{SV}_{\text{LVOT}}$$

where LVEDV and LVESV are LV volumes at the end diastole and end systole, and SV_{LVOT} is the stroke volume measured at the aortic annulus.

The PWD method uses flow at the mitral annulus as the total volume change. For that approach, PWD is sampled at the level of the mitral annulus (the regurgitant valve) with the diameter of the mitral annulus measured in diastole, and the stroke volume from a competent valve (the aortic valve) is subtracted using the following formula:

$$R_{vol} = (\pi d^2/4) \times \text{VTI}_{\text{MVI}} - \text{SV}_{\text{LVOT}}$$

where d is the diameter of the mitral annulus, VTI_{MVI} is VTI of mitral inflow measured at the annulus, and SV_{LVOT} combines diameter and PWD measured at the aortic annulus in the absence of aortic regurgitation.

The PISA method of calculating regurgitant volume begins with either the calculation or measurement of the EROA as described earlier. CWD is then used to sample the signal of MR and traced to create a VTI (stroke distance) and applied to the following formula:

$$R_{vol} = \text{EROA}_{\text{MR}} \times \text{VTI}_{\text{MR}}$$

where EROA_{MR} is either calculated from flow acceleration as above or is measured directly with 3D as the VC area, and VTI_{MR} is traced from a CWD signal of MR.

Using multiple methods in a complete assessment can assist the echocardiographer as they would ideally agree (within a few milliliters) with close agreement suggesting that the measures are more likely accurate.

Regurgitant Fraction

RF reflects the ratio of regurgitant volume to forward stroke volume, and essentially, the regurgitant volume is divided by total LV volume change. This calculation uses information already obtained to measure regurgitant volume and uses one of the following formulas:

$$\text{RF} = R_{vol}/(\text{LVEDV} - \text{LVESV})$$

$$\text{RF} = R_{vol}/[(\pi d^2/4) \times \text{VTI}_{\text{MVI}}]$$

CHALLENGES IN THE EVALUATION AND ASSESSMENT OF MITRAL REGURGITATION

Challenges in the evaluation of the mitral valve are numerous, both in the operating room (OR) and in the echocardiography lab. Imaging may be challenging, findings may be unexpected, hemodynamics may be erratic, and, most commonly, the severity assessments may not be concordant. There are data suggesting that changes in afterload result in changes in the severity of MR under general anesthesia, and while this can be partially corrected with restoration of afterload, it should be recognized that findings in the OR may be different from those in patients who are awake and not ventilated(13,18).

As seen throughout this chapter, there are numerous qualitative, semiquantitative, and quantitative methods that can be employed to evaluate the severity of MR. It is common to have some of these metrics in one category of severity and some in another. What is the conscientious echocardiographer going to report to their surgical colleague? The ideal approach in cases of known MR is to assess the severity with all necessary modalities (including transthoracic echocardiography, TEE, and magnetic resonance imaging) preoperatively with the findings thoughtfully discussed with the heart team (9). This is ideal but rarely the case. The addition of TEE to all cardiac surgical procedures has positively impacted patient outcomes, but it does provide opportunities for the discovery of previously unknown MR and, in these cases, the severity of

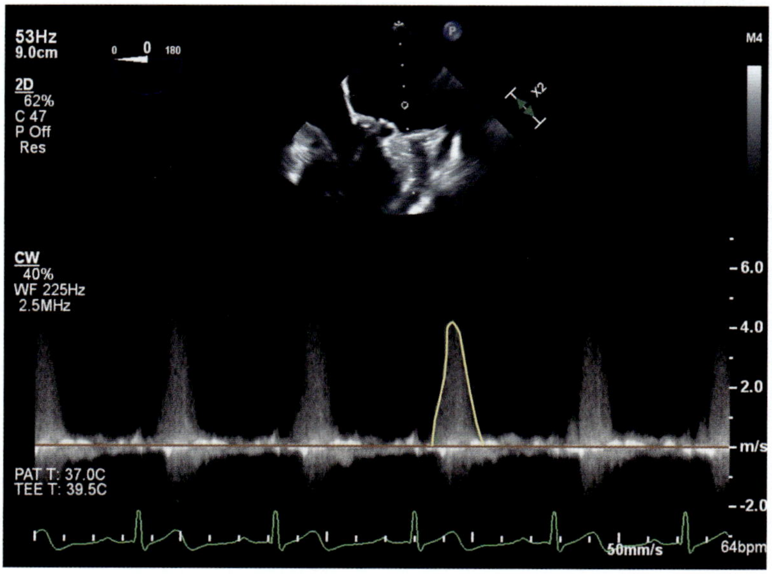

FIGURE 8.12 An example of CWD through non-holosystolic jet of mitral regurgitation from leaflet prolapse. It is critical to recognize that single-frame measurements will likely overestimate severity in these cases. Calculation of regurgitant volume and regurgitant fraction must use the actual signal of regurgitation as shown. See Video 8.10. CWD, continuous wave Doppler.

MR will impact the surgical plan and must be assessed in the moment. A reasonable approach to classifying MR in these cases, after "normalizing" hemodynamics as much as possible, is totally each metric by its severity and take the group that is most populated. Employing a routine exam sequence and having a framework for the numerous metrics for quantifying MR can assist in describing the etiology, lesion, dysfunction, severity, and consequences. In this process, the presence of high-specificity findings should be given particular priority in the determination of severity. That is to say, if there are findings such as a reversal of flow in the pulmonary veins, which have a significant physiologic impact on cardiac performance, the severity should reflect the significance of those findings.

While there are countless complexities that arise in the assessment of MR, there is a particular physiology that warrants special attention. This is the circumstance of "non-holosystolic" MR. This is typically seen in the setting of regurgitation from leaflet prolapse and corresponds to the physical exam finding of mid-systolic click with late systolic murmur. This physiology highlights the problems that can arise from "single frame" measures of severity. This includes VC width, VC area, and PISA radius. Those metrics are all extremely valuable but are only valid measures of severity in the setting of holosystolic MR. Non-holosystolic MR requires particular attention to avoid overcalling the severity, and the presence of a large EROA alone is not sufficient to diagnose severe MR. Conceptually, to create a severe volume of regurgitation would require a regurgitant orifice that is twice the size if it regurgitates for only half of systole. In these cases, it is particularly important to calculate regurgitant volume and fraction and to trace the signal of actual regurgitation rather than the entirety of systole (Video 8.10; Figure 8.12).

CONCLUSIONS

The challenge for the echocardiographer assessing the mitral valve is to be able to both identify the underlying problem with the valve and provide an assessment of the severity of regurgitation. This information will guide surgical colleagues to their best approach to the valve, whether that is through a repair, replacement, or percutaneous intervention. In some cases, it may be the heart team's conclusion that no intervention is the correct approach. The echocardiographer must have at their disposal the knowledge and skills to assess the valve using 2D, 3D, Doppler, and MPR and to assimilate the entirety of the evaluation into a succinct summary in which their assessment of the underlying cause, mechanism of dysfunction, and resulting severity of valve dysfunction is presented to a surgical colleague. Often a robust and detailed evaluation demonstrating years of cumulative knowledge and experience will be summarized in a two- or three-sentence statement about the valve. This is the goal, to take a wealth of knowledge and experience, apply it to the evaluation of the mitral valve, and deliver a summary of one's findings for the benefit of the patient.

ACKNOWLEDGMENTS

We gratefully acknowledge the contributions of the previous edition authors, Adam M. Dryden and A. Stephane Lambert, as portions of those chapters have been retained in this revision.

REFERENCES

1. Wenink ACG, Groot ACG. Embryology of the mitral valve. *Int J Cardiol.* 1986;11:75-84.
2. Carpentier A. Cardiac valve surgery—the "French correction". *J Thorac Cardiovasc Surg.* 1983;86:323-337.
3. Sidebotham DA, Allen SJ, Gerber IL, et al. Intraoperative transesophageal echocardiography for surgical repair of mitral regurgitation. *J Am Soc Echocardiogr.* 2014;27:345-366.
4. Rausch MK, Bothe W, Kvitting J-PE, et al. Characterization of mitral valve annular dynamics in the beating heart. *Ann Biomed Eng.* 2011;39:1690-1702.
5. Dal-Bianco JP, Levine RA. Anatomy of the mitral valve apparatus role of 2D and 3D echocardiography. *Cardiol Clin.* 2013;31:151-164.
6. Carpentier A, Adams DH, Filsoufi F. *Carpentier's Reconstructive Valve Surgery.* 1st ed. Saunders; 2010.
7. Zoghbi WA, Adams D, Bonow RO, et al. Recommendations for noninvasive evaluation of native valvular regurgitation: a report from the American Society of Echocardiography developed in collaboration with the Society for Cardiovascular Magnetic Resonance. *J Am Soc Echocardiogr.* 2017;30:303-371.
8. Lancellotti P, Pibarot P, Chambers J, et al. Multi-modality imaging assessment of native valvular regurgitation: an EACVI and ESC council of valvular heart disease position paper. *Eur Hear J Cardiovasc Imaging.* 2022;23:e171-e232.
9. Otto CM, Nishimura RA, Bonow RO, et al. 2020 ACC/AHA guideline for the management of patients with valvular heart disease: a report of the American College of Cardiology/American Heart Association Joint Committee on Clinical Practice Guidelines. *Circulation.* 2021;143:e72-e227.
10. Vahanian A, Beyersdorf F, Praz F, et al. 2021 ESC/EACTS guidelines for the management of valvular heart disease developed by the task force for the management of valvular heart disease of the European Society of Cardiology (ESC) and the European Association for Cardio-Thoracic Surgery (EACTS). *Eur Hear J.* 2021;43:ehab395.
11. Tribouilloy C, Rusinaru D, Grigioni F, et al. Long-term mortality associated with left ventricular dysfunction in mitral regurgitation due to flail leaflets. *Circ Cardiovasc Imaging.* 2014;7:363-370.
12. Wilkes, JO, Birmingham SG, Ellwood KRJ, Kirby BJ, eds. *Fluid Mechanics for Chemical Engineers.* 3rd ed. Prentice Hall; 2018.
13. Sanfilippo F, Johnson C, Bellavia D, et al. Mitral regurgitation grading in the operating room: a systematic review and meta-analysis comparing preoperative and intraoperative assessments during cardiac surgery. *J Cardiothorac Vasc Anesthesia.* 2017;31:1681-1691.
14. Lang RM, Badano LP, Tsang W, et al. EAE/ASE recommendations for image acquisition and display using three-dimensional echocardiography. *J Am Soc Echocardiogr.* 2012;25:3-46.
15. Thavendiranathan P, Phelan D, Collier P, et al. Quantitative assessment of mitral regurgitation how best to do it. *JACC Cardiovasc Imaging.* 2012;5:1161-1175.
16. Ashikhmina E, Shook D, Cobey F, et al. Three-dimensional versus two-dimensional echocardiographic assessment of functional mitral regurgitation proximal isovelocity surface area. *Anesth Analg.* 2015;120:534-542.
17. Buck T, Plicht B. Real-time three-dimensional echocardiographic assessment of severity of mitral regurgitation using proximal isovelocity surface area and vena contracta area method. lessons we learned and clinical implications. *Curr Cardiovasc Imaging Rep.* 2015;8:38.
18. Mihalatos DG, Gopal AS, Kates R, et al. Intraoperative assessment of mitral regurgitation: role of phenylephrine challenge. *J Am Soc Echocardiogr.* 2006;19:1158-1164.

QUESTIONS

1. For segment A2 of the mitral valve, to which papillary muscle(s) are the chordae attached?

A. Septal
B. Anterolateral
C. Posteromedial
D. Anterolateral and posteromedial

2. Which statement describes the mitral valve correctly?

A. The anterior leaflet is two-third of the area and one-third of the circumference.
B. The posterior leaflet is well supported by the annular fibrosa.
C. The posterior leaflet is two-third of the area and two-third of the circumference.
D. The major dimension of the mitral valve is along the A2-P2 axis.

3. Which congenital heart defect is most associated with a cleft of the anterior mitral leaflet?
A. Bicuspid aortic valve
B. Secundum ASD
C. Primum ASD
D. Sinus venosus ASD

4. Which of the following would be a common etiology for significant MR with Type I leaflet motion?
A. Fibroelastic deficiency (FED)
B. Endocarditis
C. Ischemic heart disease
D. Barlow valve (myxomatous valve disease)

5. Which of the following would be a common etiology for significant MR with Type IIIb leaflet motion?
A. 99% right coronary artery (RCA) lesion
B. Ruptured chordal attachments
C. Annular dilation
D. MRSA endocarditis

6. Which statement best describes the VC?
A. It is the wide section of the jet as the blood slows down.
B. It is the narrow high-pressure section of the regurgitant jet.
C. It is the narrowed section on the atrial side of the MR jet.
D. It is the segment immediately before the coaptation defect in the ventricle.

7. Which statement describes annular dilation?
A. The annulus is dilated when the ratio of the major to minor axis is 4:3.
B. The annulus dilates posteriorly away from the aortic valve.
C. The fibrous trigones within the mitral annulus are the reason why the annulus dilates.
D. When the annulus dilates, it becomes increasingly saddle shaped.

8. When calculating the *EROA* by PISA, which measurement is not required?
A. Radius of the PISA hemisphere
B. Left ventricular ejection fraction
C. Aliasing velocity of blood as it approaches the coaptation defect
D. The maximum velocity of regurgitant blood

9. Assuming a normal mitral annular size and normal LV outflow tract diameter, which of the following measurements would be consistent with severe MR?
A. MV VTI 15; LVOT VTI 18
B. MV VTI 15; LVOT VTI 15
C. MV VTI 18; LVOT VTI 13
D. MV VTI 20; LVOT VTI 14

10. Determining EROA using the VC area method is best performed using which technique?
A. CWD envelope profile and density
B. 3D CFD imaging with MPR
C. CFD color compare and biplane imaging for eccentric jets
D. 3D imaging with measurements of the visible coaptation defect

ANSWERS

1. Correct Answer: D.
Rationale: A2 has connections to both papillary muscles, and so does P2. A1 and P1 go to the anterolateral papillary muscle alone and the A3 and P3 to the posteromedial. There is no septal papillary muscle.

2. Correct Answer: A.
Rationale: The anterior leaflet is the larger of the two with the annulus representing one-third of the circumference. The posterior leaflet is not supported by any fibrous connective tissue. The largest

dimension, the major axis, is in the midcommissural plane.

3. **Correct Answer: C.**
Rationale: Primum defects arise from the same endocardial cushions that form the mitral valve during embryogenesis, resulting in associated mitral defects. Secundum ASDs are common and not associated with mitral cleft. Bicuspid aortic valve disease is the most common lesion and not associated with mitral disease. Sinus venosus lesions are associated with partial anomalous venous return.

4. **Correct Answer: B.**
Rationale: Endocarditis is the only etiology listed that is associated with normal leaflet motion. FED and Barlow are associated with Type II motion, and ischemic heart disease results in Type IIIb motion.

5. **Correct Answer: A.**
Rationale: Type IIIb motion from ischemic heart disease, RCA lesions causing inferior and inferolateral segmental wall motion abnormalities cause restrictive leaflet motion. Ruptured chordae cause Type II and annular dilation, and endocarditis cause Type I motion.

6. **Correct Answer: C.**
Rationale: The VC has a narrowing in the LA at the high-velocity low-pressure portion immediately past the orifice on the atrial size. The wide section further in the atrium or the part in the ventricle is not the VC. The VC is a low-pressure high-velocity feature and not a high-pressure one.

7. **Correct Answer: B.**
Rationale: The lack of fibrous tissue posteriorly allows for annular dilation away from the aortic valve in the posterior direction. The annulus becomes planar with a 1:1 ratio of the axes as it dilates. The fibrous trigones are near the anterior leaflet and are not associated with dilation.

8. **Correct Answer: B.**
Rationale: The equation for determining EROA by PISA is as follows:

$$\text{PISA} = (2 \times \pi \times r^2 \times V_{\text{alias}})/V_{\text{max}}$$

One needs to know the radius of the PISA hemisphere, the velocity at which the blood changes color on the screen, known as the aliasing velocity, and the peak or maximal velocity recorded using CWD as the blood is ejected through the regurgitant orifice. The ejection fraction, which can be helpful, is the overall assessment and is not required for the calculation.

9. **Correct Answer: D.**
Rationale: The ratio of mitral valve VTI to LVOT VTI can be helpful in the assessment of MR as the volume through the two regions should be the same in the absence of MR. When MR is present, more blood passes through the mitral valve and the ratio of these two measurements can reflect the relative increase in volume. A ratio of 1.4 or greater is consistent with severe MR and only the MV VTI of 20 cm and the LVOT VTI of 14 cm are consistent with a ratio of 1.4 or greater.

10. **Correct Answer: B.**
Rationale: The VC area is a narrowed region of the MR jet that is found on the LA side of the jet near the coaptation defect. While the other options can assist in qualifying and quantifying the severity of the regurgitation, only the option that uses MPR of a 3D CFD image would allow the user to align the imaging planes within MPR and focus on the VC area for measurement.

9 Mitral Valve Stenosis

Megan P. Kostibas and Mary Beth Brady

The 19th-century physician, Jean-Nicolas Corvisart, established the diagnostic value of percussion in the physical diagnosis of cardiac disorders. He described the diastolic thrill of mitral stenosis (MS) as "a peculiar rushing like water, difficult to be described, sensible to the hand applied over the precordial region, a rushing which proceeds apparently from the embarrassment which the blood undergoes in passing through an opening which is no longer proportioned to the quantity of fluid which it ought to discharge" (1). As early as 1898, DW Samways discussed the potential for performing cardiac surgery in the most severe cases of MS in an article entitled "Cardiac Peristalsis: Its Nature and Effects," published in *The Lancet* (2). In the more modern era of heart disease, cardiac catheterization traditionally provided hemodynamic information and assessment of the severity of MS, but with the expanding use of echocardiography, the need for cardiac catheterization decreased. In 1997, Popovic et al (3) investigated time-related trends in the use of preoperative invasive hemodynamic measurements in 1,985 patients with isolated valvular stenosis. During the study period, the need for invasive hemodynamic measurements acquired during catheterization dramatically decreased, superseded by noninvasive hemodynamic measurements obtained with echocardiography (3). Currently, two-dimensional (2D), three-dimensional (3D), and Doppler echocardiography have supplanted cardiac catheterization in providing a complete evaluation of patients with MS (4).

MITRAL VALVE ANATOMY

Morphologically, the mitral valve (MV) apparatus is composed of the left atrial (LA) wall, mitral annulus, anterior and posterior MV leaflets, chordal tendons, anterolateral and posteromedial papillary muscles, and left ventricular (LV) myocardium (5,6). The valvular tissue can be divided into two commissural regions, the anterolateral commissure and the posteromedial commissure, and two leaflet areas, the anterior and posterior MV leaflets. The anterior mitral leaflet is somewhat triangular in shape, with an attachment to approximately one-third of the circumference of the mitral annulus. It is attached to the fibrous skeleton of the heart, as are the left coronary cusp and half of the noncoronary cusp of the aortic valve. The attachment of the posterior mitral leaflet to the mitral annulus is lengthier than that of the anterior mitral leaflet. Clefts along the free margin of the posterior leaflet allow the identification of three individual scallops (5). Although the anterior mitral leaflet base-to-margin dimension is longer than that of the posterior mitral leaflet and the basal attachments are different for each leaflet, the two leaflets are nearly identical in their overall surface area. Chordal tendons from each papillary muscle attach to both the anterior and posterior MV leaflets. On average, 120 chordal tendons attach to the undersurface of the MV leaflets. The chordal tendons subdivide as they project from the papillary muscles toward the MV leaflets. The spaces between the chordae serve as secondary orifices between the LA and LV (6). The primary orifice is considered the space between the two MV leaflets.

The normal MV orifice area is approximately 4 to 6 cm^2. An orifice area near 2 cm^2 causes a minimal elevation in the transvalvular pressure gradient, whereas a valve area of less than 1.4 cm^2 is associated with a significant transvalvular pressure gradient and the clinical presentation of MS (7-9).

ETIOLOGY OF MITRAL STENOSIS

The causes of MS include the following: rheumatic heart disease, LA myxoma, severe mitral annular calcification, thrombus formation, parachute MV deformity, congenital MS, supravalvular mitral ring, and cor triatriatum (6,10). Figures 9.1 and 9.2 depict a large LA myxoma obstructing mitral inflow.

Throughout the world, the most common cause of MS in adults is rheumatic heart disease. In developed countries, rheumatic fever—and thus rheumatic MS—is much less common (3,6,9). Pathologic features of rheumatic MS include fusion of the commissures; contracture, scarring, and diffuse thickening of the leaflet tissue and subvalvular apparatus; and calcium deposition within the mitral leaflets. This clinically progressive process results in a diminished size of the effective valvular orifice, in addition to valve rigidity as a consequence of leaflet fibrosis and calcification. As the valve area becomes more restricted, increases in the

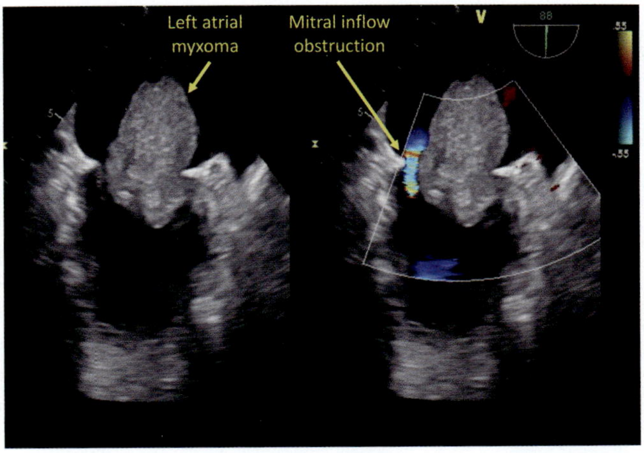

FIGURE 9.1 A transesophageal echocardiographic midesophageal two-chamber image displays a 3 × 6 cm left atrial myxoma causing symptomatic mitral stenosis. The atrial myxoma is visualized prolapsed through the mitral valve into the left ventricular cavity during diastole.

transvalvular pressure gradient and LA pressure may lead to pulmonary hypertension with tricuspid regurgitation (TR), right ventricular dysfunction, and dyspnea (6,8-10).

TRANSESOPHAGEAL ECHOCARDIOGRAPHIC EVALUATION OF MITRAL STENOSIS

A discussion of the complete diagnostic evaluation follows, and the chapter concludes with a concise summary of the recommended approach to an accurate diagnosis of MS.

Two-Dimensional Echocardiography

The anatomy of MS can be defined clearly from multiple imaging planes of 2D echocardiography. While transthoracic echocardiography (TTE) is more commonly used for the initial evaluation of possible mitral disease, transesophageal echocardiography (TEE) is superior for visualization and evaluation of morphology

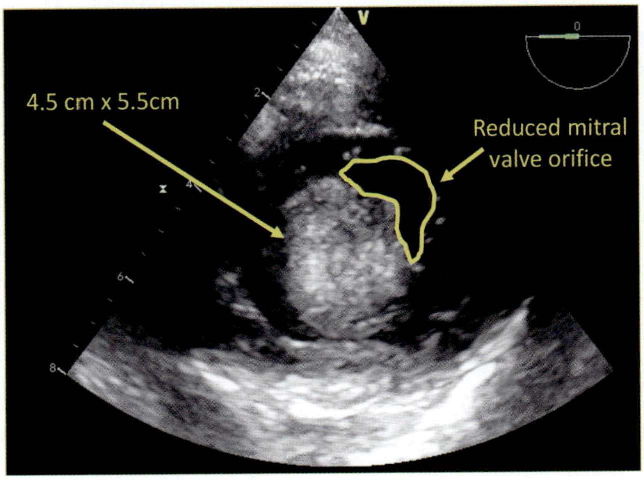

FIGURE 9.2 An atrial myxoma displayed from a transgastric basal short-axis imaging plane occupies a large portion of the mitral orifice. The mitral valve orifice measures 1.86 cm^2 in diastole.

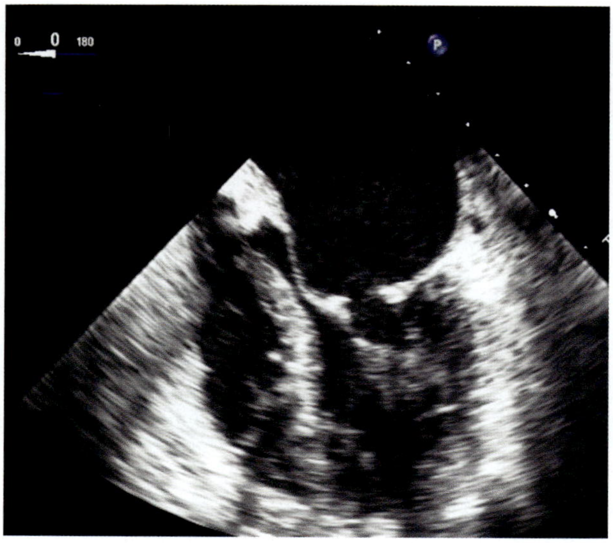

FIGURE 9.3 A midesophageal four-chamber view of rheumatic mitral stenosis displays the characteristic diastolic "doming" of the anterior mitral leaflet in diastole and an enlarged left atrium. The mitral leaflets are thickened, particularly at their margins, and appear echo bright secondary to calcium deposition.

and severity of lesions due to the more posterior location of the MV. On the basis of the pathophysiologic features of rheumatic MS, key features that must be identified include the following: degree of leaflet thickening, amount of calcium deposition, extent of subvalvular involvement, decrement in leaflet mobility, and overall changes in chamber dimensions and functions (11). Related issues, such as involvement of other valve structures, regurgitation, and pulmonary hypertension, should also be assessed.

Mitral leaflet tissue can display varying degrees of thickening and calcium deposition that cause the MV leaflets to appear "enhanced" or echo bright. The "shadow" cast by calcium may obstruct the view of the distal anatomy; one of the strengths of TEE is the ability to view the structures from another plane so that the operator can see beyond the "shadow." The standard midesophageal (ME) views (four-chamber, commissural, two-chamber, and long-axis) assist in evaluating the extent of disease. The chordal tendons can display varying degrees of thickening and contracture. The transgastric (TG) long-axis, ME four-chamber, and ME long-axis imaging planes provide helpful information with regard to the extent of subvalvular involvement in the rheumatic process. The characteristic 2D echocardiographic findings associated with rheumatic MS are represented in Figure 9.3 in an ME four-chamber view and in Videos 9.1 to 9.3. Rheumatic heart disease results in varying degrees of restricted mitral leaflet motion. In 2D TEE, restricted leaflet motion is characterized by decreased leaflet excursion and by diastolic "doming" of the anterior mitral leaflet. The appearance of "doming" is the result of fusion of the anterior and posterior leaflets along the medial and lateral commissures. The leaflets are restricted or abnormally stenotic at the tips. The maximal amplitude of motion occurs in the mobile midsection, giving the anterior mitral leaflet an arched appearance, convex toward the LV outflow tract in diastole (12,13). Figure 9.3 and Video 9.1 demonstrate the characteristic "doming" or "hockey stick" deformity of the anterior mitral leaflet in diastole.

Echocardiographic Scoring System

More than 35 years ago, Wilkins et al (11) published an echocardiographic scoring system to assess MV morphology and its relationship to the success of percutaneous balloon dilation of the MV. Each of the four components of the scoring system is graded on a scale of 0 to 4, such that total scores range from 0 to 16. The four components of the scoring system assess the MV for pathologic changes characteristically associated with rheumatic heart disease: reduced leaflet mobility, leaflet thickening, subvalvular thickening, and

TABLE 9.1 Echocardiographic Scoring System

Grade	Mobility	Subvalvular Thickening	Thickening	Calcification
1	Highly mobile valve with only leaflet tips restricted	Minimal thickening just below the mitral leaflets	Leaflets nearly normal in thickness (4-5 mm)	Single area of increased echo brightness
2	Leaflet mid and base portions have normal mobility.	Thickening of chordal structures extending up to one-third of chordal length	Mid leaflets normal, considerable thickening of margins (5-8 mm)	Scattered areas of brightness confined to leaflet margins
3	Valve continues to move forward in diastole, mainly from base	Thickening extending to the distal third of chords	Thickening extending through the entire leaflet (5-8 mm)	Brightness extending into midportion of the leaflets
4	No or minimal forward movement of the leaflets in diastole	Extensive thickening and shortening of all chordal structures extending down to papillary muscles	Considerable thickening of all leaflet tissue (>8-10 mm)	Extensive brightness throughout much of the leaflet tissue

Reproduced from Wilkins G, Weyman A, Abascal V, et al. Percutaneous balloon dilatation of the mitral valve: an analysis of echocardiographic variables related to outcome and the mechanism of dilatation. *Br Heart J*. 1988;60:299-308, with permission from BMJ Publishing Group Ltd.

calcification. These investigators reported that a high echocardiographic score (>11), representative of advanced leaflet deformity, was associated with a suboptimal outcome after balloon dilation of the MV. A low echocardiographic score (<9) was associated with an optimal outcome (11). Table 9.1 presents the scoring system and describes what each grade on the scale represents for each of the four components. Although this scoring system was developed for patients undergoing mitral balloon dilation, it can serve as a useful guide during the TEE examination of patients with rheumatic MS (see Table 9.1).

Chronic MS can alter cardiac chamber dimensions. The extent of this alteration depends on the duration and degree of MS. Typically, an increase in the LA area is associated with chronic volume and pressure overload. Additionally, because of the low-flow state of MS, LA spontaneous echo contrast or thrombus formation may be present. Daniel et al (14) characterized LA spontaneous echo contrast as "dynamic clouds of echoes curling up slowly in a circular or spiral shape within the left atrium." They found that LA spontaneous echo contrast is useful in identifying those patients with MS who are at increased risk for thromboembolic events. TEE is more sensitive than TTE in detecting LA spontaneous echo contrast. Since LA spontaneous echo contrast indicates blood stasis and may be a warning of thrombus formation, it is critical to scan the LA completely to exclude thrombus formation (14,15). Figure 9.4 displays an ME view of the LA with a thrombus in the LA appendage.

Diastolic properties of the LV are also affected in rheumatic MS. In patients with severe isolated rheumatic MS, Liu et al (16) demonstrated reduced LV diastolic compliance. The reduction in compliance appeared to be related to a functional restriction resulting from chordal tethering to a rigid valve apparatus, a finding that was immediately reversed after balloon mitral valvuloplasty. LV systolic performance in patients with severe isolated MS was nearly identical to that in age-matched controls. Chronic elevation in LA pressure can cause structural alterations in the pulmonary vasculature, leading to pulmonary hypertension and ultimately right-sided heart failure (8,9). TEE evaluation of the right side of the heart may demonstrate varying degrees of right ventricular dysfunction and TR. A comprehensive 2D, 3D, and Doppler TEE examination of the heart should be performed to exclude these associated findings and other valvular pathology.

Physiologic Assessments

Updated ACC/AHA Guidelines in 2020 emphasized a more contemporary approach to the assessment of MS (17). The central concept is that patients may present in phases of MS progression from stage A to stage D, which represents more than a simple valve area calculation or mean pressure gradient. The guideline assessment for severity includes features of MV anatomy, valve hemodynamics, patient symptoms, and disease

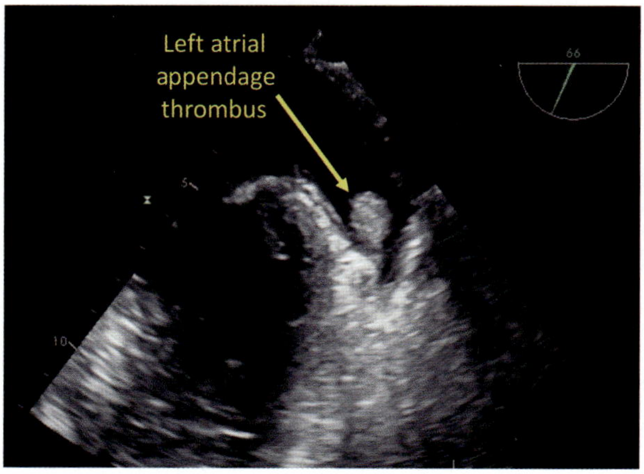

FIGURE 9.4 A left atrial appendage thrombus (arrow) is visualized from a short-axis imaging plane of the left atrium.

consequences, such as LA enlargement and elevated pulmonary artery pressures. For example, stage A: "at risk of MS" might feature mild MV diastolic doming, normal transmitral flow velocities, and no secondary hemodynamic consequences or patient symptoms; whereas stage D: "symptomatic severe MS" might feature diastolic doming, commissural fusion, valve area of less than 1.5 cm^2, pressure half-time (PHT) of 150 milliseconds or more, severe LA enlargement, elevated pulmonary artery pressure of higher than 50 mm Hg, and patient symptoms of limited exercise tolerance (Table 9.2) (17). This chapter will describe 2D and Doppler techniques for assessment and then 3D assessment.

TABLE 9.2 Stages of Mitral Stenosis From the American Heart Association/American College of Cardiology Guidelines[a]

Stage	Definition	Valve Anatomy	Valve Hemodynamics	Hemodynamic Consequences	Symptoms
A	At risk of MS	Mild diastolic doming	Normal transmitral flow velocity	None	None
B	Progressive MS	Commissural fusion, diastolic doming MVA >1.5 cm^2 via planimetry	Increased transmitral flow velocities MVA >1.5 cm^2 PHT <150 ms	Mild-moderate LAE Normal PA pressures at rest	None
C	Asymptomatic severe MS	Commissural fusion and diastolic doming MVA ≤ 1.5 cm^2 via planimetry MVA ≤ 1.0 cm^2 with very severe	MVA ≤ 1.5 cm^2 MVA ≤ 1.0 cm^2 with very severe PHT ≥ 150 ms PHT ≥ 220 ms with very severe	Severe LAE Elevated PASP >50 mm Hg	None
D	Symptomatic severe MS	Commissural fusion and diastolic doming MVA ≤1.5 cm^2 via planimetry	MVA ≤1.5 cm^2 MVA ≤1.0 cm^2 with very severe PHT ≥150 ms PHT ≥220 ms with very severe	Severe LAE Elevated PASP >50 mm Hg	Decreased exercise tolerance Exertional dyspnea

LAE, left atrial enlargement; MVA, mitral valve area; MS, mitral stenosis; PA, pulmonary artery; PASP, pulmonary artery systolic pressure; PHT, pressure half-time.

[a]From Otto CM, Nishimura RA, Bonow RO, et al. 2020 ACC/AHA guideline for the management of patients with valvular heart disease: executive summary: a report of the American College of Cardiology/American Heart Association Joint Committee on Clinical Practice Guidelines. *Circulation*. 2021;143(5):e35-e71.

Determination of the Pressure Gradient

Normal flow velocity across the MV is less than 1.3 m/s. The pressure drop across a stenotic valve can be calculated from the instantaneous flow velocity by means of the simplified Bernoulli equation (18,19):

$$\text{Pressure gradient (mm Hg)} = 4v^2$$

where v represents the instantaneous velocity.

The equation is modified from the original in that the terms that account for viscous friction and flow acceleration have been eliminated. Since the velocity distal to the obstruction is significantly greater than the velocity proximal to the obstruction, the proximal velocity term can be ignored (18,19). Continuous wave Doppler interrogation of the inflow velocities across the valve is performed with the use of the ME four-chamber, two-chamber, or long-axis view. Following manual tracing of the diastolic spectral profile, the echocardiographic machine software provides a mean gradient in millimeters of mercury. Figure 9.5 displays a mean gradient measurement across the MV in a patient with MS obtained with continuous wave Doppler in the ME four-chamber view. It is important to note that an increase in forward flow through the mitral orifice, such as that occurs in severe mitral valvular regurgitation, can result in a high transmitral gradient although the valve is only mildly stenotic. One, therefore, must be aware that the degree of MS can be overestimated in the face of significant mitral regurgitation (4). Pressure gradients are underestimated if the angle between the sampling beam and the flow vector is large (>20°) (18,20). Visualizing the inflow jet with color Doppler and aligning the sample beam with the color inflow can minimize this error (20). In general, a mean gradient of more than 10 mm Hg across a stenotic valve is considered to indicate severe stenosis (21). However, because of the variability of the mean pressure gradient with heart rate, diastolic filling period, and transvalvular forward flow, the transmitral mean pressure gradient was not included in the criteria for severity in the 2020 ACC/AHA Guidelines (17). What is of utmost importance to remember when grading severity is, according to the 2023 American Society of Echocardiography recommendations on echocardiographic evaluation of rheumatic mitral disease, "a multi-parametric approach should be used, including valve area, PHT, transmitral mean pressure gradient, taking into account both anatomic and hemodynamic consequences of the pathophysiology of MS" (21).

Calculations of Valve Area

The severity of MS is also estimated by calculating the mitral valve area (MVA). This can be done with the use of 2D, 3D, and transvalvular Doppler echocardiographic techniques.

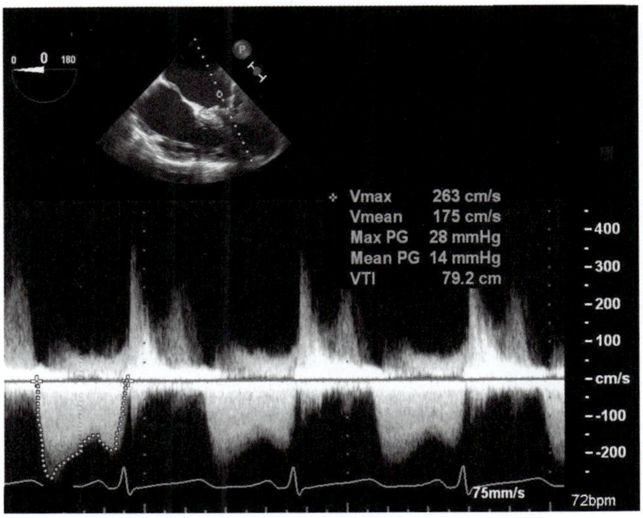

FIGURE 9.5 A diastolic spectral profile of mitral inflow has been obtained with continuous wave Doppler in this patient with mitral stenosis. The profile has been traced out, and a mean pressure gradient of 14 mm Hg has been calculated with the software available within the machine. Note that the inflow velocities are close to 2 m/s.

Planimetry Valve Area

Planimetry is a conceptually simple 2D technique used to calculate the MVA, and it is the preferred method for determining the anatomic MVA (21). It involves direct visualization of the MV orifice in diastole from a TG basal short-axis imaging plane and tracing the orifice margins to acquire a valve area measurement in square centimeters, ideally in zoom mode (21) (Figure 9.6). The results obtained with this technique have been shown to correlate well with valve area measurements acquired invasively (3,12,22). Figure 9.6 demonstrates the use of planimetry in calculating the MVA from the TG basal short-axis imaging plane in a patient with rheumatic MS. In order to optimize measurement accuracy, a number of operator "pitfalls" should be recognized when this technique is used. Instrumentation factors are critical in obtaining adequate images for planimetry. For example, if the receiver gain settings are too low, the edges of the valve may be obscured, resulting in "echo dropout," and the valve area can be overestimated (12). The opposite occurs when the gain settings are set too high, with resultant image saturation and a falsely narrowed valve orifice (21,23). Inadequate imaging plane orientation is another important measurement error with this technique. The stenotic MV looks like a funnel in diastole, the narrowest part being the commissural tip of the valve. It is critical to scan the MV orifice superiorly to inferiorly to acquire the smallest orifice area. Measuring too superiorly, in the body of the leaflets, can overestimate the valve area (22-24). In patients who have undergone mitral valvuloplasty, the valve area may be underestimated because of the inability to measure the extent of the commissural fractures with planimetry.

Pressure Half-Time

The PHT describes the pressure difference between the LA and LV and can be quantitatively related to the degree of MS. As MS becomes more severe, the rate of pressure decline between the LA and LV is proportionally slower, and consequently, the gradient between the LA and LV is maintained for a longer period of time. The PHT is the time required for the atrioventricular pressure difference to decrease from the maximum to one-half of that value. To calculate the PHT, the peak transmitral flow velocity is measured by Doppler, and the time it takes to decrease by a factor of the square root of 2 is traced and measured (3,21,25). Figure 9.7 displays the PHT measurement in a patient with MS. The signal is acquired by aligning the continuous wave Doppler beam with the mitral inflow and acquiring a transmitral flow velocity signal. The machine software automatically calculates the PHT after the operator labels the maximal and minimal velocities. The PHT increases as the severity of MS increases (21,25-27). In a normal MV, the PHT is generally

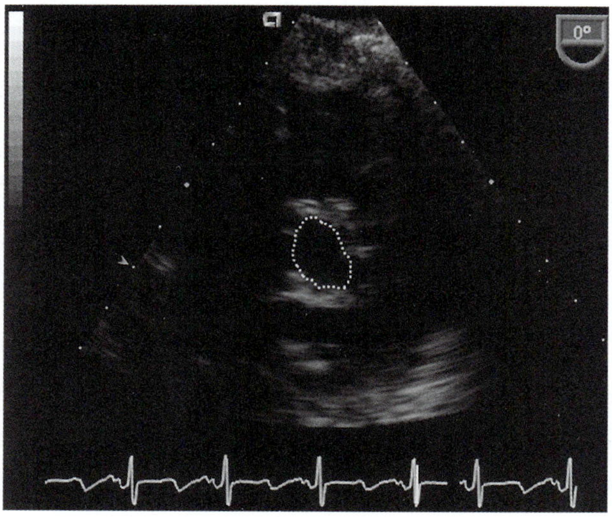

FIGURE 9.6 The mitral valve orifice assumes a "fish-mouth" appearance in a transgastric basal short-axis imaging plane in a patient with rheumatic mitral stenosis. Tracing of the orifice margins of the mitral valve during diastole resulted in a mitral valve area measurement of 1.25 cm^2.

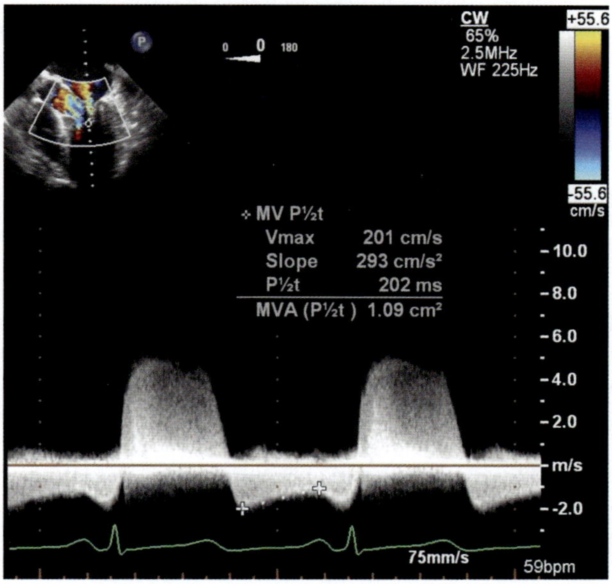

FIGURE 9.7 A diastolic spectral profile of mitral inflow obtained with continuous wave Doppler. Moderate mitral stenosis is confirmed by a pressure half-time measurement of 202 milliseconds.

less than 60 milliseconds. In mild MS, the average PHT is approximately 100 milliseconds; in moderate MS, it is approximately 200 milliseconds; and in severe MS, the average PHT measurement is more than 300 milliseconds (Table 9.3) (3,25,26).

Pressure Half-Time Calculation

The MVA can be calculated from the PHT measurement by using the following formula, originally described by Hatle and Angelsen (28):

$$\text{MVA (cm}^2) = 220/\text{pressure half-time (milliseconds)}$$

They noted that the rate of pressure decline across a stenotic MV depends on the cross-sectional area of the valvular orifice. Hence, the tighter the orifice (smaller cross-sectional area), the slower the rate of pressure decline.

The measurements obtained with the PHT method are influenced by hemodynamic factors and depend on the compliance of the LA and LV. These factors must be taken into consideration when the PHT method is applied to a stenotic MV. For example, decreased LV compliance and severe aortic regurgitation can cause a rapid rise in the LV diastolic pressure, with a resultant shortening of the PHT measurement and an overestimation of the MVA (29,30). Braverman et al (29) demonstrated the dependence of the PHT method

TABLE 9.3 Methods of Determining Mitral Valve Area

Planimetry	Trace Frozen Short-Axis View in Diastole
Pressure half-time (PHT, ms)	MVA = 220/PHT
Deceleration time (DT, ms)	MVA = 759/DT
Continuity equation	MVA = ($LVOT_{area}$ × LVOT TVI)/(MV TVI)
PISA	MVA = $2\pi r^2 \times \alpha/180 \times v_a/v_p$

α, funnel angle; LVOT, left ventricular outflow tract; MVA, mitral valve area (cm^2); PISA, proximal isovelocity surface area; TVI, time-velocity integral; v_a, aliasing velocity; v_p, peak transmitral velocity.

for calculating the MVA on hemodynamic variables, such as peak transmitral gradient and atrioventricular compliance. Conditions such as previous mitral valvuloplasty, atrial septal defect, atrial tachycardia, and restrictive cardiomyopathy also affect the accuracy of the PHT method (21,31-33).

Deceleration Time

The deceleration time is another simple means of evaluating the MVA, in which decay of the mitral inflow profile through a stenotic MV is examined. The following formula describes the relationship of the deceleration time to the MVA (20):

$$\text{MVA (cm}^2\text{)} = 759/\text{deceleration time (milliseconds)}$$

The deceleration time is the interval between the peak velocity and the time at which the extrapolated inflow velocity reaches the baseline. Figure 9.8 graphically displays the measurement of deceleration time. For profiles in which the decay is linear, the PHT is equal to 29% of the deceleration time (21,27).

Advanced Concepts That May Be Helpful in Difficult Cases

Continuity Equation

The continuity equation for calculating the area of a valve is based on the law of conservation of mass in hydrodynamics. In the absence of valvular regurgitation or shunts, flow volume at the MV should equal that at another valve according to the following equation (27,30):

$$\text{Volumetric flow} = \text{area}_1 \times \text{time} - \text{velocity integral}_1 = \text{area}_2 \times \text{time} - \text{velocity integral}_2$$

Therefore,

$$\text{Area}_2 = (\text{area}_1 \times \text{time} - \text{velocity integral}_1)/(\text{time} - \text{velocity integral}_2)$$

Flow through the MV can be calculated based on the measurements made by Doppler echocardiography as the product of the valve orifice area and the time − velocity integral of the mitral inflow. $\text{Area}_1 \times$ time − velocity integral_1 represents volumetric flow through the reference valve. The reference area (area_1) is a cross-sectional area measurement that assumes the geometric model of a circle, πr^2. The LV outflow tract or pulmonary artery is commonly used for the reference area and time − velocity integral

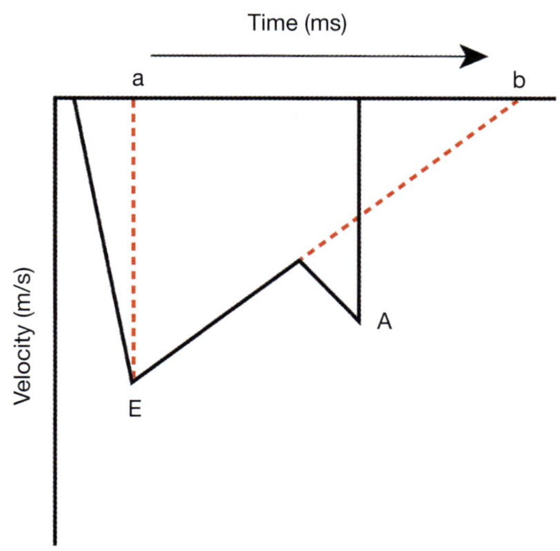

FIGURE 9.8 The deceleration time is the interval between the peak velocity (a) and the time at which the extrapolated inflow velocity reaches baseline (b). A, atrial wave; E, early wave.

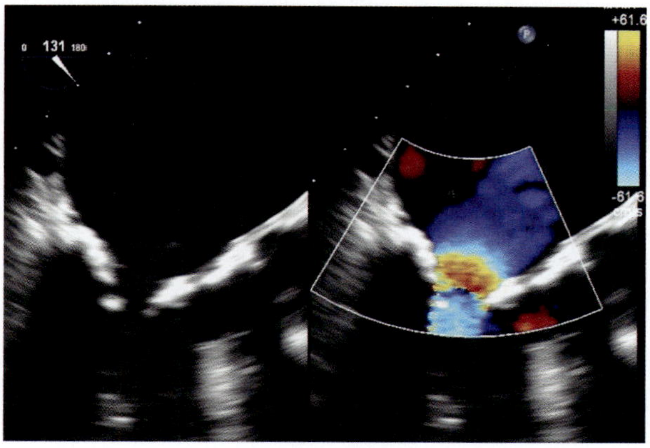

FIGURE 9.9 Color Doppler imaging from this midesophageal long-axis view of the mitral valve demonstrates proximal isovelocity surface area or flow convergence on the left atrial side of the mitral valve.

measurements. The equation is rearranged to solve for the MS area, $area_2$, as previously discussed. The continuity equation is theoretically independent of transvalvular pressure gradients, LV compliance, and changing hemodynamic conditions, such as the increased forward flow that occurs during exercise (3,29,30). The continuity equation does not apply in circumstances of regurgitation in the reference valve or the MV because the forward volumetric flows are not equal so that significant error is introduced (30,34).

Proximal Isovelocity Surface Area Method

The proximal isovelocity surface area (PISA) method, or the flow convergence method, applies the continuity principle to color flow Doppler mapping in the region of the MV orifice where flow converges from the LA. Figure 9.9 and Video 9.4 display a color flow Doppler example of proximal flow convergence in a patient with rheumatic MS.

When blood flow converges on an orifice that is small relative to the proximal chamber, it may be considered to form isovelocity "shells" with the shape of a hemisphere. The velocity of blood flow increases as blood approaches the small orifice, resulting in aliasing of the color flow signal and the creation of a large proximal flow convergence region or shell. As blood approaches the orifice, its increasing velocity is pictured by color flow imaging as progressively smaller shells. The radius of the first aliasing velocity shell is measured from the tips of the MV leaflets to the aliasing boundary (Figure 9.10) (20,35-38). The volumetric flow rate can be calculated as the product of the surface area of the hemisphere of flow and the aliasing velocity. The mitral inflow velocity profile (at the orifice) is obtained with continuous wave Doppler. The basic elements of the continuity equation can therefore be identified by this straightforward color mapping, but the calculation of a valve area requires a correction for the true shape of the mitral orifice. Truly hemispheric shells would occur if the surface of the valve were flat with the leaflets apposed at 180°. The angle α subtended by the mitral leaflets creates a funnel-shaped surface; an angle correction factor ($\alpha/180°$) adjusts the hemispheric surface area pictured by color flow mapping to calculate the volumetric flow rate more accurately. The instantaneous volumetric flow rate (Q) in this region can be calculated as the product of the surface area of a hemisphere ($2\pi r^2$) and the aliasing velocity at the shell (v_a).

$$Q = 2\pi r^2 \times \alpha/180° \times v_a$$

Flow through this region should equal flow through the restricted orifice based on the continuity principle (35-37). Once the flow rate (Q) is calculated, the MVA can be obtained with the use of the continuity equation.

$$\text{MVA (cm}^2) = Q/v_P \text{ (cm/s)}$$

where Q is the volumetric flow rate, and v_p is the peak transmitral inflow velocity.

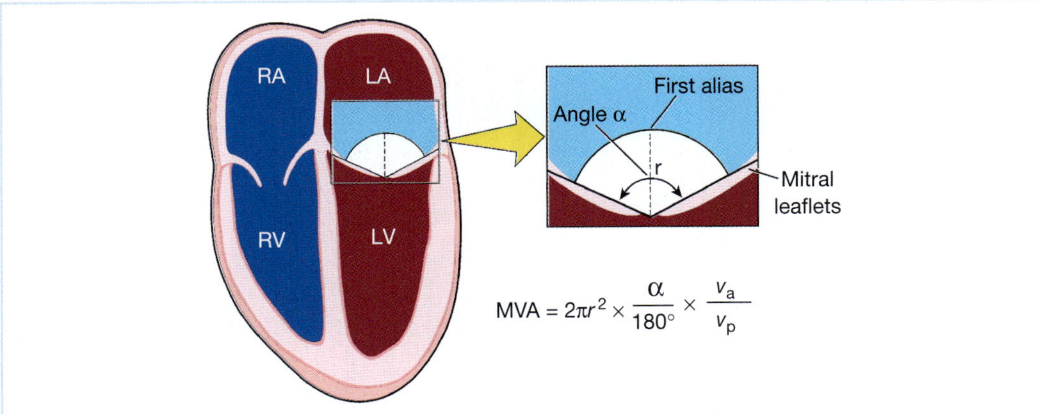

FIGURE 9.10 Midesophageal four-chamber view of the mitral valve demonstrates the measurements needed to calculate the mitral valve area by the proximal isovelocity surface area method. α/180°, angle correction factor; LA, left atrium; LV, left ventricle; MVA, mitral valve area; RA, right atrium; RV, right ventricle; v_a, aliasing velocity; v_p, peak transmitral inflow velocity. (From Rodriguez L, Thomas JD, Monterroso V, et al. Validation of the proximal flow convergence method: calculation of orifice area in patients with mitral stenosis. *Circulation.* 1993;88:1157-1165, with permission.)

Figure 9.10 illustrates the use of the flow convergence method in the calculation of MVA.

The MVA can be measured accurately with this method in the presence of mitral insufficiency. Several investigators have validated the use of the flow convergence method in the calculation of MVA by direct comparisons with anatomic and calculated measurements of orifice size (35,37,39,40). Calculation of MVA by the flow convergence method can be time-consuming; however, its accuracy is not influenced by associated mitral or aortic regurgitation. This method of calculating MVA may be the best under circumstances in which 2D planimetry is technically limited, when the continuity equation cannot be applied with the use of a reference volumetric flow, and when the PHT method is affected by hemodynamic changes (36).

A PRACTICAL APPROACH TO THE EVALUATION OF MITRAL STENOSIS

Step 1. A 2D evaluation of the MV is performed with a focus on answering the following questions: What is the appearance of the valve—that is, is the valve disfigured? Are the leaflets of normal thickness and mobility? If not, further assessment of the valve is needed to determine whether it is stenotic or regurgitant (see Chapter 8: Mitral Regurgitation). Planimetry of the MV in the TG basal short-axis view is initially performed to obtain a rough estimate of the MVA.

Step 2. After completion of the 2D examination, MV inflow interrogation with continuous wave Doppler is performed. The diastolic mitral inflow velocity profile is traced (Figure 9.5) and the mean pressure gradient is determined with the internal software of the echocardiography machine. In addition, the PHT method is used to calculate the MVA (Figure 9.7). Most TEE machines also extrapolate the flow decay and calculate the deceleration time. If the measurements are in agreement according to Table 9.2, no further evaluation is required.

Step 3. The advanced methods (continuity equation and PISA) are reserved for those patients for whom the PHT method is unreliable or unavailable.

Three-Dimensional Echocardiographic Evaluation of Mitral Stenosis

3D echocardiography has demonstrated accuracy for measuring MVA both for calcific (41) and rheumatic MS (42). 3D echocardiography measures all three spatial dimensions. Messika-Zeitoun et al (43) examined the use of real-time 3D echocardiography in the setting of percutaneous mitral commissurotomy. 3D echocardiography provided accurate and reproducible MVA measurements that were similar to 2D echocardiography. Of note, the authors found that 3D improved the "description" of valve anatomy and provided an advantage for less experienced operators as a method for MVA measurements; experienced operators

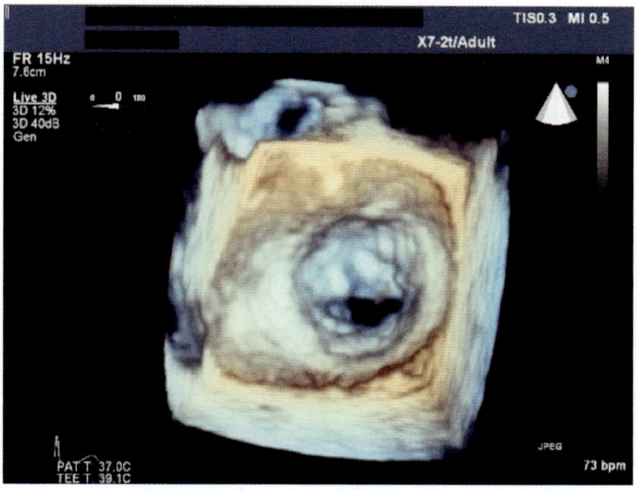

FIGURE 9.11 Three-dimensional image of a patient with rheumatic mitral stenosis.

reported similar results to 2D echocardiography findings. Shakil et al compared the use of 2D and 3D echocardiographies in the assessment of the MV subvalvular apparatus in patients with rheumatic MS. 3D echocardiography was found to be superior to 2D, particularly when assessing features such as chordal adhesion (44). In patients with rheumatic MS, Zamorano et al (42) reported that real-time 3D was not only accurate and reproducible for measurement of MVA but also the most accurate when compared to (gold standard) invasive methods. Others have described the accuracy and reproducibility of MVA measurements with the use of real-time 3D echocardiography (Figure 9.11; Videos 9.5 and 9.6) (45).

Interestingly, Anwar et al (46) validated a new echocardiographic scoring system with the use of real-time 3D echocardiography for patients with MS. The concept of the new scoring system is similar to that of the Wilkins score, yet makes use of real-time 3D echocardiography in the evaluation. The authors' new scoring system reportedly provides improved morphologic evaluation of specific aspects of the MV apparatus that relate to calcium and commissural splitting. Similar to the Wilkins score, the real-time 3D score involves an overall composite score based on the extent of valve calcification, thickening, mobility, and subvalvular involvement, with higher scores representing more advanced valve pathology. However, the 3D assessment also involves division of each leaflet into three scallops and scores them separately for thickness, calcification, and mobility; the subvalvular apparatus is graded at three levels for extent of chordal thickness and separation (Table 9.4) (46,47).

Others have utilized 3D in the assessment of MVA. Karamnov et al (48) recently compared the measurements obtained by conventional echocardiographically to assess the degree of rheumatic MS (ie, MVA determined by 2D planimetry, PHT, PISA, and continuity equation) with a novel 3D method that minimizes geometric assumptions present with 2D methods. Orifice areas with 3D were obtained offline with commercially available software. The authors found that the 3D method used to calculate MV orifice area reported a greater or more severe degree of MS compared to conventional measurement techniques (48). 3D planimetry has been reported as the most accurate method for MVA evaluation (42).

Multiplanar Reconstruction

In practice today, multiplanar reconstruction (MPR) is an effective tool that simultaneously slices 3D echocardiography and allows for simultaneous, live visualization of the MV in three different axis planes (commissural, long axis, and short axis). MPR allows for extreme localization of pathology, regurgitation severity, and orifice area. This technology can be extremely useful in transcatheter structural heart procedures. According to the 2023 American Society of Echocardiography recommendations for the use of echocardiography in the evaluation of rheumatic heart disease, 3DE multiplanar guidance should be used

TABLE 9.4 Mitral Valve Score Based on Real-Time Three-Dimensional Echocardiography

	Anterior Leaflet			Posterior Leaflet		
	■ A1	■ A2	■ A3	■ P1	■ P2	■ P3
Thickness (0-6) (0 = normal, 1 = thickened)[a]	0-1	0-1	0-1	0-1	0-1	0-1
Mobility (0-6) (0 = normal, 1 = limited)[a]	0-1	0-1	0-1	0-1	0-1	0-1
Calcification (0-10) (0 = no, 1-2 = calcified)[b]	0-2	0-1	0-2	0-2	0-1	0-2
	Subvalvular Apparatus[b]					
	■ Proximal Third		■ Middle Third		■ Distal Third	
Thickness (0-3) (0 = normal, 1 = thickened)	0-1		0-1		0-1	
Separation (0-6) (0 = normal, 1 = partial, 2 = no)	0, 1, 2		0, 1, 2		0, 1, 2	

[a]Normal = 0, mild = 1-2, moderate = 3-4, severe ≥5.
[b]Normal = 0, mild = 1-2, moderate = 3-5, severe ≥6.
Reused from Anwar A, Attia W, Nosir Y, et al. Validation of a new score for the assessment of mitral stenosis using real-time three-dimensional echocardiography. *J Am Soc Echocardiogr.* 2010;23:13-22, with permission.

when measuring MVA in eccentrically oriented or irregularly shaped MV orifice (Figure 9.12; Video 9.6) (21). Live MPR has several advantages over 2D biplane imaging including the ability to perform simultaneous measurements, reduced need to continuously maneuver the probe, and simultaneous visualization of clips during MV transcatheter edge-to-edge repair (MV-TEER) multiclip procedures when it is important to see the relationship between multiple clips. Using MPR requires a specific skillset and familiarity with this technology, and as with any 3D imaging, spatial and temporal resolution are reduced requiring regulation of sector size.

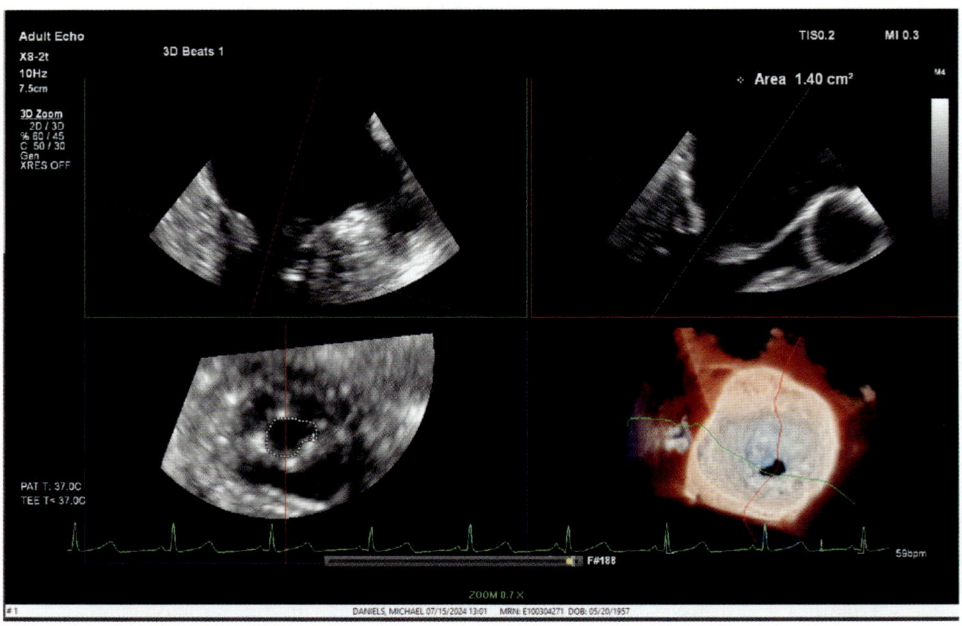

FIGURE 9.12 Multiplanar reconstruction (MPR) used to evaluate the mitral valve area (MVA = 1.4 cm²) in this mitral stenotic valve.

Use of Echocardiography for New Transcatheter Procedures

While not yet mainstream, the development of new transcatheter-based procedures to treat MS is on the horizon. A recent review article by Sarkar et al (49) described the use of transcatheter MV replacement for native and failed bioprosthetic MVs. Furthermore, the authors mentioned instances of off-label use of transcatheter MV replacement for degenerative MV stenosis as well as balloon-expandable transcatheter aortic valves for patients with severe mitral annular calcification who were deemed too high risk for surgery (49,50). Also, in the expanding world of percutaneous devices for valvular pathology, it is worthwhile to mention the potential development of MS following MV-TEER for regurgitant lesions. In a 2017 study of more than 200 patients, investigators found that procedure-related MS, quantified echocardiographically, with a pressure gradient of greater than 4.4 mm Hg predicted a significantly poorer long-term outcome (51). In a more recent study, De Felice et al looked at nearly 900 patients undergoing MV-TEER and found that those with mean gradients greater than 4 mm Hg were also at higher risk of death or heart failure hospitalization at 2 years out from the procedure (52). However, in the COAPT trial, patients with an elevated post MV-TEER gradient had similar rates of mortality, heart failure hospitalization, and measurements in functional status compared with those who did not (53). In this COAPT trial population, the clinical benefits of MR reduction were preserved despite having postprocedure gradients with a mean of 7.2 mm Hg, suggesting that the benefits of MR reduction outweigh the effects of mild to moderate MS after MV-TEER. Utsunomiya et al evaluated both 3D MVA and mean gradient after MV-TEER and found a discordance in 40% of cases. Post-TEER 3D MVA of less than 1.94 cm^2 was associated with an increased risk of all-cause mortality and hospitalization (54). This potential impact on long-term outcomes warrants careful echocardiographic MS evaluation prior to and immediately post MV-TEER placement. As these techniques become more established as a treatment option, intraprocedural echocardiography will be critical to provide important real-time information to enhance the safety and outcomes of the procedure.

SUMMARY

Echocardiography continues to be the preferred imaging modality for determining the presence, extent, and consequences of MS. Stenotic valves should be evaluated in a comprehensive approach. Table 9.3 (55) summarizes the techniques used to calculate the MVA. It is important to recognize that each technique has its limitations. Agreement between the various methods of evaluating the valve together with clinical correlation will enhance accuracy and overall judgment. Table 9.2 presents stages for the various degrees of severity of MS. In general, an MVA of greater than 1.5 cm^2 is considered to indicate mild MS and less than 1.5 cm^2 severe MS (17). It is important to recognize important elements of valve anatomy, hemodynamics, secondary hemodynamic consequences, and patient symptoms when making a severity assessment.

ACKNOWLEDGMENTS

We gratefully acknowledge the contributions of the previous edition author, Colleen G. Koch, as portions of those chapters have been retained in this revision.

REFERENCES

1. Acierno LJ. Physical examination. In: *The History of Cardiology*. Parthenon Publishing Group; 1994:461-462.
2. Acierno LJ. Surgical modalities. In: *The History of Cardiology*. Parthenon Publishing Group; 1994:627.
3. Popovic AD, Thomas JD, Neskovic AN, et al. Time-related trends in the preoperative evaluation of patients with valvular stenosis. *Am J Cardiol.* 1997;80(11):1464-1468.
4. Bruce CJ, Nishimura RA. Clinical assessment and management of mitral stenosis, valvular heart disease. *Cardiol Clin.* 1998;16(3):375-403.
5. Ranganathan N, Lam JH, Wigle ED, et al. Morphology of the human mitral valve. II. The valve leaflets. *Circulation.* 1970;41(3):459-467.
6. Roberts WC, Perloff JK. Mitral valvular disease. A clinicopathologic survey of the conditions causing the mitral valve to function abnormally. *Ann Intern Med.* 1972;77(6):939-975.
7. Kennedy JW, Yarnall SR, Murray JA, et al. Quantitative angiocardiography. IV. Relationships of left atrial and ventricular pressure and volume in mitral valve disease. *Circulation.* 1970;41(5):817-824.
8. Schlant RC, Alexander RW, O'Rourke RA, et al, eds. Mitral valve disease. In: *Hurst's the Heart.* 8th ed. McGraw-Hill; 1994:1483-1518.
9. Selzer A, Cohn KE. Natural history of mitral stenosis: a review. *Circulation.* 1972;45(4):878-890.
10. Olson LJ, Subramanian R, Ackermann DM, et al. Surgical pathology of the mitral valve: a study of 712 cases spanning 21 years. *Mayo Clin Proc.* 1987;62(1):22-34.

11. Wilkins GT, Weyman AE, Abascal VM, et al. Percutaneous balloon dilatation of the mitral valve: an analysis of echocardiographic variables related to outcome and the mechanism of dilatation. *Br Heart J.* 1988;60(4):299-308.
12. Otto C, ed. Valvular stenosis: diagnosis, quantitation, and clinical approach. In: *Textbook of Clinical Echocardiography.* 2nd ed. WB Saunders; 2000:229-264.
13. Nichol PM, Gilbert BW, Kisslo JA. Two-dimensional echocardiographic assessment of mitral stenosis. *Circulation.* 1977;55(1):120-128.
14. Daniel WG, Nellessen U, Schroder E, et al. Left atrial spontaneous echo contrast in mitral valve disease: an indicator for an increased thromboembolic risk. *J Am Coll Cardiol.* 1988;11(6):1204-1211.
15. Chen YT, Kan MN, Chen JS, et al. Contributing factors to the formation of left atrial spontaneous echo contrast in mitral valvular disease. *J Ultrasound Med.* 1990;9(3):151-155.
16. Liu CP, Ting CT, Yang TM, et al. Reduced left ventricular compliance in human mitral stenosis. Role of reversible internal constraint. *Circulation.* 1992;85(4):1447-1456.
17. Otto C, Nishimura R, Bonow R, et al. 2020 ACC/AHA guideline for the management of patients with valvular heart disease: executive summary: a report of the American College of Cardiology/American Heart Association Joint Committee on Clinical Practice Guidelines. *Circulation.* 2021;143(5):e72-e227.
18. Hatle L, Brubakk A, Tromsdal A, et al. Noninvasive assessment of pressure drop in mitral stenosis by Doppler ultrasound. *Br Heart J.* 1978;40(2):131-140.
19. Oh JK, Seward JB, Tajik AJ. Hemodynamic assessment. In: *The Echo Manual.* 2nd ed. Lippincott Williams & Wilkins; 1999:59-71.
20. Weyman AE, ed. Left ventricular inflow tract I: the mitral valve. In: *Principles and Practice of Echocardiography.* 2nd ed. Lea & Febiger; 1994:391-497.
21. Pandian NG, Kim JK, Arias-Godinez JA, et al. Recommendations for the use of echocardiography in the evaluation of rheumatic heart disease: a report from the American Society of Echocardiography. *J Am Soc Echocardiogr.* 2023;36(1):3-28.
22. Henry WL, Griffith JM, Michaelis LL, et al. Measurement of mitral orifice area in patients with mitral valve disease by real-time, two-dimensional echocardiography. *Circulation.* 1975;51(5):827-831.
23. Martin RP, Rakowski H, Kleiman JH, et al. Reliability and reproducibility of two-dimensional echocardiographic measurement of the stenotic mitral valve orifice area. *Am J Cardiol.* 1979;43(3):560-568.
24. Wann LS, Weyman AE, Feigenbaum H, et al. Determination of mitral valve area by cross-sectional echocardiography. *Ann Intern Med.* 1978;88(3):337-341.
25. Libanoff AJ, Rodbard S. Atrioventricular pressure half-time. Measure of mitral valve orifice area. *Circulation.* 1968;38(1):144-150.
26. Hatle L, Angelsen B, Tromsdal A. Noninvasive assessment of atrioventricular pressure half-time by Doppler ultrasound. *Circulation.* 1979;60(5):1096-1104.
27. Bruce C, Nishimura R. Newer advances in the diagnosis and treatment of mitral stenosis. *Curr Probl Cardiol.* 1998;23(3):125-192.
28. Hatle L, Angelsen B, eds. Pulsed and continuous wave Doppler in the diagnosis and assessment of various heart lesions. In: *Doppler Ultrasound in Cardiology: Physical Principles and Clinical Applications.* Lea & Febiger; 1982:76-89.
29. Braverman AC, Thomas JD, Lee RT. Doppler echocardiographic estimation of mitral valve area during changing hemodynamic conditions. *Am J Cardiol.* 1991;68(15):1485-1490.
30. Nakatani S, Masuyama T, Kodama K, et al. Value and limitations of Doppler echocardiography in the quantification of stenotic mitral valve area: comparison of the pressure half-time and the continuity equation methods. *Circulation.* 1988;77(1):78-85.
31. Thomas JD, Wilkins GT, Choong CY, et al. Inaccuracy of mitral pressure half-time immediately after percutaneous mitral valvotomy. Dependence on transmitral gradient and left atrial and ventricular compliance. *Circulation.* 1988;78(4):980-993.
32. Thomas JD, Weyman AE. Doppler mitral pressure half-time: a clinical tool in search of theoretical justification. *J Am Coll Cardiol.* 1987;10(4):923-929.
33. Wranne B, Msee PA, Loyd D. Analysis of different methods of assessing the stenotic mitral valve area with emphasis on the pressure gradient half-time concept. *Am J Cardiol.* 1990;66(5):614-620.
34. Karp K, Teien D, Eriksson P. Doppler echocardiographic assessment on the valve area in patients with atrioventricular valve stenosis by application of the continuity equation. *J Intern Med.* 1989;225(4):261-266.
35. Rodriguez L, Thomas JD, Monterroso V, et al. Validation of the proximal flow convergence method. Calculation of orifice area in patients with mitral stenosis. *Circulation.* 1993;88(3):1157-1165.
36. Deng YB, Matsumoto M, Wang XF, et al. Estimation of mitral valve area in patients with mitral stenosis by the flow convergence region method: selection of aliasing velocity. *J Am Coll Cardiol.* 1994;24(3):683-689.
37. Rifkin R, Harper K, Tighe D. Comparison of proximal isovelocity surface area method with pressure half-time and planimetry in the evaluation of mitral stenosis. *J Am Coll Cardiol.* 1995;26(2):458-465.
38. Vandervoort PM, Rivera JM, Mele D, et al. Application of color Doppler flow mapping to calculate effective regurgitant orifice area. An in vitro study and initial clinical observations. *Circulation.* 1993;88(3):1150-1156.
39. Degertekin M, Basaran Y, Gencbay M, et al. Validation of flow convergence region method in assessing mitral valve area in the course of transthoracic and transesophageal echocardiographic studies. *Am Heart J.* 1998;135(2 pt 1):207-214.
40. Faletra F, Pezzano A Jr, Fusco R, et al. Measurement of mitral valve area in mitral stenosis: four echocardiographic methods compared with direct measurement of anatomic orifices. *J Am Coll Cardiol.* 1996;28(5):1190-1197.
41. Chu JW, Levine RA, Chua S, et al. Assessing mitral valve area and orifice geometry in calcific mitral stenosis: a new solution by real-time three-dimensional echocardiography. *J Am Soc Echocardiogr.* 2008;21(9):1006-1009.
42. Zamorano J, Cordeiro P, Sugeng L, et al. Real-time three-dimensional echocardiography for rheumatic mitral valve stenosis evaluation: an accurate and novel approach. *J Am Coll Cardiol.* 2004;43(11):2091-2096.

43. Messika-Zeitoun D, Brochet E, Holmin C, et al. Three-dimensional evaluation of the mitral valve area and commissural opening before and after percutaneous mitral commissurotomy in patients with mitral stenosis. *Eur Heart J.* 2007;28(1):72-79.
44. Shakil SS, Ahmed CM, Khaled FI, et al. Assessment of subvalvular apparatus in patients with rheumatic mitral stenosis: comparison between 2D and 3D echocardiography. *Mymensingh Med J.* 2017;26(4):716-720.
45. Binder TM, Rosenhek R, Porenta G, et al. Improved assessment of mitral valve stenosis by volumetric real-time three-dimensional echocardiography. *J Am Coll Cardiol.* 2000;36(4):1355-1361.
46. Anwar AM, Attia WM, Nosir YF, et al. Validation of a new score for the assessment of mitral stenosis using real-time three-dimensional echocardiography. *J Am Soc Echocardiogr.* 2010;23(1):13-22.
47. Soliman OI, Anwar AM, Metawei AK, et al. New scores for the assessment of mitral stenosis using real-time three-dimensional echocardiography. *Curr Cardiovasc Imaging Rep.* 2011;4(5):370-377.
48. Karamnov S, Burbano-Vera N, Huang C, et al. Echocardiographic assessment of mitral stenosis orifice area: a comparison of a novel three-dimensional method versus conventional techniques. *Anesth Analg.* 2017;125(3):774-780.
49. Sarkar K, Reardon MJ, Little SH, et al. Transcatheter mitral valve replacement for native and failed bioprosthetic mitral valves. *Methodist Debakey Cardiovasc J.* 2017;13(3):142-151.
50. Guerrero M, Divr D, Himbert D, et al. Transcatheter mitral valve replacement in native mitral valve disease with severe mitral annual calcification: results from the first multicenter global registry. *JACC Cardiovasc Interv.* 2016;9(13):1361-1371.
51. Neuss M, Schau T, Isotani A et al. Elevated mitral valve pressure gradient after MitraClip implantation deteriorates long-term in patients with severe mitral regurgitation and severe heart failure. *JACC Cardiovascular Interv.* 2017;10(9):931-939.
52. De Felice F, Paolucci L, Musto C, et al. Outcomes in patients with high transmitral gradients after mitral valve transcatheter edge-to-edge repair for mitral regurgitation. *Am J Cardiol.* 2022;182:46-54.
53. Halaby R, Hermann H, Gertz Z, et al. Effect of mitral valve gradient after mitraclip on outcomes in secondary mitral regurgitation: results from the COAPT trial. *JACC Cardiovasc Interv.* 2021;14(8):879-889.
54. Utsunomiya H, Itabashi Y, Kobayashi S, et al. Effect of percutaneous edge-to-edge repair on mitral valve area and its association with pulmonary hypertension and outcomes. *Am J Cardiol.* 2017;120(4):662-669.
55. Falk V, Baumgartner H, Bax JJ, et al. 2017 ESC/EACTS guidelines for the management of valvular heart disease. *Eur J Cardiothorac Surg.* 2017;52(4):616-664.

QUESTIONS

1. Which among the following statements is correct concerning MV anatomy?

A. The anterior leaflet is attached to the fibrous skeleton of the heart with an attachment of approximately 1/3 of the circumference of the mitral annulus.
B. The anterior leaflet is attached to the fibrous skeleton of the heart with an attachment of approximately 1/2 of the circumference of the mitral annulus.
C. The posterior leaflet is attached to the fibrous skeleton of the heart with an attachment of approximately 1/3 of the circumference of the mitral annulus.
D. The posterior leaflet is attached to the fibrous skeleton of the heart with an attachment of approximately 1/2 of the circumference of the mitral annulus.

2. Normal MV area is:

A. 3 cm^2 or more
B. 2.5 to 3.5 cm^2
C. 4 to 6 cm^2
D. 6 to 8 cm^2

3. A valve area less than ______ is associated with a significant transvalvular pressure gradient and the clinical presentation of MS.

A. 0.9 cm^2 or less
B. 1.4 cm^2 or less
C. 2.5 cm^2 or less
D. 3.2 cm^2 or less

4. Throughout the world, the most common cause of MS is:

A. Cor triatriatum
B. BLA myxoma
C. Mitral annular calcification
D. Rheumatic heart disease

5. Which among the following statements is correct?
A. 3D echocardiography is more sensitive than TTE and TEE in detecting LA spontaneous echo contrast.
B. TTE is more sensitive than TEE in detecting LA spontaneous echo contrast.
C. TEE is more sensitive than TTE in detecting LA spontaneous echo contrast.
D. TTE and TEE are equally sensitive in detecting LA spontaneous echo contrast.

6. According to the 2020 ACC/AHA guidelines, the assessment of MS severity includes all of the following *except*:
A. LA size
B. MV anatomy
C. Patient symptoms
D. All of the above are included.

7. The severity of MS estimated by transvalvular gradient on this patient (QFigure 9.1) would:

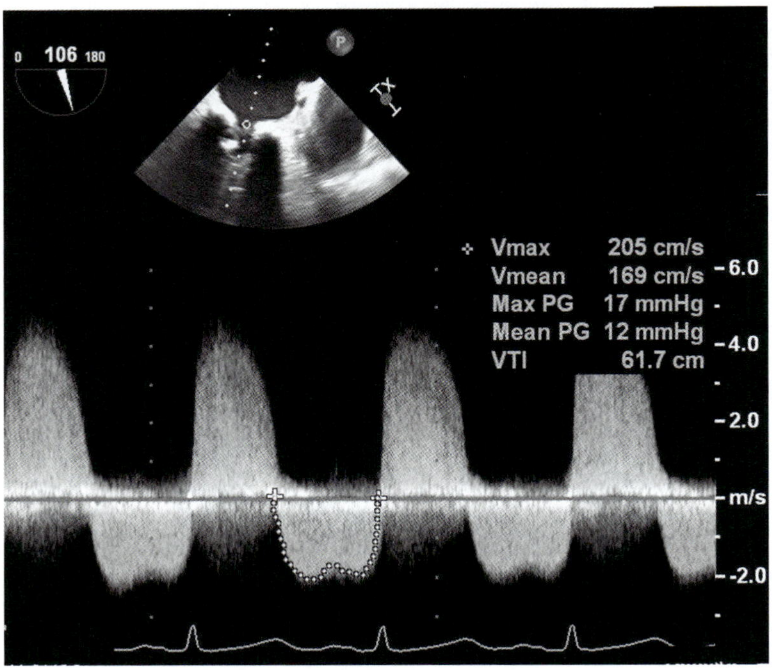

A. Accurately estimate the severity
B. Overestimate the severity
C. Underestimate the severity
D. Requires strain correction

8. Which among the following statements is correct concerning assessing MS using the continuity equation?
A. It is accurate in the setting of an ASD.
B. It is accurate in the setting of decreased cardiac output.
C. It is accurate in the setting of valvular regurgitation.
D. All of the above

9. The severity of MS estimated by PHT on this patient (QFigure 9.2) would:

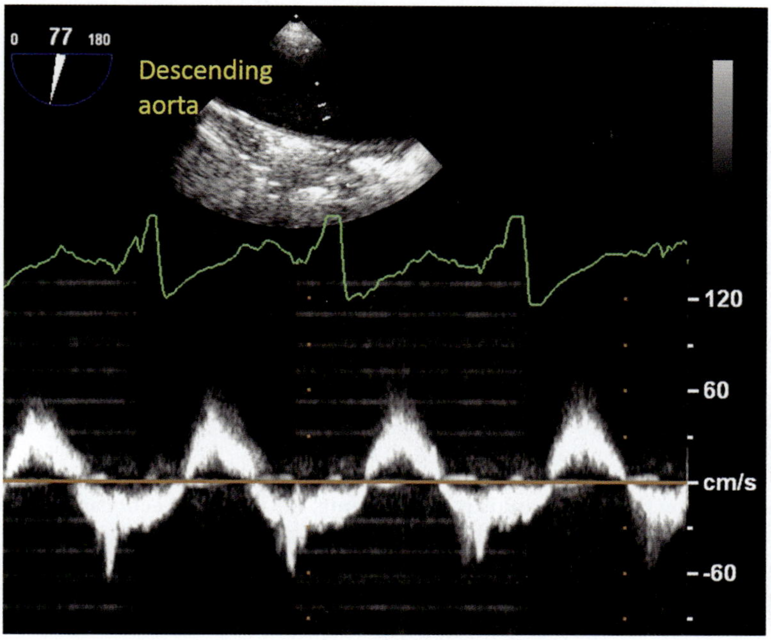

A. Accurately estimate the severity
B. Overestimate the severity
C. Underestimate the severity
D. Requires Doppler correction

10. Calculate the MV area if the PHT is 180 milliseconds.
A. 0.82 cm^2
B. 1.22 cm^2
C. 1.72 cm^2
D. 2.65 cm^2

11. Pathologic features of rheumatic MS include which among the following?
A. Doming of the anterior mitral leaflet in diastole
B. Fusion of commissures
C. Thickening of subvalvular apparatus
D. All of the above

12. Normal flow velocity across the MV is less than ____.
A. 1 m/s
B. 1.3 m/s
C. 1.5 m/s
D. 2 m/s

13. Which MV area measurement is most consistent with moderate MS?
A. Less than 1 cm^2
B. 1.2 cm^2
C. 1.5 to 1.8 cm^2
D. 2 cm^2

14. The slowly progressive symptoms of MS can result in:
A. Distention of the LA
B. Enlarged pulmonary artery
C. Paroxysmal nocturnal dyspnea
D. All of the above

15. You have calculated a MV area of 1.1 cm^2 using a deceleration time from a Doppler spectral profile. Which deceleration time would correlate with your findings?
A. 425 milliseconds
B. 680 milliseconds
C. 790 milliseconds
D. 860 milliseconds

16. Following MV-TEER, procedure-related MS has been found to be associated with worse long-term outcomes at what MV pressure gradient?
A. 3 mm Hg
B. 3.4 mm Hg
C. 4 mm Hg
D. 4.4 mm Hg

17. Compared to standard 2D echocardiographic measurements, the use of 3D echocardiography to evaluate MS is:
A. Advantageous for more experienced operators as a method of area assessments
B. Associated with less descriptive evaluation of anatomy
C. Associated with more severe degree of MS reported
D. Inferior when assessing for chordal adhesions

18. According to the ACC/AHA 2020 guidelines for the assessment of MS, stage B MS is associated with:
A. Mild-moderate LA enlargement
B. MV area of more than 1.5 cm^2
C. Normal pulmonary artery pressures at rest
D. All of the above

19. PISA is most useful in the following circumstances:
A. When there are technical limitations to the use of planimetry
B. When there is significant mitral or aortic regurgitation
C. When the continuity equation cannot be applied with the use of a reference volumetric flow
D. All of the above

20. When using the PISA method to calculate the MV area, which of the following is required?
A. $\alpha/90$
B. Aliasing velocity at the shell (v_a)
C. Diameter of the shell (d^2)
D. Mean transmitral inflow velocity (v_p)

ANSWERS

1. Correct Answer: A.
Rationale: The anterior mitral leaflet has an attachment to approximately one-third of the circumference of the mitral annulus and is attached to the fibrous skeleton of the heart. The attachment of the posterior mitral leaflet to the mitral annulus is longer than the anterior.

2. Correct Answer: C.
Rationale: The normal MV orifice area is approximately 4 to 6 cm^2.

3. Correct Answer: B.
Rationale: Once the valve area becomes less than 1.4 cm^2, a significant transvalvular pressure gradient develops, accompanied by the clinical presentation of MS.

4. **Correct Answer: D.**
Rationale: Throughout the world, the most common cause of MS remains rheumatic heart disease.

5. **Correct Answer: C.**
Rationale: TEE is more sensitive than TTE in detecting LA spontaneous echo contrast. Studies have shown that spontaneous echo contrast in those with MS is at increased risk of thromboembolic events.

6. **Correct Answer: D.**
Rationale: Because of the variability of the mean pressure gradient with heart rate, diastolic filling period, and transvalvular forward flow, the transmitral mean pressure gradient was not included in the criteria for severity in the 2020 ACC/AHA Guidelines. The guideline assessment for severity includes features of MV anatomy, valve hemodynamics, patient symptoms, and disease consequences, such as LA enlargement and elevated pulmonary artery pressures.

7. **Correct Answer: B.**
Rationale: The degree of MS can be overestimated in the face of significant mitral regurgitation, which is shown above the baseline in the Doppler image in Figure 9.1.

8. **Correct Answer: B.**
Rationale: The continuity equation is theoretically independent of transvalvular pressure gradients, LV compliance, and dynamic hemodynamic conditions. It is not accurate in the setting of regurgitation or shunts.

9. **Correct Answer: C.**
Rationale: Severe aortic regurgitation, shown in the image with holo-diastolic aortic flow reversal, causes a rapid rise in the LV diastolic pressure, with a resultant shortening of the PHT measurement and an overestimation of the MVA and therefore underestimation of MS severity.

10. **Correct Answer: B.**
Rationale: MVA (cm^2) = 220/pressure half-time (milliseconds)
MVA = 220/160
MVA = 1.22 cm^2

11. **Correct Answer: D.**
Rationale: Pathologic features of rheumatic MS include fusion of the commissures; contracture, scarring, and diffuse thickening of the leaflet tissue and subvalvular apparatus; and calcium deposition within the mitral leaflets.

12. **Correct Answer: B.**
Rationale: Normal flow velocity across the MV is less than 1.3 m/s.

13. **Correct Answer: B.**
Rationale: Severe MS by MVA is considered when MVA is less than 1 cm^2, and mild MS when greater than 1.5 cm^2.

14. **Correct Answer: D.**
Rationale: Progression of MS causes distention of the left atrium, enlarged pulmonary artery, and paroxysmal nocturnal dyspnea.

15. **Correct Answer: B.**
Rationale: MVA = 759/DT
MVA = 759/680
MVA = 1.1 cm^2

16. **Correct Answer: D.**
Rationale: In a 2017 study of more than 200 patients, investigators found that procedure-related MS, quantified echocardiographically, with a pressure gradient of greater than 4.4 mm Hg predicted a significantly poorer long-term outcome (51).

17. **Correct Answer: C.**
Rationale: It has been found that the 3D method used to calculate MV orifice area reported a greater or more severe degree of MS compared to conventional measurement techniques (48).

18. **Correct Answer: D.**
Rationale: See Table 9.2 for characteristics of stage B MS.

19. **Correct Answer: D.**
Rationale: PISA may be the best method of calculating MVA when 2D planimetry is limited, when the continuity equation cannot be applied with the use of a reference volumetric flow, when there is significant mitral or aortic regurgitation, and when the PHT method is affected by hemodynamic changes.

20. **Correct Answer: B.**
Rationale: $MVA = 2\pi r^2 \times \alpha/180 \times v_a/v_p$

10 Mitral Valve Repair

Maurice Hogan, Chirojit Mukherjee, and Jörg Ender

INDICATIONS

Mitral valve (MV) repair is the cardiac surgical procedure that relies most on echocardiography for optimal clinical management and outcomes.

MV regurgitation results from either primary (structural) or secondary (functional) heart disorders (1). Understanding the distinction between these two classes of regurgitation is one of the key factors in good clinical decision-making for MV repair. Primary MV regurgitation is most commonly caused by degenerative MV disease and implies pathology of the architecture of the mitral apparatus, that is, the valve leaflets, the chordae tendineae, the papillary muscles, the annulus, left atrial wall, and left ventricular (LV) wall. Secondary MV regurgitation implies that the MV itself is structurally normal, and this secondary regurgitation is a consequence of disease affecting the ventricle or atria (1), such as ischemic heart disease or dilated cardiomyopathy.

In these cases of secondary mitral disease, regurgitation results from displacement of the papillary muscles consequent to LV dilatation, often in combination with mitral annular dilatation. The displacement of the papillary muscles causes tethering of the valve leaflets and restricts their motion, thereby preventing coaptation (2).

Surgical repair is the optimal approach whenever feasible for patients with primary mitral regurgitation. In the developed world, most cases of primary regurgitation arise from degenerative disease (ie, either fibroelastic disease or myxomatous disease) and are very amenable to repair. Rheumatic disease however is an example of a condition that can cause primary regurgitation, and where repair is much less feasible (3). MV repair for primary disease improves long-term survival if patients are operated on early and in centers that have both low operative mortality (<1%) and high rates of repair (>90%), as opposed to valve replacement (1,4). Patients who undergo MV repair rather than valve replacement clearly demonstrate lower operative mortality, better recovery of left ventricular ejection fraction (LVEF), and better long-term survival (5). This improvement in outcome for patients treated with repair versus replacement is intuitive considering that they have lower rates of endocarditis, fewer thromboembolic events, and do not require long-term anticoagulation (unless otherwise indicated). Because their mitral apparatus is preserved, repair patients also have better LV function postoperatively (6).

The benefits of repair versus valve replacement for patients with secondary mitral regurgitation are less apparent and have not been demonstrated in clinical studies (7). In primary disease, MV repair corrects the pathology and serves as a definitive treatment for many patients. In secondary disease, an isolated valve repair does not typically modify the underlying pathology; hence, it is necessary to consider this in deciding on the treatment approach.

Chronic severe mitral regurgitation ultimately leads to LV dilatation. To maintain forward stroke volume in the face of significant regurgitant fraction, the LV chamber necessarily becomes more compliant and develops eccentric cardiac hypertrophy. Tendency for pulmonary congestion then decreases also, as the now dilated left atrium and ventricle can accommodate the regurgitant volume at a lower filling pressure. These early responses are therefore adaptive, and during this phase, the patient may remain asymptomatic. Over time, however, the progressive LV enlargement and increasing LV end-diastolic pressures lead to a reduction in LVEF. For patients with severe mitral regurgitation, a normal ejection fraction is considered as approximately 70%, and an ejection fraction less than 60% is interpreted as a deterioration in systolic function, thereby becoming a trigger for corrective surgery (Figure 10.1). With progressive left atrial dilatation, atrial fibrillation and/or pulmonary hypertension can develop, and their occurrence in patients with chronic severe mitral regurgitation constitutes an indication for surgery, even in patients with preserved LVEF and an LV end-systolic diameter less than 40 mm (1).

The recommendations for the timing of surgery in patients with chronic severe mitral regurgitation rely on patient symptoms and on echocardiographic evaluation of LV function and size (Figure 10.1) (1,3). It is noteworthy that patients with chronic severe mitral regurgitation, who are symptom free, have normal LV

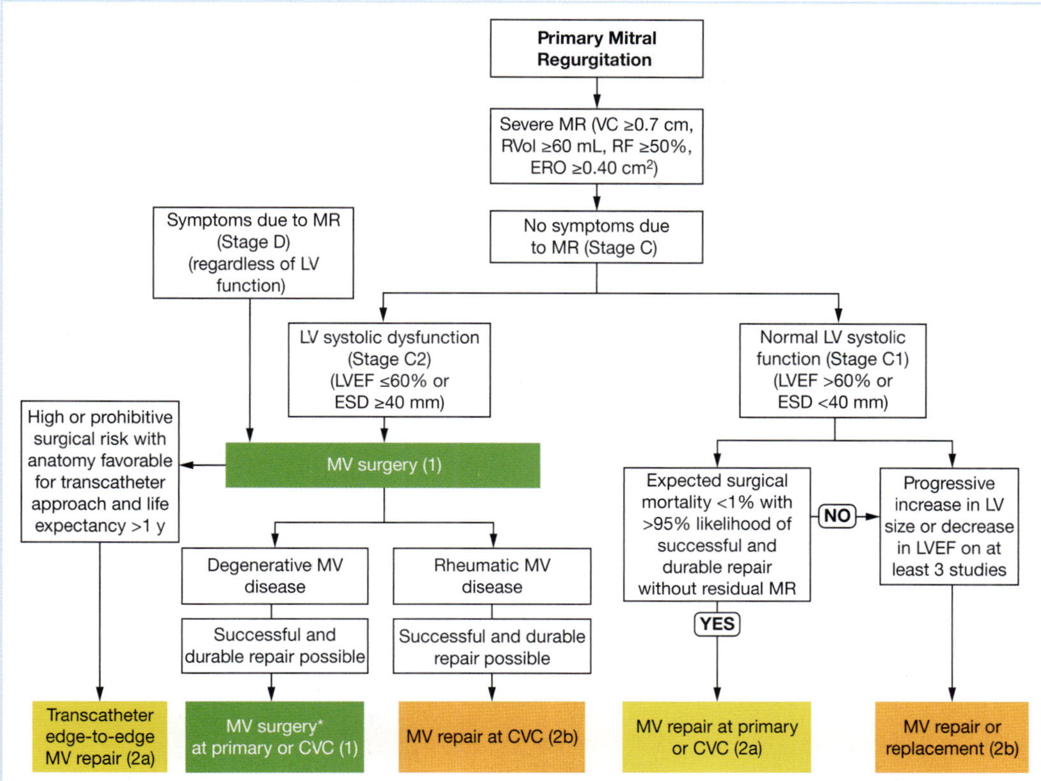

FIGURE 10.1 Guidelines for the management of patients with primary mitral regurgitation. CVC, comprehensive valve center; ERO, effective regurgitant orifice; ESD, end-systolic dimension; LV, left ventricle; LVEF, left ventricular ejection fraction; MR, mitral regurgitation; MV, mitral valve; RF, regurgitant fraction; RVol, regurgitant volume; VC, vena contracta. (Reprinted with permission from Otto CM, Nishimura RA, Bonow RO, et al. 2020 ACC/AHA guideline for the management of patients with valvular heart disease: a report of the American College of Cardiology/American Heart Association Joint Committee on clinical practice guidelines. *Circulation*. 2021;143:e72-e227. Figure 8. ©2020 American Heart Association, Inc.)

dimensions and function, and who don't have atrial fibrillation or pulmonary hypertension are only recommended to undergo valve surgery if it is likely that the valve can be repaired rather than replaced. The expectations of mitral repair surgery are high: for pathology most amenable to repair, that is, isolated posterior leaflet disease for repair and annuloplasty, there should be an almost certain repair likelihood, greater than 80% freedom from recurrent moderate or severe regurgitation at 15 to 20 years post operation, less than 1% mortality associated with the operation, and a long-term survival rate equivalent to the age-matched general population (1). In these cases, repair for most patients will be their definitive procedure and can restore them to a normal life expectancy. This explains why it is reasonable to offer early repair surgery to patients who have severe regurgitation before they develop systolic dysfunction, a dilated left ventricle, atrial fibrillation, or pulmonary hypertension. Note, however, an MV replacement is still preferable to a poor repair (1), and in cases of valve replacement, preservation of the subvalvular apparatus is favored (3).

The Society of Thoracic Surgery (STS) has released a short-term risk calculator (operative/30-day risk) specific to isolated MV repair surgery for primary mitral regurgitation and degenerative mitral etiology. This risk calculator is based on the contemporary national surgical experience from the STS Adult Cardiac Surgery Database and is designed to estimate a patient's risk for multiple outcomes: operative mortality, major morbidity, and conversion to MV replacement after attempted repair (8). Although this calculator has not yet been prospectively validated, it does at least reinforce the significance of these outcomes for patients undergoing mitral repair surgery, including the potential implications of conversion to MV replacement following attempted repair.

Guidelines on management of mitral regurgitation now incorporate a role for transcatheter edge-to-edge repair (TEER) for both primary and secondary regurgitation (Figures 10.1 and 10.2) (1). TEER is an innovative,

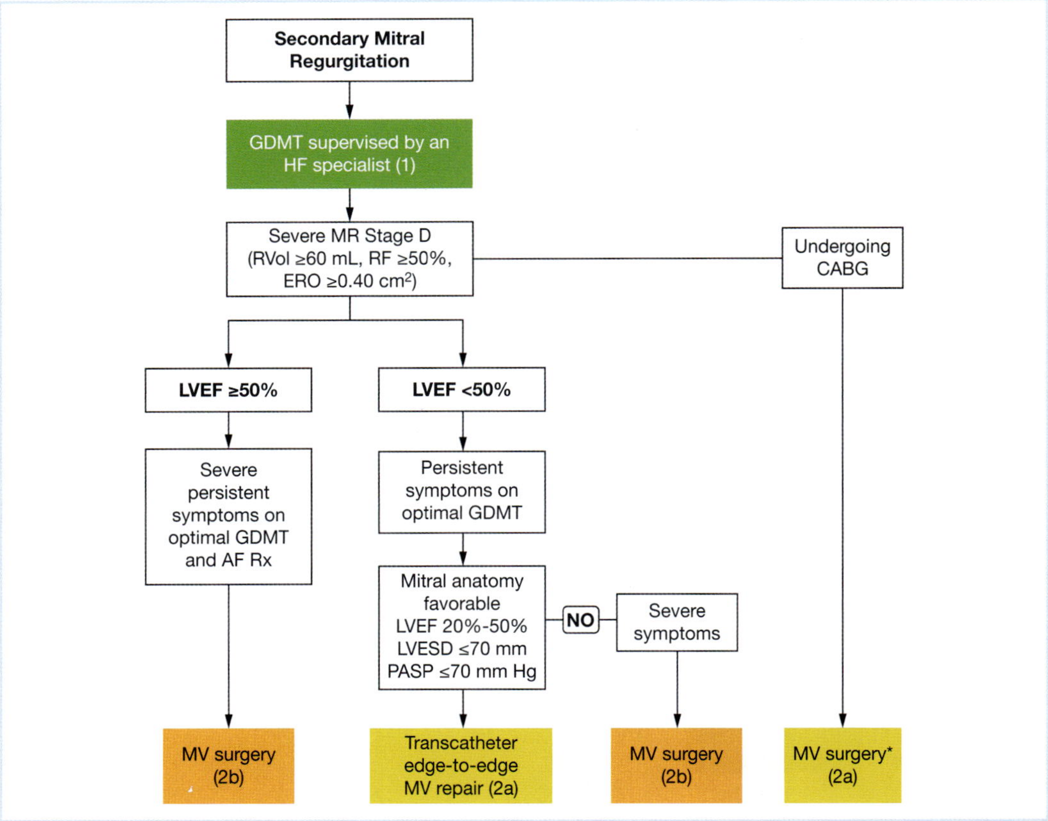

FIGURE 10.2 Guidelines for the management of patients with secondary mitral regurgitation. CABG, coronary artery bypass grafting; ERO, effective regurgitant orifice; GDMT, guideline directed medical therapy; HF, heart failure; LVEF, left ventricular ejection fraction; LVESD, left ventricular end-systolic dimension; MR, mitral regurgitation; MV, mitral valve; PASP, pulmonary artery systolic pressure; RF, regurgitant fraction; RVol, regurgitant volume; AF, atrial fibrillation; Rx, treatment. (Reprinted with permission from Otto CM, Nishimura RA, Bonow RO, et al. 2020 ACC/AHA guideline for the management of patients with valvular heart disease: a report of the American College of Cardiology/American Heart Association Joint Committee on clinical practice guidelines. *Circulation*. 2021;143:e72-e227. Figure 9. ©2020 American Heart Association, Inc.)

percutaneous, echo-guided technique of MV repair based on the open surgical edge-to-edge repair described initially by Alfieri and already established as an effective means of open MV repair (9). TEER is mainly indicated in patients considered at high or prohibitive risk for conventional open valve surgery. Patients must however have a favorable anatomy for the transcatheter approach, determined by echocardiography assessment, and have a life expectancy of greater than 1 year following the procedure (1). The percutaneous approach is a lower-risk intervention than conventional surgery, is shown to improve patients' clinical condition (10), and consequently the intervention may be offered appropriately to patients who previously would have been limited to only goal-directed medical management of their heart failure symptoms. For further discussion, see Chapter 16: Transesophageal Echocardiography for Transcatheter Interventions.

ECHOCARDIOGRAPHIC EVALUATION

The role of intraoperative echocardiography can be considered as two components: pre- and postrepair.

The Prerepair Evaluation

The prerepair examination should evaluate the:

1. structure of the MV apparatus.
2. function of the MV leaflets according to the Carpentier classification.

3. severity of the MV regurgitation.
4. the location of the circumflex artery and its relationship to the MV annulus.
5. cardiac structures for secondary or coexisting abnormalities.
6. surgical procedural considerations and guidance for minimal access surgical techniques.

This information is then summarized, and the likelihood of successful repair is discussed with the surgical team so as to be of use in planning the surgical procedure. The additional value of real-time three-dimensional (RT 3D) TEE for evaluation of the MV pathology is still a matter of debate (11,12). There is a high level of consistency between RT 3D TEE assessment of MV pathology and the findings of macroscopic surgical inspection (13). The most important potential advantage of RT 3D TEE is that it is capable of providing several unique views and images that are intuitively more understandable. RT 3D TEE is probably the method of choice when available, as it can complement the standard 2D examination (14).

1. Evaluation of the Structure of the Mitral Valve Apparatus

The MV apparatus consists of the left atrial wall, MV annulus, the MV leaflets (anterior and posterior), chordae tendineae, papillary muscles, and LV wall. The nomenclature proposed by Carpentier to describe the segments of the mitral leaflets (15) is the most commonly used and is widely accepted standard (Figures 10.3 and 10.10). The anatomy of the mitral apparatus is detailed in Chapter 8: Mitral Regurgitation. To visualize all the structures of the MV apparatus and to elucidate fully the mechanism of mitral regurgitation, and any associated pathology, several views are necessary (16).

Midesophageal (ME) four-chamber view: Normally shows the A2 and P2 segments of the MV (Figure 10.4). From there, slight withdrawal of the probe will show the A1 and P1 segments, whereas slight advancement of the probe will show the A3 and P3 segments (Figure 10.5). LV systolic function can also be assessed in this view by measuring LVEF. Interpretation of LVEF must take into account the patient's loading conditions. Patients with severe mitral regurgitation who have normal LV function demonstrate LVEF greater than or equal to 70% (1). Patients with reduced LVEF preoperatively also have reduced postoperative LVEF, higher perioperative mortality, and poorer long-term survival (17,18).

ME mitral commissural view: From the ME four-chamber view, the MV should also be scanned by forward rotation to show the P3, A2, and P1 segments (Figure 10.6). Continued forward rotation produces the ME two-chamber view with P3, A3, A2, and A1 segments (Figure 10.7) and midesophageal long-axis (ME LAX) views with the P2 and A2 segments (Figure 10.8).

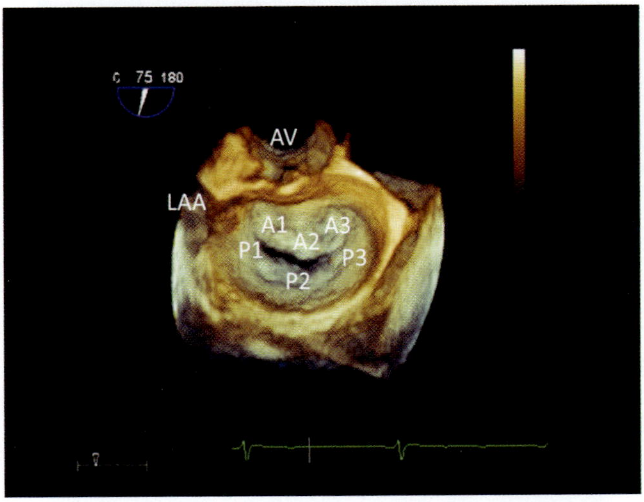

FIGURE 10.3 3D en face view looking on the mitral valve from the atrial side. Shows the aortic valve (AV) at the 12 o'clock position, and the anterior leaflet is related to this. The left atrial appendage (LAA) is also identified here and serves as another useful reference point for leaflet orientation. Using the Carpentier classification for leaflet nomenclature, the anterior leaflet is divided into A1, A2, and A3 segments, and the posterior leaflet into P1, P2, and P3 segments.

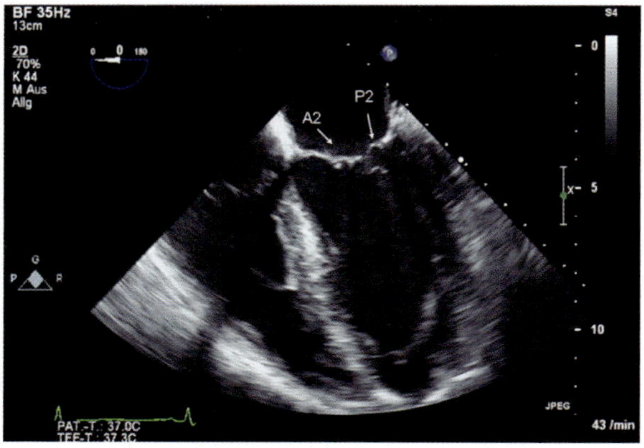

FIGURE 10.4 ME four-chamber view, with in this case P2 and A2 segments labeled. Although the typical ME four chamber most often cuts through these segments, it is possible to view A1, P1 by slight probe withdrawal, or A3, P3 by slight probe advancement (see Figure 10.5). ME, midesophageal.

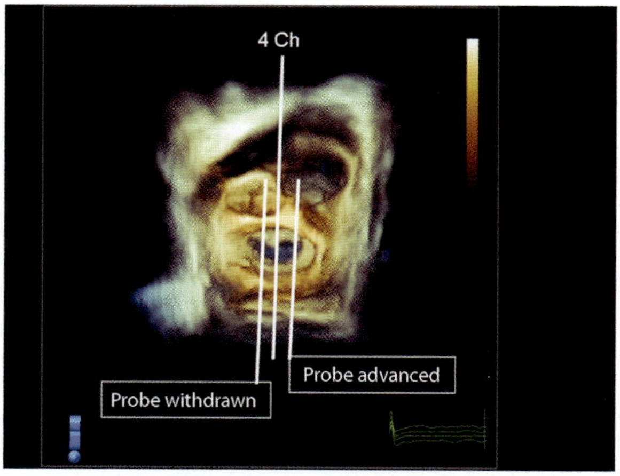

FIGURE 10.5 3D full-volume en face view of the mitral valve from the left atrium, with the aortic valve located at approximately 12 o'clock. The middle line (4Ch) shows how the typical ME four-chamber view cuts through A2, P2 segments. Probe withdrawal means the 2D probe now would cut through A1, P1, and in the corresponding 2D view, more of the aortic valve/LVOT enters the image. Probe advancement moves the 2D scan plane over A3, P3 segments. ME, midesophageal.

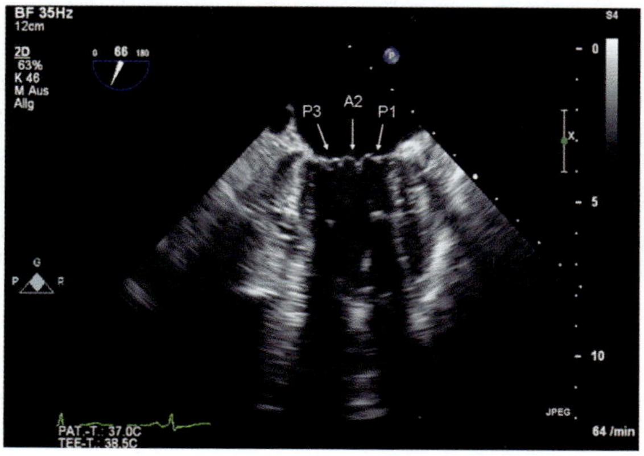

FIGURE 10.6 ME commissural view, which typically shows the P3, A2, and P1 segments. ME, midesophageal.

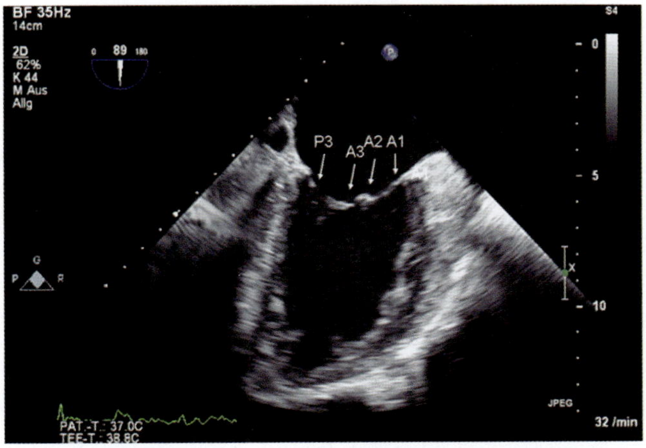

FIGURE 10.7 ME two-chamber view. Forward rotation from the ME commissural view through to approximately 90° to 100° reveals P3, A3, A2, and A1 segments.

From the ME views, the probe is advanced into the stomach to obtain the transgastric (TG) views.

TG mid short-axis (SAX) view: Regional wall motion abnormalities as well as global LV function can be assessed by measuring fractional shortening or fractional area change. This view serves as the reference view for possible new regional wall motion abnormalities that may arise due to complications of the MV repair in the postrepair examination (see postrepair examination).

TG two-chamber view: The ultrasound beam travels perpendicularly to both the papillary muscles and chordae, so these two structures are often very clearly visualized (Figure 10.9). LV diameters are measured in this view (19,20).

TG basal SAX view: Shows all segments of the mitral leaflets together with both commissures (Figure 10.10). This view allows for planimetric measurement of the MV orifice area. An existing cleft pathology in one of the leaflets can often be diagnosed in this view during diastole (Video 10.1, cleft anterior mitral leaflet). The use of color flow Doppler helps to confirm the diagnosis (Video 10.2, CFD cleft anterior mitral leaflet), and with RT 3D TEE the cleft can often be better elucidated (Video 10.3, cleft posterior mitral leaflet).

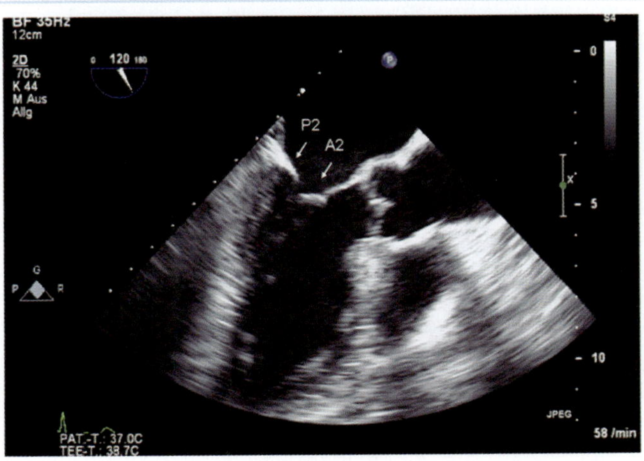

FIGURE 10.8 ME LAX view. The left atrium, left ventricle, left ventricular outflow tract, and aortic valve are viewed simultaneously, and define this view. When there is no foreshortening, the mitral segments viewed are A2 and P2. ME LAX, midesophageal long axis.

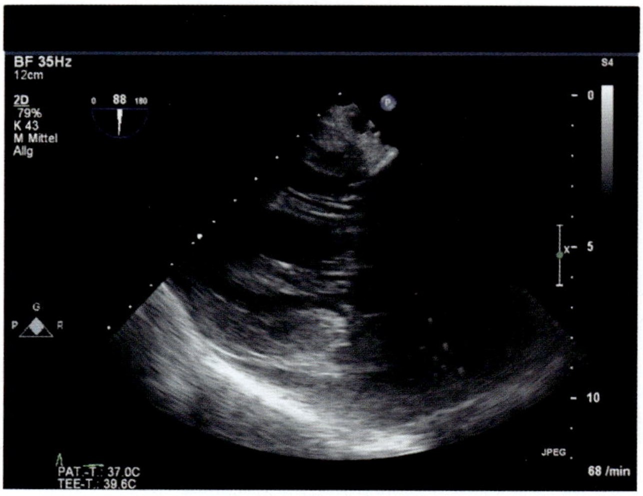

FIGURE 10.9 TG two-chamber view. This view is particularly helpful in demonstrating structural pathology of the subvalvular apparatus, as the beam travels perpendicular to these structures, enhancing their visualization. TG, transgastric.

3D Assessment of the Mitral Valve

The guidelines for image acquisition and display using 3D echocardiography (21) recommend that the MV be displayed with the aortic valve placed superiorly, regardless of whether the MV is oriented as viewed from the left atrium or left ventricle. This brings the advantage that the anterior leaflet is readily identifiable inferior to the aortic valve; the posterior leaflet must then be further inferior in this view. Viewed from the atrial side, the valve segments are named 1, 2, and 3, from left to right (Figure 10.3; Video 10.4). Cleft defects, indentations, or leaflet perforations are often distinctly better viewed in this view compared to standard 2D images.

3D color flow Doppler can also be applied and can be extremely useful in localizing regurgitation and in quantifying its severity by measuring vena contracta, or by using the proximal isovelocity surface area (PISA)

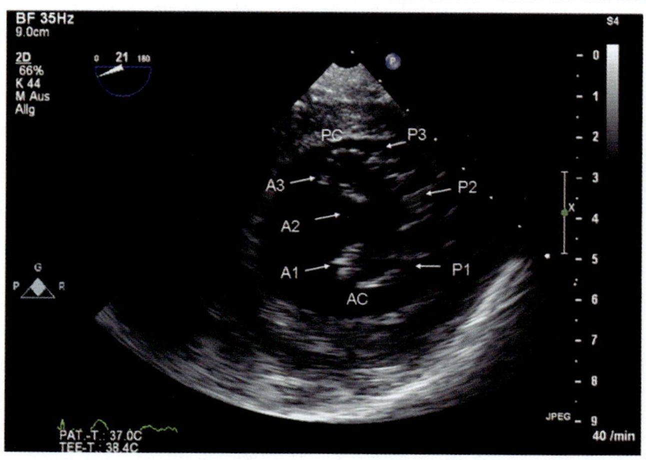

FIGURE 10.10 TG basal SAX. This view can be difficult to optimize; in its true form, it reveals the basal left ventricle in short axis, allowing basal wall motion abnormalities to be identified. In this figure, the posteromedial (PC) and anterolateral (AC) commissures are visible. All six segments of the mitral valve are also identified. Mitral valve opening area can be measured by planimetry. Applying color Doppler can often help to localize regurgitant jets. SAX, short axis; TG, transgastric.

method. 3D color flow Doppler has limitations, however; the high temporal resolution required to capture these images means that spatial resolution must be compromised, so that it is often not possible to capture the entire valve area in one image. Ironically, this can sometimes make it difficult to localize a regurgitant jet with certainty unless a distinct reference point (eg, aortic valve, left atrial appendage) is identifiable. The use of full-volume gating techniques to attempt to overcome these resolution limitations can introduce the potential problem of "stitch artifacts" obscuring the images. 3D echocardiography has shown better agreement with cardiac magnetic resonance imaging in quantifying the regurgitant volume than 2D echocardiography, particularly in eccentric, multiple, and late-systolic regurgitant jets (3).

Newer 3D modalities, including iSlice and TruVue or GlassVue, have been introduced recently. The main value of the traditional 3D en face view of the MV is that it would seem more intuitive to appreciate the nature and precise location of any MV pathology, without necessarily having advanced echocardiographic knowledge (Figure 10.11; Videos 10.5 and 10.6). iSlice is a relatively new modality that offers the capability to utilize multiplane reconstruction of images (Figure 10.12; Video 10.7), thereby facilitating precise localization of areas of interest or pathology, effectively by using a multiplanar reconstruction technique. Advanced 3D modalities are however potentially time-consuming and do require specialist understanding and competencies to acquire and optimize for presentation. In addition, TruVue and GlassVue are new variations on traditional 3D imaging, which again mainly helps those used to macroscopic rather than echocardiographic images to better appreciate MV pathology and location rather than with just traditional 2D imaging (Figure 10.13).

In examining the structure of the mitral apparatus, it is important to identify and quantify the presence and severity of calcification of the mitral apparatus, especially on the annulus and leaflets. Calcification has a characteristic echodense appearance on echo and is not difficult to identify (Figure 10.14). Because calcium gives rise to shadowing artifacts, however, it may impede visualization of other structures.

Quantitative Measurements

In the preoperative structural assessment of the mitral apparatus, a number of echocardiographic measurements should be made, as these are important first in assessing whether the valve is amenable to repair and second in helping to determine the correct repair technique.

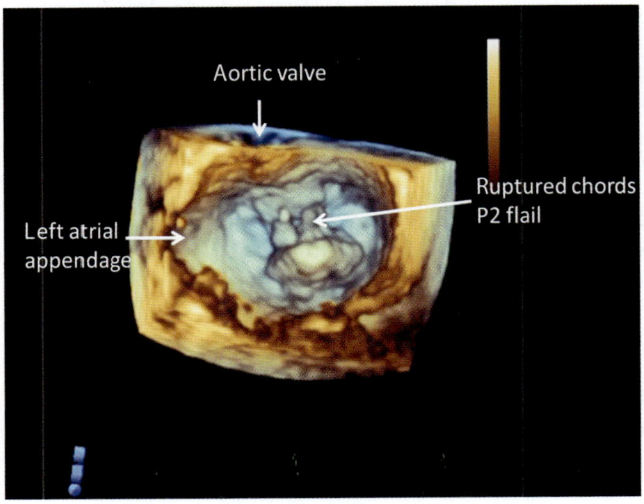

FIGURE 10.11 3D en face view of the mitral valve, looking from the atrial side. This image provides the "surgeon's view," as it represents the typical view of the valve which is seen macroscopically during open surgery. Landmarks such as the aortic valve and left atrial appendage help orientation and localization of the leaflet segments. In this case, ruptured chordae with a flail P2 segment are seen.

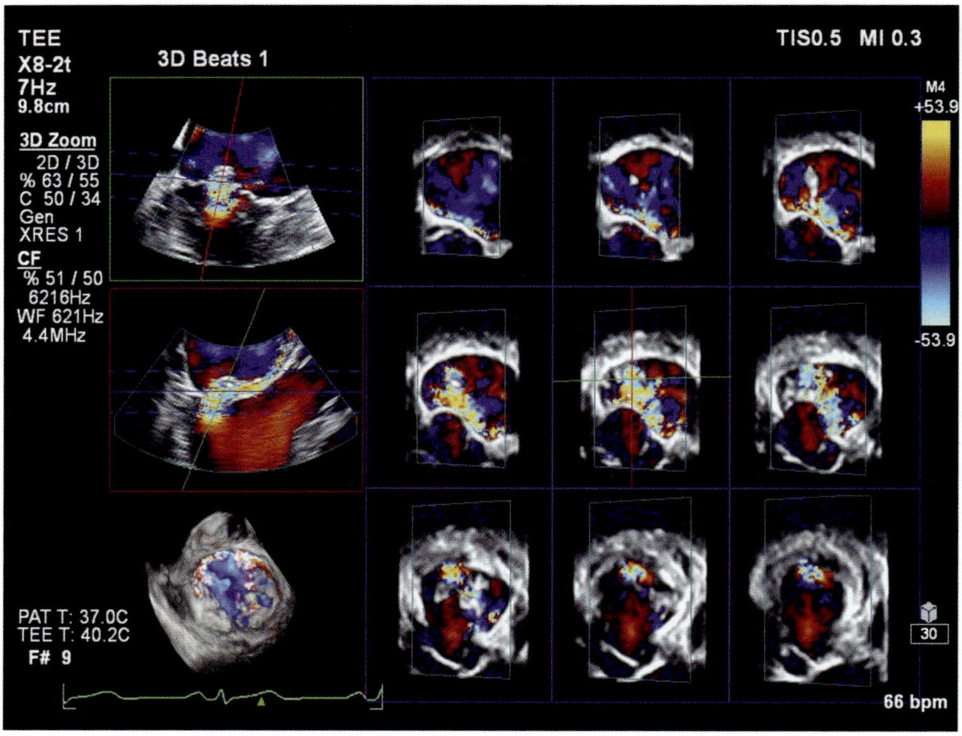

FIGURE 10.12 iSlice is a modality feature of 3D echocardiography, which allows effective simultaneous multiplanar reconstruction, in this case showing multiple 2D slices, thereby helping to identify and localize particular areas of interest.

Size of Mitral Annulus

The normal mitral annulus is not round; rather, it is described as saddle shaped, and the ratio between the transverse and anteroposterior diameters is approximately 4:3. When the annulus dilates, however, it expands predominantly in the anteroposterior direction, thus reducing the normal 4:3 ratio, as its fibroelastic skeleton is weakest around the posterior annulus. To assess mitral annular dilatation, the annulus is therefore measured in its anteroposterior diameter, between the base of the A2 and P2 segments at the level of the mitral annulus (22). This is done in diastole using the ME LAX view (Figure 10.15, D1).

Length of Anterior Mitral Leaflet

This is a particularly important measurement to make in the setting of mitral repair and is used to help determine the size of the annuloplasty ring to be implanted. The length is best measured during diastole using the ME LAX view with the measurement made from the base of the anterior leaflet (at the annulus) to its leaflet tip (Figure 10.15, D2) (22). Because of the semicircular shape of the anterior leaflet, the measurement along the A2 segment in this image plane will be the longest. Care should be taken not to include the primary chordae in the measurement, which attach to the tip of the leaflet.

Length of Posterior Mitral Leaflet

This can be measured using the same ME LAX image used for the annulus and anterior leaflet (Figure 10.15, D3). Measurement is made from the base of the leaflet at the annulus to the tip of the posterior leaflet (22). The main significance of this measurement is in predicting the likelihood of systolic anterior motion (SAM) of the anterior leaflet occurring postoperatively, as discussed later.

C-Sept Distance

The distance from the coaptation point of the mitral leaflets to the septum is also useful in the risk assessment for SAM post repair (Figure 10.16). This measurement should be made again in the ME LAX

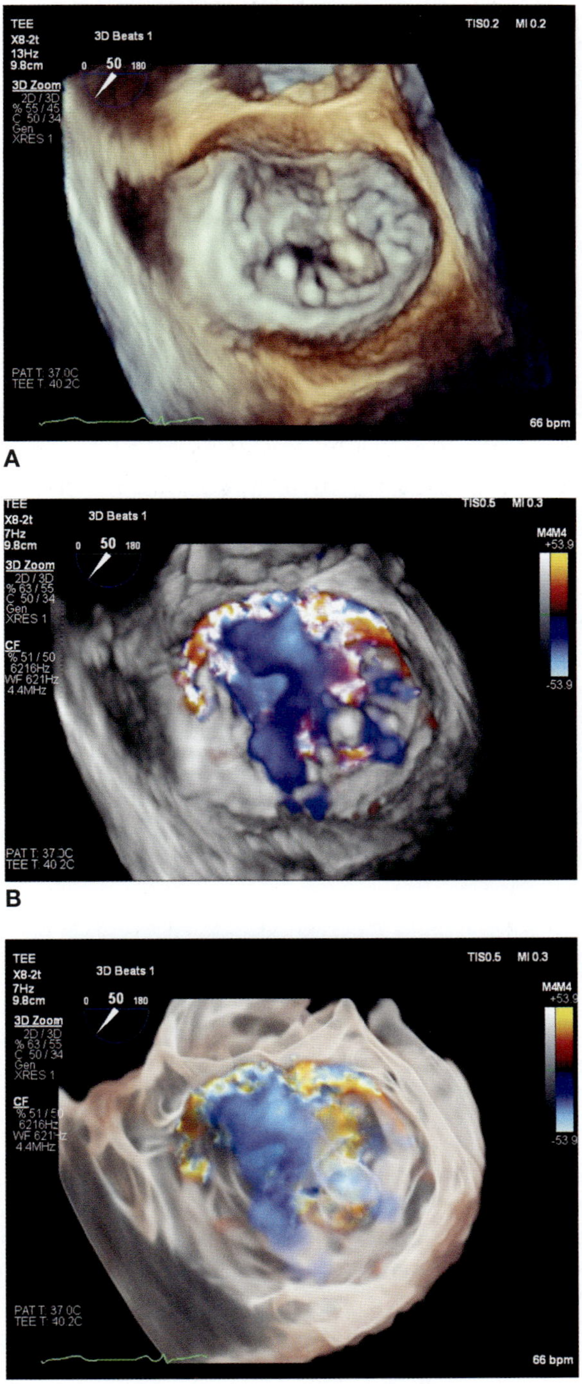

FIGURE 10.13 TrueVue is purported to provide more realistic 3D rendering, aiding interpretation by enhancing perception of depth and space compared with traditional 3D. So-called GlassVue removes the visible volume and only renders the surface. Transparency can be adjusted to provide a better view. Image A, 3D zoom shows the P2 flail clearly (white arrow). Image B by adding color Doppler does not show the origin of the regurgitant jet without cropping, whereas in Image C, by applying GlassVue, the valve is made transparent, so that the origin as well as the direction of the jet can be clearly seen (yellow arrow).

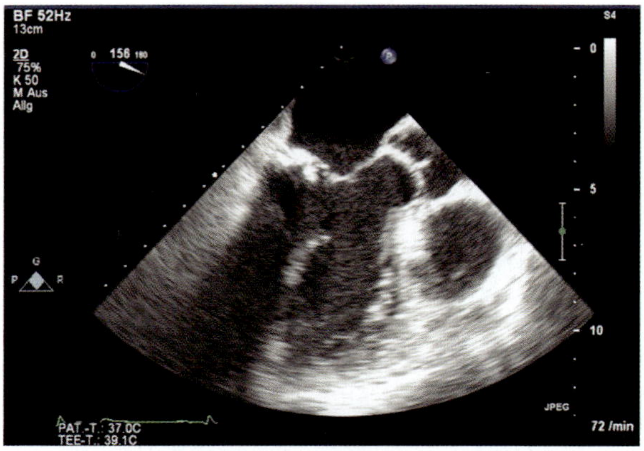

FIGURE 10.14 Calcification. This ME LAX view shows a calcified segment of the posterior leaflet, and this echodense and thickened segment of calcification creates a shadow artifact underneath which impedes visualization of underlying structures. ME, midesophageal long axis.

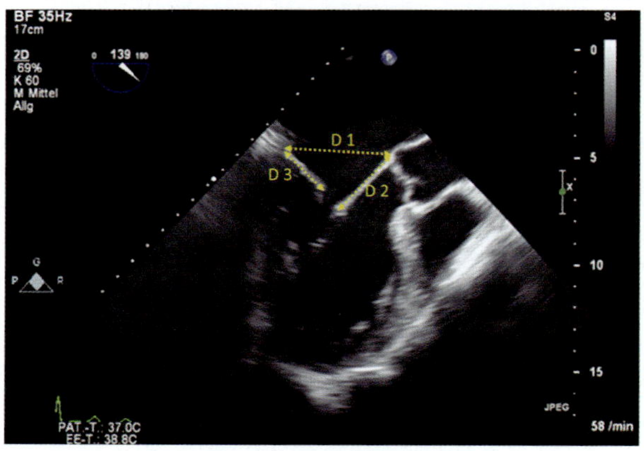

FIGURE 10.15 ME LAX view through A2, P2 segments, showing measurements made in diastole, annulus (D1), length of anterior leaflet (D2), and posterior leaflet length (D3). Optimize the image and avoid foreshortening to obtain an accurate slice. ME LAX, midesophageal long axis.

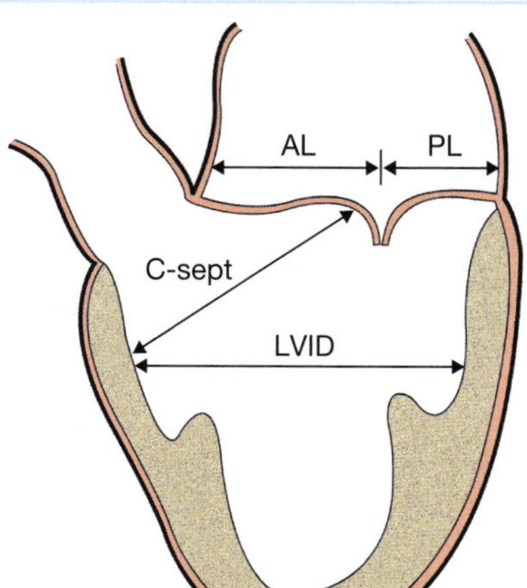

FIGURE 10.16 SAM predictors. AL, anterior leaflet; PL, posterior leaflet; LVID, left ventricular internal dimension; SAM, systolic anterior motion.

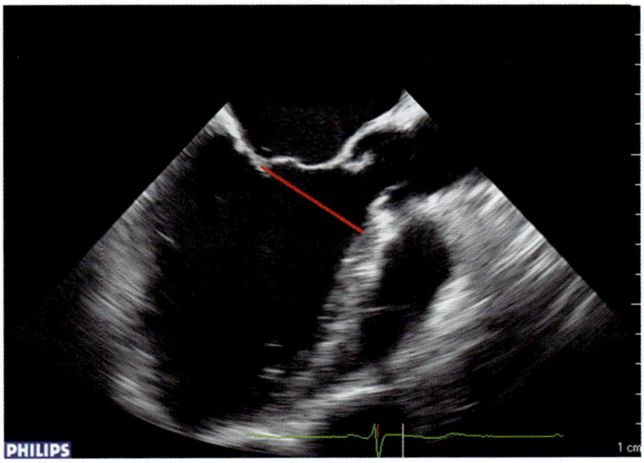

FIGURE 10.17 C-Sept distance shown here as the red line. This is measured in the ME LAX view, in systole so that the mitral leaflets coapt. ME LAX, midesophageal long axis.

view, this time in systole, so that the leaflets have coapted. The shortest direct distance from the coaptation point to the septum is measured (Figure 10.17).

Left Ventricular End-Systolic Internal Diameter

This is best measured using the TG two-chamber view, with systole timed according to MV closure. The long axis of the LV should be horizontal in the image, and measurement is made at the level of the chordae, from endocardial edge to endocardial edge (Figure 10.18). For improved accuracy, an average measurement from a number of cardiac cycles should be obtained, especially in the case of arrhythmia. A measurement greater than 40 mm defines LV dilatation. The ME two-chamber view can also be used (19,20).

Left Ventricular End-Diastolic Internal Diameter

Similar to measuring systolic internal diameter, either the TG or ME two-chamber view can be used, this time during diastole. Measurements are made at the level of the chordae, and greater than 55 mm represents LV dilatation (19,20).

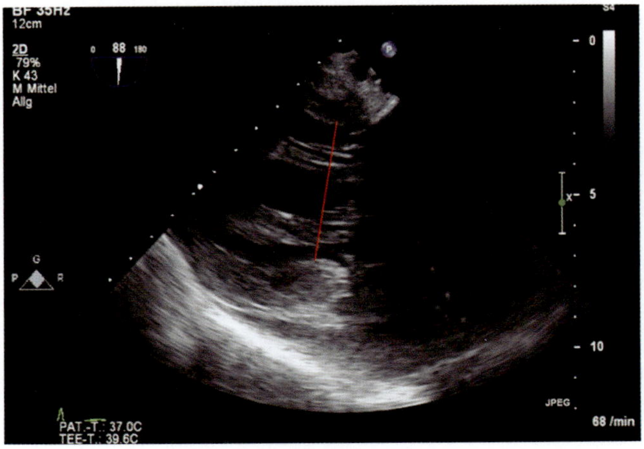

FIGURE 10.18 Left ventricular end-systolic internal diameter. Here measured in the TG two-chamber view, the ME two-chamber view is also suitable. The measurement is made in end systole, at the level of the chordae tendineae, from endocardial edge to endocardial edge, that is, the red line in this figure. ME, midesophageal; TG, transgastric.

Tenting Height

Also referred to as coaptation depth, this is a very important measurement to make, as a preoperative tenting height greater than 11 mm is associated with poor repair results, and so is usually taken as an indication for MV replacement rather than repair (23,24). This usually occurs in the setting of Carpentier type IIIb pathology, where the left ventricle is dilated and the consequent restriction of the MV leaflets in systole means that they coapt below the level of the mitral annulus. The measurement should be made in the ME LAX, or ME four-chamber views, in systole. Using the zoom function over the MV reduces the percentage error of the measurement. To make this measurement, the level of the mitral annulus is first identified by marking the annular plane. The tenting height is the perpendicular distance from this line marking the annulus level to the coaptation point (Figure 10.19).

Tenting Area

Similar to tenting height, tenting area is measured using the ME LAX view in systole. Tenting area is the area that is enclosed by the line drawn between the anterior and posterior annulus and the valve leaflets (Figure 10.20). An area of greater than 2.5 cm^2 is unfavorable for MV repair in secondary mitral regurgitation (14).

Coaptation Length

This represents the extent to which both leaflets come to oppose each other during systole. It is measured at end systole in ME LAX view (Figure 10.21). It is perhaps more important to measure post repair, as it is one of the fundamental goals of repair, and good coaptation length is associated with better repair durability and long-term results. Usually, the coaptation length is longer following implantation of artificial chords as compared to leaflet resection (25).

2. Carpentier Classification System

Functional classification of the leaflets has implications in determining the likelihood of valve repair, as will be discussed later. The functional classification of the MV is based on leaflet motion. In type I dysfunction, the motion of the leaflets is normal; in type II, it is excessive; and in type III, it is restrictive (Figure 10.22). Type III is further subclassified as type IIIa (structural) with restricted motion during both systole and diastole due to leaflet damage (calcification or rheumatic disease) and type IIIb (functional) where the restriction is limited to systole and is due to tethering of the leaflets (ischemic heart disease or dilated cardiomyopathy).

Application of color flow Doppler is helpful in determining the functional classification. In type I, the regurgitant jet is usually central. In type II, with one leaflet involved, the regurgitant jet is eccentric and directed over the noninvolved leaflet (Figure 10.23; Videos 10.8-10.13). However, if both leaflets are involved, the regurgitant jet can be central. In type III dysfunction, usually the regurgitant jet is central

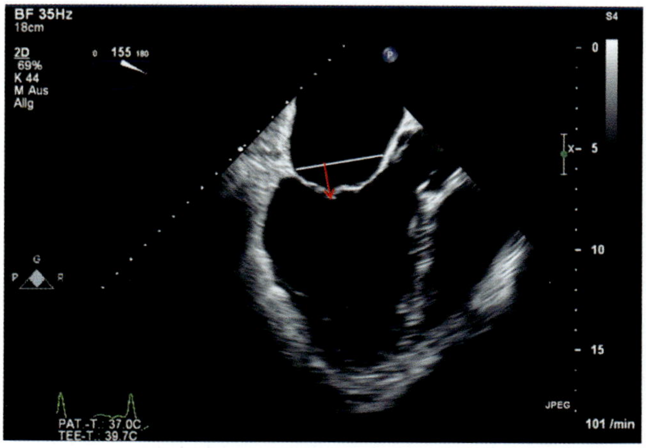

FIGURE 10.19 Tenting height. Useful in helping to determine whether a valve is repairable in functional disease. Measure in late systole using the ME LAX when the leaflets have coapted. Identify the plane of the mitral annulus (white line); the tenting height is the perpendicular distance from the coaptation point to this line (red arrow). ME LAX, midesophageal long axis.

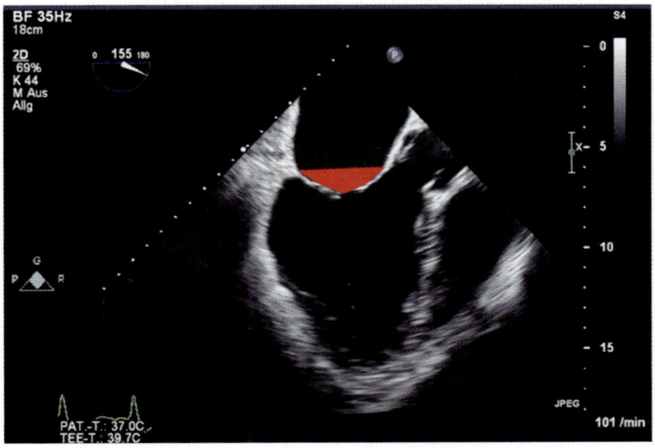

FIGURE 10.20 Tenting area. Using the same view as for tenting height, measure the area enclosed by the line along the annular plane, and the atrial sides of both valve leaflets (red triangle).

because most often both leaflets are affected (Videos 10.14-10.18). With only one leaflet involved, the regurgitant jet is eccentric and directed over the affected leaflet (Figure 10.24). Additionally, in type II dysfunction, one has to discriminate between billowing, prolapse, and flail (14,22):

1. Billowing is defined as motion of the body of the leaflets above the mitral annulus plane (Figure 10.25). To some degree, it is a normal finding. It is abnormal when greater than 2 mm in ME LAX view or greater than 5 mm in ME four-chamber view. It is generally associated with excessive tissue, chordal elongation, and possibly later occurrence of free edge prolapsed (Videos 10.19 and 10.20).
2. Prolapse describes displacement of one or both leaflet edges above the plane of the mitral annulus where the free margin is directed to the left ventricle (Figure 10.26). It is often associated with chordal elongation but can also be associated with chordal rupture (Videos 10.8-10.13). The regurgitant jet seen with color flow Doppler is always directed over the noninvolved segments in patients with type II dysfunction (Videos 10.9-10.11).
3. Flail is defined as displacement of the free edge of one or both leaflets above the mitral annular plane, where the free edge of the leaflet is also directed into the left atrium (Figure 10.27; Videos 10.21-10.23). It is often associated with chordal rupture, or even papillary muscle rupture, but can also be associated with extreme elongation of the chords.

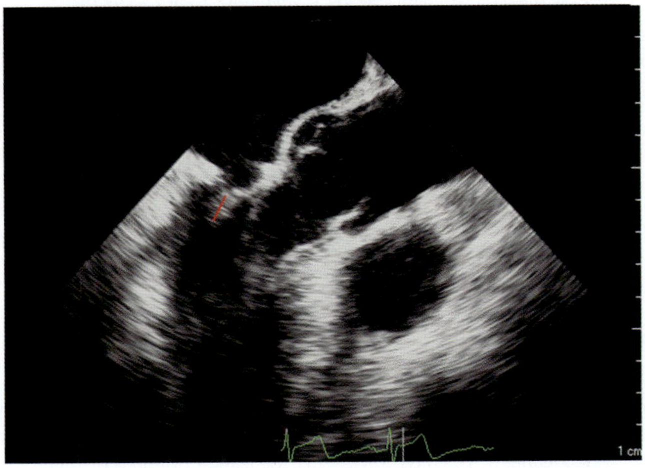

FIGURE 10.21 Coaptation length. Using either the ME LAX or ME four-chamber views, measure the length of apposition between the anterior and posterior leaflets in end systole. ME LAX, midesophageal long axis.

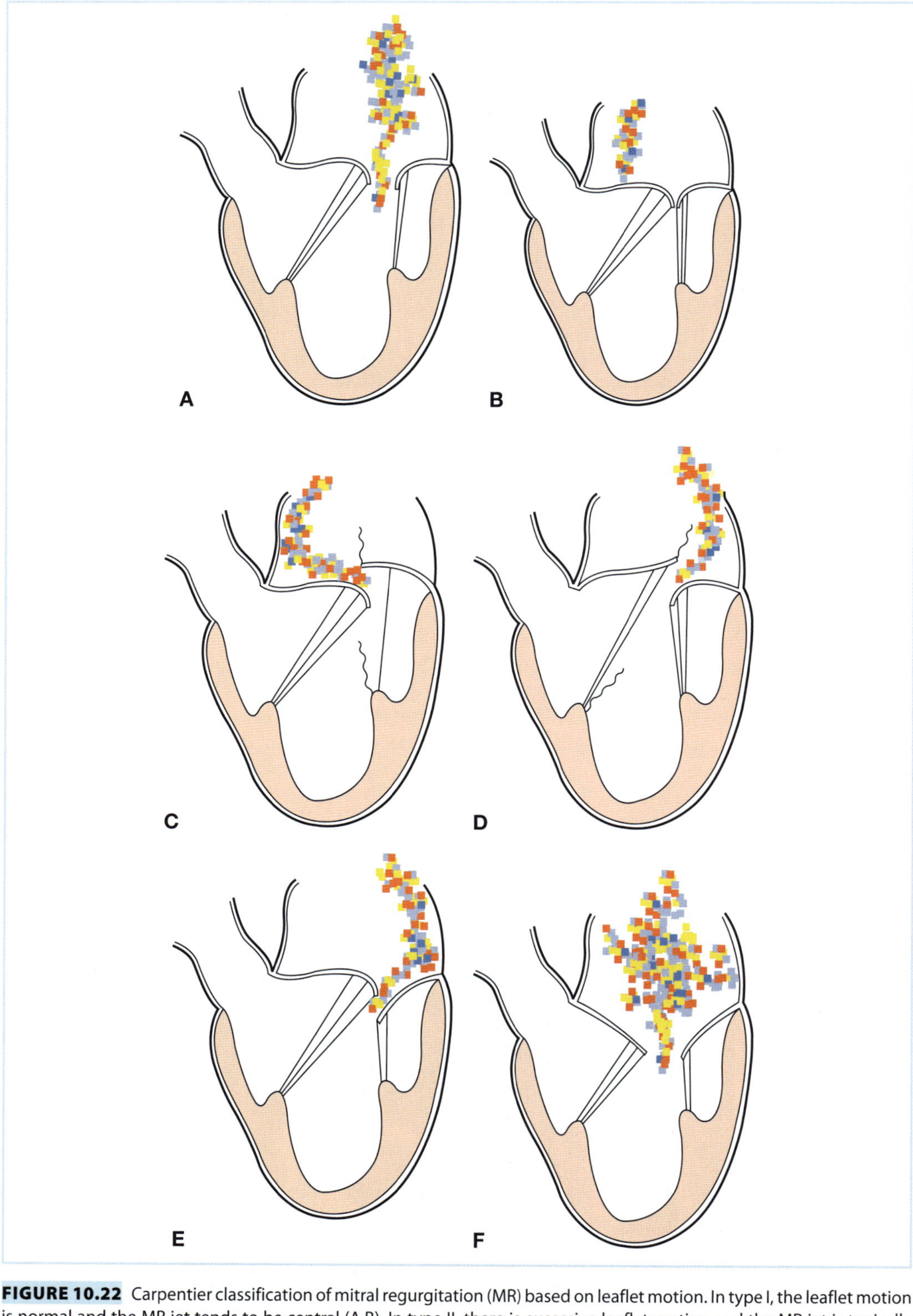

FIGURE 10.22 Carpentier classification of mitral regurgitation (MR) based on leaflet motion. In type I, the leaflet motion is normal and the MR jet tends to be central (A,B). In type II, there is excessive leaflet motion and the MR jet is typically directed away from the diseased leaflet (C, D). In type III lesions, the leaflet motion is restricted and is further subdivided into type IIIa (structural) (E), and type IIIb (functional) (F). In type III lesions the regurgitation jet may be directed toward the diseased leaflet if only one leaflet is affected, or it may be central if both mitral leaflets are equally affected. (Courtesy Dr. Gregory M. Hirschhorn).

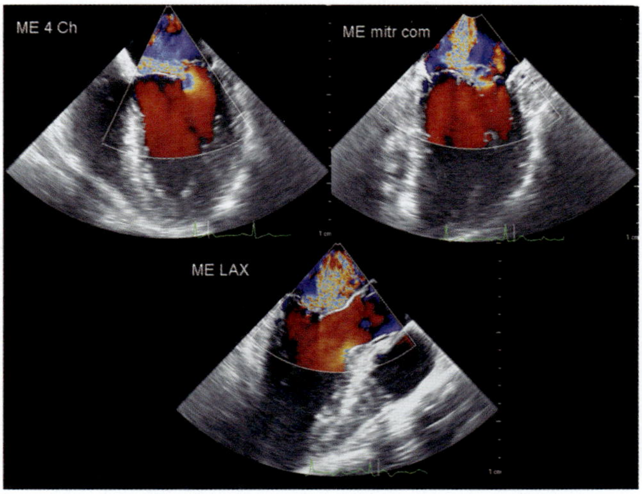

FIGURE 10.23 Color flow Doppler of type II regurgitation, caused by excessive leaflet motion, in this case prolapse affecting the P2 segment. The resulting jet is eccentric, and blood is directed over the corresponding, nonaffected (A2) leaflet. ME LAX, midesophageal long axis.

3. Assessment of the Severity of the Mitral Valve Regurgitation

The severity of the MV regurgitation is practically best assessed using the vena contracta width, the flow convergence (or PISA) method, and the pattern of pulmonary venous flow, as described in Chapter 8: Mitral Regurgitation.

4. Visualization of the Circumflex Coronary Artery and Its Relationship to the Mitral Valve Annulus

Damage or distortion of the circumflex coronary artery caused by the annuloplasty ring or prosthetic valve sutures is a well-recognized and potentially devastating complication that occurs in up to 1.8% of patients undergoing MV surgery (26-28). Visualization of the circumflex coronary artery by TEE can be accomplished in most patients by starting from the ME LAX view of the aortic valve and gradually turning the probe

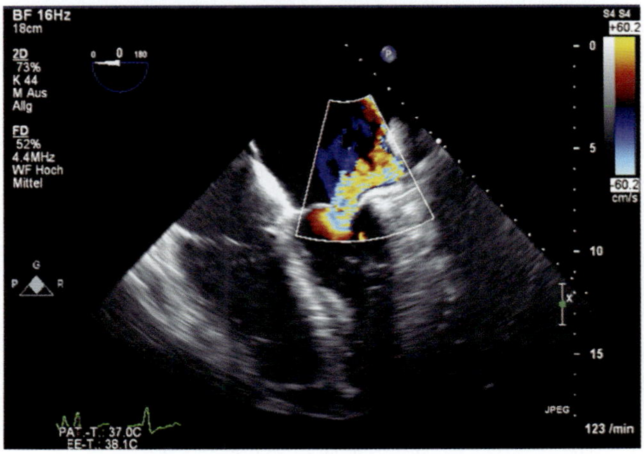

FIGURE 10.24 Color flow Doppler of regurgitation caused by restrictive leaflet motion. The posterior leaflet in this case appears restricted and does not move to coapt normally. The resulting jet is eccentric and directed over the affected posterior leaflet.

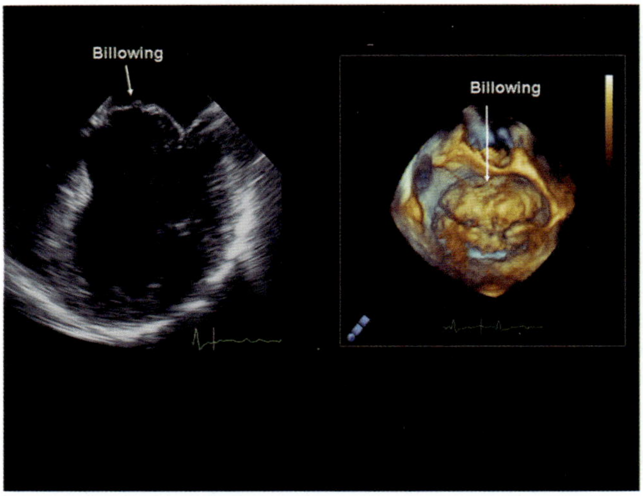

FIGURE 10.25 ME four-chamber view (left) and 3D en face view of the mitral valve from the left atrium (right) both showing extensive billowing of the anterior mitral leaflet. The body of the leaflet, but not its free edge, is pushed over the level of the mitral annulus.

to the left (29). From the origin of the left main coronary artery, one can follow the course to the bifurcation into the left anterior descending artery and the circumflex coronary artery by turning the probe to the patient's left. Further turning of the probe will visualize the course of the circumflex along the mitral annulus (Figure 10.28; Video 10.24). The circumflex coronary artery must be distinguished from the coronary sinus, a venous structure that runs in a parallel direction to it, and noting that the circumflex coronary artery decreases in diameter along its course from its point of origin, while the increases in diameter of coronary sinus will help to differentiate the two (30). The distance of the circumflex coronary artery from the mitral annulus can also be measured, and this information may directly help the surgeon. The preoperative visualization of the circumflex coronary artery acts as a reference for the postrepair visualization.

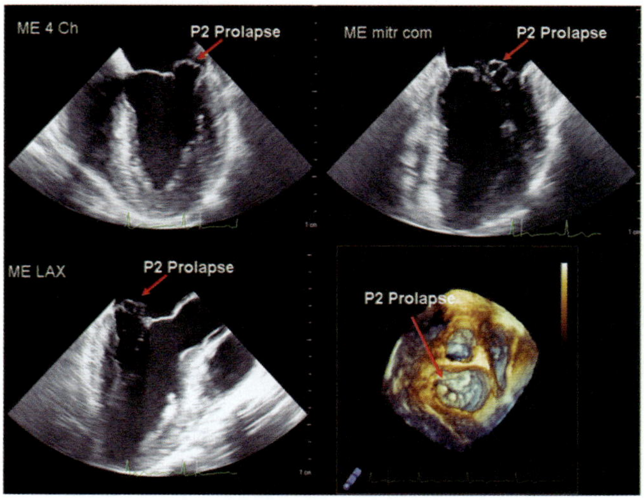

FIGURE 10.26 2D ME images; four chamber (top left), commissural (top right), LAX (bottom left), and 3D en face view of the mitral valve from the left atrium, showing prolapse of the P2 segment. The P1 segment is not visible in this 3D view. ME, midesophageal; LAX, long axis.

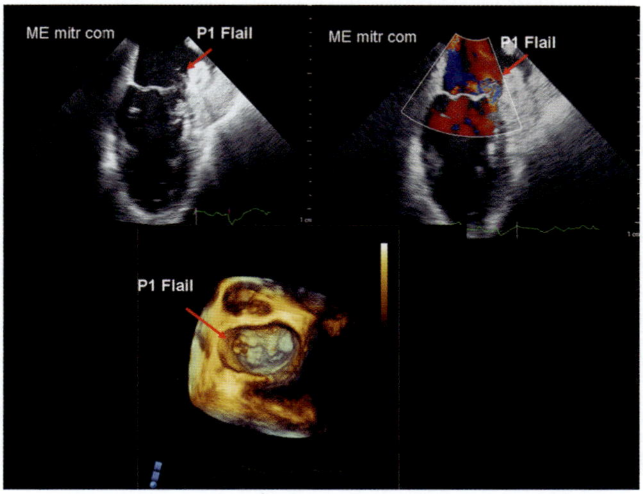

FIGURE 10.27 2D ME commissural view (above left) and with color Doppler (above right), and 3D en face view of the mitral valve from the left atrium, showing a flail P1 segment. The reason for the flail is chordal rupture; the remaining segments of chordae attached to the segment also flail over the level of the mitral annulus and point up in the direction of the left atrium. ME, midesophageal.

5. Define Secondary and Coexisting Abnormalities of Other Cardiac Structures

It is recommended that a comprehensive TEE examination be performed both pre- and postbypass in patients undergoing MV repair. In addition to defining the pathology and severity of the MV regurgitation, it is important to examine for echocardiographic evidence of secondary features of mitral regurgitation and to identify any other coexisting cardiac pathology.

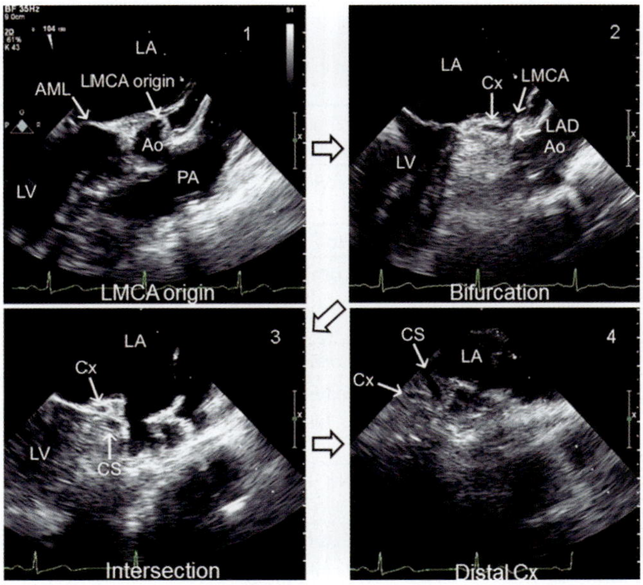

FIGURE 10.28 Visualization of the circumflex artery. AML, anterior mitral leaflet; Ao, aortic sinus; CS, coronary sinus; Cx, circumflex artery; LA, left atrium; LAD, left anterior descending; LMCA, left main coronary artery; PA, pulmonary artery. (From Ender J, Singh R, Nakahira J, Subramanian S, Thiele H, Mukherjee C. Echo didactic: visualization of the circumflex artery in the perioperative setting with transesophageal echocardiography. *Anesth Analg*. 2012;115[1]:22-6.)

Assessment of LV global and regional systolic function and chamber size has been discussed already and is important to quantify prebypass as a reference for the postoperative examination. Attention should also be paid to the aorta, specifically looking for the presence of atherosclerotic plaque, which if present increases the risk of postoperative cerebrovascular events. Ascending aortic plaque or calcification increases the risk of complications arising from aortic cannulation and cross-clamping, and if present may warrant alteration of the surgical technique (31). Plaque in the descending aorta becomes more relevant if a retrograde perfusion technique is used, as in some minimally invasive techniques.

The structure and function of the right-sided chambers should also be assessed. Tricuspid regurgitation in patients with MV disease is associated with worse outcome and predicts poorer survival, heart failure, and reduced functional capacity (32). Patients with heart failure with moderate to severe mitral regurgitation and reduced right ventricular function (tricuspid annular plane systolic excursion [TAPSE] <14 mm) had an absolute 2-year mortality that was 27% higher than similar patients who had a TAPSE greater than 14 mm (33). Patients undergoing MV surgery who also have severe tricuspid regurgitation benefit from concurrent tricuspid valve repair, and tricuspid annuloplasty may be considered for less than severe tricuspid regurgitation in patients undergoing MV repair when there is either tricuspid annular dilatation or pulmonary hypertension (1,3).

6. Surgical Procedural Considerations and Guidance for Minimal Access Surgical Techniques

Based on the TEE assessment of valve structure and function, and on the expertise of the surgeon, one can estimate the likelihood of repair. Table 10.1 describes the likelihood of successful repair based on the underlying pathology and echocardiographic features. With an isolated prolapse of the posterior leaflet, especially in the P2 segment, the success rate for repair is demonstrably more than 92% (34), and durable repair is the expectation according to current guidelines (1). More complex degenerative lesions can also be repaired with a high success rate, especially in high-volume centers, hence the guideline recommendation for either referral to or consultation with a Primary or Comprehensive Valve Center (1,3) for any patient with severe valvular disease being considered for intervention.

Degenerative valve disease is the most common cause of type II mitral regurgitation and is further subclassified as either Barlow disease or fibroelastic deficiency. Typical echocardiographic features of Barlow disease, also called diffuse myxomatous degeneration, are excessive leaflet motion, affecting usually multiple

TABLE 10.1 Probability of Successful Mitral Valve Repair in Organic Mitral Regurgitation Based on Echo Findings

Etiology	Dysfunction	Calcification	Mitral Annulus Dilatation	Probability of Repair
Degenerative	II: Localized prolapse (P2 and/or A2)	No/localized	Mild/moderate	Feasible
Ischemic/functional	I or IIIb	No	Moderate	Feasible
Barlow	II: Extensive prolapse (≥3 scallops, posterior commissure)	Localized (annulus)	Moderate	Difficult
Rheumatic	IIIa but pliable anterior leaflet	Localized	Moderate	Difficult
Severe Barlow	II: Extensive prolapse (≥3 scallops, anterior commissure)	Extensive (annulus + leaflets)	Severe	Unlikely
Endocarditis	II: Prolapse but destructive lesions	No	No/mild	Unlikely
Rheumatic	IIIa but stiff anterior leaflet	Extensive (annulus + leaflets)	Moderate/severe	Unlikely
Ischemic/functional	IIIb but severe valvular deformation	No	No or severe	Unlikely

From Lancellotti P, Moura L, Pierard LA, et al; European Association of Echocardiography. European Association of Echocardiography recommendations for the assessment of valvular regurgitation. Part 2: mitral and tricuspid regurgitation (native valve disease). *Eur J Echocardiogr*. 2010;11(4):307-332.

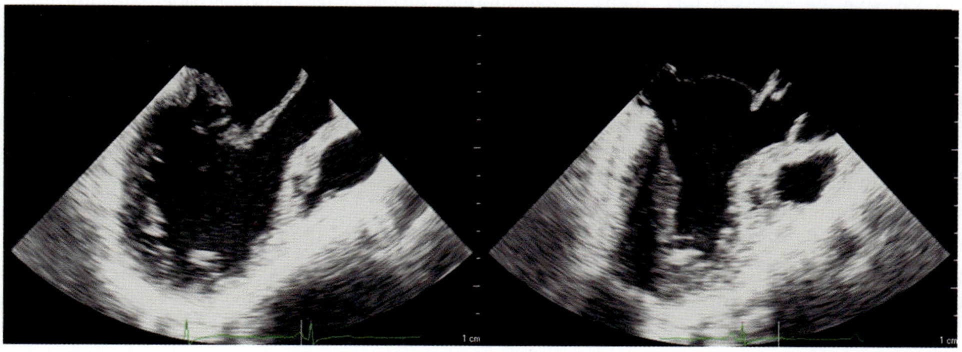

FIGURE 10.29 Typical echocardiographic appearance of a Barlow valve. Note that both leaflets are thickened, and the valve seems to have a lot of extra tissue (left). In late systole (right), the anterior leaflet prolapses, and the posterior annulus appears to tilt posteriorly.

(sometimes all) leaflet segments, with thickening of the valve leaflets, chordal elongation or rupture, and annular dilatation. Additionally, an outward displacement of the posterior mitral annulus can be observed (Figure 10.29; Video 10.25). Characteristically, there is an abundance of leaflet tissue, leading to excessive motion and ultimately regurgitation. Patients with fibroelastic deficiency of their MV tend to be older than patients with Barlow disease, and typically only a single segment of the leaflet is involved. The affected segment may be locally thickened, although this is less likely than for Barlow disease, and chordal elongation or rupture of this segment is usually evident. Valve repair of patients with Barlow disease is more challenging than for those with fibroelastic deficiency but is still the treatment of choice.

If mitral repair is to be attempted in patients with endocarditis, then the goals are durable repair with complete eradication of infected tissue. Deciding on valve repair versus replacement in cases of MV endocarditis should be based on the extent of valve destruction, the acuity of disease, and patient characteristics, as currently it cannot be concluded on the basis of available evidence that repair is superior (35). Although the presence and degree of annular and leaflet calcification can be assessed easily echocardiographically, the decision to replace the valve in patients with mitral annular calcification also relies on macroscopic inspection, as it may be possible to surgically remove some of the calcification. In all such cases, it is important to fully assess the structure and function of the mitral apparatus as outlined previously, in order to best determine the optimum surgical strategy.

Choice of repair versus replacement for mitral regurgitation arising from papillary muscle rupture is controversial, and international guidelines currently take different perspectives, with current European Society of Cardiology/European Association for Cardio-Thoracic Surgery (ESC/EACTS) opining that replacement is generally required (3), while American College of Cardiology/American Heart Association (ACC/AHA) advocate that repair should be attempted whenever possible (1). It is worth remembering, however, that mitral regurgitation secondary to papillary muscle rupture could still be classified as ischemic mitral regurgitation, a condition where repair in general has not proven superior to replacement (7); however, depending on the extent of papillary muscle damage, ventricular morphology, and surgical technique, repair may be appropriate in some cases (1). Typically, papillary muscle rupture is a mechanical complication of myocardial infarction (Videos 10.26-10.28), though it may also occur secondary to trauma. Ischemic papillary muscle rupture most commonly involves the posteromedial papillary muscle, given it has its sole blood supply from the posterior descending artery. The anterolateral papillary muscle receives its blood from both the left anterior descending and circumflex coronary arteries.

SAM of the anterior MV leaflet is a well-recognized potential complication of MV repair. Predictors of SAM after MV repair in the preoperative TEE examination are a decreased distance from mitral leaflet coaptation point to the septum (C-sept distance), a ratio of anterior to posterior mitral leaflet height of less than 1.4, and an absolute height of the posterior leaflet of greater than 1.5 cm (36,37) (Figure 10.16; Videos 10.29 and 10.30). This scenario is most likely to be seen in patients with Barlow disease, where the excess leaflet tissue often predisposes them to SAM. Septal wall hypertrophy is also associated with an increased likelihood of SAM.

The MV may be accessed for surgery via techniques other than traditional open sternotomy. These so-called minimal access surgical techniques have been defined as a reduced chest wall incision that does not include a full sternotomy. Most commonly the approach is by right anterior mini thoracotomy, with either video thoracoscopic guidance or robotic assistance.

These techniques allow for repair rates and outcomes similar to open sternotomy; however, the potential advantages of faster recovery times, less blood product administration, and a more satisfactory cosmetic result. They do however present a number of challenges and possibilities of potential complications distinct from the traditional full sternotomy.

Most significantly, perfusion cannulae are usually placed peripherally for minimal access mitral surgery as opposed to centrally for sternotomy procedure. For most patients, a single multiport venous cannula inserted via the femoral vein and secured with its tip in the superior vena cava (SVC) is adequate. For patients who weigh more than 100 kg or where the right side of the heart needs to be opened during surgery (eg, concomitant tricuspid surgery, atrial septal defect repair), then a second venous drainage cannula needs to be placed via the jugular vein. Potential complications associated with these cannulae are venous or cardiac perforation causing pericardial tamponade and needing emergency sternotomy, perforation of the interatrial septum, or malposition and consequently inadequate drainage and suboptimal flow during cardiopulmonary bypass. The risk of these complications can be reduced using echocardiography for direct real-time guidance during insertion.

As the surgeon punctures the femoral vein and advances the guidewire, this should be visualized on echo, using specifically the bicaval view (Figure 10.30). The wire needs to be seen traversing from the inferior to SVC, and free from the interatrial septum and fossa ovalis, where it may occasionally get snagged. Biplane is very useful to ensure that the wire is in the SVC. Based on the ME bicaval view and focusing on the SVC, the orthogonal plane shows the SAX view of the SVC (Figure 10.31).

When this is assured, the surgeon should then advance the cannula over the wire, under echo guidance, so that it passes smoothly and is seen in real time to advance into the SVC. As a rule, if the wire and cannula cannot be visualized, then the cannula should not be advanced, as to do so increases the risk of perforation. With the dilator still within the cannula, the cannula itself can be hard to see (Figure 10.32). After withdrawing the dilator, the cannula can be clearly seen. Again, biplane enables visualization of the cannula in SVC in LAX and SAX (Figure 10.33).

If a jugular cannula is required, then this can be placed most efficiently by the anesthetist during induction of general anesthesia, again under direct, real-time transesophageal echo guidance. The jugular vein is punctured and the wire is inserted. It should be seen coming from the SVC into the right atrium. During serial dilatation, ensure at each stage that the wire continues to move freely and has not become kinked or snagged on something. The wire should also at every stage be seen within the right atrium to move freely. Advance the multiport jugular venous cannula under direct echo guidance. Often the cannula may not be visible within the SVC, depending on its length and patient size. As it is aspirated and then flushed with saline, bubbles

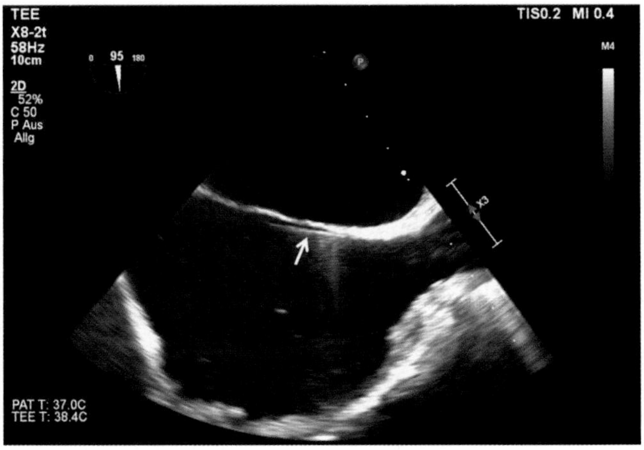

FIGURE 10.30 ME bicaval view with the guidewire (arrow) in the right atrium. ME, midesophageal.

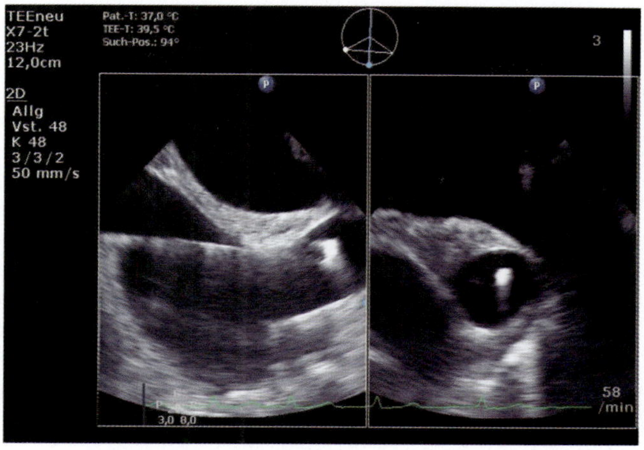

FIGURE 10.31 ME biplane bicaval view with the J tip of the guidewire in the superior vena cava.

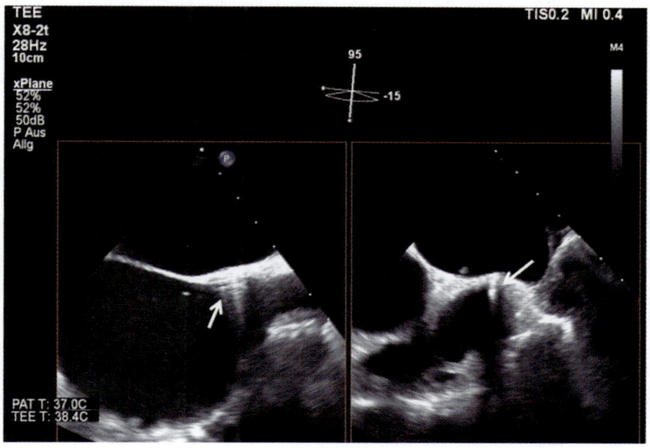

FIGURE 10.32 ME bicaval view X-plane with the cannula (arrow) in the superior vena cava. As the dilator is still in the cannula, the cannula cannot be seen clearly. ME, midesophageal.

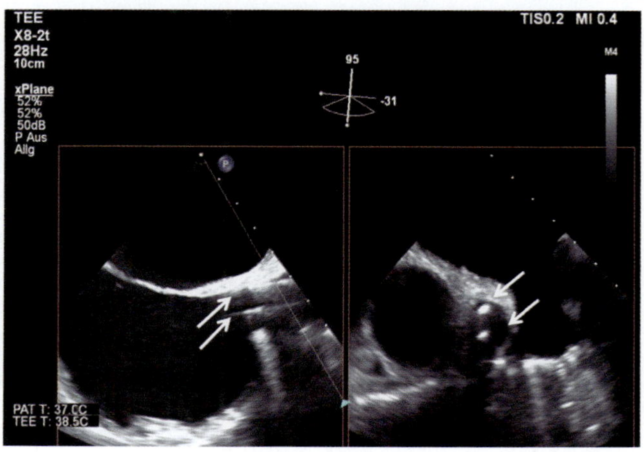

FIGURE 10.33 ME biplane bicaval view X-plane with the cannula without the dilator. The double contour of the cannula can be seen clearly (arrows). ME, midesophageal.

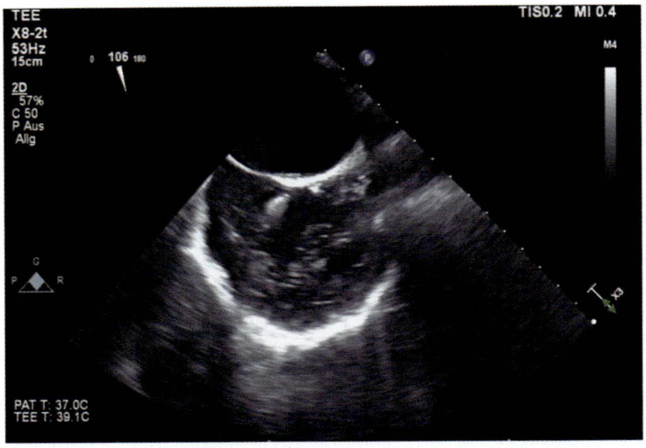

FIGURE 10.34 ME bicaval view showing bubbles in the right atrium after injection of saline via the cannula in the superior vena cava to ensure intravascular placement of the cannula. ME, midesophageal.

should be seen within the right atrium, indicating satisfactory placement (Figure 10.34). Check at the end of the procedure that there is no pericardial effusion.

For most of these minimal access cases, aortic perfusion is also peripheral, via the femoral artery. Prior to insertion, it is useful to screen the aorta for disease, atherosclerosis, aneurysm, or even chronic dissection using the transesophageal echo. The guidewire should be identified in real time as the surgeon places it, and it should be seen to move freely within the aorta (Figure 10.35). The surgeon will then advance the cannula over the guidewire, and the aortic cannula is usually not advanced high enough into the aorta to be seen on echo. As soon as bypass is initiated, it is useful to ensure that flow in the aorta is seen and that a retrograde dissection has not developed. Early identification and immediate cessation of bypass, if possible, can be lifesaving.

For most minimal access MV procedures, the aorta may be cross-clamped using a modified clamp (Chitwood clamp) inserted through a small thoracic puncture. Some centers prefer to clamp the aorta from within, using a balloon called the "endoclamp." Placement of the endoclamp relies heavily on echocardiography,

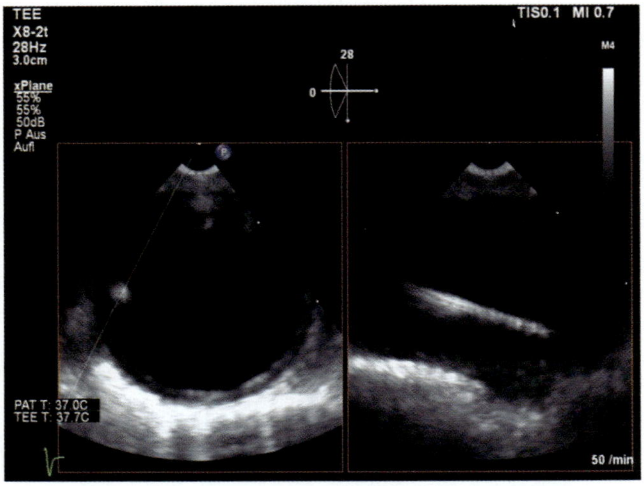

FIGURE 10.35 ME descending aorta view, biplane showing the guidewire in the descending aorta having been inserted via the femoral artery. ME, midesophageal.

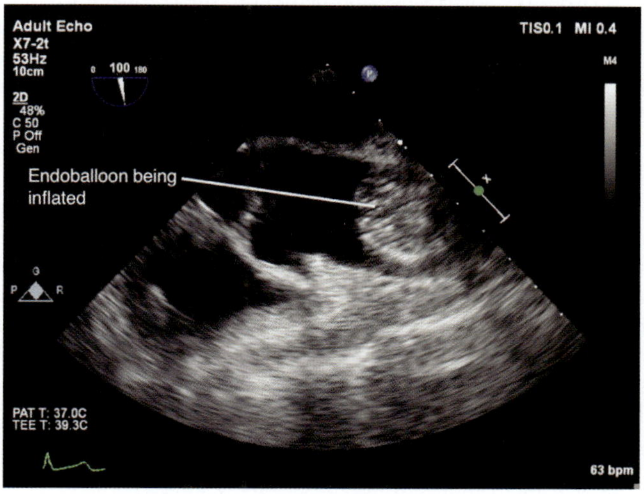

FIGURE 10.36 ME LAX view of the aortic valve, showing the endoclamp in a satisfactory position as it is being deployed and inflated. Note the right coronary ostium can be seen and is not in danger of occlusion from the balloon. ME LAX, midesophageal long axis.

and malposition during surgery can be associated with some very serious complications. A special type of femoral arterial perfusion cannula is required, with a specific port through which the endoclamp is advanced. The endo clamp should be advanced under direct echo guidance from the femoral artery up into the ascending aorta. The optimal position of the endoclamp is with its tip just distal to the sinotubular junction. Another unique feature of the endoclamp is that cardioplegia is delivered via a cannula that passes through the balloon. To initiate cardioplegic arrest, the balloon is first inflated to occlude the ascending aorta (Figure 10.36). Next cardioplegia is delivered proximal to the balloon tip, in the aortic root (Figure 10.37).

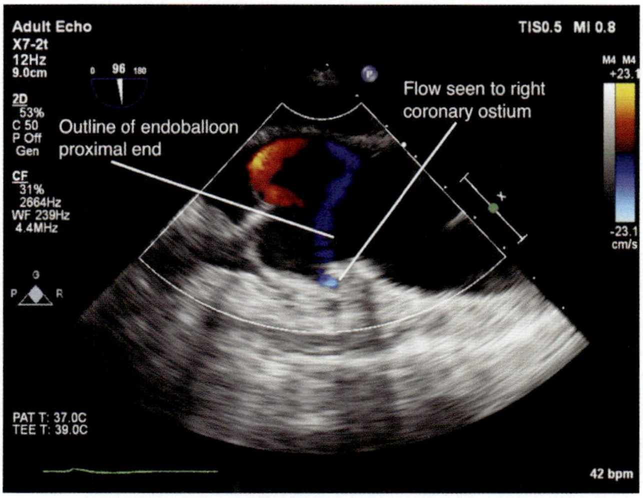

FIGURE 10.37 ME LAX of the aortic valve as the endoclamp is inflated in position, and cardioplegia is delivered. Note here that color flow Doppler with a reduction in velocity scale is applied to aid assessment of cardioplegia flow. Flow is seen at the entry to the right coronary artery. There is no evidence of aortic valve incompetence or regurgitation. The ECG is also showing asystole. Flow through the left coronary artery ostium and circumflex should be examined (not seen in this image). ECG, electrocardiogram; ME LAX, midesophageal long axis.

Pressurized cardioplegia closes the aortic valve and delivers to the coronary arteries, causing cardioplegic arrest. If the balloon has been advanced proximal to the ST junction, it may occlude the coronary arteries and prevent cardioplegia delivery. Conversely, if the pressure buildup pushes the balloon distally, occlusion of the right brachiocephalic artery can occur.

Rarely for MV surgery, placement of a pulmonary artery vent may be necessary. Essentially, this is a modified pulmonary artery catheter and is inserted in an identical manner. Echo can also provide RT guidance for passing this vent if necessary.

To help ensure that antegrade cardioplegia alone will be sufficient, it is imperative to quantify any aortic regurgitation before the procedure begins. Anything more than mild regurgitation is considered a contraindication to minimal access surgery performed under antegrade cardioplegia alone. If the surgeon intends to give retrograde cardioplegia, then this needs to be planned in advance, as the retrograde cannula also needs to be placed percutaneously via the internal jugular vein. Again, this may be performed under RT echo guidance using a number of views sequentially to visualize the coronary sinus and help with its placement and verification. This can be quite tricky, and multiple guidance techniques (eg, fluoroscopy and/or pressure transduction) may also be necessary. The majority of minimal access MV cases may be safely performed without retrograde cardioplegia, and where it is considered, it should be clearly planned beforehand.

MITRAL VALVE REPAIR TECHNIQUES

The fundamental goals of MV repair are to (38):

1. Preserve or restore full leaflet motion.
2. Create a large leaflet coaptation area.
3. Remodel and stabilize the MV annulus.

Various surgical techniques have been described, the most common of which are:

1. Annuloplasty ring implantation
2. Artificial chordae implantation
3. Chordal transfer
4. Chordal shortening or papillary muscle shortening
5. Resection of valve leaflets
6. Edge-to-edge technique (Alfieri repair)
7. Repair technique of type I valve dysfunction
8. Repair technique of type III valve dysfunction

The particular surgical technique applied and the success of MV repair depend on the particular valve pathology causing the regurgitation and the expertise and skill of the surgeon (14).

Annuloplasty

In almost all cases of open MV repair, an annuloplasty ring is implanted, and the principle behind this is to try and stabilize the annulus and restore or maintain the normal 4:3 ratio of transverse to anteroposterior distances of the MV in systole. As discussed previously, the mitral annulus dilates predominately in the anteroposterior direction because the posterior annulus is structurally the weakest point, so offers the least resistance to enlargement. Annuloplasty ring insertion normalizes the geometry of the annulus and facilitates greater coaptation between the leaflets, thereby greatly improving the durability and long-term success of the repair (39).

The most important of the many variables distinguishing the commercially available annuloplasty ring models is to select the correct size. *Generally, the optimum ring size corresponds to the length of the anterior mitral leaflet (15); however, for some type II conditions (especially Barlow disease), the ring should tend to be oversized, in order to accommodate the excessive leaflet tissue, thus allowing for good coaptation, while reducing the likelihood of postoperative SAM.* In cases of restrictive MV disease, the ring should be downsized, again to facilitate good coaptation between the leaflets. The surgeon will also verify the appropriateness of the ring size using a surgical sizer. More recently, strong correlation between annuloplasty size determined using a combination of 3D TEE imaging with superimposed computer-aided design modeling and surgically determined ring sizes has been demonstrated (40), and this approach may play a greater role in the future.

Implantation of Artificial Chordae

Implantation of artificial chordae involves the attachment of polytetrafluoroethylene (PTFE) chordae to the corresponding papillary muscle (Video 10.31), then to the free margin of the involved mitral leaflet segment (Video 10.32) and finally, the implantation of an annuloplasty ring (Video 10.33). Originally applied to repair type II defects of the anterior leaflet, this technique is now also well established for repair of posterior and bileaflet defects (41,42).

The most challenging aspect of this technique is ensuring that the length of the new artificial chordae is correct to facilitate good coaptation and normal leaflet motion. A variety of techniques have been described in order to achieve this (43), some involving the use of TEE-derived measurements (44). Prebypass TEE-derived measurements have the potential advantage that they can be made with the heart in systole, while the surgeon is limited to measuring the heart while it is arrested in diastole (34,45). The advantages of this method of repair are that it provides excellent results, can be applied to most cases of type II disease irrespective of the state of the native chordae, tissue resection can usually be avoided, and it is considered a highly reproducible technique.

Chordal Transfer

A second technique commonly applied to repair type II defects of the anterior leaflet is chordal transfer. This involves taking normal chordae with a strip of leaflet tissue from the posterior leaflet, and transferring it to the free edge of the unsupported anterior leaflet, the defect in the posterior leaflet can then be repaired, normally by quadrangular resection (46). Another option is to transfer functioning secondary chordae from the anterior leaflet to its prolapsing free edge or to fix the free edge of the anterior leaflet back onto secondary chordae with sutures. An advantage of this technique is that sizing and measurement of the transferred chordae is not required, and a disadvantage is that the technique is not always applicable, as it usually requires the posterior leaflet to be normal, which is not always the case.

Chordal Shortening, Papillary Muscle Shortening

This technique, originally described by Carpentier, has been most often applied to cases of anterior leaflet prolapse, caused by severe chordal elongation. An incision is made into the papillary muscle, and the excess chord is wrapped in a pericardial pledget, placed within the muscle, which is then oversewn, capturing the chord, and thereby effectively shortening it. In this type of repair, an annuloplasty ring is mandatory to reduce the tension on the chordae and help prevent later chordal rupture. However, the long-term results of this technique have been found to be inferior to chordal transfer, mainly due to later chordal rupture. Shortening the papillary muscle by removing a wedge-shaped section is another option aimed at correcting type II anterior leaflet prolapse.

Leaflet Resection

The majority of MV pathologies in type II disease are ruptured and elongated chords from the middle segment of the posterior leaflet. The technique of valve repair utilizing tissue resection consists of surgical inspection of the MV in cardioplegic arrest (Video 10.34), resection (so-called triangular or quadrangular resection depending on the shape of the excised section) of the involved segment (prolapse P2, Video 10.35), reconstruction of the leaflets (Video 10.36), and then implantation of an annuloplasty ring (Video 10.37). This is the technique traditionally applied to isolated segmental prolapse of the posterior leaflet and has provided excellent results; however, insertion of artificial chordae is usually a valid alternative, and in one retrospective study, the coaptation length was found to be better following repair with artificial chordae than for repair by resection in patients with type II posterior leaflet dysfunction (40). As far as possible, resection of anterior leaflet tissue should be avoided, and if performed, it should not involve more than 10% of the leaflet surface area.

Edge-to-Edge (Alfieri Stitch) Repair

This technique involves suturing the anterior and posterior leaflets together at the coaptation surfaces, classically between A2 and P2 segments, although other segments may also be sutured together. It is especially applied in cases of anterior leaflet prolapse, and also in cases of excess anterior leaflet tissue typical of Barlow disease, where it functions to reduce the likelihood of both postrepair leaflet prolapse and postoperative SAM. The Alfieri stitch presents unique challenges to the perioperative echocardiographer, in that coaptation between A2 and P2 is fixed as they are sutured together, which implies that leaflet motion in these segments is restricted, especially in diastole, and that a so-called double orifice valve is created. The total opening area of the valve will thereby be reduced (Figure 10.36; Video 10.38), so the presence or absence of postrepair mitral stenosis must be evaluated on the postoperative examination.

Repair Technique for Type I Valve Dysfunction

Type I MV dysfunction encompasses pathologies such as mitral annular dilatation, cleft MV, leaflet indentations, or leaflet perforation (trauma, endocarditis). Cleft MV is a congenital abnormality whereby a defect is seen, which extends from the leaflet tip to the annulus and is better identified in diastole. Almost exclusively this is found to affect only the anterior leaflet (Video 10.1), and then usually in the region of A2 segment, very rarely; however, the posterior leaflet may be affected (Video 10.3). Indentations are usually benign divisions found between the scallops of the posterior leaflet (Video 10.39). They do not normally extend to the annulus, and are identifiable normally during diastole, as they tend to close over during systole, and so do not cause regurgitation and are therefore not normally pathologic. Identification and differentiation of mitral cleft and indentations is one area where the use of RT 3D TEE is especially helpful (Videos 10.3 and 10.39). With a simple en face view of the MV, cleft or indentations can be directly visualized, whereas distinction of these features using standard 2D TEE is much less obvious.

Another feature of mitral cleft is that it is often found in association with other congenital cardiac defects, such as endocardial cushion defects, atrial septal defect, ventricular septal defect, or transposition of the great arteries (47). In cases of cleft MV, the TEE exam should aim to identify or exclude these defects. The repair of cleft defects or pathologic indentations is usually straightforward and can usually be successfully accomplished by direct closure, without the need for tissue resection, and with placement of an annuloplasty if annular dilatation or other indication exists.

Repair of Type III Valve Dysfunction

In type IIIa dysfunction, the MV leaflets are restricted during both systole and diastole. The most common cause worldwide is rheumatic heart disease, and in the developed world, it is calcification of the mitral apparatus. Although balloon valvuloplasty is the treatment of choice for noncalcified rheumatic mitral stenosis, many patients require open surgery for severe mitral regurgitation secondary to rheumatic heart disease. Calcium may be sometimes surgically removed in an attempt to improve leaflet mobility and to facilitate suturing of the annuloplasty ring. The presence of mitral annular calcification makes repair more difficult and increases the postoperative risk of periannular leak and also of ventricular rupture. In cases of repair of stenotic mitral lesions secondary to rheumatic heart disease, commissurotomy should be performed, as the characteristic feature of this disease process is stenosis spreading inward from the commissures. The commissurotomy incision should not extend closer than 5 mm from the annulus to avoid postoperative commissural leakage, and an annuloplasty ring will be required in the case of a dilated annulus. If the annulus is not dilated and only a commissurotomy is performed, then an annuloplasty ring is often not required.

In type IIIb dysfunction where regurgitation results from leaflet restriction in systole, TEE plays an important role in determining if a repair is feasible or not. Preoperatively, it is important to determine the size of the annulus and also the tenting height (see "The Prerepair Evaluation" section). The principle is to "downsize" the ring, in order to bring the leaflets together for better coaptation. The length of the anterior mitral leaflet is still measured as a reference, however.

Postrepair TEE Examination

The postrepair TEE examination consists of two distinct phases: the first is a shorter examination performed before final weaning from cardiopulmonary bypass and is focused specifically on identifying the circumflex artery, and on ensuring complete de-airing of the heart chambers, and the second phase consists of a comprehensive TEE examination performed after weaning from bypass, focused on the evaluation of the MV repair and on identifying any other postoperative complications.

Postrepair, Prebypass Weaning TEE Examination

1. Identification of the circumflex coronary artery and its perfusion
2. Checking for complete de-airing of the left ventricle

Postrepair, Postbypass TEE Examination

1. Localize and quantify any residual mitral regurgitation, either transvalvular or para-annular.
2. Examine for mitral stenosis secondary to the MV repair.
3. Screen for potential complications:
   a. Global and regional ventricular function
   b. SAM of the anterior MV leaflet with consecutive left ventricular outflow tract obstruction (LVOTO)
   c. New aortic valve regurgitation due to capture of the noncoronary cusp of the aortic valve with ring sutures, aortic dissection, or ventricular rupture

Identification of the Circumflex Coronary Artery Perfusion

Postoperative examination for the circumflex artery using combined 2D and color flow Doppler should be carried out as described earlier in the preoperative assessment section. As a practical tip, it is often easier to visualize while the patient is still on bypass, once the aortic cross-clamp has been removed. Identification of a patent circumflex with good flow along its course at this stage is reassuring and allows the rest of the postoperative exam to focus on identifying other potential complications. If the course of the circumflex cannot be visualized (▶ Video 10.40), having been identifiable preoperatively, then the focus should switch to looking for LV regional wall motion abnormalities, especially along the inferolateral and/or anterolateral wall, between 2 and 5 o'clock on the TG mid-SAX view, and the surgeon should be informed (▶ Video 10.41).

Checking for Complete De-Airing of the Left Ventricle

During open repair of the MV, air enters the left-sided heart chambers. If this is not vented before coming off bypass, it will embolize into the systemic circulation and be particularly problematic if it enters either the cerebral or coronary circulations. Given its more anterior origin, air will preferentially enter the right coronary artery of a supine patient (▶ Video 10.42) and then manifest as an inferior wall or right ventricular motion abnormality (48). For minimally invasive MV repairs, where exposure and access to the heart are limited, TEE assessment of intracavity air (▶ Video 10.43) and identification of new regional wall motion abnormalities are even more important. TEE assessment of intracardiac air is best performed using the ME views (four chamber, commissural, two chamber, LAX), being careful to avoid foreshortening, or shadows from the mitral annuloplasty ring, and paying particular attention to the LV apex, left atrial appendage, and left atrium, where air typically collects, and appears as an echodense bubble. As ventricular function improves, this air can be seen to dissipate on TEE and can be removed through surgical vents.

Residual Mitral Regurgitation

Immediate postrepair assessment looks at the remodeled structure of the mitral apparatus, then examines whether or not it is functionally competent, and finally checks for any new associated complications. It is important to be aware of the particular surgical technique performed, in order to be able to evaluate it properly.

ME views: Focus is directed at the motion of the MV leaflets. The anterior leaflet in particular should move freely in both systole and diastole, and depending on the particular type of repair, motion of the posterior leaflet is more likely to be limited, as in most repairs the posterior leaflet will have been pulled down somewhat to provide for a large coaptation area, one of the fundamental goals of MV repair. In normal MVs, the length of coaptation approximates 7 to 9 mm between A2 and P2 and decreases as the commissures are approached. Coaptation length postrepair should aim to be at least 5 mm, measured between A2 and P2 segments, ideally more (Figure 10.21) (25).

Another fundamental goal of MV repair, that is, restoration of normal leaflet motion, means particularly that excursion of the leaflets during systole should not exceed the annular plane, that is, no billowing, prolapse or flail, and in general neither should motion of the leaflets be restricted. This does however depend on the type of repair performed, for example, if the repair involves an Alfieri stitch (9), then P2 and A2 segments will have been sutured together to create a double orifice MV (Video 10.38). For this reason, the exact details of the surgical repair must be known. Importantly, the annular plane is not now defined by the margins of the annuloplasty ring, which will have been sutured on top of the annulus, from the atrial side, but rather by the anatomical mitral annulus.

Color Flow Doppler: The next step in the postrepair assessment is the analysis of flow through the mitral apparatus using color flow Doppler. To assess for postoperative mitral regurgitation, cardiopulmonary bypass must be completely ended. *The significance of regurgitant jets identified in patients still under mechanical circulatory support cannot be accurately interpreted, and the temptation to assess the repair while on bypass must be avoided.* For accurate assessment, it is also imperative that the Nyquist limit be set appropriately (50-60 cm/s) and that the patient's preload, afterload, and myocardial contractility are optimized. Blood flow will always follow the path of least resistance, so if systemic blood pressure and afterload are low at the time of color flow Doppler assessment, then any degree of mitral regurgitation can be underestimated, especially in the case of functional regurgitation. Baseline shift of the Nyquist limit from 50 to 37.5 cm/s leads to better intra- and interobserver variability for vena contracta measurements as well as for effective regurgitant orifice area (EROA) using PISA (49). Starting again with the ME four-chamber view, the sector scan should be rotated through 180°, this time with the color flow Doppler sector placed over the MV, left atrium, and proximal subvalvular apparatus. Once regurgitant jets are identified, they must be quantified and localized. Using RT 3D Echo with color flow Doppler more precise localization of residual mitral regurgitation is possible.

Quantification is most reliably performed by measuring the width of the vena contracta jet and using the PISA method. Evaluation of the mechanism of any residual regurgitation is relevant in deciding if rerepair is feasible. Patients who had residual mild or moderate mitral regurgitation at the end of their surgery compared to those without showed a trend toward more often requiring later reoperation, although no increased morbidity or mortality was seen (50).

Postoperative 3D assessment is particularly valuable in localizing any regurgitant jets and in distinguishing para-annular from transvalvular regurgitation. In cases where regurgitation post repair warrants a return to bypass and rerepair, it is extremely helpful to be able to identify the exact location of the leak, and of course, its pathology, as this will determine the repair strategy, and means the surgeon knows exactly where to look for the defect.

3D also provides a distinct advantage over standard 2D images in the planimetric quantification of the residual orifice opening area after an Alfieri or mitral clip repair. Using 2D imaging, it can be difficult to obtain a clear view of the MV and to be certain that it is cut at the correct level. Using 3D offline analysis, it is possible to crop the image in multiple planes so that the true orifice area is identified and measured (Figure 10.38).

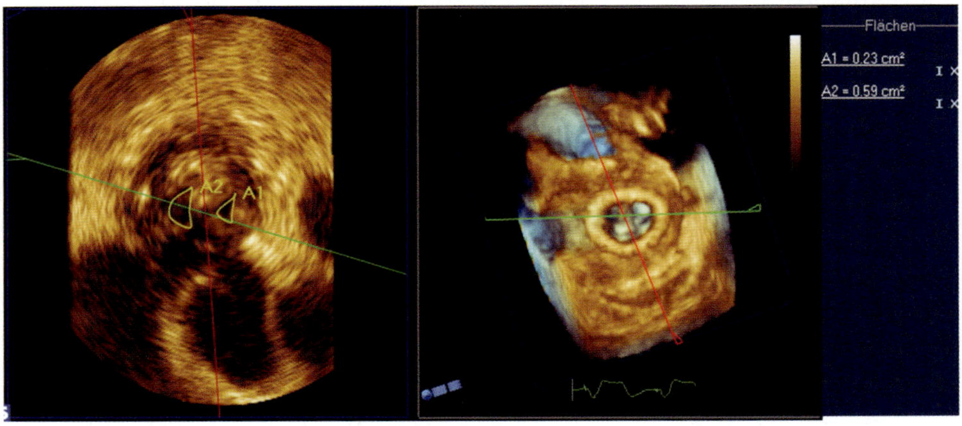

FIGURE 10.38 Offline 3D analysis of the opening area of the mitral valve in a patient post repair—in this case, an Alfieri stitch between A2 and P2, and insertion of an annuloplasty ring (right image). In the left image, the opening area of each orifice is measured individually, and the sum of both represents the total effective opening area (Area 1+ Area 2). Here the total opening area is 0.82 cm^2 (0.23 + 0.59 cm^2) representing significant stenosis and a poor result.

Even mild residual MR after repair increases the likelihood of later repair failure that would necessitate reoperation (51), so for a durable outcome, anything other than trivial residual regurgitation post repair should prompt consideration of repair revision or even replacement when a good repair is not possible (1).

Ultimately, the decision to return to bypass and attempt rerepair in cases of residual regurgitation is patient specific and should be made in collaboration between surgeon and echocardiographer.

In the case of para-annular regurgitant jets, these should also be quantified in severity, and in general, there is a lower threshold for revising the repair for anything other than very mild jets, compared to transvalvular jets. Most small para-annular jets seen directly postbypass are insignificant and disappear after protamine administration; however, persistent or larger jets may progress and lead to valvular dehiscence, hemodynamic instability, or hemolysis if not corrected.

Postrepair mitral stenosis

Mitral stenosis is a rare complication of MV repair, occurring in less than 2% of patients (52). A mean transmitral pressure gradient of greater than or equal to 7 mm Hg as measured using continuous-wave Doppler immediately following cardiopulmonary bypass is suggested as being associated with clinically significant mitral stenosis (52). *The use of pressure half-time in quantifying mitral stenosis is not reliable in the early postoperative period because of changes in left atrial and LV compliance and diastolic function.* Care should be taken in interpreting pressure gradients measured by continuous-wave Doppler in this setting. Particular difficulty may arise following an Alfieri repair. Planimetry of the MV orifice area should be performed with 2D echo in the TG basal SAX view or using 3D echo. The total valve opening area is the sum of both individual orifices (Figure 10.38). Aside from these attempts to quantify mitral stenosis, it is often helpful to eyeball the MV opening during diastole. A valve that opens freely and facilitates a clear conduit between the left atrium and ventricle is very unlikely to be associated with clinically significant stenosis. Planimetry of the MV area in the TG basal SAX view during diastole is recommended to grade the severity of mitral stenosis whenever it is feasible (see Chapter 9: Mitral Valve Stenosis) (53).

Screening for Potential Complications

Global/Regional Ventricular Dysfunction

Apart from interrupted circumflex coronary artery perfusion, other potential causes of new regional wall motion abnormalities include intracoronary air embolus, usually affecting the right coronary artery, myocardial stunning, hibernation, or ischemia post bypass, or an effect of external cardiac pacing. The TG mid-papillary view, TG basal SAX view, and ME four-chamber, two-chamber, and LAX views allow for localization of any regional wall motion abnormalities. Right ventricular function should be quantified by measuring fractional area change and TAPSE. Pulmonary artery systolic pressure also should be estimated.

Exclusion of Systolic Anterior Motion/Dynamic Left Ventricular Outflow Obstruction

The risk factors for the development of SAM of the anterior mitral leaflet and consequent dynamic left ventricular outflow tract obstruction (dLVOTO) have been discussed in the preoperative section. When these factors are identified preoperatively, the surgical repair can be tailored to minimize the risk of postoperative SAM, most commonly by using a sliding leaflet plasty with P2 resection, thereby moving the coaptation point more posteriorly, by using short artificial chords to pull the posterior leaflet straight down or by an Alfieri stitch and an annuloplasty ring that is as large as possible. If septal hypertrophy is present, then a partial septal resection can also be considered. Diagnosis of SAM and dLVOTO is made echocardiographically. The fundamental problem is that blood being compressed by the left ventricle during systole directs the anterior mitral leaflet not toward the left atrium as it should normally, but anteriorly in the direction of the left ventricular outflow tract (LVOT). This results in two problems: mitral incompetence and dLVOTO. The situation is exacerbated by some hemodynamic factors: hypovolemia, hyperdynamic circulation, tachycardia, and low afterload conditions, all of which may arise after termination of bypass.

TEE diagnosis of SAM is best appreciated using the ME LAX and five-chamber views. The anterior leaflet can be seen to be pushed in the direction of the LVOT in systole (Video 10.29). Color flow Doppler usually

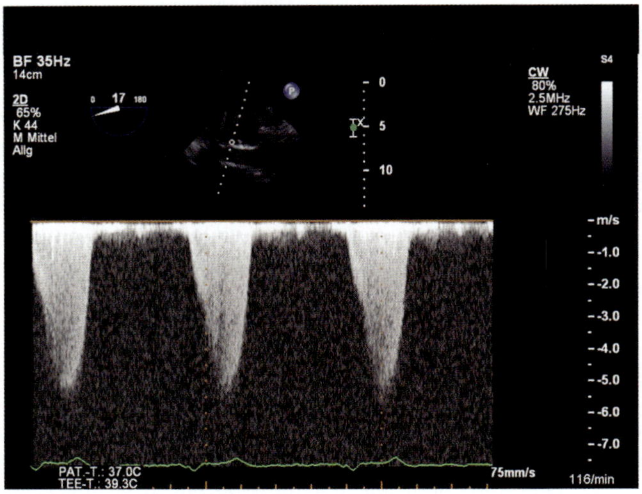

FIGURE 10.39 Continuous wave Doppler through the left ventricular outflow tract and aortic valve of a patient who developed systolic anterior motion after mitral repair. The shape of the Doppler profile is described as "dagger shaped," as the peak pressure occurs in late systole.

shows a posteriorly directed jet of mitral regurgitation toward the left pulmonary vein (Video 10.30). Continuous wave Doppler profile through the LVOT shows a characteristic dagger shape (Figure 10.39), as the obstruction and consequently the pressure gradient peaks in late systole, unlike the parabolic-shaped curve of aortic stenosis, where the pressure gradient peaks in mid systole. Dynamic LVOTO causes turbulent flow through the aortic valve and may cause the aortic leaflets to flutter in systole, and this can be demonstrated well using M-mode echocardiography with the beam directed across the aortic valve.

Once SAM with or without dLVOTO has been diagnosed, the next step is to optimize the patient's hemodynamics by ensuring adequate intravascular volume, avoiding tachycardia, increasing afterload with vasoconstrictors, and if possible eliminating inotropes. Once this has been achieved, the patient should be reevaluated for SAM, mitral regurgitation, and dLVOTO. Only rarely then may it be necessary to return to bypass and rerepair or replace the valve. The decision as to whether or not to return to bypass and attempt to improve the repair should be patient specific. SAM and dLVOTO are mixed structural and functional pathologies, so that patients predisposed to develop SAM by the structure of their mitral apparatus will likely have symptoms precipitated by functional demand, for example, with tachycardia and possibly dehydration during exercise. This must be borne in mind in evaluating the risk-to-benefit profile of returning to bypass for a particular patient.

Aortic Insufficiency/Ventricular Rupture/Aortic Dissection

New aortic valve insufficiency can occur after MV repair, particularly if the annuloplasty suture has captured either the left or noncoronary cusps of the aortic valve (Videos 10.44 and 10.45). Ventricular rupture is a potentially life-threatening though extremely rare potential complication of MV surgery (54). Patients with heavily calcified mitral annulus are most at risk. Aortic dissection likewise is a rare but potentially devastating complication (55). It is recommended that the comprehensive intraoperative TEE exam be repeated at the end of surgery to screen for these pathologies.

SUMMARY

Successful MV repair surgery relies on applying the appropriate surgical technique to the patient's particular pathology (56). Accordingly, TEE plays an integral role in success by providing an accurate diagnosis of the presence of regurgitation, classification of its pathophysiology and severity, estimation of the likelihood of valve reparability, and postoperative evaluation of the surgical result.

REFERENCES

1. Otto MC, Nishimura RA, Bonow RO, et al. 2020 ACC/AHA guideline for the management of patients with valvular heart disease: a report of the American College of Cardiology/American Heart Association Joint Committee on clinical practice guidelines. *Circulation*. 2021;143(5):e72-e227.
2. Borger AM, Alam A, Murphy PM, Doenst T, David TE. Chronic ischemic mitral regurgitation: repair, replace or rethink? *Ann Thorac Surg*. 2006;81(3):1153-1161.
3. Vahanian A, Beyersdorf F, Praz F, et al. 2021 ESC/EACTS guidelines for the management of valvular heart disease: developed by the Task Force for the management of valvular heart disease of the European Society of Cardiology (ESC) and the European Association for Cardio-Thoracic Surgery (EACTS). *Rev Esp Cardiol (Engl Ed)*. 2022;75(6):524.
4. Enriquez-Sarano M, Akins WC, Vahanian A. Mitral regurgitation. *Lancet*. 2009;373(9672):1382-1394.
5. Enriquez-Sarano M, Schaff HV, Orszulak TA, Tajik AJ, Bailey KR, Frye RL. Valve repair improves the outcome of surgery for mitral regurgitation. A multivariate analysis. *Circulation*. 1995;91(4):1022-1028.
6. Chikwe J, Goldstone AB, Passage J, et al. A propensity score-adjusted retrospective comparison of early and mid-term results of mitral valve repair versus replacement in octogenarians. *Eur Heart J*. 2011;32(5): 618-626.
7. Acker AM, Parides MK, Perrault LP, et al. Mitral-valve repair versus replacement for severe ischemic mitral regurgitation. *N Engl J Med*. 2014;370(1):23-32.
8. Badhwar V, Chikwe J, Gillinov AM, et al. Risk of surgical mitral valve repair for primary mitral regurgitation. *Ann Thorac Surg*. 2023;115(3):600-610.
9. Alfieri O, Maisano F, De Bonis M, et al. The double-orifice technique in mitral valve repair: a simple solution for complex problems. *J Thorac Cardiovasc Surg*. 2001;122(4):674-681.
10. Feldman T, Foster E, Glower DD, et al. Percutaneous repair or surgery for mitral regurgitation. *N Engl J Med*. 2011;364(15):1395-1406.
11. Grewal J, Mankad S, Freeman WK, et al. Real-time three-dimensional transesophageal echocardiography in the intraoperative assessment of mitral valve disease. *J Am Soc Echocardiogr*. 2009;22(1):34-41.
12. Mukherjee C, Tschernich H, Kaisers UX, Eibel S, Seeburger J, Ender J. Real-time three-dimensional echocardiographic assessment of mitral valve: is it really superior to 2D transesophageal echocardiography? *Ann Card Anaesth*, 2011;14(2):91-96.
13. Moustafa SE, Chandrasekaran K, Khandheria B, Tajik J, Mookadam F. Real-time three-dimensional transesophageal echocardiography assessment of the mitral valve: perioperative advantages and game-changing findings. *J Heart Valve Dis*. 2011;20(2):114-122.
14. Lancellotti P, Moura L, Pierard LA, et al. European Association of Echocardiography recommendations for the assessment of valvular regurgitation. Part 2: mitral and tricuspid regurgitation (native valve disease). *Eur J Echocardiogr*. 2010;11(4):307-332.
15. Carpentier AF, Lessana A, Relland JY, et al. The "Physio-Ring": an advanced concept in mitral valve annuloplasty. *Ann Thorac Surg*. 1995;60(5):1177-1186.
16. Hahn TR, Abraham T, Adams MS, et al. Guidelines for performing a comprehensive transesophageal echocardiographic examination: recommendations from the American Society of Echocardiography and the Society of Cardiovascular Anesthesiologists. *J Am Soc Echocardiogr*. 2013;26(9):921-964.
17. Enriquez-Sarano M, Tajik AJ, Schaff HV, et al. Echocardiographic prediction of left ventricular function after correction of mitral regurgitation: results and clinical implications. *J Am Coll Cardiol*. 1994;24(6):1536-1543.
18. Tribouilloy MC, Enriquez-Sarano M, Schaff HV, et al. Impact of preoperative symptoms on survival after surgical correction of organic mitral regurgitation. *Circulation*. 1999;99(3):400-405.
19. Lang MR, Badano LP, Mor-Avi V, et al. Recommendations for cardiac chamber quantification by echocardiography in adults: an update from the American Society of Echocardiography and the European Association of Cardiovascular Imaging. *Eur Heart J Cardiovasc Imaging*. 2015;16(3):233-271.
20. Galderisi M, Cosyns B, Edvardsen T, et al. Standardization of adult transthoracic echocardiography reporting in agreement with recent chamber quantification, diastolic function, and heart valve disease recommendations: an expert consensus document of the European Association of Cardiovascular Imaging. *Eur Heart J Cardiovasc Imaging*. 2017;18(12):1301-1310.
21. Lang MR, Badano LP, Tsang W, et al. EAE/ASE recommendations for image acquisition and display using three-dimensional echocardiography. *Eur Heart J Cardiovasc Imaging*. 2012;13(1):1-46.
22. Shah MP. Current concepts in mitral valve prolapse—diagnosis and management. *J Cardiol*. 2010;56(2):125-133.
23. Calafiore MA, Gallina S, Di Mauro M, et al. Mitral valve procedure in dilated cardiomyopathy: repair or replacement? *Ann Thorac Surg*. 2001;71(4):1146-1152.
24. Kuwahara E, Otsuji Y, Iguro Y, et al. Mechanism of recurrent/persistent ischemic/functional mitral regurgitation in the chronic phase after surgical annuloplasty. *Circulation*. 2006;114(1_supplement):I-529-I-534.
25. Falk V, Seeburger J, Czesla M, et al. How does the use of polytetrafluoroethylene neochordae for posterior mitral valve prolapse (loop technique) compare with leaflet resection? A prospective randomized trial. *J Thorac Cardiovasc Surg*. 2008;136(5):1200-1206.
26. Tavilla G, Pacini D. Damage to the circumflex coronary artery during mitral valve repair with sliding leaflet technique. *Ann Thorac Surg*. 1998;66(6):2091-2093.
27. Torres CS, Sanders JVS, Martins de Brito H, et al. Anatomical relationship between mitral valve annulus and circumflex artery and its surgical implications. *Morphologie*. 2020;104(346):182-186.
28. Aybek T, Risteski P, Miskovic A, et al. Seven years' experience with suture annuloplasty for mitral valve repair. *J Thorac Cardiovasc Surg*. 2006;131(1):99-106.
29. Ender J, Selbach M, Borger MA, et al. Echocardiographic identification of iatrogenic injury of the circumflex artery during minimally invasive mitral valve repair. *Ann Thorac Surg*. 2010;89(6):1866-1872.
30. Ender J, Singh R, Nakahira J, Subramanian S, Thiele H, Mukherjee C. Visualization of the circumflex artery in the perioperative setting with transesophageal echocardiography. *Anesth Analg*. 2012;115(1):22-26.
31. Konstadt NS, Reich DL, Kahn R, Viggiani RF. Transesophageal echocardiography can be used to screen for ascending aortic atherosclerosis. *Anesth Analg*. 1995;81(2):225-228.

32. Shiran A, Sagie A. Tricuspid regurgitation in mitral valve disease. *J Am Coll Cardiol.* 2009;53(5):401-408.
33. Dini LF, Conti U, Fontanive P, et al. Right ventricular dysfunction is a major predictor of outcome in patients with moderate to severe mitral regurgitation and left ventricular dysfunction. *Am Heart J.* 2007;154(1):172-179.
34. Seeburger J, Falk V, Borger MA, et al. Chordae replacement versus resection for repair of isolated posterior mitral leaflet prolapse: à ègalité. *Ann Thorac Surg.* 2009;87(6):1715-1720.
35. Delgado V, Ajmone Marsan N, de Waha S, et al. 2023 ESC guidelines for the management of endocarditis. *Eur Heart J.* 2023;44(39):3948-4042.
36. Maslow DA, Regan MM, Haering JM, Johnson RG, Levine RA. Echocardiographic predictors of left ventricular outflow tract obstruction and systolic anterior motion of the mitral valve after mitral valve reconstruction for myxomatous valve disease. *J Am Coll Cardiol.* 1999;34(7):2096-2104.
37. Gillinov AM, Cosgrove MD. Modified sliding leaflet technique for repair of the mitral valve. *Ann Thorac Surg.* 1999;68(6):2356-2357.
38. Carpentier A. Cardiac valve surgery—the "French correction". *J Thorac Cardiovasc Surg.* 1983;86(3):323-337.
39. Johnston RD, Gillinov AM, Blackstone EH, et al. Surgical repair of posterior mitral valve prolapse: implications for guidelines and percutaneous repair. *Ann Thorac Surg.* 2010;89(5):1385-1394.
40. Ender J, Eibel S, Mukherjee C, et al. Prediction of the annuloplasty ring size in patients undergoing mitral valve repair using real-time three-dimensional transoesophageal echocardiography. *Eur J Echocardiogr.* 2011;12(6):445-453.
41. Seeburger J, Borger MA, Doll N, et al. Comparison of outcomes of minimally invasive mitral valve surgery for posterior, anterior and bileaflet prolapse. *Eur J Cardiothorac Surg.* 2009;36(3):532-538.
42. Kuntze T, Borger MA, Falk V, et al., Early and mid-term results of mitral valve repair using premeasured Gore-Tex loops ('loop technique'). *Eur J Cardiothorac Surg.* 2008;33(4):566-572.
43. Duran CM, Pekar F. Techniques for ensuring the correct length of new mitral chords. *J Heart Valve Dis.* 2003;12(2):156-161.
44. Calafiore MA. Choice of artificial chordae length according to echocardiographic criteria. *Ann Thorac Surg.* 2006;81(1):375-377.
45. David ET. Outcomes of mitral valve repair for mitral regurgitation due to degenerative disease. *Semin Thorac Cardiovasc Surg.* 2007;19(2):116-120.
46. Gillinov AM, Cosgrove MD. Chordal transfer for repair of anterior leaflet prolapse. *Semin Thorac Cardiovasc Surg.* 2004;16(2):169-173.
47. Kondur A, Pitta S, Afonso L. Incremental utility of real-time three-dimensional echocardiography in the diagnosis and preoperative assessment of cleft mitral valve in adults. *Eur J Echocardiogr.* 2008;9(4):586-588.
48. Secknus M-A, Asher CR, Scalia GM, Cosgrove DM 3rd, Stewart WJ. Intraoperative transesophageal echocardiography in minimally invasive cardiac valve surgery. *J Am Soc Echocardiogr.* 1999;12(4):231-236.
49. Heß H, Eibel S, Mukherjee C, Kaisers UX, Ender J. Quantification of mitral valve regurgitation with color flow Doppler using baseline shift. *Int J Cardiovasc Imaging.* 2013;29(2):267-274.
50. Fix J, Isada L, Cosgrove D, et al. Do patients with less than 'echo-perfect' results from mitral valve repair by intraoperative echocardiography have a different outcome? *Circulation.* 1993;88(5 pt 2):Ii39-Ii48.
51. Suri MR, Clavel MA, Schaff HV, et al. Effect of recurrent mitral regurgitation following degenerative mitral valve repair. *J Am Coll Cardiol.* 2016;67(5):488-498.
52. Riegel KA, Busch R, Segal S, Fox JA, Eltzschig HK, Shernan SK. Evaluation of transmitral pressure gradients in the intraoperative echocardiographic diagnosis of mitral stenosis after mitral valve repair. *PLoS One.* 2011;6(11):e26559.
53. Baumgartner H, Hung J, Bermejo J, et al. Echocardiographic assessment of valve stenosis: EAE/ASE recommendations for clinical practice. *J Am Soc Echocardiogr.* 2009;22(1):1-23.
54. Deniz H, Sokullu O, Sanioglu S, et al. Risk factors for posterior ventricular rupture after mitral valve replacement: results of 2560 patients. *Eur J Cardiothorac Surg.* 2008;34(4):780-784.
55. Williams LM, Sheng S, Gammie JS, Rankin JS, Smith PK, Hughes GC. Richard E. Clark Award. Aortic dissection as a complication of cardiac surgery: report from the Society of Thoracic Surgeons database. *Ann Thorac Surg.* 2010;90(6):1812-1817.
56. Adams HD, Rosenhek R, Falk V. Degenerative mitral valve regurgitation: best practice revolution. *Eur Heart J.* 2010;31(16):1958-1966.

QUESTIONS

1. **Mitral repair versus replacement is most beneficial for patients with which underlying pathology?**
   A. Ischemic mitral regurgitation
   B. MV endocarditis with extensive anterior leaflet destruction
   C. Posterior leaflet P2 segment flail
   D. Papillary muscle rupture post-ST-elevation myocardial infarction

2. **Mitral regurgitation caused by an isolated P2 segment prolapse would be expected to demonstrate a color flow Doppler jet which is initially directed:**
   A. Anteriorly
   B. Posteriorly
   C. Centrally
   D. Around the left atrium hugging the atrial wall

3. **Which of the following conditions typically causes "secondary mitral regurgitation"?**
   A. Myxomatous (Barlow) disease
   B. Anterior leaflet cleft
   C. Dilated cardiomyopathy
   D. Ruptured MV chordae

4. **Following MV repair surgery for isolated posterior leaflet prolapse, moderate mitral regurgitation is identified on the intraoperative TEE. Select the most appropriate next action:**
   A. Reduce systemic afterload with vasodilators and reassess the severity of regurgitation.
   B. Administer protamine and reassess the severity of mitral regurgitation.
   C. Return to cardiopulmonary bypass to replace the valve.
   D. Determine the mechanism of regurgitation with a comprehensive TEE exam and discuss options for rerepair with the surgeon.

5. **Circumflex artery injury post MV surgery:**
   A. Occurs with an incidence of approximately 6% to 8%
   B. Should be suspected in any case of new wall motion abnormality or ECG signs of ischemia post-mitral surgery
   C. Cannot occur in cases of MV replacement
   D. Is of no further clinical significance

6. **Which of the following TEE measurements/findings is most likely to influence surgical technique of an MV surgery?**
   A. Tenting height
   B. Presence of a patent foramen ovale
   C. Mild aortic stenosis
   D. Moderate pulmonary hypertension

7. **Regarding mitral regurgitation caused by papillary muscle rupture, which of the following statements is true?**
   A. Rupture of the posteromedial papillary muscle is more common because it relies on a single blood supply.
   B. Papillary muscle rupture leads to restriction of the MV segments to which it is attached, and this is the mechanism of regurgitation.
   C. MV repair is clearly recommended over valve replacement for regurgitation secondary to papillary muscle rupture.
   D. Transthoracic echo is more sensitive than transesophageal echo in diagnosing papillary muscle rupture.

8. **A patient with severe mitral regurgitation due to P2 segment prolapse is scheduled for mitral repair. Which of the following repair techniques would be unacceptable?**
   A. Posterior leaflet neo chordae implantation with an annuloplasty
   B. Posterior leaflet P2 quadrangular resection with an annuloplasty
   C. Anterior leaflet A2 quadrangular resection with an annuloplasty
   D. Alfieri (double orifice) repair with suturing together of A2 and P2 segments with an annuloplasty

9. **Following an open surgical Alfieri (double orifice) repair, which of the following potential complications is relatively more likely compared with other standard repair techniques?**
   A. Circumflex artery injury
   B. Residual mitral regurgitation greater than mild severity
   C. Mitral stenosis due to reduction in valve opening area
   D. Aortic regurgitation due to right coronary cusp aortic valve damage

10. **Which of the following conditions gives rise to mitral regurgitation which would typically be associated with Carpentier type I leaflet motion?**
   A. Posterior leaflet prolapse
   B. Posterior leaflet restriction
   C. Posterior leaflet perforation
   D. Rheumatic heart disease

ANSWERS

1. **Correct Answer: C.**
Rationale: Patients with mitral regurgitation secondary to excessive leaflet motion clearly benefit from repair over replacement. This is not clear from those with ischemic mitral regurgitation where no clear benefit was seen in a randomized clinical study. Repair is a valid option to consider for patients with endocarditis; however, the emphasis should be on clearing and excising all infected material, so the decision should be made on a case-by-case basis. The optimal approach to papillary muscle rupture is uncertain, and this is reflected in current guidelines. Repair may be considered; however, the pathology may also be classified as ischemic, thus replacement may be more appropriate.

2. **Correct Answer: A.**
Rationale: The P2 segment is in the middle of the MV segments, and not directly related to the left atrial wall, so the jet would be expected to be directed anteriorly initially. Depending on its severity, it may then continue to hug the left atrial wall. Prolapse is defined by the leaflet edge being above the mitral annular plane in systole, so regurgitant blood flow is typically directed over the anterior leaflet for isolated posterior prolapse. If the anterior leaflet is also prolapsing, then the resultant regurgitant jet may actually be centrally directed.

3. **Correct Answer: C.**
Rationale: Dilated cardiomyopathy is a disease of the ventricular muscle, causing ventricular dilatation and thus impairing the ability of the mitral leaflets to coapt. There is no actual pathology of the leaflets, which themselves remain structurally normal. The other options are all pathologies of the mitral apparatus, and thereby are classified as primary causes of mitral regurgitation. This has implications in helping to determine the decision between repair versus replacement.

4. **Correct Answer: D.**
Rationale: This patient has pathology which is best treated with repair. However, moderate regurgitation seen on intraoperative TEE post repair is associated with a higher incidence of significant residual regurgitation and reoperation later and therefore is unacceptable. The expectations of repair surgery for this pathology are high. Reducing afterload may make the regurgitation appear less significant; however, this is false and not the approach to take in this scenario. Intraoperative evaluation of regurgitation must be performed with loading conditions as close to normal as possible. Protamine has no ability to alter the severity of mitral regurgitation, and this approach does not address the actual problem. Replacing the valve may ultimately be the best option, as replacement is better than a poor repair; however, the preference would be to fully evaluate the mechanism of regurgitation with TEE and plan how the repair could be improved, if possible.

5. **Correct Answer: B.**
Rationale: Circumflex artery injury is a significant potential complication of MV surgery and may be evaluated using TEE. The reported incidence generally is between 1% and 2%. It arises typically from suturing the artery close to the annulus, so it is also a risk of MV replacement surgery. Concurrent left atrial appendage suturing may also increase the risk.

6. **Correct Answer: A.**
Rationale: Tenting height may prompt consideration of valve replacement instead of repair. The presence of a patent foramen ovale is generally a benign incidental finding that can be closed easily during open surgery. Mild aortic stenosis has no influence on the approach to the MV, and pulmonary artery hypertension also does not have a direct influence on repair technique; however, as a risk factor overall for patient outcome, it may be considered in the overall approach to management.

7. **Correct Answer: A.**
Rationale: This is one area where optimal management remains unclear. The mechanism itself could be classified as Carpentier type II excessive leaflet motion, which would ordinarily favor repair. However, the underlying pathology is myocardial ischemia, a secondary cause of mitral regurgitation for which repair holds no clear advantage. In reality, there is often enough concern about the viability of the remaining papillary muscle to steer surgeons away from repair and toward replacement. The single arterial supply

of the posteromedial muscle predisposes it to damage from ischemia more than the anterolateral muscle, which has a dual blood supply. As for most pathologies of the MV, TEE is more specific and sensitive for papillary muscle rupture, with sensitivity for diagnosis approaching 85% approximately.

8. **Correct Answer: C.**
Rationale: Generally, any resection of the anterior leaflet is avoided in mitral repair surgery. Otherwise, it becomes very difficult to satisfy the goals of mitral repair, specifically to create a large leaflet coaptation area, and to preserve or restore full leaflet motion. The Alfieri approach does not have universal favor among surgeons; however, it is a technique that is proven to largely satisfy the goals of repair and importantly is technically easy to perform. It is also possibly a good second-choice technique to consider for rerepair if the first attempt is suboptimal.

9. **Correct Answer: C.**
Rationale: The double orifice technique whether open as in Alfieri's approach or percutaneous as in mitral TEER predisposes patients to have an increased MV gradient or even significant mitral stenosis and should always be considered and evaluated in patients undergoing this approach. The other options are no more likely to occur than for any other standard repair technique.

10. **Correct Answer: C.**
Rationale: Carpentier type I leaflet motion implies that the leaflets move normally; they are neither moving excessively nor restricted in their motion. A leaflet perforation is an example of type I leaflet motion.

11 Aortic Regurgitation

Praveen Mehrotra and Ira S. Cohen

The assessment of aortic regurgitation (AR) has evolved considerably with advances in echocardiographic technology since Ward et al (1) first described the use of pulsed-wave (PW) Doppler in conjunction with motion mode (M-mode) echocardiography and auscultation to detect AR. With current ultrasound technology, the exquisite sensitivity of transesophageal echocardiography (TEE) allows the physician to now detect the minute regurgitant jets engineered into the design of the St. Jude prosthetic valve to flush platelet aggregates off the valve surface and small paravalvular leaks after transcatheter aortic valve replacement (TAVR). Few studies have been performed investigating the assessment of AR primarily using TEE because of its relatively invasive nature. However, most assessments of the severity of AR are based on the assumption that transthoracic echocardiographic (TTE) approaches should be equally applicable to TEE.

ETIOLOGY AND MECHANISMS OF AORTIC REGURGITATION

The physiologic functioning of the aortic valve in diastole is dependent on the interplay of several components forming a complex that includes the aortic valve leaflets, aortic annulus, sinuses of Valsalva, and the sinotubular junction. The aortic annulus is formed by the basal insertions of the leaflets into the muscle of the left ventricular outflow tract (LVOT) and the fibrosa of the anterior mitral leaflet. The aortic valve leaflets then extend as semilunar structures along the sinuses of Valsalva to end at the sinotubular junction where the commissures are formed and whose diameter is normally 10% to 15% smaller than the diameter of the true aortic annulus (2). A delineation of the mechanisms of AR is of increasing clinical importance as the mechanism impacts on the surgical approach including determination of suitability for valve repair. A proposed classification system (Table 11.1) has been advanced that involves three functional mechanisms (Figure 11.1) (3-6):

TABLE 11.1 Etiology and Mechanisms of Aortic Regurgitation

Type 1: Normal cusp motion • **dilation of ascending aorta and sinotubular junction (STJ) (1A)** • **dilation of aortic root at sinuses of Valsalva and STJ (1B)** • **dilation of aortic annulus (1C)** • **leaflet perforation (1D)**	Congenital aortic root abnormalities Connective tissue disease (Marfan syndrome, Ehlers-Danlos syndrome, Loeys-Dietz syndrome) Bicuspid valve–associated aortopathy Acquired aortic root abnormalities Autoimmune disease (systemic lupus erythematosus, ankylosing spondylitis) Aortitis (syphilitic, Takayasu's) Aortic dissection Aortic trauma Hypertension Idiopathic Endocarditis (leaflet perforation)
Type 2: Excessive cusp motion (cusp prolapse or flail)	Bicuspid aortic valve disease Acute aortic dissection Ventricular septal defect
Type 3: Restricted cusp motion	Calcific degeneration Bicuspid aortic valve disease Radiation valvulopathy Infective endocarditis Rheumatic disease Toxin-induced valvulopathy

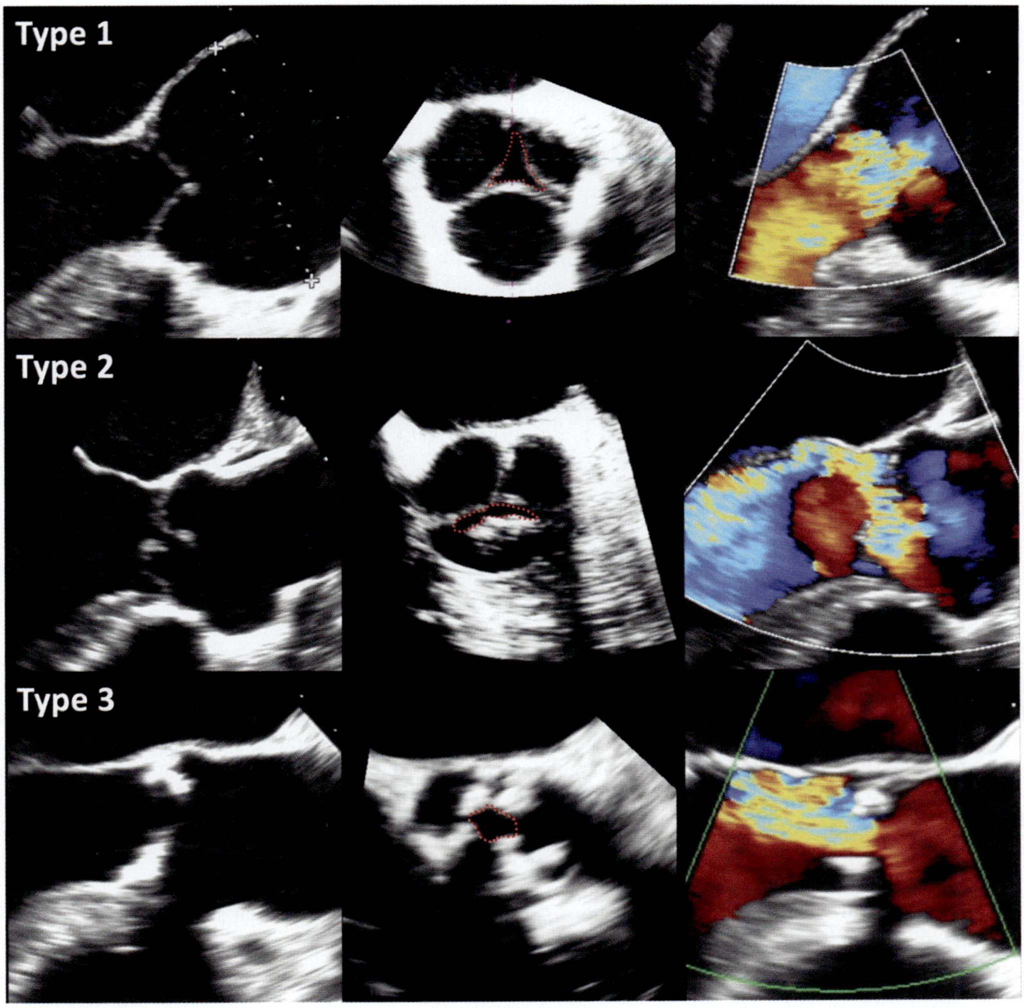

FIGURE 11.1 Examples of the various mechanisms of aortic regurgitation. Type 1: Severe dilation of the aortic root at the sinuses of Valsalva resulting in incomplete leaflet closure and severe, central aortic regurgitation (top). A central, triangular regurgitant orifice is present (dotted red tracing). Type 2: Complete prolapse of the right coronary cusp of a trileaflet aortic valve resulting in highly eccentric, severe aortic regurgitation (middle). An elliptical regurgitant orifice is present (dotted red tracing). Type 3: Severe restriction of heavily calcified aortic valve leaflets in a patient with both severe aortic stenosis and severe aortic regurgitation (bottom). A relatively circular regurgitant orifice is present (dotted red tracing).

Type 1: AR is due to the enlargement of any of the components of the aortic root or ascending aorta with normal aortic cusp motion, as seen in idiopathic annuloaortic ectasia, ascending aortic aneurysm, Marfan syndrome, aortitis, or Ehlers-Danlos syndrome (Videos 11.1 and 11.2). Aortic enlargement results in outward displacement of the commissures and leaflet tethering, which leads to incomplete leaflet closure in diastole generally resulting in a central regurgitant orifice and jet. Type 1 AR has been subdivided depending on the location of enlargement: type 1A (ascending aorta and sinotubular junction), type 1B (sinuses of Valsalva and sinotubular junction), and type 1C (aortic annulus). Type 1 AR also includes regurgitation due to aortic cusp perforation (type 1D).

Type 2: AR is due to excessive cusp motion from complete or partial prolapse or flail aortic cusp resulting in non-coaptation below the annular plane (Videos 11.3 and 11.4). Prolapse or flail cusps can occur in the setting of excessive cusp tissue (eg, bicuspid aortic valve or congenitally elongated cusp), disruption of

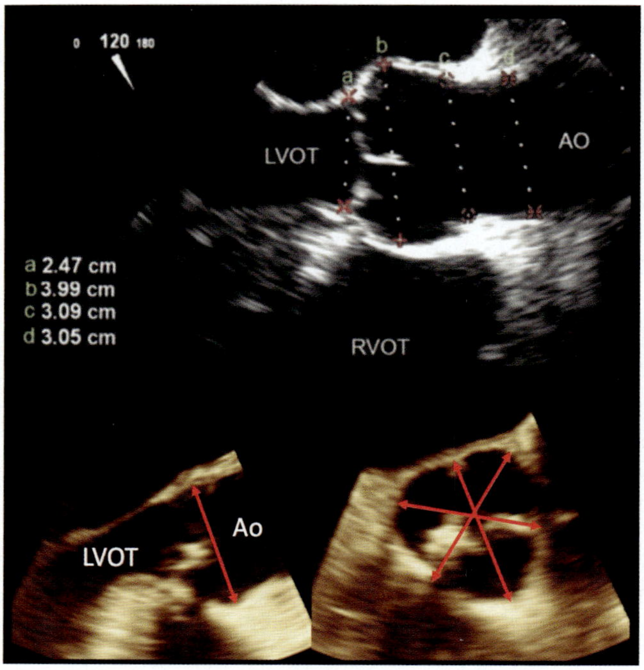

FIGURE 11.2 Midesophageal aortic valve long-axis view (top) demonstrating appropriate locations for measuring the aortic annulus (a), sinus of Valsalva (b), sinotubular junction (c), and proximal ascending aorta (d). Three-dimensional multiplanar reconstruction (bottom) demonstrating appropriate method to perform "sinus-to-commissure" aortic root measurements in the aortic root long- and short-axis views. Ao, aorta; LVOT, left ventricular outflow tract; RVOT, right ventricular outflow tract.

aortic commissures (eg, acute aortic dissection), or in the setting of a ventricular septal defect. Type 2 AR results in an eccentric regurgitant jet.

Type 3: AR is due to restricted leaflet motion and primary cusp damage resulting in poor leaflet coaptation (eg, calcific degenerative, rheumatic, radiation, quadricuspid, or bicuspid valve disease) (Videos 11.5 and 11.6). Regurgitant jets in type 3 AR may be eccentric or central.

The etiology of AR may also be multifactorial, with a single individual having AR from more than one mechanism (6). TEE evaluation has been shown to correlate very highly with surgical findings, and the evaluation of the potential mechanisms of AR should be part of the preoperative echocardiographic evaluation along with AR severity assessment (4). Lastly, the sizes of the components of the aortic root complex should be assessed prior to aortic valve surgery (Figure 11.2) not only since aortic dilation is frequently the primary cause of the AR itself but also because aortopathy is frequently present in patients with bicuspid valve disease.

HEMODYNAMICS OF AORTIC REGURGITATION

AR represents an increase in both preload and afterload to the left ventricle. The increase in preload is a result of the increased end-diastolic volume resulting from the added regurgitant volume. The increase in afterload is a function of the increased radius of the ventricle. An increase in the end-diastolic radius of a ventricle at any wall thickness causes an increase in the wall stress and the force needed to eject blood (law of Laplace). The general response of the ventricle to chronic AR is to gradually dilate and become more compliant to accommodate the extra volume and to hypertrophy in order to reduce wall stress. As the heart enlarges, the left ventricle hypertrophies primarily in a longitudinal manner with the addition of sarcomeres in series (ie, eccentric hypertrophy). Accordingly, the size of the ventricle is an index of the severity and duration of the regurgitation and should be factored into the assessment of the severity of the lesion.

Acute AR, most commonly due to a tear in the valve secondary to endocarditis, deceleration injury in a motor vehicle accident, or an acute aortic dissection, offers a contrasting clinical presentation. Acute AR is one of the least well-tolerated valvular lesions because of the limited ability of the heart to compensate for an acute increase in volume load by the mechanisms mentioned in the preceding text. Consequently, the LV diastolic pressure rises rapidly and is transmitted to the lungs, resulting in severe pulmonary congestion. Therefore, in acute AR, the chamber is often normal in size but with catastrophic hemodynamic consequences. Diagnosis of significant AR in the setting of heart failure is essential as intra-aortic balloon counterpulsation is contraindicated because diastolic pressure augmentation worsens the regurgitation.

The assessment of AR severity is complicated by the potentially dramatic effects of even transient changes in loading conditions and peripheral vascular resistance on Doppler indices. Because the operating room environment is one in which a multitude of factors affect both the preload and afterload of the ventricle, the potential impact of these changes must be borne in mind when the severity of a valvular lesion is evaluated. Acute increases in peripheral vascular resistance (eg, following surgical stimulation or the administration of vasopressors) can increase the apparent degree of valvular insufficiency by increasing systemic vascular resistance and impeding peripheral runoff. Conversely, vasodilators (eg, volatile anesthetics, angiotensin-converting enzyme inhibitors and receptor blockers, or calcium channel blockers) reduce peripheral vascular resistance and decrease the apparent degree of insufficiency, both clinically and by Doppler interrogation. The physical properties (eg, distensibility, elasticity, compliance) of the source (ie, the aorta) and recipient (ie, the left ventricle) of regurgitant flow, in addition to the size of the regurgitant orifice and the physical properties of the involved valve, are other dynamic variables that further complicate intraoperative assessment. Because of the multitude of factors influencing any assessment of the severity of AR, the estimate should be based on an integration of the results of all Doppler approaches providing technically adequate data in any given patient.

ECHOCARDIOGRAPHIC EVALUATION OF THE AORTIC VALVE

The aortic valve can be evaluated by M-mode, two-dimensional (2D), Doppler, and three-dimensional (3D) echocardiographic techniques. Transesophageal 2D echocardiographic imaging of the aortic valve is generally superior to transthoracic imaging because of the improved resolution of the higher frequency TEE probe, which makes it possible to delineate the size of regurgitant jets more accurately than with transthoracic techniques. Three-dimensional TEE also plays an important role in the assessment of AR, and reference is made to current observations utilizing 3D imaging for the assessment of regurgitant severity. Three-dimensional imaging, like 2D imaging, however, shares the limits inherent to all ultrasound techniques determined by the interrelation of sector (volume) size, frame (volume) rate, and depth on image resolution.

When imaging the regurgitant aortic valve and aortic root complex, it is, first, essential to determine the etiology of regurgitation by assessing leaflet structure, motion, and function. Two- and three-dimensional imaging of the aortic root complex should also be performed for precise measurement of dimensions of the aortic annulus, aortic root (at the sinuses of Valsalva), sinotubular junction, and ascending aorta (Figure 11.2). Following this structural assessment, a comprehensive Doppler echocardiographic assessment of the aortic valve should follow. In general, the assessment of AR severity involves an integrative approach that utilizes both qualitative and quantitative Doppler techniques. The various approaches to assessing the severity of AR with TEE will be presented in the order of their relative clinical applicability. The American Society of Echocardiography has also published detailed recommendations for the echocardiographic assessment of AR, which should be utilized as an important reference (5).

RECOMMENDED VIEWS

The most useful TEE views are generally obtained by starting from the standard midesophageal (ME) four-chamber view and changing the angle of interrogation to approximately 45° to obtain the aortic valve short-axis view. In this view, the individual aortic cusps and sinuses are visualized in exquisite detail. Anteflexing the probe in this view will bring the aortic valve into the near-field, improving the resolution of the image which is essential for 3D imaging. The angle of interrogation is then further increased to 120° to 150° to produce the ME long-axis view of the LVOT, aortic valve, and proximal aorta. Further withdrawal from this position with slight anteflexion can be used to visualize the proximal ascending aorta, while further withdrawal of the probe, decreasing the angle of interrogation to 100° or 110°, and continued anteflexion allow for visualization of the distal tubular ascending aorta. Biplane imaging of the aortic valve is also essential for simultaneous short- and long-axis imaging of the aortic valve, aortic root complex, and regurgitant jet. In addition, 3D imaging of the aortic valve can be performed either in the short-axis or long-axis view for the creation of unique en face volume renderings of the aortic valve complex and for multiplanar reconstruction of the regurgitant jet's vena contracta (VC) area.

Alternatively, but less frequently, good views can be obtained from a deep transgastric (TG) position at an angle close to 0° or greater, subject to individual variation, or from a standard midpapillary TG view at an angle of approximately 120° (TG long-axis view). These approaches have the advantage of aligning the ultrasound beam nearly parallel to the direction of blood flow, which is essential for accurate quantitative Doppler analysis of both the pressure half-time of the regurgitant jet as well as stroke volume. However, far-field beam widening and the greater distances traveled reduce spatial resolution in these views, making them a poor choice for visualizing the cross-sectional area of an AR jet immediately below the valve plane. However, they may be the only means of assessing the outflow tract in the presence of a prosthetic mitral valve (MV), which frequently causes acoustic shadowing of the aortic annulus in more standard views and, occasionally, of an aortic prosthesis when its ring obscures the outflow tract image by acoustic shadowing.

The pressure gradient between the regurgitant and recipient chambers in regurgitant valvular lesions is always high and in AR corresponds to the diastolic gradient between the aortic root and the left ventricle. By the simplified Bernoulli equation, the gradient equals 4 times the square of the peak jet velocity. In aortic regurgitant lesions, it is the rate of change in pressure gradients that provides clinically useful information unlike the peak velocity measurement used to assess stenotic lesions. While these data are best obtained in the TG views where the Doppler beam is most parallel to flow, fortunately, color Doppler techniques for the assessment of AR can also provide clinically useful information that is, to a significant degree, independent of the beam angle in relation to the regurgitant flow.

APPROACHES TO THE QUANTITATIVE ASSESSMENT OF AORTIC REGURGITATION

Color Flow Doppler

In the initial echocardiographic efforts of quantifying AR severity, color flow Doppler assessment of AR jets in the LVOT was validated against contrast aortography in human subjects (7-11), electromagnetic flow probes in animal models (12,13), intraoperative flow probes in human subjects (14), and in vitro models (15). From these studies, three main 2D techniques for color flow Doppler evaluation of AR jets were devised and are now recommended by current guidelines (5).

Ratio of Jet Height to Left Ventricular Outflow Tract Diameter

In the ME long-axis view of the aortic valve, the height of the AR jet is measured immediately below (within 1 cm of) the aortic valve plane and is then compared with the diameter of the LVOT at that same point (Figure 11.3 and Video 11.7).

The long-axis view that shows the maximal height of the color jet during diastole is selected for analysis and is identified during slow motion freeze-frame review. When performing this measurement, all three components of the jet—the proximal convergence, the VC, and distal jet—should be visualized so that an optimal measurement can be performed. A ratio of less than 25% indicates mild AR, 25% to 64% indicates moderate AR, and greater than or equal to 65% indicates severe AR (Table 11.2). Alternatively, an M-mode cursor can be placed perpendicular to the outflow tract. If color flow Doppler is then activated, the regurgitant jet will appear in color in the M-mode view of the outflow tract, and the relative dimensions can be measured from this display by using the caliper function of the ultrasound machine (Figure 11.4).

Ratio of Jet Area to the Left Ventricular Outflow Tract Area

In this second color flow Doppler technique, the short-axis area of the regurgitant jet in the LVOT is compared with the area of the LVOT at that same level (Figure 11.5 and Video 11.8).

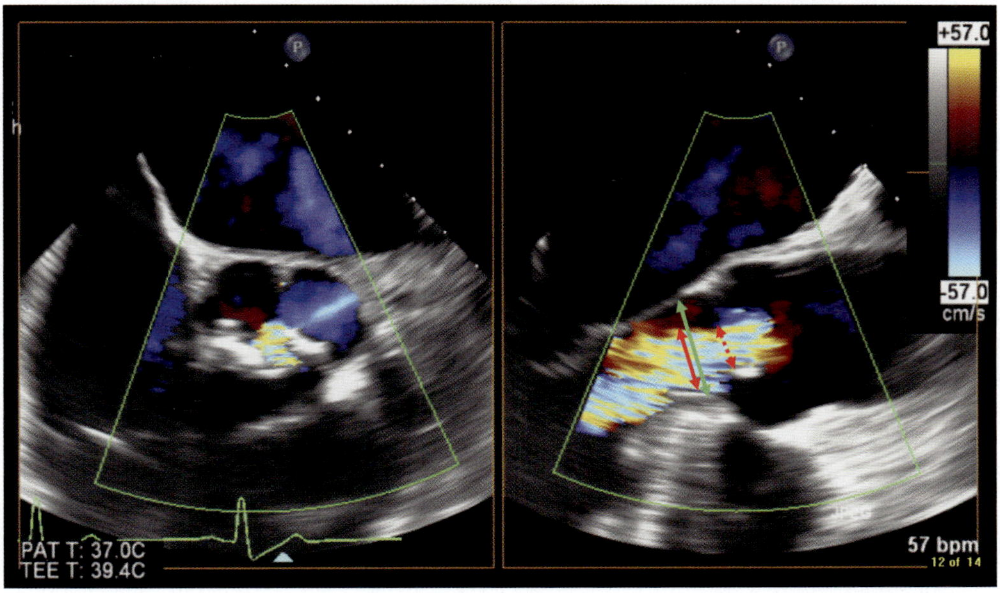

FIGURE 11.3 Midesophageal short-axis (left) and long-axis (right) views of the aortic valve with central regurgitant jet. The biplane cursor is placed through the center of the proximal flow convergence and regurgitant orifice in the short-axis view to create the corresponding long-axis view on the right. The maximal vena contracta width (dotted red line) and maximal jet height (red line) can then be measured, with the latter being compared to the LVOT diameter (green line). The vena contracta width is 8 mm. The jet height (1.4 cm) to LVOT diameter (2.1 cm) ratio is 66%. These findings are consistent with severe aortic regurgitation. LVOT, left ventricular outflow tract.

The preferred view for this approach is the ME aortic valve short-axis view, but with the probe advanced to immediately below the valve plane. Again, diastole is evaluated by slow motion freeze-frame review, and the maximal jet area is traced and compared with the area of the LVOT. Alternatively, biplane echocardiographic imaging can be utilized with the long-axis view of the LVOT as the reference plane; the biplane cursor is positioned 1 cm below the aortic valve to produce the corresponding short-axis view of the LVOT. A ratio of less than 5% indicates mild AR, 5% to 59% indicates moderate AR, and greater than or equal to 60% indicates severe AR (Table 11.2). This method is slightly more accurate than the jet height to LVOT diameter ratio method and is more easily performed with biplane imaging.

Vena Contracta Width

The third, and probably most important color Doppler technique, is the measurement of the VC width (Figure 11.3). The VC is the narrowest portion of the jet as flow converges after crossing the valve plane immediately downstream from the regurgitant orifice. The size of the VC is directly related to the size of the regurgitant orifice and is therefore considered a true measure of AR severity. Advantages of the VC measurement are that it is felt to be less dependent on the driving pressure (ie, diastolic blood pressure) and flow rate through the regurgitant orifice. In fact, changes in afterload obtained with phenylephrine or volume loading have been shown not to change the size of the VC (14). Measurements of the VC width have also been shown to have excellent correlation (better than jet height and area to LVOT ratios) with other quantitative Doppler parameters of AR severity (10).

The VC width is best measured in a zoomed ME long-axis view of the aortic valve between 120° and 150° in mid-diastole and will be smaller than the jet height that is measured downstream in the LVOT. To optimize visualization, the echo sector should be narrowed to optimize frame rate with subtle adjustments of angulation and rotation from this point to identify the largest VC width. Biplane imaging can also be utilized to identify the largest VC width (Figure 11.3). In some patients, particularly with very eccentric

TABLE 11.2 Echocardiographic Indices of Aortic Regurgitation Severity

Parameter	Mild	Moderate	Severe	Caveats
Structural Parameters				
Leaflets	Variable	Variable	Flail, wide coaptation defect	• Not reliable
LV size[a]	Normal	Variable	Usually dilated	• Enlarged in other conditions • Normal in acute AR
Quantitative Doppler Parameters[b]				
Jet/LVOT height[c] (%) Jet/LVOT area[c] (%)	<25 <5	25-45, 46-64 5-20, 21-59	≥65 ≥60	• Variable in eccentric jets • Affected by direction and shape of jets
VC width[c] (cm)	<0.3	0.3-0.6	>0.6	• Problematic with multiple jets • May be less accurate in non-circular orifice
VC area[c] (cm^2)	<0.1	0.1-0.29	≥0.30	• Measured primarily with 3D imaging
RVol (mL) RF (%) EROA (cm^2)	<30 <30 <0.1	30-44, 45-59 30-39, 40-49 0.1-0.19, 0.20-0.29	≥60 ≥50 ≥0.30	• Requires multiple measurements • Technically challenging • Time consuming
Qualitative Doppler Parameters				
Jet density	Faint	Dense	Dense	• Overlap between moderate and severe AR
Regurgitant slope (m/s^2) Pressure half-time (ms)	Slow >500	≥2 200-500	≥3 <200	• Effected by aortic and LV compliance • May be less accurate if beam is not oriented with jet
Diastolic flow reversal	Brief, early diastolic reversal	Intermediate	Prominent holodiastolic reversal	• Brief reversal is normal. • May be present in stiff aorta (in the absence of severe AR)

3D, three-dimensional; AR, aortic regurgitation; EROA, effective regurgitant orifice area; LV, left ventricular; LVOT, left ventricular outflow tract; RF, regurgitant fraction; RVol, regurgitant volume; VC, vena contracta.
[a]Left ventricular dimensions should be interpreted in the context of the patient's body surface area.
[b]Quantitative parameters allow for subclassification of moderate regurgitation into mild to moderate and moderate to severe AR.
[c]Performed at a Nyquist limit of 50-70 cm/s.

jets, visualization may still not be possible. A short-axis view of the VC can also be obtained from the ME short-axis view of the aortic valve, but precise visualization of the VC area with 2D imaging can be difficult due to cranial motion of the aortic valve complex during diastole. A VC width less than 3 mm defines mild AR, while a VC width greater than 6 mm defines severe AR (Table 11.2).

In practice, color Doppler approaches utilizing the jet height or area to LVOT ratios provide reliable estimates of severity and have consequently become widely regarded as among the best and most easily applied methods of Doppler assessment (5,7). However, they may be affected by changes in loading conditions and the size of the receiving chamber (ie, the LVOT). Moreover, severity of AR due to eccentric jets (ie, jets that are not coaxial with the long axis of the LVOT) may be underestimated by jet height and area to LVOT ratios (5). In these cases, the VC width can provide a reliable estimate of AR severity.

Three-Dimensional Vena Contracta Area

Regurgitant orifices and jets have three dimensions and their shape will affect how it is visualized in any given 2D imaging plane. If a jet arises from a narrow or "slit-like" regurgitant orifice between two aortic cusps along their line of coaptation, then interrogation perpendicular to that jet in a long-axis view may overestimate the severity of AR. In this case, a jet arising from a small regurgitant orifice may appear to fill the outflow tract in the long-axis view, while imaging of the short-axis view of the jet in the LVOT just below the aortic valve level will clarify that the jet area and VC area are, in fact, quite small. The advent of real-time 3D imaging of

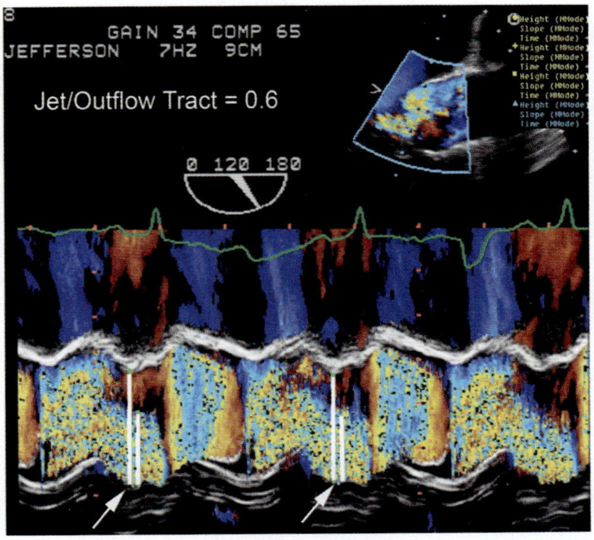

FIGURE 11.4 Color M-mode assessment of aortic regurgitation. From the midesophageal aortic valve long-axis view, the M-mode cursor is positioned perpendicular to the left ventricular outflow tract as close to the origin of the regurgitant jet as possible. The jet and the outflow tract are well delineated in the color M-mode display. Caliper measurement of the jet height is compared to that of the outflow tract (white arrows), and the resulting ratio of 60% corresponds to moderate to severe regurgitation.

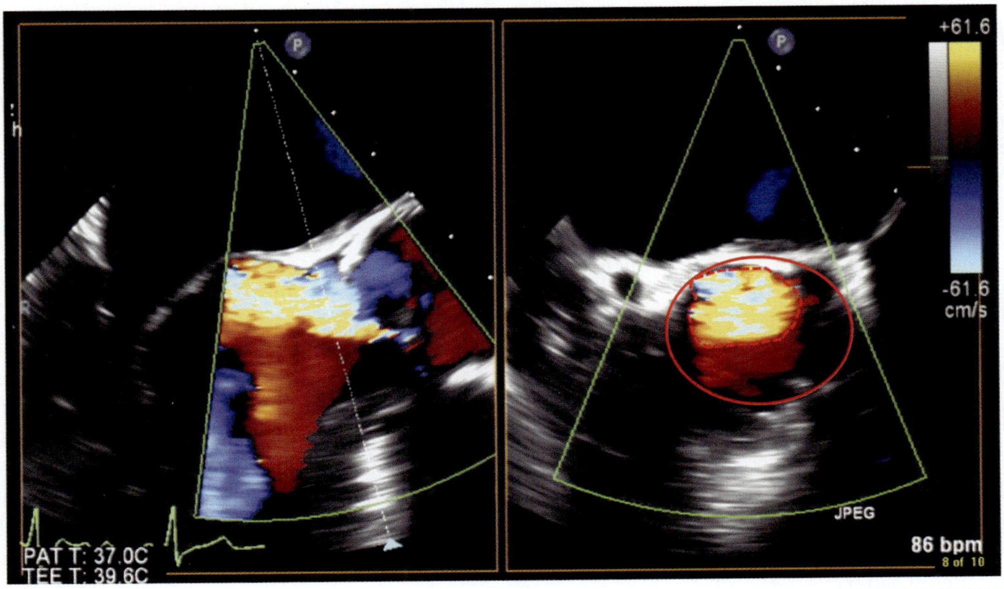

FIGURE 11.5 Midesophageal long-axis (left) and short-axis (right) views of the aortic valve with eccentric regurgitant jet. The biplane cursor is placed through the regurgitant jet approximately 1 cm below the aortic valve during diastole to create the corresponding short-axis view of the left ventricular outflow tract (LVOT; right). The jet area (dotted red tracing) to outflow tract area (solid red tracing) ratio is approximately 33% consistent with moderate to severe regurgitation. The jet height to LVOT diameter ratio of 54% is also consistent with moderate to severe regurgitation (measurements not shown). However, the eccentric jet is constrained in the LVOT; in this case, the vena contracta width and area (not shown) were consistent with severe regurgitation.

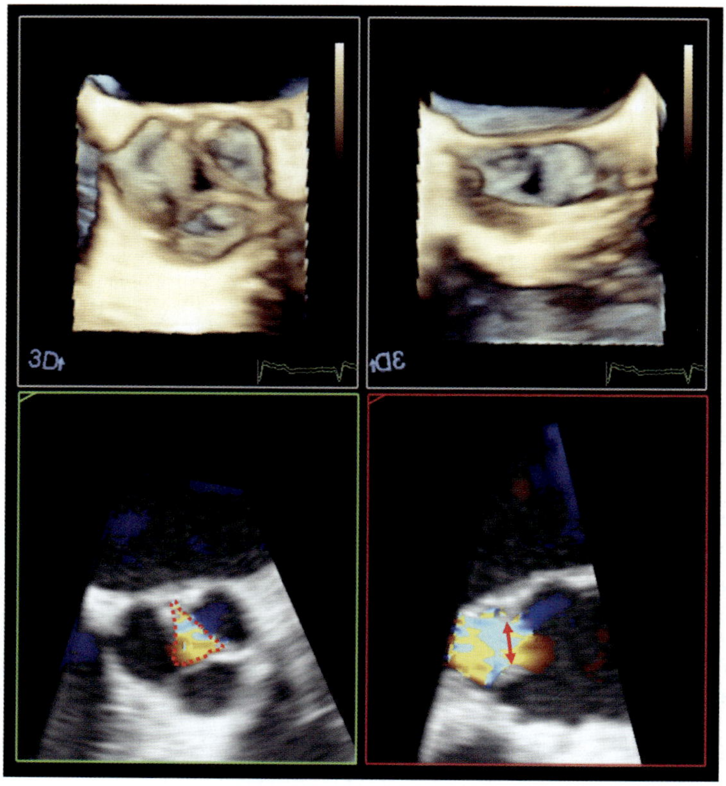

FIGURE 11.6 Three-dimensional imaging of the anatomic regurgitant orifice area and the vena contracta area. A triangular regurgitant orifice area is visualized on volume renderings from the aortic (top left) and left ventricular outflow tract (top right) views. With multiplanar reconstruction of three-dimensional color flow Doppler images, a transverse plane is positioned perpendicular to the direction of regurgitant flow at the vena contracta. A triangular vena contracta area is traced (bottom left); the vena contracta area is 0.44 cm^2 consistent with severe regurgitation. The vena contracta width can also be measured on the corresponding long-axis image (bottom right).

the VC area allows us to overcome the challenges that are presented by noncircular orifices, eccentric jets, and multiple jets, which may behave in varying manners in the LVOT.

The major potential advantage of 3D color Doppler imaging in the assessment of AR severity lies in its potential for en face imaging and direct planimetry of the VC area (Figure 11.6 and Videos 11.9-11.11), particularly in patients with eccentric jets (AR types 2 and 3) and complex orifice shapes.

The VC area obtained by 3D color Doppler imaging is considered a surrogate measurement of the effective regurgitant orifice area (EROA). While most, if not all, studies of VC area determination for AR severity assessment have been performed with 3D TTE, the superior resolution of transesophageal imaging would suggest comparable or superior utility. Furthermore, planimetry of the VC area multiplied by the time-velocity integral (TVI) obtained with continuous wave (CW) Doppler can provide an estimate of regurgitant volume.

The 3D VC area (by both TTE and TEE) has been shown to correlate well with conventional 2D quantitative color Doppler echocardiographic techniques and the 2D proximal isovelocity surface area (PISA) method (discussed later) (16-19). The 3D VC area also demonstrates excellent correlation with angiographic assessment of AR severity with little overlap between grades (19,20). Three-dimensional AR VC area–determined regurgitant volumes (ie, product of 3D VC area and AR TVI) have also been shown to correlate and agree better with regurgitant volumes obtained with cardiac magnetic resonance imaging compared to the 2D PISA method (21,22).

Three-dimensional color Doppler images of the aortic valve for planimetry of VC area are obtained and analyzed as follows:

1. Optimize the 2D short- or long-axis image of the aortic valve by optimizing probe position and using gain, compression, and overall depth controls.
2. Select the 3D zoom or full-volume color Doppler imaging option. Multi-beat mode (set to acquire at 2, 4, or 6 beats) can be used to increase spatial and temporal resolution if needed. Ensure that the LVOT and aortic sinuses are captured in the volumetric acquisition so that the proximal and distal jets are captured in the dataset.
3. The lateral and elevation widths (ie, volume size) should be optimized to include only those cardiac structures and portions of the regurgitant jet that are required for analysis and to increase spatial and temporal resolution of the volumetric acquisition. The minimum temporal resolution required for 3D analysis is generally 10 to 15 Hz.
4. Activate the imaging system's multiplanar reconstruction software package.
5. Select the appropriate mid-diastolic frame by observing for the maximal size of the AR jet in the LVOT.
6. Align the long-axis planes in the direction of the regurgitant blood flow starting from the VC.
7. Advance the transverse (ie, short-axis) plane to the level of the VC area just beyond the proximal flow convergence. Rotate/tilt the transverse planes as needed so that the plane is exactly perpendicular to regurgitant flow at the VC. The VC area may not always lie perpendicular to the long axis of the aorta (particularly for eccentric jets).
8. Move one or two frames back and then forward to visualize the motion of the leaflets, direction and behavior of the AR jet, and shape of the VC area.
9. Perform measurement using the "area" tool. Take care not to include portions of the proximal flow convergence or distal jet in the tracing. Color Doppler gain settings may need to be decreased to prevent over-measurement due to blooming of color Doppler pixels from poor spatial resolution.

Since the VC area is considered generally equivalent to the EROA, a value greater than or equal to 0.3 cm^2 indicates severe AR while a value less than 0.10 cm^2 indicates mild AR (19,23).

Calculation of Regurgitant Volume, Fraction, and Orifice Area

Volumetric Method

The AR volume can be calculated from the difference between the LVOT stroke volume and the right ventricular (RV) or mitral stroke volume in the absence of other regurgitant lesions (eg, mitral regurgitation). First, the LV stroke volume is calculated by multiplying the cross-sectional area of the LVOT (which is determined by utilizing the formula $\pi(D/2)^2$, where D is the LVOT diameter) with the TVI of LVOT flow obtained with PW Doppler either in a deep TG or TG long-axis view. The mitral stroke volume is then determined from the product of the cross-sectional area of the MV annulus (calculated from mitral annular diameter measured in the ME four-chamber view using the formula $\pi(D/2)^2$) and the mitral TVI, which is obtained by placing the PW Doppler sample volume at the mitral annulus (not at the leaflet tips) in the same view. Alternatively, the RV stroke volume is estimated from cross-sectional area of the RV outflow tract (calculated from RV outflow tract diameter) and TVI obtained in a similar fashion with the PW Doppler sample volume placed in the RV outflow tract. These calculations can be technically challenging due to the elliptical shapes of the mitral annulus and RV outflow tract and difficulty in obtaining an RV outflow tract TVI in the TG view. Finally, the LVOT stroke volume minus the mitral (or RV) stroke volume gives the aortic regurgitant volume. However, obtaining multiple, accurate measurements of the necessary parameters in an intraoperative situation is time consuming and technically challenging, so that this approach may be impractical. The regurgitant volume divided by the LVOT stroke volume provides the aortic regurgitant fraction, while the regurgitant volume divided by the AR TVI is equal to the EROA. Ranges and cutoffs for regurgitant volume, regurgitant fraction, and EROA in the assessment of AR severity are shown in Table 11.2.

Proximal Isovelocity Surface Area Method

In valvular regurgitation, blood flow converges toward the regurgitant orifice in hemispheric shells of increasing velocity and decreasing surface area; the velocity and surface area of these shells can then be used

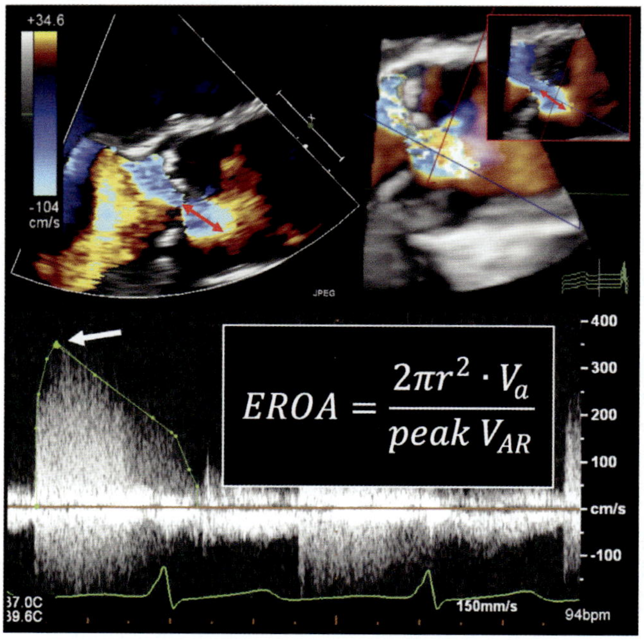

FIGURE 11.7 Proximal isovelocity surface area method for calculation of the effective regurgitant orifice area. The radius of the proximal flow convergence is measured in the midesophageal long-axis view (top left) with the baseline shifted upward in the same direction as the jet. In the case of a central jet, the radius would have to be measured in a transgastric view. The proximal flow convergence is shown with three-dimensional imaging (top right). Multiplanar reconstruction can be utilized to obtain the largest proximal flow convergence radius (inset, top right). The peak regurgitant velocity (white arrow) and time-velocity integral (bottom) are then utilized to calculate the regurgitant orifice area and regurgitant volume, respectively. EROA, effective regurgitant orifice area; *r*, radius; V_a, aliasing velocity; and peak V_{AR}, peak velocity of aortic regurgitant jet.

to calculate the regurgitant flow rate. Based on the law of conservation of mass, the flow rate can be used to determine the EROA. Compared to the assessment of mitral regurgitation, the 2D PISA method has only been studied in a limited fashion for the quantitative assessment of AR severity (24,25). The PISA method may be limited in the presence of aortic valve calcification, may not be possible in the setting of multiple jets, and may be less accurate in the presence of eccentric jets (5). Moreover, measurement of the PISA radius (Figure 11.7) for AR may not always be possible in the ME long-axis view (although the jet is better visualized here) as the proximal convergence and AR jet are likely to be perpendicular to the ultrasound beam (except in the presence of an eccentric jet). Measurement of the PISA radius is, therefore, typically performed in a zoomed TG long-axis or deep TG view. Small errors in the PISA radius measurement, however, can lead to substantial errors in the calculation of the EROA due to the squaring of the error (5).

To perform the measurements needed for the PISA calculation, the Doppler beam must be aligned in the direction of the regurgitant flow. The color baseline is shifted in the direction of the jet, and the PISA radius is measured from the point of color Doppler aliasing to the VC. The EROA by the 2D PISA method is calculated as follows:

$$\text{EROA} = \frac{2\pi r^2 \times Va}{\text{peak } V_{AR}}$$

where *r* is the PISA radius, V_a is the aliasing velocity, and peak V_{AR} is the peak velocity of the AR jet measured by CW Doppler (Figure 11.7). The 2D PISA EROA can then be multiplied by the AR TVI obtained by CW Doppler to obtain the AR regurgitant volume. The cutoffs for EROA and regurgitant volume for mild, moderate, and severe AR are the same as those determined by the volumetric method (Table 11.2).

Pulsed- and Continuous Wave Doppler

Aortic Diastolic Flow Reversal

Another early index of the severity of AR was based on the demonstration of retrograde diastolic flow in the aorta (26). Retrograde flow can be assessed by interrogating the upper esophageal view of the aortic arch, the descending thoracic aorta (Figure 11.8), and the abdominal aorta. This short-axis view of the descending thoracic or abdominal aorta is obtained by rotating the probe posteriorly to visualize the descending aorta in the ME view or TG view at 0°, respectively. Increasing the angle to 90° provides a long-axis view of the aorta with either anteflexion or retroflexion of the probe, improving the angle of insonation of the ultrasound beam with aortic flow for the assessment of flow by PW Doppler. As the probe is withdrawn into the upper esophageal position, the aortic plane elongates as the arch is cut tangentially at a point slightly deeper than 20 cm from the incisors. Angulation with firm retroflexion from this position generally allows interrogation of the high arch.

Normally, a minor retrograde flow pattern can be detected in the ascending aorta and proximal descending aorta related to runoff into the great vessels and coronary bed (5). As AR becomes more severe, the degree of apparent retrograde aortic flow relative to antegrade aortic flow increases (27). The systolic and diastolic flow curves obtained with PW Doppler can be traced, which can be used to provide a TVI ratio; the closer the diastolic TVI is to the systolic TVI, the greater the severity of the regurgitation. However, because the flow abnormality is assessed as the ratio of diastolic to systolic flow as opposed to the absolute flow velocities, the inability to assess true velocities is not a limitation. In general, the presence of holodiastolic flow reversal in the descending thoracic aorta suggests at least moderate AR, while the finding of holodiastolic flow reversal in the abdominal aorta suggests severe AR (5). The usefulness of aortic holodiastolic flow reversal as an index of severe AR is also useful particularly in the intraoperative setting in patients in whom the LVOT cannot be adequately visualized on TEE for technical reasons (eg, interposed MV prosthesis creating an acoustic shadow that obscures the LVOT). In these patients, color flow Doppler interrogation of the regurgitant jet in the LVOT is not possible (28).

Pressure Half-Time and Slope of Aortic Regurgitant Jet Decay

Analysis of a CW Doppler waveform of AR from the TG long-axis or deep TG long-axis view can be used when the Doppler beam is aligned parallel to the regurgitant jet flow. ME views of the LVOT are generally obtained at too great an angle to the flow for an accurate jet profile to be acquired. It is essential that a smooth waveform with an intact envelope be recorded for analysis to be meaningful.

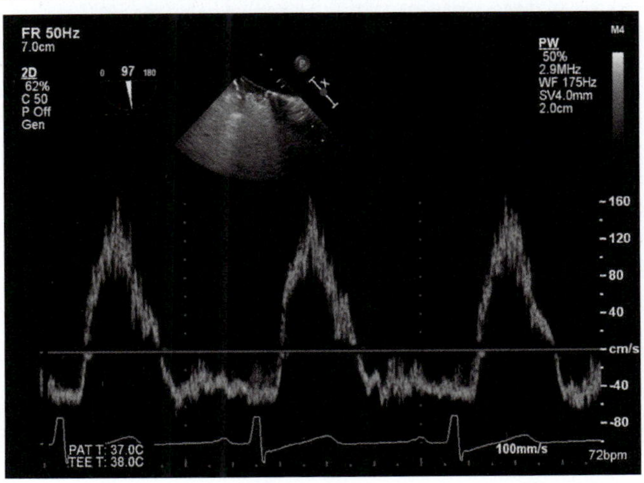

FIGURE 11.8 Pulsed-wave Doppler imaging in the midesophageal long-axis view of the descending thoracic aorta. There is evidence of holodiastolic flow reversal (below the baseline) consistent with severe aortic regurgitation.

The principle of this analysis is that the velocity of the regurgitant jet is directly related to the pressure gradient between the aortic root and the left ventricle in diastole, in accordance with the Bernoulli equation. When a large regurgitant defect is present, the pressures equalize more rapidly because more blood leaks through the valve per unit of time. Therefore, the pressure gradient between the aorta and the left ventricle decreases more rapidly in severe regurgitation and, as a result, the velocity of the jet also diminishes more rapidly. The slope or the rate of decay of this velocity and the time it takes for the pressure gradient between the aorta and left ventricle to decrement by half (ie, the pressure half-time) are measures of the severity of regurgitation. To perform these analyses on the spectral Doppler profile of the AR jet obtained with CW Doppler, the following two technical criteria must be met:

1. A smooth velocity envelope must be defined by CW Doppler.
2. It must be confirmed that the core of the regurgitant jet has been interrogated. With appropriate interrogation, the peak regurgitant jet velocity at the onset of the jet should approximate a value calculated with the Bernoulli equation ($4v^2$) as a reasonable estimate of the gradient between the measured arterial diastolic pressure and an estimate of the LV diastolic pressure.

A slope of AR velocity decay of 2 to 2.9 m/s^2 suggests moderate AR, and greater than or equal to 3 m/s^2 suggests severe AR. The computer analysis package determines the pressure half-time from the slope of the AR jet decay (Figure 11.9). A pressure half-time of less than 200 ms suggests severe AR (29,30). Factors related to left ventricular and aortic compliance and the presence of high LV diastolic pressures (heart failure, restrictive physiology, diastolic dysfunction) all potentially cause the gradient to dissipate more rapidly and may artifactually worsen the apparent severity of the lesion by these techniques. Accordingly, these two methods of analysis of the decay curve should be used mainly to confirm the color flow findings but not as a primary method of AR severity assessment. Lastly, rapid equalization of the pressure gradient can result in premature closure of the MV before the onset of ventricular systole, indicative of severe AR, or in extreme cases, premature opening of the aortic valve in diastole (29). These latter findings are generally only seen with the acute onset of severe regurgitation.

Other Doppler Findings of Aortic Regurgitation

Because the blood flow velocity is directly related to the pressure differential, the early diastolic velocity of the AR spectral Doppler profile is always high (4.0-5.0 m/s) in comparison with the systolic velocities of 1.0 to 1.7 m/s across normal valves. Typically, jet velocities are high (>4 m/s) in lesser degrees of regurgitation because the initial diastolic pressure gradient between the aorta and left ventricle is generally 60 to 80 mm

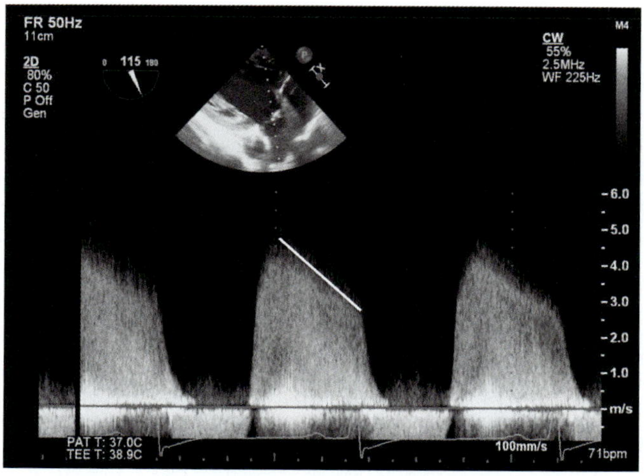

FIGURE 11.9 Continuous wave Doppler imaging in the transgastric long-axis view with nearly parallel Doppler beam alignment demonstrating the aortic regurgitant jet velocity profile. The pressure half-time is less than 200 m/s with a slope greater than 3 m/s^2 consistent with severe aortic regurgitation.

Hg. The exception is in severe acute AR, in which the aortic and LV diastolic pressures may be similar. With the exception of the latter case, lower peak velocities on the spectral display suggest that the true regurgitant jet is not being interrogated directly. High-velocity jets do not indicate that severe regurgitation is present but rather that the gradient between the aorta and left ventricle is higher. On the other hand, if the gain settings are constant, the intensity of the spectral Doppler signal is directly related to the severity of the leak. This is because the larger the regurgitant flow, the greater the number of red blood cells contained therein to reflect the ultrasound beam. Consequently, the more severe the regurgitation, the more intense the Doppler signals.

In more severe lesions, the velocity of the antegrade flow through the regurgitant valve may be increased when compared with that in normal subjects. This is a consequence of the increased stroke volume that develops because the heart must eject both the regurgitant and the normal stroke volume through the aortic annulus, which is a fairly rigid structure. The velocity of systolic flow in the LVOT increases with significant insufficiency, and outflow tract velocities equal to or above 1.5 m/s suggest "stenosis" of the outflow tract relative to the volume of blood flowing through it and support a diagnosis of significant regurgitation. The clinical corollary of this phenomenon is the development of a functional systolic ejection murmur of relative aortic stenosis, heard during auscultation of the heart in addition to the diastolic murmur of AR. However, this technique can be misleading in patients with a hyperdynamic state, who can also present with outflow tract flow velocities between 1.5 and 2.0 m/s.

Special Clinical Situations

Aortic Valve Repair

Aortic valve repair has become an established surgical option to aortic valve replacement (AVR) at experienced centers in select patients with AR (31,32). In general, type 1 and type 2 etiologies of AR are felt to be amenable to surgical repair, while type 3 etiologies are less likely to be amenable to repair due to valve calcification and frequently require AVR (4). Contraindications to aortic valve repair for AR are valves with severe calcification or fibrosis, active infection, or extremely reduced mobility (31). TEE has been shown to accurately classify AR mechanism relative to surgical inspection and, therefore, accurately predict the reparability of the aortic valve in the majority of cases (4). The intraoperative echocardiographer needs to be aware of how to make the key measurements necessary to determine if an aortic valve is amenable to aortic valve repair (Figure 11.10). A geometric leaflet height of less than 16 mm in a trileaflet valve or less than 19 mm in a bicuspid valve indicates leaflet retraction and is a contraindication to repair, while an effective height of less than 9 mm indicates the need for cusp resuspension (33). Post-repair assessment by TEE can also accurately identify patients at significant risk for recurrent AR who may require surgical revision or AVR at the time of the initial procedure. In addition to the presence of residual AR, key factors predicting a high risk of recurrence of AR after surgery are restricted leaflets, an effective leaflet height of less than 9 mm, and a leaflet coaptation length of less than 4 mm (33).

Acute Aortic Regurgitation

The condition of acute AR may be more challenging to diagnose as echocardiographic findings during its assessment may differ from those typically seen in chronic, severe AR (5). In acute, severe AR, the left ventricle has not had time to dilate due to chronic volume overload, and therefore, the left ventricle is frequently normal in size with hyperdynamic function (34). Moreover, because of the rapid equilibration of aortic pressure with LV pressure, the AR jet will have a short duration and exhibit lower velocities. Therefore, the color Doppler appearance and spectral Doppler profile of AR may terminate before the end of diastole, while the jet may not have a large appearance in the left ventricle. For the same reasons, holodiastolic flow reversal may also not be visualized in acute AR. Lastly, the sudden rise in LV end-diastolic pressure may cause premature closure of the MV (best visualized with M-mode in the TG long-axis view) and diastolic mitral regurgitation (5). Lastly, quantitative measurements may be difficult to perform in these settings especially due to the presence of marked tachycardia, but the assessment of the proximal jet (VC width and area) should remain reliable (34).

Aortic Dissection

The mechanisms of AR in cases of acute aortic dissection can be provided by TEE and then be used to guide aortic valve surgery (35,36). AR in aortic dissection occurs due to incomplete leaflet closure from aortic

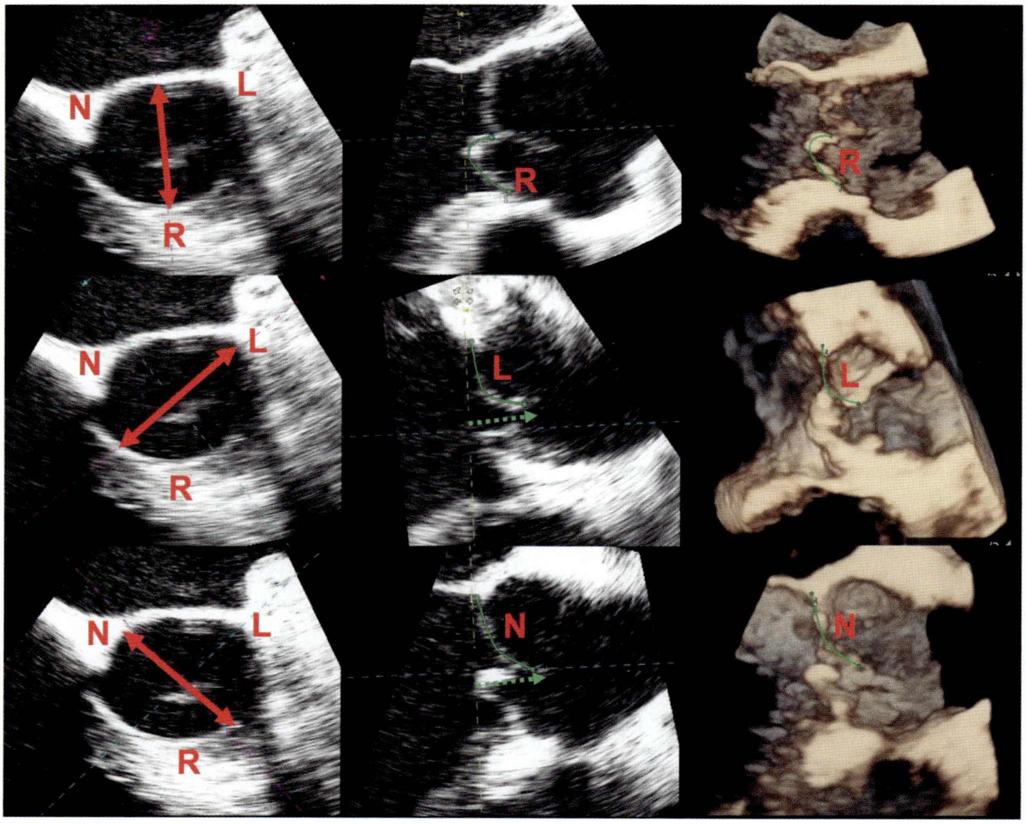

FIGURE 11.10 Three-dimensional multiplanar and volumetric imaging of aortic valve for measurement of effective and geometric leaflet heights. In the short-axis view of the LVOT (left column), the orthogonal (long-axis) plane (thick red line) is oriented in the direction of the prolapsing right coronary cusp (top row), normal left coronary cusp (center row), and normal non-coronary cusp (bottom row). The geometric leaflet height is measured using a curved distance tool (thin green line) along the length of the leaflet from its insertion at the annulus to the leaflet tip, while the effective height (dotted green line) is measured straight from the annular plane to the leaflet tip (shown only for left and non-coronary cusps). Measurements should be made on 3D multiplanar images (center column). The geometric leaflet height measurement is overlaid on the 3D volumetric image (right column). 3D, three-dimensional; L, left coronary cusp; LVOT, left ventricular outflow tract; N, non-coronary cusp; R, right coronary cusp.

dilation, aortic leaflet prolapse from disruption of aortic commissures, and dissection flap prolapse. In these cases, AR may be effectively treated with aortic valve repair by reducing the size of the sinotubular junction, resuspension of the leaflets to the aortic root, and/or resection of the intimal tear; other mechanisms of AR such as bicuspid valve disease and leaflet thickening and calcification may have to be treated with AVR (36). Multiple mechanisms, however, can be present in any given patient. In aortic dissection, both the severity of AR and degree of cusp prolapse present are directly related to the circumferential extent of annular dissection (35).

Paravalvular Aortic Regurgitation

Although TAVR is increasingly being performed without TEE and general anesthesia, the TEE assessment of paravalvular AR should still be well understood by the intraoperative echocardiographer. The presence of paravalvular AR has been shown to have negative impact on outcomes after TAVR and the accurate intraoperative assessment of its severity is, therefore, of critical importance after valve deployment. In general, paravalvular AR after TAVR occurs when there is poor apposition of the transcatheter valve in the native aortic annulus due to significant aortic valve complex calcification (eg, LVOT calcification, nodular leaflet calcification at the aortic commissures, or asymmetric leaflet calcification), significant "undersizing" of the transcatheter aortic valve (or poor expansion of the valve in the aortic annulus), annular eccentricity, or suboptimal valve positioning (37,38). The assessment of paravalvular AR, however, can be challenging due to acoustic shadowing from valvular or annular calcification and the valve stent. Moreover, these jets are frequently crescentic or irregular in shape and multiple in number; they can arise from various locations around the native annulus including the native commissures and can be directed eccentrically into the LVOT. Therefore, multiple views should be utilized to assess paravalvular AR after TAVR including the ME long-axis view with rotation of the probe from one side of the prosthesis to the other, ME short-axis view below the valve skirt, and TG views at multiple interrogation angles. Biplane imaging of the aortic valve can be particularly useful in the assessment of paravalvular AR as the biplane cursor can be carefully placed at the level of the LVOT just below the transcatheter heart valve in the ME long-axis view (reference view); an orthogonal short-axis view at or just below the ventricular aspect of the transcatheter heart valve is then created and utilized to rapidly determine the circumferential extent of AR.

According to current guidelines (23), mild paravalvular AR is defined as less than 10%, moderate paravalvular AR is defined as 10% to 30%, and severe paravalvular AR is defined as greater than 30% of the circumferential extent of the transcatheter heart valve. Care must be taken to avoid misinterpreting the high-velocity flow that may exist in the sinuses around the native leaflets after TAVR for AR; rather only flow visualized below the valve skirt in the outflow tract should be utilized when determining the presence and severity of the paravalvular AR. Unlike central jets, jet areas and heights cannot be utilized to determine AR severity because of the eccentric nature of these jets (39). Although the circumferential extent of the AR jet has been proposed to classify paravalvular AR severity, it has not been extensively validated, and it can sometimes be at odds with the angiographic grade of AR. In some cases, the radial width of a paravalvular jet may be large, resulting in significant AR despite a small circumferential extent (39). In these cases, additional methods including quantitative volumetric or 3D VC area assessment of paravalvular AR should be performed (23). Lastly, while the presence of holodiastolic flow reversal is a very specific sign for moderate or severe AR, this assessment is less accurate in the presence of coexisting aortic stenosis (9,26,40). In these patients, the presence of a noncompliant, stiff aorta may result in significant flow reversal even in the absence of significant AR; therefore, this finding may be less useful in the assessment of paravalvular AR after TAVR (39).

Iatrogenic Aortic Regurgitation After Mitral Valve Surgery

The central location of the aortic valve results in it being particularly vulnerable to iatrogenic injury at the time of cardiac surgery. In particular, the proximity and anatomic continuity of the anterior mitral leaflet with the posterior LVOT and aortic root may result in the development of iatrogenic AR after MV surgery. There are several case reports of inadvertent suture placement during mitral annuloplasty repair or replacement into aortic valve cusps, which results in cusp perforation or tethering and significant AR (41-44). Iatrogenic AR has also been described after surgical repair of atrial and ventricular septal defects (41,45).

SUMMARY

The intraoperative assessment of AR with TEE involves the assessment of the mechanisms of AR and regurgitation severity. The latter is best performed by measuring the width and/or area of the VC because this measurement is less load dependent than others, while the next most useful is the relative jet height or area in the LVOT just below the aortic valve plane. Planimetry of the VC area with 3D TEE can overcome some of the limitations of 2D imaging particularly in cases of eccentric jets and complex regurgitant orifice shapes. The assessment of diastolic flow reversal in the aorta itself remains an important adjunctive approach for the assessment of AR severity but its usefulness may be limited in patients with calcified, noncompliant aortas. The other approaches discussed in this chapter play an ancillary role, reinforcing the practitioner's confidence in making a definitive assessment. The information derived from echocardiographic imaging and analysis of the entire aortic complex can help guide the surgical approach.

REFERENCES

1. Ward JM, Baker DW, Rubenstein SA, et al. Detection of aortic insufficiency by pulse Doppler echocardiography. *J Clin Ultrasound*. 1977;5(1):5-10.
2. Underwood MJ, El Khoury G, Deronck D, et al. The aortic root: structure, function, and surgical reconstruction. *Heart*. 2000;83(4):376-380.
3. El Khoury G, Glineur D, Rubay J, et al. Functional classification of aortic root/valve abnormalities and their correlation with etiologies and surgical procedures. *Curr Opin Cardiol*. 2005;20(2):115-121.
4. le Polain de Waroux JB, Pouleur AC, Goffinet C, et al. Functional anatomy of aortic regurgitation: accuracy, prediction of surgical repairability, and outcome implications of transesophageal echocardiography. *Circulation*. 2007;116(11 suppl):I264-I269.
5. Zoghbi WA, Adams D, Bonow RO, et al. Recommendations for noninvasive evaluation of native valvular regurgitation: a report from the American Society of Echocardiography developed in collaboration with the Society for Cardiovascular Magnetic Resonance. *J Am Soc Echocardiogr*. 2017;30(4):303-371.
6. Boodhwani M, de Kerchove L, Glineur D, et al. Repair-oriented classification of aortic insufficiency: impact on surgical techniques and clinical outcomes. *J Thorac Cardiovasc Surg*. 2009;137(2):286-294.
7. Perry GJ, Helmcke F, Nanda NC, et al. Evaluation of aortic insufficiency by Doppler color flow mapping. *J Am Coll Cardiol*. 1987;9(4):952-959.
8. Rafferty T, Durkin MA, Sittig D, et al. Transesophageal color flow Doppler imaging for aortic insufficiency in patients having cardiac operations. *J Thorac Cardiovasc Surg*. 1992;104(2):521-525.
9. Zarauza J, Ares M, Vílchez FG, et al. An integrated approach to the quantification of aortic regurgitation by Doppler echocardiography. *Am Heart J*. 1998;136(6):1030-1041.
10. Tribouilloy CM, Enriquez-Sarano M, Bailey KR, et al. Assessment of severity of aortic regurgitation using the width of the vena contracta: a clinical color Doppler imaging study. *Circulation*. 2000;102(5):558-564.
11. Baumgartner H, Kratzer H, Helmreich G, et al. Quantitation of aortic regurgitation by colour coded cross-sectional Doppler echocardiography. *Eur Heart J*. 1988;9(4):380-387.
12. Ishii M, Jones M, Shiota T, et al. Quantifying aortic regurgitation by using the color Doppler-imaged vena contracta: a chronic animal model study. *Circulation*. 1997;96(6):2009-2015.
13. Ishii M, Jones M, Shiota T, et al. Evaluation of eccentric aortic regurgitation by color Doppler jet and color Doppler-imaged vena contracta measurements: an animal study of quantified aortic regurgitation. *Am Heart J*. 1996;132(4):796-804.
14. Willett DL, Hall SA, Jessen ME, et al. Assessment of aortic regurgitation by transesophageal color Doppler imaging of the vena contracta: validation against an intraoperative aortic flow probe. *J Am Coll Cardiol*. 2001;37(5):1450-1455.
15. Switzer DF, Yoganathan AP, Nanda NC, et al. Calibration of color Doppler flow mapping during extreme hemodynamic conditions in vitro: a foundation for a reliable quantitative grading system for aortic incompetence. *Circulation*. 1987;75(4):837-846.
16. Sato H, Ohta T, Hiroe K, et al. Severity of aortic regurgitation assessed by area of vena contracta: a clinical two-dimensional and three-dimensional color Doppler imaging study. *Cardiovasc Ultrasound*. 2015;13:24.
17. Abudiab MM, Chao CJ, Liu S, et al. Quantitation of valve regurgitation severity by three-dimensional vena contracta area is superior to flow convergence method of quantitation on transesophageal echocardiography. *Echocardiography*. 2017;34(7):992-1001.
18. Chin CH, Chen CH, Lo HS. The correlation between three-dimensional vena contracta area and aortic regurgitation index in patients with aortic regurgitation. *Echocardiography*. 2010;27(2):161-166.
19. Yanagi Y, Kanzaki H, Yonezawa R, et al. Diagnostic value of vena contracta area measurement using three-dimensional transesophageal echocardiography in assessing the severity of aortic regurgitation. *Echocardiography*. 2021;38:1307-1313.
20. 20 Fang L, Hsiung MC, Miller AP, et al. Assessment of aortic regurgitation by live three-dimensional transthoracic echocardiographic measurements of vena contracta area: usefulness and validation. *Echocardiography*. 2005;22(9):775-781.
21. Ewe SH, Delgado V, van der Geest R, et al. Accuracy of three-dimensional versus two-dimensional echocardiography for quantification of aortic regurgitation and validation by three-dimensional three-directional velocity-encoded magnetic resonance imaging. *Am J Cardiol*. 2013;112(4):560-566.
22. Altiok E, Frick M, Meyer CG, et al. Comparison of two- and three-dimensional transthoracic echocardiography to cardiac magnetic resonance imaging for assessment of paravalvular regurgitation after transcatheter aortic valve implantation. *Am J Cardiol*. 2014;113(11):1859-1866.
23. Zoghbi WA, Jone PN, Chamsi-Pasha MA, et al. Guidelines for the evaluation of prosthetic valve function with cardiovascular imaging: a report from the American Society of Echocardiography developed in collaboration with the Society for Cardiovascular Magnetic Resonance and the Society of Cardiovascular Computed Tomography. *J Am Soc Echocardiogr*. 2024;37(1):2-63.
24. Tribouilloy CM, Enriquez-Sarano M, Fett SL, et al. Application of the proximal flow convergence method to calculate the effective regurgitant orifice area in aortic regurgitation. *J Am Coll Cardiol*. 1998;32(4):1032-1039.
25. Pouleur AC, le Polain de Waroux JB, Goffinet C, et al. Accuracy of the flow convergence method for quantification of aortic regurgitation in patients with central versus eccentric jets. *Am J Cardiol*. 2008;102(4):475-480.
26. Diebold B, Peronneau P, Blanchard D, et al. Non-invasive quantification of aortic regurgitation by Doppler echocardiography. *Br Heart J*. 1983;49(2):167-173.
27. Quinones MA, Young JB, Waggoner AD, et al. Assessment of pulsed Doppler echocardiography in detection and quantification of aortic and mitral regurgitation. *Br Heart J*. 1980;44(6):612-620.
28. Sutton DC, Kluger R, Ahmed SU, et al. Flow reversal in the descending aorta: a guide to intraoperative assessment of aortic regurgitation with transesophageal echocardiography. *J Thorac Cardiovasc Surg*. 1994;108(3):576-582.
29. Labovitz AJ, Ferrara RP, Kern MJ, et al. Quantitative evaluation of aortic insufficiency by continuous wave Doppler echocardiography. *J Am Coll Cardiol*. 1986;8(6):1341-1347.

30. Cohen IS, Wharton TP Jr, Neill WA. Pathophysiologic observations on premature opening of the aortic valve utilizing a technique for multiplane echocardiographic analysis. *Am Heart J.* 1979;97(6):766-772.
31. Antoniou A, Harky A, Bashir M, et al. Why I choose to repair and not to replace the aortic valve? *Gen Thorac Cardiovasc Surg.* 2019;67(1):20-24.
32. Augoustides JG, Szeto WY, Bavaria JE. Advances in aortic valve repair: focus on functional approach, clinical outcomes, and central role of echocardiography. *J Cardiothorac Vasc Anesth.* 2010;24(6):1016-1020.
33. Berrebi A, Monin JL, Lansac E. Systematic echocardiographic assessment of aortic regurgitation-what should the surgeon know for aortic valve repair? *Ann Cardiothorac Surg.* 2019;8(3):331-341.
34. Stout KK, Verrier ED. Acute valvular regurgitation. *Circulation.* 2009;119(25):3232-3241.
35. Keane MG, Wiegers SE, Yang E, et al. Structural determinants of aortic regurgitation in type A dissection and the role of valvular resuspension as determined by intraoperative transesophageal echocardiography. *Am J Cardiol.* 2000;85(5):604-610.
36. Movsowitz HD, Levine RA, Hilgenberg AD, et al. Transesophageal echocardiographic description of the mechanisms of aortic regurgitation in acute type A aortic dissection: implications for aortic valve repair. *J Am Coll Cardiol.* 2000;36(3):884-890.
37. Genereux P, Head SJ, Hahn R, et al. Paravalvular leak after transcatheter aortic valve replacement: the new Achilles' heel? A comprehensive review of the literature. *J Am Coll Cardiol.* 2013;61(11):1125-1136.
38. Unbehaun A, Pasic M, Dreysse S, et al. Transapical aortic valve implantation: incidence and predictors of paravalvular leakage and transvalvular regurgitation in a series of 358 patients. *J Am Coll Cardiol.* 2012;59(3):211-221.
39. Pibarot P, Hahn RT, Weissman NJ, et al. Assessment of paravalvular regurgitation following TAVR: a proposal of unifying grading scheme. *JACC Cardiovasc Imaging.* 2015;8(3):340-360.
40. Reimold SC, Maier SE, Aggarwal K, et al. Aortic flow velocity patterns in chronic aortic regurgitation: implications for Doppler echocardiography. *J Am Soc Echocardiogr.* 1996;9(5):675-683.
41. Kolakalapudi P, Chaudhry S, Omar B. Iatrogenic aortic insufficiency following mitral valve replacement: case report and review of the literature. *J Clin Med Res.* 2015;7(6):485-489.
42. Lee AP, Walley VM, Ascah KJ, et al. A fenestrated aortic valve contributing to iatrogenic aortic insufficiency post mitral valve replacement. *Cardiovasc Pathol.* 1996;5(2):81-83.
43. Santiago M, El-Dayem MA, Dimitrova G, et al. Missed diagnosis of iatrogenic acute aortic insufficiency after mitral valve surgery. *Int Anesthesiol Clin.* 2011;49(2):26-31.
44. Babu S, Koniparambil UP, Kumar M, et al. Distortion of aortic valve from mechanical traction imposed by the mitral valve prosthesis: the three-dimensional transesophageal echocardiographic perception. *Ann Card Anaesth.* 2017;20(4):472-474.
45. Ren C, Jiang S, Wang M, et al. Iatrogenic aortic valve perforation after ventricular septal defect repair. *Ann Thorac Cardiovasc Surg.* 2018;24(1):47-50.

QUESTIONS

1. Which of the following factors can affect the degree of AR during an operative examination?
A. Administration of vasopressors
B. Use of volatile anesthetics
C. A significant change in blood pressure
D. All of the above

2. Which of the following statements is true regarding the ratio of the AR jet area to the LVOT area?
A. May not be accurate in the presence of an eccentric jet
B. Biplane imaging is not helpful.
C. The ratio that defines severe AR is greater than or equal to 50%.
D. The ratio that defines mild AR is less than 10%.

3. Which one of the following statements is true regarding aortic leaflet measurements prior to aortic valve repair?
A. A geometric leaflet height of less than 16 mm in a trileaflet valve indicates leaflet retraction.
B. A geometric height less than 19 mm in a bicuspid valve is a contraindication to repair.
C. An effective height less than 9 mm indicates the need for leaflet resuspension.
D. All of the above

4. The following statements are true about diastolic aortic flow reversal in a patient with AR *except*:
A. May be less accurate in older adult patients with concomitant aortic stenosis
B. Obtaining accurate flow velocities is essential.
C. Holodiastolic flow in the abdominal aorta generally indicates severe AR.
D. As AR becomes more severe, the degree of retrograde aortic flow relative to antegrade aortic flow increases.

5. Which one of the following statements regarding measurement of the VC width in AR is false?
A. The size of the VC is directly related to the size of the regurgitant orifice area.
B. Measurement of the VC width may not be feasible in the presence of eccentric jets.
C. The VC width is more load dependent than other Doppler indices.
D. The VC width is best measured in a zoomed ME long-axis view of the aortic valve.

6. Which of the following statements regarding measurement of the 3D VC area is false?
A. An area greater than or equal to 0.3 cm^2 indicates severe AR.
B. Is generally equivalent to the regurgitant volume
C. May be useful in patients with complex regurgitant orifice shapes
D. The 3D VC area correlates well with conventional 2D quantitative color Doppler indices.

7. Which one of the following statements regarding CW Doppler analysis of AR is false?
A. Parallel alignment with the regurgitant jet is essential.
B. The intensity of the spectral Doppler signal is proportional to the severity of the regurgitation.
C. A severe regurgitant lesion will equalize the pressure gradient between the aorta and the left ventricle more quickly.
D. The analysis should be performed in the ME view.

8. Which one of the following statements regarding the assessment of paravalvular AR is true?
A. Paravalvular AR should be assessed at the level of the prosthetic valve leaflets.
B. A circumferential extent of less than 5% indicates mild AR.
C. Risk factors for paravalvular AR include LVOT calcification, valve undersizing, and suboptimal positioning of the transcatheter valve.
D. Paravalvular AR after TAVR is not associated with adverse patient outcomes.

9. Which of the following observations regarding the PISA method for the assessment of AR severity are true:
A. The PISA radius is usually determined in a TG view.
B. The PISA radius can be determined in ME view with an eccentric jet.
C. The PISA method may be limited in the presence of valve calcification, multiple jets, and eccentric jets.
D. All of the above

10. All of the following findings indicate severe AR *except*:
A. Pressure half-time of less than 300 ms
B. Effective regurgitant orifice area greater than or equal to 0.3 cm^2
C. Ratio of AR jet height to LVOT diameter greater than or equal to 65%
D. Diastolic flow reversal in the abdominal aorta

11. Which one of the following statements is true regarding the ratio of the AR jet height to the LVOT diameter?
A. Can be performed with M-mode echocardiography
B. A ratio greater than or equal to 65% indicates severe AR.
C. A ratio of less than 25% indicates mild AR.
D. All of the above

12. Anteflexing and withdrawing the TEE probe from the ME long-axis view of the aortic valve followed by reducing the angle to 100° to 110° allows for optimal visualization of what structure?
A. The aortic valve leaflets
B. The distal tubular ascending aorta
C. The sinuses of Valsalva
D. The LVOT

13. Which of the following statements is false regarding the assessment of AR severity?
A. The AR spectral Doppler profile density is directly correlated with AR severity.
B. A VC width of less than 0.3 cm indicates mild AR.
C. The pressure half-time is the most reliable method for AR severity assessment.
D. Utilization of the volumetric method for calculation of the EROA may be impractical in the operating room.

14. Bicuspid valve disease can cause AR by which mechanism(s)?
A. Type 1, 2, 3
B. Types 1 and 2
C. Types 1 and 3
D. Type 3

15. Which of the following is a possible mechanism for AR in aortic dissection?
A. Incomplete leaflet closure from aortic dilation
B. Aortic leaflet prolapse from disruption of aortic commissures
C. Dissection flap prolapse
D. All of the above

16. The superior insertion point of the aortic leaflets is approximately at:
A. The level of the sinotubular junction where the commissures are formed
B. The level of the aortic annulus
C. The sinuses of Valsalva
D. The level of the takeoff of the right and left coronary arteries

17. Which of the following type(s) of AR are most likely to be amenable to aortic valve repair?
A. Types 1 and 3
B. Types 2 and 3
C. Types 1 and 2
D. Type 3

18. The following echocardiographic findings can be observed in patients with acute AR *except*:
A. Normal LV size
B. Smaller VC width and area
C. Premature closure of the MV
D. Diastolic mitral regurgitation

19. Following aortic valve repair for regurgitation, the following risk factors predict a high recurrence rate for significant AR *except*:
A. Restricted leaflet motion
B. Coaptation length less than 4 mm
C. Effective leaflet height greater than or equal to 9 mm
D. Residual AR after repair

20. Which one of the following statements is false regarding the pathophysiology of AR?
A. AR results in LV dilation and eccentric hypertrophy.
B. An increase in the LV radius results in a decrease in wall stress.
C. AR results in an increase in preload and afterload on the left ventricle.
D. The degree of LV dilation is a marker of AR severity and duration.

ANSWERS

1. **Correct Answer: D.**
   Rationale: A change in blood pressure from any cause including vasopressors and volatile anesthetics can affect the severity of AR and the appearance of the regurgitant jet on color Doppler images.

2. **Correct Answer: A.**
   Rationale: In an eccentric aortic regurgitant jet, the distal jet is constrained by the LVOT preventing its full expansion. Therefore, ratio of the jet area to the LVOT area may underestimate the regurgitation severity. Biplane imaging is very helpful for performing this technique. For the jet area to LVOT area method, mild and severe AR are defined as less than 5% or greater than or equal to 60%, respectively.

3. **Correct Answer: D.**
   Rationale: All of the above statements are true. A geometric height less than 16 or 19 mm for a trileaflet and bicuspid valve, respectively, indicate leaflet retraction and are a contraindication to repair. An effective height less than 9 mm indicates the need for leaflet resuspension.

4. **Correct Answer: B.**
   Rationale: Assessment of flow reversal in the descending thoracic aorta is primarily a qualitative technique. The presence of flow reversal in the descending thoracic aorta generally indicates at least moderate AR, while the presence of flow reversal in the abdominal aorta indicates severe AR. This assessment may not be accurate in patients with aortic stenosis as these patients frequently have less compliant aortas and flow reversal may be present even in the absence of significant AR. Since the ratio of the diastolic flow (ie, TVI) to systolic flow can be assessed to determine AR severity, measuring absolute flow reversal velocities is not always necessary.

5. **Correct Answer: C.**
   Rationale: The VC width is a less load-dependent index of AR severity. In fact, changes in afterload due to phenylephrine infusion or volume loading have not been shown to change the size of the VC.

6. **Correct Answer: B.**
   Rationale: The VC area is generally equivalent to the regurgitant orifice area not the regurgitant volume. The VC is the narrowest portion of the jet as flow converges after crossing the valve plane immediately downstream from the regurgitant orifice.

7. **Correct Answer: D.**
   Rationale: CW Doppler analysis of AR requires parallel alignment of the Doppler probe with the regurgitant jet. This is best achieved in a long-axis or deep TG view. The remaining statements are true.

8. **Correct Answer: C.**
   Rationale: Paravalvular AR should be assessed immediately below the level of the valve skirt ideally with the use of biplane imaging to evaluate the entire circumferential extent. A circumferential extent less than 10% indicates mild AR. Paravalvular AR after TAVR is associated with adverse patient outcomes and risk factors include LVOT calcification, valve undersizing, and suboptimal valve positioning.

9. **Correct Answer: D.**
   Rationale: The PISA method has only been studied in a limited fashion for AR evaluation. The PISA radius is generally measured in a TG view but could also be measured in ME view but only in the case of a highly eccentric jet. The PISA method may be limited in the presence of valve calcification, multiple jets, and eccentric jets.

10. **Correct Answer: A.**
    Rationale: A pressure half-time less than 200 ms indicates severe AR. All other statements are true.

11. **Correct Answer: D.**
    Rationale: The ratio of the AR jet height to the LVOT diameter can be performed with M-mode echocardiography. A ratio greater than or equal to 65% indicates severe AR, while a ratio of less than 25% indicates mild AR.

12. **Correct Answer: B.**
    Rationale: In order to visualize the distal tubular ascending aorta, the angle must be reduced to 100°-110° from the standard ME long-axis view between 120° and 150° while simultaneously anteflexing and withdrawing the TEE probe.

13. **Correct Answer: C.**
    Rationale: The pressure half-time is the least reliable method for AR severity assessment. In addition to the technical challenges of

obtaining an adequate Doppler profile, other conditions that affect LV and aortic compliance may influence the pressure half-time.

14. Correct Answer: A.
Rationale: Bicuspid valve disease can cause AR by multiple mechanisms including dilation of the aorta (type 1), aortic cusp prolapse or flail (type 2), and aortic cusp degeneration (type 3).

15. Correct Answer: D.
Rationale: In aortic dissection, AR can occur due to multiple mechanisms including aortic dilation, aortic leaflet prolapse, or dissection flap prolapse.

16. Correct Answer: A.
Rationale: The superior insertion point of the aortic leaflets is approximately at the level of the sinotubular junction where the commissures of the aortic valve are formed.

17. Correct Answer: C.
Rationale: Aortic valve repair is amenable in the setting of dilation of the aorta (type 1) and in the setting of cusp prolapse or flail (type 2).

18. Correct Answer: B.
Rationale: The VC width and area are directly related to the severity of the regurgitant orifice area. Acute AR is usually severe and poorly tolerated; therefore, the VC area will be larger (not smaller).

19. Correct Answer: C.
Rationale: An effective leaflet height of less than (not greater than or equal to) 9 mm indicates residual cusp prolapse and predicts a high recurrence rate for significant AR.

20. Correct Answer: B.
Rationale: Based on the law of Laplace, an increase in the LV radius results in an increase (not decrease) in LV wall stress.

12 Aortic Stenosis

Sophia P. Poorsattar and Jacques Neelankavil

As the leading cause of valvular heart disease worldwide, aortic stenosis (AS) is also the most common valvular lesion to require procedural intervention in individuals over 65 years of age (1). With an estimated increase in severe AS ranging from approximately 4% to 7% per year in individuals ≥65 years and an aging population, the rate of cardiac interventions for AS is expected to continuing rising in the future (2,3). The advent of transcatheter aortic valve replacement (TAVR), in addition to surgical aortic valve replacement (SAVR) has reshaped the landscape of treatment for this population, most notably, by significantly expanding treatment eligibility.

Calcific disease represents the most common etiology of AS in developed countries (4). This spectrum includes calcific degeneration of trileaflet as well as congenitally bicuspid valves. Stenosis of trileaflet valves is predominantly observed in the elderly, while bicuspid aortic valve stenosis can be seen in younger patients, particularly those aged 35 to 65 years, and may be associated with dilation of the aortic root and ascending aorta dilation as well as aortic coarctation. Rheumatic heart disease, while less common in the era of antibiotic treatment, still contributes to the global burden of AS. Rheumatic AS, which typically presents in conjunction with mitral valve involvement, can appear earlier or later in life and is characterized by commissural fusion.

Critical to the management of AS is its preoperative diagnosis, informed primarily by echocardiography, which is essential to characterize the cause and stage of the disease process. Echocardiography affords a detailed visualization of valvular morphology, quantification of stenotic severity, and assessment of resultant hemodynamic impacts, thereby informing intraoperative strategies and postprocedural evaluations. As such, the perioperative echocardiographer must be adept with the techniques used to assess the severity of AS (Table 12.1).

The clinical manifestation of AS with symptoms such as congestive heart failure (often presenting as dyspnea), syncope, and angina, or through echocardiographic evidence of left ventricular (LV) dysfunction (ie, ejection fraction <50%), constitutes a definitive indication for intervention (5). The progression of AS, while variable, underscores the necessity for timely and accurate echocardiographic assessment, guiding clinical decisions not only in symptomatic severe AS but also in moderate cases where concurrent cardiac surgeries might necessitate prophylactic aortic valve replacement.

PATHOPHYSIOLOGY OF AORTIC STENOSIS

AS represents a slowly progressive obstruction to LV outflow with a pressure gradient between the ventricle and the aorta that increases over time. As the left ventricle ejects against a narrowed aortic valve, it must generate a high intracavitary pressure to maintain stroke volume. This high intracavitary pressure increases

TABLE 12.1 Grading Severity of Aortic Stenosis

	Aortic sclerosis	Mild	Moderate	Severe
Peak velocity (m/s)	≤2.5	2.6-2.9	3.0-4.0	≥4.0
Mean gradient (mm Hg)		<20	20-40	≥40
AVA (cm^2)		>1.5	1.0-1.5	<1.0
Indexed AVA (cm^2/m^2)		>0.85	0.60-0.85	<0.6
Velocity ratio		>0.50	0.25-0.50	<0.25

AV, aortic valve; AVA, aortic valve area.

Adapted from Baumgartner H, Hung J, Bermejo J, et al. Recommendations on the echocardiographic assessment of aortic valve stenosis: a focused update from the European Association of Cardiovascular Imaging and the American Society of Echocardiography. *J Am Soc Echocardiogr*. 2017;30(4):372-392.

myocardial wall tension, to which the ventricle typically adapts with concentric hypertrophy from an increase in both muscle and fibrous tissue.

While this concentric hypertrophy serves to reduce wall tension, it also results in a chamber that is less compliant with variable degrees of diastolic dysfunction and increased filling pressures.

The pathologic changes of AS can also lead to myocardial supply–demand mismatch and angina. While obstructive coronary artery disease commonly coexists with AS and must be excluded with cardiac catheterization, angina may be present even with normal coronaries (6). The proposed mechanism of angina in AS has been a compromised coronary flow reserve from restricted dilatory capacity of penetrating coronary vessels. This is further amplified by the reduced coronary perfusion gradient in the setting of decreased aortic diastolic pressures and elevated LV filling pressures. These elevated filling pressures contribute to the significant dyspnea that may be experienced by patients with severe AS. Syncope, another ominous symptom of AS, may result from an inability to increase cardiac output in response to the peripheral vasodilation, compounded by abnormal baroreceptor responses and arrhythmia in many patients.

ECHOCARDIOGRAPHIC EVALUATION OF THE AORTIC VALVE

Echocardiography is the preferred modality for the diagnosis and grading of AS. Cardiac catheterization is not routinely recommended, except in the circumstance when echocardiography is nondiagnostic or there is a discrepancy with clinical findings (5,7). Due to the closer positioning of the valve to the transducer and lack of interference from structures in the near field, transesophageal echocardiography (TEE) is generally superior to transthoracic echocardiography (TTE) for qualitative aortic valve assessment. However, despite superior imaging of aortic valve morphology by TEE, it is important to note that hemodynamic thresholds for severe AS are based on seminal studies that used TTE (8-10). As such, TTE assessment in the awake state is the gold standard for quantitative AS assessment, and caution should be employed when relying exclusively on TEE assessment of AS for management decisions (11). Irrespective of type of echocardiography, an integrative approach using two-dimensional (2D), three-dimensional (3D), and Doppler imaging should be employed for valvular assessment (7,12).

Qualitative Assessment of Aortic Stenosis

The echocardiographic evaluation of AS begins with inspection of the valve apparatus for leaflet morphology and disease burden by both 2D and 3D. For TEE, 2D imaging of the valve should be performed in both the midesophageal aortic valve short- and long-axis views (ME AV SAX and ME AV LAX), whereas 3D datasets may be acquired from either perspective. As the 3D dataset will be used for both qualitative assessment and multiplanar reconstruction, the boundaries for image acquisition should include the left ventricular outflow tract (LVOT) proximally and aortic root distally. With each technique, visual inspection should be performed to assess leaflet number, thickness, mobility, and location and degree of calcification. While the quantification of valvular stenosis, as described further on, is critical to describing the severity of disease, the echocardiographer should not be surprised by the Doppler findings but rather should expect them based on a thorough evaluation of the valve's structure.

The distinction between trileaflet and bicuspid aortic valve morphology relies on a combination of 2D and color flow Doppler (CFD) assessment. Sclerocalcific changes, estimated by the degree of echogenicity and thickening of the leaflets, may differ between the two, with trileaflet valves developing nodular calcific masses more prominently on the basal and central aspects of each cusp and bicuspid valves having a more asymmetric pattern of calcification related to the type of cusp fusion. In the midesophageal LAX view, bicuspid aortic valves often show an asymmetric coaptation with diastolic doming in 2D. In the midesophageal SAX, bicuspid valves demonstrate an elliptical orifice in midsystole, often with the appearance of a raphe at the line of fusion between two cusps (right-left fusion in 75% of cases and right-non fusion in 14% of cases) (13). Calcified trileaflet valves have an appearance of a stellate orifice. Commissural fusion with prominent thickening at the edge of the cusps and a characteristic triangular orifice at midsystole is suggestive of rheumatic AS disease as the etiologic cause of AS. The application of CFD in the SAX view may aid in the recognition of these orifice shapes (▶ Videos 12.1-12.4). CFD use in the LAX view may demonstrate flow acceleration in the form of either an aliasing hemisphere in the LVOT proximal to the stenotic orifice or turbulent flow in the proximal aorta as blood exits the stenotic valve (Figure 12.1). Recognition of this finding should alert the echocardiographer that significant stenosis may be present and warrant further evaluation. CFD may also be

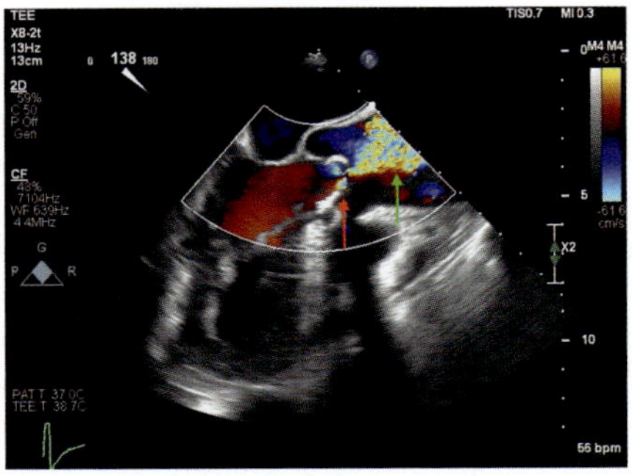

FIGURE 12.1 Midesophageal long-axis view of a stenotic trileaflet aortic valve with color flow Doppler assessment. Significant flow acceleration can be demonstrated in the form of either an aliasing hemisphere in the LVOT proximal to the stenotic orifice (red arrow) or turbulent flow in the proximal aorta as blood exits the stenotic valve (green arrow).

of use to offer a precise location of the site of increased velocity, thereby allowing the echocardiographer to discriminate between valvular, supra- or subvalvular obstructions (see further on).

Quantitative Assessment of Aortic Stenosis

The severity of AS is described with Doppler echocardiography by three primary hemodynamic parameters: peak jet velocity, mean transvalvular pressure gradient, and aortic valve area estimated by the continuity equation (Table 12.1). As with all valvular stenosis, severity represents a continuum from narrowing without hemodynamic consequences to severe flow obstruction.

While severe stenosis can be suggested by an abnormality of a single criterion, there would ideally be concordance among the criteria. When that is not the case, the findings should be integrated with additional imaging and clinical data before a determination of severity is made (7).

For each quantitative technique, it is critical to ensure that the ultrasound beam is aligned with the direction of transvalvular blood flow. An angle of more than 20° between the ultrasound beam and the direction of blood flow will result in significant underestimation of Doppler indices (14,15). Both the deep transgastric (DT) five-chamber and transgastric long-axis view (TG LAX) should be used to perform Doppler interrogation of the aortic valve and LVOT, as either may provide the optimal alignment of ultrasound beam with flow. The view with the highest recorded velocities should be used for calculations of severity. Care must be taken to avoid inadvertently sampling a jet of eccentric mitral regurgitation or dynamic LVOT obstruction.

Peak Jet Velocity

The maximum velocity (V_{max}) through the aortic valve orifice is obtained from the continuous wave Doppler (CWD) spectral profile, with the cursor carefully aligned with the stenotic jet as described previously. A smooth velocity curve with a defined outer edge and clear maximal velocity should be recorded. Attention should be paid to *avoid* fine linear signals due to transit time artifact and to adjust the gain and scale to best delineate the edge of the spectral envelope. Due to beat-to-beat variations in transvalvular blood flow, at least three beats should be used for patients in sinus rhythm and at least five beats in patients with irregular rhythms.

The V_{max} can be determined by either a point measurement at the apex of the profile or by tracing the entire outer edge of the profile to provide the highest velocity during the ejection period (Figure 12.2). The latter method will also provide the mean pressure gradient and velocity-time integral (VTI) for the continuity equation (see further on). Tracings from multiple imaging windows should be obtained with the final peak jet velocity derived from the highest velocities recorded (Table 12.1) (7).

Obtaining the highest velocity is crucial as it carries prognostic significance. In studies evaluating the relationship between V_{max} and long-term clinical outcomes in patients with severe AS, increasing V_{max} was associated with an incrementally higher risk of aortic valve-related death or heart failure hospitalization (16). The lack of significant interaction between symptoms and V_{max} on major adverse cardiac events supports the

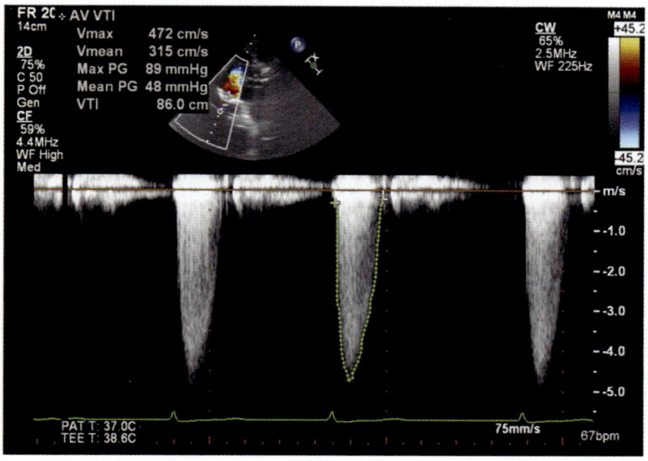

FIGURE 12.2 Deep transgastric view with parallel continuous wave Doppler beam alignment in a patient with severe aortic stenosis (AS). AS tracing is labeled with a maximal aortic valve velocity of 4.7 m/s and Bernoulli equation–derived peak and mean aortic valve gradient of 89- and 48-mm Hg, respectively. Aortic valve time-velocity integral (TVI) is 86 cm.

recommendation for AVR in asymptomatic patients with V_{max} ≥5.0 m/s regardless of LV ejection fractions or normal exercise testing. Similarly, once severe AS is present, AVR may be considered in asymptomatic patients, with a V_{max} progression of ≥0.3 m/s per year (17,18).

Mean Pressure Gradient

The mean transvalvular pressure gradient, or the pressure difference between the left ventricle and the aorta averaged across systole, is another standard parameter used to describe the severity of AS. Echocardiographic pressure gradients are derived from velocity information using the simplified Bernoulli equation, where the difference in pressure is equal to 4 times the velocity of blood flow squared (Table 12.2) (7). Because the peak velocity (V_{max}) would be used to directly calculate the peak transvalvular gradient, this additional "measurement" does not offer additional information and is not used to describe AS severity (7). In contrast, the mean pressure gradient (MPG), which has been shown to correlate better with gradients at catheterization, is always reported. By tracing the edge of the CWD derived spectral Doppler profile, the MPG is calculated with the echocardiography machine software by averaging instantaneous pressure gradients over the entire ejection period (Figures 12.2 and 12.3). It should be noted that while an equation "calculating" mean gradient from peak velocity has been described, it is not considered accurate enough for application in clinical practice.

TABLE 12.2 Doppler Equations for Aortic Transvalvular Gradients and Flow

Peak gradient (simplified Bernoulli equation)
Peak gradient (mm Hg) = $4(V_{AV})^2$
Mean gradient
Mean gradient (mm Hg) = $\Sigma\, 4(V)^2 / N$
Peak gradient with significant aortic regurgitation or high flow state (modified Bernoulli equation)
Peak gradient = $4([V_{AV}]^2 - [V_{LVOT}]^2)$
Stroke volume index
Stroke volume index (mL/m^2) = $(TVI_{LVOT} \times CSA_{LVOT}) / BSA$

AV, aortic valve; BSA, body surface area; CSA, cross-sectional area; LVOT, left ventricular outflow tract; TVI, time-velocity integral; *V*, velocity.

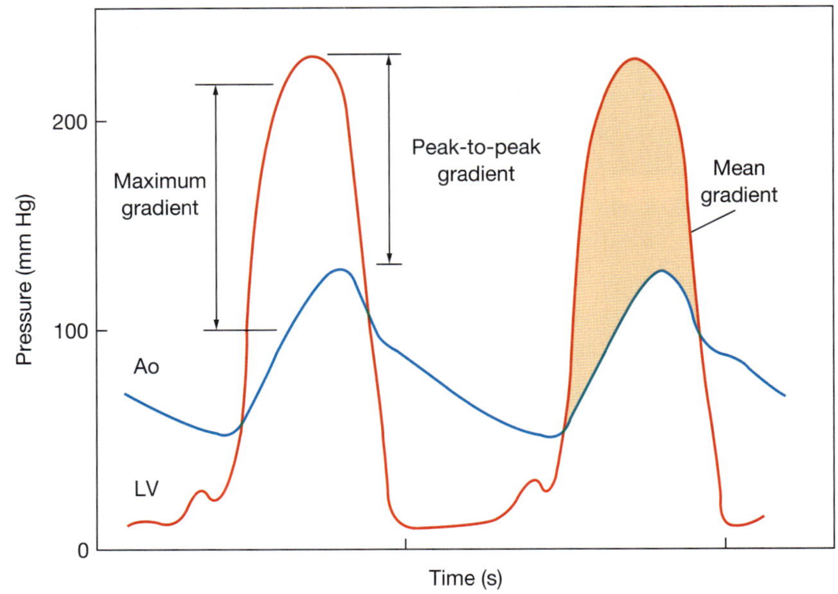

FIGURE 12.3 Example of left ventricular (LV) and aortic (Ao) pressures measured with fluid-filled catheters in a patient with severe aortic stenosis. The maximal instantaneous gradient is greater than the peak-to-peak gradient. The shaded area indicates the mean gradient.

As the simplified Bernoulli equation assumes a low proximal velocity, it cannot be applied when the LVOT velocity is >1.5 m/s, as may occur with concomitant aortic insufficiency or other high-output states. While a version of the Bernoulli equation that incorporates proximal velocity can be used to calculate *instantaneous* gradients in this situation, this equation cannot currently be applied to the instantaneous pressure gradients averaged across systole to create a mean gradient. As such, mean pressure gradients should not be reported in this situation.

Mean AV gradients of ≥40 mm Hg denote severe AS, whereas 20 to 40 mm Hg is moderate disease, and <20 mm Hg is mild (7). The exception is in patients who have a reduced stroke volume (ie, low contractility, hypovolemia, or severe mitral regurgitation). In this circumstance, the low stroke volume will be reflected by a low-pressure gradient despite having significant AS, thereby underestimating the severity (see further on). In this setting, estimating the AVA by the continuity equation is a preferred method for grading stenosis as the reduced stroke volume in both the LVOT and AV will be accounted for on each side of the equation (Table 12.3).

TABLE 12.3 Calculation of Aortic Valve Area With the Continuity Equation

Continuity equation—"What goes in must come out" LVOT stroke volume = AV stroke volume, where stroke volume = CSA × TVI Therefore, $TVI_{LVOT} \times CSA_{LVOT} = TVI_{AV} \times$ AV area AV area (cm^2) = $TVI_{LVOT} \times CSA_{LVOT} / TVI_{AV}$
Simplified continuity equation AV area (cm^2) = $V_{LVOT} \times CSA_{LVOT} / V_{AV}$
LVOT cross-sectional area LVOT CSA = $\pi (D_{LVOT} / 2)^2$

LVOT diameter is measured from inner edge to inner edge during midsystole.
AV, aortic valve; CSA, cross-sectional area; *D*, diameter; LVOT, left ventricular outflow tract; TVI, time-velocity integral; *V*, velocity.

Aortic Valve Area by Continuity Equation

While V_{max} and MPG vary with stroke volume, AVA has greater stability over a range of hemodynamic states. There are several ways to estimate the AVA; however, the preferred method is the continuity equation. This equation relies on the principle of the conservation of mass, where "what goes in must come out," and asserts that in the absence of a shunt between the two locations, the stroke volume through the LVOT must equal the stroke volume through the aortic valve (Figure 12.4). Stroke volume is determined by the product of the VTI, or the average "stroke distance" that blood travels during systole, and the cross-sectional area (CSA) of the orifice in question such that AVA is calculated as follows: $AVA = (LVOT_{CSA} \times LVOT_{VTI})/AV_{VTI}$ (Table 12.3) (12). A normal AVA is between 3 and 4 cm^2, while severe stenosis is reflected in an AVA $<$1.0 cm^2, moderate stenosis is 1.0 to 1.5 cm^2, and mild stenosis is $>$1.5 cm^2 (7).

Accurate AVA calculations rely on precise measurements, most importantly of the LVOT diameter, which is the most common source of error. The LVOT diameter is obtained in a zoomed ME AV LAX using an inner-edge to inner-edge technique at midsystole. The imaging plane is aligned through the interleaflet trigone between the left and noncoronary cusps of the AV posteriorly and the right coronary cusp anteriorly (19). Creating this precise plane may be easier using simultaneous biplane imaging from the ME AV SAX (Figure 12.5). While some recommendations suggest that LVOT diameters be measured between 5 and 10 mm from the AV annulus, this has been shown to result in a less accurate and less reproducible calculation of AVA by the continuity equation owing to the more ellipsoid or trapezoidal shape of the proximal LVOT (19,20). We recommend measuring the LVOT diameter at the level of aortic cusp insertion as this improves interobserver reproducibility, is the most circular anatomic level, and best corresponds with the "true" AVA using invasive measurements (7,12,19,22).

In cases in which there is a concern for significant LVOT diameter inaccuracies, the standard approach to echocardiographic measurement of LVOT diameter may be supplemented with an alternative measurement of $LVOT_{CSA}$ by either 3D echocardiography or computed tomography angiography, both of which have confirmed that the AV annulus and LVOT are ellipsoid rather than circular in most patients (7,23-25). Multiplanar reconstruction from a 3D image of a 2D imaging plane directly orthogonal to the LVOT can provide a more precise measurement of the $LVOT_{CSA}$ (Figure 12.5). While this method can avoid the underestimation of the true LVOT area that often occurs with the standard 2D approach, routine 3D-derived measurements of the $LVOT_{CSA}$ for continuity equation–derived AVA are not recommended, as doing so results in potentially larger AVAs and consequent erroneous assessment of disease severity (19).

Once the $LVOT_{CSA}$ is calculated, VTIs of both the LVOT and AV are obtained by using pulsed-(PWD) (Figure 12.6) and continuous wave Doppler (Figure 12.1), respectively. VTI, which is measured by integrating

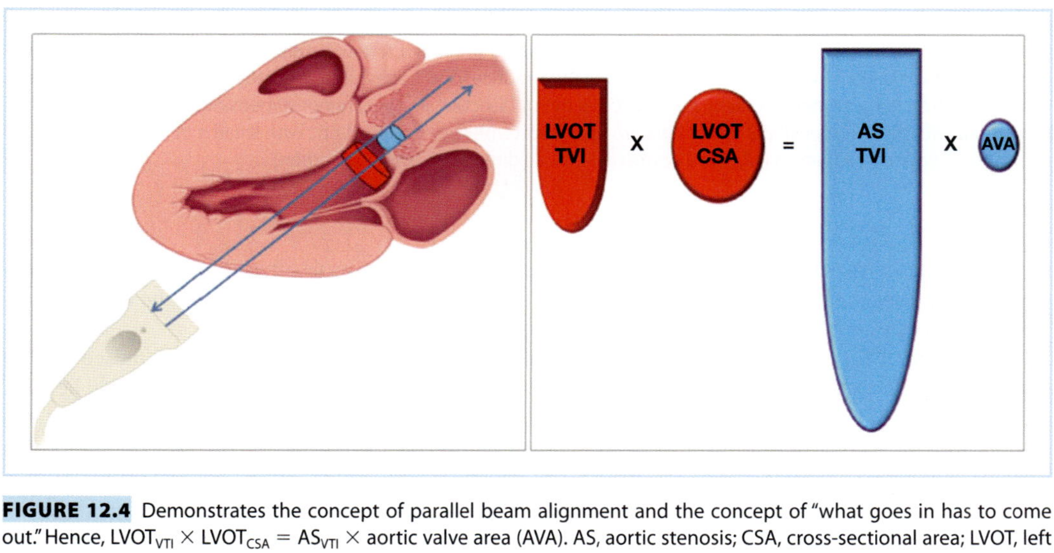

FIGURE 12.4 Demonstrates the concept of parallel beam alignment and the concept of "what goes in has to come out." Hence, $LVOT_{VTI} \times LVOT_{CSA} = AS_{VTI} \times$ aortic valve area (AVA). AS, aortic stenosis; CSA, cross-sectional area; LVOT, left ventricular outflow tract; TVI, time-velocity integral.

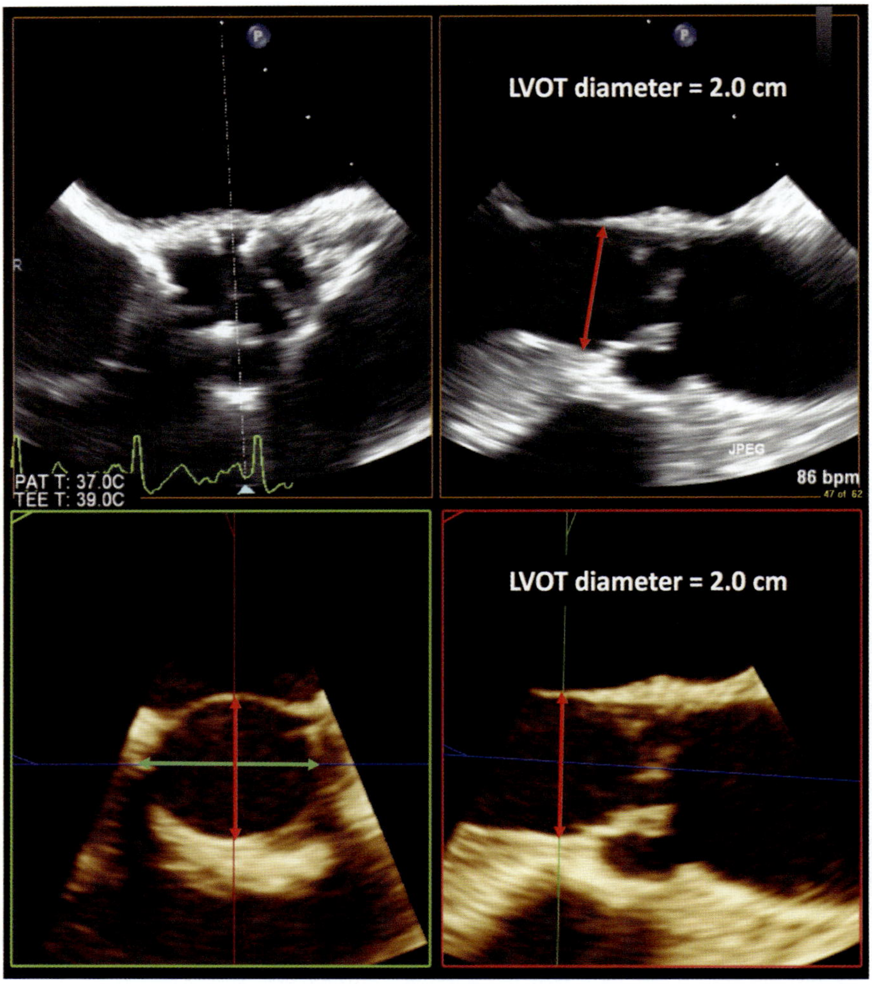

FIGURE 12.5 Midesophageal short-axis view of a stenotic trileaflet aortic valve. Biplane imaging of the aortic valve is utilized with biplane cursor positioned through commissure (between left and noncoronary sinus) and right sinus (top, left). An orthogonal view is created that generally produces the largest anteroposterior left ventricular outflow tract (LVOT) and annular measurement as the LVOT is being bisected along its minor dimension. LVOT imaging can be performed with three-dimensional multiplanar imaging (bottom). The LVOT is elliptic with small minor (anteroposterior) dimension (shown in red) and a larger major (medial-lateral) dimension (shown in green).

the area under the curve of the blood flow, is generated using computational software on the echocardiography machine after tracing the outer edge of the spectral profile. This calculation provides the distance (cm) that a blood cell travels in one systolic beat in the sampled orifice.

Once the $LVOT_{CSA}$ is calculated, VTIs of both the LVOT and AV are obtained by using pulsed-(PWD) (Figure 12.6) and continuous wave Doppler (CWD) (Figure 12.1), respectively. The $LVOT_{VTI}$ should be measured with the PWD sample gate just upstream from the systolic flow convergence at the aortic valve. Beginning with the sample gate at the level of the annulus and gradually moving it proximally until a smooth velocity profile with a narrow range of velocities is obtained suggests a good LVOT spectral profile. For the AV_{VTI}, CWD interrogation is used in the same acoustic window that was chosen for the $LVOT_{VTI}$. As CWD will measure the highest transvalvular velocities throughout systole, in the absence of a supra- or subvalvular obstruction, this will represent the spectral profile of the stenosed aortic valve orifice. Note that while the

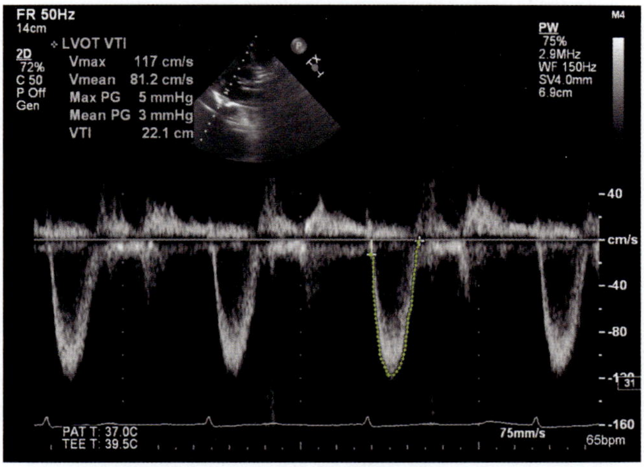

FIGURE 12.6 Deep transgastric view of the aortic valve with pulsed-wave (PW) Doppler assessment of the left ventricular outflow tract (LVOT) velocity. The LVOT time-velocity integral (TVI) is 22.1 cm. The LVOT TVI is also used to calculate the stroke volume index, which is important in the assessment of low-flow, low-gradient aortic stenosis.

LVOT signal may be seen "inside" the CWD signal of AS (called a double envelope), the LVOT measurement should not be made from this image as it includes higher velocities from the area of flow convergence (Figure 12.7).

Alternative Measures of Aortic Stenosis Severity

The following additional parameters are not required in every patient but may provide additional information for severity grading in select clinical scenarios.

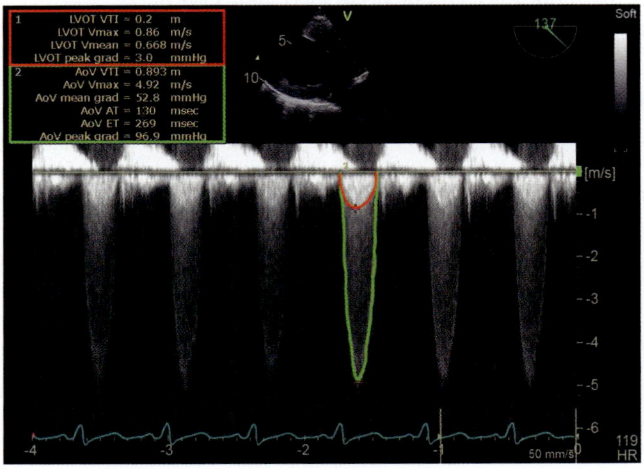

FIGURE 12.7 Transgastric long-axis view with parallel continuous wave Doppler beam alignment in a patient with severe aortic stenosis. A double envelope can be seen, with the inner envelope (red line) representing the left ventricular outflow tract (LVOT) and the outer envelope (green line) the stenosed orifice. LVOT tracing is labeled with a maximal velocity of 0.86 m/s. LVOT time-velocity integral (TVI) is 0.2 m. Aortic stenosis tracing is labeled with a maximal aortic valve velocity of 4.92 m/s and Bernoulli equation–derived peak and mean aortic valve gradient of 96.9- and 52.8-mm Hg, respectively. Aortic valve time-velocity integral (TVI) is 0.893 m.

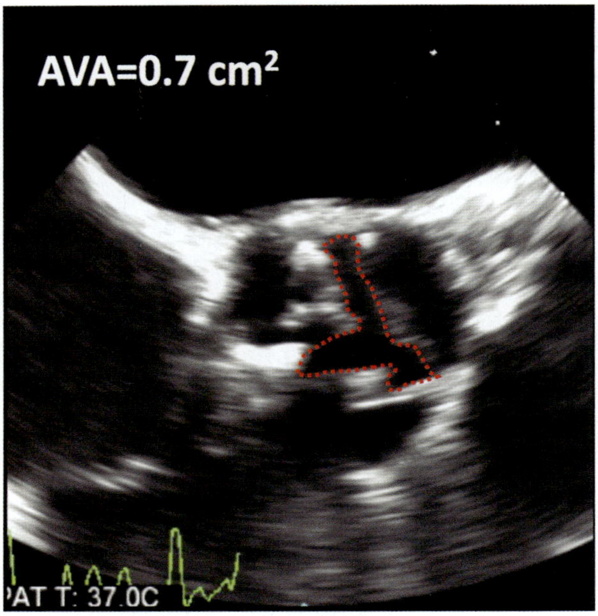

FIGURE 12.8 Two-dimensional planimetry of a stenotic aortic valve. The aortic valve area (AVA) is 0.7 cm.

Simplified Continuity Equation

The continuity equation can be simplified based on the concept that the ratio of the $LVOT_{VTI}$ and AV_{VTI} is usually very similar to the ratio of the LVOT and AV peak velocities (Table 12.3). With this assumption, the velocities of blood flow through the LVOT and AV, which may be easier to measure, are used in place of VTIs for the estimation of AVA. The limitation of this approach is that it becomes less accurate if the velocity curves are atypical. Furthermore, the inclusion of stroke volume (SV) in the assessment of severity grading is important in patients with low-gradient AS (discussed further on).

Dimensionless Index

In order to eliminate the error inherent to measuring the LVOT diameter, the dimensionless index removes $LVOT_{CSA}$ from the continuity equation to provide a ratio of the LVOT to AV VTI (or LVOT to AV peak velocity). A decreasing ratio indicates increasing obstruction of flow across the AV, with a ratio of less than 0.25 representing severe stenosis (Table 12.1). Once the dimensionless index is <0.2, the outcome is poor independent of body surface area or indexed stroke volume (26). The dimensionless index can prove useful as a simple and reliable marker of AS severity in circumstances in which image quality prevents an accurate assessment of the $LVOT_{CSA}$ or the patient has variable loading conditions (ie, low flow–low gradient AS or irregular heart rhythms) (7).

Planimetry

Planimetry is a direct measurement of the aortic valve's stenotic anatomic orifice, which can be performed with 2D or 3D imaging. While intuitively attractive, it's critical to recognize the limitations inherent to this technique, most importantly, the fundamental difference between the anatomic orifice and the effective orifice of a stenotic valve (Figure 12.8). The AVA derived from the continuity equation reflects the *effective* orifice area rather than the *anatomic* orifice, which is measured with planimetry. It is that effective orifice that has been best studied, that best reflects the clinical severity of stenosis, and upon which guidelines are based. The effective orifice will always be smaller due to the contraction of flow that occurs distal to the anatomic orifice (7,20).

While planimetry is not a first-line modality for evaluating AS, it may add value when Doppler measurements are unavailable or unreliable. Disadvantages of planimetry include the following (27):

1. Measurements may be difficult and the results inaccurate when aortic valve calcification causes acoustic shadowing or reverberation artifact.
2. It can be difficult to identify the smallest anatomic orifice, particularly with 2D imaging. If an area is measured that is proximal to the leaflet tips, the orifice area will be overestimated. This challenge can be mitigated somewhat using 3D datasets (Figure 12.9).
3. Effective orifice area is a better predictor of patient outcome than anatomic orifice area.

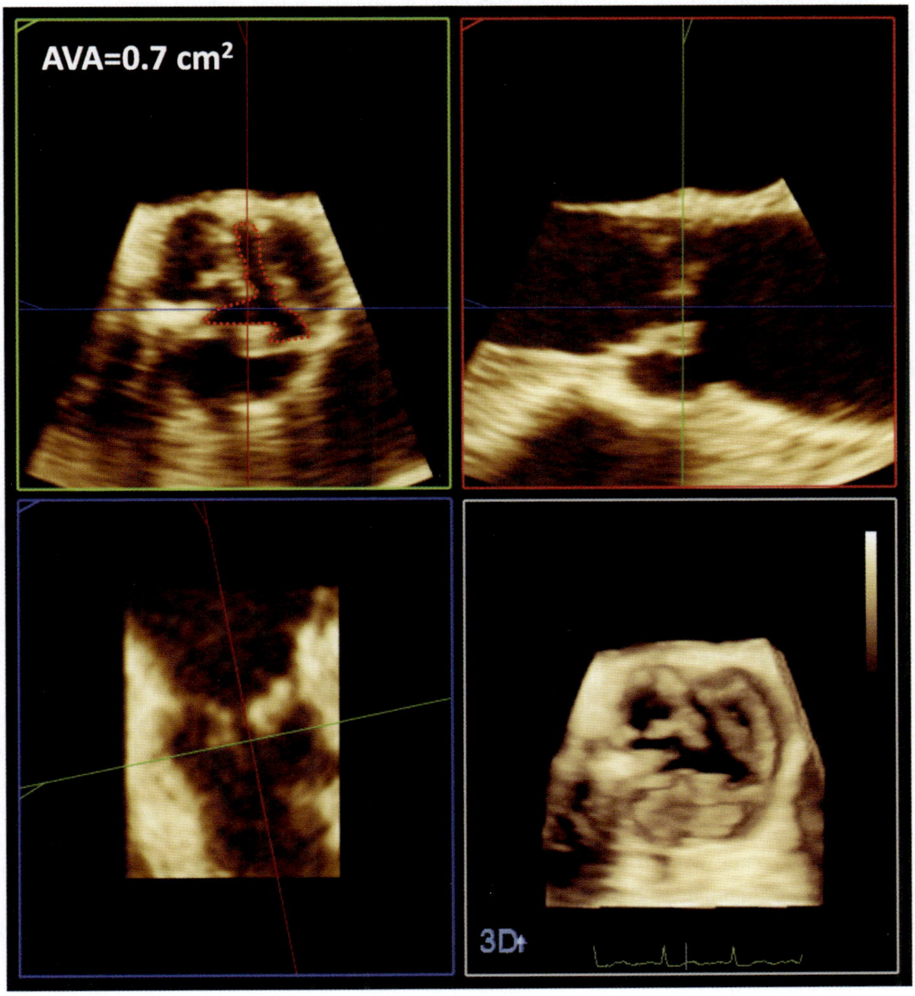

FIGURE 12.9 Three-dimensional planimetry of a stenotic aortic valve is performed with multiplanar reconstruction software. The blue and red (long-axis) planes are aligned along the direction of blow flow at the level of the aortic orifice in a midsystolic frame. The transverse (green) plane is positioned perpendicular to long-axis planes at the level of the leaflet tips. Planimetry is performed in the transverse plane (top, left). The aortic valve area is 0.7 cm^2 (same patient as in Figure 12.9). Note the stellate orifice shape seen both in the two-dimensional multiplanar image (top, left) and volume rendering (bottom, right).

Discordant Criteria in Aortic Stenosis

Ideally, there would be concordance of all the criteria listed in Table 12.1. Patients with severe AS would have a V_{max} >4.0 m/s, a MPG >40 mm Hg, and an AVA <1.0 cm^2. Unfortunately, even after excluding measurement errors, a significant minority of patients have discordance when comparing mean gradient or peak velocity to aortic valve area and require further consideration. An approach to patients with low-gradient AS (mean gradient <40 mm Hg and an aortic valve area <1.0 cm^2) is described in what follows.

Low Flow, Low Gradient Aortic Stenosis With Reduced Left Ventricular Ejection Fraction

A common cause of low-gradient AS is a reduction in flow across the aortic valve due to LV failure. Such classical low-flow, low-gradient AS will demonstrate a stroke volume index <35 mL/m^2 in the setting of reduced left ventricular ejection fraction (LVEF <50%) and in one study, was present in up to 35% of patients with AS (28). Dobutamine stress echocardiography (DSE) is a useful diagnostic test to further separate true severe from pseudosevere AS (29). During the DSE, if the mean gradient increases to >40 mm Hg with an aortic valve area <1.0 cm^2, the patient is classified as true severe AS and meets criteria for valve intervention. If the increase in flow with dobutamine results in an AVA >1.0 cm^2, this is classified as pseudosevere AS, suggesting that at low flow the valve doesn't open because the ventricle can't "push it open." These patients should be referred for heart failure therapy (28). A percentage of patients undergoing DSE for classical low flow–low gradient AS will not have a significant increase in stroke volume (<15%-20% change from baseline), and the mean gradient will remain <40 mm Hg and the valve area <1.0 cm^2. In this patient cohort with no contractile reserve, a multidetector computed tomography (MDCT) calcium score may be helpful in delineating the next steps (28).

Low-Flow, Low-Gradient Aortic Stenosis With Preserved Left Ventricular Ejection Fraction ("Paradoxical")

Paradoxical low flow, low-gradient AS has similar features to classical low flow–low gradient AS, including a valve gradient <40 mm Hg, a stroke volume index <35 mL/m^2, and an aortic valve area <1.0 cm^2. However, in paradoxical low flow–low gradient AS, the LVEF is >50%. Therefore, the decreased stroke volume is secondary to other physiologic factors, including significant concentric LV hypertrophy, diastolic dysfunction, bradycardia, tachycardia, atrial fibrillation, mitral valve regurgitation or stenosis, or right ventricular dysfunction (30).

Normal Flow, Low-Gradient Aortic Stenosis With Preserved Left Ventricular Ejection Fraction

This describes a patient with an AVA <1.0 cm^2 and a mean gradient <40 mm Hg despite a stroke volume index >35 mL/m^2 and an LVEF >50%. In this situation, it is imperative to first double-check echocardiographic measurements of the gradient and the aortic valve area and to consider indexing AVA, particularly if the patient is of small stature. The most common cause for this constellation, however, is the inconsistent cutoffs for valve area and gradient/velocity. To generate a mean gradient of 40 mm Hg at a normal flow rate, the AVA would be expected to be 0.8 cm^2 rather than 1.0 cm^2. While there is some disagreement about this issue and further data need to be collected, at present it appears that normal flow, low-gradient AS patients have outcomes similar to those with classic moderate AS. As such, the current recommendation is not to diagnose these patients as severe but rather to follow them closely and reevaluate them regularly (Figure 12.10) (20).

A Holistic Approach to Aortic Stenosis: Transthoracic Echocardiography Versus Transesophageal Echocardiography , Pressure Recovery, Combined Valve Disease, and Subaortic Obstruction

Transthoracic Echocardiography Versus Transesophageal Echocardiography

There are several factors that need to be considered when assessing patients for AS that may impact valve gradients. The mean gradient and aortic valve area that represent severe AS were established in awake spontaneous ventilated patients using TTE. For patients presenting for cardiac surgery, the echocardiographer may encounter previously undiagnosed AS. Intraoperative TEE assessment of AS for patients under general endotracheal anesthesia with positive pressure ventilation has several features that are different than

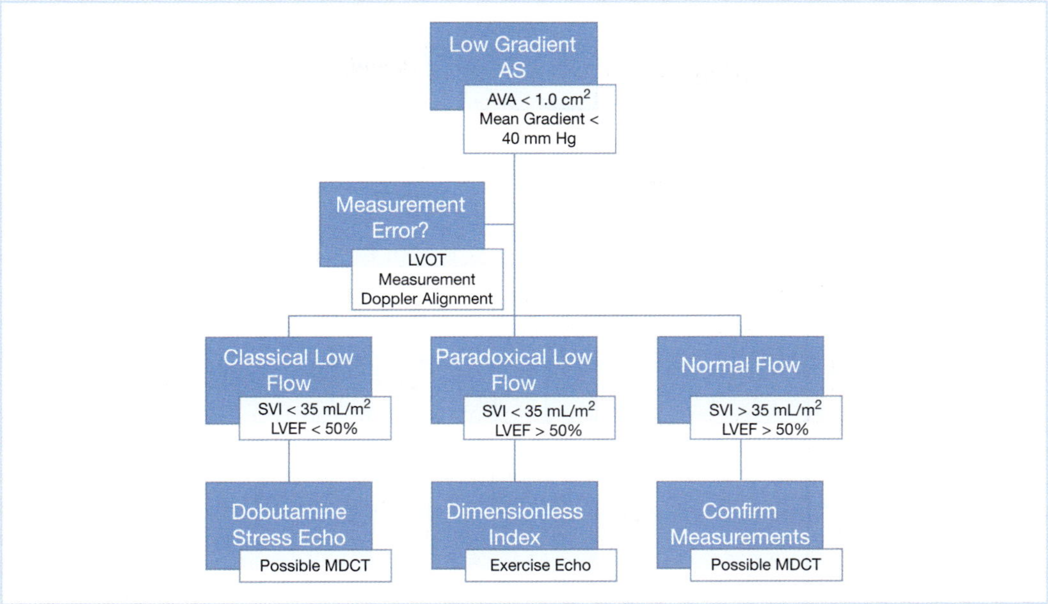

FIGURE 12.10 An approach to low-gradient aortic stenosis. After confirming accurate measurements, patients are classified and stratified based on LVEF and stroke volume index. MDCT and exercise echocardiography may help differentiate low-gradient severe aortic stenosis from less severe aortic valve disease. (Adapted from Baumgartner H, Hung J, Bermejo J, et al. Recommendations on the echocardiographic assessment of aortic valve stenosis: a focused update from the European Association of Cardiovascular Imaging and the American Society of Echocardiography. *J Am Soc Echocardiogr*. 2017;30[4]:372-392.)

preoperative TTE assessment of AS. One study that examined the difference between TTE and TEE assessment of AS demonstrated that the mean gradient on intraoperative TEE exam was 4.0 to 9.3 mm Hg lower compared to preoperative TTE, and the aortic valve area was 0.04 to 0.15 cm^2 higher on TEE compared to preoperative TTE. This can be clinically relevant as the intraoperative TEE measurements classified patients' AS as one grade lower 39.1% of the time compared to TTE (31). There are several proposed mechanisms for the discrepancy between preoperative TTE and intraoperative TEE. The physiologic effects of positive pressure ventilation may decrease stroke volume index in a similar fashion for patients with paradoxical low flow–low gradient AS. In the setting of a normal LVEF, the stroke volume index (SVI) may be reduced to <35 mL/m^2, and this could be responsible for the decreased mean gradient. Another difference between TTE and TEE is the Doppler insonation angle. There are different valve gradients secondary to different views on TTE, and the discordance between TTE and TEE may be related to Doppler alignment.

Pressure Recovery

There are other imaging modality differences that affect aortic valve mean gradients. Echocardiography uses CWD to assess the peak velocity and mean gradients in the vena contracta of the stenotic valve. When mean gradients are assessed during invasive catheter measurements, the mean gradient is measured distal to the stenotic valve. Due to pressure recovery, echocardiography Doppler gradients may be higher than catheter measured gradients. Pressure recovery is the result of flow through different-sized orifices. As blood moves through a stenotic AV, potential energy converts into kinetic energy with a resulting reduction in pressure at the vena contracta. Distal to the valve, flow in the ascending aorta results in the conversion of kinetic energy back to potential energy with recovery of pressure (Figure 12.11). Since Doppler-based methods detect the peak velocity at the vena contracta, the transvalvular gradient estimated by Doppler will be greater than that calculated from simultaneous invasive pressure measurements between the LVOT and the aortic root (Figure 12.3) (7). As the size of the aorta decreases, there is increased pressure recovery. In patients with small aortas, there may be increased discordance between Doppler and catheter gradients (32).

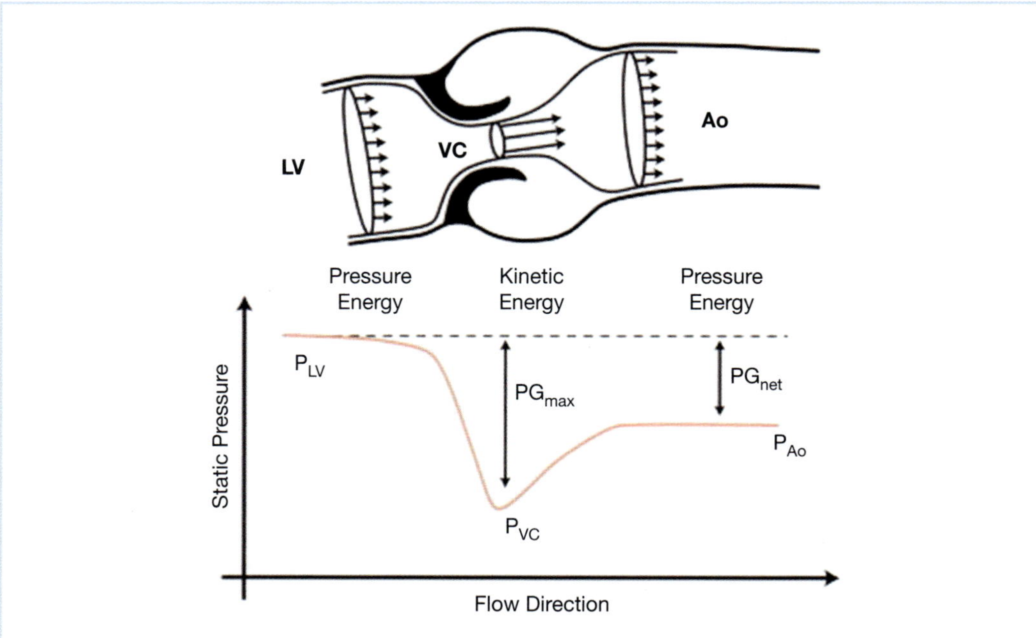

FIGURE 12.11 Pressure recovery. The convergence of flow through the stenotic aortic valve to the vena contracta converts potential (pressure) energy into kinetic energy with a resulting reduction in pressure at the vena contracta. Divergence of flow distally allows reconversion of some kinetic energy to potential (pressure) energy with recovery of a proportion of the pressure lost within a few centimeters. Ao, aortic root; LV, left ventricular; P_{Ao}, pressure in the aorta; PG_{max}, maximum pressure gradient; PG_{net}, net change in pressure gradient; P_{LV}, pressure in the left ventricular; P_{VC}, pressure at the vena contracta; VC, vena contracta.

Combined Valve Disease

Coexisting valvulopathy impacts the assessment and prognosis of AS. Significant tricuspid or mitral valve disease may contribute to paradoxical low-flow, low-gradient AS due to a decreased stroke volume index or right ventricular dysfunction in the setting of a normal LVEF. In the presence of significant aortic insufficiency, there is often an increased stroke volume and velocity across the LVOT. For these patients with AS and aortic insufficiency (AI), the mean gradient may be discordant with the degree of AS by AVA. Patients with moderate AS by valve area may have mean gradients >40 mm Hg.

Significant mitral and tricuspid regurgitation at the time of SAVR is associated with worse long-term outcomes. Results from the PARTNER trial demonstrated an increased mortality at 2 years in patients with moderate or more mitral regurgitation undergoing SAVR (33).

Serial Stenoses

Valvular AS can coexist with either dynamic LVOT obstruction from systolic anterior motion of the mitral leaflets or with fixed LVOT obstruction from a subvalvular membrane. The echocardiographer should be alert to the appearance of these causes of increased velocity.

Increased velocity from obstruction in the LVOT (either fixed or dynamic) significantly complicates the assessment of transvalvular velocity, mean gradient, and AVA by the continuity equation due to the complex hydrodynamics of serial stenoses (34). This is a situation where planimetry may be an appropriate echocardiographic technique. The classic spectral Doppler finding of dynamic LVOT obstruction is the late-peaking appearing velocity profile (Figure 12.12). While this signal is referred to as dagger-shaped this is a misnomer,

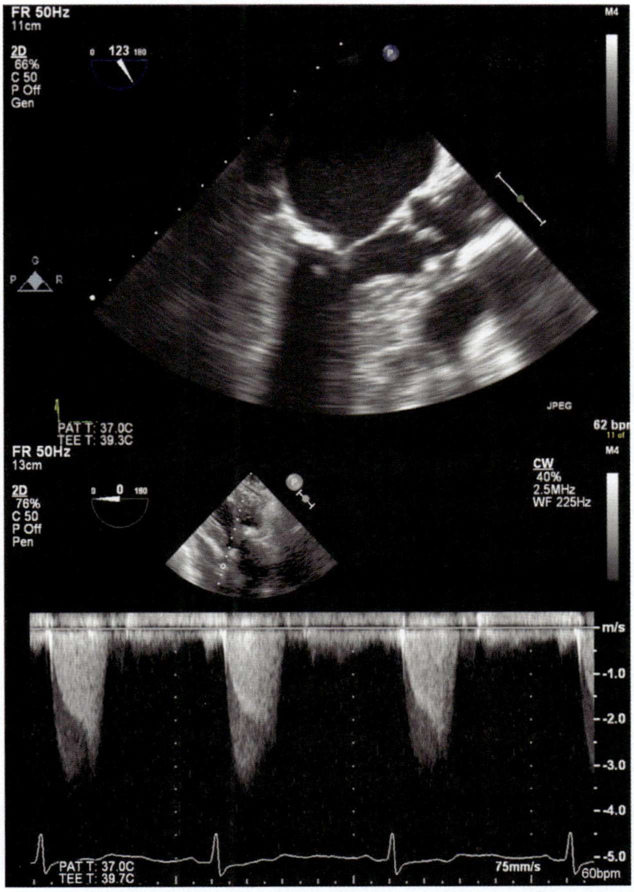

FIGURE 12.12 Midesophageal long-axis view demonstrating profound asymmetric upper septal hypertrophy in a patient with calcific aortic valve stenosis. Note the acute narrowing of the left ventricular outflow tract (LVOT) at the area of upper septal hypertrophy (top). With CWD beam aligned through the LVOT and aortic valve (performed in the deep transgastric view), two profiles are visualized: a late-peaking, dagger-shaped profile due to subaortic obstruction and a fainter signal representing flow through the stenotic aortic valve (bottom).

as daggers are characteristically symmetrical, and it is instead clip point blades that have this asymmetric, concave appearance. The spectral Doppler signal from fixed LVOT obstruction in the setting of subaortic membrane can be difficult to distinguish from that of valvular AS; however, both fixed and dynamic LVOT obstructions typically demonstrate the mosaic pattern of turbulent flow in the LVOT with CFD (which would not be expected in valvular AS).

Transesophageal Echocardiography for Transcatheter Aortic Valve Replacement

Echocardiography is a valuable tool in both the preprocedural assessment and (occasionally) for intraprocedural guidance of the TAVR procedure. Many of the goals for the preprocedural echocardiographic assessment of TAVR are similar to the prebyass assessment for surgical aortic valves. Prior to valve implantation, it is important for the echocardiographer to delineate aortic valve morphology, aortic annular dimensions, the aortic sinus and coronary artery height, and the aortic valve hemodynamics. Evidence of additional, unexpected abnormalities should also be sought. After valve deployment, the echocardiographer should assess the function of the transcatheter valve, measure the mean gradient, quantify any paravalvular leak, and seek evidence of new pericardial effusion.

Experience with TAVR has improved both the anatomic understanding of as well as the echocardiographic assessment of the aortic annulus due to the critical importance of accurate annular sizing without the availability of a manual sizer as would be used during open surgery (35,36). 2D echocardiography commonly underestimates the size of the aortic annulus both due to often improper cross sections (described previously) and because it measures the minor dimension of the elliptic annulus. 3D echocardiography is more accurate than 2D echocardiography for this evaluation and has comparable results compared to CT. There are several techniques to evaluate the aortic annulus in 3D, and a commonly used technique is called the double oblique or turnaround technique. It may be summarized thus (37):

1. The goal of the double oblique technique is to measure the virtual ring of the aortic annulus.
2. Acquire a 3D data of the aortic valve in short or long axis with TEE, and open the multiplanar reconstruction software.
3. After selecting a frame in midsystole, align the long axis view (sagittal) and orthogonal (coronal) views to be parallel with blood flow.
4. Move the short axis (transverse) plane to the level of the annulus and aim for the hinge points of the aortic valve leaflets.
5. Rotate the two orthogonal planes within the short-axis plane to confirm that the short-axis plane is at the level of all three hinge points. If the hinge point of a cusp is not aligned in the short axis, adjust the sagittal or coronal plane, and continue to rotate the two orthogonal planes until the short-axis plane intersects all three hinge points (Figure 12.13).
6. Use direct planimetry in the transverse plane to obtain the aortic annular area (Figure 12.14).

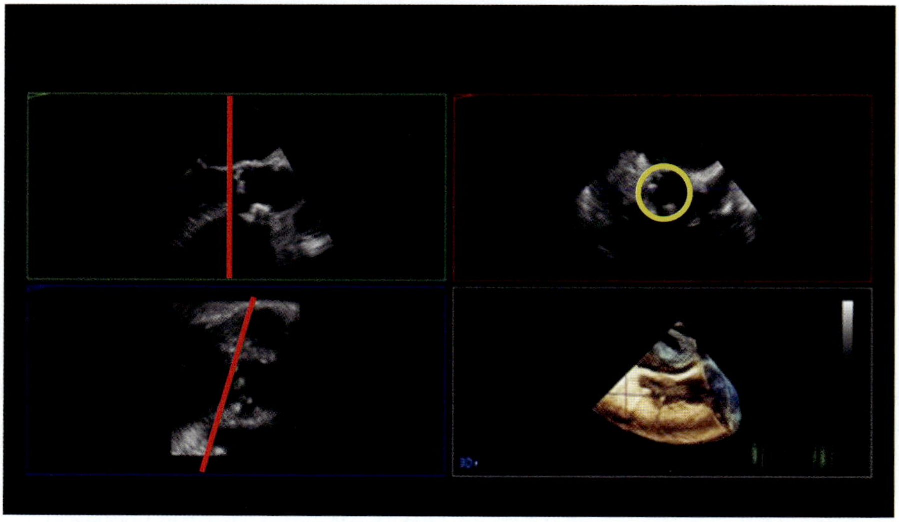

FIGURE 12.13 Multiplanar reconstruction for aortic annular measurement. The sagittal (long-axis view) is the green plane. The coronal slice is the blue plane. The short-axis view is the red plane.

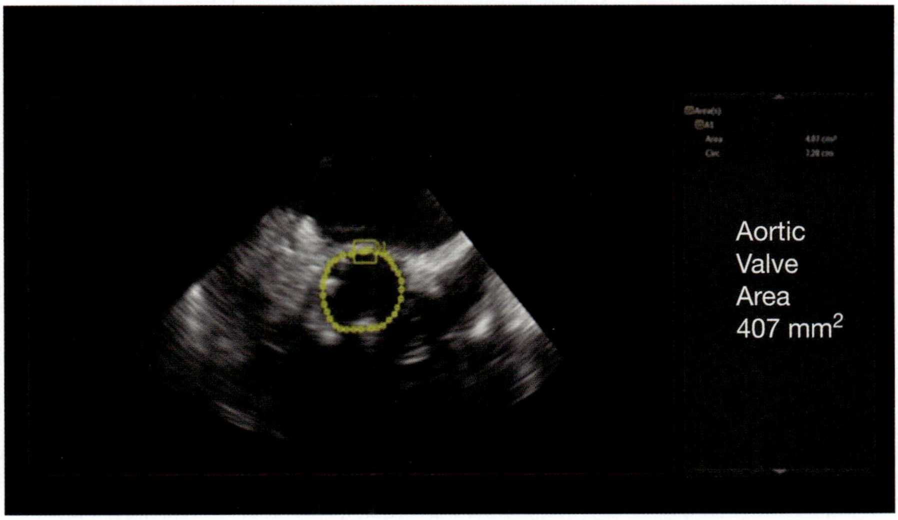

FIGURE 12.14 Area trace of aortic annulus. Planimetry area measurement of the aortic annulus. After alignment of the orthogonal planes, the turnaround technique is used to ensure the short-axis plane intersects the three hinge points of the aortic valve at the virtual annulus.

SUMMARY

AS is an important cause of cardiovascular morbidity and mortality that continues to increase in prevalence. Echocardiography is the primary modality for the assessment and risk stratification of these patients. A thorough understanding of the echocardiographic parameters used to evaluate AS is critical for all perioperative physicians caring for this patient population.

ACKNOWLEDGMENTS

We gratefully acknowledge the contributions of the previous edition authors, Praveen Mehrotra and Ira S. Cohen, as portions of those chapters have been retained in this revision.

REFERENCES

1. Lung B, Delgado V, Rosenhek R, et al; EORP VHD II Investigators. Contemporary presentation and management of valvular heart disease: the EURObservational Research Programme Valvular Heart Disease II Survey. *Circulation*. 2019;140(14):1156-1169.
2. Durko AP, Osnabrugge RL, Van Mieghem NM, et al. Annual number of candidates for transcatheter aortic valve implantation per country: current estimates and future projections. *Eur Heart J*. 2018;39(28):2635-2642.
3. Manzo R, Ilardi F, Nappa D, et al. Echocardiographic evaluation of aortic stenosis: a comprehensive review. *Diagnostics (Basel)*. 2023;13(15):2527.
4. Lindman BR, Clavel MA, Mathieu P, et al. Calcific aortic stenosis. *Nat Rev Dis Primers*. 2016;2:16006.
5. Otto CM, Nishimura RA, Bonow RO, et al. ACC/AHA guideline for the management of patients with valvular heart disease: executive summary: a report of the American College of Cardiology/American Heart Association Joint Committee on Clinical Practice Guidelines [Erratum appears in: *Circulation*. 2021;143(5):e228. Erratum appears in: *Circulation*. 2021;143(10):e784]. *Circulation*. 2021;143(5):e35-e71.
6. de Azevedo Filho AF, Accorsi TA, Ribeiro HB. Coronary artery disease in patients with aortic stenosis and transcatheter aortic valve implantation: implications for management. *Eur Cardiol*. 2021;16:e49.
7. Baumgartner H, Hung J, Bermejo J, et al. Recommendations on the echocardiographic assessment of aortic valve stenosis: a focused update from the European Association of Cardiovascular Imaging and the American Society of Echocardiography. *J Am Soc Echocardiogr*. 2017;30(4):372-392.
8. Oh JK, Taliercio CP, Holmes DR Jr, et al. Prediction of the severity of aortic stenosis by Doppler aortic valve area determination: prospective Doppler-catheterization correlation in 100 patients. *J Am Coll Cardiol*. 1988;11(6):1227-1234.

9. Otto CM, Pearlman AS, Comess KA, Reamer RP, Janko CL, Huntsman LL. Determination of the stenotic aortic valve area in adults using Doppler echocardiography. *J Am Coll Cardiol.* 1986;7(3):509-517.
10. Galan A, Zoghbi WA, Quiñones MA. Determination of severity of valvular aortic stenosis by Doppler echocardiography and relation of findings to clinical outcome and agreement with hemodynamic measurements determined at cardiac catheterization. *Am J Cardiol.* 1991;67(11):1007-1012.
11. Schwartzenberg S, Vaturi M, Kazum S, et al. Comparison of simultaneous transthoracic versus transesophageal echocardiography for assessment of aortic stenosis. *Am J Cardiol.* 2022;163:77-84.
12. Ring L, Shah BN, Bhattacharyya S, et al. Echocardiographic assessment of aortic stenosis: a practical guideline from the British Society of Echocardiography. *Echo Res Pract.* 2021;8(1):G19-G59.
13. Sievers HH, Schmidtke C. A classification system for the bicuspid aortic valve from 304 surgical specimens. *J Thorac Cardiovasc Surg.* 2007;133(5):1226-1233.
14. Hatle L, Angelsen BA, Tromsdal A. Non-invasive assessment of aortic stenosis by Doppler ultrasound. *Br Heart J.* 1980;43:284-292.
15. Zoghbi WA, Farmer KL, Soto JG, Nelson JG, Quinones MA. Accurate noninvasive quantification of stenotic aortic valve area by Doppler echocardiography. *Circulation.* 1986;73:452-459.
16. Nakatsuma K, Taniguchi T, Morimoto T, et al. Prognostic impact of peak aortic jet velocity in conservatively managed patients with severe aortic stenosis: an observation from the CURRENT AS registry. *J Am Heart Assoc.* 2017;6:e005524.
17. Vahanian A, Beyersdorf F, Praz F, et al. 2021 ESC/EACTS guidelines for the management of valvular heart disease. *Eur Heart J.* 2022;43:561-632.
18. Nishimura RA, Otto CM, Bonow RO, et al. 2014 AHA/ACC guideline for the management of patients with valvular heart disease: executive summary: a report of the American College of Cardiology/American Heart Association Task Force on Practice Guidelines [Erratum appears in *Circulation.* 2014;129(23):e650]. *Circulation.* 2014;129(23):2440-2492.
19. Clavel MA, Malouf J, Messika-Zeitoun D, et al. Aortic valve area calculation in aortic stenosis by CT and Doppler echocardiography. *JACC Cardiovasc Imaging.* 2015;8(3):248-257.
20. Hahn RT, Saric M, Faletra FF, et al. Recommended standards for the performance of transesophageal echocardiographic screening for structural heart intervention: from the American Society of Echocardiography. *J Am Soc Echocardiog.* 2022;35:1-76.
21. LaBounty TM, Miyasaka R, Chetcuti S, et al. Annulus instead of LVOT diameter improves agreement between echocardiography effective orifice area and invasive aortic valve area. *JACC Cardiovasc Imaging.* 2014;7(10):1065-1066.
22. Skjaerpe T, Hegrenaes L, Hatle L. Noninvasive estimation of valve area in patients with aortic stenosis by Doppler ultrasound and two-dimensional echocardiography. *Circulation.* 1985;72(4):810-818.
23. Ng AC, Delgado V, van der Kley F, et al. Comparison of aortic root dimensions and geometries before and after transcatheter aortic valve implantation by 2- and 3-dimensional transesophageal echocardiography and multislice computed tomography. *Circ Cardiovasc Imaging.* 2010;3(1):94-102.
24. Saitoh T, Shiota M, Izumo M, et al. Comparison of left ventricular outflow geometry and aortic valve area in patients with aortic stenosis by 2-dimensional versus 3-dimensional echocardiography. *Am J Cardiol.* 2012;109(11):1626-1631.
25. Mehrotra P, Flynn AW, Jansen K, et al. Differential left ventricular outflow tract remodeling and dynamics in aortic stenosis. *J Am Soc Echocardiogr.* 2015;28(11):1259-1266.
26. Rusinaru D, Malaquin D, Maréchaux S, Debry N, Tribouilloy C. Relation of dimensionless index to long-term outcome in aortic stenosis with preserved LVEF. *JACC Cardiovasc Imaging.* 2015;8(7):766-775.
27. Saura D, Morena G, Flores-Blanco P, et al. Aortic valve stenosis planimetry by means of three-dimensional TEE in the real clinical setting: feasibility, reliability and systematic deviations. *Echocardiography.* 2015;32(3):508-515.
28. Clavel M, Magne J, Pibarot P. Low gradient aortic stenosis. *Eur Heart J.* 2016;37:2645-2657.
29. Vahanian A, Alfieri O, Andreotti F, et al. Guidelines on the management of valvular heart disease. European Association for Cardio-Thoracic Surgery (EACTS). *Eur Heart J.* 2012;33:2451-2496.
30. Elied MF, Sorajja P, Michelena HI, et al. Flow gradient patterns in severe aortic stenosis with preserved ejection fraction: clinical characteristics and predictors of survival. *Circulation.* 2013;18:1781-1789.
31. Whitener G, Sivak J, Akushevich I, et al. Grading aortic stenosis with mean gradient and aortic valve area: a comparison between preoperative and precardiopulmonary bypass TEE. *J Cardiothorac Vasc Anesth.* 2016;30(5):1254-1259.
32. Niederberger J, Schima H, Maurer G, et al. Importance of pressure recovery for the assessment of aortic stenosis by doppler ultrasound. Role of aortic size, aortic valve area and direction of the stenotic jet in vitro. *Circulation.* 1996;94:1934-1940.
33. Barbanti M, Webb J, Hahn R, et al. Impact of preoperative moderate/severe mitral regurgitation on 2 year outcome after transcatheter and surgical aortic valve replacement: insight from the placement of aortic transcatheter valve trial cohort A. *Circulation.* 2013;128(25):2776-2784.
34. Scantlebury DC, Geske JB, Nishimura RA. Limitations of Doppler echocardiography in the evaluation of serial stenoses. *Circ Cardiovasc Imaging.* 2018;6:850-852.
35. Binder RK, Webb JG, Willson AB, et al. The impact of integration of a multidetector computed tomography annulus area sizing algorithm on outcomes of transcatheter aortic valve replacement: a prospective, multicenter, controlled trial. *J Am Coll Cardiol.* 2013;62:431-438.
36. Jilaihawi H, Kashif M, Fontana G, et al. Cross-sectional computed tomographic assessment improves accuracy of aortic annular sizing for transcatheter aortic valve replacement and reduces the incidence of paravalvular aortic regurgitation. *J Am Coll Cardiol.* 2012;59:1275-1286.
37. Hahn RT. Aortic Annular Sizing for TAVR: Echocardiographic Approaches. American College of Cardiology. January 14, 2015. Accessed June 24, 2025. https://www.acc.org/latest-in-cardiology/articles/2014/12/22/15/45/aortic-annular-sizing-for-tavr-echocardiographic-approaches-expert-analysis

QUESTIONS

1. **A 79-year-old male with a history of coronary artery disease and heart failure with reduced ejection fraction (20%) is evaluated for aortic stenosis with echocardiography. A peak systolic velocity through the aortic valve is 2.8 m/s, with a mean pressure gradient of 35 mm Hg. Which of the following is present?**
   A. Mild aortic stenosis
   B. Moderate aortic stenosis
   C. Severe aortic stenosis
   D. Unable to determine

2. **The following values are obtained during an echocardiographic examination: LVOT diameter 1.8 cm, LVOT VTI 35 cm, and AV VTI 90 cm. What is the approximate cross-sectional area of the aortic valve?**
   A. 1.0 cm^2
   B. 1.5 cm^2
   C. 2.0 cm^2
   D. 3.0 cm^2

3. **In addition to the following information (LVOT VTI 19 cm, LVOT peak velocity 74 cm/s, AV peak velocity 333 cm/s), what additional information is needed to calculate the aortic valve area?**
   A. LVOT diameter
   B. VTI of the flow proximal to the aortic valve
   C. A and B above
   D. Enough information is already provided

4. **Which of the following would be indicative of severe aortic stenosis in a patient with an indexed stroke volume of 45 mL/m^2?**
   A. Flow turbulence in the proximal aorta by color flow Doppler interrogation
   B. Mean pressure gradient of 35 mm Hg
   C. Peak pressure gradient of 55 mm Hg
   D. Peak aortic velocity of 4.2 m/s

5. **Which of the following best describes the degree of aortic stenosis as determined by the ratio of the aortic valve peak velocity: LVOT peak velocity of 0.35?**
   A. Normal
   B. Mild
   C. Moderate
   D. Severe

6. **Patients with low flow–low gradient aortic stenosis are**
   A. Classified as D1 aortic stenosis
   B. Always treated as a class I indication for SAVR
   C. Stratified with a Dobutamine Stress Echocardiogram
   D. Stratified with a TEE

7. **A 75-year-old female with an aortic valve area of 0.7 cm^2 and a mean gradient of 30 mm Hg is referred for a dobutamine stress echocardiography. She has noted an increase in her dyspnea over the past 2 months. During the exam, the patient has an increase in stroke volume of 5%. What is the next reasonable step?**
   A. Repeat the DSE with a higher dose of dobutamine
   B. Repeat a resting TTE in 6 months to assess progression of her disease
   C. Perform a left heart catheterization to assess for coronary artery disease
   D. Perform an MDCT to further risk stratify the patient

8. An 80-year-old male presents for SAVR. He has moderate to severe mitral regurgitation (MR) and tricuspid regurgitation (TR) with preserved LV and RV systolic function. His AVA and aortic mean gradient are likely to represent which type of AS?
A. D1—Severe symptomatic AS
B. D2—Classical Low Flow–Low Gradient AS
C. D3—Paradoxical Low Flow–Low Gradient AS
D. D4—Pseudosevere AS

9. A 74-year-old male presents for SAVR. On intraoperative TEE, his AVA is 1.2 cm^2, with a mean gradient of 29 mm Hg. A reason that his intraoperative gradient is discordant from his preoperative TTE includes:
A. Intraoperative TEE images are usually taken during low systemic vascular resistance and higher flow, which yield lower mean gradients compared to TTE.
B. Intraoperative TEE images are usually taken during low systemic vascular resistance and higher flow, which yield lower mean gradients compared to TTE.
C. Intraoperative TEE images are usually taken with concomitant inotropic administration, which yield lower mean gradients compared to TTE.
D. Intraoperative TEE images are usually taken with the chest open, which yield lower mean gradients compared to TTE.

10. One of the benefits of 3D planimetry assessment of the aortic valve area compared to the continuity equation for the assessment of aortic valve area includes:
A. The geometric orifice area obtained by 3D planimetry is more prognostic than the effective orifice area obtained by the continuity equation.
B. 3D planimetry assessment does not use a linear dimension for the LVOT, which leads to a more accurate assessment of AVA.
C. 3D planimetry is the assessment of choice for patients with type paradoxical low flow–low gradient aortic stenosis.
D. 3D planimetry is helpful in the assessment of AVA in patients with AS and hypertrophic obstructive cardiomyopathy (HOCM).

ANSWERS

1. Correct Answer: D.
Rationale: The use of peak aortic velocity measurements to grade the severity of aortic stenosis is subject to important limitations, most notably, factors that reduce stroke volume (ie, hypovolemia, systolic dysfunction). Since this patient has a history of heart failure with a reduced ejection fraction, he may not generate a sufficient stroke volume to create a velocity that is congruent with the severity of his aortic stenosis, which may underestimate its severity.

2. Correct Answer: A.
Rationale: The continuity equation states that the volume of blood in a single beat that is ejected through the LVOT must be the same volume that is ejected through the aortic valve in the same beat. $SV_{LVOT} = SV_{AV}$. $LVOT_{CSA} \times LVOT_{VTI} = AV_{CSA} \times AV_{VTI}$. The LVOT is assumed to be cylindrical in shape such that the $LVOT_{CSA} = \pi r^2$ or in this case, $\pi(0.9\text{ cm})^2 = 2.45\text{ cm}^2$. Multiplying this by the $LVOT_{VTI}$ gives the $LVOT_{SV}$ or $2.54\text{ cm}^2 \times 35\text{ cm} = 88.9\text{ cm}^3$. This must equal the stroke volume that travels through the aortic valve orifice (AV_{CSA}); thus, $AV_{CSA} = 88.9\text{ cm}^3/AV_{VTI} = 0.99\text{ cm}^2$ or approximately 1.0 cm^2.

3. Correct Answer: A.
Rationale: The continuity equation states that the volume of blood in a single beat that is ejected through the LVOT must be the same volume that is ejected through the aortic valve in the same beat. $SV_{LVOT} = SV_{AV}$. $LVOT_{CSA} \times LVOT_{VTI} = AV_{CSA} \times AV_{VTI}$. This equation can be further simplified based on the concept that the spectral profiles of the LVOT and AV are so similar that the ratio of the LVOT VTI and AV VTI are nearly identical to the ratio of the

LVOT peak velocity and AV peak velocity, such that $LVOT_{CSA} \times$ LVOT peak velocity = $AV_{CSA} \times$ AV peak velocity. To use this simplified continuity equation to determine aortic valve area, the only additional information that is needed is LVOT diameter.

4. Correct Answer: D.
Rationale: Peak aortic velocities of 4.0 m/s denote severe disease, whereas 3.0 to 4.0 m/s is moderate disease, and 2.6 to 2.9 m/s is mild disease. While flow turbulence in the proximal aorta by color flow Doppler may be suggestive of aortic stenosis, it is not a metric used for severity grading. Given the normal stroke volume, a mean pressure gradient of 35 mm Hg or peak pressure gradient of 55 mm Hg would be suggestive of moderate aortic stenosis.

5. Correct Answer: C.
Rationale: A low ratio indicates significant flow differences between the LVOT and the AV, with a ratio of less than 0.25 representing severe stenosis. Values of 0.25 to 0.50 suggest moderate disease, whereas values >0.5 suggest mild disease.

6. Correct Answer: C.
Rationale: Patients with low flow–low gradient are classified as D2 aortic stenosis. They may meet a class I indication for SAVR if they are found to have severe symptomatic disease after stress testing, but not all patients with low flow–low gradient AS meet criteria for SAVR. Dobutamine stress testing is helpful in differentiating severe aortic stenosis from pseudosevere aortic stenosis. Patients with low flow–low gradient stenosis are not stratified with a TEE.

7. Correct Answer: D.
Rationale: Patients with low flow–low gradient AS are referred for dobutamine stress echocardiography to further assess the disease process. A subset of patients will not see an increase in stroke volume during DSE. These patients should not have a repeat DSE if the proper protocol were followed. This patient is symptomatic and may have severe AS; therefore, she should not wait for another TTE. From the history, there does not seem to be an indication for a left heart catheterization. An MDCT may help delineate true AS depending on the calcium score.

8. Correct Answer: C.
Rationale: Patients with concomitant valvulopathy may be challenging to assess echocardiographically. Patients with severe mitral and tricuspid disease in the setting of normal LVEF and decreased SVI can be classified as paradoxical low flow–low gradient AS since the decreased SV secondary to inadequate LV end diastolic volume.

9. Correct Answer: B.
Rationale: There are several reasons why intraoperative TEE demonstrate smaller mean gradients than preoperative TTE in the same patient. Physiologic factors that decrease flow through the valve, including positive pressure ventilation and increased systemic vascular resistance may lead to smaller mean gradients compared to awake patients.

10. Correct Answer: D.
Rationale: Planimetry is a useful adjunct in the assessment of AV stenosis in patients with AS and HOCM due to the multiple Doppler signals that make the continuity equation challenging in this patient population. The downsides of planimetry include the fact that the effective orifice area is more prognostic than the geometric area. In addition, the continuity equation often uses a linear dimension for LVOT, but there are other challenging artifacts that make planimetry inaccurate.

13 Prosthetic Valves

T. Robert Feng, Albert T. Cheung, and Worasak Keeyapaj

The first successful artificial heart valves were implanted in 1960. Starr implanted a Starr-Edwards caged-ball valve in a patient with rheumatic mitral stenosis and Harken implanted the Harken caged-ball prosthesis in the subcoronary aortic position in a patient with rheumatic aortic stenosis and regurgitation. Over the next 64 years, numerous manufacturers have produced prosthetic valves of various designs for clinical use. Contemporary designs address constructing valves with improved hemodynamic performance to reduce the risk of prosthetic-patient mismatch, improved biocompatibility to decrease the risk of thromboembolism, improved durability to decrease the risk of mechanical structural failure over time, and increased resistance to calcification and immune responses to decrease the rate of degeneration over time. The production of prosthetic valves has also become a competitive business with each manufacturer creating unique products and individual cardiac surgeons developing specific preferences in their choice of valves. As a consequence, the design, construction, and marketing of prosthetic valves is an ongoing process and incremental refinements are continually being made in an effort to improve the biocompatibility, durability, hemodynamic performance, and ease of implantation that are evidenced by the frequent appearance of new models with new trade names. One of the challenges of assessing prosthetic valve function is to recognize and appreciate the distinct echocardiographic features and hemodynamic performance of each of the many varieties of prosthetic valve types, models, and sizes that have been commercially available and may be encountered in the existing patient population. Due to the aging population, the number of remaining individuals with early generation prosthetic valves are rapidly decreasing. However, echocardiographic descriptions of several of the classic early generation prosthetic valves have been included in this chapter for historical purposes.

ROLE OF TRANSESOPHAGEAL ECHOCARDIOGRAPHY IN THE EVALUATION OF PROSTHETIC CARDIAC VALVES

Multiplane transesophageal echocardiography (TEE) is considered the diagnostic technique of choice for identifying the type of prosthesis, assessing its function, and diagnosing prosthetic dysfunction (1-6). The ability of TEE to combine two-dimensional (2D) and three-dimensional (3D) with color Doppler and spectral Doppler imaging enables TEE to generate diagnostic information based on both the structure and the hemodynamic function of the prosthetic valve. However, the evaluation of prosthetic heart valves using ultrasound imaging poses special problems because mechanical valves and components of bioprosthetic valves have poor acoustic properties, making it difficult to image the valve and the surrounding soft tissues in detail. In addition, the small size of the valves and their mechanical components make detailed examination of the motion of the stent and occluder mechanisms challenging.

Despite incremental improvements in instrumentation, the imaging resolution that can be achieved using transthoracic echocardiography (TTE) does not match that achieved by TEE. The improved imaging resolution provided by TEE with the ultrasound transducer close to the cardiac valve structures permits a detailed assessment of prosthetic valve components, their function, and the ability to identify the etiology and anatomic site of prosthetic valve dysfunction. High-resolution 2D and 3D imaging can distinguish between normal and abnormal motion of the valve leaflets and occluder mechanisms. Abnormal motion of the valve stent or dehiscence of the prosthetic valve annulus can also be detected. Vegetations, calcifications, and abnormal masses on the prosthetic valve can be detected using TEE 2D imaging. TEE 3D imaging is often useful for characterizing the precise location and the extent of the defect in relation to the prosthetic valve.

Color Doppler imaging can distinguish normal closure and leakage regurgitant jets (washing jets) from pathologic transvalvular or paravalvular regurgitant jets. Quantification of blood flow velocity using spectral Doppler techniques often permits the estimation of transvalvular pressure gradients and the effective orifice area (EOA) of the prosthetic valves (1,7-10).

Clinical indications for TEE include the evaluation of the native valve prior to valve replacement, the evaluation of prosthetic valve function immediately after implantation, the diagnosis of prosthetic valve dysfunction, the assessment of prosthetic-patient mismatching, and the diagnosis of early complications associated with valve replacement (Table 13.1). When applying TEE to evaluate prosthetic heart valves, it is also important to recognize its inherent limitations. For example, acoustic shadowing prevents imaging of the distal surfaces of the prosthetic valve. The location of the TEE transducer, confined to the esophagus and stomach, may limit the ability to accurately estimate blood flow velocity or pressure gradients across specific valves. Despite high image resolution, it is still difficult to image pannus or to differentiate between pannus and thrombus using TEE.

TECHNICAL CONSIDERATIONS IN PERFORMING TEE EXAMINATIONS OF PROSTHETIC VALVES

Many of the ultrasound imaging techniques used to evaluate native valve function can be applied to the evaluation of prosthetic heart valves, but certain special considerations are necessary. Ultrasound does not penetrate through the metallic and polymeric components of mechanical and biologic valves. These material components produce highly specular echoes and impair the imaging of the distal surfaces of prosthetic components and cardiac structures distal to the prosthesis because of acoustic shadowing. Decreasing the transmit gain helps to decrease imaging artifacts and to resolve structural details in the vicinity of nonbiologic materials. To overcome some of the problems created by acoustic shadowing, it is necessary to image the prosthetic valve from different transducer positions that provide views of both the upstream and the downstream sides of the prosthetic valve. For example, the midesophageal aortic valve long-axis imaging plane will not reliably display the motion of the mechanical aortic prosthesis because of shadowing from the

TABLE 13.1 Prosthetic Heart Valves and Clinical Indications for Transesophageal Echocardiography (TEE)

TEE evaluation prior to valve replacement 1. Verify disease of native valve. 2. Assess the extent of annular calcification. 3. Estimate the annular diameter of the native valve. In aortic valve disease, a small annulus may dictate the type of valve to be implanted. 4. Evaluate the feasibility of valve repair. Considering the limitations of prosthetic valves, it is almost always preferable to repair a valve rather than replace it.
TEE evaluation immediately after valve replacement 1. Verify that the prosthetic valve apparatus is stable and well seated within the native valve annulus. 2. Verify that all leaflets or occluders move normally. 3. Verify the presence and location of characteristic transvalvular washing regurgitant jets. 4. Verify the absence of paravalvular or pathologic transvalvular regurgitation. 5. Verify that there is no left ventricular outflow tract obstruction caused by prosthetic valve struts or retained subvalvular apparatus. 6. Verify satisfactory hemodynamic function of the prosthetic valve by measuring the transvalvular pressure gradient, Doppler velocity index, and effective orifice area.
TEE evaluation to assess for collateral damage to other cardiac structures as a consequence of valve replacement 1. Mitral regurgitation from a misplaced suture through the anterior mitral valve leaflet after aortic valve replacement 2. Aortic regurgitation from a misplaced suture through an aortic valve cusp after mitral valve replacement 3. Coronary obstruction after aortic valve replacement manifested by right or left ventricular dysfunction 4. Left circumflex coronary artery injury or obstruction after mitral valve replacement manifested by left ventricular segmental wall motion abnormality 5. Ventricular or atrial septal defect after mitral or aortic valve replacement 6. Left ventricular outflow tract obstruction after mitral valve replacement
TEE diagnosis of prosthetic valve dysfunction 1. Identify prosthetic valve type 2. Detect and quantify the severity of transvalvular or paravalvular regurgitation. 3. Detect annular dehiscence. 4. Detect vegetations associated with endocarditis. 5. Detect thrombosis or pannus formation on the valve. 6. Detect and quantify valve stenosis. 7. Detect structural valvular degeneration or calcification.

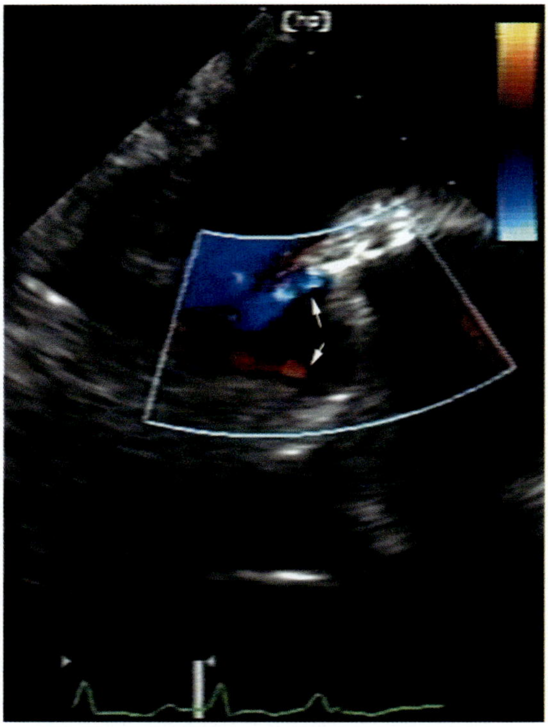

FIGURE 13.1 Bileaflet mechanical prosthesis in the aortic position. Transesophageal echocardiographic midesophageal aortic valve long-axis view at a multiplane angle of 135° in a patient with a bileaflet mechanical prosthesis in the aortic position. Color Doppler flow imaging in diastole shows the normal appearance of the two leakage regurgitant jets that originate at the leaflet hinge points (arrows). Note that ultrasound shadowing caused by the annular stent makes it difficult to assess the motion of the leaflets from this imaging angle. The transgastric long-axis or the deep transgastric long-axis views through the aortic valve are necessary to evaluate the motion of the individual leaflets.

valve sewing ring (Figure 13.1). By advancing the TEE probe to the transgastric position, prosthetic aortic leaflet motion can be observed from the apical or mid-ventricular transgastric long-axis view through the aortic valve without interference from the sewing ring (Figure 13.2). Similarly, imaging the ventricular side of mitral prosthetic valves using the transgastric mid-ventricular or deep transgastric long-axis imaging planes provides details that cannot be observed with the midesophageal views alone.

Doppler echocardiography can be used to estimate the transvalvular pressure gradient across bileaflet, tilting disc, and biologic valves that have a centrally directed, linear transvalvular flow. In contrast, for caged-ball or caged-disc valves where the occluder alters the direction of blood flow through the valve, the Bernoulli equation will not accurately estimate the transvalvular pressure gradient.

ECHOCARDIOGRAPHIC CHARACTERISTICS OF THE INDIVIDUAL PROSTHETIC CARDIAC VALVE TYPES

Each type of prosthetic valve has distinct echocardiographic features and hemodynamic characteristics. The type, shape, and motion of the structural components of the valve allow it to be identified by the TEE examination. Knowing the published and manufacturers' specifications for the normal range of motion of the valve components, the average transvalvular pressure gradient and average EOA are necessary to verify normal functioning of the prosthesis and to diagnose prosthetic dysfunction (1,8-10). In general, prosthetic valves are classified as mechanical or biologic and by the manufacturer, model number, and outside diameter of the sewing ring (Table 13.2 and Appendix D).

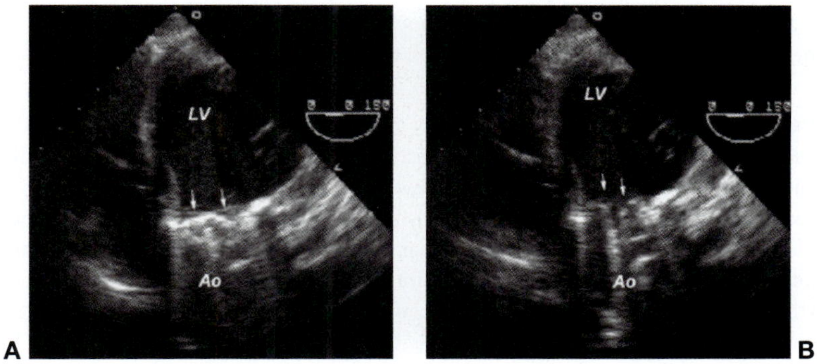

FIGURE 13.2 Bileaflet mechanical prosthesis in the aortic position. Transesophageal echocardiographic deep transgastric apical long-axis view at a multiplane angle of 0° permits imaging of prosthetic valve leaflets (arrows) and their motion. In diastole (panel A), both leaflets are in the fully closed position at an angle of 30° in relation to the plane of the valve annulus. In systole (panel B), both leaflets are in the fully open position at an angle of 90° in relation to the plane of the valve annulus. Ao, aorta; LV, left ventricle.

Mechanical Heart Valves

Mechanical heart valves are more durable than biologic valves, but their surfaces are less biocompatible, do not endothelialize, and require systemic anticoagulation to reduce the risk of thrombosis and thromboembolism. For these reasons, mechanical valves are traditionally considered for younger patients who are more likely to experience structural failure after implantation of a biologic prosthetic as a consequence of their longer life expectancy. Mechanical prosthetics may also be preferred in patients who require anticoagulation therapy for other reasons or in whom the risk of reoperation is unacceptable. The silastic, metal, and pyrolytic

TABLE 13.2 Prosthetic Valve Types

Bioprosthetic	Description
Allograft	Indistinguishable from the native valve, used only in the aortic position (CryoLife aortic allograft)
Porcine	Porcine aortic valve on polypropylene or Elgiloy mount with three support struts (eg, Hancock, Carpentier-Edwards, Medtronic Mosaic, St. Jude Bioimplant, St. Jude Medical Epic, Wessex)
Pericardial	Trileaflet valve fashioned from bovine or porcine pericardium mounted on a Dacron-covered support frame with three struts (eg, Bioflo pericardial, Carpentier-Edwards Pericardial, Labcor-Santiago pericardial, Sorin Mitroflow, Ionescu-Shiley, Sorin Pericarbon, St. Jude Medical Trifecta, Edwards Inspiris Resilia)
Stentless	Reinforced porcine aortic root (Biocor stentless, CryoLife-O'Brien stentless, Edwards Prima stentless, Medtronic Freestyle, Toronto stentless porcine valve, Medtronic ATS 3f)
Transcatheter	Trileaflet pericardial valve supported within a wireform stent for implantation through a catheter (EDWARDS SAPIEN S3 Ultra, Medtronic Evolut PRO Medtronic Avalus)
Mechanical	**Description**
Ball-in-cage	Circular sewing ring with U-shaped arches containing a silastic ball (eg, Braunwald-Cutter, Harken, Starr-Edwards)
Caged disc	Circular sewing ring with short cage containing a lightweight silastic centrally occluding disc (eg, Beall, Kay-Shiley, Kay-Suzuki, Starr-Edwards Model 6520)
Tilting disc	Eccentrically hinged single tilting disc in circular ring opening to form two orifices (eg, Björk-Shiley, Lillehei-Kaster, Medtronic Hall, Omnicarbon, Omniscience, Sorin Allcarbon monoleaflet, Wada-Cutter)
Bileaflet	Two semicircular hinged leaflets in a circular ring opening almost perpendicularly to form three orifices (eg, ATS, CarboMedics, Duromedics, Edwards MIRA, Jyros bileaflet, ON-X, St. Jude Medical, Sorin Allcarbon, Sorin Bicarbon)

carbon components of mechanical valves are poor conductors of ultrasound and cause acoustic shadowing, reverberations, and strong specular signals. The echocardiographic appearance and characteristics of mechanical prosthetic valves can be categorized based on the occluder mechanism.

Bileaflet Valves

The bileaflet mechanical valve prostheses are the most commonly implanted mechanical valves because of their outstanding record of durability and large valve orifice area in relation to sewing ring diameter. They can be implanted in the aortic, mitral, or tricuspid positions. The valves are constructed of two semicircular leaflets suspended from four hinge points in a circular annulus surrounded by a sewing ring (Figure 13.3). When the leaflets open, three separate orifices are formed within the valve annulus. Minor variations in design include the shape of the leaflets, the width of the sewing ring, and the materials used to construct the valve components.

A systematic TEE examination of the prosthetic valve includes verification of normal leaflet motion, proper seating of the prosthesis within the native valve annulus, and normal blood flow pattern through the valve. In addition, the TEE examination should verify the presence of normal washing jets and the absence of significant paravalvular or transvalvular regurgitation. Finally, TEE can be used to estimate the transvalvular pressure gradient and calculate the EOA of the valve.

1. *Confirm leaflet motion:* 2D and 3D imaging confirms the opening and closure of the two mechanical leaflets (Video 13.1). In the short-axis imaging plane, the two leaflets in the open position produce two linear shadows within a circular annulus (Figure 13.4). For valves implanted in the mitral position, leaflet motion is best examined using the midesophageal long-axis views (Figure 13.5). For bileaflet valves implanted in an anti-anatomic position, which is believed to optimize flow through the left ventricle into the left ventricular outflow tract, the TEE commissural view at a multiplane angle of 60° to 70°, with multiplane adjustments to generate a cross-sectional imaging plane that is perpendicular to the two leaflets, permits the motion of both leaflets to be observed simultaneously (Figure 13.5). The two leaflets tilt open symmetrically to an angle of 85° to 90° and close at an angle of 30° in relation to the plane of the annulus for a travel arc of approximately 60°. Leaflet motion of a valve implanted in the aortic position is more difficult to evaluate (Figures 13.1 and 13.4). Acoustic shadowing from the sewing ring and leaflets typically obscure leaflet motion in the midesophageal aortic valve long-axis view. Individual leaflet motion is better visualized in the transgastric long-axis and deep transgastric long-axis views that provide unobstructed views of the aortic valve in the far field through the left ventricle and left ventricular outflow tract (LVOT) (Figures 13.2 and 13.6; Video 13.2).

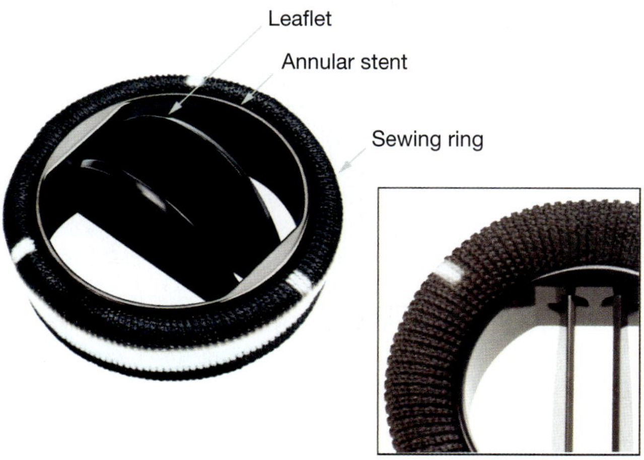

FIGURE 13.3 Photograph of a CarboMedics R-series mechanical bileaflet prosthetic aortic valve. The valve consists of two semicircular pyrolytic carbon leaflets supported within a pyrolytic carbon annular stent surrounded by the sewing ring. The inset shows a closeup of the hinge points of the leaflets. The valve is designed to permit a small amount of leakage backflow at the hinge points.

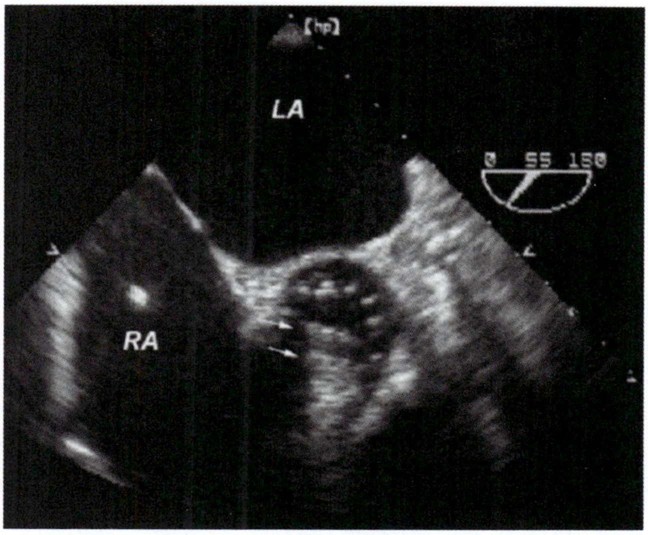

FIGURE 13.4 Bileaflet mechanical prosthesis in the aortic position. Transesophageal echocardiographic midesophageal short-axis image just above the plane of the valve annulus in systole provides cross-sectional imaging of the two parallel leaflets (arrows) of the mechanical valve in the open position. Note the acoustic shadowing caused by the mechanical leaflets in the far field making it difficult to resolve detail in the distal portion of the valve annulus. LA, left atrium; RA, right atrium.

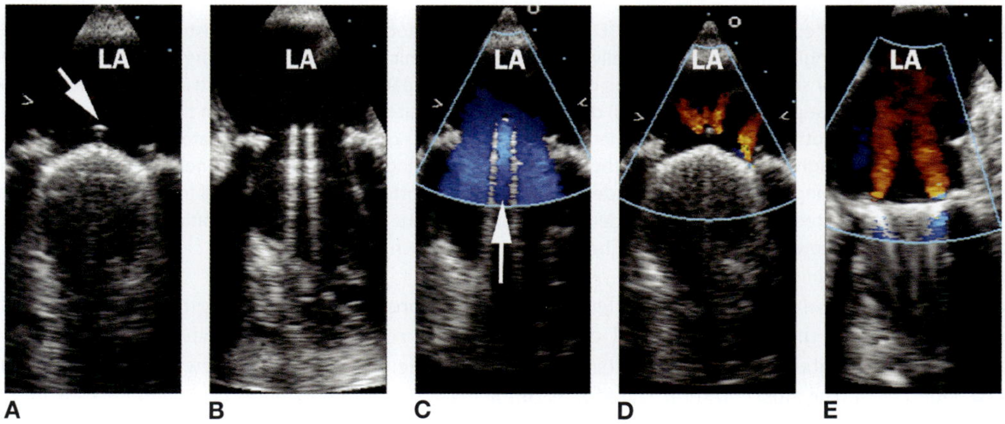

FIGURE 13.5 Multiplane transesophageal echocardiographic midesophageal images of a normally functioning bileaflet mechanical valve in the mitral position. Panels A and D show the appearance of the prosthetic valve at midsystole with both leaflets in the closed position at a multiplane angle perpendicular to the pivot axis (two-leaflet view). The arrow in panel A shows the location of the pivot guard that contains the hinge points. Panels B and C show the appearance of the prosthetic valve in diastole with both leaflets in fully opened position at a multiplane angle perpendicular to the pivot axis (two-leaflet view). The arrow in panel C shows the position of the central orifice. Doppler color flow imaging at midsystole (panels D, E) shows the typical appearance of normal regurgitant jets that originate from the hinge points or between the leaflets and the valve stent. Rotating the multiplane angle 90° forward from the two-leaflet view produces the single-leaflet view that is parallel to the pivot axis (panel E). In the single-leaflet view, Doppler color flow imaging shows the origin of the centrally directed regurgitant jets from the hinge points (panel E). (Courtesy of Drs Cheung and Streckenbach.)

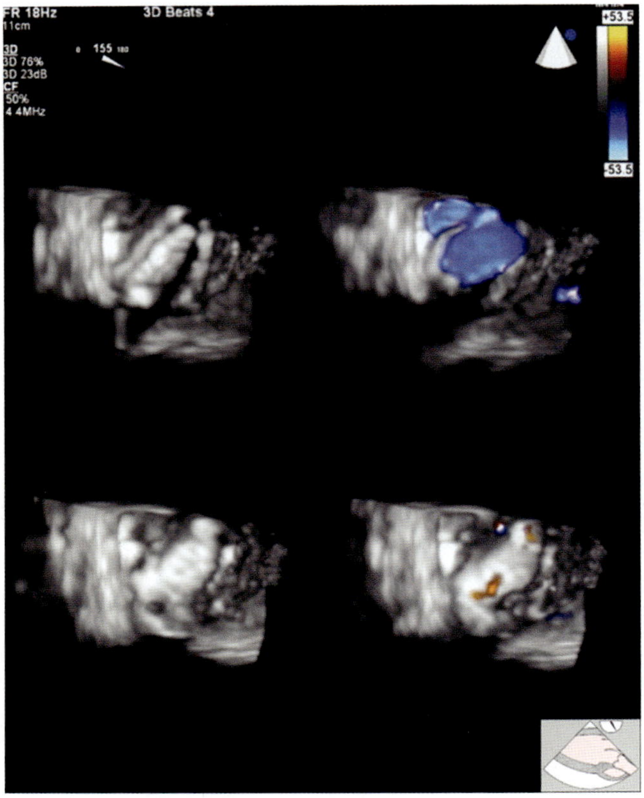

FIGURE 13.6 Doppler color flow full-volume 3D transesophageal echocardiographic transgastric aortic valve long-axis view at a multiplane angle of 155° of a normally functioning mechanical bileaflet valve in the aortic position viewed from the left ventricular side in systole with the occluders open (top panels) and in diastole with the occluders closed (bottom panels). Color suppression (left panels) demonstrates the position of the occluders in the open (top left panel) and closed positions (bottom left panel). Doppler color flow imaging (right panels) demonstrates the normal pattern of transvalvular flow through the three orifices of the prosthetic valve during systole (top right panel) and normal pattern of regurgitant jets at the hinge points of the occluders during diastole (bottom right panel). Small transvalvular regurgitant jets can often be detected between the occluder and the annular stent in a normally functioning mechanical bileaflet prosthetic valve (not shown). (Courtesy of Drs Cheung and Streckenbach.)

2. *Confirm proper valve seating:* Incomplete fixation of the prosthetic sewing ring to the native annulus or dehiscence of the sewing ring will cause paravalvular regurgitation. Paravalvular regurgitation is defined as regurgitation originating outside of the prosthetic valve annulus or sewing ring (Figure 13.7; Video 13.3). The most common cause for incomplete fixation immediately after prosthetic implantation is a severely calcified native valve annulus or an avulsed annular suture. Prosthetic endocarditis is the most common cause for late valve dehiscence and can produce a "rocking" motion of the entire valve apparatus on 2D imaging (excessive motion of the prosthetic valve annulus in relation to the native valve annulus). Proper seating of the prosthetic valve, paravalvular regurgitation, and dehiscence are best identified from the multiplane long-axis images of the valve.

   Use of biplane (X-Plane) view can be of additional value and prompts quick assessment of the valve. Scanning the entire valve using the cursor, using biplane can detect the location of leakage.
3. *Confirm normal blood flow patterns and the absence of pathologic transvalvular and paravalvular regurgitation:* Color flow Doppler imaging will demonstrate central antegrade flow through the valve annulus when the leaflets open and small characteristic regurgitant jets during leaflet closure. The use of 3D TEE color Doppler imaging is useful to characterize the precise anatomic location of individual regurgitant jets in relation to the prosthesis. A small amount of regurgitation is normal for bileaflet

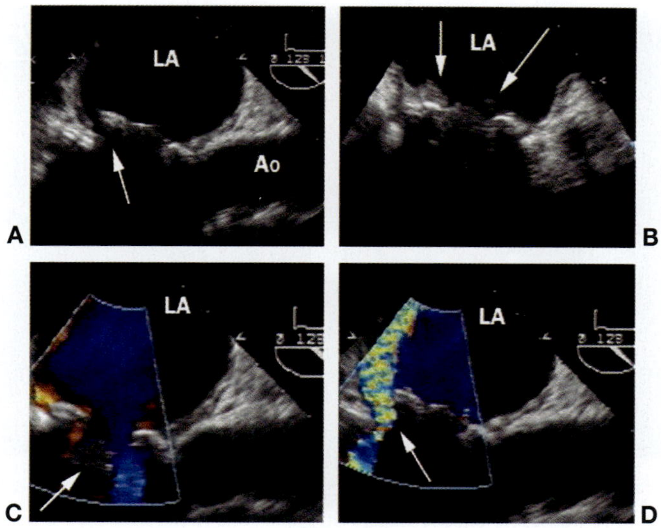

FIGURE 13.7 Transesophageal midesophageal long-axis view in a patient with a caged-ball prosthesis in the mitral position complicated by prosthetic valve endocarditis and dehiscence. Two-dimensional imaging (panel A) demonstrated a rocking motion of the prosthetic valve and separation of the sewing ring from the native annulus in the region of the posterior mitral valve annulus (arrow, panel A) that was characteristic of dehiscence. Vegetations on the prosthetic valve that were diagnostic for endocarditis were detected also by 2D imaging (arrows, panel B). Doppler color flow imaging in diastole showed antegrade flow around the open occluder into the left ventricle (arrow, panel C). Doppler color flow imaging in systole demonstrated paravalvular regurgitation in the region of dehiscence (arrow, panel D). Ao, aorta; LA, left atrium. (Courtesy of Drs Cheung and Streckenbach.)

prosthetic valves and is caused by closure backflow and leakage backflow. Closure backflow is the reversal of flow required for closure of the leaflets. Leakage backflow occurs after closure of mechanical valves, originates from the four hinge points of the leaflets and at other locations between the edges of the occluder and the prosthetic valve stent. The leakage backflow jets originating from the hinge points produces four regurgitant jets that are best visualized in the long-axis image through the prosthetic valve at a multiplane angle aligned parallel to the leaflets (Figures 13.1, 13.5, and 13.6; Videos 13.2, 13.4, and 13.5). These washing jets originate laterally near the inner border of the prosthetic annulus. The direction of washing jets is dependent on the valve models. St. Jude Medical bileaflet valves typically have convergent jets that are directed medially, whereas On-X bileaflet valves have washing jets that are nonconverging (11). The bileaflet valves are designed to permit a small amount of regurgitation at the hinge points to prevent the formation of thrombus within the hinge mechanism. Sometimes, small leakage regurgitant jets originating along the edge of the leaflet where it meets the annulus during closure can also be imaged by color Doppler imaging (Figure 13.5). Normal physiologic regurgitant jets are small, low velocity, and short in duration and can be distinguished from pathologic transvalvular regurgitation based on their size, location, velocity, direction, and duration.

Pathologic regurgitation with a jet originating within the sewing ring is called transvalvular regurgitation. Pathologic transvalvular regurgitation immediately after valve implantation indicates malfunctioning of the valve leaflets. Intraoperative causes of leaflet malfunction causing transvalvular regurgitation include retained tissue preventing valve closure, a misplaced suture interfering with leaflet motion, or debris within the hinges causing trapping of the leaflet in a fixed position (Figure 13.8). Significant regurgitant jets originating outside of the sewing ring are always pathologic and called paravalvular regurgitation.

4. *Calculate valve gradient and EOA:* The hemodynamic performance of the prosthetic valve can be assessed using Doppler echocardiography (Figure 13.9). The interpretation of Doppler-derived prosthetic valve hemodynamic parameters is complicated because even normally functioning prosthetic valves are inherently obstructive to blood flow, and blood flow velocity profiles across prosthetic valves are not uniform depending upon prosthetic valve type, model, and annular diameter. Since the blood flow

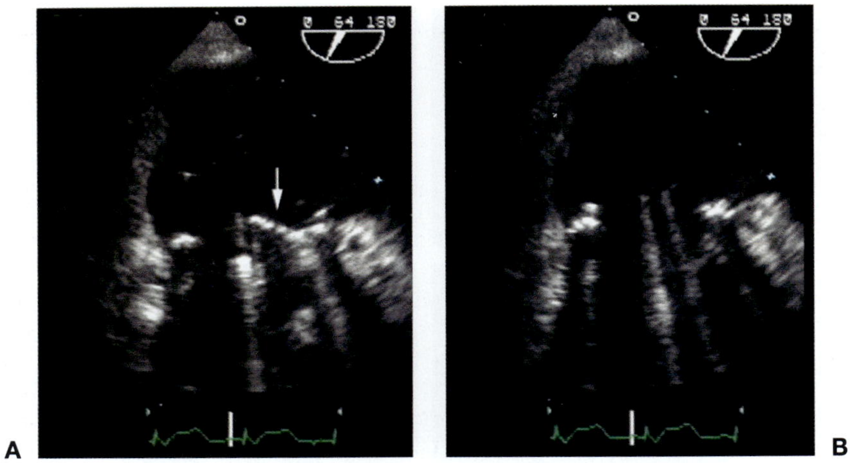

FIGURE 13.8 Intraoperative transesophageal echocardiographic (TEE) midesophageal commissural view at a multiplane angle of 64° displaying a mechanical bileaflet prosthetic in the mitral position. TEE imaging of the bileaflet view in diastole immediately after implantation demonstrated that the anterior leaflet was trapped in a closed position (arrow, panel A). TEE examination after surgical revision to free trapped leaflet showed that both leaflets were fully open in diastole (panel B) and moved normally throughout the cardiac cycle.

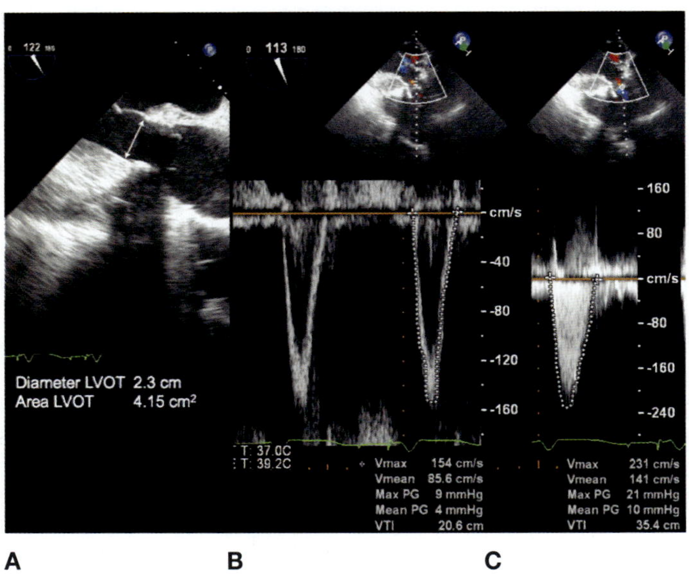

FIGURE 13.9 The functional performance of prosthetic valves implanted in the aortic position can be assessed by transesophageal echocardiography in midsystole by using 2D imaging to measure the diameter of the left ventricular outflow tract in the midesophageal aortic valve long-axis view (panel A), pulsed wave Doppler to measure the blood flow velocity in the left ventricular outflow tract in the transgastric aortic valve long-axis view (panel B), and continuous wave Doppler to measure the transvalvular blood flow velocity in the transgastric aortic valve long-axis view (panel C). In this example of a 29-mm bioprosthetic valve implanted in the aortic position, the transvalvular peak gradient was 21 mm Hg and mean gradient was 10 mm Hg using the simplified Bernoulli equation. Using the nonsimplified Bernoulli equation, the transvalvular peak gradient was 12 mm Hg and mean gradient was 6 mm Hg. The Doppler velocity index (DVI) was 0.66, and the effective orifice area was 2.4 cm^2. (Courtesy of Drs Cheung and Streckenbach.)

TABLE 13.3 Determining the Effective Orifice Area (EOA) Using the Continuity Method

$EOA = LVOT_{area} (VTI_{LVOT}/VTI_{transvalvular})$
where: EOA = effective orifice area of prosthetic valve $LVOT_{area}$ = cross-sectional area of left ventricular outflow tract (LVOT) $= \pi$ (diameter of LVOT/2)^2 $VTI_{transvalvular}$ = velocity-time integral of blood flow across valve VTI_{LVOT} = velocity-time integral of blood flow across LVOT

velocity through the central rectangular orifice is greater than the blood flow velocity through the two semicircular orifices of the bileaflet valves, some studies suggest that Doppler-derived gradients based on the Bernoulli equation may overestimate the true transvalvular gradient (12). However, the same and other studies also suggest that differences observed between Doppler- and catheter-derived gradients across prosthetic valves can be explained by localized gradients and pressure recovery downstream from the valve orifice (12,13). Based on this interpretation, differences between Doppler- and catheter-derived pressure gradients may not represent an overestimation of catheter-derived gradients, but represent instead inherent differences in measurement technique, line of interrogation, and precise location of pressure gradients relative to the prosthetic valve orifices. Furthermore, the equation used to estimate mitral valve area based on pressure half-time ($MVA = 220/PT_{1/2}$) may not apply to prosthetic valves that differ in structure and flow characteristics to the native valve. For clinical purposes of quantifying prosthetic valve function, several approaches can be applied for interpretation of Doppler-derived measurements. One approach is to report only actual values of Doppler transvalvular peak and mean flow velocities across the prosthetic valve and compare the values to established normal values for the specific type, model, and size of the prosthetic valve based on clinical reports, specifications published by the manufacturers that can be obtained from their respective websites or the package insert accompanying the prosthetic valve (9), or in the appendix of the American Society of Echocardiography guidelines for the evaluation of prosthetic valves (Appendix D) (1,10). Similarly, Doppler-derived EOAs calculated using the continuity equation for a prosthetic valve can be compared to those observed for that specific prosthetic valve type, model, and size (Table 13.3 and Appendix D) (1,10). Another variable adding to the complication of interpreting Doppler-derived hemodynamic information in patients with prosthetic valves is that Doppler-derived pressure gradients are dependent on blood flow and even blood viscosity. Decreased blood viscosity from hemodilution or increased cardiac output from inotropic support immediately after prosthetic valve implantation may lead to overestimation of prosthetic valve gradients using the simplified Bernoulli equation. One approach to address this problem of assessing aortic valve prosthetics is to index transvalvular Doppler velocity-time integral through the prosthetic valve to the velocity-time integral through the LVOT using the Doppler velocity index ($DVI = VTI_{LVOT}/VTI_{AoV}$) (Table 13.4) (1,14). For example, using the DVI or the "double-envelope" technique for assessing the function of a prosthetic valve in the aortic position, a velocity-time integral in the LVOT (VTI_{LVOT}) to transvalvular velocity-time integral (VTI_{AoV}) ratio

TABLE 13.4 Determining the Doppler Velocity Index (DVI)

Aortic valve $DVI = VTI_{LVOT}/VTI_{AoV}$ *or* $V_{maxLVOT}/V_{maxAoV}$
Mitral valve $DVI = VTI_{MV}/VTI_{LVOT}$
where: DVI = Doppler velocity index VTI_{LVOT} = Velocity-time integral for flow through the left ventricular outflow tract VTI_{AoV} = Velocity-time integral for flow across the prosthetic aortic valve $V_{maxLVOT}$ = Maximum blood flow velocity in the left ventricular outflow tract V_{maxAoV} = Maximum transvalvular blood flow through the prosthetic aortic valve VTI_{MV} = Velocity-time integral for flow across the prosthetic mitral valve VTI_{LVOT} = Velocity-time integral for flow through the left ventricular outflow tract

TABLE 13.5 Doppler Parameters for Diagnosis of Prosthetic Aortic Stenosis

Parameter	Normal	Possible Stenosis	Suggests Significant Stenosis
Peak velocity (m/s)[a]	<3	3-4	>4
Mean gradient (mm Hg)[a]	<20	20-35	>35
Acceleration time (msec)[b]	<80	80-100	>100
DVI	≥0.35	0.25-0.35	<0.25
EOA	Reference EOA ± 1 SD	<1 SD of reference EOA	<2 SD of reference EOA
Transvalvular velocity profile[b]	Triangular, early peaking	Intermediate	Rounded, symmetric contour

DVI, Doppler velocity index; EOA, effective orifice area; SD, standard deviation
In conditions of normal stroke volume (50-70 mL) through the aortic valve.
[a]These parameters are more affected by flow, including concomitant aortic regurgitation.
[b]Can be affected by LV function and heart rate.
Data from Zoghbi WA, Jone PN, Chamsi-Pasha MA, et al. Guidelines for the evaluation of prosthetic valve function with cardiovascular imaging: a report from the American Society of Echocardiography developed in collaboration with the Society for Cardiovascular Magnetic Resonance and the Society of Cardiovascular Computed Tomography. *J Am Soc Echocardiogr.* 2024;37(1):2-63.

less than 0.25 (VTI_{LVOT}/VTI_{AoV} <0.25) suggests significant prosthetic valve stenosis (Table 13.5) (1,14). Alternatively, DVI can be calculated as the ratio of the peak LVOT blood flow velocity to the peak blood flow velocity through the aortic valve and it may carry better reproducibility compared to the velocity-time integral (VTI) method (14,15). When using the DVI to estimate stenosis of prosthetic valves in the mitral or tricuspid positions, VTI or V_{max} of the LVOT is the denominator in the ratio because these valves open in diastole ($DVI = VTI_{Pr}/VTI_{LVOT}$) or ($DVI = V_{maxPr}/V_{maxLVOT}$). A transvalvular Doppler profile that is rounded and symmetrically contoured in appearance with acceleration time greater than 100 ms also suggests significant prosthetic aortic stenosis (Table 13.5) (1). Lastly, the prosthetic valve gradients can be more accurately estimated by using the nonsimplified Bernoulli equation that accounts for the velocity of blood flow on the upstream side of the valve ($[P_1 - P_2] = 4[V_2^2 - V_1^2]$). Similarly, for assessing the function of a prosthetic valve in the mitral position, a transvalvular velocity-time integral (VTI_{MV}) to LVOT velocity-time integral (VTI_{LVOT}) ratio greater than 2.5 (VTI_{MV}/VTI_{LVOT} >2.5) suggests significant prosthetic valve stenosis (Tables 13.4 and 13.6) (1).

TABLE 13.6 Doppler Parameters for Diagnosis of Prosthetic Mitral Stenosis

	Normal	Possible Stenosis[a]	Suggests Significant Stenosis[a]
Peak velocity (m/s)[b,c]	<1.9	1.9-2.5	≥2.5
Mean gradient (mm Hg)[b,c]	≤5	6-10	>10
DVI (VTI_{MV}/VTI_{LVOT}[b,c])	<2.2	2.2-2.5	>2.5
EOA (cm^2)	≥2	1-2	<1
PHT (ms)	<130	130-200	>200

DVI, Doppler velocity index; EOA, effective orifice area; PHT, pressure half-time; VTI_{LVOT}, velocity-time integral in left ventricular outflow tract; VTI_{MV}, velocity-time integral through prosthetic mitral valve.
[a]Abnormal values should prompt a closer evaluation of valve function and consideration of other conditions such as high cardiac output, tachycardia, or prosthesis-patient mismatch.
[b]Slightly higher cutoff values than shown may be seen in some bioprosthetic valves.
[c]These parameters are also abnormal in the presence of significant prosthetic mitral regurgitation.
Data from Zoghbi WA, Jone PN, Chamsi-Pasha MA, et al. Guidelines for the evaluation of prosthetic valve function with cardiovascular imaging: a report from the American Society of Echocardiography developed in collaboration with the Society for Cardiovascular Magnetic Resonance and the Society of Cardiovascular Computed Tomography. *J Am Soc Echocardiogr.* 2024;37(1):2-63.

Caged Ball

Caged-ball valves were the first prosthetic valves implanted in humans. They consist of a silastic or metal-ball occluder housed in a wire cage with three or four struts. The ball occluder casts a large acoustic shadow and its motion within the cage is best imaged in the long-axis plane of the valve (Figure 13.10). In the short-axis imaging plane, the ball occluder can be imaged within the wire struts. Doppler color flow imaging in the short-axis plane of the valve demonstrates blood flow between the wire struts through the outside perimeter of the ball occluder (Figure 13.10). These valves are no longer used given their turbulent hemodynamic profile and higher anticoagulation requirements. On rare occasions, practitioners might still encounter these valves in patients with a remote history of valvular replacement.

Tilting Disc

Tilting disc valves have been utilized in the aortic, mitral, and tricuspid positions. They consist of a single-disc occluder supported by struts. The single-disc occluder pivots open 60° to 80° to form two orifices of different size and shape with the majority of blood flowing through the major orifice. They have a low profile and offer the advantage of providing a large orifice size in relation to its stent size. Although tilting disc valves are no longer in production for implantation in the United States, there are still some patients with these mechanical valves in the population. Tilting disc mechanical valves are also part of the commercially approved total artificial heart device. The two primary models of tilting disc valves can be distinguished by the presence of a central aperture in the Medtronic Hall and the absence of a central aperture in the Björk-Shiley valve when examined by color Doppler imaging (Figures 13.11 and 13.12). In the 1980s, the Björk-Shiley valve became no longer available in the United States due to the risk of outlet strut fracture.

Echocardiographic examination includes the following:

1. Confirm proper tilting action of the occluder in the long-axis imaging plane.
2. In the short-axis imaging plane, one edge of the disc occluder should move in and out of the imaging plane as the valve tilts open.

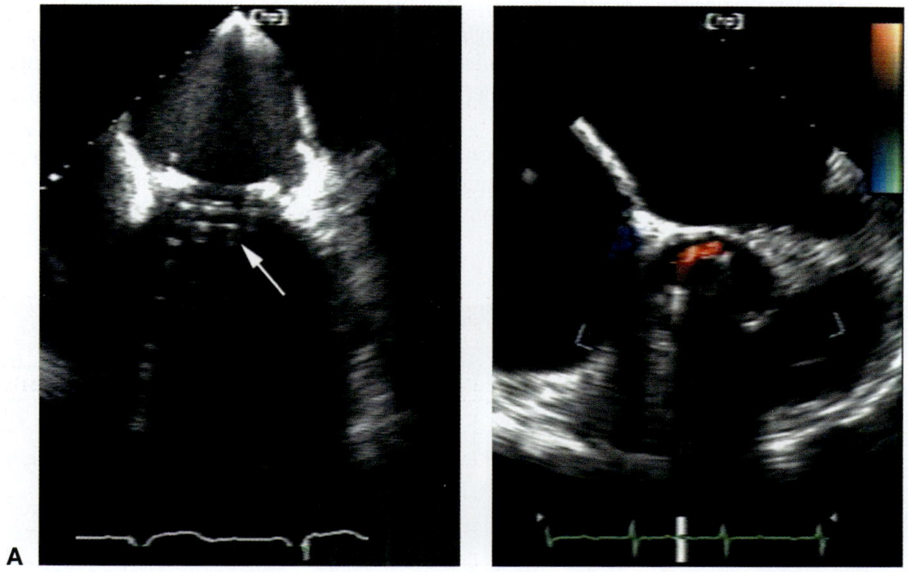

FIGURE 13.10 Starr-Edwards caged-ball mechanical valve. Panel A is a transesophageal echocardiographic midesophageal four-chamber view of a caged-ball valve prosthesis in the mitral position at end diastole. Ultrasound shadowing caused by the silastic ball occluder (arrow) contained within the wireform cage makes it difficult to image the distal side of the valve. Panel B is a TEE midesophageal aortic valve short-axis view at a multiplane angle of 50° during systole in a patient with a caged-ball valve in the aortic position. Note the three metal struts of the cage. Color Doppler flow imaging demonstrates blood flow through the valve at the perimeter of the silastic ball occluder. Again, the silastic ball occluder causes ultrasound shadowing.

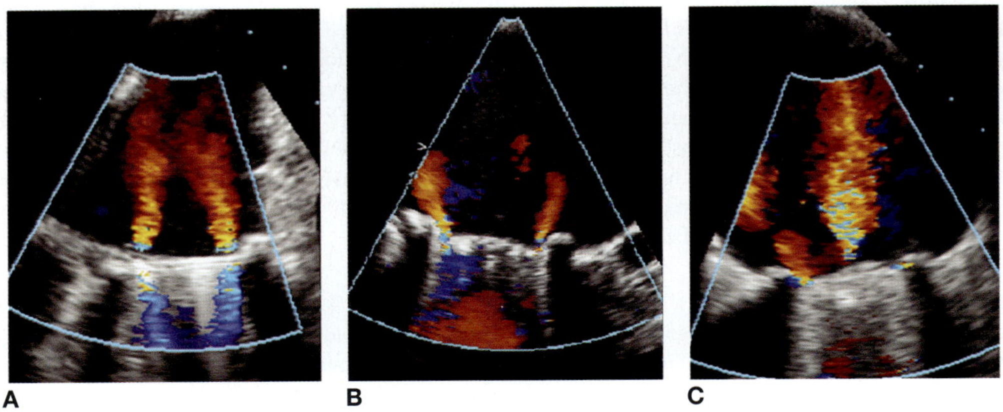

FIGURE 13.11 Transesophageal midesophageal images with color Doppler imaging in midsystole demonstrating the normal pattern of leakage regurgitant jets in patients with a bileaflet mechanical (panel A), Björk-Shiley tilting disc (panel B), and Medtronic Hall tilting disc (panel C) prosthetic valves in the mitral position. The bileaflet mechanical valve is distinguished by medially directed regurgitant jets originating from the hinge points of the occluders at a multiplane cross-sectional image parallel to the axis of rotation of the occluders (panel A). The Björk-Shiley valve is distinguished by a leakage regurgitant jet through a central orifice of the tilting disc occluder (panel C). The Medtronic Hall valve has no central orifice, but small leakage regurgitant jets originate between the tilting disc and the annular stent that are directed laterally (panel B). (Courtesy of Drs Cheung and Streckenbach.)

3. Color flow Doppler imaging showing a centrally directed leakage regurgitant jet originating from the hinge point of the disc occluder or small leakage regurgitant jets originating at the site of contact between the disc and the annular stent are normal findings for the Björk-Shiley valve (Figures 13.11 and 13.12). Two regurgitant jets originating from the inner edges of the annular stent that are directed laterally are a normal characteristic of the Björk-Shiley valve (Figure 13.11).
4. Calculate the transvalvular gradient with continuous wave Doppler. The Doppler beam alignment should travel through the major orifice of the valve in order to obtain the best estimate of the transvalvular blood flow velocity and gradient.
5. Strut fracture is a serious complication that can cause occluder malfunction and even disc embolization and is manifest by severe transvalvular regurgitation. Thrombus or pannus ingrowth on the valve can limit occluder opening or impair the occluder from closing completely, causing stenosis or transvalvular regurgitation (Figure 13.13).

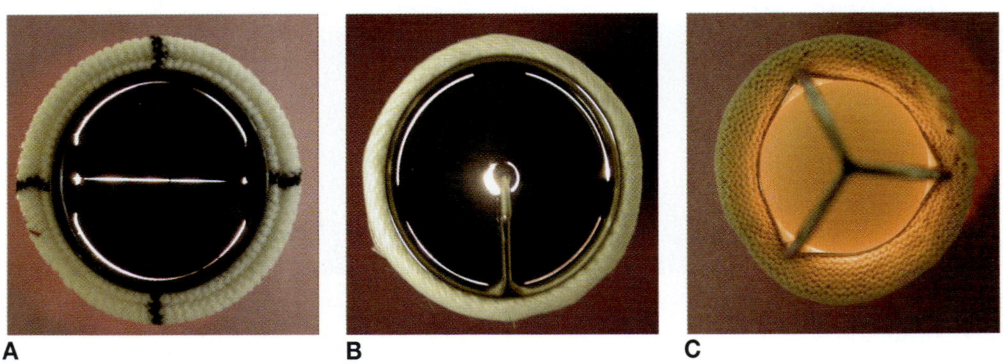

FIGURE 13.12 Transillumination of a bileaflet (St. Jude Medical, panel A), tilting disc (Medtronic Hall, panel B), and caged-ball (Starr-Edwards, panel C) mechanical prosthetic valves that demonstrate the typical sites of origin for normal washing and leakage regurgitant jets that appear on Doppler color flow imaging. (Courtesy of Drs Cheung and Streckenbach.)

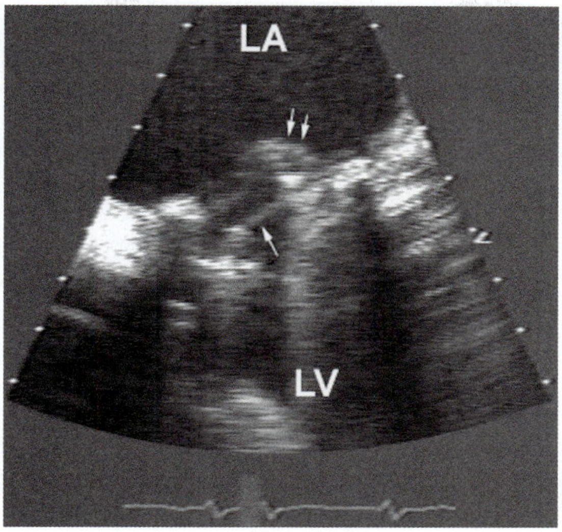

FIGURE 13.13 Pannus formation on a Björk-Shiley tilting disc mechanical prosthesis in the mitral position. Transesophageal echocardiographic midesophageal four-chamber view during systole in a patient with a tilting disc mechanical prosthesis in the mitral position. The single-disc occluder (single arrow) failed to close completely during systole and open completely during diastole (not shown). Pannus formation on the valve (double arrows) limited the motion of the disc occluder causing both prosthetic mitral stenosis and transvalvular mitral regurgitation. LA, left atrium; LV, left ventricle.

Biologic Valves or Tissue Valves

Biologic valves do not require systemic anticoagulation but have an effective life span of only 12 to 15 years. Unlike mechanical prosthetic valves, bioprosthetic valves permit future transcatheter prosthetic valve replacement to treat bioprosthetic valve dysfunction by implanting a new transcatheter prosthetic valve within the sewing ring of the existing bioprosthetic valve using a valve-in-valve (ViV) technique. The biologic components of bioprosthetic valves are susceptible to structural valvular deterioration such as leaflet calcification, tear, or perforation. Stentless bioprosthetic aortic valves are also susceptible to regurgitation from annular or aortic root dilatation. Bioprosthetic valves are traditionally preferred for older patients with a life expectancy less than 15 years or for patients who cannot tolerate anticoagulation therapy or in whom anticoagulation therapy is not feasible. With the ubiquity of transcatheter valve replacement (TAVR) techniques, bioprosthetic valves have increasingly become the valve of choice even in younger populations as they allow for future valve-in-valve TAVR, thus avoiding repeated valve surgery. The biologic components of bioprosthetic valves have favorable acoustic properties and permit imaging by ultrasound. In general, the same principles used to examine native cardiac valves can be applied to the TEE examination of biologic valve prostheses.

Stented Porcine Heterografts

Stented porcine heterografts are constructed from a glutaraldehyde-preserved porcine aortic xenograft mounted on a cloth-covered wire or polymer frame with an attached sewing ring (Figure 13.14). They can be implanted in the aortic, mitral, or tricuspid positions. In short axis, the three leaflets supported by struts open to form a central orifice in the shape of a bulging triangle. In long axis, the valve leaflets separate symmetrically when open and coapt at the center of the valve when closed. The stent struts that support the leaflets extend from the base of the annulus and point toward the downstream side of the valve. Doppler color flow imaging can sometimes detect a small closure or leakage regurgitant jet originating from the central coaptation point.

Stented Pericardial Valves

Stented pericardial valves are constructed from bovine or porcine pericardium fashioned into three leaflets supported by a wire frame with three struts attached to a sewing ring (Video 13.6). The pericardial leaflets

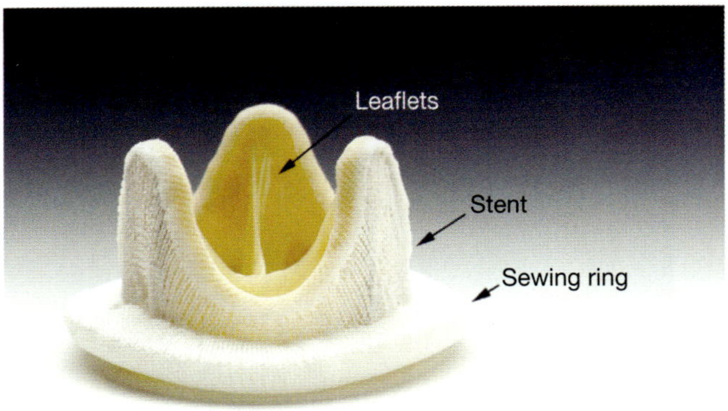

FIGURE 13.14 Photograph of a Carpentier-Edwards model 6625 porcine bioprosthetic mitral valve. The valve is constructed from a porcine aortic xenograft mounted on a wireform stent surrounded by a sewing ring.

can be mounted either on the internal side of the struts (Carpentier-Edwards PERIMOUNT) (Figure 13.15) or on the external side of the struts (Sorin Mitroflow or St. Jude Medical Trifecta) (Figures 13.16 and 13.17). In addition, the strut apparatus can be mounted above the annular sewing ring for supra-annular implantation. These modifications were designed to maximize the EOA for the prosthetic valve relative to its outside annular dimension.

Of note, the Medtronic AVALUS Valve is a next generation pericardial valve which is specifically designed for allowing a future ViV replacement. The polymer frame reduces the stress zone on the leaflets. The struts are very prominent on the TEE examination (Videos 13.7-13.9).

The pericardial bioprosthetic valves have a lower profile compared to the stented porcine bioprosthetic valves, but the echocardiographic appearance of these valves is similar, though not exactly the same as that of stented porcine aortic heterografts. Mild central transvalvular regurgitation can be normal immediately after implantation for some models of pericardial bioprosthetic valves (Figure 13.18). In addition, small transvalvular regurgitant leakage jets can sometimes be identified originating from the fabric-covered regions of the stent struts or from the region between the stent and the sewing ring (Figure 13.18). These transvalvular

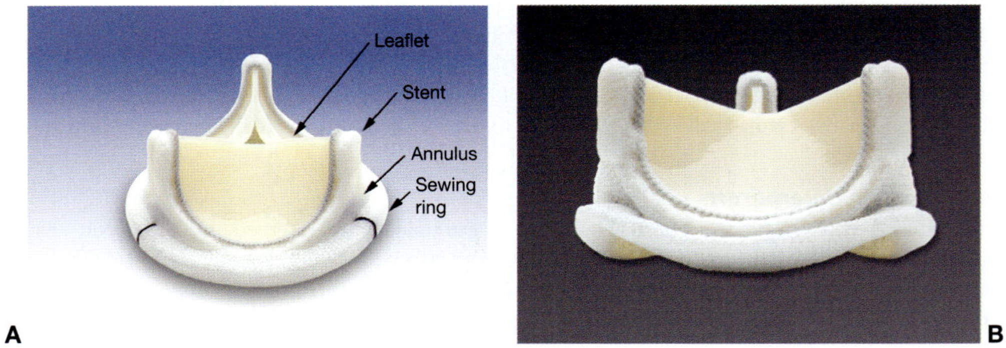

FIGURE 13.15 Photograph of a Carpentier-Edwards model 6900 bovine pericardial bioprosthetic mitral valve (panel A). The valve leaflets are constructed from bovine pericardium mounted on a wireform stent surrounded by a sewing ring. In contrast, the Carpentier-Edwards PERIMOUNT Magna valve (panel B) is a bovine pericardial bioprosthetic valve for implantation in the aortic position with a supra-annular design where the valve apparatus is mounted above the sewing ring in an effort to maximize the effective orifice area relative to the outside diameter of the sewing ring. (Courtesy of Drs Cheung and Streckenbach.)

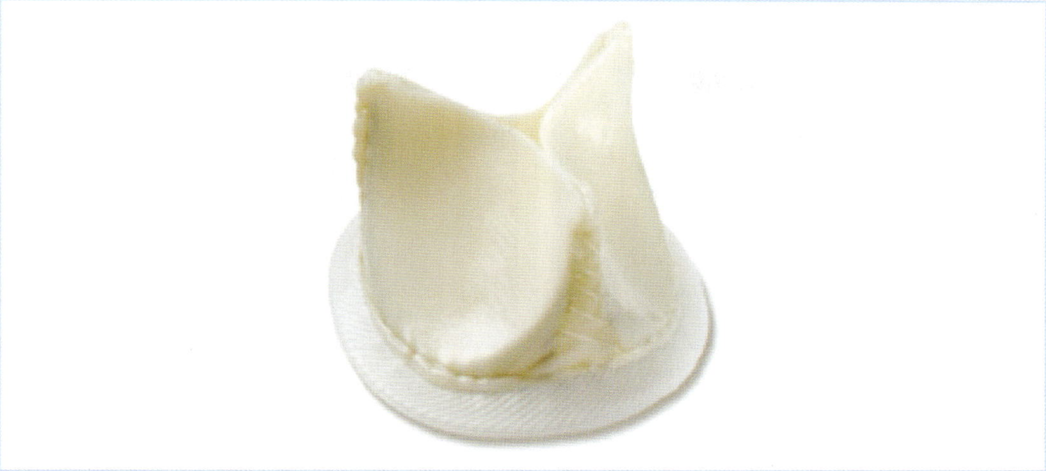

FIGURE 13.16 Photograph of a St. Jude Medical Trifecta porcine pericardial bioprosthetic aortic valve. The valve leaflets are constructed from porcine pericardium externally mounted on a titanium stent in an effort to maximize the effective orifice size relative to the outside diameter of the sewing ring. (Courtesy of Drs Cheung and Streckenbach.)

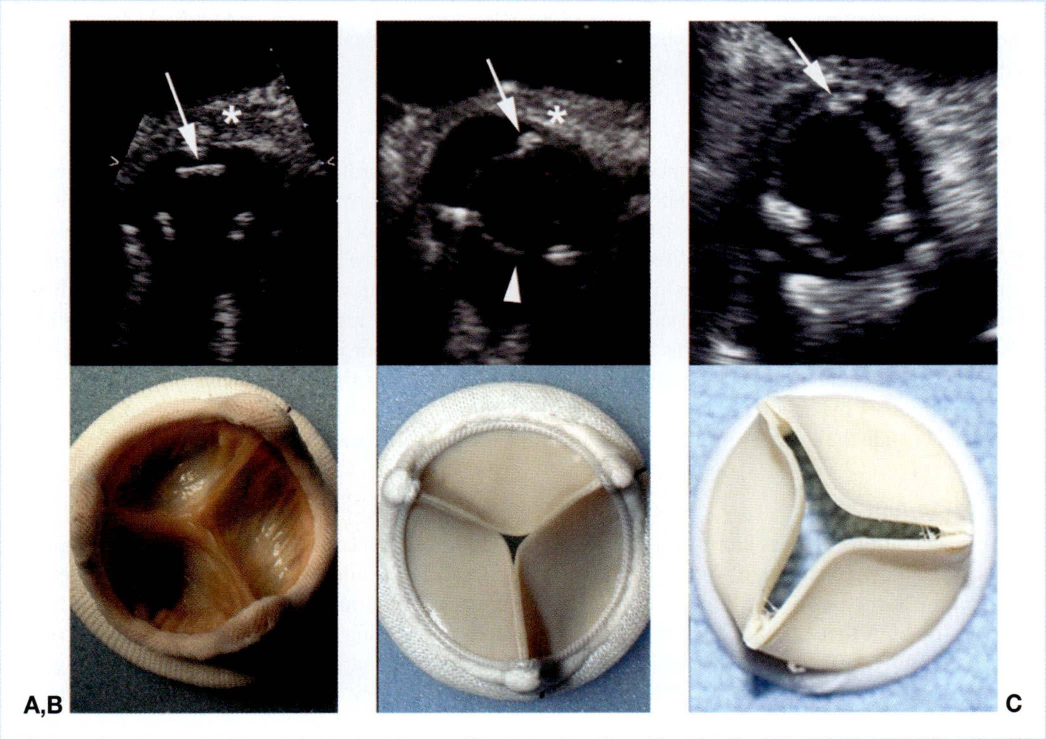

FIGURE 13.17 Transesophageal midesophageal aortic valve short-axis (panels A, B, and C) views of stented bioprosthetic valves in the aortic position with corresponding photographs of the actual prosthetic valves (lower panel). The struts protruding into the aortic root of the porcine (Hancock II) bioprosthetic valve (arrow, panel A) can be distinguished in the short-axis cross-sectional view (panel A), but acoustic shadowing from the prosthetic valve stent obscures the bioprosthetic leaflets. Both the struts (arrow, panel B) and individual leaflets (arrowhead, panel B) of a Carpentier-Edwards bovine pericardial bioprosthetic valve in systole can be imaged in the short-axis cross-sectional view (panel B). Detailed examination can distinguish that the pericardial leaflets on the Sorin Mitroflow prosthetic valve (arrow, panel C) are mounted on the external surface of the struts. Edema or thickening of the wall of the aortic root is sometimes present after aortic valve replacement (asterisks, panels A and B). (Courtesy of Drs Cheung and Streckenbach.)

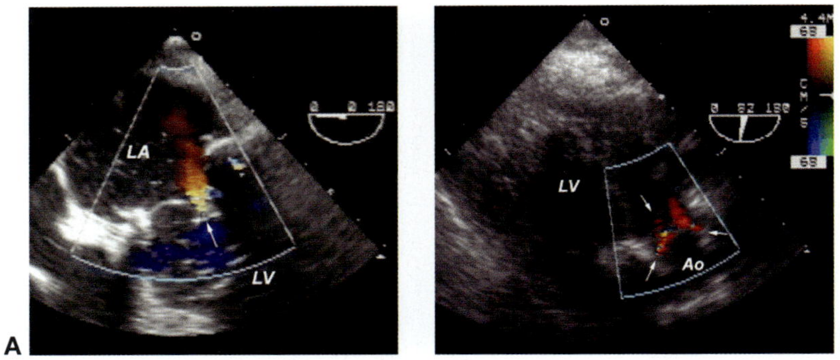

FIGURE 13.18 Mild transvalvular regurgitation can normally be detected sometimes immediately after implantation of bovine pericardial bioprosthetic valves. Midesophageal four-chamber view with color Doppler flow imaging demonstrated mild central regurgitation (arrow) through the leaflet commissures in a bovine pericardial bioprosthetic valve implanted in the mitral position (panel A). Transgastric midleft ventricular long-axis view through the aortic valve with color Doppler flow imaging detected mild regurgitation through the fabric-covered stent struts (arrows) in a bovine pericardial bioprosthetic valves implanted in the aortic position (panel B). These transvalvular regurgitant jets typically decrease in severity over time. Ao, aorta; LA, left atrium; LV, left ventricle.

regurgitant leakage jets through the fabric of bioprosthetic valves typically disappear over time as the fabric becomes sealed with cellular elements or endothelium.

Inspiris Resilia Valve

The Inspiris Resilia (Edwards Lifesciences) is an aortic bovine pericardial bioprosthetic valve that deserves special consideration, as they frequently demonstrate a transient valvular insufficiency immediately after cardiopulmonary bypass, which can be confused with a paravalvular leak (16). The Inspiris is specially designed with a unique hinge collar with "VFit" technology that allows for controlled expansion of the sewing ring diameter to accommodate a future valve-in-valve TAVR. Its wire frame (in sizes 19-25 mm) is labeled with laser-stenciled marking holes indicating the valve size, allowing fluoroscopic identification (Videos 13.10-13.12). These holes are likely the origin of this transient, signature regurgitant jet. During TEE examination of the Inspiris valve, a small regurgitant jet originating at the valve's stent post that improves quickly after separation of cardiopulmonary bypass or after protamine administration is likely this signature regurgitation, whereas any jets located outside the sewing ring at alternate locations suggest true paravalvular leakage.

Stentless Valves

The first-generation stentless bioprosthetic valves were fabric-reinforced glutaraldehyde-preserved porcine aortic heterografts constructed without the wireform frame, stents, and sewing ring. They were designed for use in the aortic position or for replacement of the aortic root. Elimination of the stent and sewing ring increases the EOA that can be achieved after valve replacement making them particularly useful in patients with a native aortic valve annulus less than 20 mm in diameter. Elimination of the stent also permits greater freedom of movement of the valve leaflets and annulus and, in theory, may decrease the risk of structural valvular degeneration. However, the competency of the stentless aortic valve is contingent on the geometry of the aortic root. Mismatching of the annular size, malalignment of the leaflets in the annular plane, or dilatation of the aortic root will alter leaflet coaptation and cause regurgitation. For this reason, it is important for the intraoperative echocardiographic examination to accurately size the native annulus and verify that the ascending aorta is not dilated and that the diameter of the sinotubular junction matches or is within 10% the diameter of the stentless valve (17).

The echocardiographic appearance of the stentless valve is virtually indistinguishable from the native aortic valve except for the presence of an acoustic shadow caused by the Dacron reinforcement at the base of the valve annulus (Figure 13.19). Implantation of the stentless valve within the native aortic root increases the thickness of the vessel wall at the region of overlap and makes paravalvular regurgitation possible

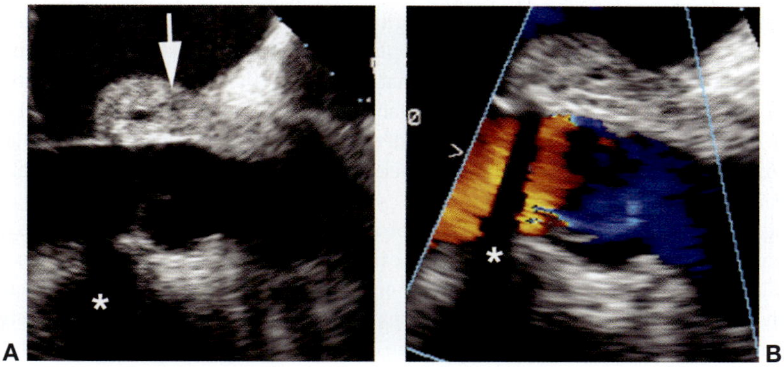

FIGURE 13.19 Intraoperative transesophageal midesophageal aortic valve long-axis view immediately after implantation of a stentless porcine bioprosthetic aortic root (Medtronic Freestyle) in the aortic position (panel A). Periaortic thickening (arrow, panel A) is common immediately after implantation and can be attributed to tissue edema. Only the cloth-reinforced annular sewing ring produces an acoustic shadow on 2D (asterisk, panel A) and Doppler color flow imaging (asterisk, panel B). (Courtesy of Drs Cheung and Streckenbach.)

(Figure 13.19). Trace or mild central aortic regurgitation is detectable up to 25% of the time immediately after implantation of the stentless bioprosthetic valve.

The Medtronic ATS 3f is a pericardial stentless valve constructed from three equine pericardial leaflets shaped in the form of a tube attached directly to a polyester annular sewing ring. After implantation within the aortic valve annulus, the three commissural tabs on the distal side of the valve attached directly to the native aortic wall and the prosthetic sewing ring can be distinguished by TEE. The absence of regurgitation by color Doppler examination after implantation is useful to ensure that the valve and the commissural suspension points are properly positioned within the aortic root.

Allograft Valves

Cryopreserved human aortic root allografts are commercially available for implantation. They are sized according to the aortic valve annulus diameter in a range from 20 to 26 mm. Absence of a stent requires that the annular size of the allograft matches the size of the native valve annulus to ensure valve competence. Implantation of an undersized or oversized allograft may result in aortic regurgitation. The echocardiographic appearance of the aortic allograft is indistinguishable from the native aortic valve and aortic root. Replacement of the aortic root and reimplantation of the coronary arteries with a human aortic root allograft, stentless porcine aortic root, or bioprosthetic or mechanical valved conduit is performed for aortic valve endocarditis with aortic root abscess, bicuspid aortic valve with dilated aortic root, Type A aortic dissection, or aneurysms involving the aortic root and ascending aorta. The aortic root allograft comes prepared as a unit with anterior mitral leaflet attached. The mitral valve leaflet is typically removed before the implantation. LVOT obstruction after allograft root implantation caused by excessive residual anterior mitral leaflet has been reported (18).

CLINICAL CAVEATS FOR THE ECHOCARDIOGRAPHIC DIAGNOSIS OF PROSTHETIC VALVE DYSFUNCTION

Prosthetic valve dysfunction can result in regurgitation, stenosis, or hemolysis. TEE is recognized as the diagnostic examination of choice for the diagnosis and evaluation of suspected prosthetic valve dysfunction.

1. *Prosthetic valve regurgitation:* When the Doppler examination reveals regurgitation in a prosthetic valve, it is important to distinguish physiologic regurgitation from pathologic regurgitation.
   a. A small amount of regurgitation is normally observed in all mechanical prosthetic valves except for caged-ball valves and in approximately 10% of bioprosthetic valves. Closure backflow is the reversal of flow required for closure of the valve. In contrast, leakage backflow occurs after closure of mechanical valves and originates from the hinges and the regions of coaptation between the occluders and the valve ring (Figures 13.1, 13.5, 13.6, 13.12, and 13.18; Videos 13.2, 13.4, and 13.5). Physiologic

regurgitation jets are small and short in duration. The leakage backflow patterns for each valve type are unique and distinct from pathologic regurgitation (Figure 13.11). Mild transvalvular regurgitation can often be detected by TEE color flow Doppler imaging in bioprosthetic valves immediately after implantation (Figure 13.18). Regurgitant jets that originate at the sites of leaflet coaptation are directed centrally. Regurgitant jets from leakage at the fabric-covered regions of the valve stent originate at the valve struts and are directed toward the center of the valve. Mild physiologic transvalvular regurgitation in bioprosthetic valves detected by TEE immediately after implantation typically decreases or even disappears by the end of the operation.

b. Pathologic transvalvular regurgitation in bioprosthetic valves is commonly associated with chronic degenerative changes that may include leaflet calcification, perforation, tears, prolapse (Figures 13.20 and 13.21), or from leaflet destruction caused by endocarditis. In mechanical prosthetic valves, pathologic transvalvular regurgitation can be caused by pannus, thrombus, vegetations, or foreign material on valve components that prevent complete closure of the occluder (Figure 13.22). The 2D and 3D imaging of leaflet or occluder motion in mechanical valves is useful for detecting transvalvular regurgitation caused by impingement of the occluder by pannus, thrombus, or vegetations (Video 13.13). Grading systems based on Doppler measurements of regurgitant fraction, regurgitant jet area, jet length, and vena contracta or jet width also apply for assessing the clinical severity of prosthetic valve regurgitation. However, the pattern and location of regurgitation associated with prosthetic valve dysfunction differ from those associated with native valvular heart disease and sometimes require an alternative or integrative approach to grade the severity of regurgitation. For example, in the case of paravalvular regurgitation, the annular extent of the defect can be used to quantify the severity of regurgitation along with regurgitant jet width, size, length, eccentricity, density, and proximal flow convergence (Tables 13.7 and 13.8).

c. Paravalvular regurgitation is always pathologic and is caused by prosthetic endocarditis, incomplete fixation of the prosthetic sewing ring to the native annulus, or dehiscence of the sewing ring. Incomplete fixation is typically caused by native annular calcification that increases the difficulty of prosthetic implantation or an avulsed annular suture. Paravalvular regurgitant jets imaged using color Doppler flow imaging originate at a point outside of the sewing ring, characteristically produce eccentric jets that track along the walls of the receiving chamber, and are usually accompanied by zones of proximal flow convergence adjacent to the site of the defect in the upstream cardiac chamber (Figure 13.7; Video 13.3). Evidence to support the best course of action in response to the TEE detection of paravalvular regurgitation immediately after prosthetic valve implantation is limited. Some clinical series suggested that intraoperative TEE was useful for detecting paravalvular regurgitation and prompted revision of the valve replacement (19). In a very small series, two out of six patients with

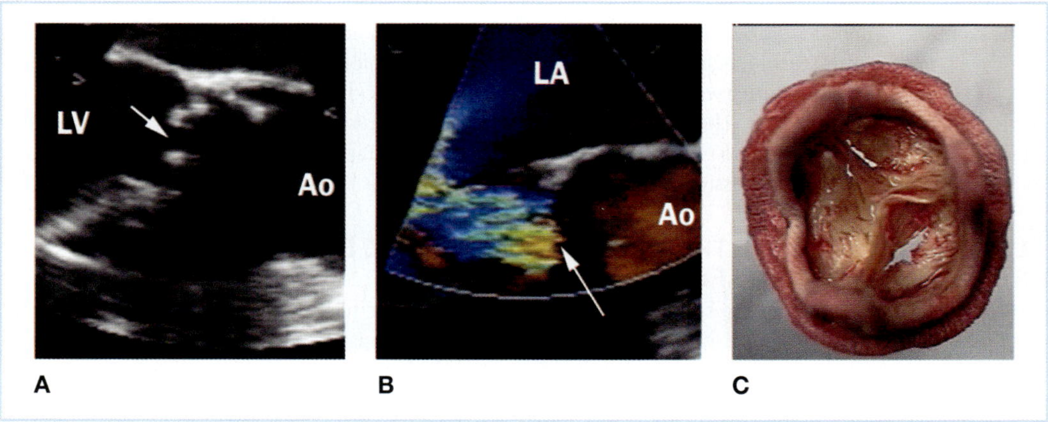

FIGURE 13.20 Transesophageal midesophageal aortic valve long-axis view of a porcine bioprosthetic valve in the aortic position demonstrating structural valvular degeneration with prolapse and perforated valve cusps (arrow, panel A). Doppler color flow imaging in diastole demonstrated severe transvalvular regurgitation through the defects (arrow, panel B) that were also apparent on the explanted prosthetic valve (panel C). Ao, aorta; LA, left atrium; LV, left ventricle. (Courtesy of Drs Cheung and Streckenbach.)

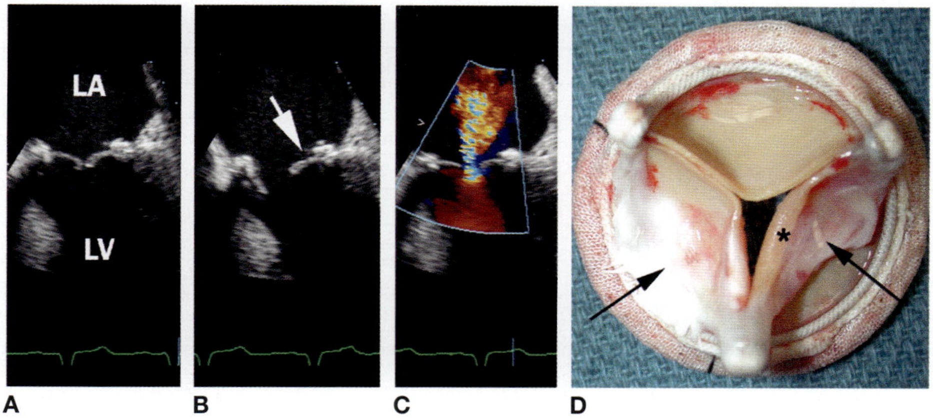

FIGURE 13.21 Transesophageal midesophageal four-chamber view of a stented bovine pericardial bioprosthetic valve implanted in the mitral position. Two-dimensional imaging demonstrated restricted leaflet motion in diastole (arrow, panel B) and incomplete coaptation in systole (panel A). Doppler color flow imaging demonstrated severe central mitral regurgitation (panel C). Pannus formation at the base of the prosthetic valve leaflets (arrows, panel D) and thickening of the leaflet edges (asterisk, panel D) causing leaflet restriction and transvalvular regurgitation was seen in the explanted specimen. LV, left ventricle; LA, left atrium. (Courtesy of Drs Cheung and Streckenbach.)

mild paravalvular regurgitation and two out of two patients with moderate paravalvular regurgitation detected by TEE immediately after mitral valve replacement had subsequent clinical deterioration (20). Another study examining 27 patients after aortic or mitral valve replacement found that small paravalvular regurgitant jets detected by TEE using Doppler color flow imaging were common after valve replacement, decreased in size and number after protamine administration, and were not associated with early postoperative morbidity (21). Finally, in a large series of 608 consecutive patients undergoing aortic or mitral valve replacement, trivial or mild paravalvular regurgitation defined as a regurgitant jet area less than 3 cm^2 by Doppler color flow imaging was detected by intraoperative TEE in 18.3% of patients (22). At early follow-up, paravalvular regurgitation had resolved in 50% of the patients. At late follow-up, only 4 out of the original 113 patients with mild paravalvular regurgitation had worsening of regurgitation. Precise characterization of the location, annular extent, and multimodal

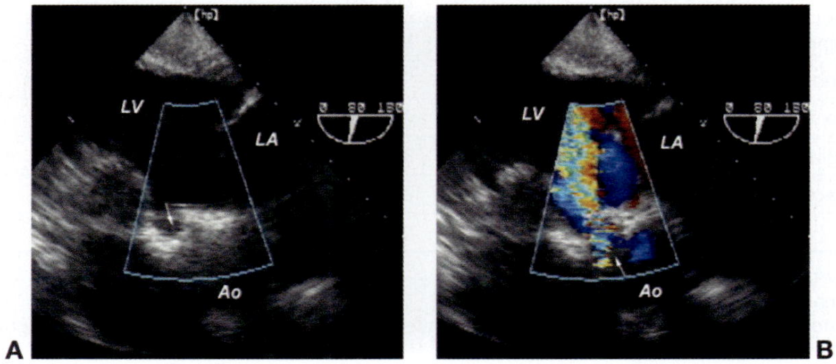

FIGURE 13.22 Severe transvalvular regurgitation caused by a leaflet trapped in the open position due to pannus ingrowth. Transgastric midleft ventricular long-axis view through the aortic valve in a patient with a bileaflet mechanical prosthetic valve in the aortic position. Two-dimensional imaging (panel A) demonstrated one of the valve leaflets was immobile and trapped in the open position (arrow). Color Doppler flow imaging (panel B) demonstrated severe transvalvular regurgitation through the region of the prosthetic valve with the leaflet trapped in the open position (arrow). Ao, aorta; LA, left atrium; LV, left ventricle.

TABLE 13.7 Echocardiographic Parameters for Grading the Severity of Prosthetic Aortic Regurgitation

Parameter	Mild	Moderate	Severe
2D and 3D parameters			
Valve stent	Normal	Abnormal[a]	Abnormal[a]
Leaflets or occluders	Normal	Abnormal[b]	Abnormal[b]
Doppler parameters			
Jet width (% LVOT diameter)[c]	Narrow (≤25)	Intermediate (26-64)	Large (>65)
Jet density (CW Doppler)	Incomplete/faint	Dense	Dense
Jet deceleration rate (PHT, ms)[d]	Slow (>500)	Variable (200-500)	Steep (<200)
Diastolic flow reversal (Desc. Ao)	Absent or brief	Intermediate	Prominent, holodiastolic
Regurgitant volume (mL/beat)	<30	30-59	≥60
Regurgitant fraction (%)	<30	30-50	≥50

CW, continuous wave; Desc. Ao, descending thoracic aorta; LVOT, left ventricular outflow tract; PHT, pressure half-time.
[a]Examples of abnormal motion include dehiscence or rocking.
[b]Examples of abnormal motion include immobile occluder, limited occluder range of travel, or prolapsed bioprosthetic leaflet.
[c]At a Nyquist limit set at 50-60 cm/s. Parameter is less accurate for eccentric jets.
[d]Influenced by left ventricular compliance.
Data from Zoghbi WA, Jone PN, Chamsi-Pasha MA, et al. Guidelines for the evaluation of prosthetic valve function with cardiovascular imaging: a report from the American Society of Echocardiography developed in collaboration with the Society for Cardiovascular Magnetic Resonance and the Society of Cardiovascular Computed Tomography. *J Am Soc Echocardiogr*. 2024;37(1):2-63.

TABLE 13.8 Echocardiographic Parameters for Grading the Severity of Prosthetic Mitral Regurgitation

Parameter	Mild	Moderate	Severe
2D and 3D parameters			
Valve stent	Normal	Abnormal[a]	Abnormal[a]
Leaflets or occluders	Normal	Abnormal[b]	Abnormal[b]
Doppler parameters			
Color flow jet[c]	Small central jet	Variable	Large central jet
	<4 cm^2	4-8 cm^2	>8 cm^2 eccentric wall-impinging jet
Flow convergence[d]	None or minimal	Intermediate	Large
Pulmonary venous flow[e]	Systolic dominance	Systolic blunting	Systolic flow reversal
Vena contracta width (cm)[f]	<0.3	0.3-0.69	≥0.7
Regurgitant volume (mL/beat)[f]	<30	30-59	≥60
Regurgitant fraction (%)[f]	<30	30-49	≥50
EROA (cm^2)[f]	<0.20	0.20-0.39	≥0.40

EROA, effective regurgitant orifice area.
[a]Examples of abnormal motion include dehiscence or rocking.
[b]Examples of abnormal motion include immobile occluder, limited occluder range of travel, or prolapsed bioprosthetic leaflet.
[c]At a Nyquist limit set at 50-60 cm/s.
[d]Minimal and large flow convergence defined as a flow convergence radius <0.4 cm and ≥0.9 cm for central jets, respectively, at a Nyquist limit of 40 cm/s; thresholds for eccentric jets may be greater.
[e]Other reasons for systolic blunting include atrial fibrillation and increased left atrial pressure.
[f]Quantitative Doppler parameters for grading prosthetic mitral regurgitation are less well validated compared to use in native mitral regurgitation.
Data from Zoghbi WA, Jone PN, Chamsi-Pasha MA, et al. Guidelines for the evaluation of prosthetic valve function with cardiovascular imaging: a report from the American Society of Echocardiography developed in collaboration with the Society for Cardiovascular Magnetic Resonance and the Society of Cardiovascular Computed Tomography. *J Am Soc Echocardiogr*. 2024;37(1):2-63.

assessment of the severity of paravalvular regurgitant jets detected by TEE after valve implantation is important for guiding intraoperative decisions as to whether surgical revision is necessary. Paravalvular regurgitation as a consequence of dehiscence is a late complication after valve replacement and is commonly associated with endocarditis. Dehiscence of part of the sewing ring may destabilize the prosthetic valve producing a "rocking" motion of the entire prosthesis and a visible separation of the native and prosthetic valve annulus detected by 2D imaging (Figures 13.7 and 13.23).

2. *Prosthetic valve stenosis:* Compared to the native valve, all prosthetic valves are mildly stenotic depending upon the valve type, size, and the hemodynamic condition of the patient. The mean pressure gradient across prosthetic valves calculated using the ***simplified*** Bernoulli equation depends on the prosthetic valve type, its position, its size, the blood flow velocity proximal to the prosthetic valve, and the cardiac output. For this reason, the package insert or published normal values that list the hemodynamic specifications for the particular valve type and model according to annular size are often used as a reference when examining the hemodynamic performance of a specific prosthetic valve (Appendix D) (1,8-10). The peak transvalvular gradient for valves in the mitral position ranges from 3 to 4 mm Hg and the peak transvalvular gradient for valves in the aortic position ranges from 10 to 30 mm Hg. Threshold values of echocardiographic parameters that suggest significant prosthetic valve stenosis are also available in published guidelines (Tables 13.5, 13.6, and 13.9) (1). The continuity method can also be used to estimate the EOA of prosthetic valves in the mitral or aortic positions (Table 13.3). The continuity method uses Doppler to measure the VTI across the prosthetic valve in relation to the cross-sectional area of the LVOT and the VTI through the LVOT. A normal value of the EOA estimated by the continuity equation is greater than or equal to 2 cm^2 for prosthetic valves in the mitral position, whereas a normal value for prosthetic valves in the aortic position depends on valve EOA reference ranges (Tables 13.5 and 13.6). The DVI is an alternative method of quantifying the severity of prosthetic valve stenosis. For prosthetic aortic valves, the DVI is the ratio of VTI in the LVOT to the VTI across the prosthetic valve. A DVI less than 0.25 is considered clinically significant aortic prosthetic stenosis, whereas a DVI between 0.25 and 0.35 may suggest possible stenosis (Table 13.5). For prosthetic mitral valves, the DVI is the ratio of the VTI across the prosthetic mitral valve to the VTI of the LVOT. In this case, a DVI greater than 2.5 suggests significant mitral stenosis, whereas a DVI between 2.2 and 2.5 may suggest possible stenosis (Table 13.6).

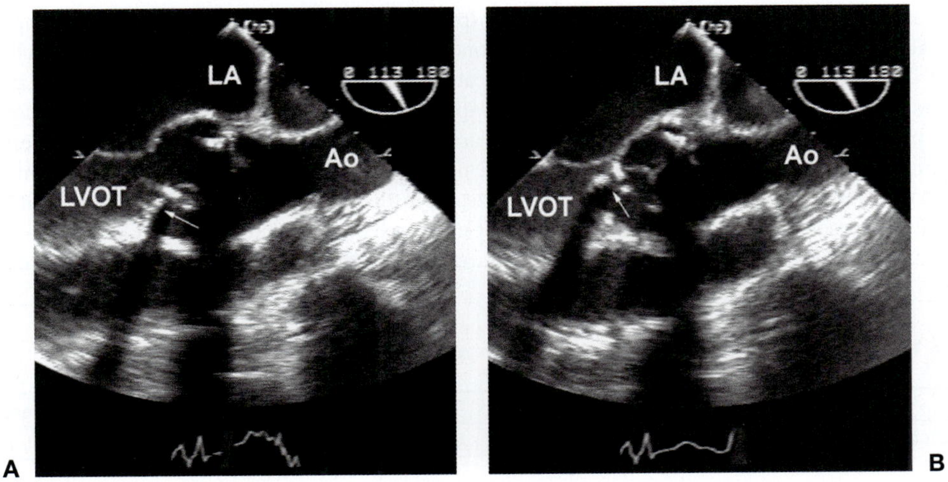

FIGURE 13.23 Transesophageal echocardiographic midesophageal aortic valve long-axis image at a multiplane angle of 113° showing dehiscence of a pericardial bioprosthesis in the aortic position. In systole (panel A), the anterior region of the prosthetic stent (arrow) is displaced toward the left ventricular side of the native aortic valve annulus. In diastole (panel B), the anterior region of the prosthetic stent is completely detached from the aortic valve annulus (arrow). Dehiscence with partial annular detachment produced a "rocking" motion of the prosthetic valve and paravalvular regurgitation in the region of separation (arrow). Ao, aorta; LA, left atrium; LVOT, left ventricular outflow tract.

TABLE 13.9 Doppler Parameters for Diagnosis of Prosthetic Tricuspid Stenosis

Parameter	Bioprosthetic	Mechanical
Peak velocity	≥2.1 m/s	≥1.9 m/s
Mean gradient	≥9 mm Hg	≥6 mm Hg
Pressure half-time	≥200 ms	≥130 ms
EOA	<1.5 cm^2	<2.0 cm^2
DVI (VTI_{PrTV}/VTI_{LVOT})[a]	≥3.3	≥2.1

PrTV, prosthetic tricuspid valve.
[a]Assess in absence of aortic regurgitation or tricuspid regurgitation. Upper normal limits vary based on valve size and type.
Data from Zoghbi WA, Jone PN, Chamsi-Pasha MA, et al. Guidelines for the evaluation of prosthetic valve function with cardiovascular imaging: a report from the American Society of Echocardiography developed in collaboration with the Society for Cardiovascular Magnetic Resonance and the Society of Cardiovascular Computed Tomography. *J Am Soc Echocardiogr.* 2024;37(1):2-63.

Other echocardiographic characteristics that indicate prosthetic aortic valve stenosis include an acceleration time exceeding 100 msec (time interval between flow initiation and peak flow) or the presence of a rounded, symmetrical, late peaking transvalvular Doppler flow profile (in contrast to an early peaking triangular Doppler flow profile) (Table 13.5). Stenosis of bioprosthetic valves is caused by chronic degenerative changes resulting in leaflet calcification, thickening, and rigidity, restricting their ability to open completely. Degenerative changes and restricted leaflet mobility can be detected by the 2D and 3D examination. In mechanical valves, stenosis can be caused by thrombus, pannus, vegetation, suture, or even retained subvalvular structures that trap the occluder mechanism in the closed position or impinge on its ability to open completely (Figures 13.8 and 13.13).

3. *Prosthesis-patient mismatch:* Prosthetic heart valves are inherently stenotic relative to native cardiac valves. Although still somewhat controversial, several clinical studies have provided evidence that implantation of a prosthetic valve that is sized too small for an individual patient has the potential to cause significant obstruction to flow (23-26). The hemodynamic consequences of flow obstruction caused by a normally functioning prosthetic valve increased the likelihood of mortality and cardiac complications after aortic valve replacement (24-26). Implantation of too small of a prosthetic valve in the aortic position for aortic stenosis has also been shown to be associated with decreased ventricular mass regression after operation (27). This condition is called prosthesis-patient mismatch and may be particularly important in patients with decreased left ventricular ejection fraction. Prosthesis-patient mismatching has been best described after aortic valve replacement because the diameter of the native aortic valve annulus limits the size of the prosthetic valve that can be implanted. However, several studies have also suggested that prosthesis-patient mismatching may also occur after mitral valve replacement and is manifested by pulmonary hypertension (28). Intraoperative TEE provides an opportunity to measure the diameter of the native aortic valve annulus to determine the size of prosthetic valve that can be implanted, and is thus helpful for predicting the risk of prosthesis-patient mismatch based on the indexed EOA (EOA_i = EOA/BSA, where EOA_i is the indexed effective orifice area, EOA is the effective orifice area of the prosthetic

TABLE 13.10 Doppler Parameters of Aortic and Mitral Valve Prosthesis-Patient Mismatch

		Normal	Moderate	Severe
Aortic Indexed EOA (cm^2/m^2)	BMI <30 kg/m^2	>0.85	0.85-0.66	≤0.65
	BMI ≥30 kg/m^2	>0.70	0.70-0.56	≤0.55
Mitral Indexed EOA (cm^2/m^2)	BMI <30 kg/m^2	>1.2	1.2-0.91	≤0.90
	BMI ≥30 kg/m^2	>1.0	1.0-0.76	≤0.75

BMI, body mass index.
Data from Zoghbi WA, Jone PN, Chamsi-Pasha MA, et al. Guidelines for the evaluation of prosthetic valve function with cardiovascular imaging: a report from the American Society of Echocardiography developed in collaboration with the Society for Cardiovascular Magnetic Resonance and the Society of Cardiovascular Computed Tomography. *J Am Soc Echocardiogr.* 2024;37(1):2-63.

valve, and BSA is the body surface area of the patient in m^2) (Table 13.3). Prosthesis-patient mismatch is considered severe after aortic valve replacement if the EOA_i is less than or equal to 0.65 cm^2/m^2, moderate if the EOA_i is between 0.66 and 0.85 cm^2/m^2, and not significant if the EOA_i is greater than or equal to 0.85 cm^2/m^2 (Table 13.10) (24). Prosthesis-patient mismatch is considered moderate after mitral valve replacement if the EOA_i is less than or equal to 1.2 cm^2/m^2 and severe if the EOA_i is less than or equal to 0.9 cm^2/m^2 (Table 13.10) (1, 24). If intraoperative TEE measurements detect a small aortic valve annulus prior to aortic valve replacement, operative options to decrease the risk of prosthesis-patient mismatch include implanting the prosthetic valve in the supra-annular position, choosing a prosthetic valve model with the greatest EOA for the given annular diameter, performing an aortic root enlargement procedure to permit implantation of a larger prosthetic valve, or replacing the aortic root.

4. *Thrombosis and pannus:* Acute thrombosis, usually as a result of inadequate anticoagulation, can cause stenosis or regurgitation by obstructing blood flow through the valve or by interfering with occluder opening and closure. Stenosis or regurgitation can also be caused by ingrowth of pannus, which is a subacute condition. The 2D and 3D imaging may demonstrate abnormal masses attached to the prosthetic valve sometimes interfering with or limiting the range of motion of the occluder device (Figure 13.13). Pannus, with its fibrous composition, is echo dense and firmly fixed to the valve apparatus. Thrombus tends to be more mobile, larger in size, and sometimes associated with spontaneous echo contrast in the cardiac chambers indicating regions of low flow (29). Color flow Doppler imaging may demonstrate transvalvular regurgitation or an eccentric inflow pattern across the affected leaflet (Figure 13.22). Sometimes, pannus ingrowth is diagnosed only indirectly via TEE by demonstrating significant prosthetic valve stenosis or abnormal patterns of regurgitation.
5. *Hemolysis:* Hemolysis is unusual with modern valve prostheses, but hemolysis can occur when blood is subjected to high-peak shear stresses. These hydrodynamic conditions can occur when blood accelerates rapidly or decelerates rapidly upon collision or impingement with prosthetic material (30). Regurgitant jets associated with hemolysis often exhibit patterns of flow fragmentation, collision, or rapid acceleration by color flow Doppler imaging. Free regurgitant jets or jets that decelerate gradually are less likely to produce hemolysis.
6. *Endocarditis:* Prosthetic endocarditis occurs in approximately 3% to 6% of patients after valve replacement and has a mortality that ranges between 20% and 80% (3). TEE is currently the best diagnostic technique for detecting vegetations, dehiscence, or annular abscess for the diagnosis of prosthetic endocarditis (Figures 13.7 and 13.24) (31). Because of acoustic shadowing artifacts, it is important to use both

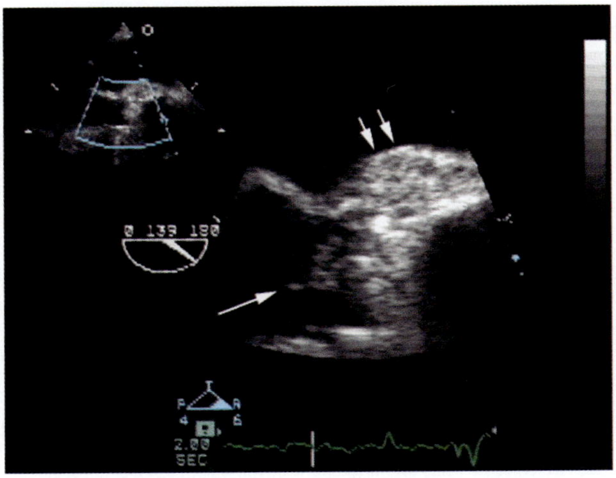

FIGURE 13.24 Endocarditis and aortic root abscess, mechanical bileaflet valve, aortic position. Transesophageal echocardiographic midesophageal aortic valve long-axis image at a multiplane angle of 139° demonstrating prosthetic endocarditis in a patient with a mechanical bileaflet valve in the aortic position. A vegetation attached to the prosthetic valve was imaged in the left ventricular outflow tract during diastole (single arrow). Thickening of the posterior wall of the aortic root (double arrows) suggested aortic root abscess.

TABLE 13.11 General Principles for Applying Transesophageal Echocardiography (TEE) in Valve Replacement Procedures

1. Know the make and models of prosthetic valves used in your hospital and their characteristic 2D, 3D, and Doppler echocardiographic features.
2. Perform and record a baseline (prebypass) complete standardized TEE examination.
3. Watch and listen to the surgeons as they implant the prosthetic valve.
4. Start TEE assessment of the prosthetic valve before separation from bypass.
5. Use TEE to assist with de-airing the cardiac chambers.
6. Become an expert at examining the cardiac valves from the transgastric views.
7. Use 2D, 3D, zoom, and slow-motion replay to examine a prosthetic valve.
8. Use Doppler echocardiography to quantify the hemodynamic performance of the prosthetic valve.
9. Get a second opinion to confirm a difficult diagnosis.
10. Have available reference of the hemodynamic specifications for commonly used prosthetic valve models and sizes.

midesophageal and transgastric imaging planes to examine both sides of the prosthetic valve for the presence of vegetations.

7. *LVOT obstruction:* LVOT obstruction causing subvalvular aortic stenosis is an uncommon but recognized complication of mitral valve replacement (32-34). After *mitral* valve replacement performed using valve sparing or chordal sparing techniques, residual mitral valve leaflet or chordal apparatus remaining in the LVOT can cause LVOT obstruction. LVOT obstruction can also be caused by a bioprosthetic valve in the mitral position with a strut protruding into the LVOT causing obstruction to left ventricular outflow. Leaflet displacement of the anterior mitral leaflet toward the LVOT and narrowing of the LVOT after deployment can also cause LVOT obstruction in up to 13% of patients undergoing transcatheter mitral valve replacement (TMVR) (35). The transgastric long-axis view provides a means to image the LVOT after mitral valve replacement and to estimate the LVOT pressure gradient using continuous wave Doppler (Video 13.14).

CONCLUSION

The evaluation of prosthetic heart valves, the diagnosis of prosthetic valve dysfunction, and the detection of complications associated with valve replacement are important clinical applications of TEE. A systematic approach to the TEE examination in patients undergoing valve replacement operations and in patients with prosthetic cardiac valves is necessary to verify the proper functioning of the prosthetic valves and to diagnose prosthetic valve dysfunction or complications associated with valve replacement procedures (Table 13.11).

REFERENCES

1. Zoghbi WA, Jone PN, Chamsi-Pasha MA, et al. Guidelines for the evaluation of prosthetic valve function with cardiovascular imaging: a report from the American Society of Echocardiography developed in collaboration with the Society for Cardiovascular Magnetic Resonance and the Society of Cardiovascular Computed Tomography. *J Am Soc Echocardiogr.* 2024;37(1):2-63.
2. Seward JB, Labovitz AJ, Lewis JF, et al. ACC position statement. Transesophageal echocardiography. *J Am Coll Cardiol.* 1992;20:506.
3. Vongpatanasin W, Hillis LD, Lange RA. Medical progress: prosthetic heart valves. *N Engl J Med.* 1996;335:407-416.
4. Daniel WG, Mugge A, Grote J, et al. Comparison of transthoracic and transesophageal echocardiography for detection of abnormalities of prosthetic and bioprosthetic valves in the mitral and aortic positions. *Am J Cardiol.* 1993;71:210-215.
5. Khandheria BK, Seward JB, Oh JK, et al. Value and limitations of transesophageal echocardiography in assessment of mitral valve prostheses. *Circulation.* 1991;83:1956-1968.
6. Karalis DG, Chandrasekaran K, Ross JJ Jr, et al. Single-plane transesophageal echocardiography for assessing function of mechanical or bioprosthetic valves in the aortic position. *Am J Cardiol.* 1992;69:1310-1315.
7. Chambers J, Fraser A, Lawford P, et al. Echocardiographic assessment of artificial heart valves: British Society of Echocardiography position paper. *Br Heart J.* 1994;71(4 suppl):6-14.
8. Panidis IP, Ross J, Mintz GS. Normal and abnormal prosthetic valve function as assessed by Doppler echocardiography. *J Am Coll Cardiol.* 1986;8:317-326.

9. Reisner SA, Meltzer RS. Normal values of prosthetic valve Doppler echocardiographic parameters: a review. *J Am Soc Echocardiogr*. 1988;1:201-210.
10. Rosenhek R, Binder T, Maurer G, et al. Normal values for Doppler echocardiographic assessment of heart valve prostheses. *J Am Soc Echocardiogr*. 2003;16:1116-1127.
11. Chaudhary R, Garg J, Krishnamoorthy P, et al. On-X Valve. *Cardiol Rev*. 2017;25(2):77-83.
12. Baumgartner H, Khan S, DeRobertis M, et al. Discrepancies between Doppler and catheter gradients in aortic prosthetic valves in vitro. A manifestation of localized gradients and pressure recovery. *Circulation*. 1990;82:1467-1475.
13. Bech-Hanssen O, Gjertsson P, Houltz E, et al. Net pressure gradients in aortic prosthetic valves can be estimated by Doppler. *J Am Soc Echocardiogr*. 2003;16:858-866.
14. Maslow AD, Haering JM, Heindel S, et al. An evaluation of prosthetic aortic valves using transesophageal echocardiography: the double-envelope technique. *Anesth Analg*. 2000;91:509-516.
15. Sacchi S, Dhutia NM, Shun-Shin MJ, et al. Doppler assessment of aortic stenosis: a 25-operator study demonstrating why reading the peak velocity is superior to velocity time integral. *Eur Heart J Cardiovasc Imaging*. 2018;19(12):1380-1389.
16. Vanneman MW, Dalia AA. Perioperative and echocardiographic considerations for the Inspiris Resilia aortic valve—current and future. *J Cardiothorac Vasc Anesth*. 2020;34(10):2807-2812.
17. Guarracino F, Zussa C, Polesel E, et al. Influence of transesophageal echocardiography on intraoperative decision making for Toronto stentless prosthetic valve implantation. *J Heart Valve Dis*. 2001;10:31-34.
18. Kumar PA, McGrath T, Griffin BP, et al. Aortic valve homograft: a rare cause of left ventricular outflow tract obstruction. *Anesth Analg*. 2009;109(2):361-363.
19. Shapira Y, Vaturi M, Weisenberg DE, et al. Impact of intraoperative transesophageal echocardiography in patients undergoing valve replacement. *Ann Thorac Surg*. 2004;78:579-583.
20. Movsowitz HD, Shah SI, Ioli A, et al. Long-term follow-up of mitral paraprosthetic regurgitation by transesophageal echocardiography. *J Am Soc Echocardiogr*. 1994;7:488-492.
21. Morehead AJ, Firstenberg MS, Shiota T, et al. Intraoperative echocardiographic detection of regurgitant jets after valve replacement. *Ann Thorac Surg*. 2000;69:135-139.
22. O'Rourke DJ, Palac RT, Malenka DJ, et al. Outcome of mild periprosthetic regurgitation detected by intraoperative transesophageal echocardiography. *J Am Coll Cardiol*. 2001;38:163-166.
23. Koch CG, Khandwala F, Estafanous FG, et al. Impact of prosthesis-patient size on functional recovery after aortic valve replacement. *Circulation*. 2005;111:3221-3229.
24. Blais C, Dumesnil JG, Baillot R, et al. Impact of valve prosthesis-patient mismatch on short-term mortality after aortic valve replacement. *Circulation*. 2003;108:983-988.
25. Tasca G, Mhagna Z, Perotti S, et al. Impact of prosthesis-patient mismatch on cardiac events and midterm mortality after aortic valve replacement in patients with pure aortic stenosis. *Circulation*. 2006;113:570-576.
26. Mohty-Echahidi D, Malouf JF, Girard SE, et al. Impact of prosthesis-patient mismatch on long-term survival in patients with small St. Jude Medical mechanical prostheses in the aortic position. *Circulation*. 2006;113:420-426.
27. Tasca G, Brunelli F, Cirillo M, et al. Impact of valve prosthesis-patient mismatch on left ventricular mass regression following aortic valve replacement. *Ann Thorac Surg*. 2005;79:505-510.
28. Li M, Dumesnil JG, Mathieu P, et al. Impact of valve prosthesis-patient mismatch on pulmonary arterial pressure after mitral valve replacement. *J Am Coll Cardiol*. 2005;45:1034-1040.
29. Barbetseas J, Nagueh SF, Pitsavos C, et al. Differentiating thrombus from pannus formation in obstructed mechanical prosthetic valves: an evaluation of clinical, transthoracic, and transesophageal echocardiographic parameters. *J Am Coll Cardiol*. 1998;32:1410-1417.
30. Garcia MJ, Vandervoort P, Stewart WJ, et al. Mechanisms of hemolysis with mitral prosthetic regurgitation. Study using transesophageal echocardiography and fluid dynamic simulation. *J Am Coll Cardiol*. 1996;27:399-406.
31. Piper C, Korfer R, Horstkotte D. Prosthetic valve endocarditis. *Heart*. 2001;85:590-593.
32. Jett GK, Jett MD, Banhart GR, et al. Left ventricular outflow tract obstruction with mitral valve replacement in small ventricular cavities. *Ann Thorac Surg*. 1986;41:70-74.
33. Come PC, Riley MF, Weintraub RM, et al. Dynamic left ventricular outflow tract obstruction when the anterior leaflet is retained at prosthetic mitral valve replacement. *Ann Thorac Surg*. 1987;43:561-563.
34. Gallet B, Berrebi A, Grinda JM, et al. Severe intermittent intraprosthetic regurgitation after mitral valve replacement with subvalvular preservation. *J Am Soc Echocardiogr*. 2001;14:314-316.
35. El Sabbagh A, Al-Hiji M, Wang DD, et al. Predictors of left ventricular outflow tract obstruction after transcatheter mitral valve replacement in severe mitral annular calcification: an analysis of the transcatheter mitral valve replacement in mitral annular calcification global registry. *Circ Cardiovasc Interv*. 2021;14:e010854.

▶QUESTIONS

1. A 68-year-old female underwent aortic valve replacement for severe aortic stenosis with a bioprosthetic valve prosthesis. Continuous wave Doppler echocardiography measured a peak velocity of 213 cm/s and a mean velocity of 121 cm/s across the prosthetic valve. Pulsed wave Doppler echocardiography measured a peak velocity of 135 cm/s and a mean velocity of 74 cm/s in the LVOT. The DVI across the bioprosthetic aortic valve is:

A. 0.57
B. 0.63

C. 0.55
D. 0.34
E. 1.58

2. A 72-year-old male presents for follow-up 5 years after a bioprosthetic tricuspid valve replacement for tricuspid stenosis from carcinoid syndrome. In his follow-up visit, his echocardiogram demonstrated a tricuspid valve velocity-time integral (VTI_{PrTV}) of 25 cm. His LVOT diameter measured 2.2 cm and he had no aortic regurgitation. Assuming he has a normal stroke volume of 80 mL, what is the DVI of his prosthetic tricuspid valve?

A. 0.8
B. 0.2
C. 1.2
D. 4.8
E. 3.3

3. A 55-year-old patient presents for follow-up after aortic valve replacement for bicuspid aortic stenosis. Which of the following findings on echocardiography would be suggestive of significant prosthetic aortic valve stenosis?

A. DVI 0.36
B. Acceleration time 75 ms
C. Jet velocity 2.8 m/s
D. EOA 1.2 cm^2
E. Mean gradient 36 mm Hg

4. A 45-year- old female underwent aortic valve replacement for aortic stenosis. On intraoperative TEE examination, her aortic valve annulus was measured to be 20 mm in diameter and a 19-mm bioprosthetic valve with an EOA of 1.5 cm^2 was implanted in the aortic position. This patient would be expected to be at greatest risk of prosthetic-patient mismatch if:

A. The patient had an estimated body mass index (BMI) of 37 kg/m^2.
B. The patient had an estimated BSA of 1.7 m^2.
C. The preoperative aortic valve mean gradient was 55 mm Hg.
D. The preoperative left ventricular ejection fraction was 35%.
E. A 19-mm mechanical prosthetic valve had been implanted in the aortic position instead of the bioprosthetic valve.

5. A 62-year-old patient undergoes mitral valve replacement for rheumatic mitral stenosis. Postoperative echocardiographic evaluation of the mitral prosthesis demonstrates an indexed effective orifice area (EOA_i) of 1.1 cm^2/m^2. This finding is consistent with:

A. No prosthesis-patient mismatching.
B. Mild prosthesis-patient mismatching.
C. Moderate prosthesis-patient mismatching.
D. Severe prosthesis-patient mismatching.
E. Cannot be determined by the information provided

6. A 47-year-old male with unknown history presents to the operating room with a type-A dissection. Intraoperative transesophageal echocardiography demonstrates a prosthetic valve in the aortic position. Examination of the aortic prosthesis in the deep transgastric view demonstrates low-velocity convergent jets originating from within the sewing ring. Which of the following aortic valves does the patient most likely have?

A. On-X bileaflet prosthesis
B. St. Jude Medical bileaflet prosthesis
C. Medtronic Hall tilting disc prosthesis
D. Starr-Edwards caged-ball prosthesis
E. Carpentier-Edwards bioprosthesis

7. A 59-year- old female underwent bioprosthetic mitral valve replacement for myxomatous mitral valve disease. Following implantation, which of the following regional wall motion abnormalities is most likely to be seen?

A. Inferior wall hypokinesis
B. Inferolateral wall hypokinesis
C. Anterior wall hypokinesis
D. Anterolateral wall hypokinesis
E. Anteroseptal wall hypokinesis

8. A 67-year-old patient underwent aortic valve replacement 10 years ago for severe aortic regurgitation. Echocardiography demonstrates an aortic valve area of 1.0 cm^2 and DVI of 0.24. Given these findings, what is the most likely acceleration time in this patient?

A. 60 ms
B. 80 ms
C. 100 ms
D. 120 ms
E. Cannot be determined based on the information provided

9. In contemporary practice, the implantation of mechanical prosthetic valves has decreased over time due to all of the following EXCEPT:

A. Patient preference.
B. An aging population.
C. Increased number of patients undergoing TAVR compared to surgical aortic valve replacement (SAVR).
D. The ability to perform transcatheter valve-in-valve implantation.
E. Increased mortality as a consequence of the need for systemic anticoagulation.

10. A 63-year-old female underwent a bioprosthetic tricuspid valve replacement 8 years ago for tricuspid valve endocarditis. Continuous wave Doppler echocardiography reveals a peak velocity of 1.9 m/s, a mean gradient across the valve of 6 mm Hg, and a pressure half-time of 180 ms. These findings are consistent with:

A. A normally functioning prosthetic valve.
B. Possible stenosis of the prosthetic valve.
C. Significant stenosis of the prosthetic valve.
D. Significant stenosis of the prosthetic valve if the cardiac output is normal.
E. Cannot be determined from the information given.

▶ANSWERS

1. Correct Answer: B.

Rationale: DVI for the aortic valve is calculated using the formula DVI = VTI_{LVOT}/VTI_{AoV}, where VTI is velocity-time integral. Alternatively, DVI can also be calculated as DVI = $V_{maxLVOT}/V_{maxAoV}$, where V is velocity. Typically, either the VTI or peak velocities are used, with the LVOT measurement in the numerator and the aortic valve measurement in the denominator. Other answer choices use the incorrect velocities in the numerator or denominator.

2. Correct Answer: C.

Rationale: Unlike the DVI of the aortic valve, the DVI of a prosthetic tricuspid valve or mitral valve is calculated with the VTI of the prosthetic valve (VTI_{Pr}) in the numerator and VTI_{LVOT} in the denominator because these valves open during diastole. In the presence of significant aortic regurgitation, the right ventricular outflow tract VTI can be used instead of the VTI_{LVOT}. In this example, VTI_{LVOT} can be calculated by dividing the cardiac stroke volume by the LVOT area ($\pi r^2 = \pi*[1.1 \text{ cm}]^2$ or $80/[3.14*(1.1)^2]$ that equals to 21 cm. Therefore the DVI of the prosthetic tricuspid valve is equal to 25/21 or 1.2.). This can then be used to calculate the DVI of the tricuspid valve using the equation VTI_{PrTV}/VTI_{LVOT}. Answer (A) incorrectly uses the DVI equation for an aortic prosthetic valve, with the VTI of the valve in the denominator and VTI of the LVOT in the numerator. The remaining answers represent incorrect calculations.

3. Correct Answer: E.

Rationale: A mean gradient greater than 35 mm Hg indicates significant prosthetic aortic stenosis. An EOA of 1.2 cm^2 is considered normal for a prosthetic aortic valve. A DVI of 0.25 to 0.35, an acceleration time of 80 to 100 ms, or a mean transvalvular mean gradient of 20 to 35 mm Hg indicate possible stenosis for prosthetic aortic valves and warrant further investigation.

4. **Correct Answer: D.**
Rationale: Severe aortic prosthetic-patient mismatch is defined as a prosthetic valve with an EOA indexed to body surface area (EOA_i = EOA/BSA) of less than or equal to 0.65 cm^2/m^2. Prosthetic-patient mismatch is considered moderate if the EOA_i is between 0.65 and 0.85 cm^2/m^2 and not significant if the EOA_i is greater than or equal to 0.85 cm^2/m^2. The BMI is not typically used to index the EOA, but when BMI is taken into consideration, a BMI greater30 kg/m^2 and an EOA_i less than 55 cm^2/m^2 would be considered severe prosthetic-patient mismatch. A BSA of 1.7 m^2 would result in an EOA_i of 0.88 cm^2/m^2 for a prosthetic valve with an EOA of 1.5 cm^2 and would not result in severe prosthetic-patient mismatch. For any given valve size, the EOA of mechanical prosthetic valves is similar to the EOA of bioprosthetic valves and do not pose an added risk for prosthetic-patient mismatch. Patients with reduced left ventricular ejection fraction or significant aortic stenosis with a low transvalvular pressure gradient are at increased risk for prosthetic-patient mismatch.

5. **Correct Answer: C.**
Rationale: Prosthesis-patient mismatch is considered moderate after mitral valve replacement if the EOA_i is less than or equal to 1.2 cm^2/m^2 and severe if less than or equal to 0.9 cm^2/m^2.

6. **Correct Answer: B.**
Rationale: Low-velocity jets from within the sewing ring are likely representative of washing jets, or leakage backflow jets. Convergence of washing jets is suggestive of a St. Jude Medical bileaflet mechanical prosthesis. The On-X bileaflet prosthesis would demonstrate nonconverging washing jets. Medtronic Hall tilting disc prosthesis is characterized by a single central jet, whereas the Starr-Edwards caged-ball prosthesis would demonstrate closure backflow, but no washing jets. Bioprosthetic valves are not characterized by washing jets.

7. **Correct Answer: A.**
Rationale: Inferior wall hypokinesis secondary to air embolism is the most likely regional wall motion abnormality after mitral valve replacement and is usually transient and caused by intracardiac air entry into the right coronary ostium. Inferolateral wall hypokinesis or akinesis caused by injury, ligation, or obstruction of the left circumflex coronary artery that is adjacent to the mitral valve annulus is a recognized complication of mitral valve surgery, but is relatively rare. Left anterior descending coronary artery injury or air embolism into the left main coronary ostium causing anterior or anteroseptal hypokinesis is less likely.

8. **Correct Answer: D.**
Rationale: This patient demonstrates echocardiographic findings suggestive of prosthetic aortic valve stenosis. Stenotic aortic valves typically demonstrate an acceleration time greater than 100 ms. The acceleration time is measured using Doppler echocardiography as the time interval between the onset of flow and the peak flow velocity across the prosthetic valve. A rounded, symmetrical, late peaking Doppler transvalvular velocity profile is also a characteristic finding of a stenotic prosthetic aortic valve. A normal prosthetic aortic valve has a triangular, early peaking transvalvular Doppler velocity profile.

9. **Correct Answer: E.**
Rationale: The overall survival among patients undergoing valve replacement with mechanical or bioprosthetic valves is no different despite the need for systemic anticoagulation for mechanical prosthetic valves and the limited durability of bioprosthetic valves due to structural valvular degeneration. Percutaneous valve-in-valve replacement can be performed to treat structural valvular degeneration in patients with bioprosthetic valves but not in patients with mechanical valves. Bioprosthetic valves are also often chosen for older patients who are unlikely to outlive the durability of the bioprosthetic valve and in whom the risk of systemic anticoagulation is a consideration.

10. **Correct Answer: A.**
Rationale: The included Doppler parameters are consistent with a normally functioning bioprosthetic valve in the tricuspid position. Cutoff values suggestive of bioprosthetic tricuspid valve stenosis are: peak E velocity greater than or equal to 2.1 m/s, mean gradient greater than or equal to 9 mm Hg, and pressure half-time greater than or equal to 200 ms.

14 Right Ventricle, Right Atrium, Tricuspid and Pulmonic Valves

Etienne J. Couture, Lars Grønlykke, and André Y. Denault

Right ventricular (RV) dysfunction is a common concern in the perioperative period. Inadequate myocardial protection, increased pulmonary vascular resistance, air embolism to the right coronary artery (RCA), volume overload, and acute valvular dysfunction can compromise RV performance. This chapter surveys the echocardiographic approaches for evaluating the right side of the heart including the tricuspid valve (TV) and pulmonic valve (PV).

RIGHT VENTRICLE

Anatomy

From a functional perspective, the RV consists of inflow and outflow tracts separated by the trabeculated apical myocardium. The RVs nongeometric, asymmetric shape complicates echocardiographic evaluation. Morphologically, the RV is described in terms of three components: (1) the inlet, which comprises the TV, chordae tendineae, and papillary muscles; (2) the trabeculated apical myocardium; and (3) the infundibulum, or conus, which corresponds to the smooth myocardial outflow region (Figure 14.1). RV regional function is further categorized into anterior, lateral, and inferior walls; infundibulum; as well as basal, mid, and apical sections. The infundibulum and the anterior wall have dual blood supply from the RCA and left anterior descending artery. The lateral wall has a single blood supply from the acute marginal artery of the RCA. The RV inferior wall is perfused by the posterior descending artery and ventricular branches of the distal RCA. Three prominent muscular bands divide the RV: the parietal, the septal, and the moderator band (Figure 14.2).

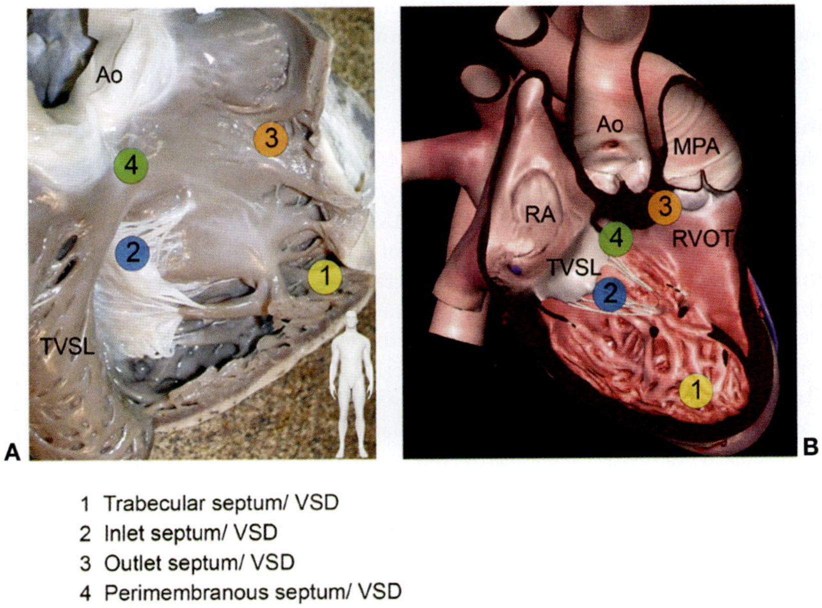

FIGURE 14.1 Interventricular septum. (A, B) Anatomic photo and schematic representation of the ventricular septum appears from the RV perspective. The anatomic classification divides the ventricular septum into membranous, trabecular, inlet, and outlet portions. Abbreviations: Ao, aorta; LA, left atrium; MPA, main pulmonary artery; RA, right atrium; RV, right ventricle, RVOT, right ventricular outflow tract; TVSL, tricuspid valve septal leaflet. (© 2025 André Y. Denault. From the Denault AY, Couture P, Julien M, Couture É, et al. *Transesophageal Echocardiography Multimedia Manual: A Perioperative Transdisciplinary Approach*. 3rd ed. Taylor & Francis/CRC Press; 2025. Reproduced by permission of Taylor and Francis Group, LLC, a division of Informa plc.)

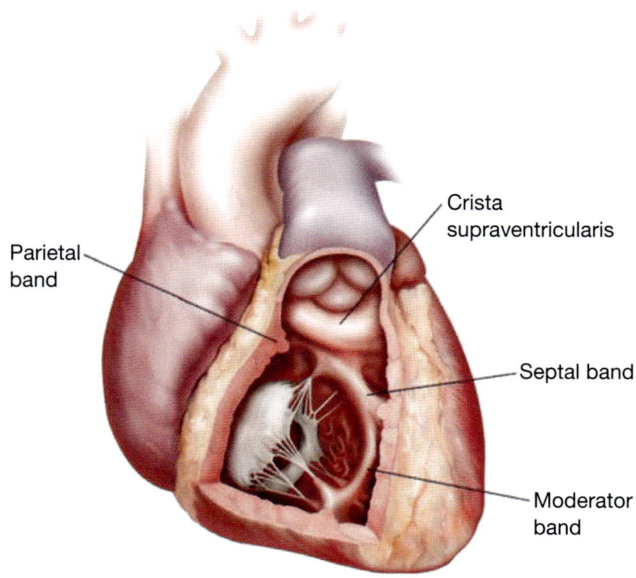

FIGURE 14.2 Schematic drawing of anatomic structures in the right ventricle.

The most apical portion with the distinctive moderator band is often well visualized with transesophageal echocardiography (TEE). The moderator band is a muscular trabeculation containing the right bundle branch, extending from the lower interventricular septum to the anterior papillary muscle of the RV lateral wall and serves as an anchoring structure for the tricuspid papillary muscles.

Transesophageal Echocardiographic Views

1. **Midesophageal (ME) RV-focused four-chamber (4C) view.** This long-axis (LAX) view of the RV allows assessment of all three segments, from apex to base, of the RV lateral wall. In this view, the RV appears triangular in comparison to the elliptic left ventricle (LV). RV length is approximately two-thirds that of the LV. This view is recommended for rapid assessment of RV systolic and diastolic function (Figure 14.3 #5).
2. **ME RV inflow-outflow view.** Often termed the "wrap around" view as the right atrium (RA), RV, PV, and pulmonary artery (PA) appear to wrap around the aortic valve (AoV) and left atrium, creating a 270° arc from left to right of the TEE monitor display. This view is favored for diagnosis of RV outflow tract obstruction (RVOTO) and assessment of lateral, anterior, and infundibular wall function (Figure 14.3 #6).
3. **Transgastric (TG) basal and midpapillary short-axis (SAX) views.** The anterior, lateral, and inferior RV walls and the interventricular septum are evaluated from these views (Figure 14.3 #10-12). These views are particularly useful for evaluating the interventricular septum to determine the presence of RV volume or pressure overload (see later).
4. **TG RV inflow view.** Analogous to the two-chamber view of the LV, this view is acquired by advancing the multiplane angle 90° from the TG SAX view of the RV or until the RA and RV are seen in LAX, with the RV inflow and TV centered in the image. Alternatively, one can develop the TG two-chamber view of the left atrium and LV and then turn the probe clockwise (rightward) until the two right-sided chambers are displayed. Both techniques should result in similar images of the RV inflow tract and the LAX of the RA and the RV with the anterior and inferior RV walls (Figure 14.3 #13). This view can be useful in evaluating basal RV function.
5. **Deep TG RV outflow and inflow-outflow views.** Due to the angulation of the ultrasound beam, these views are optimal for interrogating the tricuspid annulus with pulsed-wave Doppler (PWD) or tissue Doppler imaging (TDI) (Figure 14.3 #14-15). These views can be useful for diagnosing TV pathology and measuring pressure gradients across the TV and PV. They can also be used to evaluate RV diastolic function through interrogation of the basal inferior segment using TDI.

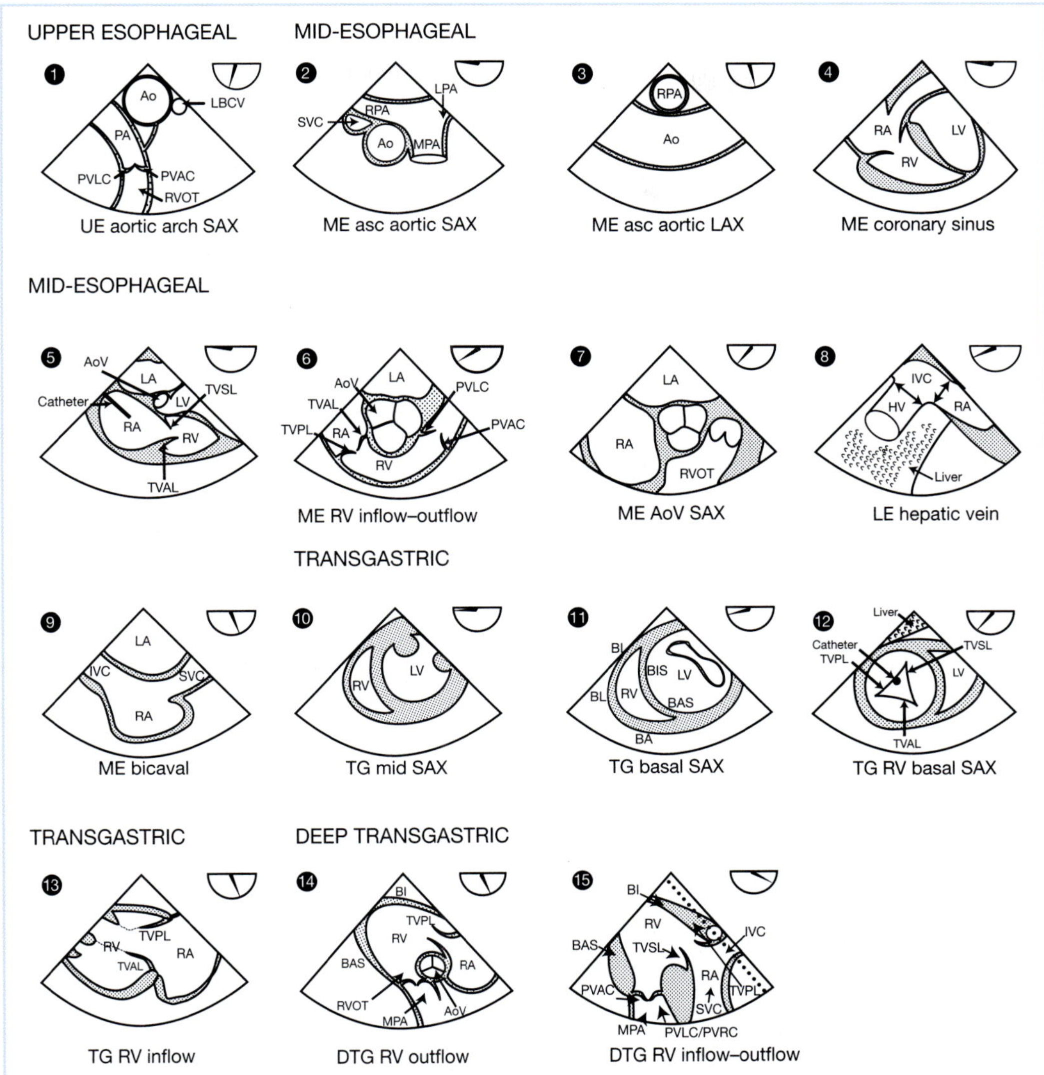

FIGURE 14.3 Transesophageal echocardiographic views to evaluate right-sided structures. Upper esophageal (UE), midesophageal (ME), transgastric (TG), and deep TG views are useful in the evaluation of right ventricular function. Ao, aorta; AoV, aortic valve; asc, ascending; BA, basal anterior; BAS, basal anteroseptal; BI, basal inferior; BIS, basal infero-septal; BL, basal lateral; CS, coronary sinus; DTG, deep transgastric; HV, hepatic vein; IVC, inferior vena cava; LA, left atrium; LAX, long axis; LE, lower esophageal; LPA, left pulmonary artery; LBCV, left brachiocephalic vein; LV, left ventricle; MPA, main pulmonary artery; PA, pulmonary artery; PV, pulmonic valve; PVAC, pulmonic valve anterior cusp; PVLC, pulmonic valve left cusp; PVRC, pulmonic valve right cusp; RA, right atrium; RPA, right pulmonary artery; RV, right ventricle or ventricular; RVOT, right ventricular outflow tract; SAX, short axis; SVC, superior vena cava; TV, tricuspid valve; TVAL, tricuspid valve anterior leaflet; TVPL, tricuspid valve posterior leaflet; TVSL, tricuspid valve septal leaflet. (Reproduced and adapted by permission of Taylor and Francis Group, LLC, a division of Informa plc from Denault AY, Couture P, Vegas A, Buithieu J, Tardif JC. *Transesophageal Echocardiography Multimedia Manual, Second Edition: A Perioperative Transdisciplinary Approach*. Informa Healthcare; 2011.)

Assessment of Right Ventricular Structure

Right Ventricular Wall Thickness

The normal thickness of the RV lateral wall is less than 5 mm at end diastole (1-3). RV hypertrophy is present when the RV lateral wall thickness exceeds 5 mm, indicating RV systolic pressure overload due to elevated PA pressure, chronic thromboembolic pulmonary hypertension, RVOTO or pulmonic stenosis (PS) (4). The inferior or lateral walls of the RV are the preferred locations for measurement since, in contrast to the anterior wall, they are not invested with as much epicardial fat that must be excluded from RV wall thickness measurement (5). The inferior wall of the RV is best assessed in TG views performed at 0°, whereas the RV lateral wall is best measured in the ME 4C view. Because the RV wall is thinner and more trabeculated than the LV wall, precise measurements are more difficult to obtain. In patients with chronic cor pulmonale, the RV wall thickness may exceed 10 mm while intracavitary trabecular patterns become more prominent, particularly at the apex. Certain conditions are associated with RV wall thinning, such as RV myocardium infarction, Uhl syndrome, or arrhythmogenic RV cardiomyopathy. In arrhythmogenic RV cardiomyopathy, aneurysms typically occur in the anterior infundibulum, basal inferior wall, and apex. There are no accepted echocardiographic criteria to define an abnormally thin RV wall (3,6).

Right Ventricular Dimension

RV dimension is best estimated at end diastole from an ME RV-focused 4C view (Figure 14.4). Care should be taken to obtain an RV-focused image demonstrating its maximal diameter without foreshortening. This can be accomplished by making sure that the crux and apex of the heart are in view. Diameter greater than 41 mm at the base and greater than 35 mm at the mid-level indicates RV dilatation. Similarly, longitudinal dimension, from the apex to tricuspid annulus, greater than 83 mm indicates RV enlargement (2,3). RV dilation can occur with RV volume or pressure overload. Normally, the RV end-diastolic cross-sectional area is approximately 60% of the area of the LV. As the RV dilates, its shape changes from triangular to round. In addition, the cardiac apex, which should be made up solely of the LV, may be equally shared between the ventricles or even dominated by the RV, indicating significant RV dilation. With mild RV dilation, the RV area exceeds 70% of the LV area on two-dimensional (2D) imaging. With moderate RV dilation, the RV area may equal that of the LV, and with severe RV enlargement, the RV area exceeds that of the LV (7).

Interventricular Septum and Eccentricity Index

The analysis of interventricular septum may provide useful insights into RV pathology. Examination of interventricular septal motion can help distinguish RV volume overload from RV pressure overload. Normally, the interventricular septum functions as part of the LV and maintains a concave shape throughout the cardiac cycle. As the RV dilates or becomes hypertrophic, the septum flattens and paradoxical septal motion develops. Normally, during systole and subsequently during diastole, the inward and outward motion of all the walls of the LV will be seen. If there is an opposite motion of the interventricular wall during diastole, this is referred to as paradoxical motion. It can be seen in an ME 4C view or the TG midpapillary SAX view. The eccentricity index, a measure of septal curvature, represents the ratio of the LV minor axis diameter (parallel to the septum) to its perpendicular axis (Figure 14.5; Videos 14.1 and 14.2). In normal subjects, the index is approximately one at both end diastole and end systole. Acquired pressure overload situations such as pulmonary hypertension or PS displace the interventricular septum toward the LV at end diastole leading to a D-shaped LV with an eccentricity index of less than 1. The septal displacement reflects the pressure gradient between the two ventricles. In early stages of RV volume overload, diastolic pressure in RV exceeds that in the LV thus pushing the septum toward LV cavity in diastole only. With severe RV pressure overload, the LV exhibits a D-shape in both diastole and systole (1,8).

Assessment of Right Ventricular Systolic Function

Quantitative assessment of RV systolic function can be done with volumetric and non-volumetric assessment. However, its volumetric function evaluation is limited by its unique geometry, while variations in shape occur readily with changes in RV volume. RV ejection is a complex process involving three components: inward motion of the RV lateral wall, longitudinal shortening of the RV with systolic descent of the tricuspid annulus, along with contributions from the right ventricular outflow tract (RVOT) (1,4). Signs of RV dysfunction include severe hypokinesis or akinesis of the RV lateral wall, RV enlargement, change in shape of the RV from crescent to round, and flattening or bulging of the interventricular septum toward the left side.

Volumetric Function Assessment

Volumetric evaluation is commonly estimated by the RV fractional area change (RVFAC) defined as (end-diastolic area − end-systolic area)/end-diastolic area × 100 assessed from the ME 4C view. Diagnostic cutoff for RV dysfunction is made by RVFAC of less than 35%, and its severity can be described as mild, moderate,

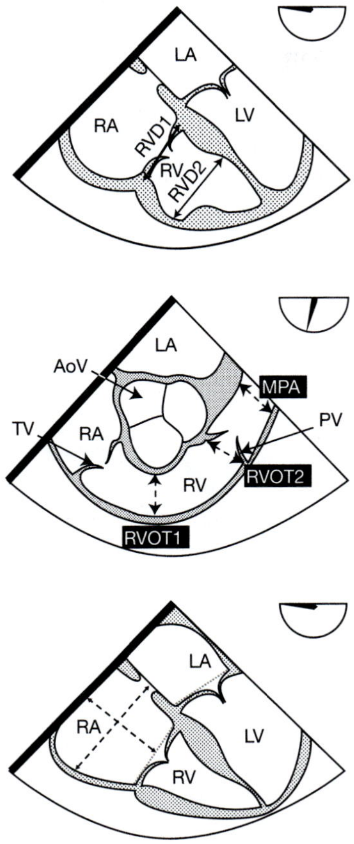

A

Normal value for 2D RV chamber size

Parameter	Mean ± SD	Normal range
RVD1 (mm)	33 ± 4	25–41
RVD2 (mm)	27 ± 4	19–35
RV wall thickness (mm)	3 ± 1	1–5

B

Normal value for 2D RV chamber size

Parameter	Mean ± SD	Normal range
RVOT1 (mm)	28 ± 3.5	21–35
RVOT2 (mm)	22 ± 2.5	17–27
MPA (mm)	21 ± 3	11–31

C

Normal value for RA and LA size

RA size	Women	Men
RA minor axis dimension (cm/m^2)	1.9 ± 0.3	1.9 ± 0.3
RA major axis dimension (cm/m^2)	2.5 ± 0.3	2.4 ± 0.3
2D echocardiographic RA volume (mL/m^2)	21 ± 6	25 ± 7

FIGURE 14.4 Basic transesophageal echocardiography (TEE) measurements. A: TEE measurements, at end diastole, of various right ventricular diameters (RVD) obtained from a midesophageal four-chamber view optimized to the maximum right ventricular (RV) size by varying angles 0° to 20°. The table shows normal and abnormal values for RVD1, RVD2, RVD3, and RV wall thickness. B: TEE measurements, taken at end diastole, of the right ventricular outflow tract (RVOT) at two levels (RVOT1, RVOT2) and the main pulmonary artery (MPA) from the midesophageal right ventricular inflow/outflow view. C: TEE measurements, at ventricular end systole, of the right atrium (RA) from the midesophageal four-chamber view optimally positioned to visualize both chambers. The minor axis of the RA should be measured in the midesophageal four-chamber view as the distance between the lateral RA wall and interatrial septum, at the midatrial level, which is defined by half of the RA long or major axis. Table of normal and abnormal values for ventricular and atrial dimensions (mm ± standard deviation [SD]) and volumes (mL/m^2) as absolute values and indexed to body surface area (BSA). AoV, aortic valve; LA, left atrium; PV, pulmonic valve; TV, tricuspid valve. (Adapted from Lang RM, Badano LP, Mor-Avi V, et al. Recommendations for cardiac chamber quantification by echocardiography in adults: an update from the American Society of Echocardiography and the European Association of Cardiovascular Imaging. *J Am Soc Echocardiogr.* 2015;28[1]:1-39 e14; reproduced by permission of Taylor and Francis Group, LLC, a division of Informa plc; Denault AY, Couture P, Vegas A, Buithieu J, Tardif JC. *Transesophageal Echocardiography Multimedia Manual, Second Edition: A Perioperative Transdisciplinary Approach*. Informa Healthcare; 2011.)

or severe for values of 25 to 35, 18 to 25, and 18% or less, respectively (Figure 14.6) (1). A limitation of this approach is that RVFAC does not examine the contribution of the RVOT that corresponds to approximately 20% of the ejected RV volume.

NON-VOLUMETRIC FUNCTION ASSESSMENT

Right Ventricular Myocardial Performance Index

Global assessment of RV function can be done by right ventricular myocardial performance index (RVMPI or Tei index) using PWD or TDI at the lateral tricuspid annulus. It represents an estimate of both RV systolic

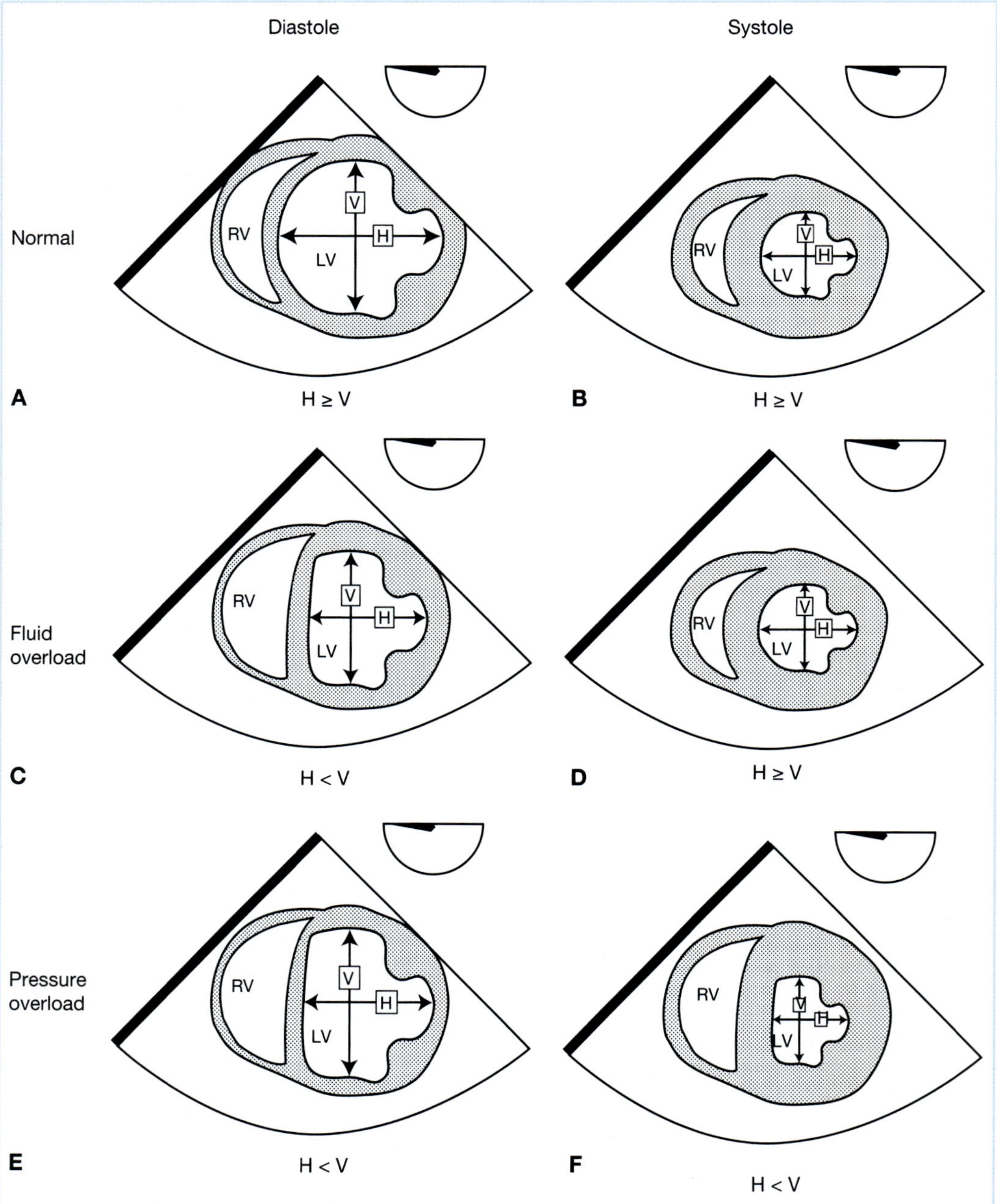

FIGURE 14.5 Eccentricity index. A,B: Using the transgastric mid-short-axis view, the eccentricity index (EI) is calculated as the ratio of the vertical (V) to horizontal (H) diameter of the left ventricle (LV). C,D: In volume overload, the H dimension is smaller than V dimension only during systole but E,F in pressure overload, it remains smaller in both systole and diastole (Videos 14.1 and 14.2). RV, right ventricle. (Reproduced by permission of Taylor and Francis Group, LLC, a division of Informa plc from Denault AY, Couture P, Vegas A, Buithieu J, Tardif JC. *Transesophageal Echocardiography Multimedia Manual, Second Edition: A Perioperative Transdisciplinary Approach*. Informa Healthcare; 2011.)

and diastolic function. It is based on the relationship between ejection and non-ejection work of the heart. The RVMPI is defined as the ratio of isovolumetric time divided by ejection time (ET), or ([isovolumetric relaxation time (IVRT) + isovolumetric contraction time (IVCT)]/[ET]). Presence of RV dysfunction is characterized by an RVMPI of greater than 0.43 in PWD and of greater than 0.54 in TDI (2). The Tei index

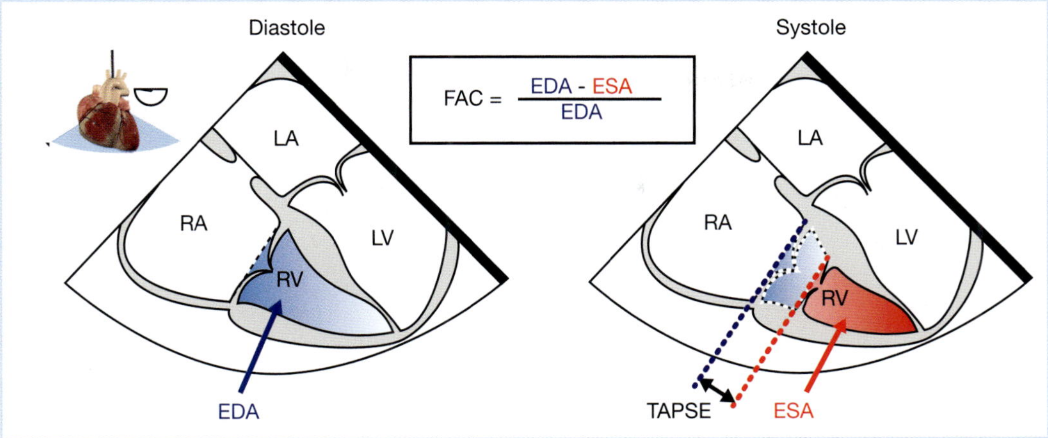

FIGURE 14.6 RV systolic function assessment. The right ventricular (RV) fractional area change (FAC) corresponds to the difference of the RV end-diastolic area (EDA) minus the RV end-systolic area (ESA) divided by the RV EDA. Tricuspid annular plane systolic excursion (TAPSE) represents the systolic excursion of the lateral tricuspid annulus. TAPSE can be measured as the change in the distance (arrow) in diastole between the apex and the lateral tricuspid annulus. Normal TAPSE should be greater than 17 mm (3). LA, left atrium; LV, left ventricle; RA, right atrium. (Reproduced by permission of Taylor and Francis Group, LLC, a division of Informa plc from Denault AY, Couture P, Vegas A, Buithieu J, Tardif JC. *Transesophageal Echocardiography Multimedia Manual, Second Edition: A Perioperative Transdisciplinary Approach*. Informa Healthcare; 2011.)

has been shown to be independent of the loading condition, heart rate, and atrioventricular valvular regurgitation (9). However, a major pitfall should be highlighted: severe RV diastolic dysfunction can significantly reduce IVRT, thus preventing the increase of Tei index in the presence of severe systolic dysfunction. One should keep in mind that a normal Tei index does not exclude either RV systolic or diastolic dysfunction. In valvular surgery, RVMPI is an independent predictor of difficult weaning from cardiopulmonary bypass (CPB), mortality, circulatory failure, duration of hospitalization, and intensive care unit stay (10) (Figure 14.7).

Tricuspid Annular Plane Systolic Excursion

LAX systolic excursion of the lateral aspect of the tricuspid annulus represents an easily recognizable longitudinal movement on echocardiography and may be used as an indicator of RV systolic function. Typically measured in M-mode and corrected for angulation of interrogation, TAPSE (tricuspid annular plane systolic excursion) is defined as the total excursion of the tricuspid annulus from end diastole to end systole. Normal TAPSE is 20 to 25 mm with less than 17 mm suggestive of RV dysfunction and less than 15 mm being considered significantly depressed (3). The angle of excursion is toward the cardiac apex and is slightly greater than normal mitral annular plane excursion (1). The tricuspid annulus tilts toward the apex, whereas the mitral annulus moves more symmetrically toward the apex, somewhat like a piston, emphasizing the importance of measuring motion at the lateral tricuspid annulus (4). Depressed TAPSE measurements suggest depressed RV systolic function from a variety of causes. TAPSE has been correlated to right ventricular ejection fraction (RVEF). However, it is important to note that TAPSE has several limitations in the intraoperative period. First, the annular motion vector is oblique to the ME 4C view which results in angle-related errors. TAPSE is load dependent and not reliable after pericardectomy. Also, it reflects only the longitudinal displacement of a single segment of the complex RV three-dimensional (3D) structure (Figure 14.8; Video 14.3). Lastly, it does not assess the contribution to ejection from the inward motion of the free wall and the RVOT.

Tissue Doppler Peak Velocity at the Tricuspid Annulus

Tissue Doppler peak velocity at the tricuspid annulus (S′) (Figure 14.9; Video 14.4) of less than 9.5 cm/s is a sign of RV dysfunction as it represents the basal RV lateral wall function. RV acceleration during isovolumic acceleration is also measured by TDI at the lateral tricuspid annulus. Right ventricular acceleration during isovolumic contraction (RVIVA) is defined as the peak isovolumic myocardial velocity divided by time-to-peak velocity. This parameter is rate dependent and appears to be less load dependent than RVMPI. A value less than 2.2 m/s^2 is considered to be indicative of RV dysfunction.

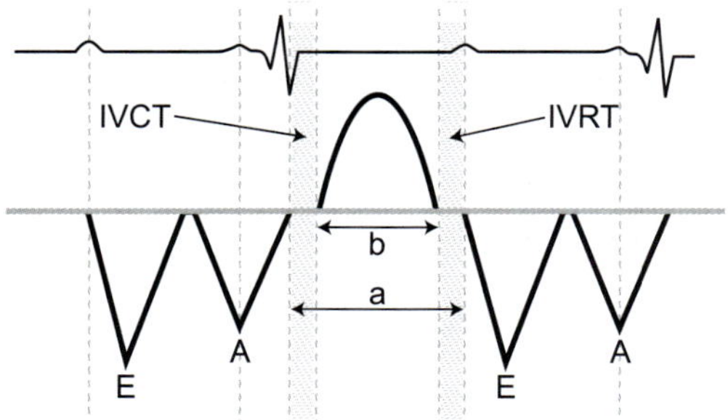

$$a = IVRT + IVCT + ET$$

$$b = ET$$

$$MPI = \frac{a - b}{b} = \frac{IVRT + IVCT}{ET}$$

Normal value: LV = 0.39 ± 0.05
RV = 0.28 ± 0.04

FIGURE 14.7 Myocardial performance index. To calculate the myocardial performance index (MPI) or Tei index of the left ventricle (LV), the transmitral flow is used for measurement of the duration "*a*" from the end of atrial contraction (A wave) to the beginning of LV filling (E wave). The ejection time (ET) or "*b*" is measured from a deep transgastric long-axis view using a Doppler assessment of the left ventricular outflow tract. The MPI of the right ventricle (RV) is similarly obtained using the transtricuspid flow and the midesophageal ascending aorta short-axis view for the RV outflow tract. A, peak late diastolic TMF velocity; E, peak early diastolic TMF velocity; IVCT, isovolumic contraction time; IVRT, isovolumic relaxation time. (Reproduced by permission of Taylor and Francis Group, LLC, a division of Informa plc from Denault AY, Couture P, Vegas A, Buithieu J, Tardif JC. *Transesophageal Echocardiography Multimedia Manual, Second Edition: A Perioperative Transdisciplinary Approach*. Informa Healthcare; 2011.)

Assessment of Right Ventricular Diastolic Function

Presence of tricuspid regurgitation (TR) or irregular RR intervals renders the analysis of diastolic dysfunction difficult immediately after CPB weaning. However, in the absence of these conditions, gradation of diastolic RV function can be achieved through transtricuspid flow (TTF) and hepatic venous flow (Figure 14.10).

Transtricuspid Flow

Early and late filling wave velocities (E and A wave, respectively) and E deceleration time recorded by PWD in the TTF and the lateral tricuspid annulus velocity during early filling (E′) recorded by TDI allows diastolic categorization of RV function. A tricuspid E/A ratio of less than 0.8 suggests impaired relaxation, a tricuspid E/A ratio of 0.8 to 2.1 with an E/E′ ratio of greater than 6 or diastolic flow predominance in the hepatic veins suggests pseudonormal filling, and a tricuspid E/A ratio of greater than 2.1 with a deceleration time of less than 120 milliseconds suggests restrictive filling (11) (Figure 14.10).

Right Ventricular Strain and Strain Rate

Deformation indices such as strain and strain rate have been shown to be useful parameters for estimating RV global and regional systolic function (2). Longitudinal strain is a percentage of systolic shortening of the RV lateral wall that should be measured in the ME RV-focused 4C view. This measurement is still dependent on RV loading conditions and RV size and shape. Peak global longitudinal strain of the RV lateral wall (also termed RV free wall strain in the literature) has been shown to be more sensitive and specific for detection of RV systolic dysfunction than other evaluation modalities (12). It has also been reported to have prognostic value in various disease states such as heart failure, acute myocardial infarction, pulmonary hypertension, amyloidosis, and to predict RV failure after LV assist device implantation. Current reference values have been published (2). Global longitudinal RV lateral wall strain of 20% or less in absolute value is considered abnormal.

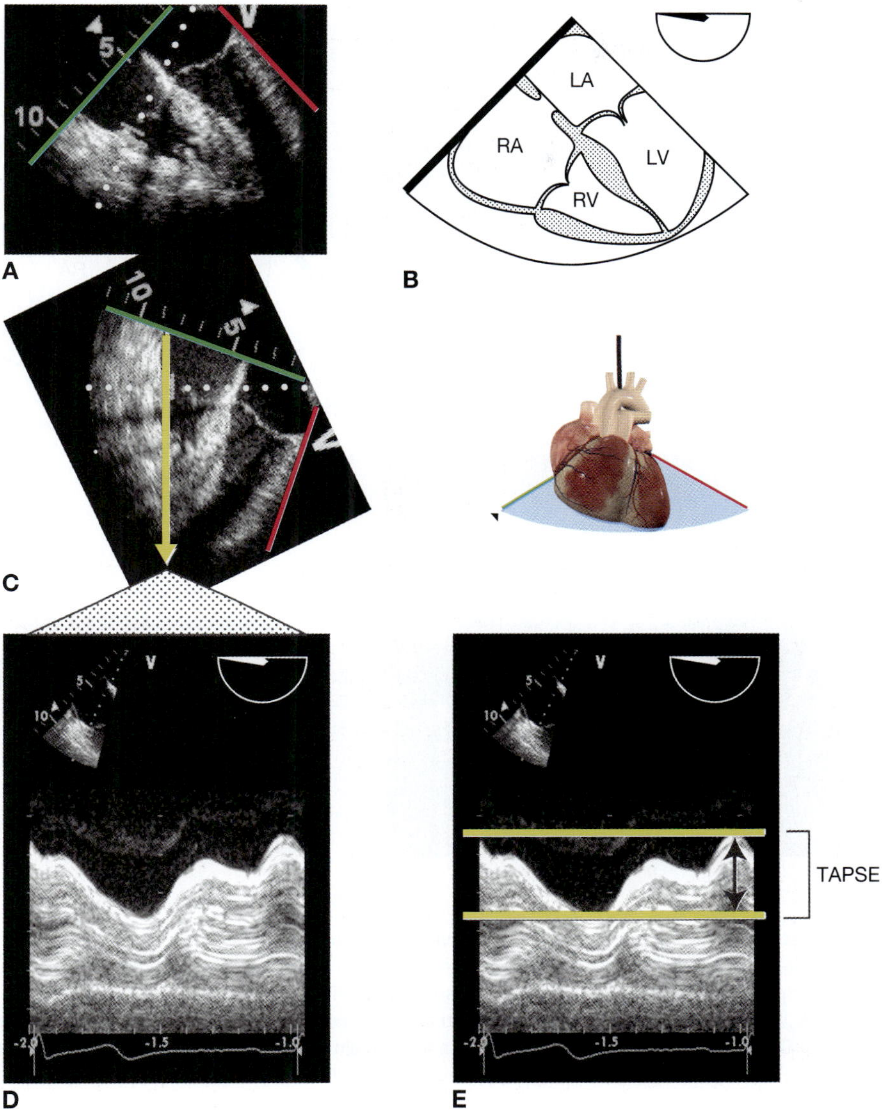

Normal values for TAPSE

Parameter	Mean ± SD	Abnormality threshold
TAPSE (mm)	24 ± 3.5	< 17

F

FIGURE 14.8 TAPSE. A-E: Steps in the measurement of the tricuspid annular plane systolic excursion (TAPSE) using anatomic M-mode are shown. A,B: First, a midesophageal four-chamber view is acquired and the M-mode cursor is positioned along the plane of the TAPSE motion to obtain the M-mode image of this displacement (D). The lower point corresponds to the maximal systolic excursion and the upper point is the atrial contraction (E). The TAPSE is equal to the total systolic displacement of the tricuspid annulus which is normally 20 to 25 mm. F: Normal values from Lang RM, Badano LP, Mor-Avi V, et al. Recommendations for cardiac chamber quantification by echocardiography in adults: an update from the American Society of Echocardiography and the European Association of Cardiovascular Imaging. *J Am Soc Echocardiogr*. 2015;28(1):1-39 e14 (Video 14.3). LA, left atrium; LV, left ventricle; RA, right atrium; RV, right ventricle; SD, standard deviation. (From Lang RM, Badano LP, Mor-Avi V, et al. Recommendations for cardiac chamber quantification by echocardiography in adults: an update from the American Society of Echocardiography and the European Association of Cardiovascular Imaging. *J Am Soc Echocardiogr*. 2015;28[1]:1-39.e14; Reproduced by permission of Taylor and Francis Group, LLC, a division of Informa plc. From Denault AY, Couture P, Vegas A, Buithieu J, Tardif JC. Transesophageal Echocardiography Multimedia Manual: A Perioperative Transdisciplinary Approach. 2nd ed. Informa Healthcare; 2011.)

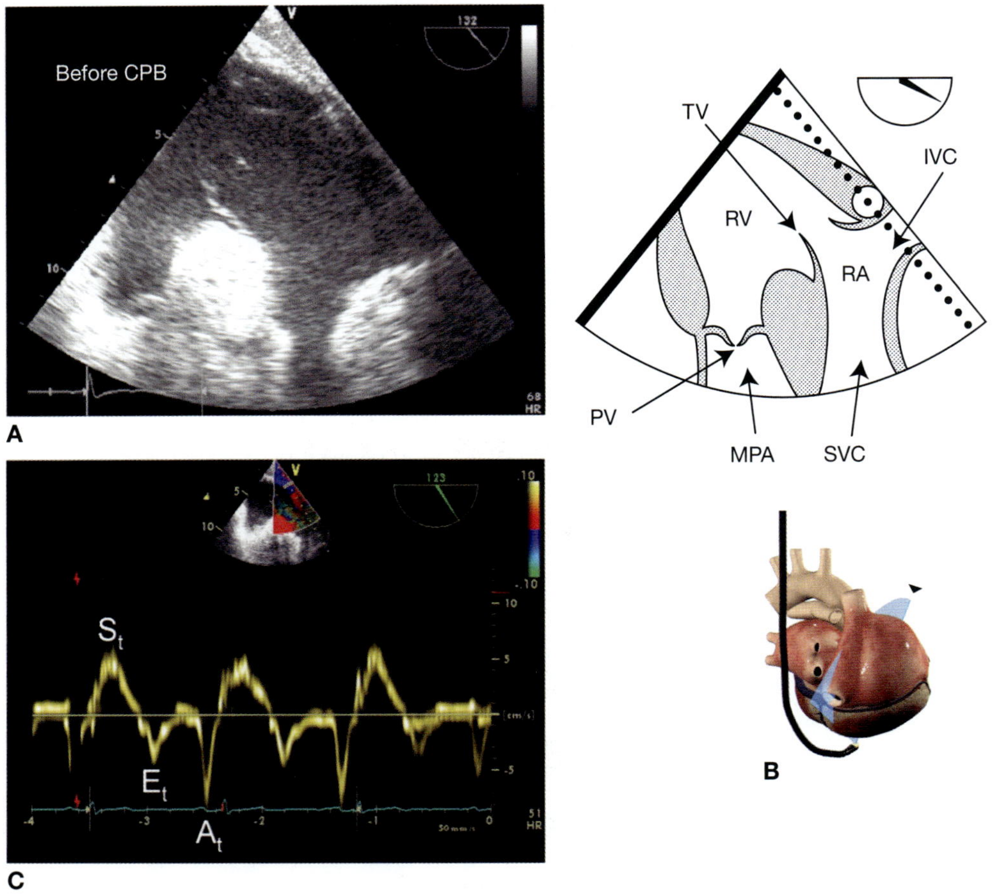

FIGURE 14.9 Tissue Doppler imaging (TDI) for right ventricular function. A,B: Deep transgastric right ventricular inflow/outflow long-axis view allows the evaluation of both the pulsed-wave Doppler interrogation of the tricuspid valve and TDI of the tricuspid annulus along the dotted line. C: Tissue Doppler signal obtained at the base of the tricuspid annulus. (Video 14.4). A_t, tricuspid late diastolic filling (during atrial contraction) tissue Doppler velocity; E_t, tricuspid early diastolic filling tissue Doppler velocity; IVC, inferior vena cava; MPA, main pulmonary artery; PV, pulmonic valve; RA, right atrium; RV, right ventricle; S_t, tricuspid systolic tissue Doppler velocity; SVC, superior vena cava; TV, tricuspid valve. (Adapted with permission from Haddad F, Couture P, Tousignant C, Denault AY. The right ventricle in cardiac surgery, a perioperative perspective: II. Pathophysiology, clinical importance, and management. *Anesth Analg*. 2009;108(2):422-433.)

Three-Dimensional Right Ventricular Ejection Fraction

3D echocardiographic RVEF is a global measure of RV systolic function and performance. This newer modality has been extensively validated against cardiovascular magnetic resonance (2). It has been described as being of particular value in patients after cardiac surgery when conventional indices of RV function are generally reduced and no longer a real representation of the overall RV performance. The limitations of the 3D RVEF are load dependency, interventricular changes affecting septal motion (RV pacing), poor acoustic windows, and irregular rhythms. Keeping this in mind, the latest American Society of Echocardiography guidelines on chamber quantification published in 2015 recommend 3D RVEF as a method to quantify RV systolic function. An RVEF of less than 45% reflects abnormal RV systolic function. Limitation of 3D RVEF is that it is not available in real time in most current TEE platforms.

Assessment of Regional Right Ventricular Function

RV perfusion is supplied primarily by the RCA. Its first branch, the conus artery, is responsible for the blood supply to a small portion of the anterior and infundibular wall as well as to the conus of the main

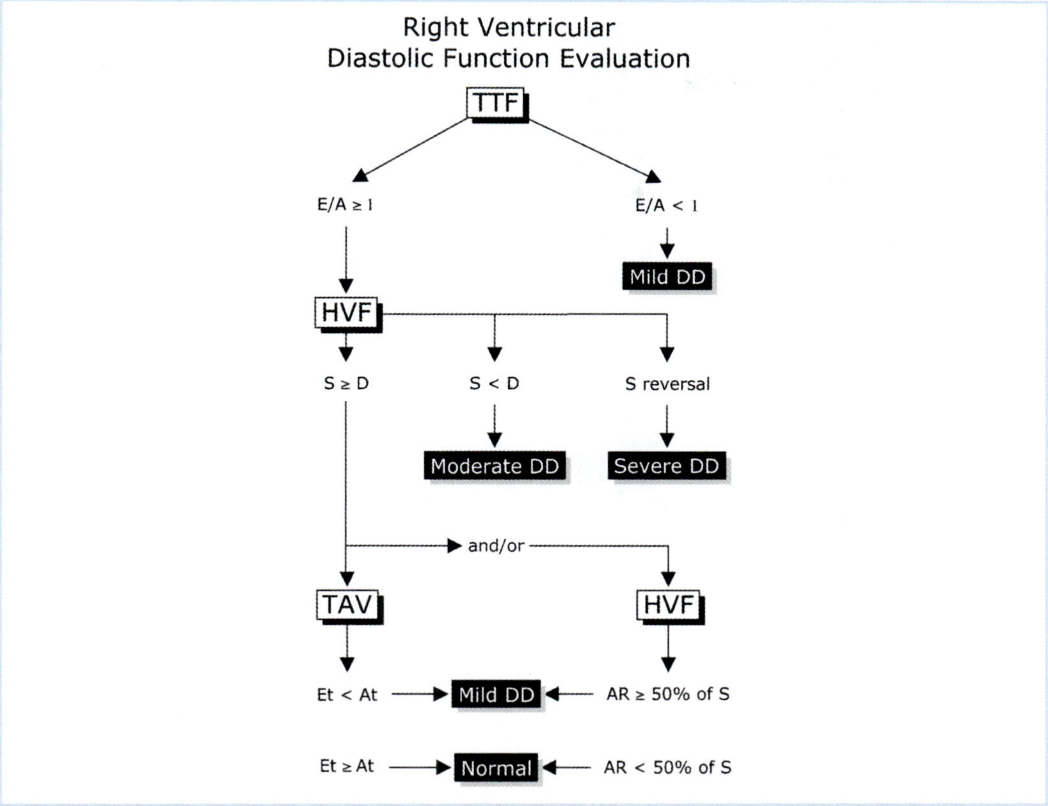

FIGURE 14.10 Right ventricular diastolic dysfunction (DD) algorithm. Diastolic function is classified by pulsed-wave Doppler of the transtricuspid flow (TTF), hepatic venous flow (HVF), and tissue Doppler imaging of the tricuspid annular velocity (TAV). Patients with a pacemaker, atrial fibrillation, non-sinus rhythm, moderate-to-severe tricuspid regurgitation, and tricuspid annuloplasty are excluded from analysis. A, atrial component TTF; AR, atrial reversal HVF; A_t, atrial TAV; D, diastolic HVF; E, early filling TTF; E_t, early TAV; S, systolic HVF. (Reproduced by permission of Taylor and Francis Group, LLC, a division of Informa plc from Denault AY, Couture P, Vegas A, Buithieu J, Tardif JC. *Transesophageal Echocardiography Multimedia Manual, Second Edition: A Perioperative Transdisciplinary Approach*. Informa Healthcare; 2011.)

PA. RCA is dominant in 85% of the population, which, in addition to supplying blood flow to the RV lateral wall, supplies the inferior wall of the LV and the posterior third of the septum. In the minority of patients, the RCA is nondominant where the infundibular, anterior, and inferior walls are perfused from both right and left contributions. However, the lateral wall is perfused only by the RCA (13). Since the thin-walled RV is a volume-dependent chamber, the RVEF is extremely sensitive to changes in afterload. In contrast, the thick-walled LV is a pressure-dependent chamber, and its LV ejection fraction is largely preserved over large changes in afterload demand. Furthermore, the irregularity and asymmetry of the RV make changes in inotropic function difficult to detect or quantify. More dramatic changes in function such as akinesia or dyskinesia are more readily identified and are sensitive indicators of RV infarction. Less common findings associated with RV infarction include RV dilation, papillary muscle dysfunction, TR, and paradoxical motion of the interventricular septum (4,14). It is also important to mention that the RV is perfused in both systole and diastole (15).

Hemodynamic and Extracardiac Manifestation of Right Ventricular Dysfunction

The use of RV and RA pressure waveform monitoring (Figure 14.11) is another method for detecting diastolic RV dysfunction (16). Interestingly, these waveforms correlate with the extracardiac consequences of RV dysfunction on intraabdominal organs. These effects can be identified using TG abdominal ultrasound to evaluate hepatic, portal, or splenic and renal venous flow (17-19).

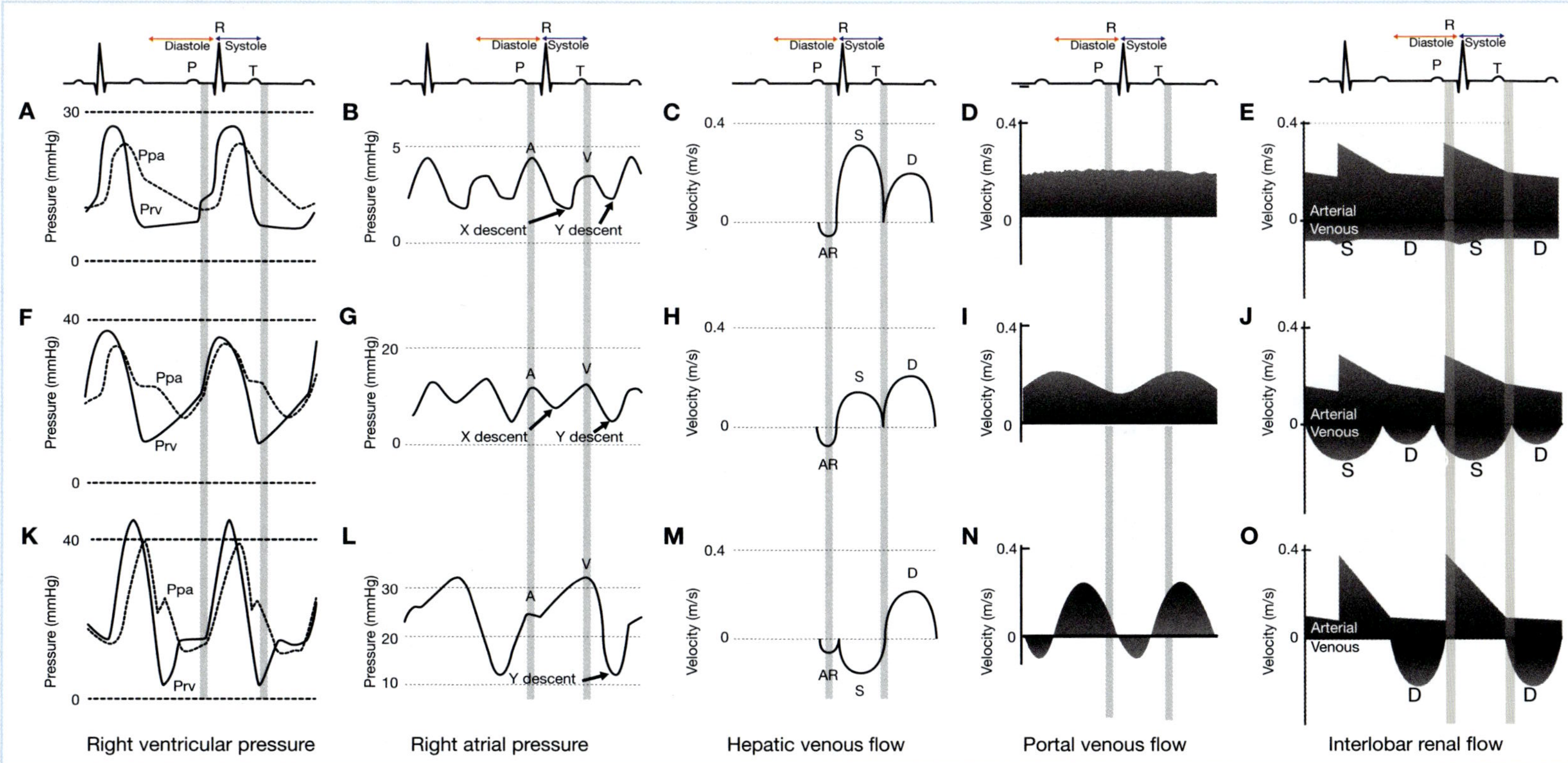

FIGURE 14.11 Right ventricular pressure (Prv), right atrial pressure, hepatic venous flow (HVF), portal venous flow, and interlobar arterial and venous renal flow in normal patients (A-E) and typical patterns commonly observed in patients with mild (F-J) and severe (K-O) right ventricular dysfunction. AR, atrial reversal HVF velocity; D, diastolic HVF Doppler velocity; Ppa, pulmonary artery pressure; S, systolic HVF velocity. (Adapted from Amsallem M, Kuznetsova T, Hanneman K, Denault A, Haddad F. Right heart imaging in patients with heart failure: a tale of two ventricles. Curr Opin Cardiol. 2016;31(5):469-482; Denault AY, Beaubien-Souligny W, Elmi-Sarabi M, et al. Clinical significance of portal hypertension diagnosed with bedside ultrasound after cardiac surgery. Anesth Analg. 2017;124(4):1109-1115.)

Hepatic Venous Flow Patterns

Examination of flow velocity patterns with PWD during different phases of the cardiac cycle can contribute with useful information about RV function. Normal hepatic venous flow is directed away from the liver to the RA and fluctuates during the cardiac cycle (Figure 14.11C).

Normal hepatic venous flow patterns have four phasic components: AR corresponding to atrial reversal, S corresponding to ventricular contraction and movement of the tricuspid annulus toward the RV apex, and D corresponding to early ventricular filling. Initial forward flow during systole is associated with atrial relaxation and apical movement of the TV during RV systole and corresponds to the x-descent in atrial pressure measurements. Subsequent diastolic flow, associated with early ventricular filling, corresponds to the y-descent. Two small retrograde hemodynamic waves are often detectable; one corresponding to atrial contraction at end diastole (A), and a small V-wave at end systole corresponding to the end-systolic phase prior to the y-descent.

Systolic flow is normally of higher velocity than diastolic flow. This correlates with the x-descent being naturally larger than the y-descent. This is due to the downward motion of the tricuspid annulus during ventricular systole resulting in a rapid filling of the RA. In patients with RV dysfunction, decreased TAPSE and/or TR during ventricular systole will lead to a reduction of the S wave velocity and to a systolic-to-diastolic ratio of less than 1 (S/D <1) as shown in Figure 14.11H. In severe RV dysfunction or severe TR, the S wave appears completely reversed with backward flow in the hepatic veins during systole causing a negative systolic-to-diastolic ratio (S/D <0) as shown in Figure 14.11M (20).

Portal and Splenic Venous Flow Patterns

Flow in the portal and splenic veins can be assessed using TEE but more easily with transthoracic echocardiography (TTE) (17,19). Due to the fact that the splenic vein is a direct tributary of the portal vein, its assessment provides the same information. Imaging of the portal vein is accomplished by means of a TG SAX cut of the liver by turning the probe to the right side of the patient. A multiplane angle rotation of 90° to 120° leads to a cranio-caudal plane of the liver. The portal vein is usually within a few centimeters of the transducer and the inferior vena cava (IVC) is usually not visible in the same 2D view (Figure 14.12; ▶ Video 14.5).

Alternatively, assessment of splenic vein flow can also be done with TG scanning. This view can be obtained by turning the probe to the left side of the patient and by performing a multiplane angle rotation of 90°. This will bring the splenic hilum into view. In this view, venous blood flow travels toward the probe resulting in positive velocities during Doppler examination (Figure 14.13A-C). An alternative view can be obtained by positioning the probe toward the posterior aspect of the body, while maintaining the multiplane angle rotation at 0°. In this position, the splenic vein is located anterior to the descending aorta and venous flow will be traveling away from the probe leading to negative Doppler velocities (Figure 14.13D-F; ▶ Videos 14.6 and 14.7). Based on clinical experience, the success rate for splenic vein flow assessment using TEE is believed to be as good or better than portal flow assessment.

Venous flow through the portal or splenic vein has a low velocity (20 cm/s) because this circulation is isolated from the systemic circulation by the liver sinusoids and splanchnic capillary bed. Therefore, portal venous flow exhibits minimal variations through the cardiac cycle (Figure 14.11D). A difference of more than 50% between systolic and diastolic velocities, known as the pulsatility fraction (PF), is considered abnormal and is referred to as pulsatile portal flow (17) (Figure 14.11I,N).

Pulsatile blood flow is a sign of posthepatic portal hypertension and has been studied as a marker of severity in patients with congestive heart failure. The presence of abnormal portal pulsatility has been shown to predict increased central venous pressure (CVP) and worse functional class in patients with heart failure. Venous congestion resulting from congestive heart failure begins with an elevation of the CVP and dilatation of the IVC and its main tributaries such as the hepatic veins. As dilatation becomes severe, the venous compliance of the IVC is decreased leading to pressure transmission through the hepatic sinusoids to the portal system. This results in a decrease in velocities in the portal system or, in severe cases, a complete absence or reversal of portal flow. The PWD interrogation of the portal flow can be used as a marker of end-organ venous congestion (21-23). For portal flow to actually be a reflection of central venous congestion, other causes of portal hypertension, such as cirrhosis and portal thrombosis, must not be present. A PF of more than 50% has also been reported in some individuals with low body mass index and normal cardiac function. However, other signs of elevated CVP such as IVC dilatation/non-collapsibility and abnormal hepatic vein flow waveform should support this finding. In cardiac surgery patients who are at high risk, portal PF of more than 50% detected in the operating room before CPB was associated with a longer duration of life support therapy such as mechanical ventilation, after surgery (24).

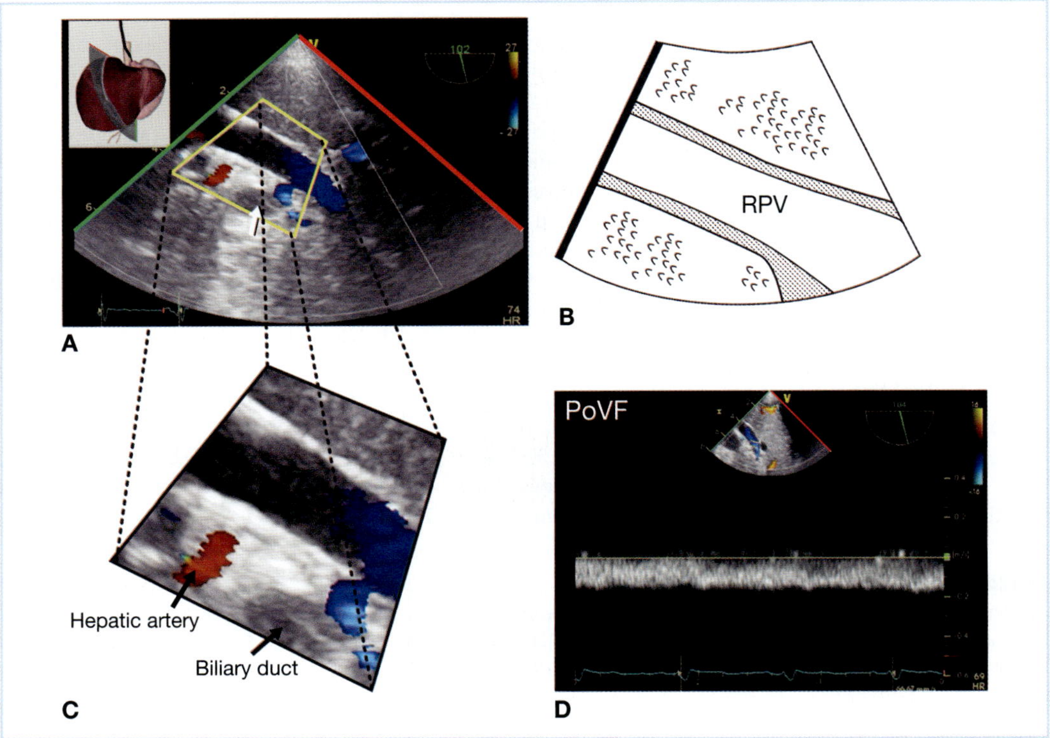

FIGURE 14.12 Portal vein. A-C: Transesophageal echocardiography transgastric views with right-sided rotation show the main branch of the right portal vein (RPV). Note the portal vein has a hyperechoic sheath around the vein as opposed to the inferior vena cava or the hepatic vein whose wall is barely seen. The hyperechoic sheath is a result of the proximity of the biliary duct and the hepatic artery which forms the portal triad. D: Pulsed-wave Doppler of portal vein shows low resistance continuous, monophasic low-velocity portal venous flow (PoVF) (Video 14.5). (Reproduced by permission of Taylor and Francis Group, LLC, a division of Informa plc from Denault A, Vegas A, Lamarche Y, Tardif J, Couture P. *Basic Transesophageal and Critical Care Ultrasound*. Taylor and Francis, CRC Press; 2018.)

Renal Vascular Flow Evaluation

The impact of elevated CVP on intrarenal hemodynamics can be assessed by PWD using TG TEE (25). In physiologic conditions, blood flow in the interlobar veins is continuous during the cardiac cycle (Figure 14.11E). With high CVP, venous flow transforms into a discontinuous biphasic pattern similar to the PWD pattern seen in the hepatic veins (Figure 14.11J). With severe RV dysfunction, venous flow transforms into a discontinuous monophasic pattern with flow restricted to the diastole (Figure 14.11O). Discontinuous flow in the interlobar renal veins can be linked to the CVP waveform during the cardiac cycle. As CVP increases and the IVC becomes noncompliant, the CVP waveform is transmitted backward to the renal parenchyma. Flow in the interlobar vein can be observed during the systolic and diastolic filling of the RA (during the x- and y-descent on CVP waveform). As RV dysfunction worsens, intrarenal venous flow becomes restricted to diastole reflecting the predominance of the y-descent of the CVP waveform. This change is analogous to the variation in the systolic-to-diastolic ratio in the hepatic vein waveform with decreased filling of the RA during systole. Abnormal intrarenal venous flow is a significant predictor of rehospitalization and mortality in patients with heart failure (26). Abnormal intrarenal venous patterns after cardiac surgery have been associated with acute kidney injury (27).

RIGHT ATRIUM

Anatomy

The RA is a thin-walled, irregularly shaped structure with the superior vena cava entering near the anterior portion of the superior wall and the IVC entering near the right posterior portion of the inferior wall. The tricuspid annulus forms the inferior portion of the RA, and the coronary sinus opens into the RA just above this

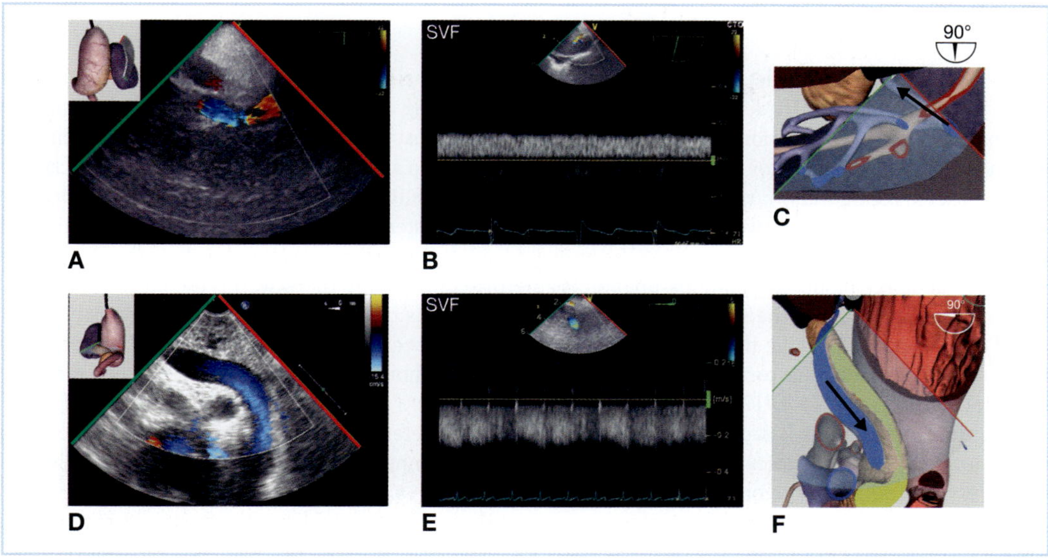

FIGURE 14.13 Splenic Doppler flow. A: Transesophageal echocardiography (TEE) transgastric view at 90° of the spleen with color Doppler (Nyquist 22 cm/s) shows flow in the splenic vessels. B,C: In this view, a monophasic splenic venous flow (SVF) velocity using pulsed-wave spectral Doppler will be seen. Note that the Doppler signal from the splenic hilum is toward the transducer. D: TEE transgastric view at 0° with color Doppler (Nyquist 15 cm/s) shows flow in the splenic vessels. E,F: Note that from this transducer position, the Doppler signal is away from the transducer (Videos 14.6 and 14.7). (Reproduced by permission of Taylor and Francis Group, LLC, a division of Informa plc from Denault A, Vegas A, Lamarche Y, Tardif J, Couture P. *Basic Transesophageal and Critical Care Ultrasound.* Taylor and Francis, CRC Press; 2018.)

structure. The eustachian valve and Chiari network are typically attached to the orifice of the IVC. Failure of regression of the right or inferior valve of the sinus venosus during gestation may result in a persistent eustachian valve. The Chiari network is a fenestrated, strand-like structure within the RA cavity. Although it most often arises from the orifice of the IVC, it may originate from the RA lateral wall, the coronary sinus, or interatrial septum (28). The upper limit of normal for end-systolic RA size is 18 cm^2, or 5.3 cm × 4.4 cm (3). Normal RA volume is 21 ± 6 mL/m^2 for women and 25 ± 7 mL/m^2 for men (2) (Figure 14.4C).

The RA appendage is often used as the entry point of the venous cannula for CPB. Thrombus formation has been described in this structure. Thus, it is prudent to exclude an RA appendage thrombus before insertion of the venous cannula in patients with a low-flow state or procoagulant conditions (29,30).

Transesophageal Echocardiographic Views

Due to the proximity to the TEE probe, RA is difficult to image in ME position.

1. **ME AoV SAX.** This view is useful for assessing the presence of a patent foramen ovale by decreasing the Doppler color scale (Figure 14.3 #7).
2. **ME RV inflow-outflow view.** This view allows a rapid evaluation of the RA, TV, and RV inflow tract. The interatrial septum with the septum secundum and septum primum flap can also be visualized (Figure 14.3 #6).
3. **ME bicaval view.** In this view, the left atrium is seen in the near field, while the smooth-walled part of the RA and its lateral wall are seen in the far field. The IVC and superior vena cava are displayed on the left and right sides of the image, respectively. Some modification of the sectors around the 90° angle may be required to align the scanning plane with both vena cavae. If inferior structures are seen on the left of the screen, a filamentous mass at the junction of the IVC and the RA is most likely a Chiari network, and if it appears ridgelike, it is more likely a eustachian valve. The crista terminalis is seen at the junction of the superior vena cava and the RA on the right of the sector (Figure 14.3 #9). It is a ridge that separates the venous component of the RA and the contractile portion.

TRICUSPID VALVE

Anatomy

The TV consists of valve leaflets, chordae tendineae, papillary muscles, an annular ring, and the RV myocardium. Typically, the TV is trileaflet in 54% of the cases, featuring anterior, septal, and posterior leaflets of unequal size, with the anterior leaflet being the largest and most mobile (Figure 14.14). The presence of several anatomic variations for TV leaflet configuration has led to a recent nomenclature scheme to classify the TV leaflet configuration: type I form by three leaflets; type II form by two leaflets; type III form by four leaflets (type IIIA with two anterior, type IIIB with two posterior, and type IIIC with two septal); and type IV has more than four leaflets (31). The anterior leaflet attached to the lateral wall of the RV and its anteroseptal or anterosuperior commissure points anterolaterally toward the AoV. It is the most cranial leaflet and is not attached to the septal wall. The posterior leaflet is distinguished by its caudal position and a scalloped appearance. Like the anterior leaflet, it is not attached to the septum. The septal leaflet is the smallest and most difficult to visualize. It has multiple septal chordal attachments to the interventricular septum (28,32) (Figure 14.3 #12).

The tricuspid annulus is saddle-shaped with the major diameter in the anteroposterior orientation and the minor diameter perpendicular to this orientation. Tricuspid annulus dilatation is defined by end-diastolic diameter of 40 mm or more or greater than 21 mm/m^2 (Figure 14.15; Videos 14.8-14.11). The anterior papillary muscle is the largest and originates from the moderator band, while the chordae tendineae connect the papillary muscles to the tricuspid leaflets. The TV annulus is larger and located in a slightly more apical position than the mitral valve annulus.

Transesophageal Echocardiographic Views

TEE evaluation of the TV focuses on the same standard views as for the RV.

1. **ME RV-focused 4C view.** From the standard ME 4C view, slight rightward (clockwise) turning of the probe moves the TV to the center of the scan plane; advancing and withdrawing the transducer allows imaging of the entire TV. This view demonstrates the anterior leaflet attached next to the RV lateral wall and septal leaflet next to the septal border (Figure 14.3 #5). However, a deeper scan will show the septal and posterior leaflet.

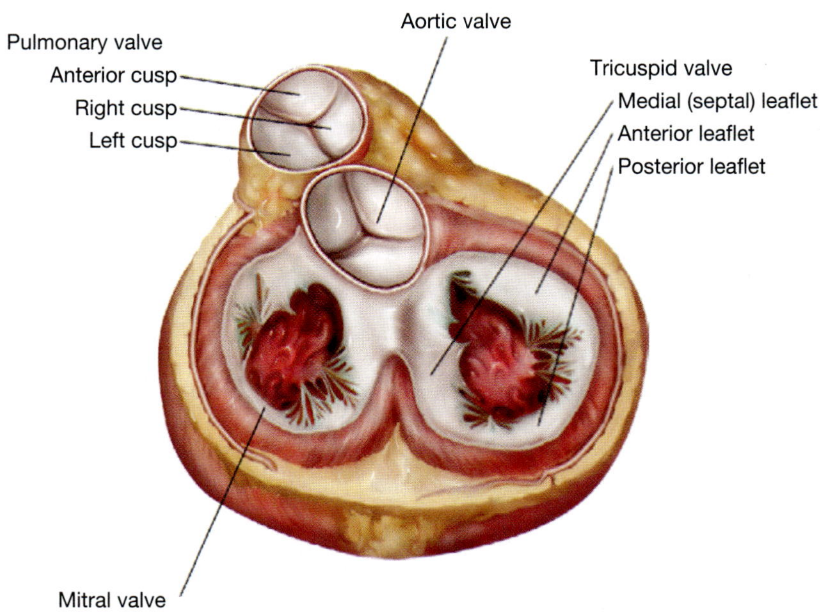

FIGURE 14.14 Schematic drawing of the tricuspid valve anatomy.

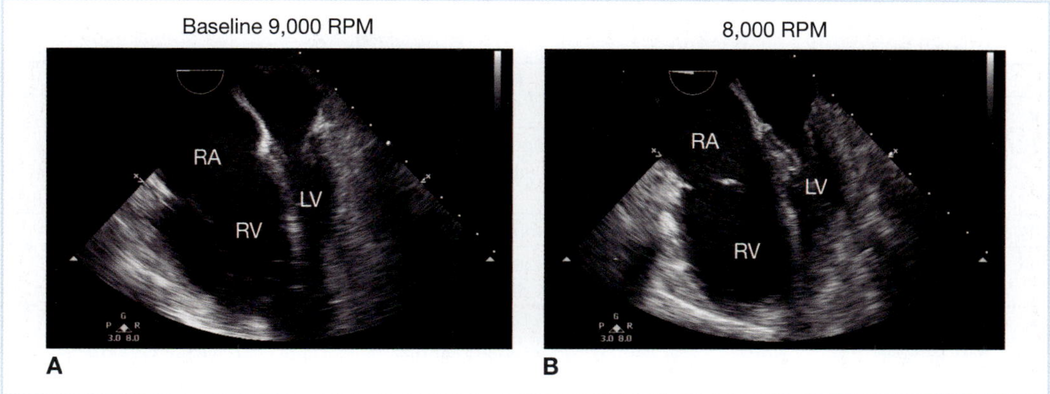

FIGURE 14.15 Dilated tricuspid valve annulus and right ventricle (RV) in a patient with a left ventricular assist device. A: Midesophageal four-chamber view baseline view with 9,000 revolutions per minute (RPM). Note the small left ventricle (LV). B: As RPM is reduced, there is little change in RV dimension (Videos 14.8-14.11). RA, right atrium.

2. **ME RV inflow-outflow view.** This view provides a nearly orthogonal view of the TV, with the orifice aligned nearly parallel to the ultrasound beam. As a result, quantitative measurements of TV flow velocities are optimized (Figure 14.3 #6).
3. **ME-modified bicaval view.** From the standard ME bicaval view at approximately 120°, the multiplane angle is increased slightly until the TV appears in the far left of the display. This view provides the best alignment of the ultrasound beam and the direction of the regurgitant tricuspid jet, minimizing errors in continuous or PWD measurements (Figure 14.3 #9).
4. **TG views.** The TG views used to evaluate the RV also provide useful windows for imaging the TV. Turning the TEE transducer right (ie, clockwise) from the TG mid-SAX view of the LV provides a good view of the TV in SAX, allowing identification of its septal, anterior, and posterior leaflets. The TG RV inflow view provides the best image of the chordae tendineae and RV papillary muscles supporting the TV (Figure 14.3 #10-13). The deep TG views can also be used to see the TV (Figure 14.3 #14-15).

Tricuspid Regurgitation

TR is the most common right-sided valvular lesion in adults. Primary TR is typically due to a structural abnormality of the valve, which can include valve degeneration, congenital heart disease, radiation-induced heart disease, trauma, or damage from previous heart biopsies. Secondary or functional TR is due to pathology that originates from the atrium in case of atrial fibrillation or from the ventricle in case of RV dysfunction, RV infarction, pulmonary hypertension, or chronic RV pacing for example. In most cases, it is caused by tricuspid annular dilation secondary to RV enlargement. Echocardiographic features of TR include RA, RV, and tricuspid annular dilation causing incomplete TV closure or even TV leaflet prolapse (Figure 14.15).

TR severity is most easily assessed using color flow (CF) Doppler (Table 14.1). Severe dysfunction is defined by one or more of the following measurements: an abnormal CF signal filling of 33% or more of the RA, TR jet area of a larger than 10 cm^2, or a TR jet length of more than 4.5 cm in the RA. When the regurgitant jet is directed toward the atrial septum, it is important to distinguish it from normal caval inflow or flow through an atrial septal defect. Severe TR may also be documented by the presence of a dense, early-peaking, triangular envelope by continuous-wave Doppler (CWD) due to rapid pressure equalization between RV and RA. This assessment can be complemented by evaluating reversed or retrograde systolic hepatic vein flow (Figure 14.16; Video 14.12). In 2017, a new expanded 5-grade scale including massive and torrential TR was proposed to better characterize the severity of TR treated with various transcatheter platforms (33).

Tricuspid Stenosis

Visualization of structural abnormalities of the TV leaflets and quantified by CWD examination of TTF flow are the first steps to evaluate TS. Features consistent with TS include increased echo density of the thickened

TABLE 14.1 Grading the Severity of Chronic Tricuspid Regurgitation by Echocardiography

	Mild	Moderate	Severe		
Structural					
TV morphology	Normal or mildly abnormal leaflets	Moderately abnormal leaflets	Severe valve lesions (eg, flail leaflet, severe retraction, large perforation)		
RV and RA size	Normal	Normal/mild dilation	Usually dilated[a]		
IVC diameter	Normal, <2 cm	Normal to mildly dilated, 2.1-2.5 cm	Dilated, >2.5 cm		
Qualitative Doppler					
Color flow jet area[b]	Small, narrow, central	Moderate central	Large central jet or eccentric wall-impinging jet of variable size		
Flow convergence zone	Not visible, transient or small	Intermediate in size and duration	Large throughout systole		
CWD jet	Faint/partial/ parabolic	Dense, parabolic, or triangular	Dense, often triangular		
Semiquantitative					
Color flow jet area (cm^2)[b]	Not defined	Not defined	>10		
VCW (cm)[b]	<0.3	0.3-0.69	Severe	Massive	Torrential
			0.7-1.3	1.4-2.0	≥2.1
PISA radius (cm)[c]	≤0.5	0.6-0.9	>0.9		
Hepatic vein flow[d]	Systolic dominance	Systolic blunting	Systolic flow reversal		
Tricuspid inflow[d]	A-wave dominant	Variable	E wave, >1.0 m/s		
Quantitative					
EROA (cm^2)	<0.20	0.20-0.39[e]	Severe	Massive	Torrential
			0.40-0.59	0.60-0.79	≥0.80
RVol (mL/beat)	<30	30-44[e]	≥45		
3D VCA or quantitative EROA[f] (cm^2)			Severe	Massive	Torrential
			0.75-0.94	0.95-1.14	≥1.15

Bolded signs are considered specific for their tricuspid regurgitation grade.
2D, two-dimensional; 3D, three-dimensional; CWD, continuous-wave Doppler; EROA, effective regurgitant orifice area; IVC, inferior vena cava; PISA, proximal isovelocity surface area; RA, right atrium; RV, right ventricle; RVol, regurgitant volume; TV, tricuspid valve; VCA, vena contracta area; VCW, vena contracta width.
[a]RV and RA size can be within normal range in patients with acute severe tricuspid regurgitation.
[b]With Nyquist limit of greater than 50 to 70 cm/s.
[c]With baseline Nyquist limit shift of 28 cm/s.
[d]Signs are nonspecific and are influenced by many other factors (RV diastolic function, atrial fibrillation, RA pressure).
[e]There are little data to support further separation of these values.
[f]3D VCA and quantitative Doppler EROA cutoffs may be larger than PISA EROA.
Adapted from Zoghbi WA, Adams D, Bonow RO, et al. Recommendations for noninvasive evaluation of native valvular regurgitation: a report from the American Society of echocardiography developed in collaboration with the society for cardiovascular magnetic resonance. *J Am Soc Echocardiogr*. 2017;30(4):303-371; Davidson LJ, Tang GHL, Ho EC, et al. The tricuspid valve: a review of pathology, imaging, and current treatment options: a scientific statement from the American Heart Association. *Circulation*. 2024;149(22):e1223-e1238.

leaflets, diastolic leaflet doming, and decreased size of the tricuspid orifice. Indirect signs include right atrial enlargement and dilated IVC (Table 14.2) (34).

Being the largest of the cardiac valves, TTF velocities are often very low, typically less than 0.7 m/s. Although normal prosthetic valves in the tricuspid position may demonstrate peak velocities nearly twice normal, peak flow velocity of greater than 1.5 m/s suggests TS. As with any suspected valve dysfunction, the effective orifice area should be calculated to confirm peak flow estimates of severity (3) Although not validated, pressure half-time (PHT) can be used to estimate TV area (TVA = 190/PHT) (34).

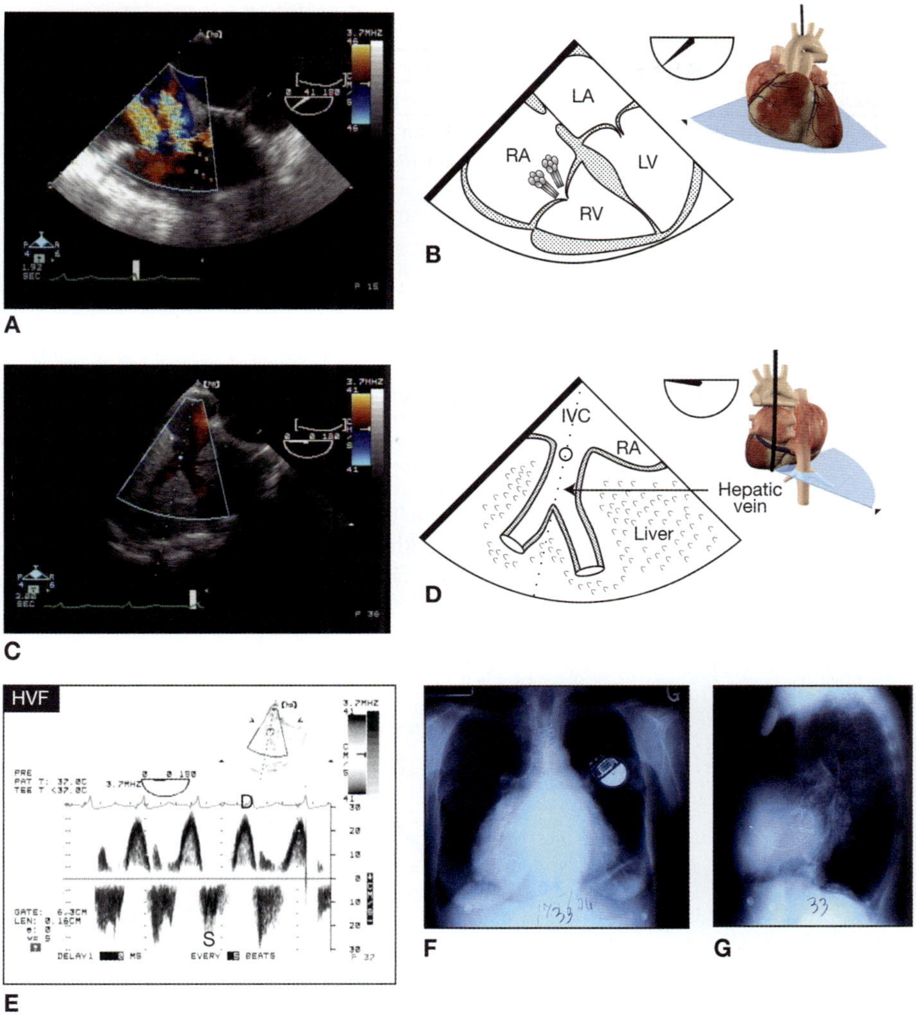

FIGURE 14.16 Tricuspid regurgitation. A,B: Color Doppler midesophageal four-chamber view shows severe TR in a 77-year-old woman before tricuspid annuloplasty. C,D: Transgastric IVC long-axis view indicates dilated hepatic veins. E: Pulsed-wave Doppler of HVF shows systolic flow reversal. F,G: Chest radiography confirms the abnormal right heart border consistent with dilated right-sided structures (Video 14.12). D, peak diastolic HVF velocity; HVF, hepatic venous flow; IVC, inferior vena cava; LA, left atrium; LV, left ventricle; RA, right atrium; RV, right ventricle; S, peak systolic HVF velocity; TR, tricuspid regurgitation. (Reproduced by permission of Taylor and Francis Group, LLC, a division of Informa plc from Denault AY, Couture P, Vegas A, Buithieu J, Tardif JC. *Transesophageal Echocardiography Multimedia Manual, Second Edition: A Perioperative Transdisciplinary Approach*. Informa Healthcare; 2011.)

Etiology of Tricuspid Valve Disease

Annular Dilation

Annular dilation generally occurs in the anterolateral direction because of the septal support made from the fibrous skeleton of the heart. Annular dilation results in decreased leaflet coaptation and progressive TR. The severity of the regurgitation is directly related to the degree of annular dilation and may be treated with ring annuloplasty (Figure 14.15).

TABLE 14.2 Findings Indicative of Hemodynamically Significant Tricuspid Stenosis

■ **Specific Findings**	
Mean pressure gradient	≥5 mm Hg
Inflow time-velocity integral	>60 cm
Pressure half-time	≥190 ms
Valve area by continuity equation[a]	≤1 cm^{2a}
■ **Supportive Findings**	
Enlarged right atrium ≥ moderate Dilated inferior vena cava	

[a]Stroke volume derived from left or right ventricular outflow. In the presence of more than mild tricuspid regurgitation, the derived valve area will be underestimated. Nevertheless, a value 1 cm^2 or less implies a significant hemodynamic burden imposed by the combined lesion.
Adapted from Baumgartner H, Hung J, Bermejo J, et al. Echocardiographic assessment of valve stenosis: EAE/ASE recommendations for clinical practice. *J Am Soc Echocardiogr*. 2009;22(1):1-23; quiz 101-102.

Rheumatic Disease

Rheumatic disease is the most common cause of acquired TS, resulting in fibrosis and scarring of the TV leaflets, doming, and eventually frank commissural fusion. Rheumatic tricuspid disease often includes regurgitation, and the mitral valve is almost uniformly involved (Figure 14.17; Videos 14.13 and 14.14).

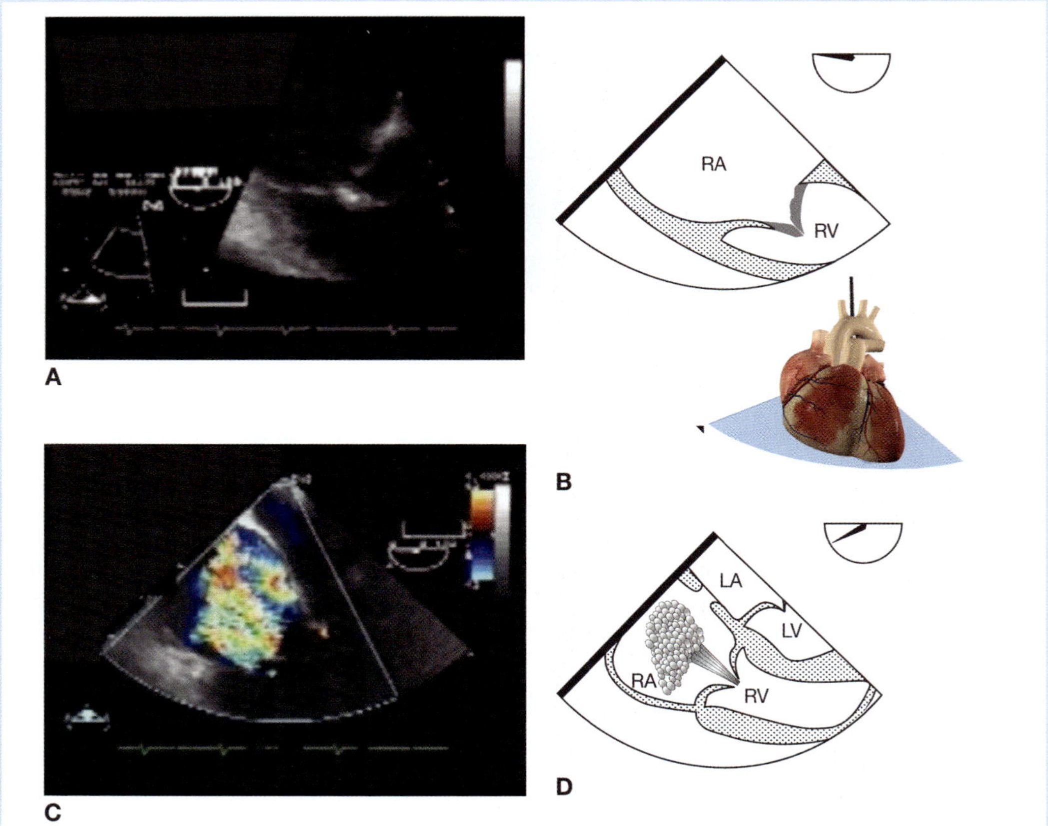

FIGURE 14.17 Rheumatic TV. Zoomed midesophageal four-chamber view (A,B) of the TV shows restricted motion from chordal shortening and fusion with severe tricuspid regurgitation (C,D) (Videos 14.13 and 14.14). LA, left atrium; LV, left ventricle; RA, right atrium; RV, right ventricle; TV, tricuspid valve. (Reproduced by permission of Taylor and Francis Group, LLC, a division of Informa plc; Denault AY, Couture P, Vegas A, Buithieu J, Tardif JC. *Transesophageal Echocardiography Multimedia Manual, Second Edition: A Perioperative Transdisciplinary Approach*. Informa Healthcare; 2011.)

Endocarditis

TV vegetations are usually oscillating, echo-dense masses attached to the leaflets or the annulus. Typically, they involve the atrial surface of affected leaflets and are often larger and bulkier than those found on the left side. Leaflet destruction may eventually result in flail segments and severe TR (Figure 14.18; Video 14.15).

Carcinoid Syndrome

Carcinoid tumors typically occur in the distal small bowel and secrete serotonin, bradykinins, histamine, and prostaglandins. Damage from these substances is usually limited to right-sided valvular structures as they are inactivated by monoamine oxidase abundantly present in normal lung tissue. Typical features of carcinoid heart disease include TV and/or PV leaflet thickening and fibrosis with moderate-to-severe TR, mild TS, and PS (14). TR is caused primarily by restricted leaflet mobility preventing adequate coaptation of the leaflet tips. In contrast to rheumatic heart disease, carcinoid syndrome does not result in tricuspid leaflet doming or commissural fusion (Figure 14.19; Videos 14.16 and 14.17).

Ebstein Anomaly

Ebstein anomaly is a congenital condition in which a malformed TV arises from a location abnormally displaced toward the RV apex. Typically, the anterior leaflet is redundant, often fenestrated and "sail-like," while the septal and posterior leaflets are either rudimentary or completely absent. Ebstein anomaly should be suspected when the LAX separation between the mitral and tricuspid annular planes exceeds 8 mm/m^2. This marked apical displacement of the TV causes a portion of the morphologic RV to become atrialized.

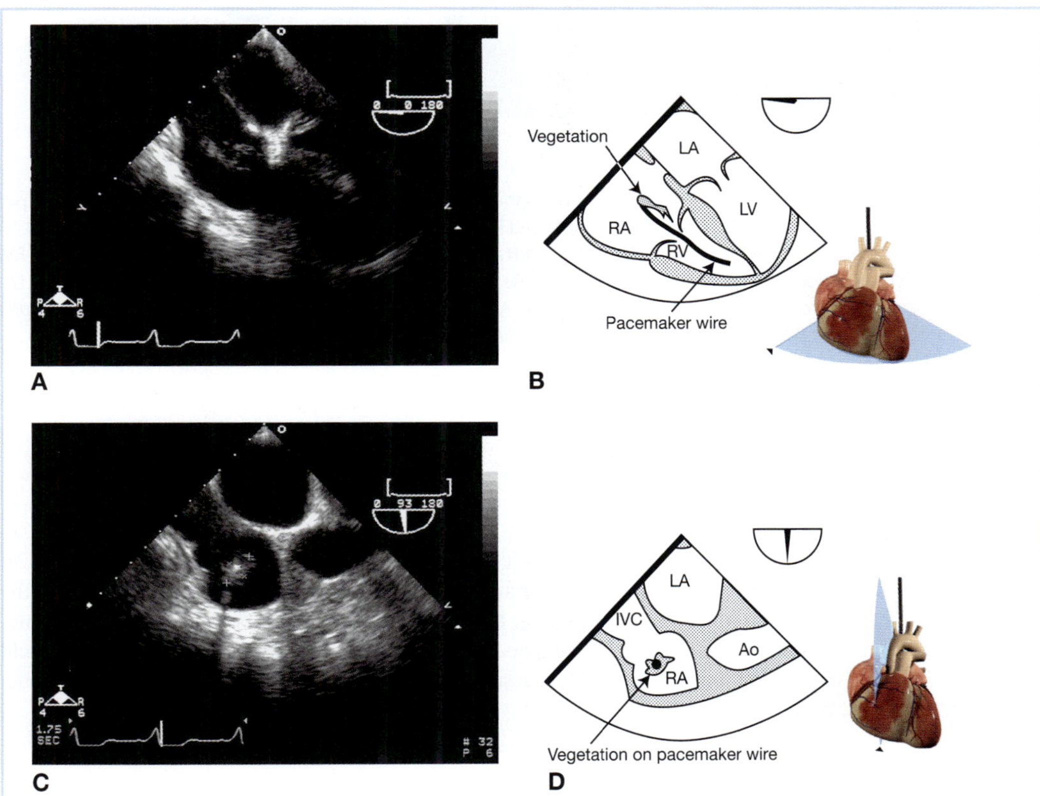

FIGURE 14.18 TV endocarditis. Echogenic material attached to a pacemaker lead is seen in midesophageal four-chamber (A,B) and 90° views (C,D) (Video 14.15). Ao, aorta; IVC, inferior vena cava; LA, left atrium; LV, left ventricle; RA, right atrium; RV, right ventricle; TV, tricuspid valve. (Reproduced by permission of Taylor and Francis Group, LLC, a division of Informa plc from Denault AY, Couture P, Vegas A, Buithieu J, Tardif JC. *Transesophageal Echocardiography Multimedia Manual, Second Edition: A Perioperative Transdisciplinary Approach*. Informa Healthcare; 2011.)

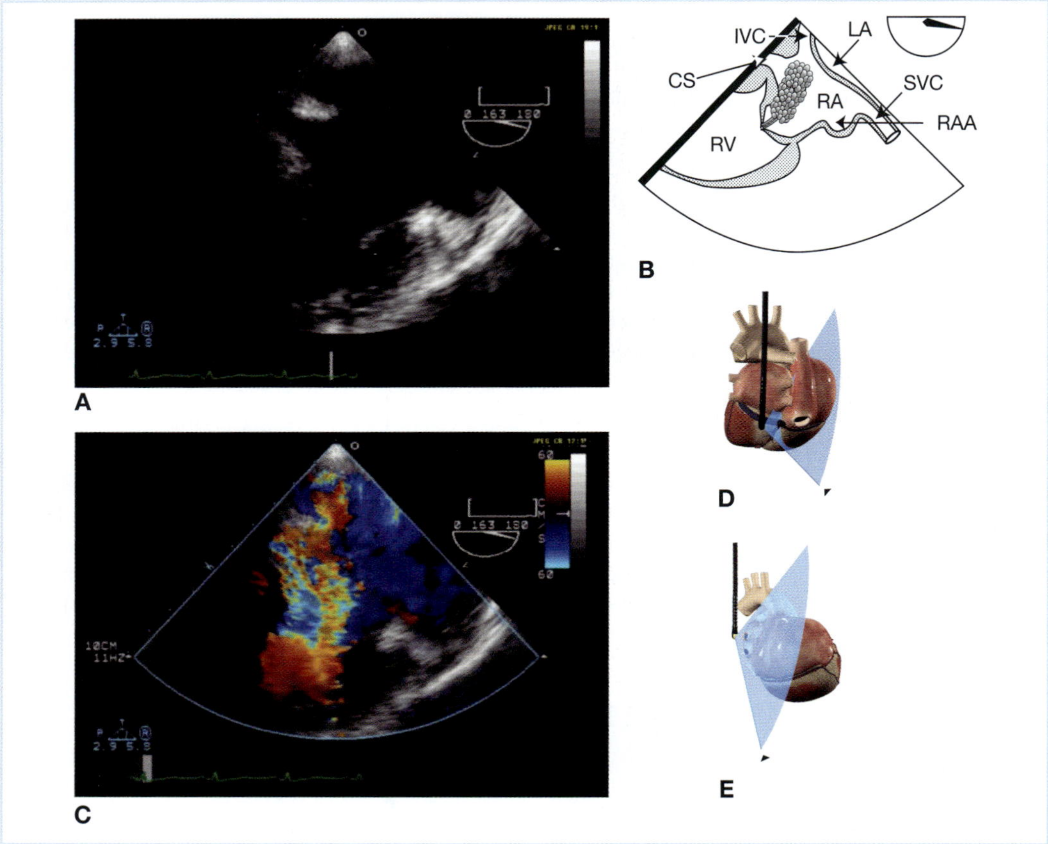

FIGURE 14.19 Carcinoid heart disease of TV. (A-E) Midesophageal views with rightward rotation show severe tricuspid regurgitation with a huge regurgitant orifice due to thickened TV leaflets retracted in the open position (Videos 14.16 and 14.17). CS, coronary sinus; IVC, inferior vena cava; LA, left atrium; RA, right atrium; RAA, right atrial appendage; RV, right ventricle; SVC, superior vena cava; TV, tricuspid valve. (Reproduced by permission of Taylor and Francis Group, LLC, a division of Informa plc from Denault AY, Couture P, Vegas A, Buithieu J, Tardif JC. *Transesophageal Echocardiography Multimedia Manual, Second Edition: A Perioperative Transdisciplinary Approach*. Informa Healthcare; 2011.)

Associated features include an atrial septal defect, impaired RV function, conduction abnormalities, and TR (35) (Figure 14.20; Video 14.18).

PULMONIC VALVE

Anatomy

The PV is a trileaflet valve with anterior, right, and left posterior semilunar cusps (Figures 14.2 and 14.21; Videos 14.19 and 14.20). The leaflets are thinner than the AoV leaflets and are directly connected to the musculature of the RV. The pulmonary annulus is larger than the aortic annulus; as a result, the normal time-velocity integral will be lower in that of the left ventricular outflow tract (28). Evaluation of the PV should always be conducted in conjunction with a complete assessment of the right heart structures to evaluate the repercussions of the primary disease.

Transesophageal Echocardiographic Views

Because of its anterior position, high-resolution images of the PV are difficult to obtain with TEE. In addition to visualizing the valvular anatomy, the aims of imaging the PV apparatus should include inspection of the RVOT, PV annulus, main PA, and proximal branches.

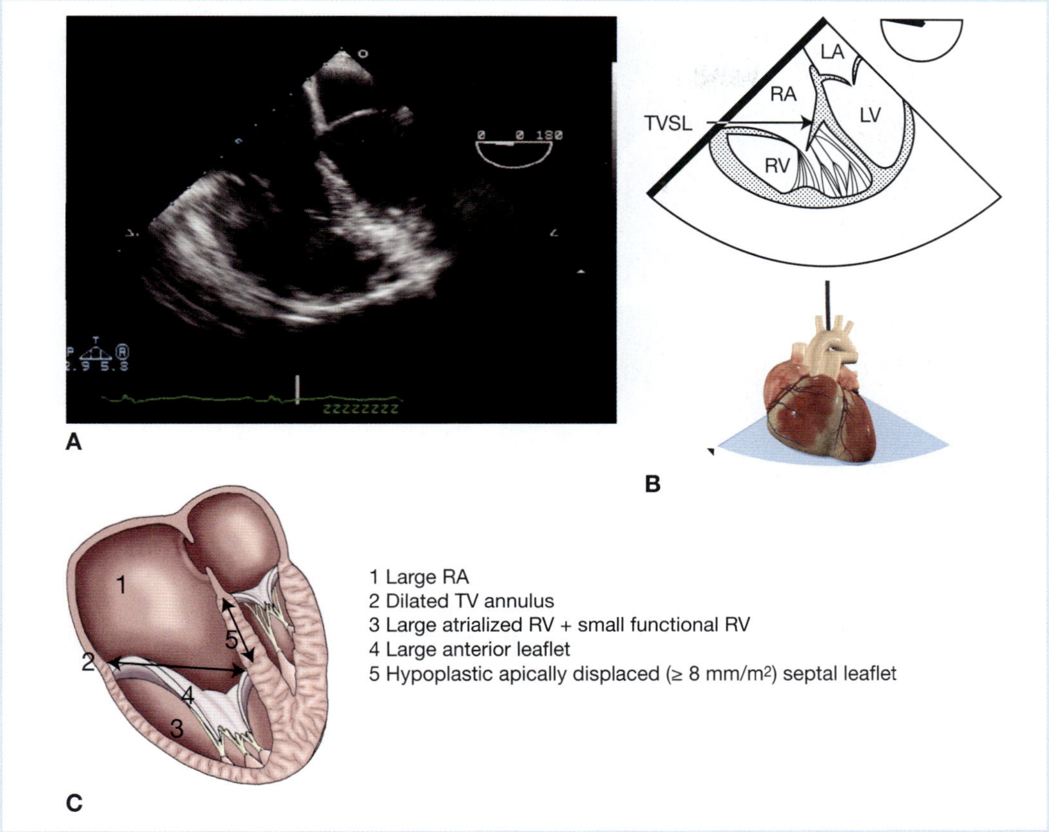

FIGURE 14.20 Ebstein anomaly. A,B: Midesophageal four-chamber view in a patient with Ebstein anomaly shows a number of key findings as illustrated in the diagram (C) (Video 14.18). LA, left atrium; LV, left ventricle; RA, right atrium; RV, right ventricle; TV, tricuspid valve; TVSL, tricuspid valve septal leaflet. Source: Part C with permission, copyright of Gian-Marco Busato. (Reproduced by permission of Taylor and Francis Group, LLC, a division of Informa plc from Denault AY, Couture P, Vegas A, Buithieu J, Tardif JC. *Transesophageal Echocardiography Multimedia Manual, Second Edition: A Perioperative Transdisciplinary Approach*. Informa Healthcare; 2011.)

1. **ME RV inflow-outflow view.** The most consistent TEE scan plan for imaging the PV is the ME RV inflow-outflow view. Since the PV is oriented at approximately 90° to the AoV, it is usually viewed in LAX when the AoV is seen in SAX (Figure 14.3 #6).
2. **ME AoV SAX.** With gradual withdrawal of the probe from the ME AoV SAX position, the PV will come into view. In LAX it is possible to visualize the PV adjacent to the AoV, but also with a significant portion of the main PA and even its bifurcation into right and left branches in the extreme near field (commonly known as the Y-view) (Figure 14.3 #7).
3. **Upper esophageal aortic arch SAX/PV LAX view.** This view may be reached by rotating the transducer angle to 90° from either an LAX of the aortic arch or from the Y-view described earlier. The close alignment of blood flow with the ultrasound signal vector makes this an excellent position from which to detect pulmonic regurgitation (PR) or quantify PS with CWD (Figures 14.3#1 and 14.21).
4. **Deep TG RV outflow and inflow-outflow view.** From the TG LV midpapillary SAX view, the probe is turned to the right and the transducer is rotated at 110° to 140°, the RVOT and PV in LAX will appear in the far field. This view is useful for obtaining PWD measurements of cardiac output from the RVOT (Figure 14.3 #14).

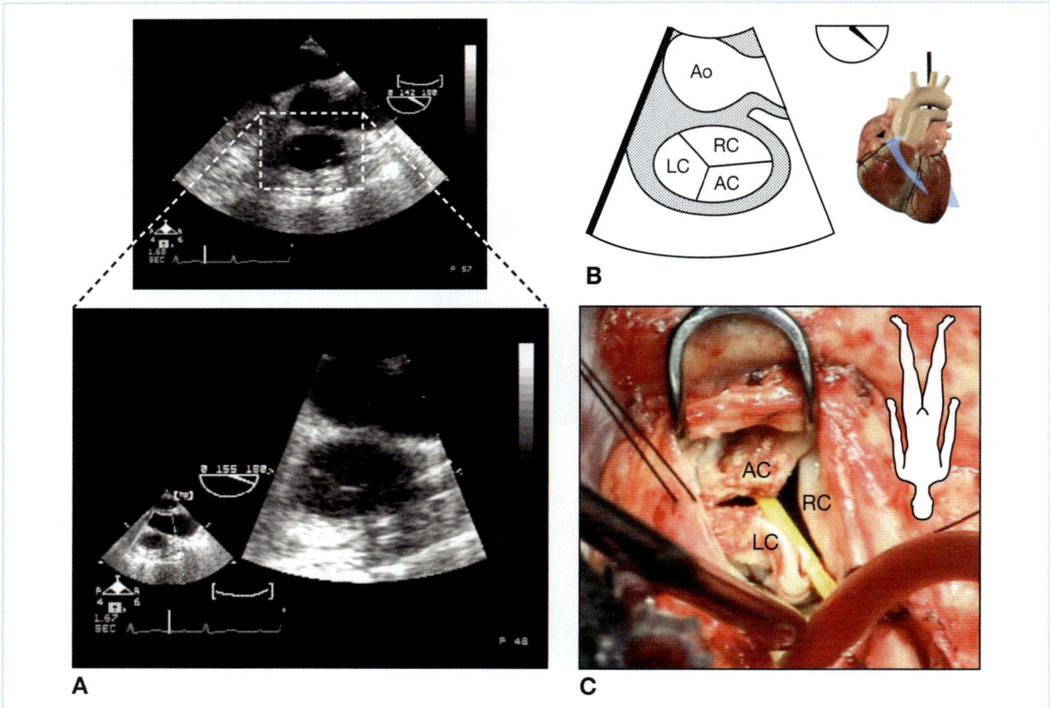

FIGURE 14.21 Normal pulmonic valve. A,B: Modified midesophageal long-axis view at 142° shows a transverse view of a normal PV. C: Corresponding intraoperative view is shown (Videos 14.19 and 14.20). AC, anterior cusp; Ao, aorta; LC, left cusp; PV, pulmonic valve; RC, right cusp. (Reproduced by permission of Taylor and Francis Group, LLC, a division of Informa plc from Denault AY, Couture P, Vegas A, Buithieu J, Tardif JC. *Transesophageal Echocardiography Multimedia Manual, Second Edition: A Perioperative Transdisciplinary Approach*. Informa Healthcare; 2011.)

Pulmonic Regurgitation

Mild PR, similar to TR, is a common finding, reported in up to 75% of the population and is generally of little hemodynamic significance (36). The severity of PR is usually quantified by CF Doppler mapping (Table 14.3). PA catheters have a minimal effect on the severity of PR or TR (37). Primary PR due to abnormal cusp structure from congenital heart disease and after balloon valvuloplasty for PS is more common than acquired valve disease. Significant acquired PR is rare, occurring in less than 1% of patients. When it does occur it

TABLE 14.3 Grading the Severity of Pulmonic Regurgitation by Echocardiography

	Mild	Moderate	Severe
Structural			
PV morphology	Normal	Normal or abnormal	Abnormal
RV size	Normal[a]	Normal or dilated	Dilated[b]
Jet size, color Doppler[c]	Thin (usually <10 mm in length) with a narrow origin	Intermediate	Broad origin; variable depth of penetration
Ratio of PR jet width/ pulmonary annulus			>0.7[d]
Jet density and contour (CWD)	Soft	Dense	Dense; early termination of diastolic flow
Deceleration time of the PR spectral Doppler signal			Short, <260 ms

TABLE 14.3 Grading the Severity of Pulmonic Regurgitation by Echocardiography *(continued)*

	Mild	Moderate	Severe
Pressure half-time of PR jet			<100 ms[e]
PR index[f]		<0.77	<0.77
Diastolic flow reversal in the main or branch of PA (PWD)			Prominent
Pulmonic systolic flow (VTI) compared to systemic flow (LVOT VTI) by PWD[g]	Slightly increased	Intermediate	Greatly increased
RF[h]	<20%	20%-40%	>40%

CMR, cardiovascular magnetic resonance; CWD, continuous-wave Doppler; LVOT, left ventricular outflow tract; PA, pulmonary artery; PR, pulmonic regurgitation; PV, pulmonic valve; PWD, pulsed-wave Doppler; RF, regurgitation fraction; RV, right ventricle; RVol, regurgitant volume; VTI, velocity-time integral.
[a]Unless there are other reasons for RV enlargement.
[b]Exception: acute PR.
[c]At a Nyquist limit of 50 to 70 cm/s.
[d]Identifies a CMR-derived PR fraction 40% or more.
[e]Not reliable in the presence of high RV end-diastolic pressure.
[f]Defined as the duration of the PR signal divided by the total duration of diastole, with this cutoff identifying a CMR-derived PR fraction more than 25%.
[g]Cutoff values for RVol and fraction are not well validated.
[h]RF data primarily derived from CMR with limited application with echocardiography.
Adapted from Zoghbi WA, Adams D, Bonow RO, et al. Recommendations for noninvasive evaluation of native valvular regurgitation: a report from the American Society of echocardiography developed in collaboration with the society for cardiovascular magnetic resonance. *J Am Soc Echocardiogr*. 2017;30(4):303-371.

often causes pulmonary hypertension, annular dilation, or other structural distortions and can be seen in adults with pathologies such as rheumatic heart disease, endocarditis, carcinoid valve disease, or pergolide-induced disease. In rare cases, blunt chest trauma may lead to leaflet disruption and prolapse. Secondary PR is most common in patients with elevated PA pressure, although the volume of regurgitation is usually small. By definition, the PV cusps are normal with secondary PR. There is limited literature on the quantitation of PR severity using Doppler echocardiography. Since no single parameter is precise enough to correctly quantify PR severity, an integrative approach combining color, PWD, and CWD methods should be used in the grading of PR. The simplest and most robust method is PR jet width, vena contracta, and the duration of PR over the total diastolic time (<0.77) (36) (Figure 14.22; Videos 14.21 and 14.22).

Pulmonic Stenosis

PS is most commonly congenital but may also stem from rheumatic or carcinoid heart disease, or infective endocarditis. Severity of PS is quantified with 2D examination of leaflet motion, CF Doppler appearance of transvalvular flow, and transpulmonary pressure gradient. Estimation of PV area by planimetry is not achievable since the required image plane is generally not available. Continuity equation or proximal isovelocity surface area method is feasible but has not been validated in PS (34). Measurement of a pressure gradient across the PV is a simple method to assess severity (Figure 14.23; Videos 14.23 and 14.24).

Two-Dimensional Echocardiography

Features of PS include initial abnormal systolic leaflet motion and subsequent doming of stenotic leaflets into the PA. Other common findings are RV hypertrophy and RA enlargement. Doppler features of PS include increased flow velocities through the stenotic valve and post stenotic turbulence (Table 14.4).

Ross Procedure

In 1967, Donald Ross described the replacement of a diseased AoV using the patient's native PV (ie, pulmonary autograft). In this procedure, TEE is important in establishing candidate suitability by assessing for PR

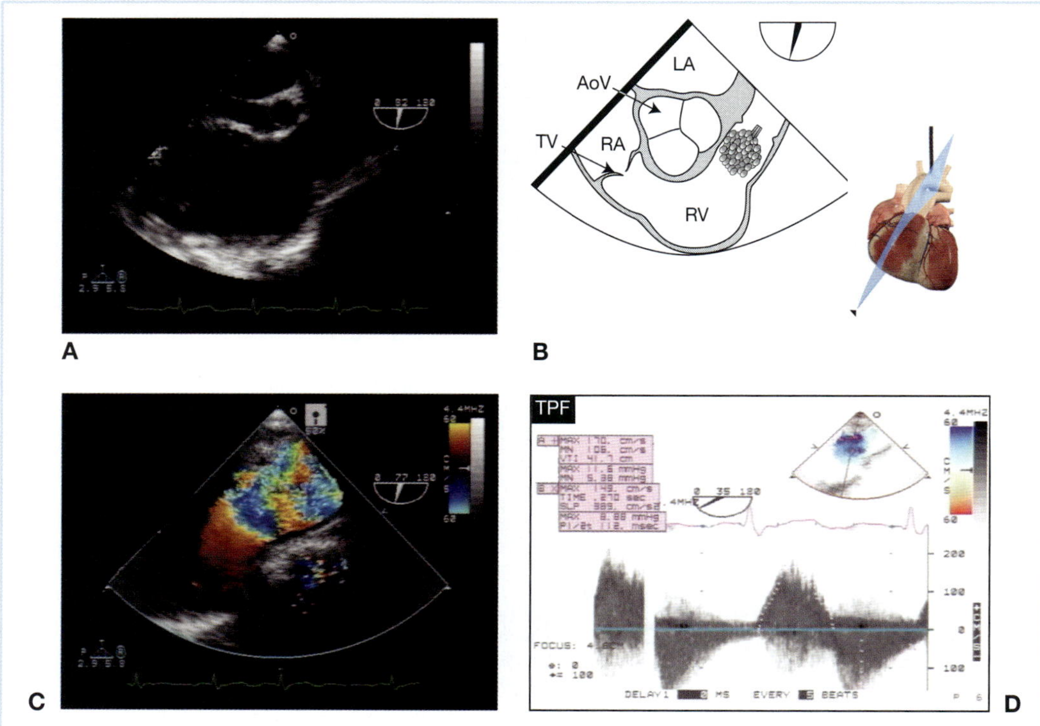

FIGURE 14.22 Severe pulmonic regurgitation. Severe pulmonic regurgitation (PR) is present in a patient with prior TOF repair. A,B: Midesophageal right ventricular inflow-outflow tract view shows an almost complete absence of the PV. C: Color Doppler imaging demonstrates that the low-velocity wide-open severe PR is associated with a high stroke volume across the PV and secondary aliased flow during systole. D: Using continuous-wave Doppler of the TPF, a 5 mm Hg mean systolic gradient is measured across the PV (Videos 14.21 and 14.22). AoV, aortic valve; LA, left atrium; PR, pulmonic regurgitation; PV, pulmonic valve; RA, right atrium; RV, right ventricle; TOF, tetralogy of Fallot; TPF, transpulmonic flow; TV, tricuspid valve. (Reproduced by permission of Taylor and Francis Group, LLC, a division of Informa plc from Denault AY, Couture P, Vegas A, Buithieu J, Tardif JC. *Transesophageal Echocardiography Multimedia Manual, Second Edition: A Perioperative Transdisciplinary Approach*. Informa Healthcare; 2011.)

and providing dimensions of PV and AoV. In addition, new intraoperative LV septal wall motion abnormalities may indicate ligation of a septal coronary artery branch during dissection and excision of the PV. Postoperatively, the patients are followed for development of aortic insufficiency, an early sign of autograft failure.

Estimation of Pulmonary Artery Systolic Pressure

The presence of TR allows for the use of a simplified Bernoulli equation ($\Delta P = 4v^2$; v = peak TR jet velocity) to estimate the tricuspid transvalvular pressure gradient, which when added to the RA pressure yields an estimate of RV systolic pressure. In the absence of RV outflow obstruction, this calculated RV systolic pressure provides a good estimate of the PA systolic pressure. It is critical, however, to align the ultrasound beam with the direction of regurgitant jets to avoid an underestimation error.

Conceptually similar, PA diastolic pressure can be estimated from the velocity at the end of PR, while PA mean pressure can be derived from the maximal velocity of the PR. RA pressure is added to these two previous measurements to obtain the estimate. PA mean pressure can be estimated by the PA acceleration time (AT) (PA mean pressure = 79 – [0.45 × AT] and PA mean pressure = 90 – [0.62 × AT] if AT <120 milliseconds) or derived from the systolic and diastolic pressures (PA mean pressure = 1/3[PA systolic pressure] + 2/3 [PA diastolic pressure]) (Figure 14.24; Video 14.25).

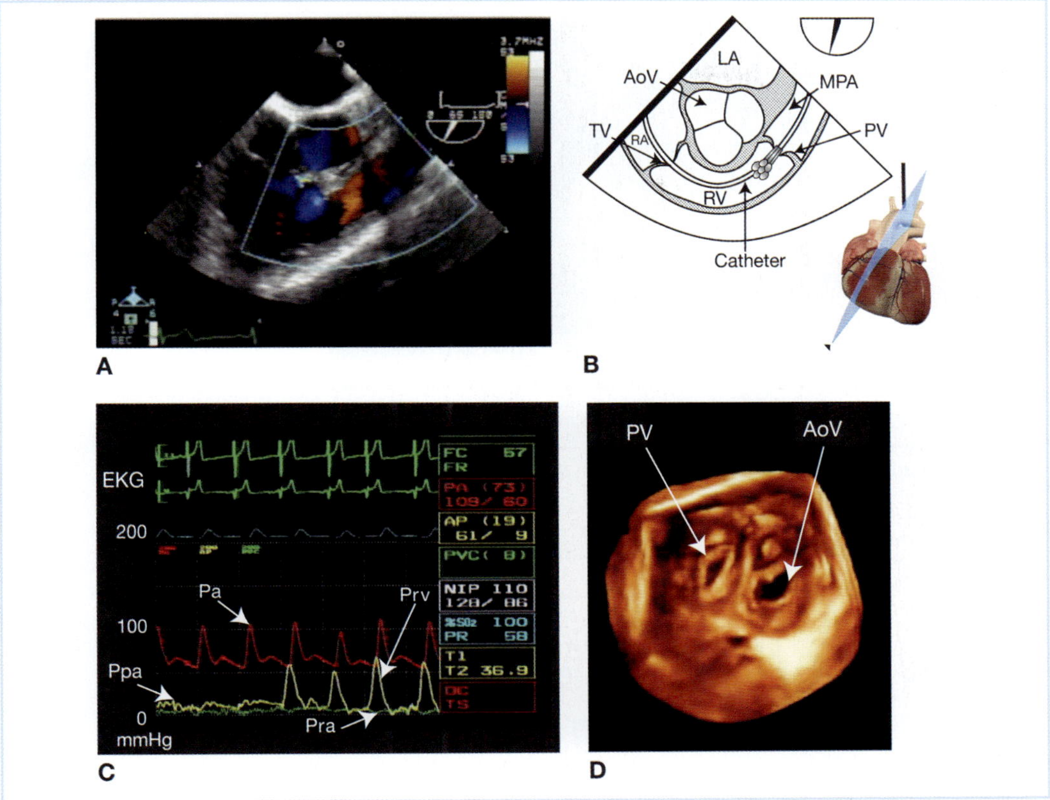

FIGURE 14.23 PV stenosis. A 29-year-old man presents with a stenotic bicuspid PV before open commissurotomy. A,B: Color Doppler midesophageal right ventricular inflow-outflow view shows pulmonic regurgitation. C: Measurement of the gradient between the Ppa and the Prv from a PAC. The Prv was obtained through the paceport lumen of the PAC. D: Intraoperative epicardial 3D echocardiogram of PV stenosis viewed from the pulmonary artery (Videos 14.23 and 14.24). AoV, aortic valve; ECG, electrocardiogram; LA, left atrium; MPA, main pulmonary artery; Pa, arterial pressure; PAC, pulmonary artery catheter; Ppa, pulmonary artery pressure; Pra, right atrial pressure; Prv, right ventricular pressure; PV, pulmonic valve; RA, right atrium; RV, right ventricle; TV, tricuspid valve. Source: Photo D courtesy of Philips Healthcare. (Reproduced by permission of Taylor and Francis Group, LLC, a division of Informa plc from Denault AY, Couture P, Vegas A, Buithieu J, Tardif JC. *Transesophageal Echocardiography Multimedia Manual, Second Edition: A Perioperative Transdisciplinary Approach*. Informa Healthcare; 2011.)

REAL-TIME THREE-DIMENSIONAL TRANSESOPHAGEAL ECHOCARDIOGRAPHY

The use of 3D echocardiography to evaluate RV function necessitates identifying end-diastolic RV volume and end-systolic RV volume to calculate RVEF. 3D RVEF of less than 45% is highly suggestive of RV dysfunction. End-diastolic volumes of more than 87 mL/m^2 for men and more than 74 mL/m^2 for women are indicative of RV enlargement. Intraoperative RVEF assessment with 3D TEE is feasible and reproducible in patients with both normal RV size and in patients with dilated RV without being excessively time consuming (38) (Figure 14.25; Video 14.26). Real-time 3D transesophageal echocardiography (RT 3D TEE) using zoom

TABLE 14.4 Gradation of Pulmonic Stenosis

	Mild	Moderate	Severe
Peak velocity (m/s)	<3	3-4	>4
Peak gradient (mm Hg)	<36	36-64	>64

Adapted from Baumgartner H, Hung J, Bermejo J, et al. Echocardiographic assessment of valve stenosis: EAE/ASE recommendations for clinical practice. *J Am Soc Echocardiogr*. 2009;22(1):1-23; quiz 101-102.

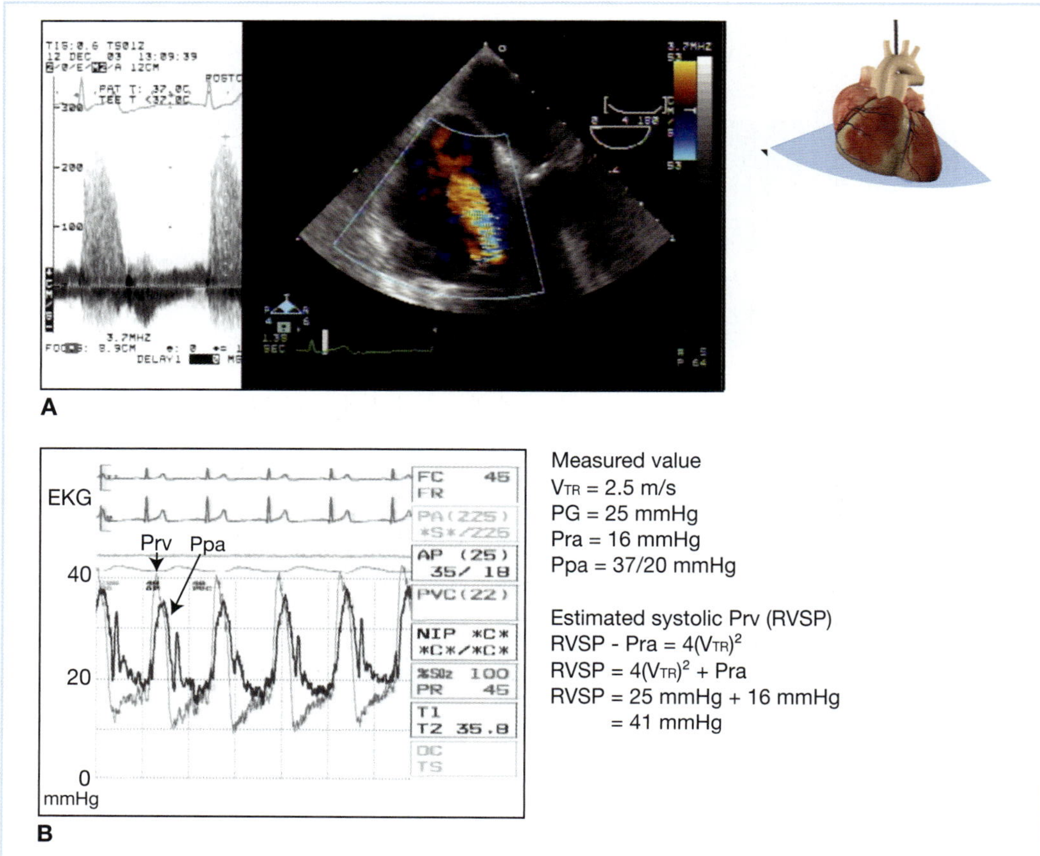

FIGURE 14.24 Right ventricular systolic pressure. A: Estimation of RVSP using the PG obtained from TR and RAP. B: Note that the RVSP is higher than the systolic pulmonary artery pressure (Ppa) due to a small gradient across the pulmonic valve (Video 14.25). ECG, electrocardiogram; LA, left atrium; LV, left ventricle; PG, pressure gradient; RA, right atrium; RAP or Pra, right atrial pressure; RV, right ventricle; RVSP or Prv, right ventricular systolic pressure; TR, tricuspid regurgitation; V, velocity; V_{TR}, peak tricuspid regurgitant velocity. (Reproduced by permission of Taylor and Francis Group, LLC, a division of Informa plc from Denault AY, Couture P, Vegas A, Buithieu J, Tardif JC. *Transesophageal Echocardiography Multimedia Manual, Second Edition: A Perioperative Transdisciplinary Approach*. Informa Healthcare; 2011.)

and full-volume modalities has proven useful for imaging right-sided cardiac structures, including detailed views of the TV leaflets and subvalvular supporting structures. RT 3D TEE can help in estimating the severity of TR using CF Doppler, by measuring the area of vena contracta of the TR jet and cropping the RT 3D TEE CF Doppler data set with imaging planes exactly parallel to the TV orifice. This is especially useful in advanced stages of TR, as the valve's natural saddle shape becomes rounder and flatter (39,40). In the stenotic valve, the orifice may be more easily visualized and measured using planimetry from RT-3D TEE (Figure 14.23).

Conventional 2D imaging techniques support RV volumetric assessments but provide only surrogates of EF. However, with RT 3D TEE capability, rapid acquisition of a 3D RV data set is becoming more feasible and has been shown to be reproducible over a wide range of RV dimensions. Furthermore, it appears to be less prone to underestimation of both end-systolic and end-diastolic volume measurements, yielding more accurate measurements of chamber volumes and EF than 2D techniques. At present, although RV quantification software exists, integration into clinical practice is still not standardized. Significant limitations to 3D TEE are the variable quality of available acoustic windows, especially for the PV, education, and the time required for data collection and analysis (3). 3D assessment improves measurement precision of left and right heart structures. Numerous other indications will grow as anesthesiologists familiarize themselves with this essential technology in cardiac imaging.

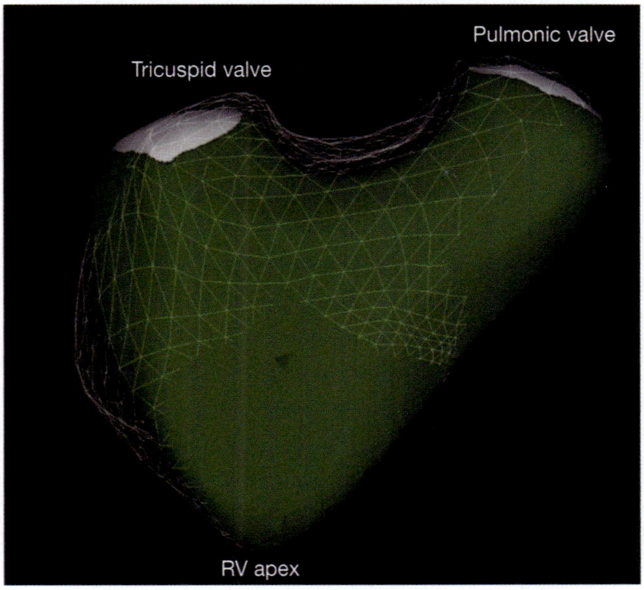

FIGURE 14.25 3D right ventricular (RV) function (Video 14.26).

ACKNOWLEDGMENTS

We gratefully acknowledge the contributions of the previous edition authors, Ying Tung Sia and Georges Desjardins, as portions of those chapters have been retained in this revision.

REFERENCES

1. Haddad F, Couture P, Tousignant C, Denault AY. The right ventricle in cardiac surgery, a perioperative perspective: I. Anatomy, physiology, and assessment. *Anesth Analg.* 2009;108(2):407-421.
2. Lang RM, Badano LP, Mor-Avi V, et al. Recommendations for cardiac chamber quantification by echocardiography in adults: an update from the American Society of Echocardiography and the European Association of Cardiovascular Imaging. *J Am Soc Echocardiogr.* 2015;28(1):1-39 e14.
3. Rudski LG, Lai WW, Afilalo J, et al. Guidelines for the echocardiographic assessment of the right heart in adults: a report from the American Society of Echocardiography endorsed by the European Association of Echocardiography, a registered branch of the European Society of Cardiology, and the Canadian Society of Echocardiography. *J Am Soc Echocardiogr.* 2010;23(7): 685-713; quiz 786-788.
4. Horton KD, Meece RW, Hill JC. Assessment of the right ventricle by echocardiography: a primer for cardiac sonographers. *J Am Soc Echocardiogr.* 2009;22(7):776-792; quiz 861-862.
5. Cacho A, Prakash R, Sarma R, Kaushik VS. Usefulness of two-dimensional echocardiography in diagnosing right ventricular hypertrophy. *Chest.* 1983;84(2):154-157.
6. Haddad F, Couture P, Tousignant C, Denault AY. The right ventricle in cardiac surgery, a perioperative perspective: II. Pathophysiology, clinical importance, and management. *Anesth Analg.* 2009;108(2):422-433.
7. Vitarelli A, Terzano C. Do we have two hearts? New insights in right ventricular function supported by myocardial imaging echocardiography. *Heart Fail Rev.* 2010;15(1):39-61.
8. Ryan T, Petrovic O, Dillon JC, Feigenbaum H, Conley MJ, Armstrong WF. An echocardiographic index for separation of right ventricular volume and pressure overload. *J Am Coll Cardiol.* 1985;5(4):918-927.
9. Karatzis EN, Giannakopoulou AT, Papadakis JE, Karazachos AV, Nearchou NS. Myocardial performance index (Tei index): evaluating its application to myocardial infarction. *Hellenic J Cardiol.* 2009;50(1):60-65.
10. Haddad F, Denault AY, Couture P, et al. Right ventricular myocardial performance index predicts perioperative mortality or circulatory failure in high-risk valvular surgery. *J Am Soc Echocardiogr.* 2007;20(9):1065-1072.
11. Denault AY, Couture P, Buithieu J, et al. Left and right ventricular diastolic dysfunction as predictors of difficult separation from cardiopulmonary bypass. *Can J Anesth.* 2006;53(10):1020-1029.

12. Focardi M, Cameli M, Carbone SF, et al. Traditional and innovative echocardiographic parameters for the analysis of right ventricular performance in comparison with cardiac magnetic resonance. *Eur Heart J Cardiovasc Imaging.* 2015; 16(1):47-52.
13. Crystal GJ, Pagel PS. Right ventricular perfusion: physiology and clinical implications. *Anesthesiology.* 2018;128(1):202-218.
14. Bruce CJ, Connolly HM. Right-sided valve disease deserves a little more respect. *Circulation.* 2009;119(20):2726-2734.
15. Silverton NA, Gebhardt BR, Maslow A. The intraoperative assessment of right ventricular function during cardiac surgery. *J Cardiothorac Vasc Anesth.* 2022;36(10):3904-3915.
16. Amsallem M, Kuznetsova T, Hanneman K, Denault A, Haddad F. Right heart imaging in patients with heart failure: a tale of two ventricles. *Curr Opin Cardiol.* 2016;31(5):469-482.
17. Denault AY, Beaubien-Souligny W, Elmi-Sarabi M, et al. Clinical significance of portal hypertension diagnosed with bedside ultrasound after cardiac surgery. *Anesth Analg.* 2017;124(4):1109-1115.
18. Tang WH, Kitai T. Intrarenal venous flow: a window into the congestive kidney failure phenotype of heart failure? *JACC Heart Fail.* 2016;4(8):683-686.
19. Denault AY, Roberts M, Cios T, et al. Transgastric abdominal ultrasonography in anesthesia and critical care: review and proposed approach. *Anesth Analg.* 2021;133(3):630-647.
20. Scheinfeld MH, Bilali A, Koenigsberg M. Understanding the spectral Doppler waveform of the hepatic veins in health and disease. *Radiographics.* 2009;29(7):2081-2098.
21. Tremblay JA, Beaubien-Souligny W, Elmi-Sarabi M, Desjardins G, Denault AY. Point-of-care ultrasonography to assess portal vein pulsatility and the effect of inhaled milrinone and epoprostenol in severe right ventricular failure: a report of 2 cases. *A A Case Rep.* 2017;9(8):219-223.
22. Beaubien-Souligny W, Bouchard J, Desjardins G, et al. Extracardiac signs of fluid overload in the critically ill cardiac patient: a focused evaluation using bedside ultrasound. *Can J Cardiol.* 2017;33(1):88-100.
23. Beaubien-Souligny W, Eljaiek R, Fortier A, et al. The association between pulsatile portal flow and acute kidney injury after cardiac surgery: a retrospective cohort study. *J Cardiothorac Vasc Anesth.* 2018;32(4):1780-1787.
24. Denault A, Couture EJ, De Medicis E, et al. Perioperative Doppler ultrasound assessment of portal vein flow pulsatility in high-risk cardiac surgery patients: a multicentre prospective cohort study. *Br J Anaesth.* 2022;129(5):659-669.
25. Bandyopadhyay S, Kumar Das R, Paul A, Sundar Bhunia K, Roy D. A transesophageal echocardiography technique to locate the kidney and monitor renal perfusion. *Anesth Analg.* 2013;116(3):549-554.
26. Iida N, Seo Y, Sai S, et al. Clinical implications of intrarenal hemodynamic evaluation by Doppler ultrasonography in heart failure. *JACC Heart Fail.* 2016;4(8):674-682.
27. Beaubien-Souligny W, Benkreira A, Robillard P, et al. Alterations in portal vein flow and intrarenal venous flow are associated with acute kidney injury after cardiac surgery: a prospective observational cohort study. *J Am Heart Assoc.* 2018; 7(19):e009961.
28. Tan CO, Harley I. Perioperative transesophageal echocardiographic assessment of the right heart and associated structures: a comprehensive update and technical report. *J Cardiothorac Vasc Anesth.* 2014;28(4):1100-1121.
29. Subramaniam B, Riley MF, Panzica PJ, Manning WJ. Transesophageal echocardiographic assessment of right atrial appendage anatomy and function: comparison with the left atrial appendage and implications for local thrombus formation. *J Am Soc Echocardiogr.* 2006;19(4):429-433.
30. Ozer O, Sari I, Davutoglu V. Right atrial appendage: forgotten part of the heart in atrial fibrillation. *Clin Appl Thromb Hemost.* 2010;16(2):218-220.
31. Hahn RT, Weckbach LT, Noack T, et al. Proposal for a standard echocardiographic tricuspid valve nomenclature. *JACC Cardiovasc Imaging.* 2021;14(7):1299-1305.
32. Davidson LJ, Tang GHL, Ho EC, et al. The tricuspid valve: a review of pathology, imaging, and current treatment options: a scientific statement from the American Heart Association. *Circulation.* 2024;149(22):e1223-e1238.
33. Hahn RT, Zamorano JL. The need for a new tricuspid regurgitation grading scheme. *Eur Heart J Cardiovasc Imaging.* 2017;18(12):1342-1343.
34. Baumgartner H, Hung J, Bermejo J, et al. Echocardiographic assessment of valve stenosis: EAE/ASE recommendations for clinical practice. *J Am Soc Echocardiogr.* 2009;22(1):1-23; quiz 101-102.
35. Attenhofer Jost CH, Connolly HM, Dearani JA, Edwards WD, Danielson GK. Ebstein's anomaly. *Circulation.* 2007; 115(2):277-285.
36. Zoghbi WA, Adams D, Bonow RO, et al. Recommendations for noninvasive evaluation of native valvular regurgitation: a report from the American Society of Echocardiography developed in collaboration with the society for cardiovascular magnetic resonance. *J Am Soc Echocardiogr.* 2017;30(4):303-371.
37. Goldman ME, Guarino T, Fuster V, Mindich B. The necessity for tricuspid valve repair can be determined intraoperatively by two-dimensional echocardiography. *J Thorac Cardiovasc Surg.* 1987;94(4):542-550.
38. Fusini L, Tamborini G, Gripari P, et al. Feasibility of intraoperative three-dimensional transesophageal echocardiography in the evaluation of right ventricular volumes and function in patients undergoing cardiac surgery. *J Am Soc Echocardiogr.* 2011;24(8):868-877.
39. David TE. Functional tricuspid regurgitation: a perplexing problem. *J Am Soc Echocardiogr.* 2009;22(8):904-906.
40. Hai T, Amador Y, Mahmood F, et al. Changes in tricuspid annular geometry in patients with functional tricuspid regurgitation. *J Cardiothorac Vasc Anesth.* 2017;31(6):2106-2114.

QUESTIONS

1. **What would be the estimation of the systolic PA pressure if the TR maximal velocity is 4 m/s in a patient with a measured CVP of 12 mm Hg?**
   A. 76 mm Hg
   B. 64 mm Hg
   C. 16 mm Hg
   D. 52 mm Hg

2. **Among the following factors, which one is highly suggestive of TS?**
   A. Small RA
   B. Increased echo density of TV thickened leaflets
   C. Enlarged RVOT
   D. Peak TTF velocity of 0.5 m/s

3. **Which finding is not associated with the condition shown in QFigure 14.1?**

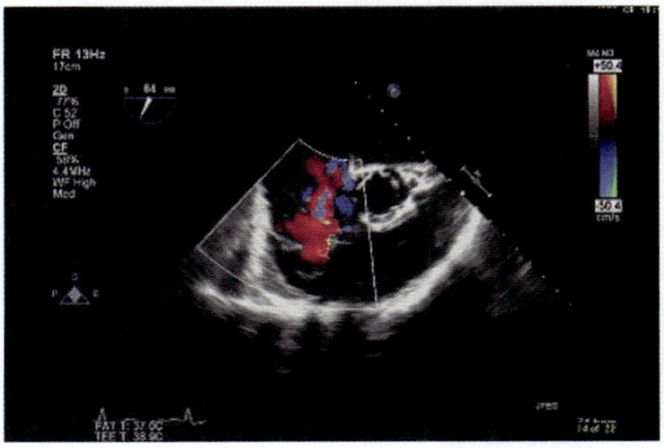

   A. Right atrial dilation
   B. Tricuspid annular dilation
   C. TV leaflet prolapse
   D. Collapsed IVC

4. **Which of the following conditions is not associated with the condition shown in QFigure 14.2?**

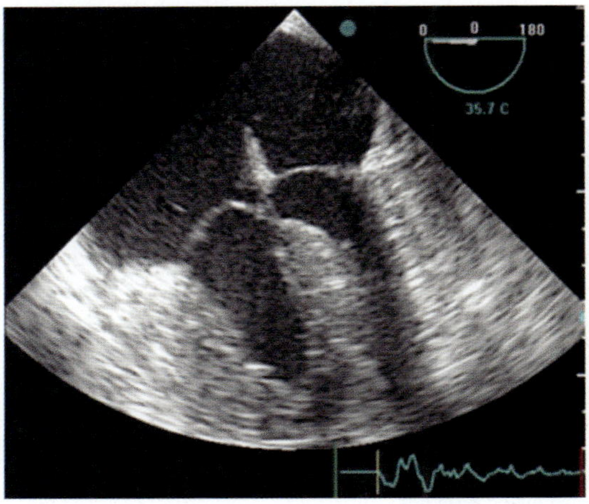

   A. Chronic thromboembolic pulmonary hypertension
   B. Pulmonary arterial hypertension associated with scleroderma
   C. Pulmonic stenosis
   D. Arrhythmogenic right ventricular cardiomyopathy

5. The eccentricity index can be used to characterize the LV shape during different parts of the cardiac cycle to identify abnormal motion of the interventricular septum in different conditions of the right ventricular overload. Which of the following sentence proposes the best description for its use?

A. The eccentricity index is the ratio of the vertical diameter over the horizontal diameter of the LV taken from a transgastric short-axis view.
B. The eccentricity index is the ratio of the vertical length of the LV over the horizontal diameter of the LV taken from a ME 4C view.
C. The eccentricity index is the ratio of the end-diastolic right ventricular area over the end-diastolic LV area taken from a ME 4C view.
D. The eccentricity index is the ratio of the vertical diameter over the horizontal diameter of the right ventricle taken from a transgastric short-axis view.

6. In QFigure 14.3, which of the following best describes the echocardiographic finding?

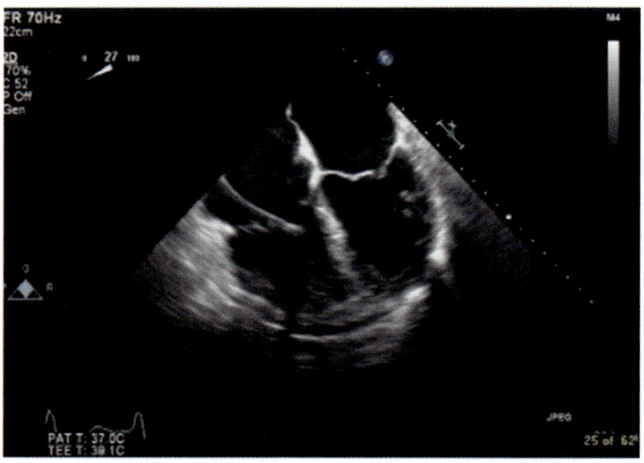

A. Eustachian valve
B. Crista terminalis
C. Chiari network
D. PA catheter

7. Which condition can be associated with the finding on Figure 14.4 pulse wave Doppler interrogation of the hepatic veins?

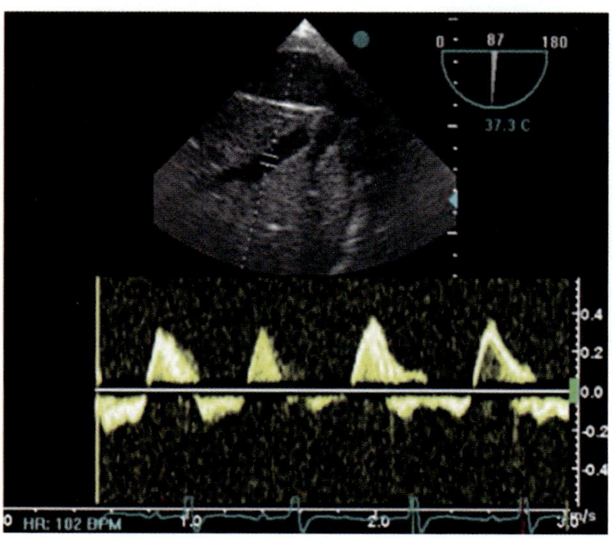

A. Type 1 atrioventricular block
B. Severe bradycardia
C. Severe TR
D. Hypovolemia

8. **Using QFigure 14.5, which of the following can be assessed using PWD?**

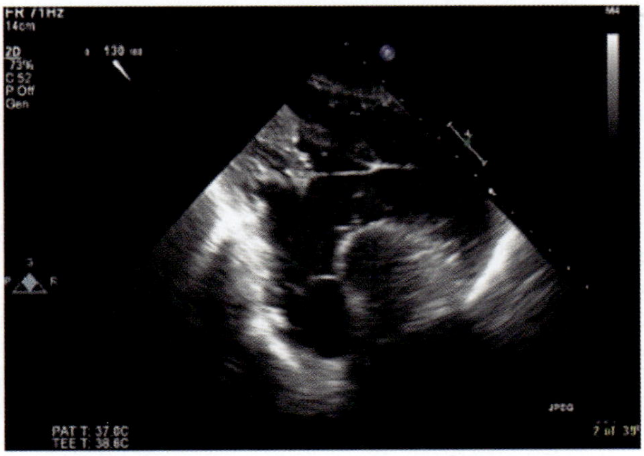

A. Right atrial pressure
B. Cardiac output
C. Aortic regurgitation severity
D. AoV area

9. **Which of the following does not refer to the use of RVFAC for assessment of right ventricular systolic function?**
A. Normal right ventricular systolic function is defined by RVFAC of more than 35%.
B. RVFAC corresponds to a percentage change in the right ventricular area from end diastole to end systole.
C. RVFAC considers the entire right ventricle.
D. A global appraisal of right ventricular systolic function

10. **TAPSE can be used to assess right ventricular systolic function. Which of the following represents a misconception related to its use?**
A. Tricuspid annular plane motion should be assessed using the angle correction features available on echocardiography machines.
B. It is not reliable after pericardectomy.
C. It is an easily recognizable longitudinal movement on echocardiography.
D. It is a global function parameter that considers the entire right ventricular structure.

ANSWERS

1. **Correct Answer: A.**
Rationale: Maximal TR jet velocity obtained by using CWD gives the maximal systolic pressure difference between the right ventricle and the RA when using the modified Bernoulli equation. Thus, by using the flowing equation: $P = 4$ (maximal TR jet velocity)^2, where P corresponds to a pressure difference on which the right atrial pressure must be added to obtain an estimation of the right ventricular systolic pressure. By using this concept, probability of pulmonary hypertension can be estimated based on the maximal TR jet velocity; 2.8 m/s or less being low probability, 2.9 to 3.4 m/s being intermediate probability, and greater than 3.4 m/s being high probability.

2. **Correct Answer: B.**
Rationale: Two-dimensional features consistent with TV stenosis include increased echo density of thickened leaflets of the TV, diastolic TV leaflet doming in addition to

decreased size of the tricuspid orifice. Indirect signs associated with the presence of TV stenosis include right atrial enlargement and dilated IVC. TTF velocities are typically very low, inferior to 0.7 m/s. On the counterpart, peak flow velocity greater than 1.5 m/s is suggestive of TV stenosis. As with any suspected valve dysfunction, the effective orifice area should be calculated to confirm peak flow estimates of severity. Although not validated, PHT can be used to estimate TVA using the following formula: TVA = 190/PHT.

3. **Correct Answer: D.**
Rationale: TR is the most common right-sided valvular lesion in adults. TR is commonly associated with dilatation of RA, tricuspid annular dilation secondary to right ventricular enlargement, incomplete TV closure in addition to TV prolapse. IVC is often dilated due to increased right atrial pressure and venous congestion.

4. **Correct Answer: D.**
Rationale: Right ventricular hypertrophy is seen when the right ventricular lateral wall thickness exceeds 5 mm. This can be associated with a situation of right ventricular systolic pressure overload due to elevated PA pressure, chronic thromboembolic pulmonary hypertension, RVOT obstruction, or PS. Inversely, certain conditions are associated with right ventricular wall thinning, such as right ventricular myocardium infarction, Uhl syndrome, or arrhythmogenic right ventricular cardiomyopathy. In arrhythmogenic RV cardiomyopathy, aneurysms typically occur in the anterior infundibulum, basal inferior wall, and apex. There are no accepted echocardiographic criteria to define an abnormally thin RV wall.

5. **Correct Answer: A.**
Rationale: The eccentricity index has been described as a modality to evaluate interventricular septal motion through the cardiac cycle. It is the ratio of the vertical diameter over the horizontal diameter of the LV taken from a transgastric short-axis view. The vertical diameter corresponds to the anterior to inferior diameter, and the horizontal diameter corresponds to the septal to lateral diameter. These diameters are measured at end diastole and end systole. Under normal pressure and volume loading conditions, the eccentricity index is 1. The ratio will increase over 1 during systole and diastole in right ventricular pressure overload. Volume overload will be associated with a ratio greater than 1 only during end diastole, when the right ventricle is being overfilled and distended.

6. **Correct Answer: D.**
Rationale: The eustachian valve and Chiari network are typically attached to the orifice of the IVC. Failure of regression of the right or inferior valve of the sinus venosus during gestation may result in a persistent eustachian valve. The Chiari network is a fenestrated, strand-like structure within the right atrial cavity. Although it most often arises from the orifice of the inferior vena cave, it may originate from the lateral wall of the RA, the coronary sinus, or the interatrial septum. A ridgelike structure located at the junction between IVC and the RA is most likely to be the eustachian valve which is a consequence of a failure of regression of the right or inferior valve of the sinus venosus during gestation. The crista terminalis can be seen at the junction of the superior vena cava and the RA. It represents a ridge that separates the venous component of the RA and the contractile portion.

7. **Correct Answer: C.**
Rationale: The pulse wave Doppler interrogation of the hepatic veins shows an inverted systolic (S) wave. This finding can be associated with right ventricular diastolic dysfunction that leads to a decrease of the systolic hepatic vein flow velocity and eventually, a systolic-to-diastolic ratio less than 1 (S/D <1) that may progress to blunting of the S wave before it became completely reversed. Systolic retrograde flow in the hepatic veins during systole can also be due to significant TR.

8. **Correct Answer: B.**
Rationale: Deep transgastric RVOT view can be used to obtain measurement of cardiac output. Pulse wave Doppler interrogation to obtain velocity-time integral (VTI) of the ejection phase combined with measurement of the diameter to obtain the area of the RVOT can be used according to the following formula to obtain cardiac output: Right ventricular output = Heart rate × $Area_{RVOT}$ × VTI_{RVOT}.

9. **Correct Answer: C.**
Rationale: RVFAC is defined as the difference between end-diastolic and end-systolic right ventricular area compared to the end-diastolic right ventricular area; (RV end-diastolic area – RV end-systolic right ventricular area)/end-diastolic right ventricular area × 100. RVFAC is obtained by tracing the right ventricular endocardium in diastole and systole from the lateral portion of the tricuspid annulus, along the lateral wall to the apex, and then to the septal portion of the tricuspid annulus, all along the interventricular septum.
A limitation of RVFAC is that it does not examine the contribution of the RVOT that corresponds to approximately 20% of the ejected RV volume. The lower reference value for normal right ventricular systolic function for RVFAC is 35%. Some references grade the severity of right ventricular dysfunction based on RVFAC according to the following: mild (RVFAC 25%-31%), moderate (RVFAC 18%-24%), and severe (RVFAC <18%). RVFAC provides an estimate of global RV systolic function as it has been shown to correlate with RVEF by magnetic resonance imaging.

10. **Correct Answer: D.**
Rationale: LAX systolic excursion of the lateral aspect of the tricuspid annulus represents an easily recognizable longitudinal movement on echocardiography and may be used as an indicator of RV systolic function. TAPSE is measured in M-mode and it must be corrected for angulation of interrogation due to the tricuspid annulus motion vector that is oblique when assessed using the ME 4C view. Important limitations must be considered concerning the use of the TAPSE in cardiac surgery patients. First, the annular motion vector is oblique to the ME 4C view which results in angle-related errors. TAPSE is load dependent and not reliable after pericardectomy. It reflects only the longitudinal displacement of a single segment of the complex right ventricular three-dimensional structure as it does not assess the contribution to ejection from the inward motion of the free wall and the RVOT.

IV Clinical Challenges

15 Transesophageal Echocardiography for Coronary Revascularization and Mechanical Support

Justiaan Swanevelder, Ettienne Coetzee, and Edwin Turton

Transesophageal echocardiography (TEE) has evolved into an indispensable tool in the perioperative management of patients undergoing coronary artery bypass grafting (CABG) and mechanical circulatory support (MCS). While early literature emphasized its role in intraoperative monitoring and identification of unrecognized cardiac pathology, recent literature has solidified TEE's impact on surgical decision-making, hemodynamic optimization, and improved patient outcomes (1-3). Previous guidelines consistently endorsed the use of TEE for hemodynamically unstable patients (2-5). However, current recommendations now further advocate its routine use in all patients undergoing CABG and those requiring MCS, unless contraindications exist (1,6). This shift reflects growing evidence demonstrating TEE's critical role in optimizing intraoperative decision-making, assessing ventricular function, guiding hemodynamic management, and improving overall patient outcomes.

TEE provides real-time assessment of ventricular function, preload status, regional wall motion abnormalities (RWMAs), and intraoperative ischemia, which are particularly relevant in CABG patients with impaired left ventricular (LV) function. Historically, studies demonstrated that preoperative transthoracic echocardiography (TTE) was often inadequate in detecting subtle cardiac pathology, particularly in patients with poor acoustic windows. The superiority of TEE in perioperative assessment has further increased its routine use in CABG, with studies reporting significant alterations in surgical planning based on intraoperative findings (7). TEE plays a pivotal role in both on-pump and off-pump procedures by guiding graft placement, assessing the adequacy of revascularization, and detecting intraoperative complications such as embolic events, aortic pathology, or unexpected valvular disease. Recent large-scale retrospective analyses suggest that TEE use during CABG is associated with lower operative mortality, particularly in high-risk patients (1). The ability to immediately reassess cardiac function postrevascularization allows for tailored hemodynamic management, including optimized fluid resuscitation, inotropic support, and, when necessary, initiation of MCS. TEE has identified previously unrecognized cardiac pathology in 20% to 33% of patients, prompting modifications in surgical management in 10% to 25% of cases (8). By providing real-time, clinically relevant data, TEE influences surgical decision-making, leading to changes before and after bypass, ultimately optimizing perioperative management and patient outcomes (9-12) (Table 15.1). The new information provided and subsequent interventions have also been shown to be cost effective (13). Preoperative assessments in the cardiology clinic may not always provide an accurate representation of a patient's pathology due to limitations in TTE, incomplete or inaccurate reporting, and/or the progression of underlying disease (11,14).

The use of TEE enables clinicians to correlate measured pressures (such as central venous- or pulmonary artery pressure) with actual cardiac filling status, which can guide postoperative management in the intensive care unit. This is especially valuable in patients with hypertension or ventricular systolic and diastolic dysfunction, where venous pressure measurements alone may not accurately reflect intracardiac volume or preload status (15,16).

Beyond CABG, TEE has become critical in the perioperative management of patients requiring mechanical support, including intra-aortic balloon pumps (IABPs), left ventricular assist devices (LVADs),

TABLE 15.1 Role of Transesophageal Echocardiography in Patients Undergoing Coronary Artery Bypass Grafting

To supplement cardiac workup
• Confirm diagnosis and evaluate cardiac function for patients undergoing emergent surgery. • Provide an updated examination of cardiac and valvular functions. • Evaluate potential target sites of coronary revascularization by administration of contrast agents (evaluate coronary perfusion) or dobutamine (stress test to evaluate viability).
To diagnose impact of previously unrecognized pathology on surgical procedure

• Valvular pathology:
  • Aortic insufficiency—distension of the ventricle during cardiopulmonary bypass
  • Mitral regurgitation (MR)—dynamic MR, ischemic MR
  • Aortic stenosis—previously undetected, underestimated, or disease progression
• Patent foramen ovale/atrial septal defect
• Emboli, thrombus, or mass
• Persistent left superior vena cava
• Regional wall motion abnormalities—pre- or postbypass
• Aortic dissection—iatrogenic or previously undetected
• Atherosclerotic disease

To assist the surgeon in the conduct of circulatory management
Positioning/placement of: • Aortic cross-clamp • Coronary sinus cardioplegia catheter • Intra-aortic balloon pump • Femoral venous cannula Port access (endoaortic catheter, venous cannula, coronary sinus catheter) • Ventricular assist device
To facilitate the conduct of circulatory management or surgical procedure
• Redo sternotomy • Conduct bypass: assess left ventricle chamber size for distension • Plan management strategies for separation from cardiopulmonary bypass for patients with poor cardiac function • Separation from cardiopulmonary bypass (titration of volume and pharmacologic or mechanical support)
To diagnose cause of acute cardiovascular compromise
• New myocardial ischemia • New valvular lesions • Ventricular failure • Ventricular filling

and extracorporeal membrane oxygenation (ECMO). The rapid assessment of LV and right ventricular (RV) function, as well as dynamic monitoring of device function, enables early detection of complications such as thrombosis, inadequate unloading, and RV failure (7). Advanced modalities such as real-time three-dimensional (RT3D) echocardiography and strain imaging further enhance the precision of ventricular function assessment, particularly in cases of dyssynchrony or regional ischemia (17).

Modern guidelines now advocate for routine TEE use in high-risk cardiac surgery, including CABG and MCS implantation (7). The shift from its traditional role in diagnostic assessment to a real-time, decision-guiding modality underscores the expanding capabilities of intraoperative echocardiography.

In summary, the role of TEE in coronary revascularization and mechanical support has transitioned from an adjunct monitoring tool to an essential component of perioperative cardiac decision-making and patient management. Its ability to refine surgical planning, enhance hemodynamic optimization, and improve patient outcomes ensures its continued integration into modern cardiac anesthetic and surgical practice.

SAFETY AND COMPLICATIONS

The risk of major complications, notably perforation of the esophagus, remains small, with an incidence reported between 0.01% and 0.02% in earlier studies (18,19). However, recent audits suggest that the incidence may be slightly higher, at approximately 0.08%, particularly in patients undergoing complex or extended procedures (20). Minor complications such as sore throat and odynophagia are relatively common but can often be minimized through careful probe insertion and the use of a laryngoscope. Antibiotic prophylaxis is generally not indicated but may be considered in high-risk scenarios, such as ventilated patients with prosthetic valves in intensive care settings, where oropharyngeal bacterial translocation poses a concern (21). Careful patient selection is crucial, as contraindications, including recent esophageal surgery, significant esophageal pathology, or a history of esophagectomy, present substantial risks (6,22). In the eyes of many experts, absolute contraindications should be strictly adhered to with a multidisciplinary approach recommended for complex cases.

PREBYPASS EXAMINATION

The prebypass intraoperative examination should target the pathology at hand, be performed in a systematic manner, and organized into a comprehensive study. In contrast, the post-cardiopulmonary bypass (post-CPB) examination is usually targeted toward assessing the results of the intervention, although a routine examination should also be performed to troubleshoot the possible complications. Preoperative digital echo loops should be recorded as part of the medical record and to review and compare with examination findings during the postbypass period. The preoperative ventricular status often undergoes significant changes during the coronary revascularization procedure, and may result in altered ventricular function postoperatively. In addition to the recorded images, a TEE examination should always include a written report for the patient's records and a discussion of the findings with the cardiac surgeon.

Assessment of Ventricular Function

Traditionally, LV filling and cardiac output (CO) have been quantified by using a PAC. Intraoperative TEE often supplements or replaces these measures in current practice. Real-time echo images allow accurate qualitative evaluation of CO, quantification of ventricular and valvular functions (Video 15.1), intraoperative hemodynamic assessment, and most importantly contractility. Hypovolemia or severe LV dysfunction is easy to detect but various degrees of RWMAs can often be subtle as well as subjective and operator dependent. The standard views used to evaluate global LV function or regional ischemia (23) are discussed in Chapter 4: Diagnosis of Myocardial Ischemia. Table 15.2 summarizes the other TEE tools available to assess cardiac function.

New Advances in Intraoperative Assessment of Global and Regional Cardiac Function

Recent advancements in myocardial deformation imaging techniques, such as tissue Doppler imaging (TDI) and RT3D echocardiography, have greatly enhanced our understanding of ventricular function and ischemic

TABLE 15.2 Assessment of Cardiac Function by Transesophageal Echocardiography

Preload
LV end-diastolic area
LV end-diastolic pressure (estimated from AI jet)
LA pressure (estimated from pulmonary vein flow)
Contractility
Fractional area change (calculated)
Ejection fraction (visual estimate)
Segmental wall motion
Fractional shortening
Tissue Doppler
Quantitative hemodynamics
Stroke volume/cardiac output
Systemic vascular resistance
RV systolic pressure
Diastolic function
Mitral inflow velocities
Pulmonary vein blood flow velocities

AI, aortic insufficiency; LA, left atrium; LV, left ventricle; RV, right ventricle.

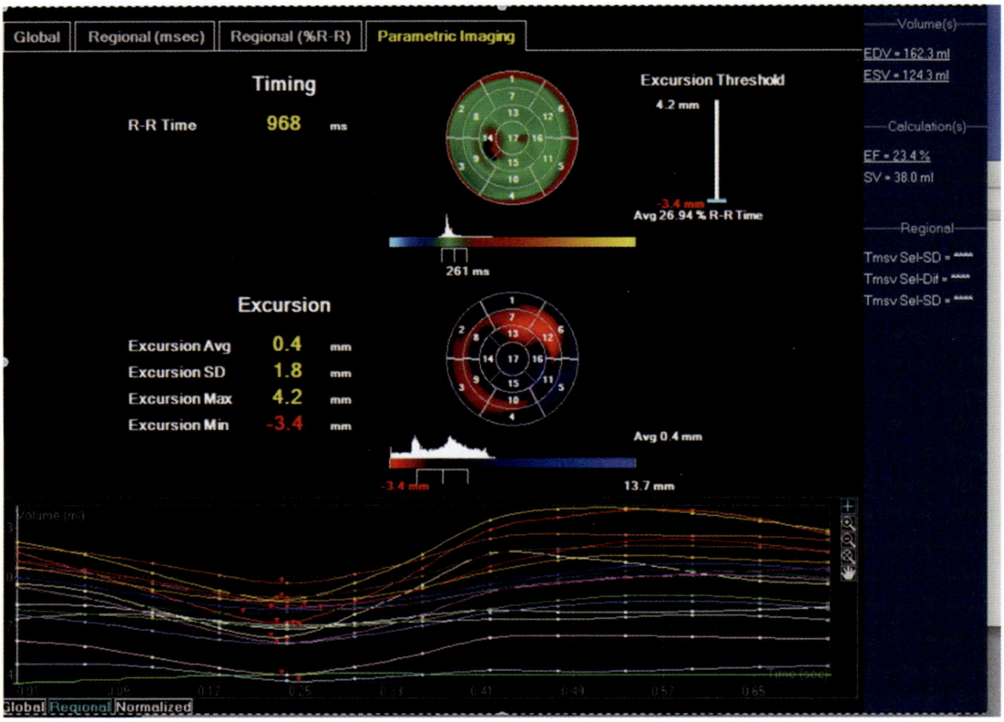

FIGURE 15.1 The "bull's eye" depicts the standard deviation of time taken by individual segments in cross-section to contract maximally. This may aid resynchronization therapy.

changes. These improvements have markedly increased our ability to quantify ischemia, offering more precise assessments of intraoperative cardiac function (24). Because of angle dependency, fast-changing hemodynamic conditions, and lack of accurate validation studies, intraoperative TDI has never found its way into routine intraoperative TEE practice and has been replaced by other techniques such as RT3D strain analysis to display myocardial deformation.

RT3D is useful to search for myocardial ischemia in high-risk surgical patients, in addition to assessing LV volumes and ejection fraction (EF) (25). Multiple slices from the apex to the base can now be displayed simultaneously (26,27). A computer-generated endocardial cast can graphically display the timing of contraction of each of the 17 segments to detect delays that may represent myocardial ischemia (Figures 15.1 and 15.2). Evaluation of RWMAs with RT3D is still qualitative, and with the newer tools available, the observer bias can be minimized. Initial studies of RT3D using dobutamine stress echo suggest that these multislice displays are highly specific for the detection of angiographically confirmed ischemic myocardial regions (27). There are other quantitative methods of detecting myocardial ischemic deformation. For example, strain measured by speckle tracking uses two-dimensional (2D) images and analyzes the movement of stable acoustic markers (speckles) between frames which are now more available rather than used for research (26-28). RT3D enables tracking of myocardial strain in three dimensions, overcoming limitations of 2DE, such as out-of-plane motion (29). However, reproducibility remains a challenge. Automated approaches to cardiac chamber quantification align RT3D results more closely with MRI standards, addressing prior issues of underestimation and overcoming the 2D limitations of fractional shortening of the ventricles (29).

Monitoring of Ischemia

Visualizing the Aortic Root, Coronary Arteries, and Coronary Blood Flow

TEE imaging of the coronaries is discussed in detail in Chapter 4: Diagnosis of Myocardial Ischemia. As the aortic root runs oblique to the sagittal plane, the origin of the left coronary artery (LCA) is interrogated in

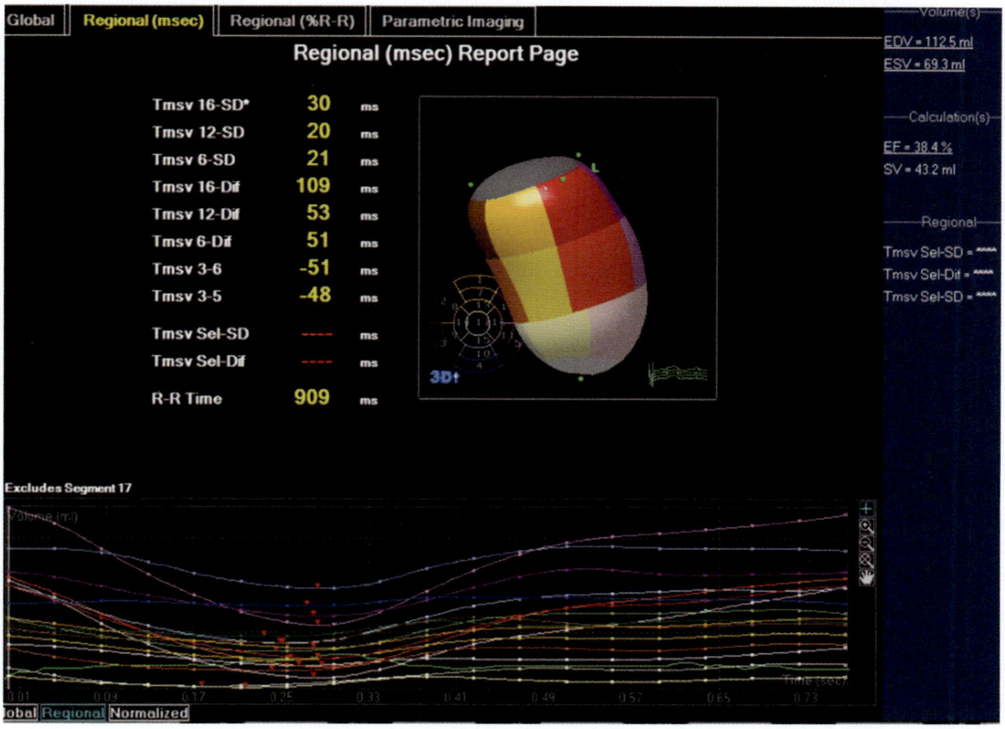

FIGURE 15.2 Complete 3D regional wall motion map. The regional segments' movements are displayed in milliseconds.

a more superior (cephalad) plane than the right coronary artery (RCA) in TEE short-axis (SAX) views. TEE visualizes approximately 70% to 88% of the left (Video 15.2) and 25% to 50% of the RCA ostia (30). Although difficult to quantify, flow can often be visualized with TEE in more distal branches of the larger coronary arteries, that is, the circumflex coronary artery in the atrioventricular groove (Figure 15.3; Video 15.3) (31). It is important to recognize, both for ischemia detection and revascularization procedures, the patient variability in the coronary blood supply to the various myocardial segments (Figure 4.2).

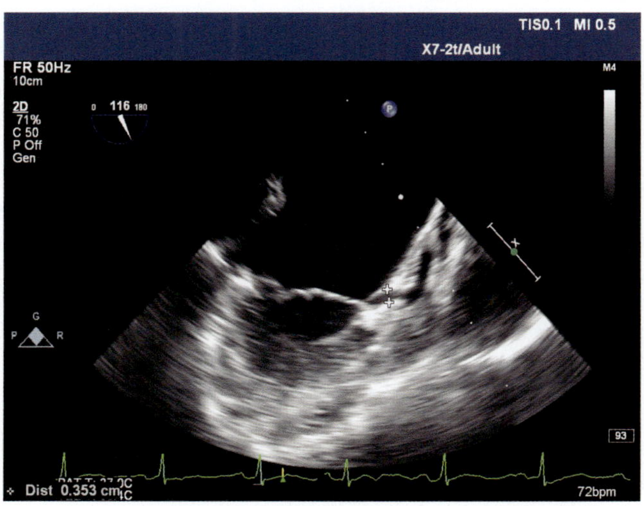

FIGURE 15.3 A 2D demonstration of the circumflex coronary artery visualized in the atrioventricular groove (Video 15.3).

TABLE 15.3 Segmental Scores in Increasing Order of Severity

Normal—1
Hypokinesis—2
Akinesis (negligible wall thickening)—3
Dyskinesis (paradoxical systolic motion)—4
Aneurysmal (diastolic deformation)—5

It is important to score any myocardial segments with RWMAs prior to bypass and evaluate post-CABG for improvement (Table 15.3). Unfortunately, not all RWMAs benefit from coronary revascularization. Most akinetic and dyskinetic regions are the result of transmural myocardial infarction and thus represent nonviable myocardium. In general, hypokinetic segments are viable and may represent active ischemia.

Shortcomings of Transesophageal Echocardiography

RWMAs can be difficult to quantify because the ventricle twists when contracting, causing different myocardial segments to move in and out of the imaging plane during one cardiac cycle. The endocardial and epicardial borders cannot always be completely identified, limiting accurate quantification of wall thickening. Bear in mind that interpreting regional wall motion is an operator-dependent skill, therefore very subjective. RWMAs may also occur in the absence of coronary artery disease, for example, when paced.

NEW REGIONAL WALL MOTION ABNORMALITY AFTER CARDIOPULMONARY BYPASS

What Does It Signify?

In two classic studies by Roizen and Smith, the occurrence of postoperative myocardial infarction was increased in patients who exhibited new RWMAs during CABG or aortic vascular surgery (32,33). The incidence of postoperative infarction was more strongly associated with new RWMAs than with new electrocardiographic changes. Swaminathan confirmed worsening RWMA immediately after CABG was associated with a 2-fold increase in long-term major adverse cardiac events (34). Although TEE may be sensitive in diagnosing ischemia, a new RWMA does not always predict myocardial infarction. In the study of Leung et al (35), a myocardial infarction was subsequently diagnosed in only one of eight patients in whom a new, persistent RWMA had developed. This apparent discrepancy is consistent with the concept of "myocardial stunning," in which an acute episode of myocardial ischemia can result in wall motion abnormalities that later resolve without any permanent injury. RWMAs can be experienced sometimes post CPB owing to accumulation of air due to incomplete de-airing before separating from bypass. RT3D is a valuable modality for precise quantification of regional wall motion during revascularization procedures (17).

What Should We Do?

The appearance of new RWMAs after bypass is common, but they may be caused by factors other than acute graft occlusion. These include transient ischemia resulting from the distal coronary embolization of air or debris, spasm of the left internal mammary artery, low coronary perfusion pressure, increased oxygen demand due to inotropic drugs, myocardial stunning, myocardial inflammation and surgical trauma, electrolyte disturbance, cardiac pacing, and conduction abnormalities. Any apparent dyskinesia due to conduction abnormalities can be differentiated from ischemia by looking for myocardial thickening. Although some investigators have suggested that the detection of new RWMAs warrants further surgical intervention, the sensitivity and specificity of new RWMA to predict graft failure confirmed by angiography in a large retrospective analysis do not support such an aggressive approach (36); this has to be on an individual case basis. The additional morbidity/mortality associated with the resumption of bypass to place another graft would likely outweigh the potential benefit in most cases. A more progressive approach is presented in Table 15.4.

The surgeon can assess graft patency and flow by visual inspection to confirm the absence of graft kinking or torsion, by stripping the vein graft to confirm refill, by palpation, by transit time flow measurements (37),

TABLE 15.4 Strategy for Management of a New Regional Wall Motion Abnormality After Separation From Cardiopulmonary Bypass

Increase the coronary perfusion pressure.
Restore normal conduction pathways (sinus rhythm, A-pace, biventricular pace A-V sequential).
Normalize electrolytes and arterial blood gases.
Inspect coronary grafts: Visual inspection and stripping Doppler flow examination Echo contrast examination
Return to cardiopulmonary bypass. Consider more invasive cardiac support (intra-aortic balloon counterpulsation (91), ventricular assist devices or extra corporeal membrane oxygenation).

and using an epicardial surface Doppler flow probe. Decreased flow in an arterial conduit can result from poor distal runoff, a compromised anastomosis, or vasospasm that can be effectively treated with nitroglycerin, papaverine, or a calcium channel antagonist such as nicardipine or nifedipine.

Ventricular septal hypokinesis and dyskinesia are common immediately after separation from CPB and usually recover within 10 to 15 minutes. The abnormal conduction progression inherent with RV pacing results in contractile dyssynchrony, which may be interpreted as a septal RWMA. Temporary atrioventricular or biventricular pacing may be considered to restore contractile synchrony (38,39). If septal dyskinesia persists or suddenly appears after a significant time postbypass, then the surgeon should be advised to check the LAD and RCA grafts if present. RWMAs in other areas of the LV need the patency of the graft to be checked sooner. If an RWMA persists or, more commonly, global dysfunction is seen with TEE, then circulatory support should be started either with inotropes or by inserting a circulatory assist device. The level of assist depends on the dysfunction seen. TEE aids placement of the devices and monitoring of recovery.

Differentiation between poor perfusion and stunned myocardium is more difficult. Possible strategies include epicardial scanning and the administration of a contrast agent to determine coronary flow patterns. If the area demonstrates flow of the contrast agent, the RWMA may resolve with time. The absence of contrast agent suggests a technical problem at the anastomosis or distal obstruction in the native coronary. Such information can help guide any possible surgical intervention. The technique of contrast perfusion can also be performed before bypass. If a specific area is likely to be infarcted, as demonstrated by the absence of contrast flow and significant wall thinning, surgical interventions are not likely to be of value. Both these techniques are uncommonly applied in routine operative practice, and their impact remains to be determined.

ACUTE CARDIAC DYSFUNCTION: ASSESSMENT AND MANAGEMENT

Cardiac dysfunction may develop at any time during the perioperative period. TEE examination of the heart and great vessels can provide a quick assessment of the primary factors related to hypotension: preload, afterload, myocardial contractility, valvular function, and integrity of the aorta. TEE can significantly affect the surgical and anesthetic management, especially in high-risk patients or in patients with acute hemodynamic collapse. The reader is reminded that post-CPB cardiac function must be interpreted in the context of the prebypass examination findings and the occurrence of any significant bypass events. The myocardial performance index (MPI) has been shown to be a useful predictor of postoperative outcomes following revascularization, with elevated preoperative MPI values strongly correlating with increased postoperative inotropic and vasopressor requirements. Additionally, the need for an IABP to sustain CO postrevascularization aligns closely with both reduced preoperative left ventricular ejection fraction (LVEF), higher MPI values and mortality outcome (40).

The TEE examination quickly provides data that guide pharmacologic therapy and volume resuscitation. In several studies, TEE significantly modified both surgical and hemodynamic decision-making during the perioperative period (41-43). The echocardiographic findings associated with common causes of hypotension and cardiac dysfunction are presented in Table 15.5 and discussed below. Mechanical cardiac displacement

TABLE 15.5 Echocardiographic Findings in Hypotension and Cardiac Dysfunction

	LVEDA	LVESA	FAC	CO
Decreased LV preload	↓	↓	0	↓↓
Decreased LV afterload	0	↓↓	↑↑	↑
Increased LV afterload	↑	↑	↓	↓
LV dysfunction	↑	↑↑	↓↓	↓
RV dysfunction	↓	↓	↓/0	↓
Acute mitral regurgitation LV distension	↑↑	0/↑	↓	↓

↑, increased; ↓, decreased; 0, unchanged; CO, cardiac output; FAC, fractional area change; LV, left ventricle; LVEDA, left ventricular end-diastolic area; LVESA, left ventricular end-systolic area; RV, right ventricle.

is often necessary for successful off-pump coronary artery surgery (OPCAB). This can lead to transient biventricular systolic and diastolic dysfunction. The use of transesophageal echocardiography is essential to evaluate hemodynamic disturbances associated with cardiac displacement, such as ventricular interdependence, dyskinesia, significant mitral regurgitation (MR), and LV outflow tract obstruction. These conditions, if present, may compromise hemodynamic stability and are not well-tolerated during grafting procedures (41).

Hypovolemia

Hypovolemia, a common cause of hypotension, is often related to the obstruction of venous return as a consequence of venous cannula placement. After separation from bypass, hypovolemia can be caused by reequilibration of volume as well as bleeding. The assessment of LV chamber size by TEE has been shown to be a sensitive measure of LV preload. The quantitative analysis of changes in the transgastric short-axis (TG SAX) area could reliably detect even a 2.5% decrease in intravascular volume (44). Left ventricular end-diastolic volume (LVEDV) reflects ventricular preload, while left ventricular end-systolic volume (LVESV) assesses systolic function by measuring postcontraction volume. TEE allows direct visualization of diastolic chamber size for assessment of fluid status. 3D echocardiography offers more accurate volumetric data, especially in the abnormal ventricle. While TEE enhances visualization, it has limitations in standardizing chamber dimensions compared to TTE (45).

After separation from CPB, the LV is usually stunned and noncompliant, especially when the LV is hypertrophic. This makes assessment of filling difficult when relying on a pressure reading from a CVP or PAC as higher pressures will be necessary to achieve optimal preload. Similarly, many dynamic indicators of fluid responsiveness such as pulse pressure variation (PPV) rely on heart-lung interaction and are not valid in the postischemic ventricle and "open chest" though PPV remains useful in the postoperative period (42,46,47). In addition, volume responsiveness can be assessed by tilting the patient head down and confirming an increase in CO by aortic valve (AV) VTI in this situation. An interatrial septum that remains curved toward the right throughout the cardiac cycle is another indicator of raised left atrial (LA) pressure and ventricular dysfunction (48).

Dynamic Mitral Regurgitation

LV dysfunction, often from ischemia, can lead to distension of the LA and LV and papillary muscle dysfunction. In addition, excessive volume resuscitation or increased afterload can also result in LV or LA distension resulting in incomplete coaptation of the mitral leaflets and a dynamic central jet of regurgitation. Significant MR may require mitral valve (MV) surgery or hemodynamic management, such as adjusting the systemic vascular resistance, administering inotropic agents, or decreasing the LV preload. LA volume index is a strong predictor of dynamic changes in MR after CABG. Intraoperative LV and LA function is important in postoperative MR progression, suggesting that early detection could help predict MR changes over time (49).

Right Ventricular Dysfunction

The development of tricuspid regurgitation (TR) can occur in the presence of increased pulmonary pressures and RV failure. RV dysfunction is a common contributor to perioperative low CO and hypotension. The RV can be affected by pathology of the LV and vice versa. Following myocardial infarction, this ventricular interdependence can affect the shape, size, and function (pressure-volume relationship) of the other ventricle, and is a predictor of outcome. RV dysfunction is associated with RV dilation, TR, an abnormal "D-shaped" septal wall (septal shift), and decreased LV chamber size. Management includes checking for ischemia (especially right coronary region of perfusion), optimizing the pulmonary vascular resistance (PVR), maintaining the systemic perfusion pressure and enhancing contractility. One should avoid rapid volume expansion of the right ventricle to reduce the risk of RV failure. An additional risk will be the sole use of retrograde cardioplegia often associated with inadequate RV protection, as the balloon on the cannula can obstruct the right cardiac vein, preventing cardioplegia reaching the territory drained by it.

RV systolic dysfunction following CABG is commonly diagnosed by 2D echo images using midesophageal (ME) four-chamber, ME RV inflow/outflow, the TG SAX views, as well as the TG RV view and TG RV inflow-outflow 130° (50). Of note, tricuspid annular plane systolic excursion (TAPSE) is not a reliable indicator of RV dysfunction postbypass due to the open pericardium. After open heart surgery, any residual intraventricular air is more likely to enter the RCA because of its ostium's anterior position, causing temporary RV ischemia and dysfunction. While the chest is open, a distended and impaired RV wall can easily be visualized directly. Cardiac dysfunction and recovery after CPB can be monitored by TEE. This can be managed instituting cardiac rest (reinitiating CPB), initiating inotropic agents to support the RV (eg, norepinephrine in conjunction with milrinone and/or dobutamine) and adjusting PVR by titration of pulmonary vasodilators (eg, nitric oxide, prostaglandin E_1, or nitroglycerin) (Videos 15.4 and 15.5).

Low Ejection Fraction

Patients presenting for surgery who have reduced LVEF are often on β-blockers. Ventricular function may initially appear sluggish on TEE during and after separation from bypass, often requiring temporary inotropic or chronotropic support as the heart recovers from post cross-clamp stunning. TEE monitoring helps assessment of contractility and filling and facilitates weaning of inotropes. Patients with a prebypass LVEF less than 30% are likely to require inotropic support postbypass. If dysfunction persists in spite of optimal hemodynamic management, insertion of an IABP may be indicated. Failing this, the institution of venoarterial extracorporeal membrane oxygenation (VA ECMO) or a ventricular assist device (VAD) is the next consideration for temporary support.

Unexpected Diagnosis of Coexisting Problems

Unexpected intraoperative findings secondary to interval disease progression or previously undetected findings are not uncommon in patients who have undergone a standard workup, (11,14). Diagnosis of previously undetected pathologies can dramatically alter the surgical plan, for example, additional insertion of a mitral ring for severe MR, or closure of a significant patent foramen ovale (PFO).

Intracardiac Shunts; Patent Foramen Ovale or Atrial Septal Defect

Up to 25% of adult cardiac surgical populations have an intracardiac shunt which can affect the surgical plan and long-term prognosis. If a patent foramen ovale is found incidentally during CABG surgery, this may be considered a risk for paradoxical air embolism and could affect neurologic outcome. The decision regarding closure, including surgical versus interventional approaches, usually depends on the size and direction of the shunt as well as individual surgical preference (51). When an open-chamber procedure is performed in conjunction with CABG surgery or in a patient with a stroke history, an incidental PFO should be closed. Postoperatively identified PFO is associated with a significantly increased risk of ischemic stroke, worse respiratory outcomes, and prolonged hospitalization (52).

A PFO can be most reliably detected when the interatrial septum is examined with color flow Doppler (CFD). The color scale should be adjusted down to allow accurate detection of the low-flow velocity difference between the left and right atrium across the PFO. Release of Valsalva breath following agitated air contrast injection in the ME four-chamber and bicaval views, the presence of contrast bubbles in the left atrium within five cardiac cycles confirms the diagnosis of a PFO.

Intraoperative detection of a previously unsuspected PFO has relevance to ICU management and emphasizes the need for an accurate echocardiographic report in the medical record and communication with the ICU staff. For example, if atelectasis develops post-CABG surgery resulting in an increase in pulmonary pressures and RV afterload, the increase in right heart pressures can cause the shunt direction to change or exacerbate an existing right-to-left intracardiac shunt, with subsequent worsening hypoxemia.

Pleural Effusions

Iatrogenic pleural effusions often develop when the pleura is opened during internal mammary artery harvesting and may be already present in patients with cardiac failure. This may have a marked effect on post-CPB ventilation and oxygenation, as well as the hemodynamic status of a patient with borderline cardiac function. Ultrasound can easily detect both left- and right-sided pleural effusions. Left pleural effusions can be seen in the ME descending aortic SAX view. Right-sided effusions are seen by turning the probe from the ME four-chamber view to the right (Videos 15.6 and 15.7).

Previously Unknown Aortic Valve Pathology

Intraoperative TEE is instrumental in detecting previously undiagnosed AV disease during CABG. Its use has been associated with lower operative mortality, particularly in higher-risk patients, and an increased likelihood of unplanned valve procedures, underscoring its value in intraoperative surgical decision-making (1). Quantification of AV disease and the decision when to perform a combined CABG and aortic valve replacement (AVR) procedure can be difficult, especially when LV function is compromised, and loading conditions may be altered. Evidence shows that a subsequent AVR after a previous CABG has a higher mortality than a single combined procedure (53). The degree of calcification is important because the progression of the disease process even in the patient without symptoms may be rapid. Progression is quite variable, with a decrease in effective valve area ranging from approximately 0.1 to 0.3 cm^2/y. In a primary CABG procedure, it is therefore recommended that AVR should be considered in a patient with even moderate AS. Best practice dictates that patients are adequately investigated prior to surgery and decisions about concomitant AV surgery and risk are discussed before the patient is scheduled for surgery. The development of TAVR means that future progression of AS can be treated without the need for redo surgery, although it has its own associated risks.

A patient with coronary artery disease may need insertion of an IABP during ischemic or unstable periods after CPB. If aortic regurgitation is diagnosed intraoperatively, the use of an IABP is contraindicated due to its effect increasing the LV end-diastolic volume and wall tension.

Coexisting Mitral Valve Regurgitation—Combined Coronary Artery Bypass Grafting and Mitral Valve Surgery

Patients presenting for CABG often have coexisting functional or ischemic MR (eg, Carpentier classes I and III) of a mild or moderate degree. The team needs to decide whether or not to surgically address the MV pathology during the coronary operation. The altered loading conditions under anesthesia should be taken into consideration when quantifying MR. The reduction in ventricular chamber size, systemic vascular resistance, and blood pressure that typically occurs in anesthetized patients can significantly reduce the degree of mitral incompetence compared to the awake state. In order to gain more reliable information, it is advised to simulate awake loading conditions by increasing both preload and afterload with a vasopressor.

In patients with mild functional ischemic MR (graded 1-2), the MV is usually left untouched. For moderate ischemic MR (>2+ under anesthesia), the controversy regarding surgical intervention persists (Figure 15.4; Video 15.8); however, recent guidelines indicate that MV surgery is reasonable when CABG is performed for myocardial ischemia (Class 2a, Level of Evidence B-NR), emphasizing an individualized approach (53). In severe ischemic MR (≥3+), MV intervention remains recommended, with chordal-sparing mitral valve replacement (MVR) increasingly favored over downsized annuloplasty in patients with chronic severe secondary MR and persistent symptoms despite guideline-directed medical therapy. While prior studies have not demonstrated a survival benefit for adding MV surgery to CABG in moderate MR, the guidelines suggest that surgical intervention may still be considered on a case-by-case basis. The final decision whether to proceed with mitral surgery in the setting of ischemic heart disease depends on the surgeon. Importantly, moderate MR secondary to a structural leaflet abnormality (eg, Carpentier class II) should be corrected as the disease is progressive and revascularization alone will not improve valve function.

In summary, the 2020 ACC/AHA guidelines continue to support a conservative approach for mild functional ischemic MR (1-2+), recommending that the MV remain untouched as LV function may improve with CABG alone. Compared to previous recommendations, the 2020 update leans slightly more in favor of MV surgery for select patients with moderate MR and strengthens support for chordal-sparing MVR over annuloplasty in severe MR requiring intervention. The overall approach remains consistent, with an emphasis on avoiding unnecessary MV surgery in mild MR, reinforcing the role of CABG in improving LV function and MR severity.

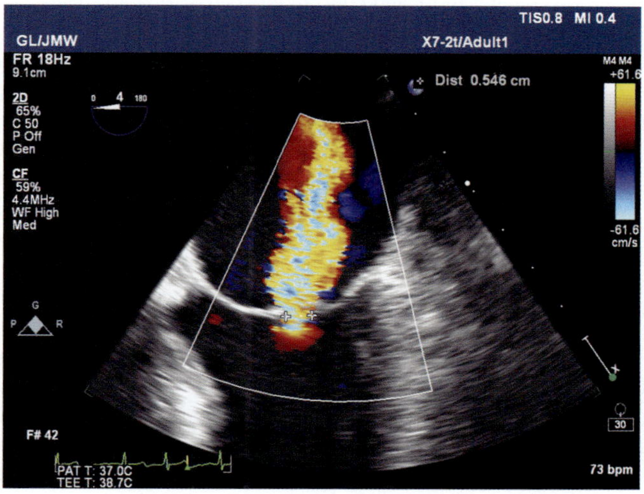

FIGURE 15.4 Midesophageal four-chamber view of a patient with a central jet of moderate mitral regurgitation based on vena contracta of 0.546 cm (Video 15.8).

Proposals about concomitant MV surgery are best considered before the patient is scheduled for surgery. The introduction of MitraClip inserted for functional MV disease is a controversial point, but can be performed at a later time if severe MR progresses or persists.

Use of 3D Echo in Coronary Artery Revascularization

RT3D TEE has become an essential tool for evaluating ventricular function, offering superior volumetric assessment compared to traditional 2D imaging. Initially, its application during CABG was limited, but it is now routinely integrated into revascularization procedures. RT3D TEE enhances the assessment of cardiac chamber volumes, regional ischemia, and CO by eliminating some of the geometric assumptions inherent in 2D imaging, thereby improving accuracy and reducing subjectivity (29,54-56).

Three-dimensional LVEF and volume measurements are typically derived from the ME four-chamber and two-chamber views. To ensure accurate full-volume acquisition and minimize foreshortening, the echocardiographer must ensure that the entire LV is within the imaging field. A full-volume image is considered optimal when the mitral annulus, septal and lateral walls, and apex are clearly visualized. Ventilation can briefly be paused to reduce stitch artifacts in multibeat 3D imaging. Recent technologic advancements have improved single-beat volume imaging allowing higher frame rates and reduced artifact generation, particularly beneficial for patients with arrhythmias or hemodynamic instability. Additionally, the new-generation matrix-array transducer now combines 2D and 3D imaging, improving workflow efficiency in perioperative settings.

The integration of artificial intelligence (AI) and machine learning into 3D echocardiographic imaging has significantly improved real-time image acquisition, automated border detection, and chamber quantification. AI-driven segmentation tools minimize operator dependency, enhance chamber alignment, and reduce foreshortening error (56).

Machine learning models trained on large echocardiographic datasets assist in artifact reduction, improve stitching accuracy in multibeat acquisitions, and enhance volume-rendered imaging by intelligently selecting optimal frames. These developments are paving the way for highly automated, faster, and more reliable perioperative 3D echocardiographic assessments.

There is a high correlation between 3D echocardiographic volume reconstructions and cardiac MRI, with 3D echo generally underestimating LV volumes due to challenges in detecting endocardial trabeculae. AI-based automated border detection algorithms are reducing these discrepancies.

Compared to 2D imaging, 3D echocardiography provides superior surface rendering, eliminating geometric assumptions that can impact accuracy—particularly in cases where LV aneurysms or RWMAs are present. Postrevascularization changes in EF and contractility can be quantitatively measured which can aid in clinical decision-making and post-CABG patient management.

Segmental wall function can be assessed using both 3D volume reconstruction and time tracking of the 17 myocardial segments, where each segment is color coded to indicate the time required to reach minimum volume (maximum contraction). Ideally, all segments should contract synchronously, but any delay in contraction timing suggests LV dyssynchrony, which may indicate underlying conduction abnormalities or regional ischemia. The systolic dyssynchrony index (SDI) quantifies the variability in systolic timing across different segments of the left ventricle (57). It is calculated as the standard deviation (SD) of segmental contraction times, expressed as a percentage of the total cardiac cycle. A higher SDI indicates greater ventricular dyssynchrony, while a lower SDI reflects more synchronized contraction. Expressing SDI as a percentage, rather than in milliseconds, allows for standardized comparisons between patients with varying heart rates.

The echocardiography machine can then automatically generate a comprehensive report, featuring a bull's eye map that visually represents the 17 myocardial segments as parametric images, with color shading to highlight timing disparities in contraction (see Figure 15.1). This automated analysis facilitates rapid identification of segments with delayed contraction, aiding in the diagnosis of ischemia. Following revascularization, the same imaging is repeated to objectively assess regional wall motion recovery.

The RV is particularly susceptible to ischemia during coronary revascularization. Due to its crescentic shape and complex contraction patterns, 2D echocardiography often fails to accurately measure RV size, function, and volume. The 3D echocardiography is now considered an essential tool for RV evaluation, providing direct volumetric quantification without geometric assumptions (▶ Video 15.9) (56,58). Compared to 2D imaging, the 3D TEE provides improved accuracy in assessing RV strain, regional wall motion, and dyssynchrony, particularly in patients with RCA disease involvement. Validation against cardiac MRI has demonstrated high correlation in RV volume measurements, reinforcing the role of 3D echocardiography in perioperative RV assessment.

Recent advancements in 3D rendering technologies have introduced new visualization techniques (56,58). Photorealistic vision rendering uses virtual light sources and shadowing enhancements to improve depth perception and structural visualization, particularly useful for valvular assessment. Glass mode transparency rendering aims to improve visualization of underlying anatomic relationships, aiding in preoperative planning for CABG and complex valvular procedures.

In summary, 3D echocardiography has become a useful modality for perioperative assessment in CABG patients, enabling evaluation of ventricular function, RWMAs, and ischemia. Developments in AI-driven quantification, automated image acquisition, and advanced visualization techniques have enhanced real-time 3D TEE, supporting intraoperative cardiac imaging and surgical decision-making.

Transesophageal Echocardiography for Specific Surgical Situations

Redo Sternotomy

TEE can be useful in detecting adherence of the RV to the sternum. This is best viewed in the ME RV inflow-outflow plane where restriction of the free wall of the RV can be seen. Femoral cannulation may be a preferred option in these circumstances.

Off-Pump Coronary Artery Bypass Graft

TEE intraoperative evaluation has aided off-pump coronary artery bypass (OPCAB) graft or minimally invasive direct coronary artery bypass (MIDCAB) surgery techniques (59,60). Patient tolerance to the procedure can be monitored in real time with TEE as patients undergoing OPCAB are susceptible to cardiovascular instability, especially when the myocardial stabilizer is applied. Application of the stabilizer and displacement of the heart can also cause transient occlusion of the coronary arteries and ischemia, which can be detected by TEE. Intraoperative detection of moderate to severe MR may indicate that the OPCAB approach is not warranted.

RWMA during OPCABG: TG images are often lost when the heart is displaced to access the right and circumflex coronary arteries. However, evaluating the ME four-chamber, two-chamber, and LAX views, during OPCAB surgery, allows for more than 14 segments to be evaluated for new RWMAs (61). Placement of a sterile glove filled with saline instead of lap pads (saline bags) posterior to the heart has been shown to improve image acquisition of the TG views (62). If a new RWMA is detected, repositioning of the stabilizer or insertion of an intercoronary perfusion shunt may be beneficial. Persistent abnormalities may predict postoperative problems and graft patency (▶ Video 15.10).

MR during OPCABG: This can be a new development when the heart is displaced, and the annulus distorted. It is easily detected by CFD in ME views. Preexisting MR may preclude OPCAB surgery as it increases the risk of progressing to severe persistent MR and pulmonary edema (Video 15.11).

IABP insertion during OPCABG: An IABP is used occasionally to support the heart during OPCAB surgery, especially if the LV function is poor or the patient has unstable angina. TEE guidance is useful for insertion as the OPCAB approach is commonly selected in patients with severe atheromatous disease of the aorta.

Preload assessment during OPCABG: Diastolic filling can be impaired when using a myocardial stabilization suction system, and compression of the right atrium (RA) can occur when the heart is elevated. The Trendelenburg position helps maintain ventricular filling and TEE can distinguish between hypovolemia and impaired cardiac function.

Conversion to CPB during OPCABG: This decision can be elective or an emergency response. TEE can anticipate deterioration of ventricular function, persistent RWMAs requiring graft revision, or development of severe MR, before sudden hemodynamic collapse occurs. New information, for example, valvular abnormalities or atrial septal defects, indicating a need for CPB may also be found in these patients. Early elective conversion is advisable rather than emergency conversion, due to worse outcomes associated with sudden instability (59).

Graft patency during OPCABG: The patency of the grafts is assessed with TEE by looking for normal function and resolution of RWMAs prior to chest closure. The intraoperative use of myocardial contrast echocardiography may differentiate causes of LV dysfunction immediately following revascularization by looking at regional flow patterns. Hence, TEE can modify OPCAB cases and may improve morbidity and mortality in these patients (63).

Role of Transesophageal Echocardiography in Vascular Cannulations

Aortic cannula: As part of a complete examination during coronary revascularization, the ascending and descending aorta should be examined for atheromatous plaques or calcification. This will influence surgical decision-making when instrumentation of the aorta is considered, for example, aortic cannula, aortic cross-clamp, or intra-aortic balloon counterpulsation. Detection of severe atheromatous disease of the ascending aorta is a risk factor for poor outcome, and modification of surgical technique may be warranted. Changing the aortic cannulation and cross-clamp sites, avoiding an aortic side-clamp by performing all proximal and distal coronary anastomoses during one single ischemic cross-clamp period, can be used to reduce embolic consequences. Currently, no strong evidence supports the use of endoaortic balloon occlusion in OPCAB patients with aortic atherosclerosis, while alternative approaches such as no-touch OPCAB and selective use of epiaortic ultrasound may be more effective in reducing stroke risk (64). Furthermore, OPCAB surgery or CABG under hypothermic circulatory arrest can also be considered.

The ME ascending aorta LAX and SAX, the ME AV LAX, UE aortic arch SAX and LAX views examine the ascending aorta and arch, and the ME descending aorta SAX and LAX views examine the descending aorta. Due to the anatomic location of the trachea and the left main stem bronchus, which lies between the esophagus and the aortic arch, TEE only visualizes 50% to 80% of the ascending aorta. If it is important to visualize the distal ascending aorta, insertion of a saline-filled balloon in the left main bronchus can overcome this "blind spot" (65) or epiaortic scanning should be considered. Atheroma is measured perpendicularly from the outer vessel wall to the intimal surface and graded 1 to 4 depending on the thickness. Grade 5 is a mobile plaque (Figure 15.5; Videos 15.12 and 15.13).

Comparison of Katz Classification and ASE/EACVI Guidelines for Aortic Atheroma Grading (66,67).

Grade	Katz Classification (1992)	ASE/EACVI Guidelines (2015)
I	Normal aorta	Intimal thickness <2 mm
II	Extensive intimal thickening	Focal or diffuse intimal thickness 2-3 mm
III	Sessile atheroma extending <5 mm into the lumen	3-5 mm (no mobile/ulcerated components)
IV	Sessile atheroma protruding >5 mm	>5 mm (no mobile/ulcerated components)
V	Mobile atheroma	Complex grade 2-4 atheroma plus mobile or ulcerated components

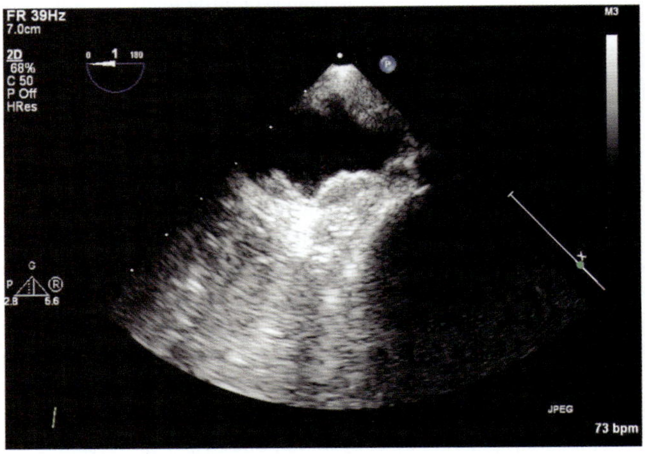

FIGURE 15.5 Grade 4 plaques in the arch of the aorta. This changed the operation from on-pump to off-pump coronary artery bypass grafting to avoid the "sandblasting" effect. The patient woke up neurologically intact.

Severe atheroma (grades 4-5) found in the descending aorta has been correlated with the presence of a similar grade atheroma in the ascending aorta. Detection of severe or mobile plaques in the aortic arch may change the surgical plan converting an on-pump coronary revascularization to OPCAB procedure to avoid the "sandblasting" effect of the aortic inflow cannula disrupting plaque and sending it into the systemic circulation as emboli (68,69). Aortic cannula assessments are made to check for iatrogenic dissection originating from the aortic cannulation and antegrade cardioplegia sites, as well as the proximal vein graft sites.

1. *Cardioplegia.* Cardioplegia is given either by antegrade and/or retrograde routes. Prior to placement of the antegrade cardioplegia cannula, TEE and epiaortic imaging are used to check for the presence of atheroma in the ascending aorta, arch, and descending aorta. Aortic dissection is a rare complication of antegrade cardioplegia cannulation but may be detected by TEE in the ME ascending aorta LAX view.

   TEE is useful to guide and confirm placement of the retrograde cannula in the coronary sinus. The ME four chamber with slight retroflexion and advancement of the probe provides the most reliable view of the coronary sinus (Figure 15.6). Alternatively, the coronary sinus can be visualized in a modified bicaval view with the imaging plane at approximately 130°. The presence of a valve at the entrance to the coronary sinus (thebesian valve) may complicate insertion of the retrograde cardioplegia cannula. In the presence of an enlarged coronary sinus, a persistent left-sided superior vena cava (SVC) must be

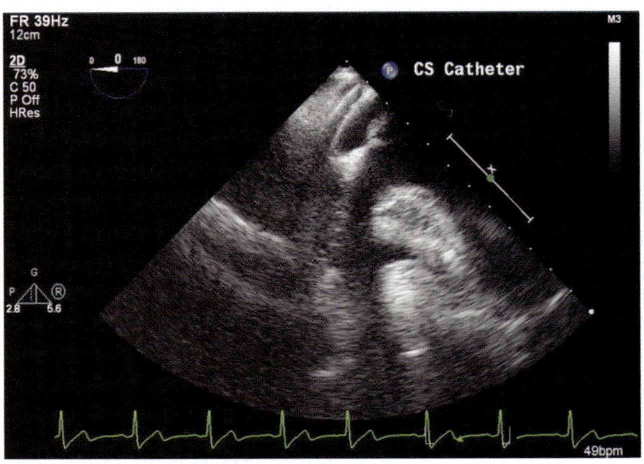

FIGURE 15.6 Insertion of a retrograde cannula for cardioplegia showing the coronary sinus catheter within the coronary sinus in midesophageal four-chamber view with slight probe retroflexion.

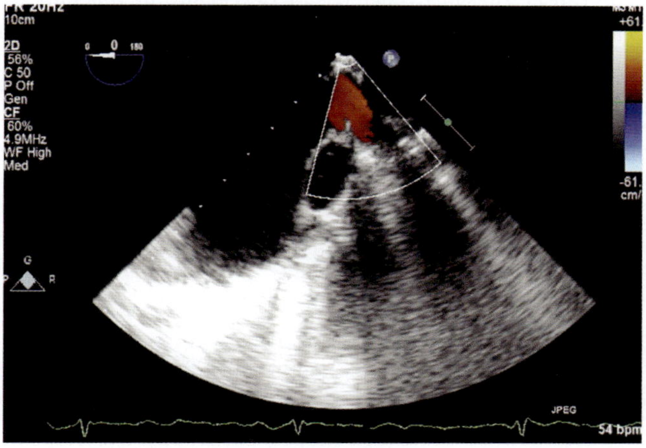

FIGURE 15.7 Patient with a persistent left superior vena cava seen in this view anterior to the left upper pulmonary vein.

suspected and actively excluded, as its presence can render retrograde cardioplegia ineffective. This persistent left-sided SVC is best seen in the ME four-chamber view with the probe slightly withdrawn next to the left upper pulmonary vein (LUPV), although an enlarged coronary sinus showing positive contrast echo from left-sided peripheral IV access is more reliable (Figure 15.7).

2. *IABP.* IABP remains an essential tool to stabilize patients with coronary artery disease and unstable angina prior to surgery, as well as intraoperatively in patients with deteriorating ventricular function. TEE is useful to ensure correct placement and avoid associated complications. First, confirm proper intraluminal position of the guide wire. Second, guide correct IABP position from the ME descending aorta SAX view with the tip positioned just distal (2-3 cm) to the left subclavian artery.
3. *Femoral vascular cannulation.* Arterial and venous femoral lines are inserted for a variety of clinical indications including aortic surgery and coronary artery bypass surgery. Severe atheromatous disease or dilation of the ascending aorta can preclude cannulation at this site. Redo surgery is now more prevalent and femoral cannulation allows decompression of the heart prior to sternotomy, decreasing risk of injury to the RV when attached to the posterior surface of the sternum by adhesions. It also reduces the need for anatomic dissection around the heart that conventional cannulation requires. The femoral vessels are exposed, and guide wires are passed up the aorta and inferior vena cava (IVC). Dissection is ruled out by the presence of the wire within the lumen of the aorta and is visualized in the ME descending aorta SAX and LAX views. The wire has bright echogenicity. The femoral venous wire is passed up into the RA and is best seen in the ME bicaval view (Video 15.14). SVC cannulation can also be performed under echo guidance with the wire passing down from the right internal jugular vein (RIJV) into the RA. This is best seen in the ME bicaval view and the tip of the cannula is adjusted to allow isolation of the cava if necessary.

Endoscopic Vein Harvesting

Recent advances in harvesting the long saphenous vein endoscopically, while reducing morbidity from the leg incision and increasing early mobility, have produced its own problems. The insufflation of carbon dioxide (CO_2) to facilitate harvesting has resulted in reports of CO_2 embolism. The ME bicaval and TG views of the hepatic veins and the IVC are used to detect the presence of bubbles in the RA (70). Rapid diagnosis by TEE allows prompt treatment. The incidence has been reported to be between 0.5% for severe and 3.5% for moderate emboli.

Failure to Wean From Cardiopulmonary Bypass

Echo in Extracorporeal Membrane Oxygenation

Postcardiotomy cardiogenic shock (PCCS) remains a significant challenge, often necessitating advanced circulatory support strategies. Extracorporeal life support (ECLS), particularly venoarterial extracorporeal membrane oxygenation (VA ECMO), has emerged as rescue therapy in the management of refractory PCCS.

Patients undergoing CABG are at particularly high risk for developing intraoperative and postoperative cardiogenic shock. Early identification and intervention with MCS to prevent hemodynamic deterioration is essential. While VA ECMO has been increasingly utilized in the postoperative period, its impact on long-term survival remains inconclusive, with mixed evidence regarding overall mortality and morbidity reduction (71). The AHA has issued guidelines in 2017 regarding the management of this condition (72). TEE is invaluable in assessing cardiogenic shock which is a possible complication of CABG. Veno-venous (V-V) ECMO is used for refractory respiratory failure with preserved cardiac function and both the inflow and outflow cannulas are placed in the venous system, preferably under imaging guidance. V-A ECMO is used when there is inadequate cardiac function associated with respiratory failure and as support for the RV following LVAD placement. A comprehensive TEE is used to determine if V-V ECMO will be sufficient or if V-A ECMO is indicated depending on cardiac function.

1. *Cannulation placement.* TEE is invaluable in assessing patient selection, cannula insertion, correct placement, detection of complications, monitoring improvement, and weaning from VA ECMO by assessing recovery of cardiac function (73). Prior to cannulation, a TEE should be performed to check any structural abnormalities, for example, a PFO, ASD, large eustachian valve, Chiari network, or TV pathology, which may impede the placement of the inflow cannula. Proper management or closure of any intracardiac right-to-left shunt can eliminate the need for ECMO. For V-V ECMO, dual lumen cannulas are now available and are inserted into the SVC via the RIJV. Blood from the SVC and IVC enter one lumen. This lumen is positioned just above the IVC entry into the RA and provides inflow to the oxygenator. Oxygenated blood is then returned via a separate lumen, positioned so that flow is directed through the tricuspid valve into the RV. TEE is essential for the correct placement and positioning of this double lumen cannula. CFD from the ME views is used to adjust the position of the outflow port toward the TV (Figure 15.8). If it is incorrectly positioned, the outflow of oxygenated blood instead of passing into the RV is taken back to the oxygenator by the inflow port and recirculation occurs. A marked difference between the color of the blood in the dual lumens assists in confirming correct position, so that recirculation is minimized.

   Separate cannulas may be inserted, with the inflow lumen positioned at the junction of the IVC and RA, and the outflow cannula placed above the TV. Large patients (over 100 kg) often need a second oxygenator. The second inflow cannula is usually placed in the femoral vein. TEE is used to visualize the guide wire in the RA, as it is placed via the RIJV into the SVC, passing through the heart down the IVC. Alternatively, the guidewire can be placed from the femoral vein into the IVC. The SVC approach is the most common route for placement of the cannula.

   In V-A ECMO, TEE is used to assess the ascending aorta to exclude aortic dissection before proceeding. The ME AV LAX, UE aortic arch, and ME descending aorta SAX and LAX views are used during cannulation to check for the location of the guide wire and to rule out the presence of aortic atheroma.

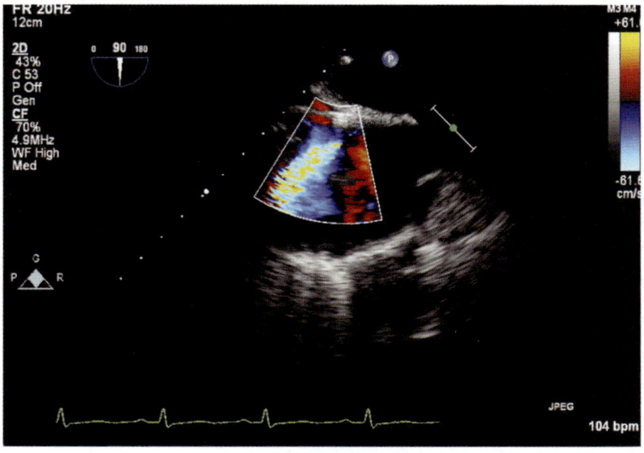

FIGURE 15.8 Extracorporeal membrane oxygenation cannula showing color flow Doppler with outflow opening positioned in-line with the tricuspid valve.

TEE evaluation of ventricular decompression is made in the ME and TG views. Once ECMO is established, TEE is used to monitor the effect on the heart. With V-A ECMO, preload is decreased but afterload is increased due to the pressurized arterial return. In severe LV dysfunction, this can lead to further LV failure, severe MR, and the AV not opening at all. Spontaneous echo contrast from stasis can lead to thrombosis and this should be excluded in the LV, aorta, and pulmonary veins. When stasis is visualized, anticoagulation needs to be increased and flow reduced until the spontaneous echo contrast improves. If it does not, then an LVAD may be more appropriate than ECMO.

In V-V ECMO, there are fewer hemodynamic changes. The increase in oxygen content of the returned blood will decrease PVR and therefore improve RV and LV function.

2. *ECMO complications.* Diagnosing tamponade on VA ECMO can be challenging, as typical clinical signs may be obscured due to the patient being on partial bypass, which assist perfusion pressures. If ECMO flow is maintained, tamponade may only be detected by TEE (74). Thrombosis is a concern and the presence of venous casts, when the cannulas are removed, should be evaluated in the ME bicaval and four-chamber views. TEE can show complications of cannula displacement, for example, migration across the atrial septum or through the TV. TEE is used to assess ventricular filling and function, and aids repositioning of cannulas if required. Another recognized problem is difficulty in removing the SVC cannula after being in situ for a prolonged period. TEE is valuable for confirming that the cannula remains free and untethered within the ventricle.
3. *ECMO weaning.* TEE is not very useful for separation from V-V ECMO due to the fact that weaning is primarily determined by improvement in pulmonary compliance and oxygenation. However, in V-A ECMO, TEE is useful to assess the recovery of LV and RV function and the timing when to wean. Being on ECMO alters the physiology and myocardial recovery. The unloaded ventricle makes functional assessment more challenging. No single parameter is superior; rather, a combination of measurements and clinical experience is typically required (60,73,75,76). A similar approach is applied during VAD weaning. Echocardiographic criteria for successful weaning include an LVEF greater than 25%, LVOT VTI greater than 10 cm, mitral annular S wave velocity greater than 6 cm/s and the absence of LV dilation as pump flow is gradually reduced (77).

   RV function should also be assessed while weaning pump flows. RV dysfunction is diagnosed when at least two of the following criteria persist: RVEDD greater than 35 mm, TAPSE less than 12 mm, sTDI of the tricuspid annulus less than 10 cm/s, poor RVEF, or severe functional TR.

   Daily echocardiographic assessments should be performed in patients on VA ECMO to monitor AV opening, LV distention, and thrombus formation (77). TEE is valuable to guide various LV decompression techniques (atrial septostomy, percutaneous transaortic venting, Impella device) when addressing LV distension during VA ECMO, avoiding pulmonary edema and thrombus formation.

Impella Endovascular Devices

The Impella is a temporary device to support the LV or RV. It serves as rescue therapy and can be inserted without the need for CPB. This miniaturized axial pump is inserted via the femoral artery or centrally for left heart assist, or through the RIJV for right assist. It is passed through the AV into the LV cavity or through the TV into the RV cavity. It uses microaxial flow forces to draw blood from the LV and delivers it into the ascending aorta or from RV into the pulmonary artery, providing continuous, nonpulsatile cardiac support. As there is minimal contact with blood, the level of anticoagulation required is low. ACT target is 170 to 200 seconds, with a reduced systemic inflammatory response. The Impella relies on some residual LV or RV ejection—CO greater than 1.5 L/min or LVEF greater than 20% as it cannot provide full CO. Echocardiography is essential to ensure correct placement of the device.

Prior to insertion, TEE is essential to exclude the presence of aortic stenosis, obstructive cardiomyopathy, or hypertrophy of the LV septum, LV aneurysm, or a billowing anterior MV leaflet, which may all impede filling. TEE should also exclude severe atherosclerosis. A multiparametric approach—combining fluoroscopy (30° right anterior oblique view), automated Impella controller (AIC) waveforms, and a TEE three-chamber view for precise depth assessment—is ideal to detect malpositioning (78).

TEE is used to guide Impella insertion through the AV and position it approximately 3.0 to 3.5 cm from the AV plane. The device outflow should be placed 1.5 to 2.0 cm from the sinus of Valsalva. To prevent obstruction, it should remain clear of the LV wall. If available, RT3D is particularly useful for spatial alignment. Postinsertion TEE is performed to evaluate ventricular recovery (Figure 15.9; Video 15.15 and 15.16).

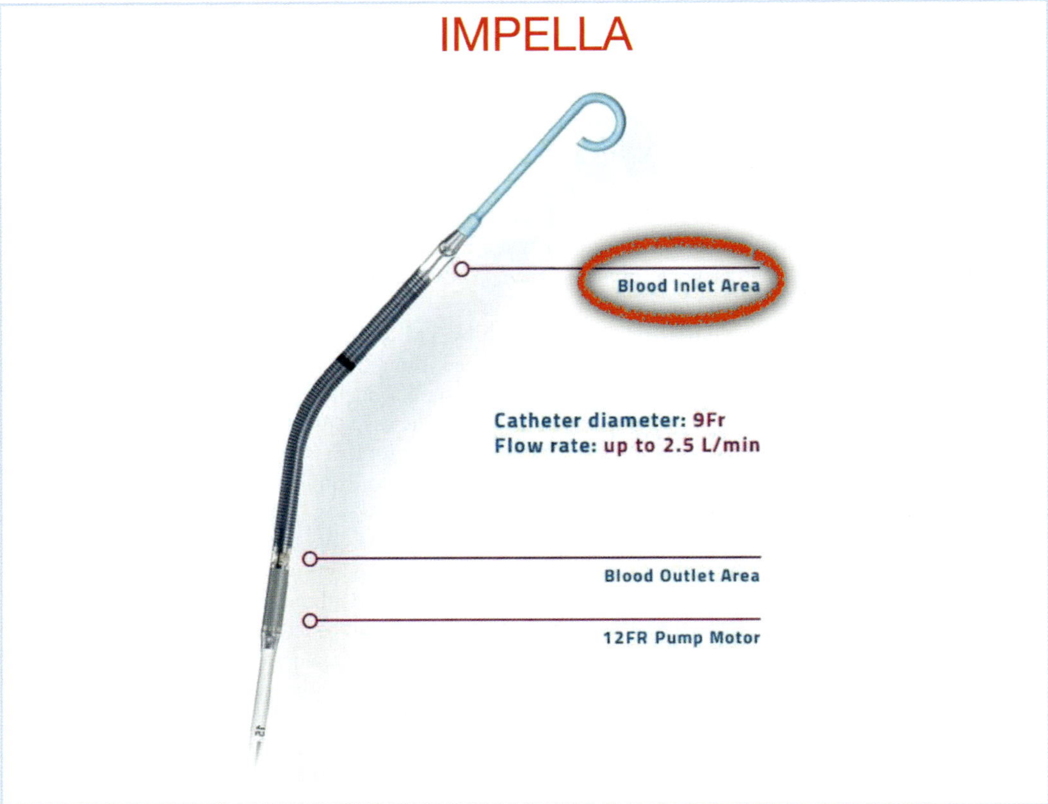

FIGURE 15.9 Impella device. The inlet to the motor is visualized as a teardrop shape in midesophageal aortic valve long axis. The inlet should stay 3.5 cm below the aortic valve. Impella 5.5, requires that the inflow port is 5 cm below the aortic valve annulus. (© 2025 ABIOMED. All rights reserved.)

Ventricular Assist Devices

The use of VADs is becoming increasingly common as rescue therapy, a bridge to transplant, or destination therapy. The use of TEE to assist implantation and management is a category I indication (4). LVADs are the most frequently implanted, but right ventricular assist device (RVAD) and biventricular assist devices (BIVADs) are also used occasionally. Echocardiography is an essential tool for pre-, peri-, and postoperative assessments (73,76,79,80). RT3D TEE is increasingly useful to guide spatial positioning of cannulas and assess problems (80). Prior to implantation, it is necessary to quantify baseline ventricular function and to exclude various pathologies. A comprehensive examination should be performed, with special attention to the following:

1. *Intracardiac, ventricular, or atrial thrombus*. Sluggish flow will be evident in both chambers confirming the underlying need for circulatory support. Ventricular aneurysms and scarred ventricular regions may contain thrombi and should be avoided during insertion of the inflow cannula. Thrombus may occlude the inflow cannula when placed at the ventricular apex, the most common site. Alternative sites include the left atrium or pulmonary veins; however, while drainage and ventricular unloading may be less effective, decannulation may be more straightforward. (Figures 15.10 and 15.11; Videos 15.17 and 15.18).
2. *Intracardiac shunts (PFO, ASD).* PFOs are common in up to 27% of the population. Undiagnosed PFO or ASD can exacerbate hypoxemia and increase the risk of stroke.

   Identifying a PFO is critical, as it may remain undetectable in a failing LV with elevated LA pressure. The PFO often becomes apparent only after LVAD implantation and once ventricular decompression has occurred. After cannula placement, it is crucial to reassess for a PFO, as LV and LA decompression may cause it to open. If a significant shunt is detected, closure should be performed, either surgically or percutaneously.

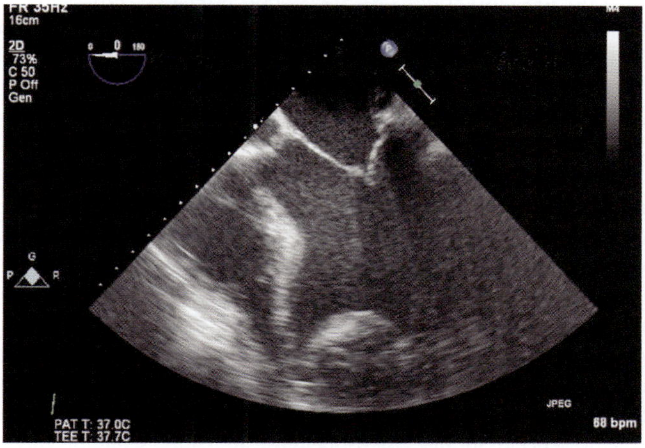

FIGURE 15.10 Two-dimensional transesophageal echocardiography four-chamber view demonstrating thrombus in the left ventricular apex in a patient scheduled for left ventricular assist device placement.

3. *Valvular abnormalities.* AR decreases forward flow from the LVAD and increases recirculation as aortic blood returns to the LV. Because of reduced gradients in failing ventricles, AR should be reevaluated on CPB as it can be underestimated on the initial examination. If significant, the AV may need to be replaced if the LVAD is for bridging, or sutured shut if it is for destination therapy. Intermittent AV opening, achieved by reducing LVAD support under TEE guidance, helps minimize stasis and thrombosis risk. Similarly, pulmonary insufficiency should be evaluated before RVAD placement to ensure optimal function.

   MR is common in end-stage heart failure and should improve with LVAD placement. In contrast, mitral stenosis (MS) restricts LVAD filling when positioned in the LV. This limitation can be avoided by placing the device in the atrium or pulmonary veins, or by performing a mitral valvotomy before insertion.
4. *RV function.* While LVAD implantation reduces LV afterload and may improve RV function, RV failure remains common, occurring in up to 40% of patients (81). Increased RV preload can exacerbate its failure, and the leftward septal shift following LVAD placement may further impair RV function.

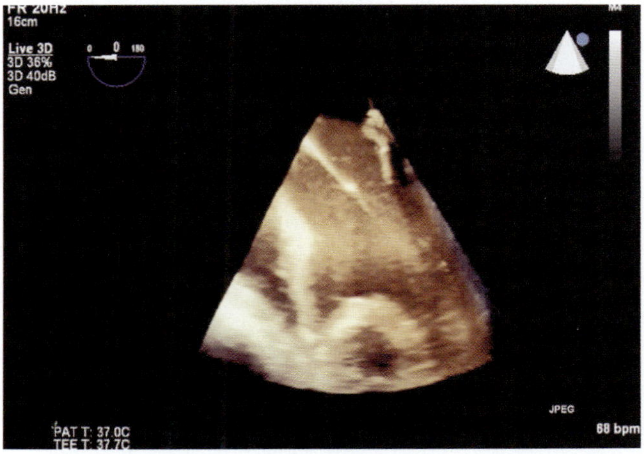

FIGURE 15.11 Three-dimensional transesophageal echocardiography four-chamber view demonstrating thrombus in the left ventricular apex in a patient scheduled for left ventricular assist device placement (Video 15.18).

If RV function deteriorates and requires RVAD support after LVAD implantation, the prognosis significantly worsens with mortality up to 30%. Therefore, assessment of RV function is essential prior to LVAD implantation. Indicators of good RV function include normal or mildly hypokinetic free wall motion and the absence of severe TR. Additional predictors include fractional shortening of the RVOT exceeding 20% and a TAPSE between 10 and 15 mm (81). Severe TR can reduce filling of the LV and impair LVAD function.

Predicting RV failure after LVAD implantation is challenging, but key indicators include (81-87):

- TAPSE less than 7.5 mm
- RV to LV diameter ratio greater than 7.5
- Eccentricity index of the RV greater than 0.6
- RVEDD greater than 50 mm
- Peak longitudinal strain of the RV greater than 0.6
- Pulmonary artery pulsatility index (PAPI) less than 1.85
- Low Load-Adaptation Index (LAIRV)

At present there is no long-term RVAD available.

5. *Aortic atheroma.* The presence of mobile atheroma in the arch and ascending aorta is associated with an increased risk of stroke following LVAD placement. Although part of the ascending aorta is not well seen, atheroma in the proximal ascending-, arch, and descending aorta is associated with cerebral dysfunction.
6. *Positioning of VAD cannulas.*
   a. *Inflow cannula.* As previously mentioned, the inflow cannula can be in various positions. The most common is through the LV apex for LVADs and the RV or RA for RVADs (Figure 15.12; Videos 15.19 and 15.20).
   b. *LVAD inflow examination.* On 2D TEE, the LV inflow cannula should be aligned with the mitral inflow and not obstructed by any ventricular wall (Figure 15.13). The 2D TEE, using at least two orthogonal views, for example, ME four-chamber and two-chamber, is useful to assess proper placement. RT3D TEE is useful in checking the orientation of the cannula (80). CFD should demonstrate unidirectional laminar flow with pattern specific to the particular device. Pulsatile LVADs such as HeartMate I, Thoratec, and Novacor will have a pulsatile pattern of flow where normal velocities should be less than 2.3 m/s with and flow rates of 65 mL/s (compatible with a 16-mm cannula). Impeller-driven axial flow devices (eg, HeartMate II, Jarvik 2000) are not microaxial. They use larger axial flow pumps designed for long-term circulatory support, whereas the Impella is a microaxial flow pump designed for temporary, short-term support. The impeller-driven axial flow devices are implanted directly through the LV apex and have no inflow cannula. They show continuous inflow throughout the cardiac cycle as well as a pulsatile pattern that synchronizes with the ECG (79,82,88). These axial

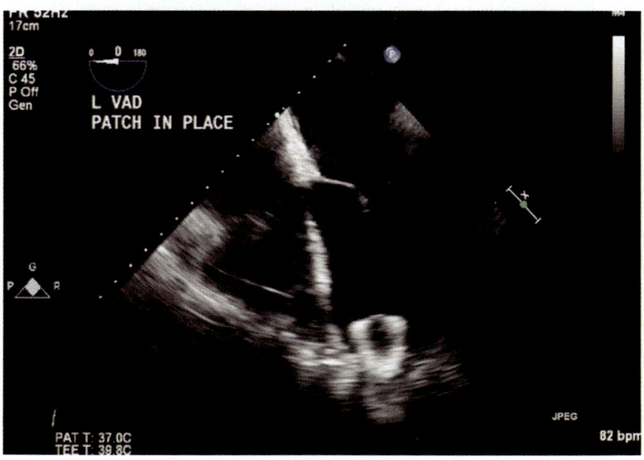

FIGURE 15.12 Midesophageal four-chamber view of inflow cannula at the left ventricular apex.

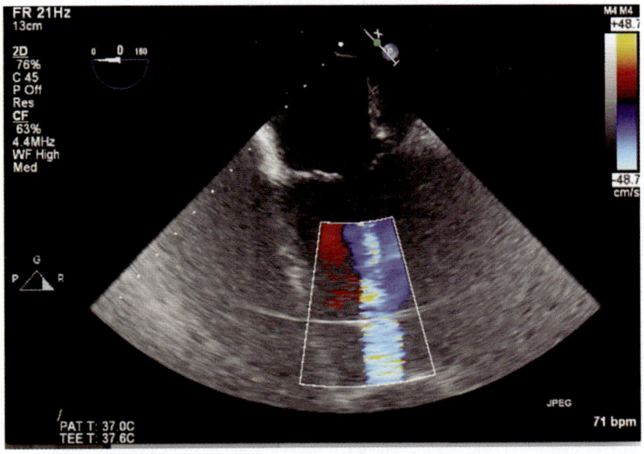

FIGURE 15.13 Midesophageal four-chamber view showing left ventricular assist device inflow via color Doppler.

flow devices have peak-filling velocities of 1 to 2 m/s depending on the preload and residual CO from the LV. Inflow cannula malfunction is identified by elevated PWD velocities within the LV cavity and incomplete LV emptying. Additionally, high-velocity flow through the AV with frequent AV opening suggest improper function. Under normal LVAD operation, minimal flow should pass through the AV, which remains mostly closed.

A "suckdown effect" results when hypovolemia and/or rapid decompression from excessive LVAD flow causes intermittent obstruction of the inflow cannula. This situation can occur during weaning of CPB to LVAD support. There is a prominent bowing of the interventricular septum toward the LV which may occlude the inflow cannula (Figures 15.14 and 15.15; Videos 15.21 and 15.22). When faced with this effect in a hemodynamically unstable patient, it is important not to increase LVAD speed to improve flow and blood pressure, but rather to decrease LVAD speed and increase preload. Later, progressive increases in LVAD support can be initiated. Another cause of reduced LV cavity size on TEE is an intracavity thrombus.

Cannula obstruction in RVADs may be caused by the TV anterior leaflet, subvalvular apparatus, or an aneurismal interatrial septum.

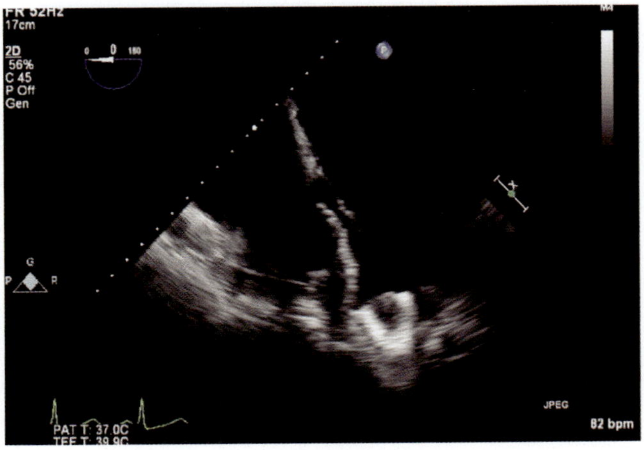

FIGURE 15.14 Two-dimensional Midesophageal four-chamber view of "suckdown" where the intraventricular septum bows toward left ventricular inflow cannula, potentially causing obstruction.

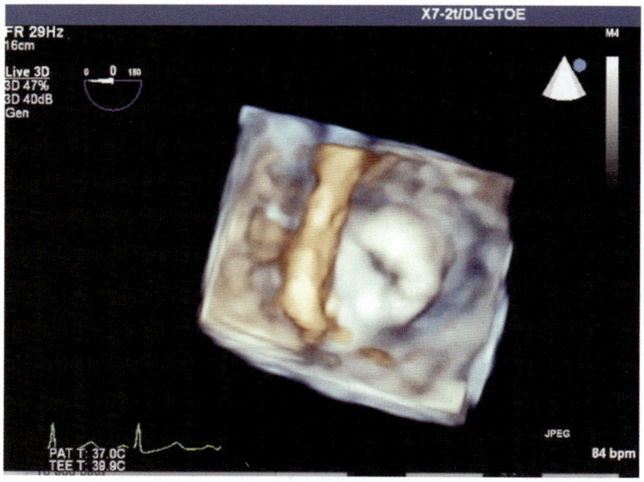

FIGURE 15.15 Three-dimensional image of the intraventricular septum encroaching on left ventricular assist device-left ventricular inflow cannula (Video 15.22).

c. *Outflow cannula.* The most common position for the LVAD outflow cannula is the ascending aorta. This cannula should be perpendicular to the ascending aorta and is assessed by CFD, looking for laminar aortic flow in the ME AV LAX view (Figure 15.16).

For RVADs, the PA is the most common position site for the outflow cannula, using either direct anastomosis or via RV through the PV. Assessment is performed using the ME ascending aortic SAX and ME RV inflow/outflow views. These views provide critical imaging for evaluating RVAD function and detecting inflow outflow cannula malposition or dysfunction (Figures 15.17 and 15.18; Videos 15.23 and 15.24). Normal peak velocities typically range from 1.7 to 2.5 m/s; however, lower velocities between 1.0 and 2.0 m/s are considered acceptable. These values are measured using PWD at 1 cm proximal to pulmonary artery position (79,82).

Obstruction of the outflow cannula or incompetence of the AV or PV may be diagnosed by increased flow velocity measured proximally in the graft. Causes of outflow obstruction may include thrombus, vegetations, extrinsic compression by mediastinal hematoma, or kinking of the graft during sternal closure. Other indications of obstruction are rightward septal deviation, LV dilation, and

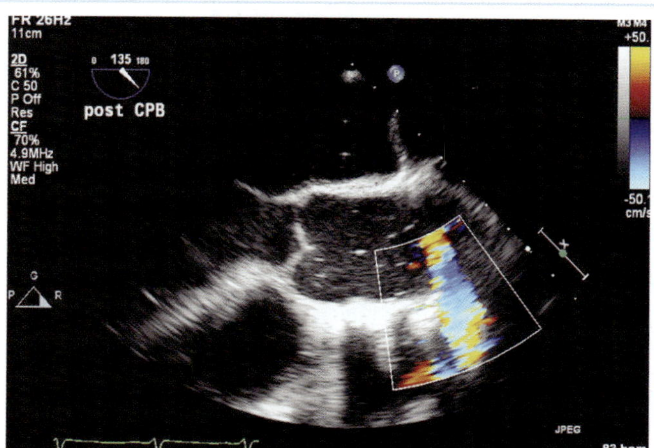

FIGURE 15.16 Two-dimensional midesophageal long axis showing color flow out of the outflow aortic cannula of left ventricular assist device.

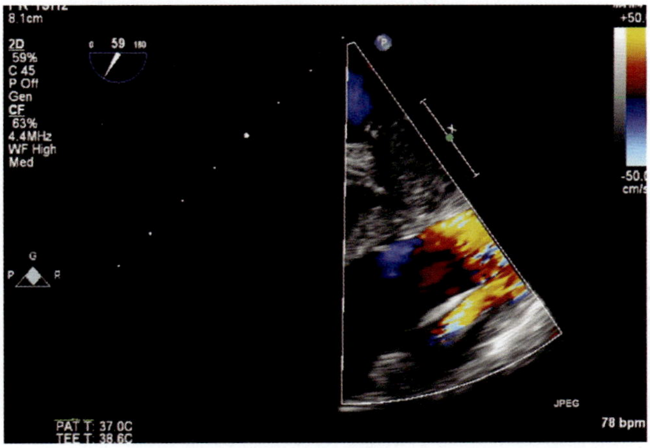

FIGURE 15.17 Two-dimensional midesophageal right ventricle inflow-outflow view of the right ventricular outflow tract showing the outflow cannula for right ventricular assist device going into pulmonary artery (Video 15.23).

increased MR. Acute increases in afterload can result in decreased LV unloading and present with high Doppler velocities. Table 15.6 summarizes post-VAD implantation checks and complications.

In patients with V-A ECMO or an LVAD, hemodynamic instability or abnormal flow requires prompt evaluation. Echocardiography is invaluable in identifying potential causes and guiding management. Incidence of tamponade ranges from 11% to 48%, with up to 30% of patients needing to return to theater for evacuation. Tamponade diagnosis may be masked, because the LV is mechanically supported (74).

7. *VAD follow-up and device dysfunction.* Regular follow-up is needed as device failure and malfunction can be as high as 35% (82,89). For pulsatile LVADs, inflow regurgitation secondary to mechanical failure of the inflow valve is the most common cause of LVAD dysfunction. Inflow cannula regurgitation results in turbulent flow at the inflow cannula during LVAD ejection. Doppler examination will detect a biphasic inflow pattern as opposed to the unidirectional laminar flow seen in the normally functioning LVAD. PWD demonstrates flow reversal in the inflow cannula during LVAD ejection as well as decreased peak velocities ($<$1.8 m/s) in the outflow cannula. Other indications of a malfunctioning inflow cannula with a pulsatile LVAD are a full or dilated LV and frequent opening of the AV.

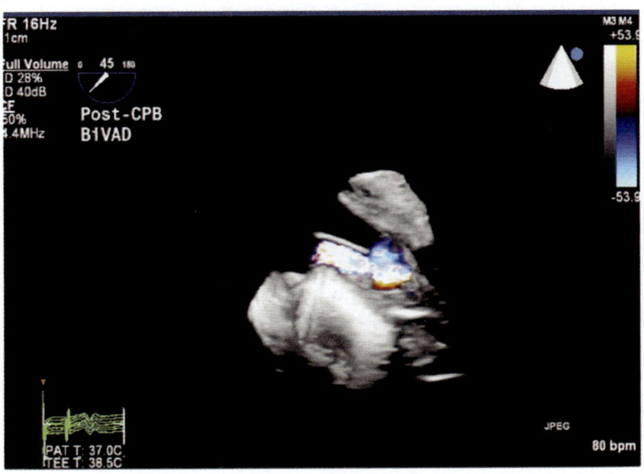

FIGURE 15.18 Three-dimensional long-axis image of right ventricular assist device outflow cannula into pulmonary artery (Video 15.22).

TABLE 15.6 Summary of Post Ventricular Assist Device Implantation Checks and Complications

- De-airing, both intracardiac and device
- Reevaluation for PFO
- Presence of MR, this should be reduced, if not then it possibly indicates poor positioning of the inflow cannula.
- Frequent arrhythmias are also a sign of poor cannula positioning
- Decompression of the LV
- Septal position should be neutral. Right shift indicates inadequate emptying. Left shift can result from excessive decompression due to excessive pump speeds or hypovolemia.
- Right ventricular failure
- Rule out cardiac tamponade
- Doppler interrogation of the cannulas
- Aortic valve opening. This can be intermittent with axial flow devices but in pulsatile devices it should be closed at all times.
- Aortic valve regurgitation. This can become apparent at a later stage postoperatively and result in pulmonary edema.

LV, left ventricle; MR, mitral regurgitation; PFO, patent foramen ovale.

Axial flow VAD designs (Jarvik 2000 and HeartMate II and III) eliminate the use of valves. Diastolic regurgitation through the outflow graft from the aorta through the VAD and into the LV secondary to pump failure is associated with an abnormal retrograde apical flow pattern on Doppler. Thromboembolic problems can occur and result in inflow obstruction. Detection inside the devices is not possible with TEE but thrombi in the LAA, LV apex, and intraventricular septum, as well as around the cannula, may indicate intradevice thrombi. Measured flow is generally accurate; however, it may be artificially elevated if the inflow cannula is obstructed. This obstruction can create false readings masking true hemodynamic status (90). For pulsatile pumps, a peak inflow velocity greater than 2.3 m/s or interruptions of the usual laminar inflow pattern is consistent with inflow cannula obstruction. With continuous flow devices, inflow obstruction is suggested by turbulent flow and Doppler-derived peak inflow velocities of greater than 2 m/s. Aortic dissection can occur as there is increased stress on the aortic intima by the blood being reinfused at high velocities against the aortic wall. Endocarditis may develop resulting in vegetations on native valves, and conduits may cause obstruction and even rupture in extreme cases.

8. *Weaning from VADs.* As with ECMO, the criteria for weaning from VADs are still not fully defined, but involve a combination of TEE and clinical features. Recovery of the LV can occur and is assessed visually and objectively: LVEF greater than 45% and LV end-diastolic diameter lea than 45 mm. RVAD support following LVAD insertion is usually only needed for 2 to 4 weeks and can be discontinued when recovery of the RV occurs. However, appropriate RVAD weaning is more difficult to assess than LVAD weaning. The PVR must be optimized, and support from the RVAD gradually weaned, while monitoring the RV function visually. The ME four-chamber and ME RV inflow/outflow views are used for assessment of RV function while continuing to monitor venous pressures and LV function.

SUMMARY

TEE can significantly influence clinical management and improve patient outcome in coronary revascularization. Recent recommendations from both sides of the Atlantic support its routine use in all patients undergoing coronary revascularization. As surgical approaches to revascularization develop along with associated technologies, TEE has proven to be an increasingly valuable tool for patient care.

TEE plays a critical role in the perioperative management of coronary revascularization by providing real-time assessment of ventricular function, RWMAs, CO, and hemodynamic stability. Current North American and European guidelines endorse its routine use in all patients undergoing CABG and other revascularization procedures due to its ability to optimize surgical decision-making and improve outcomes.

TEE is particularly valuable for assessing myocardial function before and after CPB, detecting new RWMAs that may indicate ischemia or graft failure, and guiding interventions such as fluid resuscitation, inotropic support, and IABP placement. It enhances the diagnosis of unexpected valvular or structural pathology which can impact surgical planning. In OPCAB, TEE helps monitor cardiac displacement effects and anticipate the need for conversion to CPB.

Recent advancements in 3D TEE and myocardial deformation imaging have further improved intraoperative assessments by enhancing the quantification of LVEF, ischemic changes, and myocardial dyssynchrony aligning with cardiac MRI standards.

Beyond CABG, TEE is essential for guiding MCS, including ECMO, VADs, and the Impella, ensuring correct device placement, assessing myocardial recovery, and optimizing weaning strategies. It is also used to evaluate vascular cannulation sites, detect aortic atheroma, and monitor complications such as tamponade and thrombosis.

As surgical techniques and technology evolve, TEE remains an indispensable tool for optimizing perioperative care, enhancing decision-making, and improving long-term cardiac outcomes in patients undergoing coronary revascularization and MCS.

ACKNOWLEDGMENT

We gratefully acknowledge the contributions of previous edition authors, Donna L. Greenhalgh and Henry J. Skinner, as portions of those chapters have been retained in this revision.

REFERENCES

1. Metkus TS, Thibault D, Grant MC, et al. Transesophageal echocardiography in patients undergoing coronary artery bypass graft surgery. *J Am Coll Cardiol.* 2021;78(2):112-122.
2. Swanevelder J, Chin D, Kneeshaw J, et al. Accreditation in transoesophageal echocardiography: statement from the Association of Cardiothoracic Anaesthetists and the British Society of Echocardiography Joint TOE Accreditation Committee. *Br J Anaesth.* 2003;91(4):469-472.
3. Kolev N, Brase R, Swanevelder J, et al. The influence of transoesophageal echocardiography on intra-operative decision making. A European multicentre study. *Anaesthesia.* 1998;53(8):767-773.
4. American Society of Anesthesiologists and Society of Cardiovascular Anesthesiologists Task Force on Transesophageal Echocardiography. Practice guidelines for perioperative transesophageal echocardiography. An updated report by the American Society of Anesthesiologists and the Society of Cardiovascular Anesthesiologists Task Force on Transesophageal Echocardiography. *Anesthesiology.* 2010;112(5):1084-1096.
5. Flachskampf FA, Badano L, Daniel WG, et al. Recommendations for transoesophageal echocardiography: update 2010. *Eur J Echocardiogr.* 2010;11(7):557-576.
6. Hauser ND, Swanevelder J. Transoesophageal echocardiography (TOE): contra-indications, complications and safety of perioperative TOE. *Echo Res Pract.* 2018;5(4):R101-R113.
7. Nicoara A, Skubas N, Ad N, et al. Guidelines for the use of transesophageal echocardiography to assist with surgical decision-making in the operating room: a surgery-based approach. *J Am Soc Echocardiogr.* 2020;33(6):692-734.
8. Yu S, Peffley S, Fabbro M, Mohammed AN. A narrative review of the 2020 guidelines for use of transesophageal echocardiography to assist with surgical decision—making by the cardiac anesthesiologist in the operating room. *J Cardiothorac Vasc Anesth.* 2022;36(1):258-274.
9. Eltzschig HK, Rosenberger P, Löffler M, Fox JA, Aranki SF, Shernan SK. Impact of intraoperative transesophageal echocardiography on surgical decisions in 12,566 patients undergoing cardiac surgery. *Ann Thorac Surg.* 2008;85(3):845-852.
10. Qaddoura FE, Abel MD, Mecklenburg KL, et al. Role of intraoperative transesophageal echocardiography in patients having coronary artery bypass graft surgery. *Ann Thorac Surg.* 2004;78(5):1586-1590.
11. Klein AA, Snell A, Nashef SAM, Hall RMO, Kneeshaw JD, Arrowsmith JE. The impact of intra-operative transoesophageal echocardiography on cardiac surgical practice. *Anaesthesia.* 2009;64(9):947-952.
12. Desjardins G, Cahalan M. The impact of routine transoesophageal echocardiography (TOE) in cardiac surgery. *Best Pract Res Clin Anaesthesiol.* 2009;23(3):263-271.
13. Fanshawe M, Ellis C, Habib S, Konstadt SN, Reich DL. A retrospective analysis of the costs and benefits related to alterations in cardiac surgery from routine intraoperative transesophageal echocardiography. *Anesth Analg.* 2002;95(4):824-827.
14. Skinner HJ, Mahmoud A, Uddin A, Mathew T. An investigation into the causes of unexpected intra-operative transoesophageal echocardiography findings. *Anaesthesia.* 2012;67(4):355-360.
15. Schwann NM, Hillel Z, Hoeft A, et al. Lack of effectiveness of the pulmonary artery catheter in cardiac surgery. *Anesth Analg.* 2011;113(5):994-1002.
16. Guarracino F. [The role of transesophageal echocardiography in intraoperative hemodynamic monitoring]. *Minerva Anestesiol.* 2001;67(4):320-324.

17. Aggarwal N, Unnikrishnan KP, Biswas I, Karunakaran J, Suneel PR. Intraoperative assessment of transient and persistent regional left ventricular wall motion abnormalities in patients undergoing coronary revascularization surgery using real time three-dimensional transesophageal echocardiography: a prospective observational study. *Echocardiography.* 2017;34(11):1649-1659.
18. Ramalingam G, Choi S-W, Agarwal S, et al. Complications related to peri-operative transoesophageal echocardiography—a one-year prospective national audit by the Association of Cardiothoracic Anaesthesia and Critical Care. *Anaesthesia.* 2020;75(1):21-26.
19. Purza R, Ghosh S, Walker C, et al. Transesophageal echocardiography complications in adult cardiac surgery: a retrospective cohort study. *Ann Thorac Surg.* 2017;103(3):795-802.
20. Patel KM, Desai RG, Trivedi K, Neuburger PJ, Krishnan S, Potestio CP. Complications of transesophageal echocardiography: a review of injuries, risk factors, and management. *J Cardiothorac Vasc Anesth.* 2022;36(8):3292-3302.
21. Kitkungvan D, Kalluru D, Lunagariya A, et al. Safety of transesophageal echocardiography in patients with thrombocytopenia. *J Am Soc Echocardiogr.* 2019;32(8):1010-1015.
22. Smith BB, Rehfeldt KH, Meinhardt JR, Smith MM. Safety and feasibility of transesophageal echocardiography in patients with prior esophageal surgery. *Echocardiography.* 2020;37(9):1430-1435.
23. Shanewise JS, Cheung AT, Aronson S, et al. ASE/SCA guidelines for performing a comprehensive intraoperative multiplane transesophageal echocardiography examination: recommendations of the American Society of Echocardiography Council for Intraoperative Echocardiography and the Society of Cardiovascular Anesthesiologists Task Force for Certification in Perioperative Transesophageal Echocardiography. *Anesth Analg.* 1999;89(4):870-884.
24. Nabeshima Y, Seo Y, Takeuchi M. A review of current trends in three-dimensional analysis of left ventricular myocardial strain. *Cardiovasc Ultrasound.* 2020;18(1):23.
25. Ng A, Swanevelder J. Perioperative monitoring of left ventricular function: what is the role of recent developments in echocardiography? *Br J Anaesth.* 2010;104(6):669-672.
26. Vegas A, Meineri M. Three-dimensional transesophageal echocardiography is a major advance for intraoperative clinical management of patients undergoing cardiac surgery: a core review. *Anesth Analg.* 2010;110(6):1548-1573.
27. Lang RM, Badano LP, Tsang W, et al. EAE/ASE recommendations for image acquisition and display using three-dimensional echocardiography. *J Am Soc Echocardiogr.* 2012;25(1):3-46.
28. Saito K, Okura H, Watanabe N, et al. Comprehensive evaluation of left ventricular strain using speckle tracking echocardiography in normal adults: comparison of three-dimensional and two-dimensional approaches. *J Am Soc Echocardiogr.* 2009;22(9):1025-1030.
29. Lang RM, Addetia K, Narang A, Mor-Avi V. 3-dimensional echocardiography: latest developments and future directions. *JACC Cardiovasc Imaging.* 2018;11(12):1854-1878.
30. Ballal RS, Nanda NC, Gatewood R, et al. Usefulness of transesophageal echocardiography in assessment of aortic dissection. *Circulation.* 1991;84(5):1903-1914.
31. Ender J, Singh R, Nakahira J, Subramanian S, Thiele H, Mukherjee C. Visualization of the circumflex artery in the perioperative setting with transesophageal echocardiography. *Anesth Analg.* 2012;115(1):22-26.
32. Roizen MF, Beaupre PN, Alpert RA, et al. Monitoring with two-dimensional transesophageal echocardiography. *J Vasc Surg.* 1984;1(2):300-305.
33. Smith JS, Cahalan MK, Benefiel DJ, et al. Intraoperative detection of myocardial ischemia in high-risk patients: electrocardiography versus two-dimensional transesophageal echocardiography. *Circulation.* 1985;72(5):1015-1021.
34. Swaminathan M, Morris RW, De Meyts DD, et al. Deterioration of regional wall motion immediately after coronary artery bypass graft surgery is associated with long-term major adverse cardiac events. *Anesthesiology.* 2007;107(5):739-745.
35. Leung JM, O'Kelly B, Browner WS, Tubau J, Hollenberg M, Mangano DT. Prognostic importance of postbypass regional wall-motion abnormalities in patients undergoing coronary artery bypass graft surgery. *Anesthesiology.* 1989;71(1):16-25.
36. De Mey N, Couture P, Laflamme M, et al. Intraoperative changes in regional wall motion: can postoperative coronary artery bypass graft failure be predicted? *J Cardiothorac Vasc Anesth.* 2012;26(3):371-375.
37. D'Ancona G, Karamanoukian HL, Ricci M, Schmid S, Bergsland J, Salerno TA. Graft revision after transit time flow measurement in off-pump coronary artery bypass grafting. *Eur J Cardiothorac Surg.* 2000;17(3):287-293.
38. Russell SJ, Tan C, O'Keefe P, et al. Optimized temporary bi-ventricular pacing improves haemodynamic function after on-pump cardiac surgery in patients with severe left ventricular systolic dysfunction: a two-centre randomized control trial. *Eur J Cardiothorac Surg.* 2012;42(6):e146-e151.
39. García-Bengochea JB, Fernández AL, Calvelo DS, Escudero JA, Gude F, Juanatey JRG. Temporary epicardial left ventricular and biventricular pacing improves cardiac output after cardiopulmonary bypass. *J Cardiothorac Surg.* 2012;7(1):113.
40. Shitole A, Kothiwale V, Patil S, et al. Evaluating impact of surgical myocardial revascularization on global left ventricular systolic function and immediate postoperative outcome using transesophageal echocardiography. *J Sci Soc.* 2024;51(4):522-530.
41. Shim JK, Kim KS, Couture P, et al. Hemodynamic management during off-pump coronary artery bypass surgery: a narrative review of proper targets for safe execution and troubleshooting. *Korean J Anesthesiol.* 2023;76(4):267-279.
42. Kramer A, Zygun D, Hawes H, Easton P, Ferland A. Pulse pressure variation predicts fluid responsiveness following coronary artery bypass surgery. *Chest.* 2004;126(5):1563-1568.
43. Bergquist BD, Leung JM, Bellows WH. Transesophageal echocardiography in myocardial revascularization: I. Accuracy of intraoperative real-time interpretation. *Anesth Analg.* 1996;82(6):1132-1138.
44. Cheung AT, Savino JS, Weiss SJ, Aukburg SJ, Berlin JA. Echocardiographic and hemodynamic indexes of left ventricular preload in patients with normal and abnormal ventricular function. *Anesthesiology.* 1994;81(2):376-387.
45. Lang RM, Badano LP, Mor-Avi V, et al. Recommendations for cardiac chamber quantification by echocardiography in adults: an update from the American Society of Echocardiography and the European Association of Cardiovascular Imaging. *J Am Soc Echocardiogr.* 2015;28(1):1-39.e14.

46. Albano P, Habana I. Prediction of fluid responsiveness in the immediate post-operative period of cardiac surgery. *J Anesth Crit Care Open Access*. 2021;13(1):35-45.
47. De Waal EEC, Rex S, Kruitwagen CLJJ, Kalkman CJ, Buhre WF. Dynamic preload indicators fail to predict fluid responsiveness in open-chest conditions. *Crit Care Med*. 2009;37(2):510-515.
48. Haji DL, Ali MM, Royse A, Canty DJ, Clarke S, Royse CF. Interatrial septum motion but not Doppler assessment predicts elevated pulmonary capillary wedge pressure in patients undergoing cardiac surgery. *Anesthesiology*. 2014;121(4):719-729.
49. Wang H, Zhang B, Wu WC, Zhu ZH, Wang H. Changes and predictors of secondary mild mitral regurgitation after coronary artery bypass grafting. *Rev Cardiovasc Med*. 2022;23(2):78.
50. Kasper J, Bolliger D, Skarvan K, Buser P, Filipovic M, Seeberger MD. Additional cross-sectional transesophageal echocardiography views improve perioperative right heart assessment. *Anesthesiology*. 2012;117(4):726-734.
51. Sukernik MR, Goswami S, Frumento RJ, Oz MC, Bennett-Guerrero E. National survey regarding the management of an intraoperatively diagnosed patent foramen ovale during coronary artery bypass graft surgery. *J Cardiothorac Vasc Anesth*. 2005;19(2):150-154.
52. Laghlam D, Coroyer L, Martial PJ, Estagnasie P, Squara P, Nguyen LS. Risk factors and complications associated with intra-operative or post-operative identification of a PFO in cardiac surgery patients: a cohort study. *Front Neurol*. 2023;13:1057479.
53. Otto CM, Nishimura RA, Bonow RO, et al. 2020 ACC/AHA guideline for the management of patients with valvular heart disease: executive summary. *J Am Coll Cardiol*. 2021;77(4):450-500.
54. Hur DJ, Sugeng L. Integration of three-dimensional echocardiography into the modern-day echo laboratory. *Echocardiography*. 2022;39(7):985-1000.
55. Turton EW, Ender J. Role of 3D echocardiography in cardiac surgery: strengths and limitations. *Curr Anesthesiol Rep*. 2017;7(3):291-298.
56. Efrimescu CI, Ng WCK, Vegas A. Perioperative 3D transoesophageal echocardiography. Part 1: fundamental principles. *BJA Educ*. 2024;24(6):217-226.
57. El Missiri AM. Echocardiographic assessment of left ventricular mechanical dyssynchrony—a practical approach. *Egypt Heart J*. 2014;66(3):217-225.
58. Faletra FF, Agricola E, Flachskampf FA, et al. Three-dimensional transoesophageal echocardiography: how to use and when to use—a clinical consensus statement from the European Association of Cardiovascular Imaging of the European Society of Cardiology. *Eur Heart J Cardiovasc Imaging*. 2023;24(8):e119-e197.
59. Bianco V, Kilic A, Gelzinis T, et al. Off-pump coronary artery bypass grafting: closing the communication gap across the ether screen. *J Cardiothorac Vasc Anesth*. 2020;34(1):258-266.
60. Kapoor PM, Chowdhury U, Mandal B, Kiran U, Karnatak R. Trans-esophageal echocardiography in off-pump coronary artery bypass grafting. *Ann Card Anaesth*. 2009;12(2):167.
61. Wang J, Filipovic M, Rudzitis A, et al. Transesophageal echocardiography for monitoring segmental wall motion during off-pump coronary artery bypass surgery. *Anesth Analg*. 2004;99(4):965-973.
62. Kim SH, Yeo JS, Yoon TG, Kim TY, Chee HK. Placing a saline bag underneath the displaced heart enhances transgastric transesophageal echocardiographic imaging during off-pump coronary artery bypass surgery. *Anesth Analg*. 2009;109(4):1038-1040.
63. Gurbuz AT, Hecht ML, Arslan AH. Intraoperative transesophageal echocardiography modifies strategy in off-pump coronary artery bypass grafting. *Ann Thorac Surg*. 2007;83(3):1035-1040.
64. Knol WG, Budde RPJ, Mahtab EAF, Bekkers JA, Bogers AJJC. Intimal aortic atherosclerosis in cardiac surgery: surgical strategies to prevent embolic stroke. *Eur J Cardiothorac Surg*. 2021;60(6):1259-1267.
65. van Zaane B, Nierich AP, Buhre WF, Brandon Bravo Bruinsma GJ, Moons KGM. Resolving the blind spot of transoesophageal echocardiography: a new diagnostic device for visualizing the ascending aorta in cardiac surgery. *Br J Anaesth*. 2007;98(4):434-441.
66. Katz ES, Tunick PA, Rusinek H, Ribakove G, Spencer FC, Kronzon I. Protruding aortic atheromas predict stroke in elderly patients undergoing cardiopulmonary bypass: experience with intraoperative transesophageal echocardiography. *J Am Coll Cardiol*. 1992;20(1):70-77.
67. Goldstein SA, Evangelista A, Abbara S, et al. Multimodality imaging of diseases of the thoracic aorta in adults: from the American Society of Echocardiography and the European Association of Cardiovascular Imaging. *J Am Soc Echocardiogr*. 2015;28(2):119-182.
68. Gold JP, Torres KE, Maldarelli W, Zhuravlev I, Condit D, Wasnick J. Improving outcomes in coronary surgery: the impact of echo-directed aortic cannulation and perioperative hemodynamic management in 500 patients. *Ann Thorac Surg*. 2004;78(5):1579-1585.
69. Evered LA, Silbert BS, Scott DA. Postoperative cognitive dysfunction and aortic atheroma. *Ann Thorac Surg*. 2010;89(4):1091-1097.
70. Lin TY, Chiu KM, Wang MJ, Chu SH. Carbon dioxide embolism during endoscopic saphenous vein harvesting in coronary artery bypass surgery. *J Thorac Cardiovasc Surg*. 2003;126(6):2011-2015.
71. Jung C, Bruno RR, Jumean M, et al. Management of cardiogenic shock: state-of-the-art. *Intensive Care Med*. 2024;50(11):1814-1829.
72. Van Diepen S, Katz JN, Albert NM, et al. Contemporary management of cardiogenic shock: a scientific statement from the American Heart Association. *Circulation*. 2017;136(16):e232-e268.
73. Platts DG, Sedgwick JF, Burstow DJ, Mullany DV, Fraser JF. The role of echocardiography in the management of patients supported by extracorporeal membrane oxygenation. *J Am Soc Echocardiogr*. 2012;25(2):131-141.
74. Catena E, Tasca G. Role of echocardiography in the perioperative management of mechanical circulatory assistance. *Best Pract Res Clin Anaesthesiol*. 2012;26(2):199-216.
75. Pappalardo F, Pieri M, Arnaez Corada B, et al. Timing and strategy for weaning from venoarterial ECMO are complex issues. *J Cardiothorac Vasc Anesth*. 2015;29(4):906-911.

76. Cavarocchi NC, Pitcher HT, Yang Q, et al. Weaning of extracorporeal membrane oxygenation using continuous hemodynamic transesophageal echocardiography. *J Thorac Cardiovasc Surg*. 2013;146(6):1474-1479.
77. Douflé G, Roscoe A, Billia F, Fan E. Echocardiography for adult patients supported with extracorporeal membrane oxygenation. *Crit Care*. 2015;19(1):326.
78. Baldetti L, Beneduce A, Chieffo A, Scandroglio AM. Technical tips for inserting and positioning the Impella device. *Card Interv Today*. 2023;17(4):60-65.
79. Chumnanvej S, Wood MJ, MacGillivray TE, Melo MFV. Perioperative echocardiographic examination for ventricular assist device implantation. *Anesth Analg*. 2007;105(3):583-601.
80. Castillo JG, Anyanwu AC, Adams DH, Nyirenda T, Fischer GW. Real-time 3-dimensional echocardiographic assessment of current continuous-flow rotary left ventricular assist devices. *J Cardiothorac Vasc Anesth*. 2009;23(5):702-710.
81. Hsu PL, Parker J, Egger C, Autschbach R, Schmitz-Rode T, Steinseifer U. Mechanical circulatory support for right heart failure: current technology and future outlook. *Artif Organs*. 2012;36(4):332-347.
82. Sheinberg R, Brady MB, Mitter N. Intraoperative transesophageal echocardiography and ventricular assist device insertion. *Semin Cardiothorac Vasc Anesth*. 2011;15(1-2):14-24.
83. Lampert BC, Teuteberg JJ. Right ventricular failure after left ventricular assist devices. *J Heart Lung Transplant*. 2015;34(9):1123-1130.
84. Puwanant S, Hamilton KK, Klodell CT, et al. Tricuspid annular motion as a predictor of severe right ventricular failure after left ventricular assist device implantation. *J Heart Lung Transplant*. 2008;27(10):1102-1107.
85. Kato TS, Jiang J, Schulze PC, et al. Serial echocardiography using tissue Doppler and speckle tracking imaging to monitor right ventricular failure before and after left ventricular assist device surgery. *JACC Heart Fail*. 2013;1(3):216-222.
86. Kang G, Ha R, Banerjee D. Pulmonary artery pulsatility index predicts right ventricular failure after left ventricular assist device implantation. *J Heart Lung Transplant*. 2016;35(1):67-73.
87. Dandel M, Hetzer R. Echocardiographic assessment of the right ventricle: impact of the distinctly load dependency of its size, geometry and performance. *Int J Cardiol*. 2016;221:1132-1142.
88. Nicoara A, Mackensen GB, Podgoreanu MV, Milano CA, Mathew JP, Swaminathan M. Malpositioned left ventricular assist device cannula: diagnosis and management with transesophageal echocardiography guidance. *Anesth Analg*. 2007;105(6):1574-1576.
89. Kirkpatrick JN, Wiegers SE, Lang RM. Left ventricular assist devices and other devices for end-stage heart failure: utility of echocardiography. *Curr Cardiol Rep*. 2010;12(3):257-264.
90. Allen SJ, Sidebotham D. Postoperative care and complications after ventricular assist device implantation. *Best Pract Res Clin Anaesthesiol*. 2012;26(2):231-246.
91. Grieshaber P, Schneider T, Oster L, et al. Prophylactic intra-aortic balloon counterpulsation before surgical myocardial revascularization in patients with acute myocardial infarction. *Perfusion*. 2018;33(5):390-400.

QUESTIONS

1. A 65-year-old patient undergoing CABG is being monitored with TEE. In the ME LAX view, the LVOT VTI is noted to be significantly reduced after separation from CPB. What is the most likely cause?

A. AR
B. Low CO due to myocardial stunning
C. RV failure
D. Pericardial tamponade

2. Which of the following echocardiographic findings is most suggestive of ischemia-related RWMA during coronary revascularization?

A. Global hypokinesis
B. Septal paradoxical motion
C. Dyskinesis of an apical segment
D. Hypokinesis in a coronary artery distribution

3. A patient undergoing OPCAB suddenly develops severe MR when the stabilizer is applied. What is the most likely mechanism?

A. Rupture of a mitral chordae tendineae
B. Myocardial stunning
C. Annular distortion due to cardiac displacement
D. Acute MI

4. During TEE examination of a patient requiring MCS with VA ECMO, which finding suggests that the LV is inadequately unloading?
A. AV opening in every cardiac cycle
B. LV distention with spontaneous echo contrast
C. Small LV EDD
D. Normal MV Doppler inflow pattern

5. A 70-year-old male undergoing CABG has persistent RV dysfunction postoperatively. Which of the following would best guide fluid management?
A. RA pressure
B. PA systolic pressure
C. IVC collapsibility index
D. TG RV end-diastolic area (EDA)

6. Which TEE finding is most indicative of significant AR?
A. PWD diastolic flow reversal in the descending aorta
B. Increased MV E velocity
C. RV dilation
D. Hyperdynamic LV function

7. During CABG, a patient experiences persistent hypotension despite aggressive fluid resuscitation and inotropic support. TEE is performed. Which of the following findings would be most concerning for ongoing myocardial ischemia?
A. Increased LVOT VTI
B. RWMA in an anterolateral segment
C. Preserved global LV function
D. Hyperdynamic LV function with reduced LV ESV

8. A patient after CABG on VA ECMO develops worsening hypoxemia despite adequate oxygenation settings. TEE is performed to evaluate the cause. Which of the following findings would suggest the presence of a PFO contributing to right-to-left shunting?
A. ME four-chamber view with CFD showing left-to-right shunting
B. ME bicaval view with contrast injection demonstrating bubbles in the LA within three cardiac cycles
C. TG SAX view showing a hyperdynamic LV
D. ME AV SAX view demonstrating laminar aortic flow

9. A patient on VA ECMO after CABG is evaluated with TEE. Which of the following findings would indicate a need to modify ECMO support?
A. LV distention with spontaneous echo contrast
B. AV opening with each cardiac cycle
C. Small LV cavity with reduced MV inflow
D. Normal septal motion and contractility

10. During CABG, a patient suddenly develops hemodynamic instability after grafting the LAD. TEE is performed. Which of the following findings would be most concerning for graft failure?
A. New severe MR with eccentric jet
B. Hyperdynamic LV function with reduced LV ESV
C. New akinesis of the anterior wall
D. Increased AV opening frequency

ANSWERS

1. **Correct Answer: B.**
Rationale: Option A: AR would typically present with a widened PP and holodiastolic flow reversal in the descending aorta on PWD. Option B: Myocardial stunning is common post-CPB due to ischemia-reperfusion injury. This results in transient myocardial dysfunction, often with low CO and reduced LVOT VTI. Option C: RV failure primarily affects right-side hemodynamics and may result in septal flattening but would not directly explain the reduction in LVOT VTI. Option D: Pericardial tamponade would result in a classic diastolic collapse of the RA and RV, as well as exaggerated respiratory variation in MV and TV inflows.

2. **Correct Answer: D.**
Rationale: Option A: Global hypokinesis suggests a systemic issue such as hypoperfusion or cardiomyopathy rather than focal ischemia. Option B: Septal paradoxical motion is often due to RV pacing or post-CPB changes rather than ischemia. Option C: Dyskinesis of an apical segment may be seen in Takotsubo cardiomyopathy but is not the classic sign of new ischemia. Option D: Hypokinesis in a coronary artery distribution is the hallmark of ischemia and is used to diagnose intraoperative ischemic changes.

3. **Correct Answer: C.**
Rationale: Option A: Rupture of a mitral chordae tendineae typically causes acute severe MR but is rare during OPCAB. Option B: Myocardial stunning can cause transient LV dysfunction but does not directly lead to severe MR. Option C: Annular distortion from heart positioning with stabilizers during OPCAB is a well-recognized cause of transient MR. Option D: Acute MI may cause ischemic MR, but it is not the most common cause in this intraoperative setting.

4. **Correct Answer: B.**
Rationale: Option A: AV opening in every cardiac cycle indicates that the LV is ejecting some volume, reducing concerns of inadequate unloading. Option B: LV distention with spontaneous echo contrast suggests blood stasis due to inadequate decompression, increasing the risk of thrombosis. Option C: A small LV EDD suggests excessive unloading rather than inadequate unloading. Option D: A normal MV inflow pattern would indicate preserved diastolic function, which is unlikely in a failing LV on VA ECMO.

5. **Correct Answer: D.**
Rationale: Option A: RA pressure may not accurately reflect preload due to ventricular interdependence. Option B: PA systolic pressure can be elevated due to primary pulmonary hypertension rather than volume status. Option C: IVC collapsibility index is unreliable in cardiac surgical patients due to mechanical ventilation effects. Option D: The TG RV EDA is a direct measure of RV preload and is most useful in assessing fluid responsiveness.

6. **Correct Answer: A.**
Rationale: Option A: PWD diastolic flow reversal in the descending aorta is a hallmark of severe AR, as retrograde flow occurs due to significant regurgitant volume. Option B: Increased MV E velocity is associated with elevated LV filling pressures but is not specific for AR. Option C: RV dilation may be seen in chronic left heart failure but is not a primary feature of AR. Option D: Hyperdynamic LV function can be seen in compensated AR but does not confirm severity.

7. **Correct Answer: B.**
Rationale: Option A: Increased LVOT VTI is generally associated with improved stroke volume and not a sign of ischemia. Option B: RWMA suggests ongoing ischemia or graft failure and is a critical intraoperative finding in CABG patients. Option C: Preserved global LV function would not indicate significant ischemia requiring immediate intervention. Option D: Hyperdynamic LV function with reduced LV ESV suggests hypovolemia or high catecholamine state rather than ischemia.

8. **Correct Answer: B.**
Rationale: Option A: ME four-chamber view with CFD showing left-to-right shunting does not confirm a right-to-left shunt, which is the cause of hypoxemia in this setting. Option B: ME bicaval view with contrast injection demonstrating bubbles in the LA within three cardiac cycles confirms a right-to-left shunt through a PFO, which can cause systemic desaturation in a post-CABG patient on VA ECMO. Option C: TG SAX view showing a

hyperdynamic LV is nonspecific and does not assess intracardiac shunting. Option D: ME AV SAX view demonstrating laminar aortic flow focuses on aortic valve function and is unrelated to detecting a PFO.

9. **Correct Answer: A.**
Rationale: Option A: LV distention with spontaneous echo contrast suggests inadequate unloading, which increases the risk of thrombosis and may require LV venting or increased ECMO flow adjustments. Option B: AV opening with each cardiac cycle indicates that the LV is ejecting blood, suggesting that ECMO flow may be appropriately balanced. Option C: A small LV cavity with reduced MV inflow suggests excessive unloading rather than a need for increased ECMO support. Option D: Normal septal motion and contractility would indicate that ECMO is adequately supporting cardiac function.

10. **Correct Answer: C.**
Rationale: Option A: New severe MR with eccentric jet may indicate papillary muscle dysfunction but is not a direct sign of graft failure. Option B: Hyperdynamic LV function with reduced LV ESV suggests hypovolemia or catecholamine surge rather than graft failure. Option C: New akinesis of the anterior wall strongly suggests ischemia due to LAD graft failure, which requires urgent assessment and possible revision. Option D: Increased AV opening frequency indicates improved CO and is not a sign of graft failure.

16

Transesophageal Echocardiography for Transcatheter Interventions

Massimiliano Meineri, Chirojit Mukherjee, and Anna Flo Forner

PART A: MITRAL VALVE INTERVENTIONS

Mitral valve regurgitation (MR) remains the second most common valve pathology in Europe and North America (1). Surgical mitral valve (MV) repair remains the gold standard (2), up to 50% of symptomatic patients do not have access to it due to unfavorable anatomy, excessive perioperative risk, or lack of consent (3).

Transcatheter interventions offer a therapeutic option for patients at excessive risk for conventional surgery who remain symptomatic despite optimal medical therapy. They include: edge-to edge repair, NeoChord implantation, and transcatheter MV implantation.

TRANSCATHETER EDGE-TO-EDGE REPAIR

Transcatheter edge-to-edge repair (TEER) has become a well-established option for patients with symptomatic MR at high risk for surgical repair (4,5).

The technique consists in "clipping" the MV leaflets together, creating a double-orifice valve as achieved surgically by an "Alfieri" stitch (6). Despite only addressing the leaflet contribution to MR, it offers good long-term results for primary MR and secondary MR (SMR).

Surgical repair remains the standard of care for primary MR (2); for a comparable mortality it provides lower rates of MR recurrence (4).

In inoperable patients however, 1-year mortality seems to be in favor of MV TEER (5). In this subset of patients, TEER is to be considered with a Class IIa level of evidence (2) according to the European and American guidelines (1).

While this evidence is based on first-generation devices and initial experience, ongoing trials (MITRA MR and REPAIR MR) are comparing current devices with surgical repairs based on current experience.

For SMR, in the large COAPT trials, MV TEER after guideline-directed medical therapy (GDMT) (7) and cardiac resynchronization proved to reduce the incidence of heart failure (HF)-related hospitalization and all-cause mortality (8). The same year another large randomized trial, the MITRA-FR (6), failed to confirm these results. One of the possible explanations is that in the COAPT trial, the MR was "disproportionate" to the degree of left ventricular (LV) dilation while in the MITRA-FR trial it was not, and in the latter, patients had more dilated LV (9). The real-world COAPT post-approval study clearly defined on 5,000 patients the efficacy of MV TEER in SMR with an increased quality of life and decreased HF-related hospitalization at 1 year using both abovementioned study enrollment criteria (10).

Current European surgical guidelines (2) suggest MV TEER for patients with SMR who remain symptomatic despite GDMT and fulfill the COAPT trial (8) criteria (Class I level of evidence). The American guidelines suggest MV TEER for suitable anatomy and a LV ejection fraction between 20 and 50, LV end systolic diameter (LVESD) of 70 mm or less, and pulmonary systolic pressure of 70 or less (Class IIa level of recommendation) (Table 16.1).

Advanced HF symptoms (New York Heart Association [NYHA] Class III and IV) are correlated with poor outcome after MV TEER for SMR (2) as well as decreased right ventricular (RV) function (11), pulmonary hypertension (12), chronic obstructive pulmonary disease (13), and chronic kidney disease (14).

PREPROCEDURAL EVALUATION

A comprehensive transesophageal echocardiography (TEE) examination (15) is a Class I indication for the preprocedural screening of patients undergoing MV TEER (1).

A structured approach to the assessment of the MV and the feasibility of TEER has been proposed by Hahn et al (16) and include the following steps:

1. Assessment of MV anatomy
2. Definition of MR mechanism
3. Quantification of MR

TABLE 16.1 Criteria for TEER in Secondary MR

	ACC/AHA Guidelines (1)	ASC/EACTS Guidelines (2)	
	Inclusion	Inclusion (COAPT Criteria)	Exclusion
LVEF	<50%	25%-50%	Moderate/severe RVF
LVESD	≤70 mm	≤70 mm	COPD on oxygen or steroids
PAPS	≤70 mm Hg	<70 mm Hg	CAD or TV disease requiring surgery
	Symptoms despite GDMT		Hypertrophic, restrictive, or infiltrative cardiomyopathy
			Hemodynamic instability

ACC/AHA, American College of Cardiology/American Heart Association; ASC/EACTS, American Society for Cardiovascular Surgery/European Association for Cardio-Thoracic Surgery; CAD, coronary artery disease; COPD, chronic obstructive pulmonary disease; GDMT, guideline-directed medical therapy; LVEF, left ventricular ejection fraction; LVESD, left ventricular end systolic diameter; MR, mitral regurgitation; PAPS, pulmonary artery pressure systolic; RVF, right ventricular failure; TEER, transcatheter edge-to-edge repair; TV, tricuspid valve.

4. Assessment of TEER feasibility
5. Assessment of the interatrial septum (IAS) and the left atrial appendage (LAA)

Assessment of Mitral Valve Anatomy

A complete assessment of the MV anatomy includes the following 2D views:

Midesophageal (ME) four-chamber view, mitral commissural, long-axis (LAX) view, and transgastric (TG) basal short-axis (SAX) view.

From the mitral commissural view where the MV coaptation can be assessed, a secondary plane can be activated and allows simultaneous display of the perpendicular LAX view (multiplane view) with and without color Doppler and shows the leaflet morphology and motion (Figures 16.1 and 16.2; Videos 16.1 and 16.2). In this view the anteroposterior and mediolateral annulus can be simultaneously measured. The secondary plane can be tilted left and right to scroll through the entire MV commissure from medial to lateral and identify the exact location of the pathology responsible for the MR.

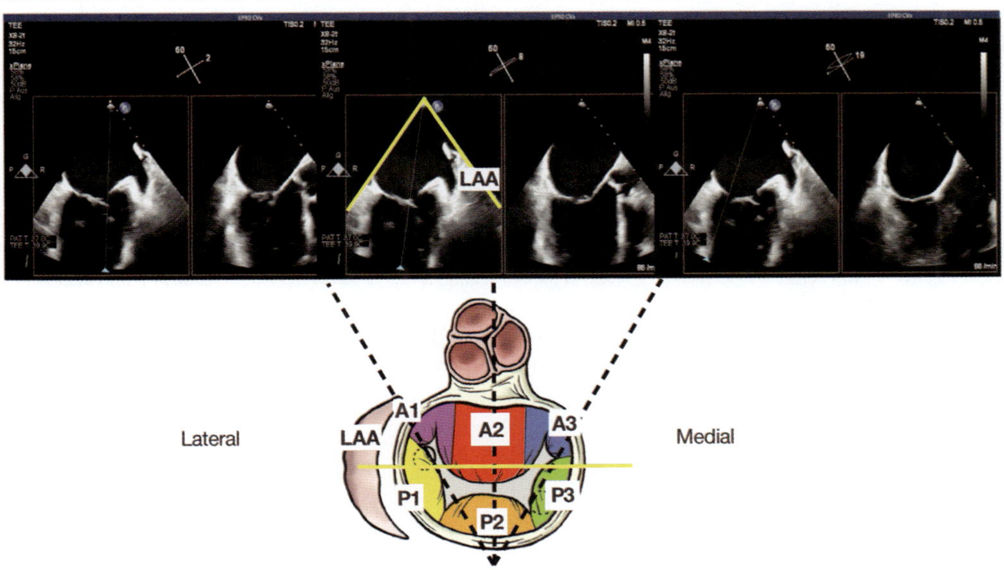

FIGURE 16.1 Multiplane view mitral valve (MV) scanning. Midesophageal (ME) mitral commissural (MC) view with the simultaneous perpendicular ME long-axis (LAX) view on the secondary plane to the right cutting in the middle of the MV and displaying A2-P2 scallops. The secondary plane can be moved laterally toward the left atrial appendage (LAA) and cut through A1-P1 or in the opposite direction medially to display A3-P3 scallops.

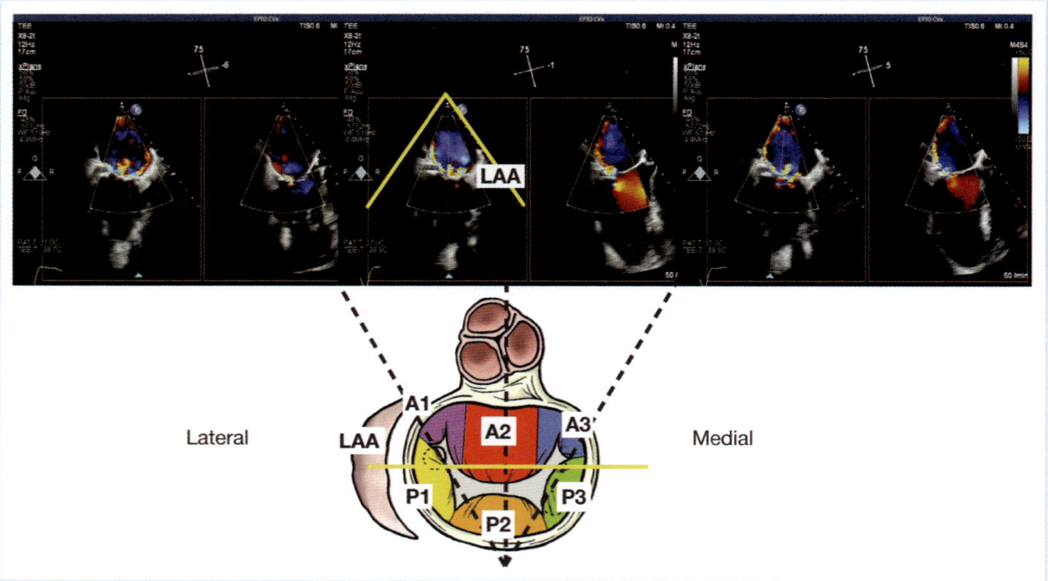

FIGURE 16.2 Multiplane view mitral valve (MV) scanning with color Doppler. Multiplane mode can be used also with color Doppler at the cost of a lower temporal resolution. LAA, left atrial appendage.

Definition of Mitral Regurgitation Mechanism

From the multiplane view a 3D zoom view can be obtained by placing the region of interest on the two perpendicular views including the entire MV annulus (Figure 16.3; Video 16.3). After orienting the 3D dataset in the surgical orientation (en face view) color Doppler can be activated to confirm the origin of the regurgitation jet. Apnea should be performed to allow multibeat electrocardiogram (ECG)-gated acquisition to increase the temporal resolution of the 3D, especially color 3D datasets. TEE should then define the pathophysiology of MR according to the Carpentier classification (17).

In *primary* MR, the mechanism of MR is excessive leaflet motion (Type II). It is important to define whether this is due to Barlow disease, with excessive tissue "baggy" leaflets and extensive prolapse or fibroelastic deficiency, leading to leaflet thinning and chordal rupture with more localized pathology (Figure 16.3;

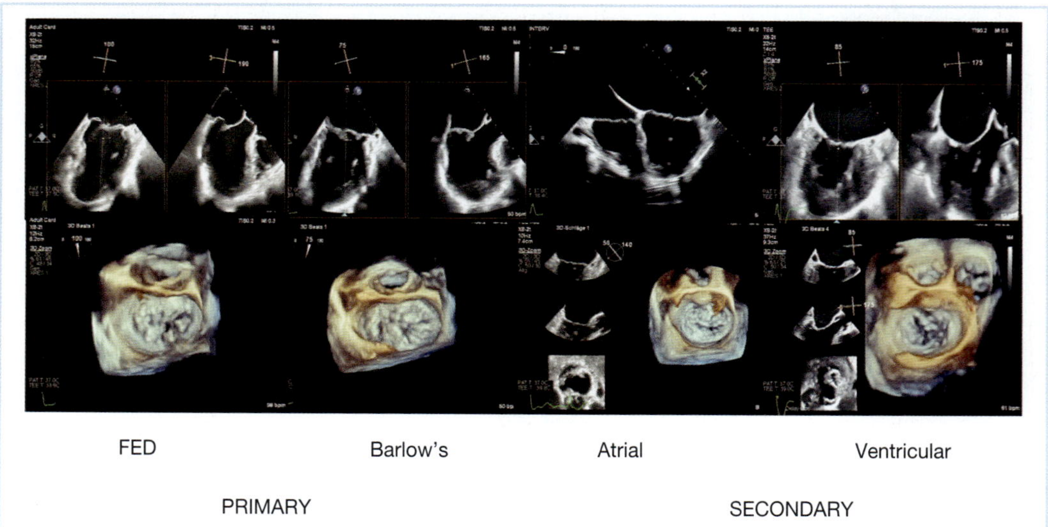

FIGURE 16.3 Mitral regurgitation etiology.

Video 16.3) (18). **The presence of leaflet indentations or clefts (indentations that involve the entire leaflet length until the annulus) should be carefully assessed in the 3D MV en face view (19) as they cannot be addressed with TEER intervention.**

In SMR (functional) the leaflets are morphologically normal, and the MR is due to either annular dilation (Type I) secondary to chronic atrial fibrillation (20) or LV dilation and systolic leaflet tethering (Type IIIb) (21).

Evaluating the presence and size of leaflet and annular calcification is very important to determine TEER feasibility.

Quantification of Mitral Regurgitation

Quantification of MR is performed according to current guidelines and should include 2D and 3D echocardiography to define quantitative parameters (22). In SMR the effective regurgitant orifice area (EROA) is typically not round (23) (Figure 16.4A,B; Video 16.4); therefore, the quantification based on proximal isovelocity surface area (PISA) and 2D vena contracta underestimates the degree of MR. In this patient population, it is key to obtain a 3D color Doppler vena contracta area at baseline to then assess the results postintervention.

Assessment of Transcatheter Edge-to-Edge Repair Feasibility

Intraoperative preprocedural MR evaluation carries the challenge of a chanced physiologic milieu in comparison to preprocedural assessment. General anesthesia (GA) and positive pressure ventilation lead to vasodilation and reduced preload (24). For proper evaluation of the degree of MR it is key to attempt to reproduce "awake" preoperative conditions by increasing the arterial blood pressure to preoperative values with vasoconstrictors, reproduce preoperative LV end diastolic volumes by administering fluids, and pause positive pressure ventilation (Figure 16.4C,D; Video 16.4).

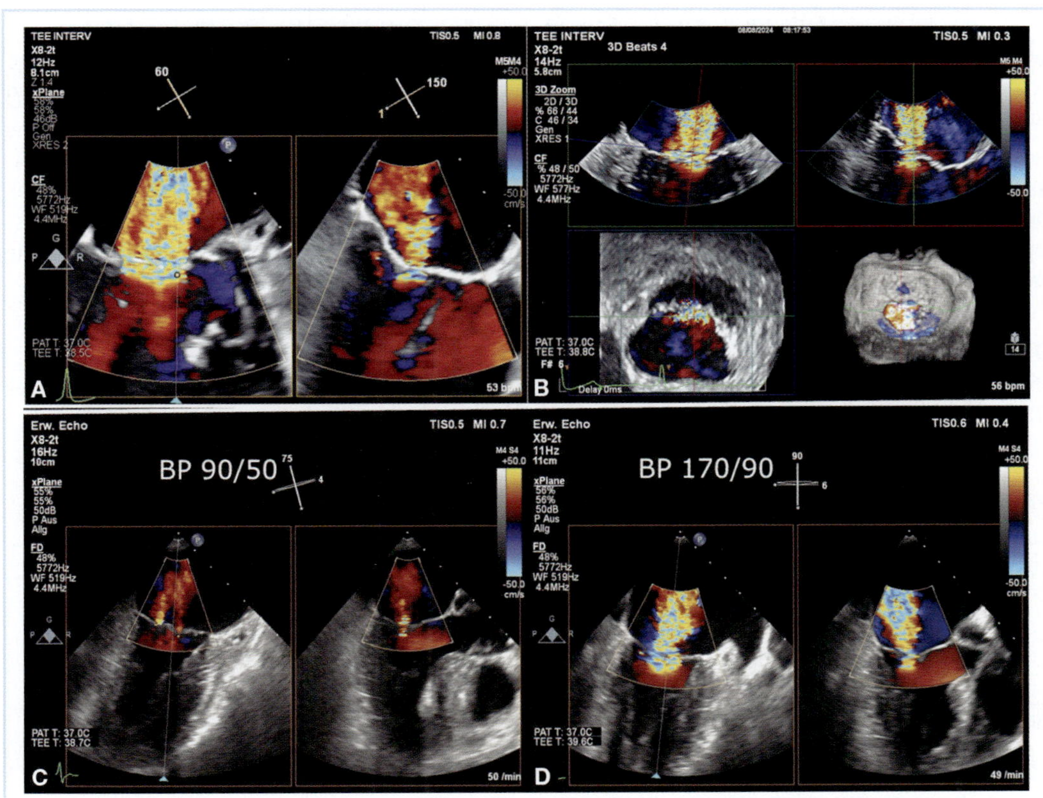

FIGURE 16.4 Intraoperative evaluation of secondary mitral regurgitation (MR). A: Midesophageal (ME) mitral commissural (MC) view displaying a much larger jet than the perpendicular ME long-axis (LAX) view. B: Secondary MR results in an oval regurgitant orifice as demonstrated by the vena contracta (VC) displayed in the lower left panel. C,D: In this patient the degree of MR is minimal with lower blood pressure and severe hypertension.

TABLE 16.2 MV TEE Feasibility Definition According to the Expert Consensus

	Favorable	Less Favorable or Unfavorable
Pathology location	Medial	Commissure, leaflet perforation or clefts
Calcification	None or minimal	Severe leaflet at the grasping zone Severe annular
Mean MV gradient	<4 mm Hg	>5 mm Hg
MV area	>4 cm^2	<4 cm^2
Grasping zone	>10 mm	<7 mm
Primary MR	Flail width <15 mm, flail gap <10 mm Single segment pathology	Flail width >15 mm, flail gap >10 mm Multisegment pathology Severe leaflet thickening (>5 mm) Redundant leaflets LVESD >50 mm
Secondary MR	Tenting height <11 mm Coaptation (overlap) length >2 mm	LVESD >70 mm

LVESD, left ventricular end systolic diameter; MR, mitral regurgitation; MV, mitral valve; TEE, transesophageal echocardiography. Reprinted from Bonow RO, O'Gara PT, Adams DH, et al. 2020 focused update of the 2017 ACC expert consensus decision pathway on the management of mitral regurgitation: a report of the American College of Cardiology Solution Set Oversight Committee. *J Am Coll Cardiol*. 2020;75(17):2236-2270. With permission from Elsevier.

Assessment of the MV orifice area by 3D and pressure gradients using continuous-wave Doppler is key to plan transcatheter intervention.

The number, location, and size of the regurgitant jets will play a significant role in planning of the transcatheter approach and the use of a single or multiple clips. Feasibility of MV TEER was defined in the updated expert consensus decision pathway document summarized in Table 16.2 (25). The consensus also pointed out that in experienced large volume centers TEER can still be performed in less favorable MV anatomy.

Assessment of the Interatrial Septum and the Left Atrial Appendage

Finally, the assessment of IAS using ME bicaval view and multiplane display to identify the optimal transseptal puncture location as well as the assessment of LAA to rule out thrombi should be integrated in the preintervention assessment.

DEVICE SELECTION

There are three different devices available in the market: the Pascal, the Mitraclip, and the Dragonfly devices (Table 16.3).

TABLE 16.3 Clip Types

Type of Device	Mitral Clip G4	Pascal Precision	Dragonfly
	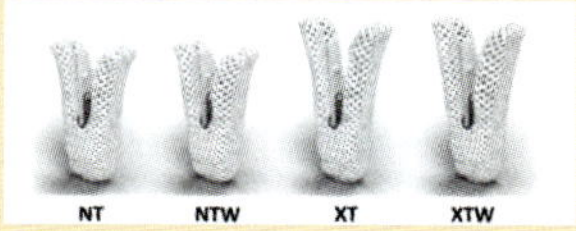	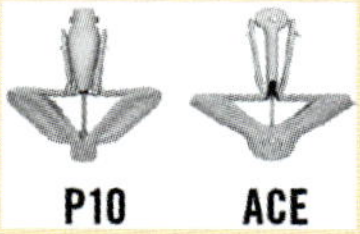	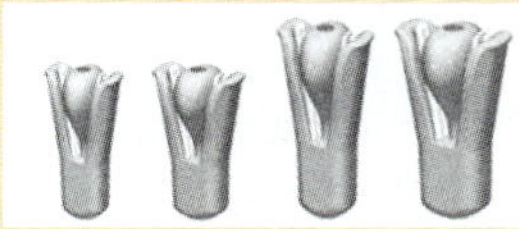
Sizes	NT NTW XT XTW	P10 ACE	SN0409 XN0412SW0609 XW0612
Frame	Cobalt-chromium	Nitinol	Cobalt-chromium
Closure	Active	Passive	Active
Arms	Rigid	Flexible	Rigid
Spacer	No	Yes (P10)	Adjustable
Independent grasping	Yes	Yes	Yes

The Mitraclip system was the first to be introduced into the market (26) and has reached its fourth generation (27). It consists of two rigid cobalt-chromium frames and two flexible independent nitinol-based grippers equipped with small hooks. The closing mechanism is active and applies force to the arms to pull the leaflets together. It comes in two sizes, a classic NT (9 mm arms) and XT (12 mm arms), which come in a thinner version (NT, XT 4 mm width) or a thicker version (NTW, XTW 6 mm width). In case of difficulties in extracting the clip from underneath the valve, the arms can be reverted.

The Pascal system was first described in 2016 (28) and is now in its second generation of devices (Precision). It offers two types of clips: the P10 and the ACE. The P10 clip consists of a nitinol frame with two 26-mm curved paddles held open at 180° and two 10-mm grippers with small hooks. When released, after grasping, the two paddles close due to the passive recoil of the nitinol frame against a central bullet-shaped spacer. The ACE clip has the same characteristics of the P10 but has no spacer, allowing placement of two clips next to one another.

The newly described Dragonfly system (29) is a hybrid of the two earlier mentioned systems. It comes in four sizes and consists of a rigid cobalt-chromium frame and two flexible independent nitinol-based grippers equipped with small hooks. After active closure of the arms, a central adjustable spacer that can be filled with a variable amount of saline fills eventual gaps between the arms. Approval for clinical use in Europe and North America is still pending.

Head-to-head comparison (30) showed noninferiority of the Pascal versus the Mitraclip system for primary MR. There are no clear guidelines on clip selection, and it is mostly based on institutional experience. As a general rule, bigger and rigid clips tend to generate more tension on the leaflets than smaller clips carrying a higher risk of leaflet tears and single-leaflet attachment. However, retrospective analyses failed to show a difference between the Mitraclip NT and XT (31).

Smaller clips may be indicated in cases of localized disease, after failed surgical repair, for multiple and more commissural lesions (32).

The reduction of MV area (MVA) after clipping has been reported as 47% for the Pascal P10 clips, 52% for the Mitraclip NT, and 57% for the Mitraclip XT. The reduction is more pronounced when the clip is placed centrally (33).

For proper clip selection we need to consider the following factors:

1. Pathophysiology (primary MR vs SMR)
2. Leaflet morphology and dynamics
3. MVA and gradient
4. Single or combined procedures
5. Center experience

Center volume and operator experience play an important role in procedural success (34). More complex valve anatomy should be referred to high-volume centers (35).

INTRAPROCEDURAL GUIDANCE

Intraprocedural guidance for MV TEER requires special training (36) and relies on continuous effective communication between the interventionalist and the echocardiographer. Ideally both should be able to continuously and easily view the fluoroscopy (to see the catheter position with respect to the TEE probe) and the echocardiographic images. The placement of the device requires a stepwise approach to TEE guidance and includes

1. Transseptal puncture
2. Introduction of the clip delivery catheter
3. Positioning of clip to grasping location
4. Leaflet grasping and clip closure
5. Assessment of results
6. Clip release

Transseptal Puncture

The IAS is punctured in the fossa ovalis, which is punctured in the superior-posterior corner. The aim is for the catheter to cross high from the MV in the intersection of an imaginary vertical line from the posteromedial commissure that intersects the superior rim of the fossa ovalis. This will allow the best trajectory and enough room for catheter maneuvers.

Optimal transseptal puncture is key for success and carries a high risk of iatrogenic injury such as atrial and aorta perforation (37). Fusion imaging may be used to possibly reduce procedural time and increase precision and safety (38).

One starts with the ME bicaval view that allows visualization of the superior and inferior end of the fossa ovalis close to the superior (SVC) and inferior vena cava (IVC), respectively. Biplane imaging is activated to display the anterior (close to the aortic valve) and posterior aspect of the fossa ovalis. When the bicaval view is obtained at more than 90° the perpendicular modified ME RV inflow-outflow view is right left inverted. The puncture catheter is positioned in the SVC and the needle stylet is then advanced. The catheter is retracted and rotated against the IAS. As soon as the superior rim of the fossa ovalis is reached in the ME bicaval view, the needle is pushed against the septum, resulting in an indentation (Figure 16.5A; Video 16.5). The anteroposterior position is evaluated in the perpendicular view. The puncture site should be between 4 and 5 cm from the coaptation plane. The puncture height is measured in the ME four-chamber view (Figure 16.5B). From the ME four-chamber view, a 3D zoom view can be obtained to visualize en face the site of puncture and its relation to the posteromedial commissure (Figure 16.5C; Video 16.5). The needle is then advanced through the septum for a maximum of 1 cm to allow the catheter to the left atrium (LA). Needle electrification allows crossing of fibrotic septa and better control during this procedure.

Introduction of the Clip Delivery Catheter

Through the catheter a wire is advanced and inserted in the upper pulmonary vein (Figure 16.5D,E; Video 16.5). Over the wire the guiding sheath with a pointed and long dilator is advanced through the septum under echo guidance (Figure 16.5F; Video 16.5) and after removal of the dilator and wire, the catheter's tip is to be positioned approximately 2 cm in the LA.

The clip delivery catheter is advanced through the guiding sheath into the LA (Figure 16.6A; Video 16.6). The advancement of the clip can be followed on fluoroscopy. The clip tip should be immediately identified on TEE as it comes out of the delivery catheter (Figure 16.6B; Video 16.6) and followed the whole time until it reaches the MV annular plane (Figure 16.6C; Video 16.6) in order to avoid contact with the

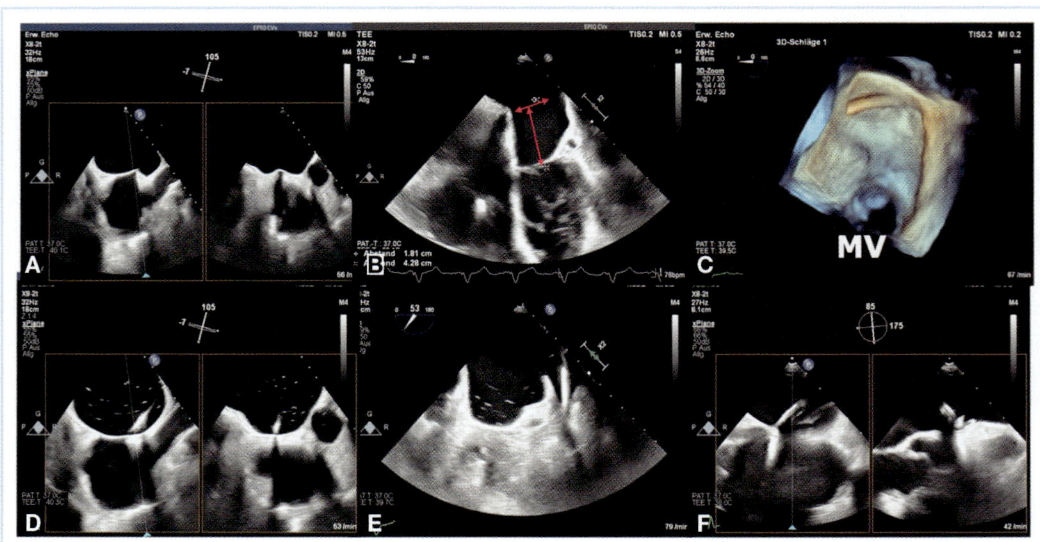

FIGURE 16.5 Transseptal puncture. A: Midesophageal (ME) bicaval view: ideal tenting of the transseptal puncture needle in the upper part of the fossa ovalis and posterior with respect to the aorta in the perpendicular view. B: ME four-chambered view: measurement of puncture height with respect to the mitral valve (MV) coaptation. C: 3D live view of the delivery catheter with respect to the medial MV commissure. D: Multiplane view of the interatrial septum (IAS): crossing of the catheter. E: Modified mitral commissural (MC) view: wire in the left upper pulmonary vein. F: Multiplanar view of the IAS: position of the delivery catheter.

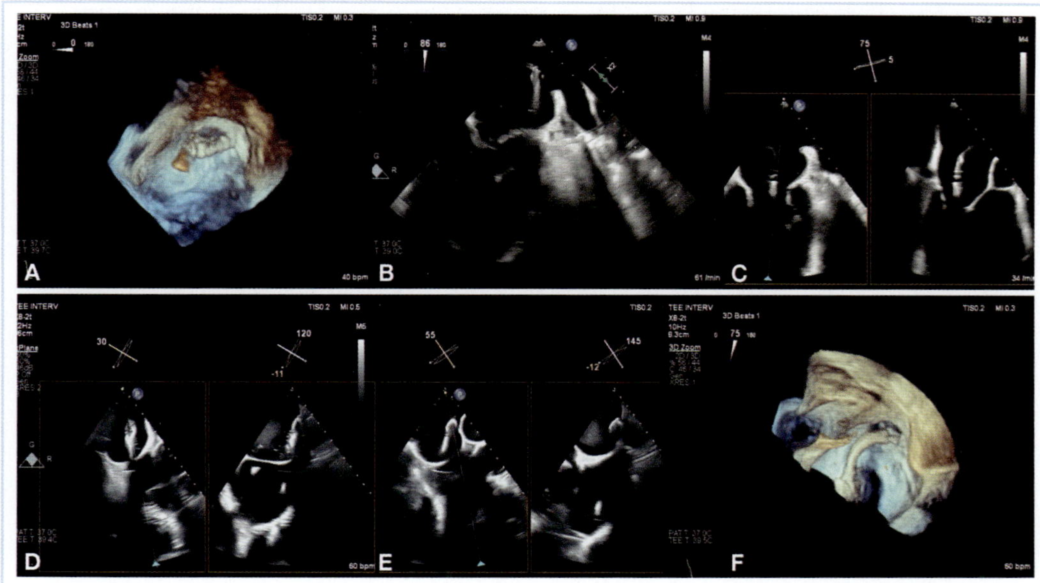

FIGURE 16.6 Positioning of the clip. A: Live 3D view of the interatrial septum (IAS) from the left atrium (LA): position of the delivery catheter with respect to the mitral valve (MV). B: Modified midesophageal (ME) two-chamber view: clip tip aiming at the Coumadin ridge. C: ME mitral commissural (MC) and simultaneous ME long-axis (LAX) views: clip above the MV leaflets. D: Multiplane view of the IAS: clip coming out of the delivery catheter. E: Multiplane view of the LA: the clip advancing toward the aorta. F: 3D live view of the MV from the LA: clip above the MV leaflets.

atrial wall and potential injury. The Pascal system comes out of the guiding sheath elongated (Figure 16.6D; Video 16.6) and must immediately be loaded (Figure 16.6C) with direct TEE visualization. For this purpose, the ME mitral commissural view with multiplane imaging can be used or live 3D modes (narrow sector or zoom) (Figure 16.6; Video 16.6).

Positioning of Clip to Grasping Location

In the ME mitral commissural view the clip is moved medial and lateral to be positioned above the lesion. Biplane imaging is activated and the secondary plane aligned along the clip delivery catheter. The clip is then opened, and the arms are to be viewed only in the secondary LAX plane (Figure 16.7A). At this point a 3D zoom view is activated to confirm the position of the clip with respect to the MV commissure. The clips can be further rotated to be perpendicular to the commissure (Figure 16.7B-D; Video 16.7). Color flow Doppler can be activated to confirm that the clip lies within the regurgitant jet. The clip is then advanced into the LV (Figure 16.7D; Video 16.7). The correct clip positioning should be confirmed in the ME mitral commissural view and the secondary plane positioned along the clip delivery catheter. 3D zoom can be obtained including enough depth to include the clip and the gain reduced to make the leaflets transparent to further confirm the correct clip positioning (Figure 16.7E; Video 16.7).

Leaflet Grasping and Clip Closure

The clip is then gently withdrawn to load the leaflets into the arms (Figure 16.8).

Ideally at least 4 mm of leaflet should be loaded and the leaflet tips (Figure 16.9; Video 16.8) should reach the arm's hinge point in order to minimize the risk of single-leaflet attachment and optimize results (39). The graspers are then put down and the clips closed. Leaflet grasping and clip closure can be recorded as a long loop to document their effect on MV leaflet by creating tension and pulling them together (Figure 16.8). The same steps are followed for the Pascal device (Figure 16.10; Video 16.9). In case of large gaps or challenging grasping, ventilation can be stopped and positive end-expiratory pressure (PEEP) applied. The effect of intrathoracic pressure on clip positioning follows the "EMIL" principle: expiratory = medial; inspiratory = lateral. Other techniques have also been used such as rapid pacing or adenosine-induced bradycardia.

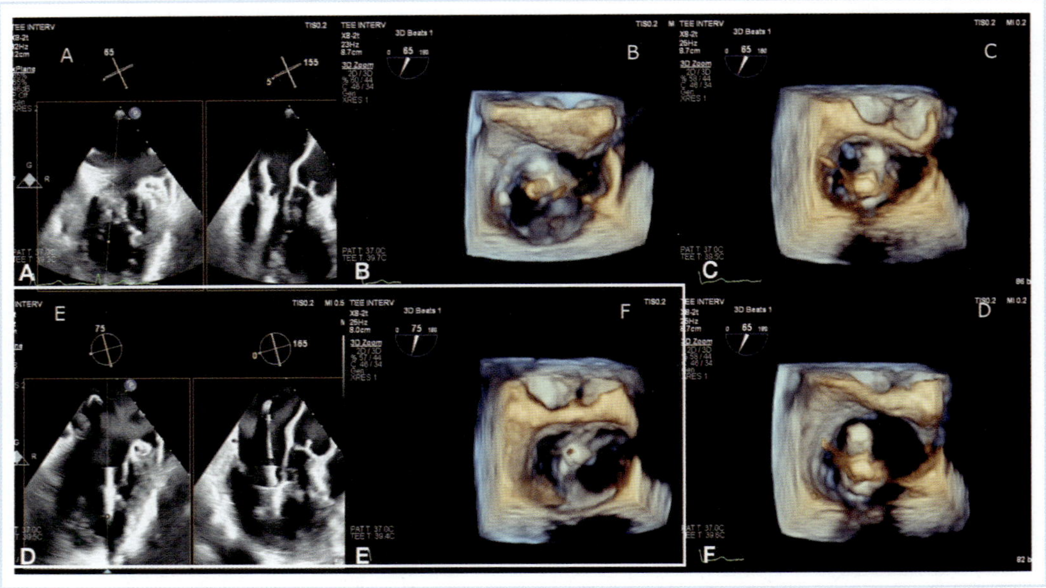

FIGURE 16.7 Leaflet grasping. A: Midesophageal (ME) mitral commissural (MC) and simultaneous ME long-axis (LAX) views: clip opening above the mitral valve (MV). B: 3D en face view of the MV: clip oriented at 11 to 5 o'clock. C: 3D en face view of the MV: clip rotated to 1 to 7 o'clock. D: 3D en face view of the MV: clip open at 12 to 6 o'clock and displaced laterally. E: ME MC and simultaneous ME LAX views: clip advanced into the left ventricle (LV). F: 3D en face view of the MV: clip advanced into the LV.

Assessment of Results

At this point a comprehensive evaluation of MV function should be performed. A gradient of more than 5 mm Hg should be ruled out as well as residual MVA of less than 1.5 cm^2.

Residual MR should be evaluated and in case of multiple jets the respective vena contracta area (VCA) areas on 3D color Doppler should be added (40).

Residual MR is a common unwanted finding following MV TEER. After MV TEER for primary MR, patients with residual MR less than mild seem to have a better outcome when compared to those with a residual MR more than moderate (41). On the other hand, the COAP trial failed to show a outcome difference in patients with different grades of residual MR (12).

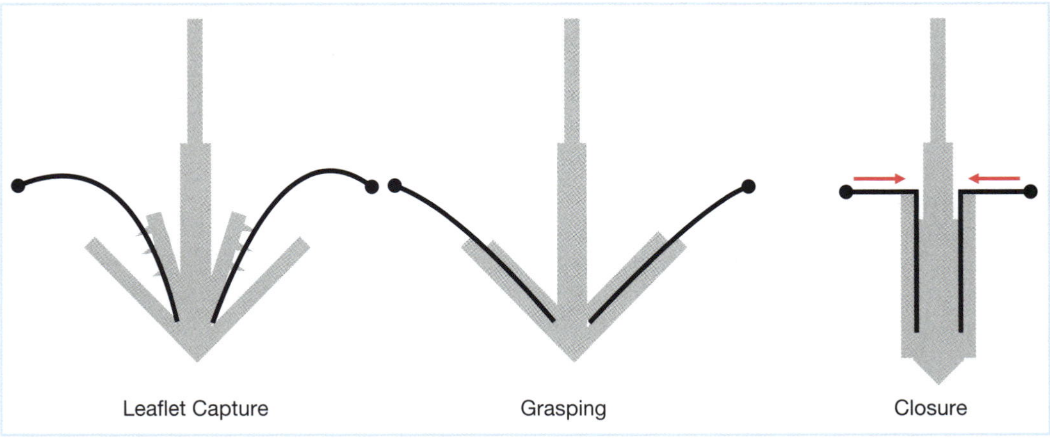

FIGURE 16.8 Leaflet grasping. Ideal leaflet grasping position. The red arrow symbolizes the leaflet tension.

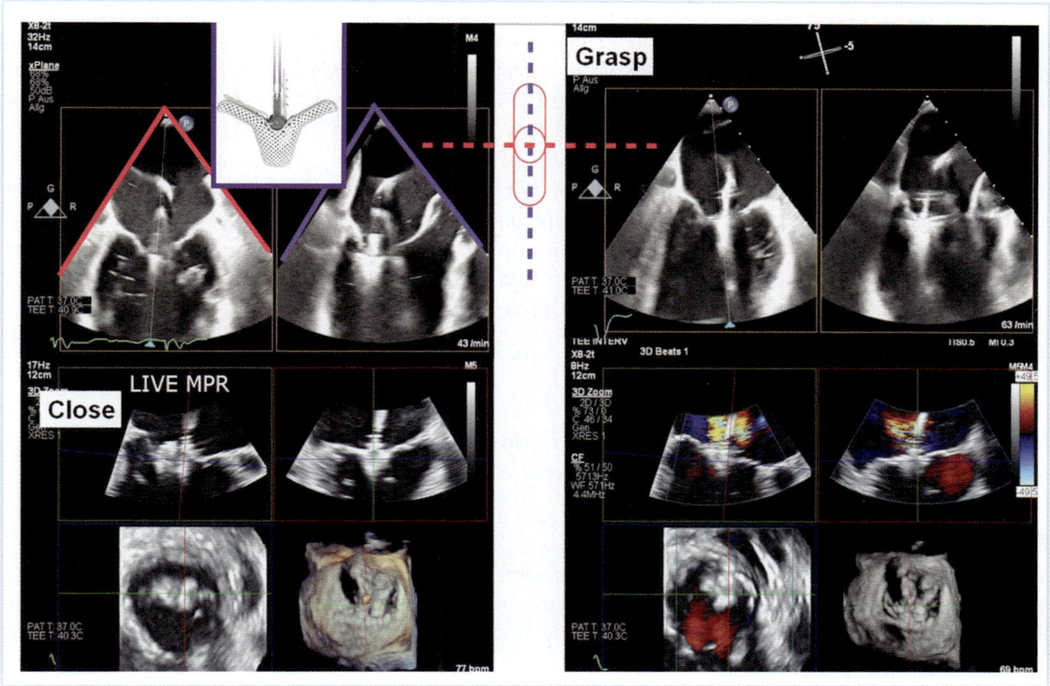

FIGURE 16.9 Leaflet grasping, Mitraclip. Midesophageal (ME) mitral commissural (MC) and simultaneous ME long-axis (LAX) views: clip in grasping position and grasp closure; live multiplanar reconstruction after clip closure with and without color Doppler. The green and the red planes have been aligned with the clip.

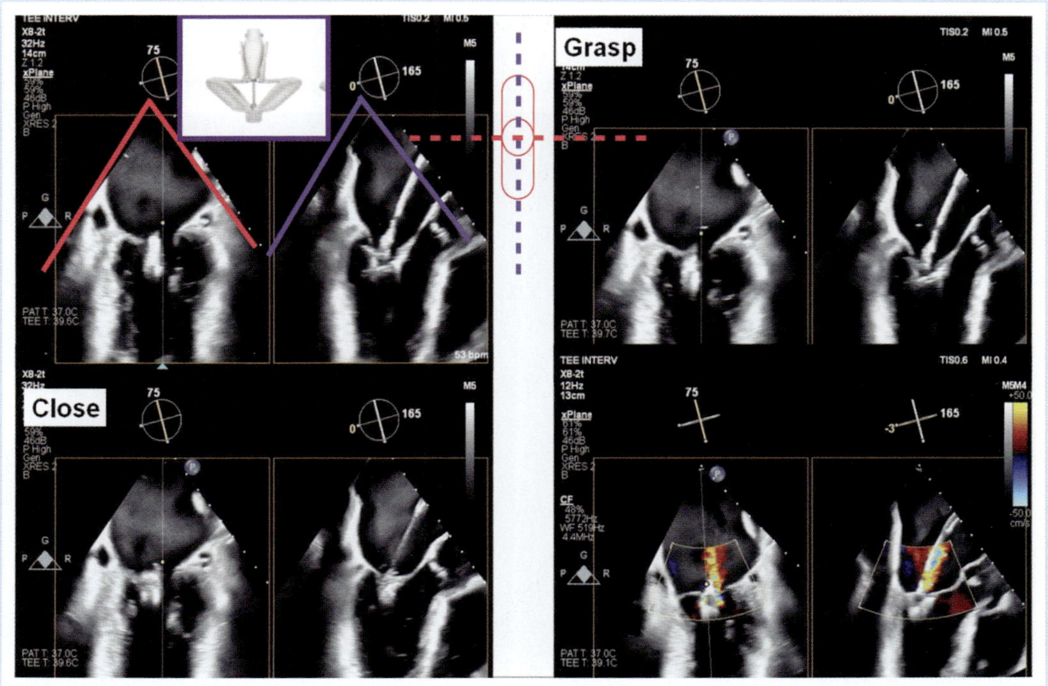

FIGURE 16.10 Leaflet grasping, Mitraclip Pascal. Midesophageal (ME) mitral commissural (MC) and simultaneous ME long-axis (LAX) views: clip in grasping position and grasp closure followed by clip closure and color Doppler assessment of residual mitral regurgitation (MR).

In challenging cases, MR reduction should be balanced against increased gradients and reduction of mitral valve orifice area (MVOA). A post-implant mean gradient of more than 5 mm Hg (42) and a MVOA of less than 1.9 cm^2 (43) are associated with worse outcomes and failed reduction of pulmonary congestion. While pressure gradients highly depend on loading and hemodynamic conditions, residual MVA should be quantified using multiplanar reconstruction (MPR) on a 3D MV dataset (Figure 16.11; Video 16.10).

The clip delivery catheter allows for direct measure of LA pressure. The decrease in LA pressure has been used as an indirect measure of MR reduction and TEER success (44). Similarly, the pulmonary vein flow analysis seams to correlate to MR recurrence and outcomes (45).

In case of suboptimal results, after grasping the clip can be released and withdrawn (failed procedure or change of strategy with new size clip), reopened, and repositioned or the grasping can be optimized by regrasping one of the leaflets and slightly rotating the clip (32).

Clip Release

In case of acceptable residual MR and no stenosis the clip is released. Valve function and presence of residual MR must be reevaluated since the clip is no longer held by the delivery catheter, follows the leaflets movement, and worsening of MR can at times be observed.

POSTPROCEDURAL COMPLICATION

Residual interatrial septal defect in the location of septal puncture is always observed after MV TEER. In most cases, the shunt is left to right and has no acute consequences on oxygenation and hemodynamics and the defect often closes spontaneously (46) over time. In case of concomitant tricuspid regurgitation (TR) or increased right atrial (RA) pressure, removal of the delivery catheter results in a sudden right to left shunt and sudden desaturation. In this case, percutaneous closure should be performed as soon as possible.

Large residual commissural or inter-clip MR jets have been addressed with the implantation of occluder devices (47) despite the risk of embolization and residual stenosis.

Single-leaflet attachment has been reported in 3.5% of cases (48). Intraoperatively, it has been addressed with a second or third stabilizing clip when feasible. Postoperative occurrence results inevitably in the recurrence of severe MR. In this scenario a new transcatheter approach has been described and consists in clip excision and percutaneous MV implantation (49).

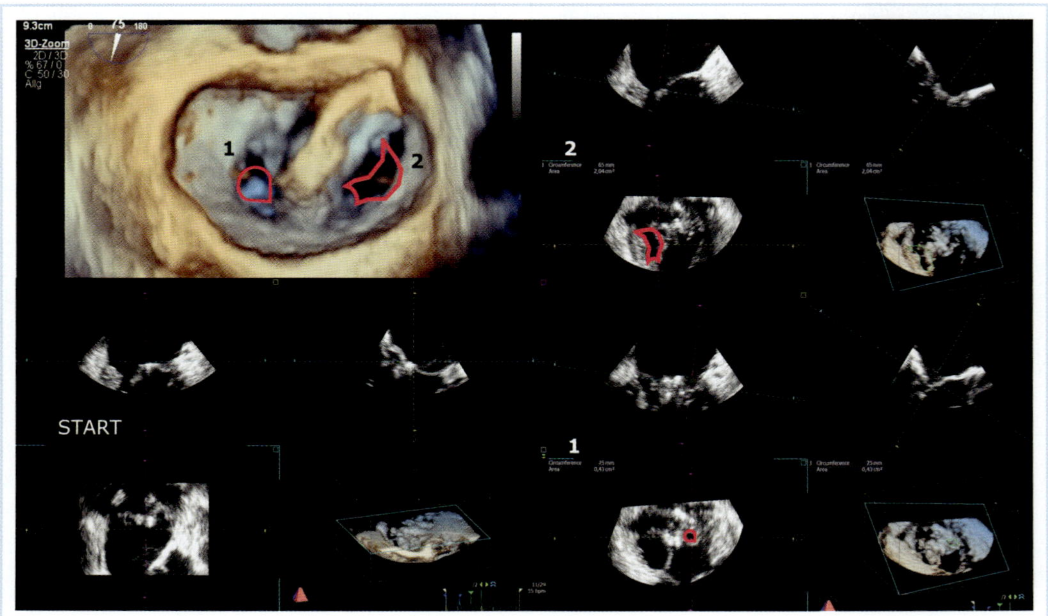

FIGURE 16.11 3D mitral valve area. 3D live en face view after clip closure and offline multiplanar measurement of individual orifice areas for the two openings. The purple and the yellow planes are oriented perpendicular to the orifice and the blue plane is positioned at the leaflet tip.

Other possible but less formally reported complications following MV TEER include: RV failure due to air embolism during clip placement, pericardial effusion secondary to LA perforation, and LV afterload mismatch after elimination of MR in patients with severely reduced LV function. An ME four-chamber view at the end of the procedure should be obtained to document absence of pericardial effusion and identify worsening LV and RV function.

TRANSAPICAL CHORD IMPLANTATION

This method consists of repairing the MV by implanting artificial neochordae on a beating heart between the edge of the MV leaflets and the LV apex. It is suitable for patients with Carpentier Type II disease without annulus dilation and increased surgical risk. It carries the downsides of the apical approach and requires a left lateral thoracotomy, and its popularity has been partially overcome by TEER. However, it results in a more physiologic outcome and carries a minimal risk of MV stenosis. There are two delivery systems available for this procedure: the NeoChord DS1000 and the Harpoon. The NeoChord system has proven good results (50) in favorable anatomy and long-term durability (51). The Harpoon system came later on the market but also proved its feasibility (52) and durability to affect LV remodeling at 1 year (53).

Preoperative assessment should focus on the assessment of feasible anatomy (Figure 16.12A-C; Video 16.11; Table 16.4) (54). This includes identification of calcification and lack of leaflet redundancy that contraindicates this procedure.

Intraprocedural guidance starts with identification of LV apex by surgical digital palpation following chest opening in the ME mitral commissural view and the multiplane perpendicular LAX view (Figure 16.12D; Video 16.11). The same view guides device positioning of the NeoChord delivery system to the affected scallop (Figure 16.12E,F; Video 16.11). The polytetrafluoroethylene (PTFE) suture of the NeoChord is retracted after color-coded optics verifies leaflet grasping and perforation. The Harpoon system approaches the leaflet from the ventricular side and perforates it with a needle through which a double helix knot holds the NeoChord on the atrial side of the leaflet. For both systems, again in the ME mitral commissural view and the multiplane perpendicular LAX view with and without color Doppler the chord tension is adjusted to

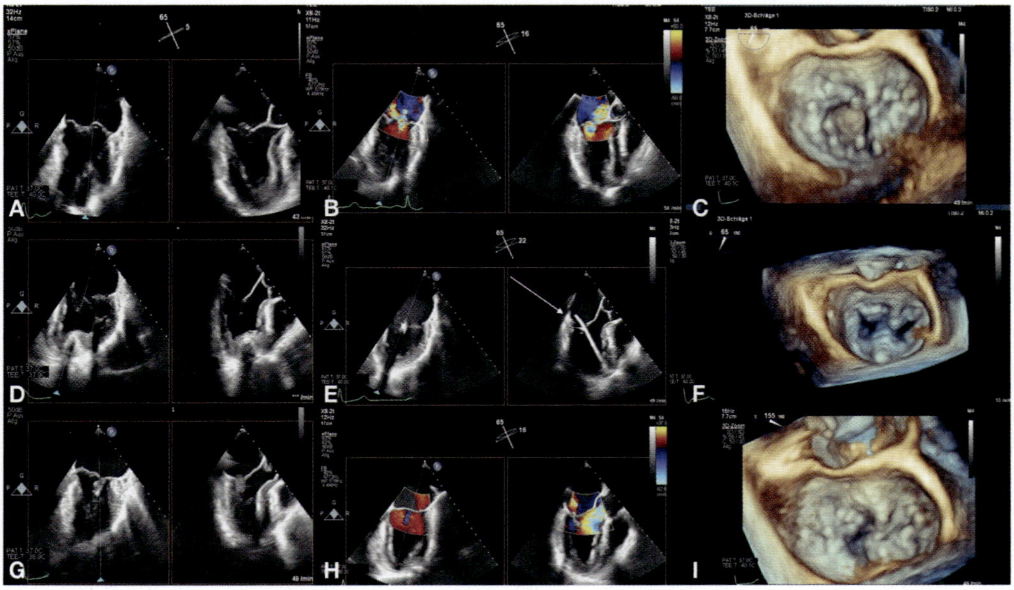

FIGURE 16.12 Transapical chordal implantation. A: Midesophageal (ME) mitral commissural (MC) and simultaneous ME long-axis (LAX) views: P2-P1 prolapse. B: ME MC and simultaneous ME LAX views with color Doppler: P2-P1 flail with anteriorly directed jet. C: 3D mitral valve (MV) en face view: P2-P1 flail. D: ME MC and simultaneous ME LAX views: digital palpation of the LV apex. E: ME MC and simultaneous ME LAX views: positioning of delivery system. F: 3D MV en face view: delivery system in place. G: ME MC and simultaneous ME LAX views: after NeoChord implantation. H: ME MC and simultaneous ME LAX views with Color Doppler after NeoChord implantation. I: 3D MV en face view after NeoChord implantation.

TABLE 16.4 Feasible Anatomy Assessment for Neo-Chordae Implantation

	Ideal	Intermediate	Unsuitable
Prolapse location	P2	Other than P2	Commissural
Flail width	10-20 mm	20-30 mm	<8 mm
Indexed left ventricular systolic volume	12-30 mL	30-55 mL	>55 mL

achieve best leaflet coaptation (Figure 16.12G,H; Video 16.11). The 3D en face view (Figure 12I; Video 16.11) should confirm effective leaflet coaptation. At this point the NeoChord is tightened with knots on the epicardium of the LV apex. Multiple chordae can be implanted to address large leaflet pathology and to distribute tension.

TRANSCATHETER MITRAL VALVE IMPLANTATION

While transcatheter options have become a standard of care for the management of aortic stenosis in patients at intermediate and high surgical risk (2), the development of transcatheter prostheses for the MV has not followed at the same pace due to intrinsic challenges of MV anatomy and physiology (55). They include the nonplanar saddle-shaped MV annulus, the complex subvalvular apparatus, the dynamic forces applied to native leaflets and the proximity to the left ventricular outflow tract (LVOT), and the risk of LVOT obstruction.

Transcatheter MV implantation (TMVI) may be an alternative option for patients referred to MV TEER with unfavorable anatomy. A common contraindication to surgical MV intervention or TEER is the presence of annular and leaflet calcification. MV annular calcification (MAC) involves the entire circumference in 1% of cases (56) and most commonly the posterior part (57). Valve calcium scoring has been proposed and correlated to the risk of valve embolization (58).

A direct comparison with TEER is currently under investigation. TMVI seems to provide a superior reduction of MR and improvement of symptoms despite a higher mortality (59). A small LV end diastolic diameter (<47 mm) is a contraindication to TMVI. Reduced LV function mandates anticoagulation after TMVI.

Preprocedural Evaluation

Preprocedural planning includes a comprehensive transthoracic echocardiogram (TTE) and TEE to assess valve morphology and quantify the pathology. Particular attention should be dedicated to valve calcification, baseline gradients, and LVOT patency and gradients. 3D computed tomography (CT) has become the standard imaging modality to plan these procedures and fulfill the following tasks:

- Quantify annular dimensions and area.
- Measure the papillary muscle to annulus distance.
- Identify location of calcifications.
- Define the best LV apical puncture site and approach angle with respect to papillary muscle.
- Assess the risk of LVOT obstruction.

The latter is assessed through computer simulation of valve implantation and quantification of residual neo-LVOT diameter. A post-deployment LVOT diameter less than 1.7 cm^2 may result in significant obstruction. Several interventions have been described to address an increased risk of LVOT obstruction and include:

- Prophylactic alcohol septal ablation (60)
- Laceration of the anterior MV leaflet to prevent LVOT obstruction (LAMPOON procedure) (61)

Device Selection and Approach

There are several specific devices available for implantation in the mitral position with different fixation systems to be delivered using the transseptal or the transapical approach (60). Table 16.5 summarizes the most commonly available devices.

The latter is more common due to the valve and delivery catheter sizes.

TAVI systems can also be used in the MV position and delivered transseptally (62).

TABLE 16.5 Transcatheter Mitral Valves

Type of Valve	Access	Design	Sizes	Anchoring System
Tendyne	Transapical	D shape, self-expandable	35-40 mm septolateral and 34-50 mm intercommissural diameter	External apical pad
Tiara	Transapical	D shape, self-expandable	35- and 40-mm mediolateral diameter	Three subannular anchors
Intrepid	Transapical/ transseptal	Circular, self-expandable	43-, 46-, and 50-mm outer frame	Annular anchoring cleats and radial force
EVOQUE	Transseptal	Circular, self-expandable	44 and 48 mm	Subvalvular anchors and radial force
Sapien M3	Transseptal	Balloon expandable	29 mm	Radial force and docking
Sapien TAVI	Transseptal	Balloon expandable	20, 23, 26, 29 mm	Radial force

Intraprocedural Guidance

For the *transapical* approach, TEE must confirm the correct site for apical puncture. This is performed in the ME mitral commissural view and in the multiplane perpendicular LAX view by identifying the invagination of LV apex by surgical digital palpation (Figures 16.13E and 16.14C; Videos 16.12 and 16.13). In the same view, a needle is seen in the LV and a wire is followed through the MV into the LA (Figure 16.14D; Video 16.13). Over the wire a balloon-tipped catheter is inserted with the balloon inflated to test the path into the LA (flossing or lollypop technique) (Figure 16.14E [*arrow*]; Video 16.13). The delivery catheter is then advanced in the LA (Figure 16.4F-H; Video 16.13) and the atrial end of the valve released (Figure 16.13F-H

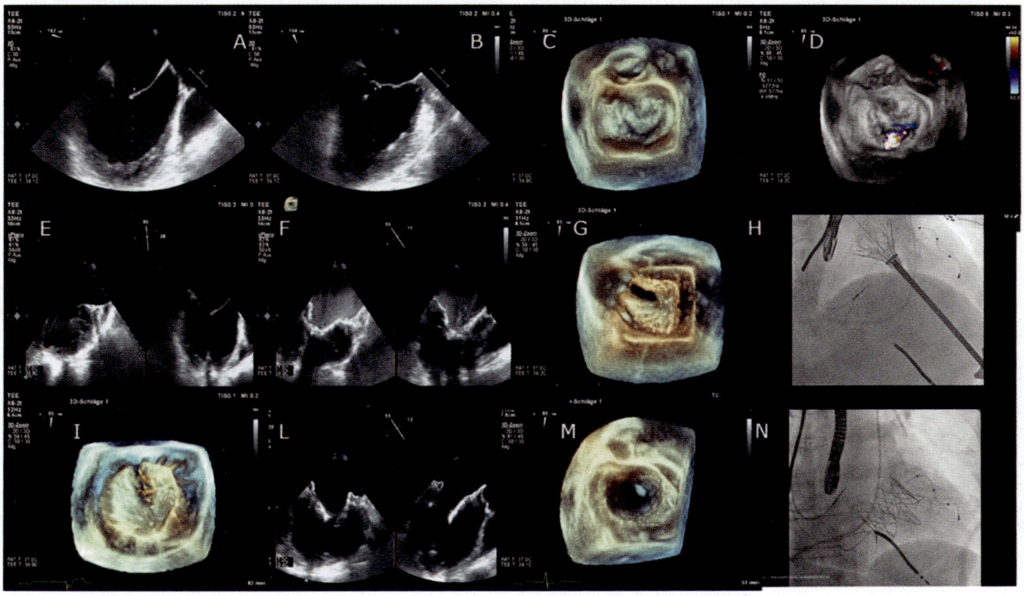

FIGURE 16.13 Mitral valve (MV) implantation: Tiara valve. A: Midesophageal (ME) long-axis (LAX) view: restrictive MV leaflets. B: ME two-chamber View: restrictive MV leaflets. C: 3D en face view: restrictive MV leaflets. D: 3D en face view with color Doppler: broad posteriorly directed mitral regurgitation (MR) jet. E: ME mitral commissural (MC) and simultaneous ME LAX views: digital palpation of left ventricular (LV) apex. F: ME MC and simultaneous ME LAX views: valve deployment, note "smoke" in left atrium due to stagnant flow. G: 3D MV en face view: valve deployment. H: Fluoroscopy: valve deployment. I: 3D MV en face view: valve deployment. L: G: 3D MV en face view: after deployment. M: 3D MV en face view: after deployment. N: Fluoroscopy: after deployment.

and 16.14E-L; Videos 16.13 and 16.14). A 3D en face view is useful to guide this step. The Tendyne valve is rotated to position the higher part of the valve at 12 o' clock anteriorly (Figure 16.14E-L; Video 16.13). For all valves, while pulling the valve toward the LV apex, the annular and ventricular end is released (Figure 16.13E-N; Video 16.12). For the Tendyne valve the tension on the valve string connected to the apical pad (Figure 16.14N [arrow]) can be modulated to optimize sealing and minimize paravalvular leaks before being locked in the final position. Before release of the retention system, the valve can be retrieved.

For the *transseptal* approach transseptal puncture (Figure 16.15C; Video 16.14) is performed as described for TEER; the puncture height from the MV annulus varies from model to model and is typically lower than that for TEER. For most delivery systems, dilation is not enough, and a balloon dilation of the septum is necessary to allow the large delivery catheter safely enter the LA (Figure 16.15D; Video 16.14).

For the EVOQUE system in the 3D MV en face view, using live MPR, the nine subvalvular anchors are deployed underneath the MV leaflets to grasp the annulus before the atrial part is released.

The Sapien M3 valve includes a docking system (like a ring) that provides a wider and safer anchoring to a Sapien 3 TAVI balloon-expandable valve. The Sapien valve can also be deployed transseptally directly in a MV bioprosthesis (valve-in-valve) (Figure 16.15A-H; Video 16.14) in a MV ring after MV repair (valve-in-ring) (Figure 16.16; Video 16.15) or in a heavily calcified MV annulus (valve-in-calcium) (Figure 16.15I-N; Video 16.14).

TEE guidance includes positioning of a wire through the MV into the LV (Figure 16.15E-L; Video 16.14) and guidance of the delivery catheter above the MV. This can be achieved with the ME mitral commissural view and with the multiplane perpendicular LAX view as well as with a tilted 3D en face view of the MV (Figure 16.16E-L; Video 16.15). The Sapien valve can then be positioned into the MV maintaining the top of the valve a few millimeters above the MV annulus.

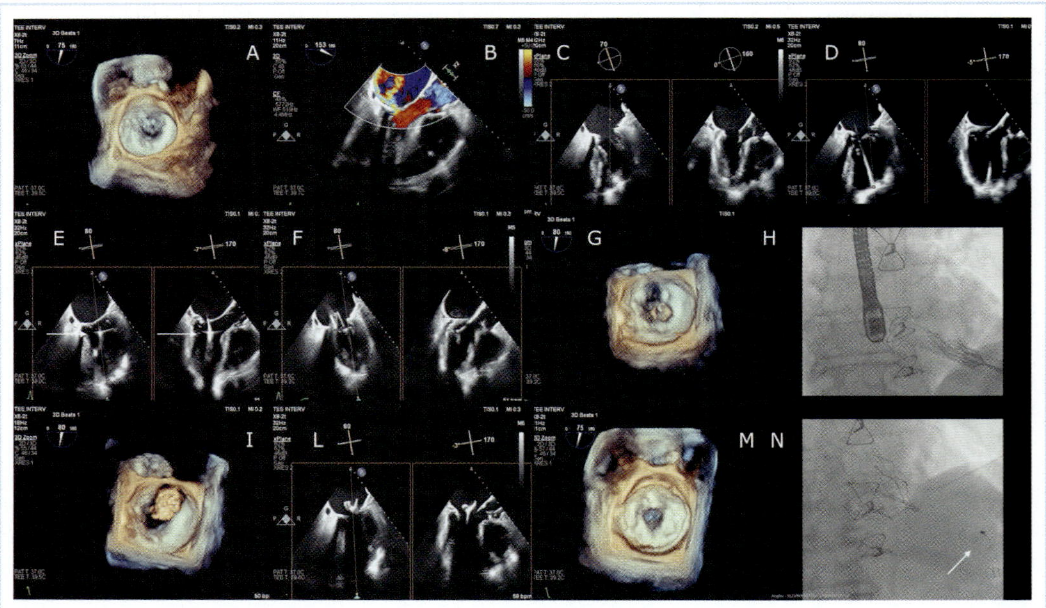

FIGURE 16.14 Mitral valve (MV) implantation: Tendyne valve. A: 3D MV en face view: mitral annular calcifications. B: Midesophageal (ME) long-axis (LAX) view with color Doppler: posteriorly directed mitral regurgitation (MR) jet. C: ME mitral commissural (MC) and simultaneous ME LAX views: digital palpation of left ventricular (LV) apex. D: ME MC and simultaneous ME LAX views: wire advancement through the MV. E: ME MC and simultaneous ME LAX views: balloon (arrow) flossing through the LV and MV. F: ME MC and simultaneous ME LAX views: positioning of the delivery system through the MV. G: 3D MV en face view: delivery system in place. H: Fluoroscopy: delivery system in place with crimped valve inside. I: 3D MV en face view: valve deployment. L: ME MC and simultaneous ME LAX views: valve deployment. M: 3D MV en face view: post-deployment. N: Fluoroscopy: post-deployment.

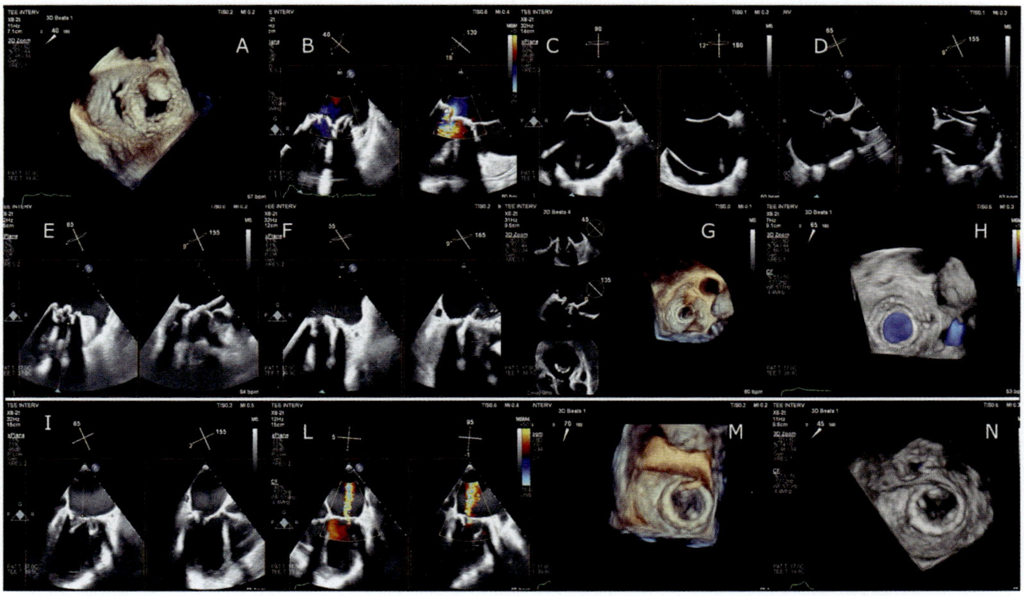

FIGURE 16.15 Mitral valve (MV)-in-valve and valve-in-ring: A: 3D MV en face view: degenerated MV bioprosthesis. B: Midesophageal (ME) mitral commissural (MC) and simultaneous ME long-axis (LAX) views with color Doppler: turbulent flow through the MV in diastole. C: ME bicaval view: ideal tenting of the transseptal puncture needle in the upper part of the fossa ovalis and anterior to the aorta in the perpendicular view. D: Multiplane view of the interatrial septum (IAS): balloon dilation of the puncture site. E: ME MC and simultaneous ME LAX views: valve positioning. F: ME MC and simultaneous ME LAX views: valve deployment. G: 3D MV en face view: post-deployment. H: 3D MV en face view with color Doppler: post-deployment. I: ME MC and simultaneous ME LAX views: calcified MV ring and restricted leaflet motion. L: ME MC and simultaneous ME LAX views with color Doppler: central MR jet. M: 3D MV en face view: post-deployment. N: 3D MV en face view with color Doppler: post-deployment.

The LAMPOON procedure consists of the Laceration of the Anterior Mitral leaflet to Prevent Outflow ObtructioN. After splitting the anterior MV leaflet, the two leaflet's halves will be pushed on the side of the LVOT by the MV prosthesis implantation, minimizing flow obstruction under the aortic valve.

The LAMPOON procedure can be performed transseptally from the LA (Figure 16.16B-H; Video 16.15) and transaortically or transapically from the LV. A catheter is positioned at the base of the A2 scallop of the MV using the 3D MV en face view and multiplane from the ME mitral commissural view (Figure 16.16B,C; Video 16.15). Through the catheter a wire is advanced and electrified to perforate the leaflet. A loop awaits on the other side to retrieve the wire and pull it into a second catheter (Figure 16.16D-H; Video 16.15). At this point the wire is electrified and pulled to split the anterior MV leaflet in half. **The resulting acute MR may lead to hemodynamic instability;** therefore, prompt valve deployment (Figure 16.16I-N; Video 16.15) is necessary to reestablish hemodynamic stability.

Postprocedural Assessment and Complication

Postprocedural TEE should aim at assessment of paravalvular leaks and MV gradients. For some valves (eg, Sapien 3) post-deployment balloon dilation may reduce their severity, and for the Tendyne valve more tension on the apical pad may achieve the same result.

Careful assessment of LVOT includes measurement of gradient and 3D cross-sectional area. Acute LVOT obstruction can lead to hemodynamic instability and can be addressed by LVOT ballooning or deployment of a LVOT stent or stented TAVI.

Post-deployment pericardiac effusion and LV failure should also be ruled out.

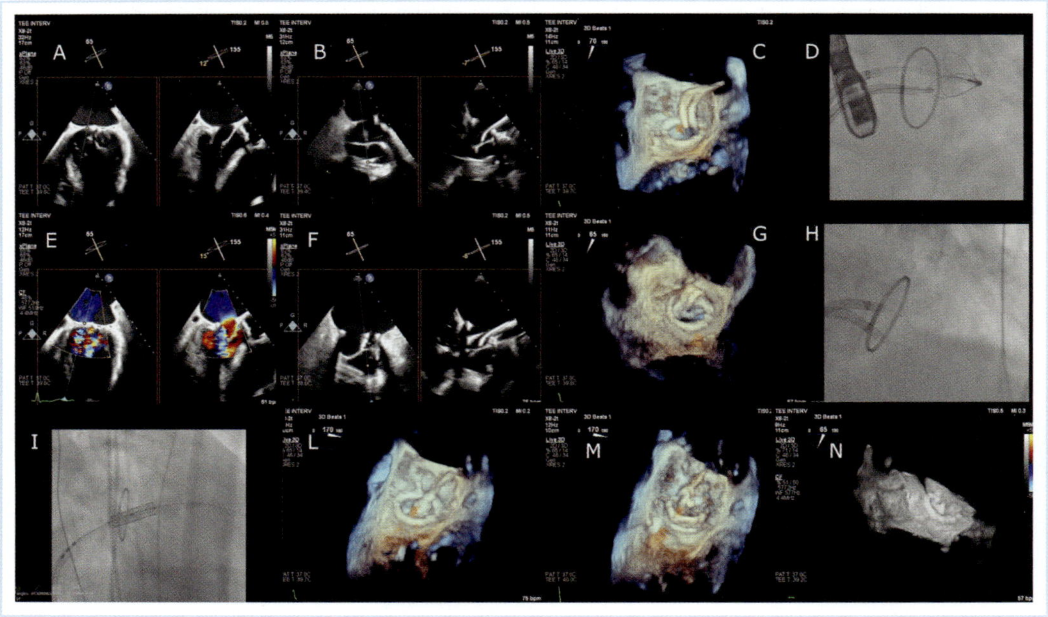

FIGURE 16.16 LAMPOON procedure. A: Midesophageal (ME) mitral commissural (MC) and simultaneous ME long-axis (LAX) views: post-mitral valve (MV) repair. B: ME MC and simultaneous ME LAX views: catheter positioning at the base of the MV anterior leaflet. C: MV 3D side view: puncturing catheter at the base of the MV anterior leaflet and catching catheter in the left ventricle (LV). D: Fluoroscopy: catching the puncturing catheter with a loop in the LV. E: ME MC and simultaneous ME LAX views with color Doppler: eccentric recurrent mitral regurgitation (MR) jet. F: ME MC and simultaneous ME LAX views: wire positioned through the MV anterior leaflet. G: MV 3D side view: wire positioned through the MV anterior leaflet. H: Fluoroscopy: wire positioned through the MV anterior leaflet. I: Fluoroscopy: valve positioning in the MV ring. L: MV 3D side view: valve positioning in the MV ring. M: MV 3D side view: post-deployment. N: MV 3D side view with color Doppler: post-deployment.

SUMMARY

TEE plays a key role in the planning and guidance of transcatheter MV procedures.

Current guidelines clearly define the steps for preoperative MV pathology quantification and planning of the intervention (15,16). Special training is required (36).

Intraoperative guidance has been described by several authors (39,63-65) and may vary slightly from center to center. It also requires understanding of the technology used.

Transcatheter MV procedures and especially MV TEER has placed the echocardiographer on the main seat and his contribution to the team plays a significant role in procedural success (66).

PART B: TRICUSPID VALVE INTERVENTIONS

TR is a common valvular heart disease, the prevalence and severity of which increases with advanced age (67). A TR grade of more than mild is commonly associated with elevated morbidity and mortality and decreased quality of life (68). TR is generally asymptomatic until advanced stages of the disease occur and includes pedal edema and systemic congestion secondary to liver and renal dysfunction. In these conditions, surgical approach of TR is associated with a high or prohibitive mortality and often remains untreated (69-72).

Transcatheter tricuspid valve therapies (TTVTs) have evolved as an attractive alternative to treat patients with severe symptomatic TR, who are otherwise considered inoperable (73). Different interventional devices (devices for leaflet approximation, annuloplasty devices, orthotopic and heterotopic valve replacement) have been recently developed (74-78). Early feasibility studies validate that TTVT is efficacious in reducing TR and is associated with a low incidence of complications. As compared with complications associated with conservative goal-directed medical therapy, patients with TTVT demonstrate improvement in symptoms and quality of life (79-85). Successful outcomes are dependent upon the etiology and initial severity of TR, associated comorbidities, and ultimately the degree of TR reduction (86).

A proper evaluation of tricuspid valve (TV) anatomy, morphology, etiology, and the severity of TR is essential for transcatheter device selection and guidance (16,22,87-91,92-95). Although multimodality imaging is usually required in the preoperative screening and during intraprocedural device implantation guidance, TEE remains the mainstay of intraoperative guidance (78,92,96-98).

ETIOLOGY OF TRICUSPID REGURGITATION

TR is a result of four etiologies:

1. Primary (depicts less than 10% of TR)
2. Related to cardiac implantable electronic device (CIED)
3. Atrial secondary TR and
4. Ventricular secondary TR (94,99)

When a CIED interacts with the subvalvular apparatus or causes TV leaflet impingement, TTVT may result in a suboptimal outcome (97).

Secondary TR is the most frequent cause of TR and may be associated with left-sided heart disease (valve disease or LV dysfunction), pulmonary arterial (PA) hypertension, or RV disease or dysfunction. It is usually associated with RV dilation, displacement of the papillary muscles, and tethering of TV leaflets.

Atrial secondary TR is concomitant with preserved LV and RV function with TV annulus and RA dilation, and irrelevant leaflet tethering associated with tethering of one, two, or all three leaflets. It is usually associated with atrial fibrillation or heart failure with preserved ejection fraction (HFpEF) and diastolic dysfunction. With the progression of the disease, secondary ventricular TR is eminent owing to volume overload, tethering, and dilation of RV elucidating mixed valve pathology (99).

TYPES OF DEVICES

There are numerous TTVT devices presently available in the market. Currently the following are approved in Europe:

1. TEER:
    a. Pascal device (Edwards Lifesciences)
    b. TriClip (Abbott Vascular)
2. Direct transcatheter annuloplasty—Cardioband (Edwards Lifesciences)
3. Orthotopic valve replacement—EVOQUE (Edwards Lifesciences).

The key predictors of procedural success are interrelated to the anatomy of the valve, proper device selection, and periprocedural guidance using quality TEE images (99-102). Although for TEER procedures TEE plays a major role in planning, there is an additional value of CT for all other TTVT interventions.

The largest experience to date is with edge-to-edge repair with no substantial differences between TriClip and Pascal devices (78). Both devices in randomized controlled trials showed promising results by achieving implant success, TR reduction, and improvement in patient's functional capacity and quality of life. With a 2-year follow-up, the TriClip TRILUMINATE study in 85 patients shows a TR reduction to moderate or less in 60% of patients, a reduction of at least 1° of TR severity compared to preintervention in 85.4%, and all-cause mortality in 18.7% (30 days 0%, 1 year 7.3%) (85). With a 1-year follow-up, the Pascal CLASP TR study demonstrated in 65 patients a TR reduction to moderate or less in 86% of patients, a reduction of at least 1° of TR severity in 100%, and all-cause mortality in 4.8% (30 days 3.1%) (82).

Identified predictors of procedural success for TEER include:

- Trileaflet TV morphology,
- Septolateral coaptation gap of 7 mm or less (not recommended when ≥8.5 mm even using the new models with extended arms),
- Anteroseptal or central TR jet position,
- TR severity less than torrential, and
- Absence of CIED leaflet impingement, excessive annular dilation, severe leaflet tethering, and severe RA volume enlargement (83,99,101).

Although tricuspid annuloplasty is the standard surgical procedure for TR, transcatheter tricuspid annuloplasty device implantation is a complex procedure with challenging intraprocedural imaging guidance and the potential risk of coronary artery injury (103). Cardiac CT anatomy is optimally performed in addition to echocardiography. Cardiac CT allows for annular sizing, exclusion of annular calcification that may prevent optimal anchoring, and size adjustment; evaluation of distance from the annular hinge points to the right coronary artery (RCA) all around the annulus perimeter. These measurements are necessary to avoid iatrogenic injury to RCA during anchoring. A distance of less than 2 mm between anchoring annular point and RCA increases the risk of impingement and is more common at the level of the posterior leaflet (104). A 2-year follow-up of the TRI-REPAIR study (Cardioband device) has been published (84). Cardioband implantation shows a 100% technical success, TR reduction to moderate or less of 72% (63% at 1 year), with major adverse events in 20%, survival rate of 83% at 1 year and 73% at 2 years, and improvement in functional capacity at follow-up (84). Although promising, this technique has a significant learning curve and is highly dependent on expertise of intraoperative echo imaging and the interventional team.

Favorable anatomic criteria for procedural success using transcatheter annuloplasty include:

- annular dilation as primary mechanism of TR,
- not exceeding device size (120 mm − circumference of annulus measured from anteroseptal commissure to the end of coronary sinus),
- central TR jet position,
- TR severity less than torrential,
- absence of reduced RV function,
- absence of pronounced RV remodeling with tethering height less than 0.76 cm, tenting area less than 1.63 cm^2, tenting volume (3D) less than 2.3 mL,
- absence of CIED leaflet impingement,
- adequate tissue for anchor placement, and
- sufficient distance of annular anchor point to the RCA (79,99,102,104).

Patients with no suitable valve anatomy for TV repair, including large coaptation gaps, short or extremely tethered septal leaflets, torrential TR or noncentral regurgitant jets, may benefit from percutaneous transfemoral TV replacement (105). The EVOQUE valve is a self-expanding bovine valve with circumferential anchors that use the native apparatus for stabilization. The TRISCEND safety and performance study evaluated the 1-year outcomes using the EVOQUE (Edwards Lifesciences) valve in a prospective study (81). It demonstrated a procedural success of 93%, with TR grade reduction to mild regurgitation or less of 97.6%. Major adverse events reported severe bleeding of 25.5% and cardiovascular mortality of 9.1% at 1 year. Thirteen percent of patients required the placement of a permanent pacemaker. Patients experienced marked improvements in symptoms and functional as well as quality-of-life outcomes (81).

Unfavorable anatomic criteria for procedural success using transcatheter TV replacement include: annulus size that exceeds available valve size, small RV size that prevents the proper positioning of the device, severe RV function, and too acute IVC to RA angle that is challenging for device placement toward the tricuspid annulus (TA) (78,99).

A SYSTEMATIC APPROACH TO IMPLANTATION

Transcatheter Edge-to-Edge Repair Step-by-Step Deployment

TEER interventions are performed using fluoroscopic and TEE guidance under GA or deep sedation (106). When estimating the TR severity, the hemodynamic effects of GA must be taken into consideration (107-109). To draft a clipping plan with the interventionist, a detailed examination of the TV anatomy including the leaflet and subvalvular apparatus configuration as well as the distribution, localization, and severity of the TR is required (16,89,93,94,96,110) (Figure 16.17; Videos 16.16A,B).

Given the large area of the TV, especially in the advanced stages of severe TR, multiple device placements are typically planned. The approximation of the anteroseptal commissure line with one or more devices has proven to be technically feasible and has been observed to provide annular size reductions with substantial TR improvement (111). It is possible to attach the posterior and septal leaflets in a central position or near the commissure. It is also possible to clip the anterior and the posterior leaflets using the same view (Figure 16.18A,B; Videos 16.17A,B) (83,112).

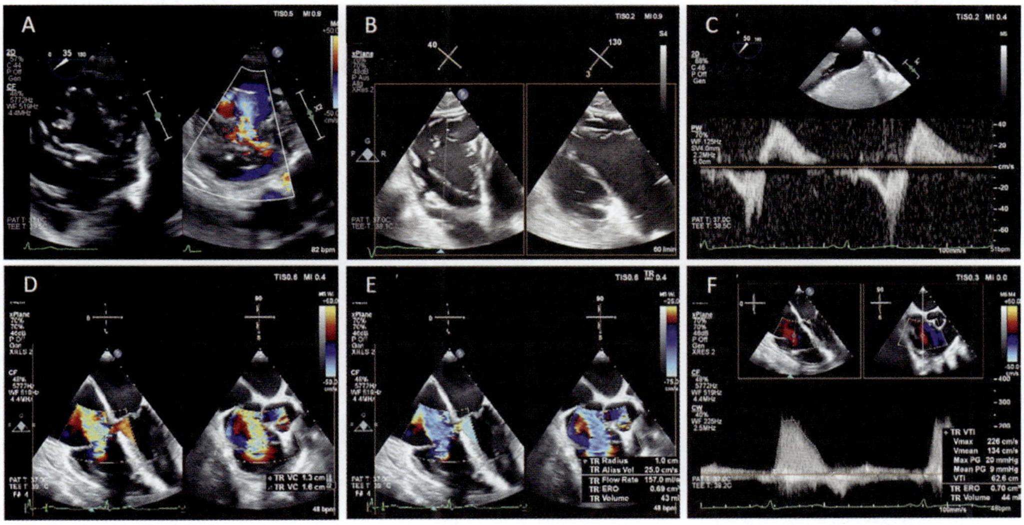

FIGURE 16.17 Preprocedural estimation of tricuspid regurgitation (TR). A: Transgastric (TG) short-axis (SAX) leaflet anatomy and TR localization. B: Leaflet and papillary muscle anatomy. C: Hepatic vein reversal flow. D: Vena contracta (VC) measurement in midesophageal (ME) four-chambered and biplane view. E and F: Radius measurement, maximal velocity, and velocity-time integral (VTI) of TR continuous-wave (CW) Doppler for assessment of effective regurgitation orifice area (EROA) and regurgitant volume by proximal isovelocity surface area (PISA) method.

When planning a multiple device strategy, it is advisable to start placing the devices from an anterior position to avoid device shadowing in the subsequent deployment.

There are two different devices available for TEER:
Pascal Transcatheter Mitral Valve Repair (TMVr) System (Edwards Lifesciences) and TriClip Transcatheter Tricuspid Valve Repair system (Abbott Structural Heart). Despite the differences between the two available systems, the required approach and the procedural image protocols are similar (96-98,113-115). Optimal TEE imaging of the TR leaflets in the supine position from mid- or deep esophageal views is important to succeed with the TEER procedure.

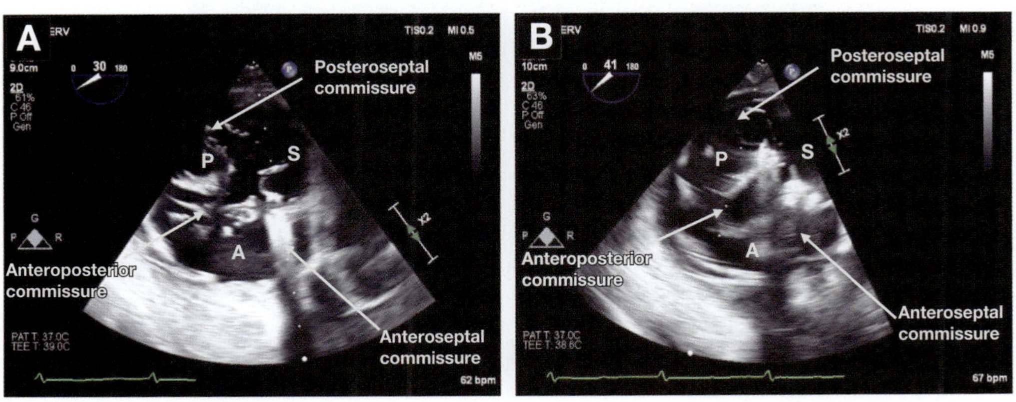

TEER device in the anteroseptal commissure

TEER device in the anteroseptal and in the posteroseptal commissure

FIGURE 16.18 A: First device in anterior and septal leaflet. B: Second device in posterior and septal leaflet.

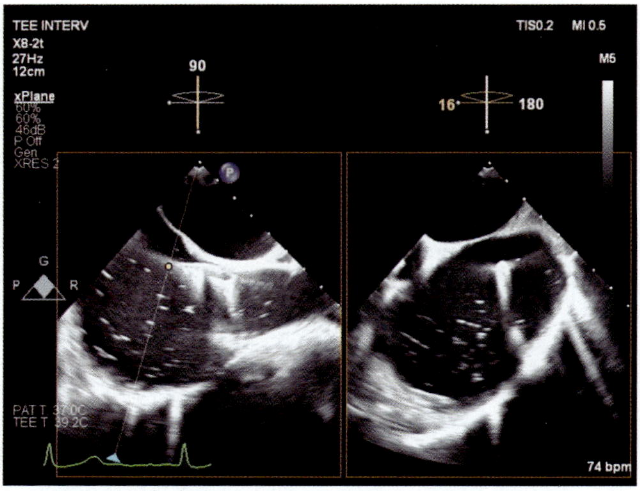

Biplanar ME bicaval view - introduction of the steerable catheter and device delivery system into the RA

FIGURE 16.19 Biplanar image of the bicaval view to guide the introduction of the steerable catheter and device delivery system into the right atrium (RA).

Step 1

One starts at the ME bicaval view using biplane technology to guide the introduction of the steerable catheter and device delivery system into the RA. The device delivery system is then retracted to position the tip of the device away from the IAS into the RA (Figure 16.19; Video 16.18).

Step 2

Next, one turns the probe in an anticlockwise rotation from the initial biplanar bicaval view to observe the tip of the device. One then follows the anteroinferior movement of the device toward the TV (on the bottom of Figure 16.20). Continuous visualization of the device and its relationship to the IAS, RA appendage, and coronary sinus should be maintained (Figure 16.20; Video 16.19).

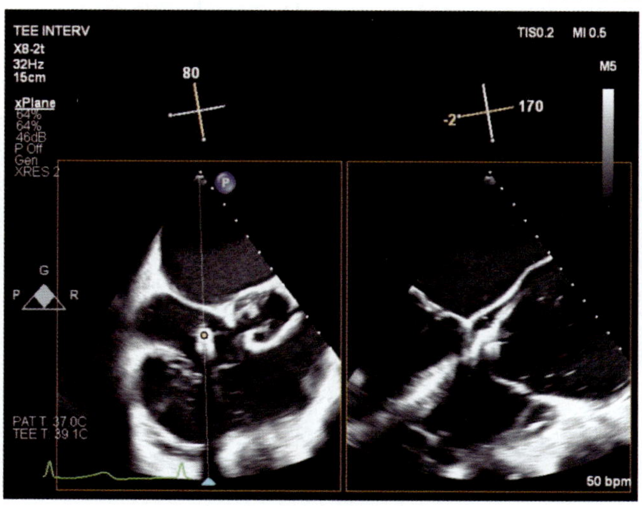

Biplanar view to follow the device towards the TV

FIGURE 16.20 Midesophageal (ME) right ventricular (RV) inflow-outflow and biplanar view. Movement of device toward the tricuspid valve (TV).

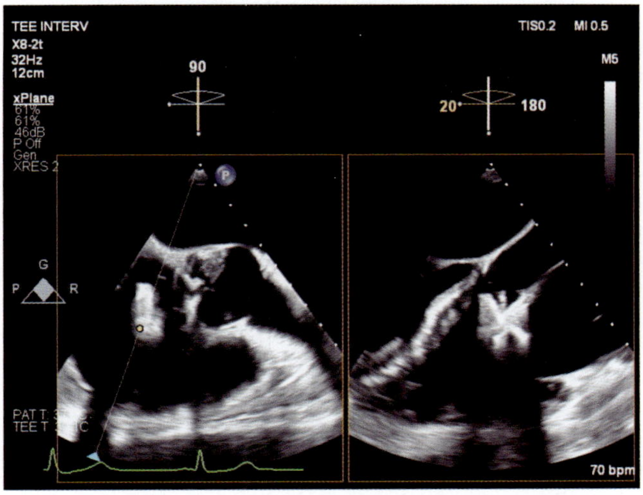

Movement and identification of the arms and clasps of the device

FIGURE 16.21 Midesophageal (ME) right ventricular (RV) inflow-outflow and biplanar view. Identification movement of the arms and clasps of the device.

Step 3

Adjust the mechanical rotation between 60° and 90° to obtain a ME or deep RV inflow-outflow view of the TV to control the anteroposterior trajectory of the device. On the biplanar image, an inverse ME or deep esophageal four-chambered view is displayed, which permits visualization of the medial to lateral movement of the device. The objective is to position the device as perpendicular as possible to the TV annulus and in the middle of the valve. Correct movement and identification of the arms and clasps of the device can be verified using TEE or fluoroscopy (Figure 16.21; Video 16.20).

Step 4

Device guidance through the TV can be followed using biplanar ME or TG views. It is important to rule out any interaction with the subvalvular apparatus to avoid entrapment of chordae or leads (Figure 16.22; Video 16.21).

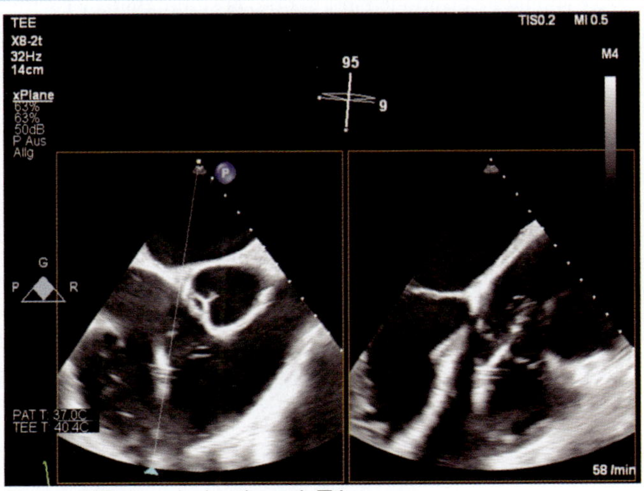

Biplane ME view-device through TV

FIGURE 16.22 Midesophageal (ME) right ventricular (RV) inflow-outflow and biplanar view. Device guiding through the tricuspid valve (TV).

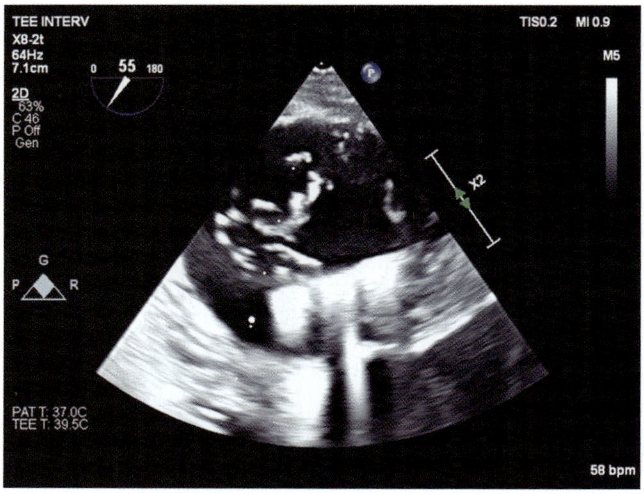

TG SAX view of the TV - location and orientation of the open device arms perpendicular to the anteroseptal coaptation linie

FIGURE 16.23 Transgastric (TG) short-axis (SAX) tricuspid valve (TV). Location and the orientation of the open device arms are perpendicular to the coaptation line.

Step 5

The TG SAX view of the TV (from the ventricular side) allows for visualization of the device implant location and the orientation of the open device arms perpendicular to the desired coaptation line. The device is then pulled back from the ventricle side to be placed under the leaflets (Figure 16.23; Video 16.22).

Step 6

The RV inflow-outflow view in biplane mode can be utilized to assess the optimal depth to visualize both the arms of the device in the orthogonal plane. Usually the septal leaflet is difficult to visualize in this view and hence rotating the transducer prevents shadowing of the septal leaflet. Once all the leaflets are visualized, both the arms of the device should be positioned in a central position, thereby creating a restricted motion of the leaflets (Figure 16.24).

Step 7

The clasps are lowered to capture the leaflet (Video 16.23). With separate leaflet grasping, the anterior leaflet is usually grasped first followed by the septal leaflet.

Step 8

There should be confirmation of proper orientation, localization, and leaflet capture in the TG SAX view.

Step 9

Gradual closure of the device arms should be assessed either in the same TG (Figure 16.25; Video 16.24) or in the ME view (Figure 16.26; Video 16.23).

Step 10

Prior to final device deployment, the following should be assessed (Figure 16.27; Video 16.25A,B):

- confirmation of proper grasping of both leaflets with adequate tissue bridging and leaflet insertion,
- satisfactory location of the device,

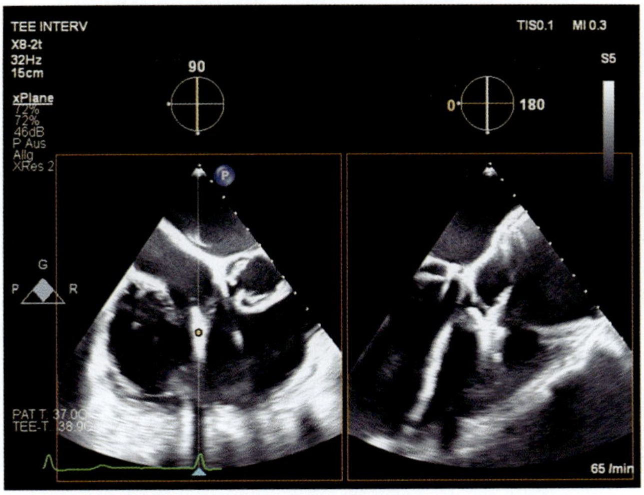

Biplanar ME view—visualization of both arms of the device in the orthogonal plane under the leaflets of TV

FIGURE 16.24 Midesophageal (ME) right ventricular (RV) inflow-outflow and biplanar view. Leaflets image positioned on the device arm.

- residual TR severity,
- mean gradient across the TV,
- hepatic venous flow.

Adequate leaflet insertion and tissue bridging can be challenging and multiple views at different levels should be used to confirm the appropriate positioning of the device. Recording a long loop of leaflet grasping and measuring the shortening of the leaflets after device closure may support the verification of a successful grasping. This can prevent leaflet detachment after grasping and the need for repositioning of the device.

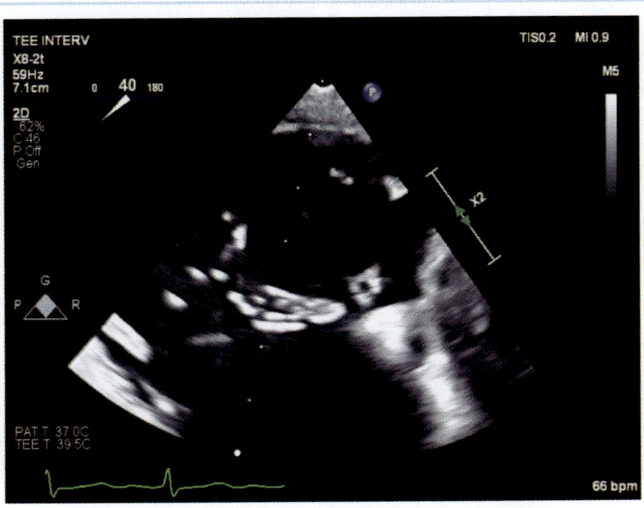

TG SAX view of the TV – closed device in the anteroseptal commisure

FIGURE 16.25 Transgastric (TG) view. Closure of the device arms.

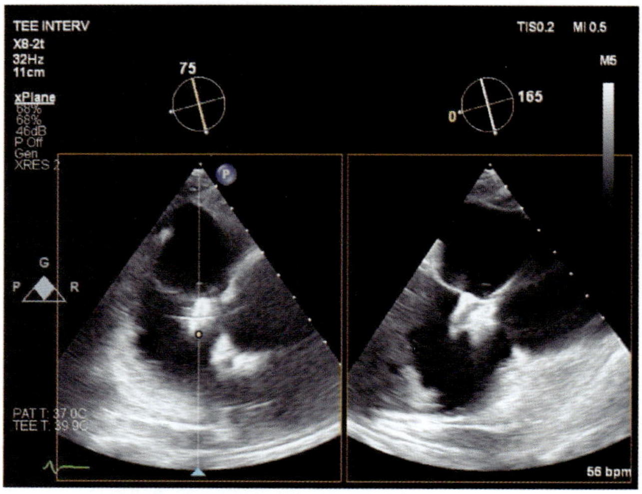

Biplanar ME view of the TV -closed device

FIGURE 16.26 Deep midesophageal (ME) biplanar view. Closure of the device arms.

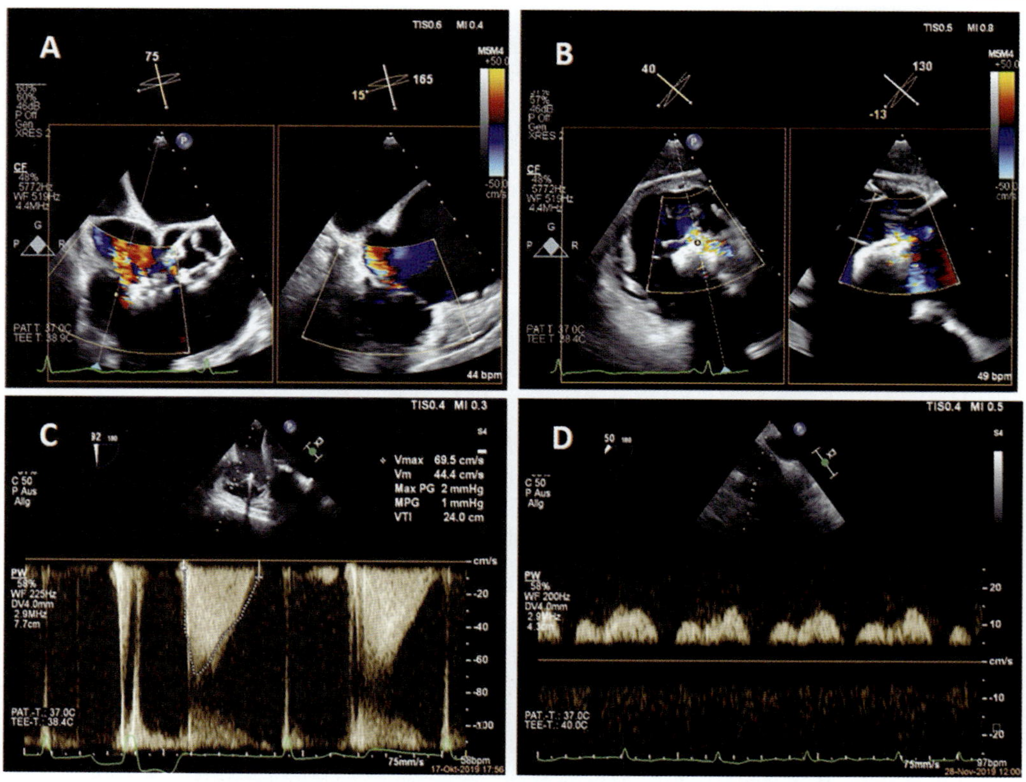

FIGURE 16.27 Assessment of results after device deployment. A: Midesophageal (ME) right ventricular (RV) inflow-outflow and biplanar view with color to assess residual tricuspid regurgitation (TR). B: Transgastric (TG) biplanar view with color to assess residual TR. C: Doppler across the tricuspid valve (TV) to assess transvalvular gradient; D: Hepatic vein flow.

If the quality of esophageal imaging is inadequate, the whole process of leaflet grasping can be visualized using TG TV view alone (116). In case of high-quality esophageal imaging, it is possible to do the procedure using 3D en face or 3D MPR imaging from the ME or deep esophageal views, displaying simultaneously the three orthogonal 2D planes (117) (Figure 16.28; Video 16.26A-C). If the quality of 3D MPR images is acceptable, advancing the probe from ME to TG can be avoided. That is especially useful in case of poor TG imaging or in patients with esophageal and stomach pathologies.

Step 11

Biplanar ME views are used at the end of the procedure for retraction of the delivery system into the steerable guide catheter.

Post-Deployment Assessment

An evaluation of the TV is again performed to ensure device stability. Quantitative assessment of TV residual regurgitation severity should be obtained from multiple views using the PISA, volumetric, and/or 3D vena contracta area methods. Changes in the hepatic venous flow pattern further allows one to assess the reduction in TR from the clipping procedure.

Localization and severity of the residual regurgitation using the TG TV SAX view or 3D color Doppler MPR, assessing the remaining leaflet surface to be eventually grasped and evaluation of mean gradient across the TV, are used to assess if and where subsequent clips should be attempted. Finally, the presence of pericardial effusion has to be ruled out.

Cardioband Step by Step

Percutaneous annuloplasty is performed using a flexible polyester band deployed through a steerable catheter from the atrial side of the TV annulus. The device (Cardioband®, Edwards Lifesciences) is attached using up to 17 stainless steel anchors inserted along the perimeter of the TV annulus from the anteroseptal commissure to the coronary sinus in a clockwise direction (104). After band anchoring, the perimeter size can be adjusted in a reversible fashion to reduce the TV annulus diameter and increase the leaflet coaptation under real-time fluoroscopic and TEE monitoring to obtain a satisfactory reduction of TR.

A preprocedural study describing the course and localization of the RCA using cardiac CT and the TV annulus dimensions using CT and 3D echocardiography is necessary in order to assess the feasibility of the procedure (Figure 16.29).

Intraprocedural deployment is done under GA. The guidance requires both fluoroscopy and TEE, particularly 3D TEE with multiplanar reconstructions.

Step 1

Under fluoroscopy a wire is placed into the RCA. This allows the course of the RCA to be visualized during implantation and will serve as a marker to assess the distance between anchors and the RCA. It also assists in determining the anterolateral aspect of the annulus (implant landing zone localization).

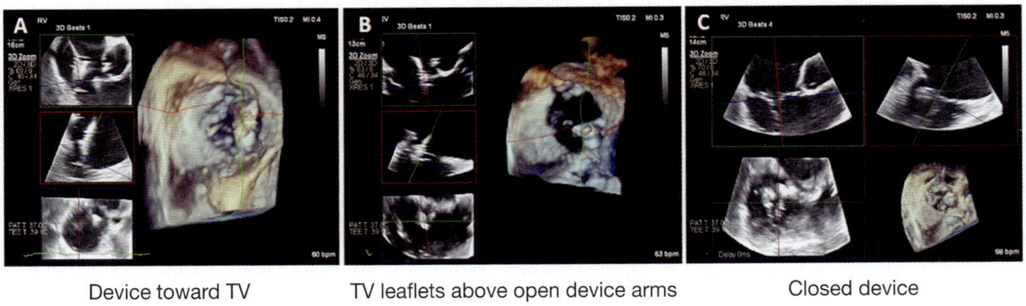

FIGURE 16.28 Multiplanar reconstruction (MPR) device guidance. A: Device alignment. B: Device positioning. C: Device stability. Cardioband.

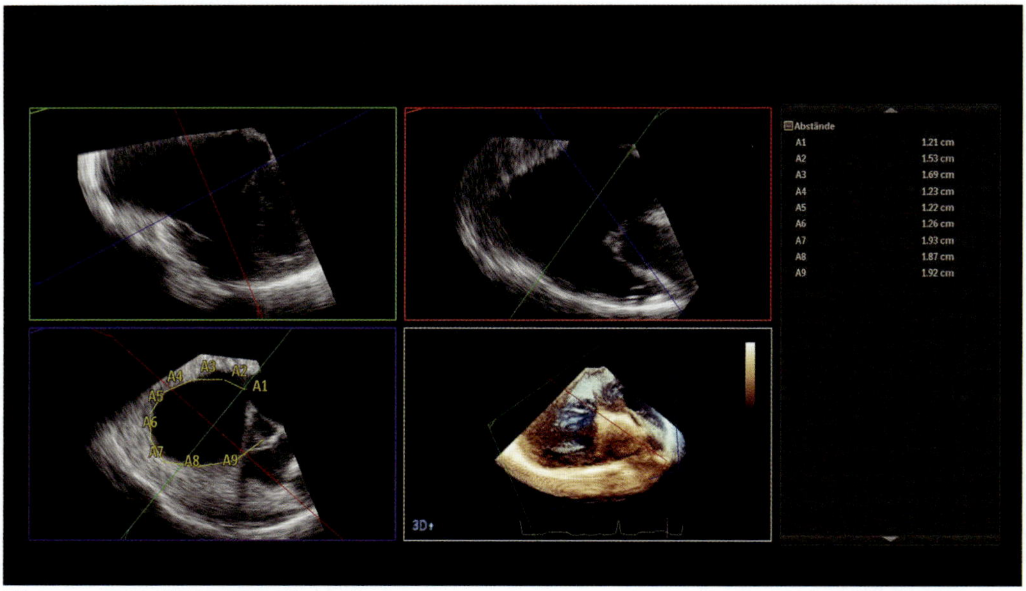

3D assessment of TV annulus dimension

FIGURE 16.29 Multiplanar reconstruction (MPR) measurement of tricuspid annulus.

Step 2

One starts at the ME bicaval view using biplane technology to guide the introduction of the steerable catheter and device delivery system from the IVC into the RA and toward the TV, avoiding interactions with IAS and other structures in the RA.

Step 3

Rotating the TEE probe anticlockwise, the TV is visualized on the bottom of the image and the device catheter is oriented to the anterior portion of the TV annulus.

Step 4

Using both fluoroscopy and TEE (ME RV inflow-outflow view, TG RV basal view, TG RV inflow view), the first anchor is placed at the anteroseptal commissure as close as possible to the aortic root, which is crucial (Figure 16.30).

The position of the tip of catheter with adequate tissue contact can be well visualized in MPR mode as well as in biplane mode. Since the tip of the catheter should be at the level of the annulus of the TV, the MPR mode is advantageous to align the catheter tip orthogonal to the annular plane (Figure 16.31).

Before deployment of the anchor, any contact of the anchor with the TV leaflets, aortic annulus, and/or the RCA must be ruled out. The anchor should be as orthogonal as possible into the annular tissue and neither too shallow nor tightly fixed. Before releasing the anchor, a simple pull and push test allows the confirmation of device stability.

Step 5

The anterior, lateral, and posterior TV annulus visualization has to be optimized to continue with the implantation. The anchors are placed in a stepwise fashion in a clockwise direction. The anterior TV annulus is imaged in TG RV SAX and ME inflow-outflow views. Visualization of the lateral and posterior TV annulus

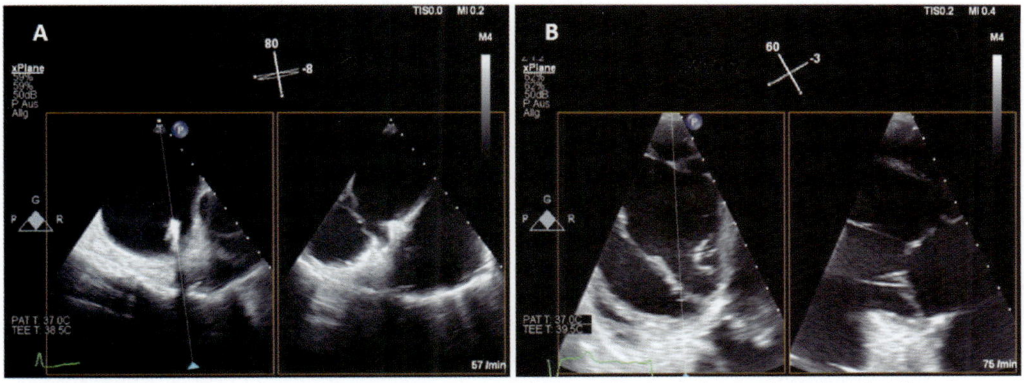

Biplanar ME view—first anchor placed at the anteroseptal commissure

Biplanar TG view—first anchor placed at the anteroseptal commissure

FIGURE 16.30 First anchor at anteroseptal commissure. A: Deep esophageal and biplanar view. B: TG and biplanar view.

is more challenging and multiple biplanar views and MPR analysis may be required to identify the right position and angulation. The coronary sinus must be identified to place the last anchor. Biplanar deep esophageal views may be very useful.

During every anchor placement, a simple series of safety steps should be checked, which include, confirming the distance of the anchor to the RCA, its correct angulation and orientation by fluoroscopy, demonstrating adequate tissue capture, and ruling out contact with TV leaflets using TEE. **Performing the pull and push test before deploying the device is mandatory.** When the last anchor is deployed in the posteroseptal commissure, the implant device system is retrieved.

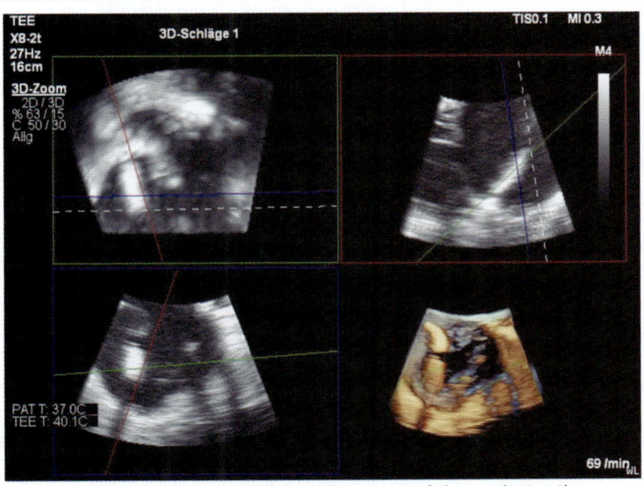

MPR mode—assessment of the alignment of the catheter tip orthogonal to the annular plane

FIGURE 16.31 Multiplanar reconstruction (MPR) analysis to determine the correct coaxial angulation and position of the tip.

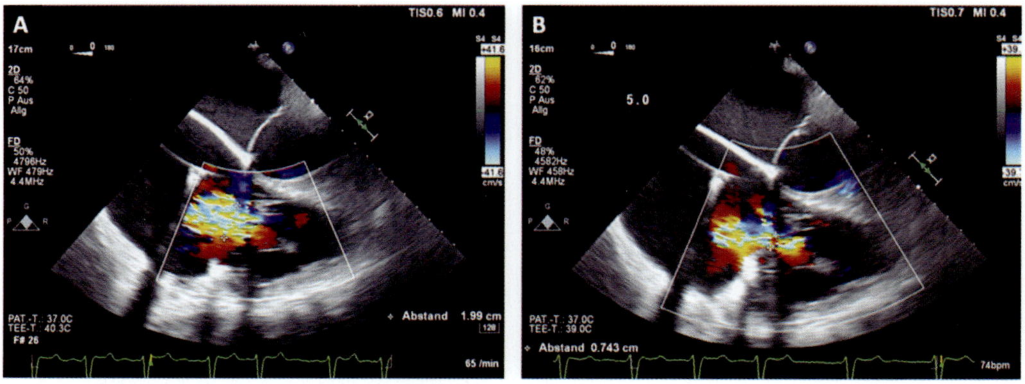

TR before (A) and after (B) cinching the annular band

FIGURE 16.32 Tricuspid regurgitation (TR) before (A) and after (B) cinching tricuspid annulus (TA) 5 cm.

Step 6

The size adjustment tool is introduced over a wire to cinch the band and reduce the TV annular diameter under fluoroscopic and echocardiographic control. Changes in annular dimensions, coaptation gap, TR, and transvalvular gradient have to be assessed to find the optimal effective result (Figure 16.32). During band contraction, fluoroscopy has to rule out any deformation of the RCA that could compromise coronary flow. Once cinching is completed, the delivery system is pulled back and a final check-up is repeated including RV function and ruling out the presence of a pericardial effusion.

Orthotopic Tricuspid Valve Replacement Step by Step

Procedural implantation for the EVOQUE TV (Edwards Lifesciences) is performed under GA using fluoroscopy and TEE imaging guidance. The best TEE view may allow an optimal 3D TV en face image and its MPR analysis to show the properly aligned orthogonal LAX planes (105).

Step 1

One starts with insertion of sheath from the IVC into RA with TEE guidance and insertion of the guidewire across the TV into the RV apex ensuring freedom of interactions with the TV subvalvular apparatus. The guidewire motion should be evaluated in multiple TEE views.

Step 2

Under TEE guidance the steerable delivery catheter is positioned across the TV annulus and the EVOQUE valve is introduced into the RV (Figure 16.33; Video 16.27).

Step 3

The proper position and depth of the device between the tricuspid leaflets and the heads of papillary muscles are then confirmed through TEE (Figure 16.34; Video 16.28A,B).

Step 4

Partial retraction of the delivery system is done to expose the nine anchors in a U shape. Using 3D MPR imaging, rotating the orthogonal views along the TV annulus, every anchor has to be localized and visualized confirming the position of the leaflet above the anchor in systole without interaction with the papillary muscle or cords (Figure 16.35; Video 16.29).

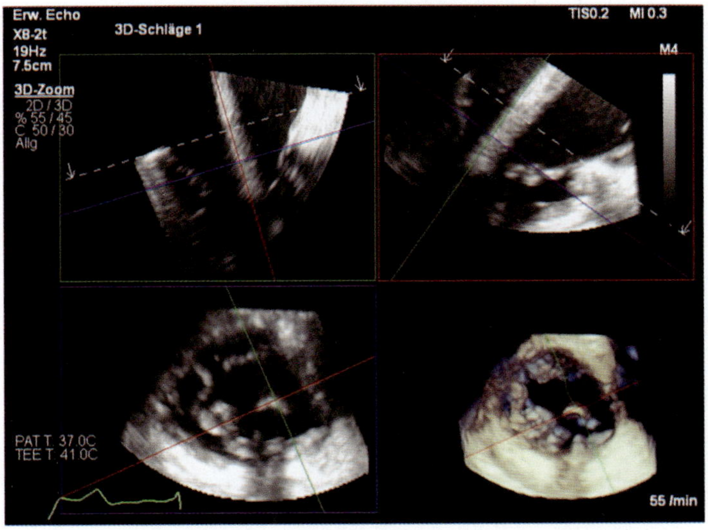

MPR mode - steerable delivery catheter positioned across the TV annulus

FIGURE 16.33 Multiplanar reconstruction (MPR) guidance. Steerable delivery catheter across the tricuspid annulus (TA).

Step 5

The valve is progressively expanded allowing the anchors to capture the leaflets (Figure 16.36; Video 16.30). 3D MPR imaging must be repeated to confirm that all the anchors are attached to the TV annulus. An anchor positioned under a commissure or fold may be unable to capture leaflet tissue. No more than two sequential anchors should be closed without adequate grasping of the TV tissue. This prevents device migration and paravalvular regurgitation.

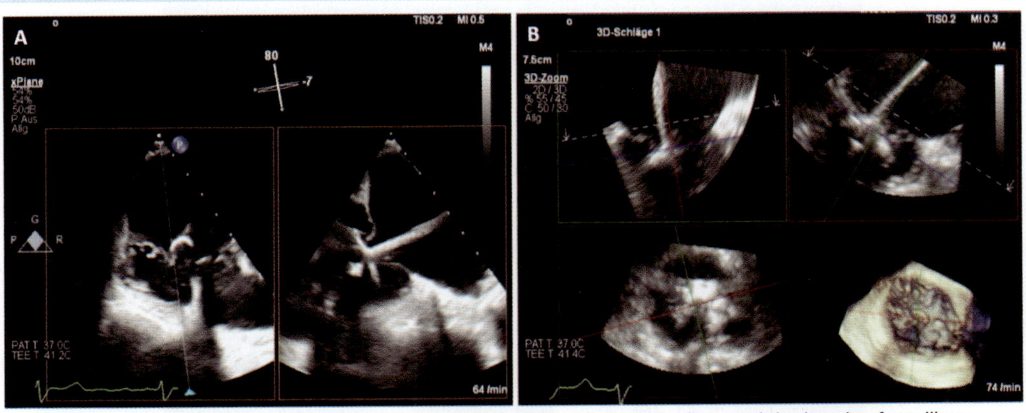

Assessment of position and depth of the device between the tricuspid leaflets and the heads of papillary muscles: A –biplanar ME view; B –MPR mode

FIGURE 16.34 Confirmation of proper position and depth of the device. A: Deep esophageal and biplane guidance; B: Multiplanar reconstruction (MPR) guidance.

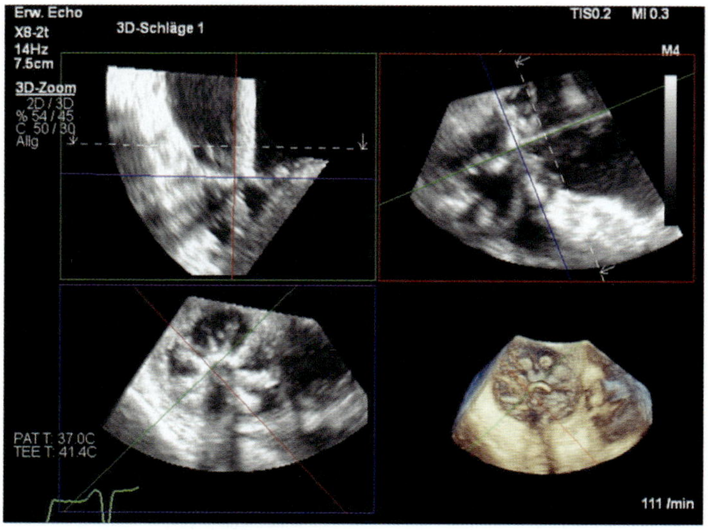

MPR mode–exposure of the anchors in a U shape

FIGURE 16.35 Multiplanar reconstruction (MPR) guidance. Exposure of the nine anchors.

Step 6

Expansion of the device and thereafter further release of the valve from the delivery system is done. Finally, TEE assessment of results should include valve stability, the evaluation for central or paravalvular regurgitation, valve orifice area, calculation of transvalvular gradients, RV size, RV function, and the absence of a new pericardial effusion (Figure 16.37; Video 16.31).

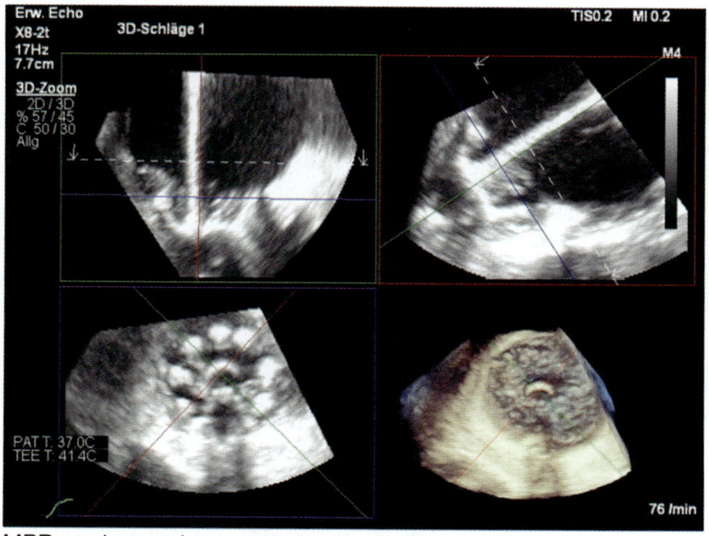

MPR mode - anchors capturing the leaflets

FIGURE 16.36 Multiplanar reconstruction (MPR) guidance. Expanded anchors to capture leaflets.

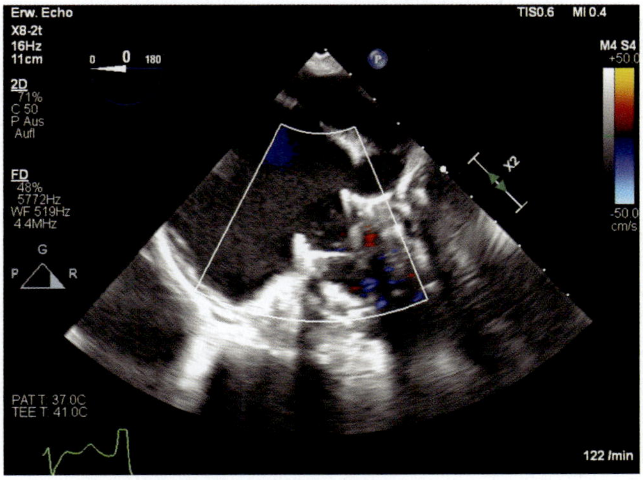

Assessment of results after valve release

FIGURE 16.37 Color Doppler assessment of results.

SUMMARY

The options for TTVT are rapidly developing and needs an individualized tailored approach for successful outcome. TV pathology needs to be clearly understood for device selection and TEE-guided intervention including preoperative multimodular imaging is imperative for clinical decision-making and patient selection.

REFERENCES

1. Otto CM, Nishimura RA, Bonow RO, et al. 2020 ACC/AHA guideline for the management of patients with valvular heart disease: a report of the American College of Cardiology/American Heart Association Joint Committee on Clinical Practice Guidelines. *Circulation*. 2021;143(5):e72-e227.
2. Vahanian A, Beyersdorf F, Praz F, et al. 2021 ESC/EACTS Guidelines for the management of valvular heart disease: developed by the Task Force for the management of valvular heart disease of the European Society of Cardiology (ESC) and the European Association for Cardio-Thoracic Surgery (EACTS). *Rev Esp Cardiol (Engl Ed)*. 2022;75(6):524.
3. Iung B, Delgado V, Rosenhek R, et al. Contemporary presentation and management of valvular heart disease: the EURObservational Research Programme Valvular Heart Disease II survey. *Circulation*. 2019;140(14):1156-1169.
4. Feldman T, Kar S, Elmariah S, et al. Randomized comparison of percutaneous repair and surgery for mitral regurgitation: 5-year results of EVEREST II. *J Am Coll Cardiol*. 2015;66(25):2844-2854.
5. Lim DS, Reynolds MR, Feldman T, et al. Improved functional status and quality of life in prohibitive surgical risk patients with degenerative mitral regurgitation after transcatheter mitral valve repair. *J Am Coll Cardiol*. 2014;64(2):182-192.
6. Alfieri O, Maisano F, De Bonis M, et al. The double-orifice technique in mitral valve repair: a simple solution for complex problems. *J Thorac Cardiovasc Surg*. 2001;122(4):674-681.
7. Buzzatti N, Van Hemelrijck M, Denti P, et al. Transcatheter or surgical repair for degenerative mitral regurgitation in elderly patients: a propensity-weighted analysis. *J Thorac Cardiovasc Surg*. 2019;158(1):86-94.e1.
8. Stone GW, Lindenfeld J, Abraham WT, et al. Transcatheter mitral-valve repair in patients with heart failure. *N Engl J Med*. 2018;379(24):2307-2318.
9. Grayburn PA, Sannino A, Packer M. Proportionate and disproportionate functional mitral regurgitation: a new conceptual framework that reconciles the results of the MITRA-FR and COAPT trials. *JACC Cardiovasc Imaging*. 2019;12(2):353-362.
10. Goel K, Lindenfeld J, Makkar R, et al. Transcatheter edge-to-edge repair in 5,000 patients with secondary mitral regurgitation: COAPT post-approval study. *J Am Coll Cardiol*. 2023;82(13):1281-1297.
11. Caiffa T, De Luca A, Biagini E, et al. Impact on clinical outcomes of right ventricular response to percutaneous correction of secondary mitral regurgitation. *Eur J Heart Fail*. 2021;23(10):1765-1774.
12. Ben-Yehuda O, Shahim B, Chen S, et al. Pulmonary hypertension in transcatheter mitral valve repair for secondary mitral regurgitation: the COAPT trial. *J Am Coll Cardiol*. 2020;76(22):2595-2606.
13. Saxon JT, Cohen DJ, Chhatriwalla AK, et al. Impact of COPD on outcomes after MitraClip for secondary mitral regurgitation: the COAPT trial. *JACC Cardiovasc Interv*. 2020;13(23):2795-2803.
14. Sisinni A, Munafo A, Pivato CA, et al. Effect of chronic kidney disease on 5-year outcome in patients with heart failure and secondary mitral regurgitation undergoing percutaneous MitraClip insertion. *Am J Cardiol*. 2022;171:105-114.

15. Hahn RT, Abraham T, Adams MS, et al. Guidelines for performing a comprehensive transesophageal echocardiographic examination: recommendations from the American Society of Echocardiography and the Society of Cardiovascular Anesthesiologists. *J Am Soc Echocardiogr.* 2013;26(9):921-964.
16. Hahn RT, Saric M, Faletra FF, et al. Recommended standards for the performance of transesophageal echocardiographic screening for structural heart intervention: from the American Society of Echocardiography. *J Am Soc Echocardiogr.* 2022;35(1):1-76.
17. Filsoufi F, Carpentier A. Principles of reconstructive surgery in degenerative mitral valve disease. *Semin Thorac Cardiovasc Surg.* 2007;19(2):103-110.
18. Anyanwu AC, Adams DH. Etiologic classification of degenerative mitral valve disease: Barlow's disease and fibroelastic deficiency. *Semin Thorac Cardiovasc Surg.* 2007;19(2):90-96.
19. Narang A, Addetia K, Weinert L, et al. Diagnosis of isolated cleft mitral valve using three-dimensional echocardiography. *J Am Soc Echocardiogr.* 2018;31(11):1161-1167.
20. Deferm S, Bertrand PB, Verbrugge FH, et al. Atrial functional mitral regurgitation: JACC review topic of the week. *J Am Coll Cardiol.* 2019;73(19):2465-2476.
21. Nielsen SL, Nygaard H, Mandrup L, et al. Mechanism of incomplete mitral leaflet coaptation—interaction of chordal restraint and changes in mitral leaflet coaptation geometry. Insight from in vitro validation of the premise of force equilibrium. *J Biomech Eng.* 2002;124(5):596-608.
22. Zoghbi WA, Adams D, Bonow RO, et al. Recommendations for noninvasive evaluation of native valvular regurgitation: a report from the American Society of Echocardiography developed in collaboration with the Society for Cardiovascular Magnetic Resonance. *J Am Soc Echocardiogr.* 2017;30(4):303-371.
23. Goebel B, Heck R, Hamadanchi A, et al. Vena contracta area for severity grading in functional and degenerative mitral regurgitation: a transoesophageal 3D colour Doppler analysis in 500 patients. *Eur Heart J Cardiovasc Imaging.* 2018;19(6):639-646.
24. Mihalatos DG, Gopal AS, Kates R, et al. Intraoperative assessment of mitral regurgitation: role of phenylephrine challenge. *J Am Soc Echocardiogr.* 2006;19(9):1158-1164.
25. Bonow RO, O'Gara PT, Adams DH, et al. 2020 focused update of the 2017 ACC expert consensus decision pathway on the management of mitral regurgitation: a report of the American College of Cardiology Solution Set Oversight Committee. *J Am Coll Cardiol.* 2020;75(17):2236-2270.
26. Feldman T, Wasserman HS, Herrmann HC, et al. Percutaneous mitral valve repair using the edge-to-edge technique: six-month results of the EVEREST Phase I Clinical Trial. *J Am Coll Cardiol.* 2005;46(11):2134-2140.
27. Chakravarty T, Makar M, Patel D, et al. Transcatheter edge-to-edge mitral valve repair with the MitraClip G4 system. *JACC Cardiovasc Interv.* 2020;13(20):2402-2414.
28. Praz F, Spargias K, Chrissoheris M, et al. Compassionate use of the PASCAL transcatheter mitral valve repair system for patients with severe mitral regurgitation: a multicentre, prospective, observational, first-in-man study. *Lancet.* 2017;390(10096):773-780.
29. Liu X, Chen M, Han Y, et al. First-in-human study of the novel transcatheter mitral valve repair system for mitral regurgitation. *JACC Asia.* 2022;2(3):390-394.
30. Zahr F, Smith RL, Gillam LD, et al. One-year outcomes from the CLASP IID randomized trial for degenerative mitral regurgitation. *JACC Cardiovasc Interv.* 2023:S1936-8798(23)01358-4.
31. Asch FM, Grayburn PA, Siegel RJ, et al. Echocardiographic outcomes after transcatheter leaflet approximation in patients with secondary mitral regurgitation: the COAPT trial. *J Am Coll Cardiol.* 2019;74(24):2969-2979.
32. Hausleiter J, Stocker TJ, Adamo M, Karam N, Swaans MJ, Praz F. Mitral valve transcatheter edge-to-edge repair. *EuroIntervention.* 2023;18(12):957-976.
33. Kassar M, Praz F, Hunziker L, et al. Anatomical and technical predictors of three-dimensional mitral valve area reduction after transcatheter edge-to-edge repair. *J Am Soc Echocardiogr.* 2022;35(1):96-104.
34. Chhatriwalla AK, Vemulapalli S, Szerlip M, et al. Operator experience and outcomes of transcatheter mitral valve repair in the United States. *J Am Coll Cardiol.* 2019;74(24):2955-2965.
35. Chhatriwalla AK, Vemulapalli S, Holmes DR Jr, et al. Institutional experience with transcatheter mitral valve repair and clinical outcomes: insights from the TVT Registry. *JACC Cardiovasc Interv.* 2019;12(14):1342-1352.
36. Hahn RT, Mahmood F, Kodali S, et al. Core competencies in echocardiography for imaging structural heart disease interventions: an expert consensus statement. *JACC Cardiovasc Imaging.* 2019;12(12):2560-2570.
37. Mijangos-Vazquez R, Garcia-Montes JA, Zabal-Cerdeira C. Aortic iatrogenic perforation during transseptal puncture and successful occlusion with Amplatzer ductal occluder in a case of mitral paravalvular leak closure. *Catheter Cardiovasc Interv.* 2016;88(2):312-315.
38. Afzal S, Veulemans V, Balzer J, et al. Safety and efficacy of transseptal puncture guided by real-time fusion of echocardiography and fluoroscopy. *Neth Heart J.* 2017;25(2):131-136.
39. Guarracino F, Baldassarri R, Ferro B, et al. Transesophageal echocardiography during MitraClip® procedure. *Anesth Analg.* 2014;118(6):1188-1196.
40. Gruner C, Herzog B, Bettex D, et al. Quantification of mitral regurgitation by real time three-dimensional color Doppler flow echocardiography pre- and post-percutaneous mitral valve repair. *Echocardiography.* 2015;32(7):1140-1146.
41. Sorajja P, Vemulapalli S, Feldman T, et al. Outcomes with transcatheter mitral valve repair in the United States: an STS/ACC TVT Registry report. *J Am Coll Cardiol.* 2017;70(19):2315-2327.
42. Neuss M, Schau T, Isotani A, Pilz M, Schopp M, Butter C. Elevated mitral valve pressure gradient after MitraClip implantation deteriorates long-term outcome in patients with severe mitral regurgitation and severe heart failure. *JACC Cardiovasc Interv.* 2017;10(9):931-939.
43. Utsunomiya H, Itabashi Y, Kobayashi S, et al. Effect of percutaneous edge-to-edge repair on mitral valve area and its association with pulmonary hypertension and outcomes. *Am J Cardiol.* 2017;120(4):662-669.
44. Taramasso M, Gavazzoni M, Kuwata S, Meier P, Maisano F. From color to hemodynamic assessment: is it time to change the paradigm in judging MitraClip outcomes? *JACC Cardiovasc Interv.* 2019;12(2):151-154.

45. Ikenaga H, Yoshida J, Hayashi A, et al. Usefulness of intraprocedural pulmonary venous flow for predicting recurrent mitral regurgitation and clinical outcomes after percutaneous mitral valve repair with the MitraClip. *JACC Cardiovasc Interv.* 2019;12(2):140-150.
46. Hart EA, Zwart K, Teske AJ, et al. Haemodynamic and functional consequences of the iatrogenic atrial septal defect following Mitraclip therapy. *Neth Heart J.* 2017;25(2):137-142.
47. Nakajima Y, Kar S. First experience of the usage of a GORE CARDIOFORM septal occluder device for treatment of a significant residual commissural mitral regurgitation jet following a MitraClip procedure. *Catheter Cardiovasc Interv.* 2018;92(3):607-610.
48. Mangieri A, Melillo F, Montalto C, et al. Management and outcome of failed percutaneous edge-to-edge mitral valve plasty: insight from an international registry. *JACC Cardiovasc Interv.* 2022;15(4):411-422.
49. Bartkowiak J, Reineke D, Tomii D, et al. Electrosurgical laceration and stabilization of MitraClip followed by valve implantation for iatrogenic mitral stenosis. *JACC Cardiovasc Interv.* 2022;15(1):110-112.
50. Colli A, Manzan E, Aidietis A, et al. An early European experience with transapical off-pump mitral valve repair with NeoChord implantation. *Eur J Cardiothorac Surg.* 2018;54(3):460-466.
51. D'Onofrio A, Fiocco A, Nadali M, et al. Outcomes of transapical mitral valve repair with neochordae implantation. *J Thorac Cardiovasc Surg.* 2023;165(3):1036-1046.e4.
52. Gammie JS, Bartus K, Gackowski A, et al. Beating-heart mitral valve repair using a novel ePTFE cordal implantation device: a prospective trial. *J Am Coll Cardiol.* 2018;71(1):25-36.
53. Gammie JS, Bartus K, Gackowski A, et al. Safety and performance of a novel transventricular beating heart mitral valve repair system: 1-year outcomes. *Eur J Cardiothorac Surg.* 2021;59(1):199-206.
54. Bergonzoni E, D'Onofrio A, Mastro F, Gerosa G. Microinvasive mitral valve repair with transapical mitral neochordae implantation. *Front Cardiovasc Med.* 2023;10:1166892.
55. Hensey M, Brown RA, Lal S, et al. Transcatheter mitral valve replacement: an update on current techniques, technologies, and future directions. *JACC Cardiovasc Interv.* 2021;14(5):489-500.
56. Carpentier AF, Pellerin M, Fuzellier JF, Relland JY. Extensive calcification of the mitral valve anulus: pathology and surgical management. *J Thorac Cardiovasc Surg.* 1996;111(4):718-729; discussion 729-730.
57. Van Mieghem NM, Piazza N, Anderson RH, et al. Anatomy of the mitral valvular complex and its implications for transcatheter interventions for mitral regurgitation. *J Am Coll Cardiol.* 2010;56(8):617-626.
58. Guerrero M, Wang DD, Pursnani A, et al. A cardiac computed tomography-based score to categorize mitral annular calcification severity and predict valve embolization. *JACC Cardiovasc Imaging.* 2020;13(9):1945-1957.
59. Ludwig S, Kalbacher D, Ali WB, et al. Transcatheter mitral valve replacement or repair for secondary mitral regurgitation: a propensity score-matched analysis. *Eur J Heart Fail.* 2023;25(3):399-410.
60. Guerrero M, Wang DD, Eleid MF, et al. Prospective study of TMVR using balloon-expandable aortic transcatheter valves in MAC: MITRAL Trial 1-year outcomes. *JACC Cardiovasc Interv.* 2021;14(8):830-845.
61. Lisko JC, Babaliaros VC, Khan JM, et al. Tip-to-base LAMPOON for transcatheter mitral valve replacement with a protected mitral annulus. *JACC Cardiovasc Interv.* 2021;14(5):541-550.
62. Urena M, Himbert D, Brochet E, et al. Transseptal transcatheter mitral valve replacement using balloon-expandable transcatheter heart valves: a step-by-step approach. *JACC Cardiovasc Interv.* 2017;10(19):1905-1919.
63. Bushari LI, Reeder GS, Eleid MF, et al. Percutaneous transcatheter edge-to-edge mitraclip technique: a practical "step-by-step" 3-dimensional transesophageal echocardiography guide. *Mayo Clin Proc.* 2019;94(1):89-102.
64. Wollborn J, Schuler A, Sheu RD, Shook DC, Nyman CB. Real-time multiplanar reconstruction imaging using 3-dimensional transesophageal echocardiography in structural heart interventions. *J Cardiothorac Vasc Anesth.* 2023;37(4):570-581.
65. Nyman CB, Mackensen GB, Jelacic S, Little SH, Smith TW, Mahmood F. Transcatheter mitral valve repair using the edge-to-edge clip. *J Am Soc Echocardiogr.* 2018;31(4):434-453.
66. Grayburn PA, Mack MJ, Manandhar P, et al. Comparison of transcatheter edge-to-edge mitral valve repair for primary mitral regurgitation outcomes to hospital volumes of surgical mitral valve repair. *Circ Cardiovasc Interv.* 2024;17(4):e013581.
67. Chorin E, Rozenbaum Z, Topilsky Y, et al. Tricuspid regurgitation and long-term clinical outcomes. *Eur Heart J Cardiovasc Imaging.* 2020;21:157-165.
68. Offen S, Playford D, Strange G, et al. Adverse prognostic impact of even mild or moderate tricuspid regurgitation: insights from the National Echocardiography Database of Australia. *J Am Soc Echocardiogr.* 2022;35:810-817.
69. Axtell AL, Bhambhani V, Moonsamy P, et al. Surgery does not improve survival in patients with isolated severe tricuspid regurgitation. *J Am Coll Cardiol.* 2019;74:715-725.
70. Badhwar V, Rankin JS, He M, et al. Performing concomitant tricuspid valve repair at the time of mitral valve operations is not associated with increased operative mortality. *Ann Thorac Surg.* 2017;103:587-593.
71. Bar N, Schwartz LA, Biner S, et al. Clinical outcome of isolated tricuspid regurgitation in patients with preserved left ventricular ejection fraction and pulmonary hypertension. *J Am Soc Echocardiogr.* 2018;31:34-41.
72. Kilic A, Saha-Chaudhuri P, Rankin JS, et al. Trends and outcomes of tricuspid valve surgery in North America: an analysis of more than 50,000 patients from the Society of Thoracic Surgeons database. *Ann Thorac Surg.* 2013;96:1546-1552; discussion 1552.
73. Vahanian A, Alfieri O, Andreotti F, et al. Guidelines on the management of valvular heart disease (version 2012): the Joint Task Force on the Management of Valvular Heart Disease of the European Society of Cardiology (ESC) and the European Association for Cardio-Thoracic Surgery (EACTS). *Eur J Cardiothorac Surg.* 2012;42:S1-S44.
74. Ambrosino M, Sangoi M, Monzer N, et al. Tricuspid regurgitation: a review of current interventional management. *J Am Heart Assoc.* 2024;13:e032999.
75. Blusztein DI, Hahn RT. New therapeutic approach for tricuspid regurgitation: transcatheter tricuspid valve replacement or repair. *Front Cardiovasc Med.* 2023;10:1080101.
76. Chen V, Altisent OA, Puri R. A comprehensive overview of surgical and transcatheter therapies to treat tricuspid regurgitation in patients with heart failure. *Curr Opin Cardiol.* 2024;39:110-118.

77. Hagemeyer D, Ong G, Peterson MD, et al. Transcatheter tricuspid valve intervention: to repair or to replace? *Curr Opin Cardiol.* 2022;37:495-501.
78. Maisano F, Hahn R, Sorajja P, et al. Transcatheter treatment of the tricuspid valve: current status and perspectives. *Eur Heart J.* 2024;45:876-894.
79. Davidson CJ, Lim DS, Smith RL, et al. Early feasibility study of cardioband tricuspid system for functional tricuspid regurgitation: 30-day outcomes. *JAAC Cardiovasc Interv.* 2021;14:41-50.
80. Gray WA, Abramson SV, Lim S, et al. 1-year outcomes of cardioband tricuspid valve reconstruction system early feasibility study. *JAAC Cardiovasc Interv.* 2022;15:1921-1932.
81. Kodali S, Hahn RT, Makkar R, et al. Transfemoral tricuspid valve replacement and one-year outcomes: the TRISCEND study. *Eur Heart J.* 2023;44:4862-4873.
82. Kodali SK, Hahn RT, Davidson CJ, et al. 1-year outcomes of transcatheter tricuspid valve repair. *J Am Coll Cardiol.* 2023;81:1766-1776.
83. Lurz P, Besler C, Schmitz T, et al. Short-term outcomes of tricuspid edge-to-edge repair in clinical practice. *J Am Coll Cardiol.* 2023;82:281-291.
84. Nickenig G, Weber M, Schuler R, et al. Tricuspid valve repair with the Cardioband system: two-year outcomes of the multicentre, prospective TRI-REPAIR study. *EuroIntervention.* 2021;16:e1264-e1271.
85. von Bardeleben RS, Lurz P, Sorajja P, et al. Two-year outcomes for tricuspid repair with a transcatheter edge-to-edge valve repair from the transatlantic TRILUMINATE trial. *Circ Cardiovasc Interv.* 2023;16:e012888.
86. Dreyfus J, Galloo X, Taramasso M, et al. TRI-SCORE and benefit of intervention in patients with severe tricuspid regurgitation. *Eur Heart J.* 2024;45:586-597.
87. Hahn RT, Thomas JD, Khalique OK, et al. Imaging assessment of tricuspid regurgitation severity. *JACC Cardiovasc Imaging.* 2019;12:469-490.
88. Hahn RT. State-of-the-art review of echocardiographic imaging in the evaluation and treatment of functional tricuspid regurgitation. *Circ Cardiovasc Imaging.* 2016;9:e005332.
89. Hahn RT, Weckbach LT, Noack T, et al. Proposal for a standard echocardiographic tricuspid valve nomenclature. *JACC Cardiovasc Imaging.* 2021;14:1299-1305.
90. Hahn RT, Zamorano JL. The need for a new tricuspid regurgitation grading scheme. *Eur Heart J Cardiovasc Imaging.* 2017;18:1342-1343.
91. Kitamura M, Kresoja KP, Besler C, et al. Impact of tricuspid valve morphology on clinical outcomes after transcatheter edge-to-edge repair. *JAAC Cardiovasc Interv.* 2021;14:1616-1618.
92. Lancellotti P, Pibarot P, Chambers J, et al. Multi-modality imaging assessment of native valvular regurgitation: an EACVI and ESC council of valvular heart disease position paper. *Eur Heart J Cardiovasc Imaging.* 2022;23:e171-e232.
93. Nguyen TKH, Rudski LG. Optimal echocardiographic approach to the evaluation of tricuspid regurgitation. *Curr Cardiol Rep.* 2020;22:108.
94. Hahn RT, Badano LP, Bartko PE, et al. Tricuspid regurgitation: recent advances in understanding pathophysiology, severity grading and outcome. *Eur Heart J Cardiovasc Imaging.* 2022;23:913-929.
95. Ancona F, Agricola E, Stella S, et al. Interventional imaging of the tricuspid valve. *Interv Cardiol Clin.* 2018;7:13-29.
96. Agricola E, Meucci F, Ancona F, et al. Echocardiographic guidance in transcatheter structural cardiac interventions. *EuroIntervention.* 2022;17:1205-1226.
97. Ram P, Shekiladze N, Xie J, et al. Echocardiographic imaging of the tricuspid valve: preprocedural planning and intraprocedural guidance. *Interv Cardiol Clin.* 2022;11:11-25.
98. Hungerford SL, Rye EE, Hansen PS, et al. Key echocardiographic considerations for tricuspid valve transcatheter edge-to-edge repair. *J Am Soc Echocardiogr.* 2023;36:366-380.e1.
99. Muraru D, Badano LP, Hahn RT, et al. Atrial secondary tricuspid regurgitation: pathophysiology, definition, diagnosis, and treatment. *Eur Heart J.* 2024;45:895-911.
100. Dahou A, Levin D, Reisman M, et al. Anatomy and physiology of the tricuspid valve. *JACC Cardiovasc Imaging.* 2019;12:458-468.
101. Besler C, Orban M, Rommel KP, et al. Predictors of procedural and clinical outcomes in patients with symptomatic tricuspid regurgitation undergoing transcatheter edge-to-edge repair. *JACC Cardiovasc Interv.* 2018;11:1119-1128.
102. Praz F, Muraru D, Kreidel F, et al. Transcatheter treatment for tricuspid valve disease. *EuroIntervention.* 2021;17:791-808.
103. Gerçek M, Rudolph V, Arnold M, et al. Transient acute right coronary artery deformation during transcatheter interventional tricuspid repair with the Cardioband tricuspid system. *EuroIntervention.* 2021;17:81-87.
104. Mariani M, Bonanni M, D'Agostino A, et al. Multimodality imaging approach for planning and guiding direct transcatheter tricuspid valve annuloplasty. *J Am Soc Echocardiogr.* 2024;37:449-465.
105. Fam NP, von Bardeleben RS, Hensey M, et al. Transfemoral transcatheter tricuspid valve replacement with the EVOQUE system: a multicenter, observational, first-in-human experience. *JACC Cardiovasc Interv.* 2021;14:501-511.
106. Haurand JM, Kavsur R, Ochs L, et al. Deep sedation vs. general anesthesia for transcatheter tricuspid valve repair. *Front Cardiovasc Med.* 2022;9:976822.
107. Kuwajima K, Kagawa S, Yamane T, et al. Comparison of residual tricuspid regurgitation severity assessed by intraprocedural and postprocedural echocardiography in patients undergoing transcatheter tricuspid valve repair. *J Cardiothorac Vasc Anesth.* 2022;36:4555-4557.
108. Zoller JK, Gregory SH. Anesthetic considerations for transcatheter tricuspid valve repair. *J Cardiothorac Vasc Anesth.* 2020;34:1942-1951.
109. Wang H, Oran A, Butler CG, et al. Preoperative tricuspid regurgitation is associated with long-term mortality and is graded more severe than intraoperative tricuspid regurgitation. *J Cardiothorac Vasc Anesth.* 2023;37:1904-1911.
110. Donal E, Sitges M, Panis V, et al. Characterization of tricuspid valve anatomy and coaptation gap in subjects receiving tricuspid transcatheter edge-to-edge repair: observations from the bRIGHT TriClip study. *JACC Cardiovasc Imaging.* 2024;37:397-404.

111. Russo G, Hahn RT, Alessandrini H, et al. Effects of tricuspid transcatheter edge-to-edge repair on tricuspid annulus diameter—data from the TriValve registry. *Int J Cardiol*. 2024;405:131934.
112. Mehr M, Taramasso M, Besler C, et al. 1-year outcomes after edge-to-edge valve repair for symptomatic tricuspid regurgitation: results from the TriValve registry. *JAAC Cardiovasc Interv*. 2019;12:1451-1461.
113. Aman E, Atsina KB. Tricuspid valve transcatheter edge-to-edge repair guidance with transesophageal echocardiography and intracardiac echocardiography. *JAAC Cardiovasc Interv*. 2024;13:1-10.
114. Hahn RT, Nabauer M, Zuber M, et al. Intraprocedural imaging of transcatheter tricuspid valve interventions. *JAAC Cardiovasc Interv*. 2019;12:532-553.
115. Hahn RT, Kodali SK. State-of-the-art intra-procedural imaging for the mitral and tricuspid PASCAL Repair System. *JAAC Cardiovasc Interv*. 2022;23:e94-e110.
116. da Rocha ESJG, Ruf TF, Hell MM, et al. Transgastric imaging-the key to successful periprocedural TEE guiding for edge-to-edge repair of the tricuspid valve. *Echocardiography*. 2021;38:1948-1958.
117. Wollborn J, Schuler A, Sheu RD, et al. Real-time multiplanar reconstruction imaging using 3-dimensional transesophageal echocardiography in structural heart interventions. *J Cardiothorac Vasc Anesth*. 2023;37:570-581.

PART A: QUESTIONS

1. **Transcatheter MV edge-to-edge repair is indicated in which of the following conditions?**
   A. Degenerative MV stenosis
   B. Degenerative MV prosthesis
   C. Mitral regurgitation and prohibitive surgical risk
   D. All cases of MR

2. **Post-MV edge-to-edge repair, what would be an acceptable result?**
   A. A mean gradient of 6 mm Hg
   B. An MVA of 1.7 cm^2
   C. A mean gradient of 5 mm Hg
   D. An MVA of 2.5 cm^2

3. **Which of the following features contraindicates MV edge-to- edge repair in secondary MR?**
   A. A posterior leaflet length of 12 mm
   B. An anterior leaflet length of 15 mm
   C. A flail gap of 9 mm
   D. LV end diastolic diameter of 100 mm

4. **Which of the following features constitutes a favorable anatomy for MV edge-to-edge repair?**
   A. A posterior leaflet less than 10 mm
   B. Leaflet calcifications
   C. A coaptation gap of 11 mm
   D. A tenting height of 15 mm

5. **Which of the following is a common complication of MV edge-to-edge repair?**
   A. Mitral stenosis
   B. LVOT obstruction
   C. Pulmonary valve insufficiency
   D. Aortic dissection

6. **According to the Carpentier classification, which of the following causes of MR can be addressed with NeoChord implantation?**
   A. I
   B. II
   C. IIIa
   D. IIIb

7. **Which of the following complications may occur after transcatheter mitral valve implantation?**
   A. Aortic dissection
   B. Coronary artery obstruction
   C. LVOT obstruction
   D. Pulmonary vein obstruction

8. Which of the following findings may contraindicate the implantation of transcatheter MV?
A. Mitral annular calcification
B. Mitral stenosis
C. LV end diastolic diameter of 40 mm
D. Aortic insufficiency

9. To address paravalvular leak after deployment of a Tendyne valve, which of the following maneuvers should be performed?
A. Post-balloon dilation
B. Placement of an Amplatzer occluder
C. Increase tension on the anchoring system
D. Valve rotation

10. Which of the following level of expertise is advised to guide MV transcatheter interventions?
A. Basic TEE certification
B. TEE and TTE certification
C. Special training in transcatheter interventions
D. Comprehensive TEE certification

PART A: ANSWERS

1. Correct Answer: C.
Rationale: According to current guidelines, surgical mitral valve repair remains the standard of care for MR. In high-risk patients, transcatheter edge-to-edge repair is a valuable option when the anatomy allows it.

2. Correct Answer: C.
Rationale: An MVA >1.9 cm^2 is considered as an acceptable result by most authors.

3. Correct Answer: D.
Rationale: According to the COAPT trial inclusion criteria, a LVESD of 70 mm is the cutoff for TEER in secondary MR.

4. Correct Answer: C.
Rationale: According to expert consensus a coaptation gap less than 15 mm poses for a favorable anatomy for edge-to-edge repair.

5. Correct Answer: A.
Rationale: TEER causes a reduction of MVA and may result in MV stenosis. The clip is delivered through the IAS; therefore, lesions of the aorta, LVOT, and pulmonary valve are very uncommon.

6. Correct Answer: B.
Rationale: Carpentier classification Type II depicts excessive MV leaflet motion and can be addressed by NeoChord by pulling the leaflets edge down into the ventricle and resolve flail.

7. Correct Answer: C.
Rationale: Deployment of a prosthetic MV causes displacement of anterior mitral valve leaflet and may cause LVOT obstruction. Lesion of the aorta and coronary arteries is extremely uncommon.

8. Correct Answer: C.
Rationale: Transcatheter MV implantation may not be possible is a small LV due to a high risk of LVOT obstruction. Mitral stenosis is often the indication for implantation. Mitral annular calcification is a favorable feature allowing good valve seating.

9. Correct Answer: C.
Rationale: Increasing the tension on the string that connects the valve to the apical pad will cause a better valve sealing.

10. Correct Answer: C.
Rationale: Current guidelines advise special training in structural heart interventions for cardiologists and anesthesiologists who already hold a certification in advanced perioperative TEE.

PART B: QUESTIONS

1. **Which statement is false regarding TR (one or more):**
   A. TR is a rare valvular heart disease in advanced age.
   B. TR is asymptomatic until advanced stages.
   C. Prognosis of TR is mild during the asymptomatic period.
   D. Surgical approach is the best approach in symptomatic patients with TR.

2. **Regarding TTVTs, which statement is true (one or more):**
   A. TTVT has shown to be efficacious in reducing TR.
   B. TTVT is associated with a high incidence of complications.
   C. TTVT has shown to improve quality of life independently of TR reduction.
   D. TR etiology and TV anatomy are determinant for TTVT device selection.

3. **Which statement regarding TR etiology is true (one or more):**
   A. Primary TR is the common cause of TR in advanced age.
   B. CIEDs can cause leaflet impingement.
   C. Atrial secondary TR is associated with RV dilation and leaflet tethering.
   D. Ventricular secondary TR is associated with RA and tricuspid annulus dilation.

4. **Which statement regarding TTVTs is true**
   A. TEE is useful in planning the proper device but not for its guidance.
   B. With a good quality preoperative CT intraprocedural fluoroscopy is not necessary
   C. Cardioband shows the best results in ventricular secondary TR.
   D. Orthotopic valve replacement shows the best results regarding TR reduction.

5. **Which statement regarding predictors of procedural success for TEER is true:**
   A. All TV anatomies are suitable to be treated with TEER.
   B. TEER shows best procedural success in posteroseptal TR jets.
   C. TEER is particularly useful in TR with leaflet tethering.
   D. TEER by torrential TR with leaflet impingement shows poor performance results.

6. **Which statement regarding TEER procedure is true:**
   A. Bicaval view is necessary to guide IAS puncture.
   B. 3D imaging of the TR is not useful in TEER guiding.
   C. Fluoroscopy alone may be sufficient for TEER guiding.
   D. TG views of TV alone may be sufficient for TEER guiding.

7. **Which echocardiographic view is not useful in guiding TEER?**
   A. Bicaval view
   B. Deep ME RV inflow-outflow tract
   C. ME LAX view
   D. TG RV LAX view

8. **Regarding echocardiography in TEER:**
   A. Biplanar imaging is essential in guiding leaflet grasping.
   B. Transvalvular gradient is not to be assessed before deployment of every device.
   C. ME RV four-chambered view is the recommended view to assess TEER results.
   D. 3D vena contracta area of residual TR is not reliable.

9. **Transcatheter tricuspid annuloplasty:**
   A. has the potential risk of severe bleeding.
   B. does not need fluoroscopy support during procedure.
   C. preprocedure cardiac CT anatomy is necessary to assess procedure feasibility.
   D. is the procedure of choice in TR with leaflet tethering.

10. The orthotopic valve replacement
A. is not indicated for torrential TR.
B. shows the higher TR grade reduction with lower incidence of major complications.
C. has the potential risk of RCA injury.
D. 3D echocardiography is necessary for its guiding.

▶PART B: ANSWERS

1. **Correct Answer: A, C, and D are false.**
Rationale: Prevalence of TR increases with advanced age and when more than mild is associated with increased morbidity and mortality even when asymptomatic. TR become generally symptomatic when the disease is already in an advanced stage and the surgical approach is then associated with high risk of mortality.

2. **Correct Answer: A and D are true.**
Rationale: TTVT has shown to be efficacious in reducing TR with a low incidence of complications. TR etiology and TV anatomy are the main determinants for proper device selection. Successful outcomes are related to TR decrease, between others.

3. **Correct Answer: B is true.**
Rationale: Primary TR is due to TV pathology and is rare. In advanced age atrial secondary TR is common, associated with TV annulus dilation due to atrial fibrillation and TR due to CIED. Ventricular secondary TR is associated with left-sided heart disease, pulmonary hypertension, and RV dysfunction with RV dilation and TV leaflet tethering.

4. **Correct Answer: D is true.**
Rationale: TEE is useful for planning and necessary in guiding the device performance. Fluoroscopy is indispensable in Cardioband and EVOQUE implantation and useful in TEER. Cardioband shows the best results in annular dilation without leaflet tethering (atrial secondary TR) and EVOQUE shows the best TR reduction.

5. **Correct Answer: D is true.**
Rationale: Trileaflet anatomy with anterolateral or central jet and no tethering is a good predictor of TEER success. Torrential TR and leaflet impingement together with excessive annular and RA dilation are poor predictors of success.

6. **Correct Answer: D is true.**
Rationale: It is not necessary to go through IAS, and 3D technology is essential in guiding TEER (biplanar imaging, 3D live en face of TV and MPR). Fluoroscopy does not allow to visualize TV anatomy, leaflet grasping, or TR, among others.

7. **Correct Answer: C is true.**
Rationale: All ME, deep ME, and TG views showing TV and RV may be necessary to guide TEER. LAX is not necessary.

8. **Correct Answer: A is true.**
Rationale: It is necessary to assess transvalvular gradient before and after every device deployment to avoid TV stenosis. To assess TEER results, multiple views are necessary to ensure device stability and residual regurgitation. 3D vena contracta is very useful to assess residual eccentric regurgitant jets.

9. **Correct Answer: C is true.**
Rationale: The most feared risk of transcatheter tricuspid annuloplasty is RCA injury, which is why a preprocedure cardiac CT and an intraoperative fluoroscopy with RCA cannulation are necessary to guide the procedure. Annular dilation without tethering is among the predictor of procedural success.

10. **Correct Answer: D is true.**
Rationale: 3D echocardiography with MPR imaging is the only possibility to control the attachment of all the anchors to the TA. Orthotopic valve replacement is indicated in patients with no suitable anatomy for TV repair such as torrential TR, leaflet tethering, or leaflet impingement. Although orthotopic valve replacement shows the highest TR reduction, it also shows the highest incidence of complications. The most common complication in orthotopic valve replacement is bleeding.

17

Transesophageal Echocardiography of the Thoracic Aorta

Michele L. Sumler and Roman M. Sniecinski

Although simple in structure, the thoracic aorta is a crucial component of the routine perioperative transesophageal echocardiography (TEE) examination. Pathologies such as atheroma, aneurysms, and dissections can be readily diagnosed and inspected in the operating room. Likewise, TEE can help guide the insertion of cannulas, stents, and intraaortic balloon pumps (IABPs), both in the operating room and the intensive care unit. It is therefore imperative that the perioperative echocardiographer has a firm grasp on both the anatomy and potential abnormalities of this vital blood vessel.

ANATOMY AND TRANSESOPHAGEAL ECHOCARDIOGRAPHY IMAGING

The basic structure of the aorta is similar to that of an upside-down letter "J," albeit with a slight twist (Figure 17.1). The aortic valve annulus, leaflets, and sinuses of Valsalva comprise the beginning of the thoracic aorta, collectively known as the aortic root. The ascending aorta, which is the start of the tubular portion, begins at the sinotubular junction (STJ), travels cephalad, and extends to the origin of the innominate (aka brachiocephalic) artery. The aortic arch begins at this point and travels horizontally to the origin of the left subclavian artery (LSCA). The descending aorta begins just distal to the LSCA, at a region known as the aortic isthmus, and travels caudad going through the diaphragm.

It is important to keep this shape of the aorta in mind during its examination. The vertical nature of the descending portion explains why a short-axis (SAX) view of this section is typically obtained at an angle of around 0°, while the SAX view of the arch, which is horizontal in nature, is at 90°. The reverse is true of the long-axis views, with the descending and arch portions of the aorta obtained at 90° and 0°, respectively. It is also important to recognize that the relationship between the esophagus and aorta changes as these structures travel from the thoracic cavity into the abdomen. At the level of the diaphragm, the aorta is posterior to the esophagus, while at the level of the arch, the aorta is anterior. As a result, the TEE probe is typically turned as it is withdrawn from the stomach to the upper esophagus in order to keep the aorta in the imaging field. Designating anterior/posterior and left/right while examining the descending aorta is also challenging.

The thoracic aorta has been divided into "segments" and "zones" that have varied with time and surgical approach (1,2,3). The currently described "landing zones" begin with zone 0 that starts at the STJ and ends just past the innominate artery. The remainder of the aorta is divided into 11 zones terminating after the takeoff of the external iliac arteries (Figure 17.1). Due to the interposition of the trachea and left main stem bronchus, TEE cannot reliably image the distal ascending aorta or proximal arch, which is the rationale for performing epiaortic scanning (see section that follows).

Because of the sheer length of the structure, the thoracic aorta can be viewed in many of the standard imaging planes. However, a systematic approach to its examination is recommended to ensure all possible sections are visualized. One common method is to begin its examination after obtaining the transgastric views of the left ventricle and turning the probe to the left until the descending aorta is seen in SAX at 0°. From here, the depth is typically set to 6 to 8 cm (to ensure simultaneous visualization of the left pleural space) and the probe is withdrawn, following the aorta until the circular view of the descending aorta in SAX becomes the tubular view of the arch in long axis (▶ Video 17.1). The omniplane angle can then be adjusted to about 90° to obtain the SAX of the arch and the probe advanced, following the descending aorta down to the diaphragm in long axis (▶ Video 17.2). The process can be repeated using color flow Doppler to help visualize dissections or coarctations of the descending aorta.

The ascending aorta can be visualized by first obtaining a midesophageal long axis of the aortic valve at a typical omniplane angle of 110° to 140°, and slowly withdrawing the probe to visualize the proximal ascending aorta. The omniplane angle can then be decreased by 90° to obtain a SAX of the ascending aorta and the probe advanced to follow the aortic root down to the aortic valve in SAX (▶ Video 17.3). The views used to scan the thoracic aorta are provided in Figure 17.1, and while their order of acquisition is not important, all are required for a complete examination.

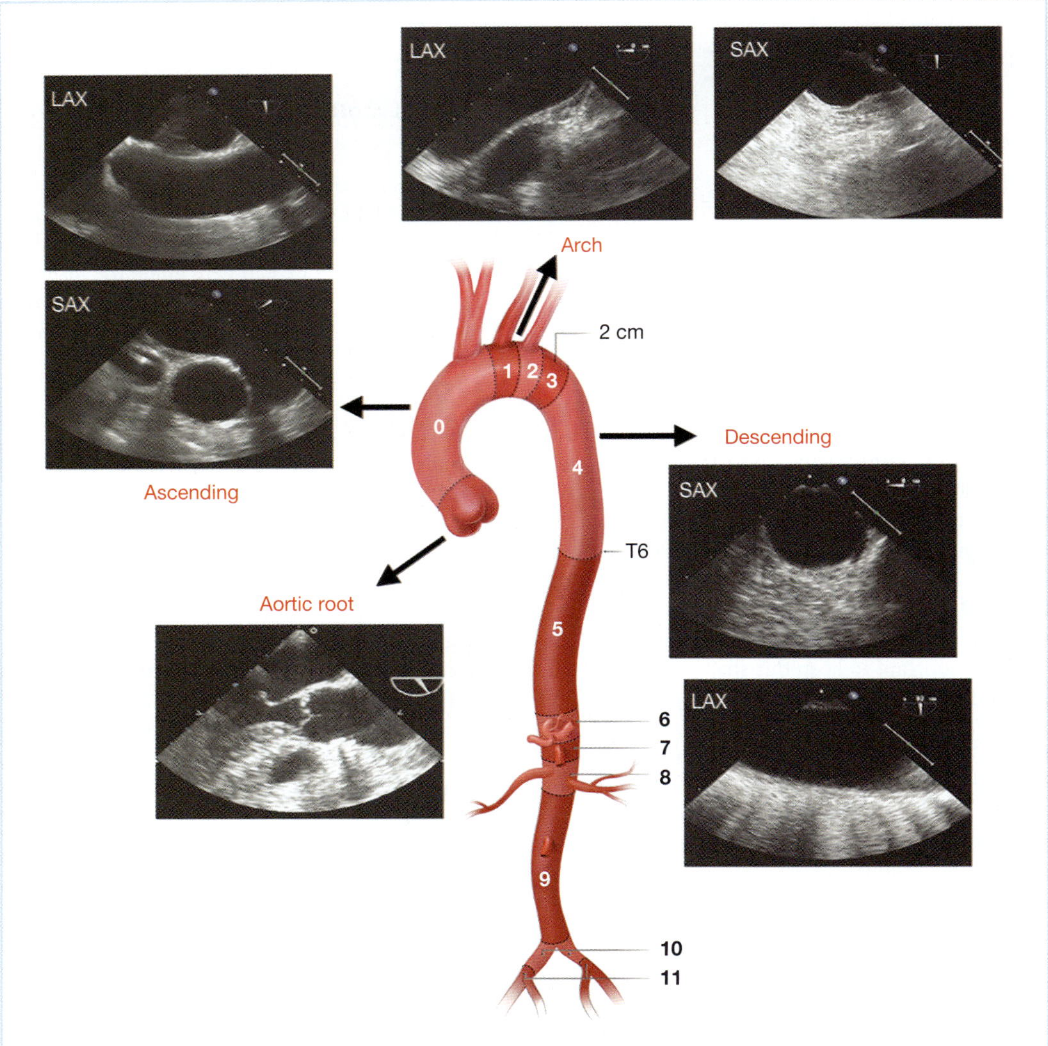

FIGURE 17.1 The thoracic aorta resembles a slightly twisted "J." It can be broadly divided into the aortic root (from the aortic annulus to the sinotubular junction, STJ), the ascending aorta (from the STJ to the innominate artery), the aortic arch (from the innominate to the left subclavian artery), and the descending aorta (from the left subclavian artery to the diaphragm). Also included are the numbered aortic landing zones (numbered 0 through 11), used most commonly in endovascular stent-grafting. LAX, long axis; SAX, short axis. (Reprinted from Czerny M, Schmidli J, Adler S, et al. Current options and recommendations for the treatment of thoracic aortic pathologies involving the aortic arch: an expert consensus document of the European Association for CardioThoracic surgery [EACTS] and the European Society for Vascular Surgery [ESVS]. *Eur J Cardiothorac Surg*. 2019;55:133-162, by permission of Oxford University.)

ACUTE AORTIC SYNDROMES

Acute aortic syndromes are a collection of life-threatening conditions including thoracic aortic dissection (TAD), intramural hematoma (IMH), and penetrating atherosclerotic ulcer (PAU). Pathology that involves the ascending aorta has a higher mortality than pathology that does not (4), although the presence and type of malperfusion also have a great influence on survival (5). Timely diagnosis is critical so that appropriate intervention, either surgical or medical, can be instituted. While computed tomography is recommended as the initial diagnostic modality in suspected acute aortic syndromes, TEE still plays an essential role in confirming the diagnosis and guiding surgical repair (6). Important aspects for the intraoperative echocardiographer to address during the examination are summarized in Table 17.1 (7,8).

TABLE 17.1 Role of Intraoperative TEE in Acute Ascending Aortic Dissection

(1) Confirm the diagnosis	• Visualize the intimal flap in two separate imaging planes. • Determine the proximal extent of the flap.
(2) Identify the entry points	• Color flow Doppler to see flow from true to false lumen. • There may be multiple tears.
(3) Determine coronary involvement	• Look for flap extending into the aortic root and coronary ostia. • Look for regional wall motion abnormalities. • Assess ventricular function.
(4) Assess aortic valve	• Grade severity of any aortic regurgitation. • Determine if aortic valve may be repairable.
(5) Look for effusions	• Pericardial and pleural effusions are common.
(6) Rule out additional cardiac pathology	• Preoperative workup is often minimal due to the urgency of the surgery—a complete examination is essential.

TEE, transesophageal echocardiography.
Adapted from Meredith EL, Masani ND. Echocardiography in the emergency assessment of acute aortic syndromes. *Eur J Echocardiogr*. 2009;10(1):i31-i39. By permission of Oxford University.

Acute Aortic Dissection

An aortic dissection begins with a tear in the intimal layer of the aorta. The tear allows blood to enter and separate the intima from the media or adventitia, creating a "flap" of tissue separating the true aortic lumen from the false lumen. TADs are commonly classified by either the Stanford or DeBakey systems (Figure 17.2). While the DeBakey system is based upon the location and extent of the tear, the Stanford system is based upon whether the ascending aorta either is (type A) or is not (type B) involved. Dissections in the aortic arch are typically extensions of those originating from the descending aorta and generally share the same management and prognosis as type B TADs (9).

The hallmark of an acute aortic dissection on TEE is the visualization of the intimal flap. It is usually irregularly shaped and highly mobile (Video 17.4). Visualizing the flap in two separate imaging planes (Figure 17.3) is important in order to distinguish artifacts from true dissection flaps.

One such confounder is the presence of a pulmonary artery (PA) catheter, which can create reverberation artifacts mimicking a flap (Figure 17.4). When in doubt, this can be remedied by pulling the catheter back and seeing if the "flap" remains. Other sources of linear artifacts include calcifications on the aortic valve or root, and atherosclerosis of the ascending aorta (10). They can typically be distinguished from a true dissection by their lack of rapid, oscillatory movement, their tendency to cross known anatomic boundaries, and their indistinct structural borders.

Once the dissection flap is visualized, it is useful to determine where the break in the intima (aka the "tear" or "entry point") has occurred, since one of the primary aims of surgical treatment is to excise this region. Color flow Doppler is often used to visualize a turbulent jet flowing from the true lumen into the false lumen (Figure 17.5). This separation, or "margination," of flow can also be helpful in distinguishing a true dissection from an artifact that has no margination of color flow Doppler. The true lumen can usually be differentiated from the false lumen due to its expansion during systole (Video 17.5). Additionally, the false lumen is often larger and frequently has spontaneous echo contrast or thrombus within it, particularly in the descending aorta.

Intramural Hematoma

While the initiating event for the classical aortic dissection is a break in the intimal layer, the underlying cause of an IMH is thought to be a rupture of vasa vasorum in the medial layer, although very small breaks in the intima may be present (11). Blood accumulation causes a thickening of the medial layer, which may progress to intimal fracture, and subsequent flap formation or frank aortic rupture. The mortality from IMH is dependent on the location (ie, ascending or descending aorta) and is similar to that of classic TAD. As such, the Stanford classification system is applied, with type A considered a surgical emergency.

Unlike the classic aortic dissection, there is no intimal flap. On TEE imaging, IMH appears as a thickening of the medial layer of the aorta (Figure 17.6; Video 17.6). In the absence of blood flow, thickening of

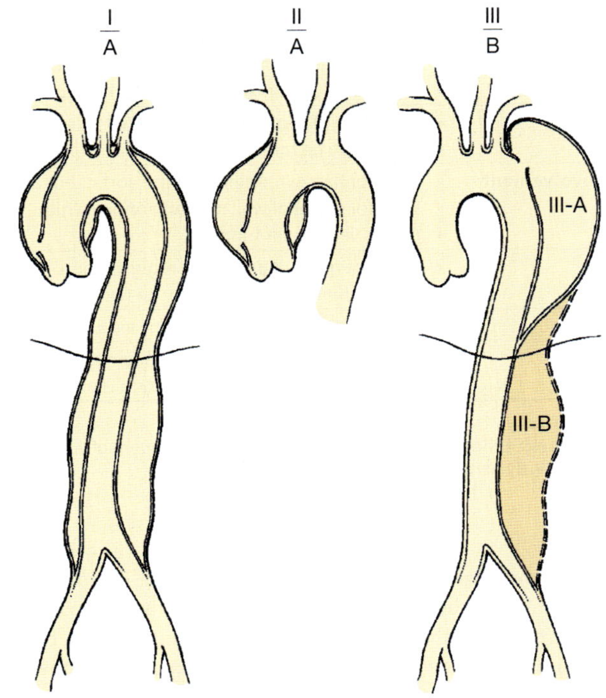

FIGURE 17.2 Stanford (A & B) and DeBakey (I, II, III) classifications of aortic dissection. DeBakey type III is further classified into those extending below the diaphragm (III-B) or not (III-A). (From Crawford ES, Crawford JL. *Diseases of the Aorta*. Williams & Wilkins; 1984:174.)

more than 5 mm is diagnostic of IMH (12). Other features may include echolucency within the medial layer and medial displacement of calcium in the intimal layer. It is important to note that atherosclerotic plaques appear above the intimal layer, while IMHs occur below the intimal layer.

Penetrating Atherosclerotic Ulcer

Of the acute aortic syndromes, PAU is the least common, accounting for somewhere between 2% and 7% of cases (12,13). While most atherosclerotic disease protrudes above the intimal layer into the vessel lumen, PAU consists of plaque that has eroded through the internal elastic lamina into the aortic media. No dissection flap is created, but the localized erosion of the medial wall can lead to aneurysm formation. A PAU may be associated with IMH, leading to a high risk of rupture. Current guidelines recommend urgent repair when this occurs in the ascending aorta (6). However, even in the descending aorta, where most PAUs occur, it may be reasonable to undergo urgent repair when a PAU is associated with IMH in the thoracic region (6). Similar to TAD, isolated PAUs can cause pain, which is another indication for urgent repair (6).

No dissection flap or false lumen is generally visualized on TEE in cases of PAU. Instead, there is a crater-like ulcer with jagged edges and possible echolucent areas within the plaque (Figure 17.7). The erosion into the medial layer can make it difficult to clearly see the exact borders of the aortic lumen. There are typically extensive surrounding areas of atherosclerotic disease, and adjacent effusions or fluid collections are common.

Following Repair

Following the repair of an ascending aortic dissection, efforts should be made to identify both the proximal and distal ends of the graft. Most synthetic grafts are made from either a polyester fiber (eg, Dacron) or polytetrafluoroethylene. On TEE, these materials can usually be distinguished from native tissue by their

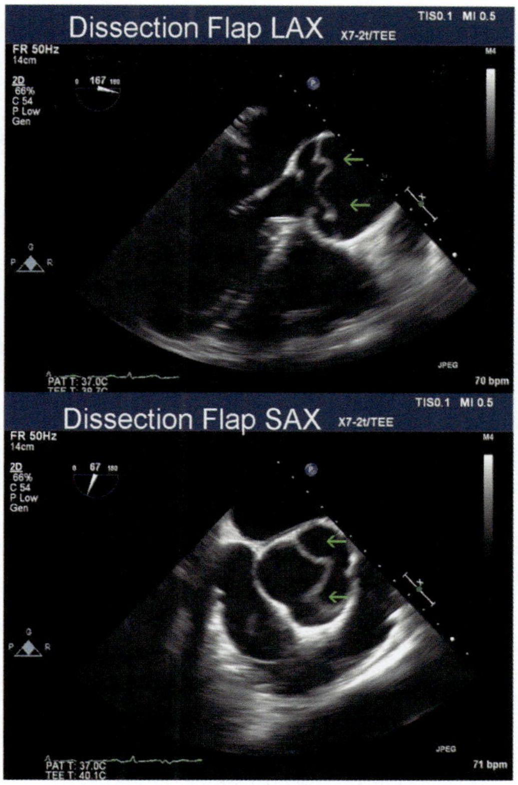

FIGURE 17.3 Dissection flap in the ascending aorta. A dissection flap (green arrows) is irregularly shaped and typically mobile. It should be visualized in two separate views to minimize the chance of mistaking an artifact for a flap. LAX, long axis; SAX, short axis.

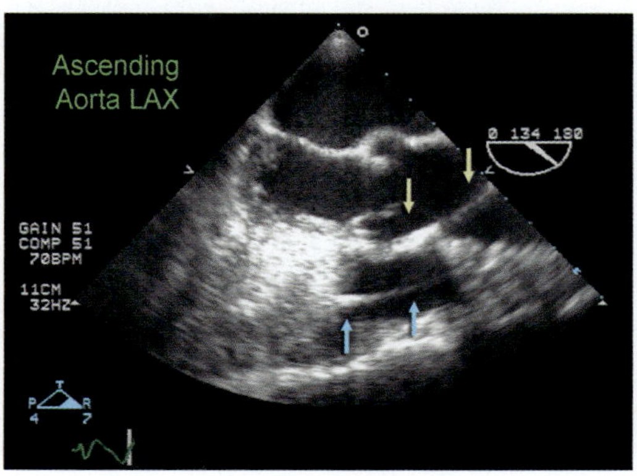

FIGURE 17.4 Pulmonary artery catheter mimicking aortic dissection flap. The false appearance of a dissection flap in the ascending aorta is often due to the presence of a pulmonary artery catheter in the right ventricle (delineated by blue arrows) causing a reverberation artifact (delineated by yellow arrows). LAX, long axis.

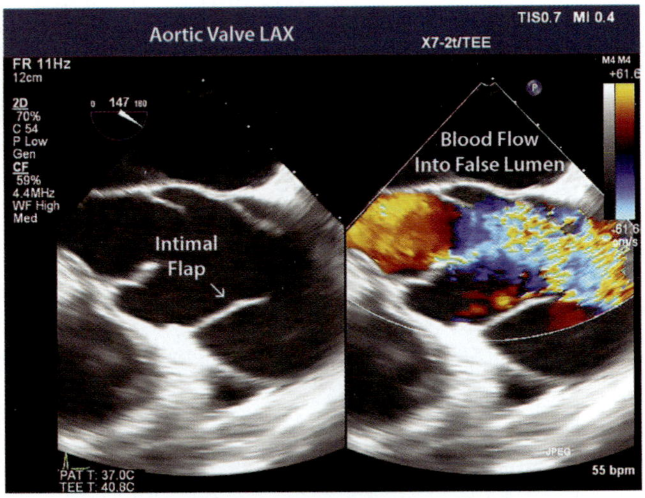

FIGURE 17.5 Blood flow into the false lumen. Color flow Doppler usually demonstrates flow into the false lumen at the point of the intimal tear. Note that there is margination. LAX, long axis.

striated appearance (Figure 17.8). Interrogation of the aortic valve should be performed as per usual practice following any valvular intervention. It should be noted, however, that prosthetic valves or resuspended native valves are typically sewn within the aortic graft.

Thoracic Aortic Aneurysms

Dilatation of the thoracic aorta can occur due to a variety of clinical conditions including altered flow dynamics, underlying connective tissue disorders, and atherosclerosis. The presence of a bicuspid aortic valve (BiAV) is commonly associated with aortic dilation. It is therefore useful to provide measurements of the

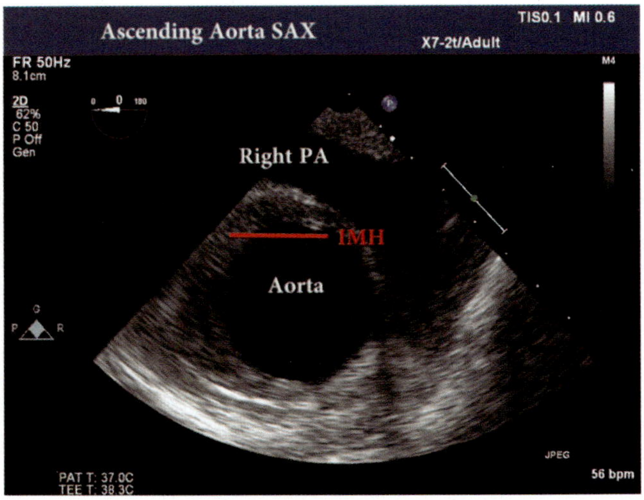

FIGURE 17.6 Intramural hematoma of the ascending aorta. In this short-axis (SAX) view of the ascending aorta, the intramural hematoma is designated "IMH." The thickening occurs beneath the intimal layer, giving a smooth appearance. This contrasts with atherosclerotic plaques which are typically irregularly shaped and protrude into the lumen of the artery. PA, pulmonary artery.

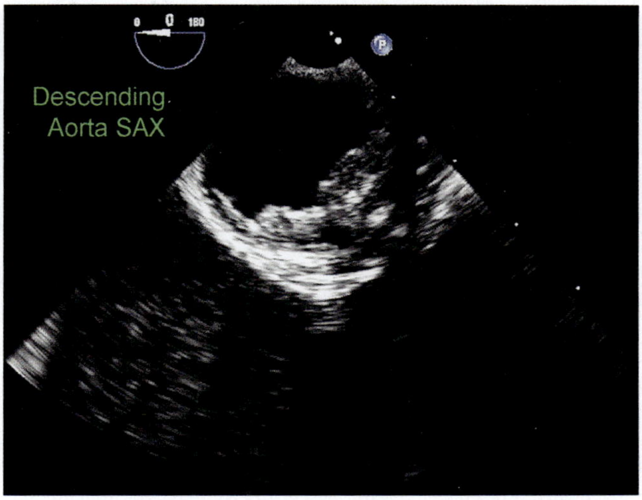

FIGURE 17.7 Penetrating atherosclerotic ulcer in the descending aorta. Note the craterlike appearance and echolucent areas of the atherosclerotic plaque. Disruption of the medial layers has made it difficult to determine where the adventitia layer is. SAX, short axis.

aortic root and ascending aorta as part of a complete examination. These TEE measurements are illustrated in Figure 17.9. 2D measurements should be taken using the "leading edge-to-leading edge" technique at end diastole, though it's likely reasonable to consider inner edge-to-inner edge measurements if the views are created with multiplanar reconstruction of 3D data sets. Although there is some debate about whether measurements should be indexed to either body surface area or height, diameters of greater than 4.0 cm are generally considered "dilated" for most patients. Diameters of 4.5 cm or more are more properly termed an "aneurysm" (6).

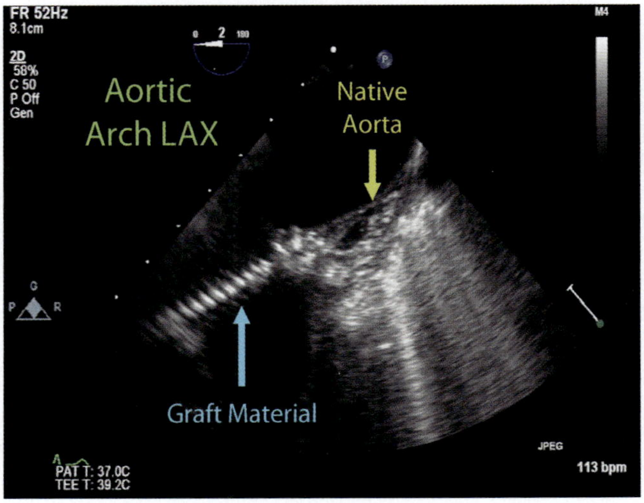

FIGURE 17.8 Distal end of an aortic hemiarch repair. Note the serrated appearance of the synthetic graft material compared to the native aortic tissue. LAX, long axis.

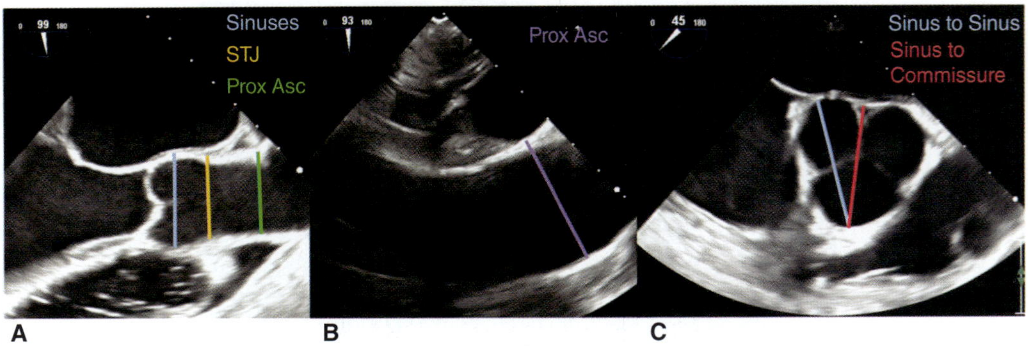

FIGURE 17.9 Typical measurements of the aorta obtained in the operating room. All are measured at end diastole. A: From the ME AV LAX view, the maximum sinus (blue line), sinotubular junction (yellow line), and proximal ascending aorta diameters (green line) are obtained using the leading edge-to-leading edge technique. B: From the ME ascending aorta LAX view, the maximal diameter (purple line) is measured, also leading edge-to-leading edge. C: From the ME AV SAX view, the sinus to sinus (blue line) and sinus to commissure (red line) diameters are measured. These measurements will likely be most accurate when created using multiplanar reconstruction of a 3D data set and can then be measured inner edge-to-inner edge. AV, aortic valve; LAX, long axis; ME, midesophageal; Prox Asc, proximal ascending aorta; SAX, short axis; STJ, sinotubular junction.

Aneurysms can be broadly divided into either *saccular*, meaning a focal outpouching, or *fusiform*, meaning cylindrical and affecting the entire circumference of the aorta. Aneurysms of the ascending aorta are typically fusiform. The dilatation can be proximal to the STJ, in which case it is called a "root" aneurysm, or it can start distal to the STJ, in which case it is known as a "supracoronary" aneurysm (14). The distinction is important because root-type aneurysms typically require coronary artery reimplantation and possible aortic valve repair/replacement, while supracoronary aneurysms frequently do not. Diffuse dilation involving both the aortic root and ascending aorta is referred to as "tubular" and typically results in effacement of the STJ (Figure 17.10).

The timing of surgical intervention for ascending aneurysm repair depends not only upon measurements but also on the underlying etiology, patient symptoms, and the need for concomitant heart surgery. Current guidelines recommend repair of the aorta in asymptomatic patients without genetic risk factors when the maximal diameter is 5.5 cm or more and consider repair by experienced teams reasonable with diameters of 5.0 cm or more (6). This threshold is lowered for patients with known connective tissue disorders such as Marfan syndrome, Loeys-Dietz syndrome, or certain genetic defects; surgical intervention can be considered at measurements as low as 4.0 cm in some of these patient populations (6). In patients undergoing cardiac surgery for other indications, particularly those with a BiAV, it is reasonable to surgically address ascending aortic aneurysms with diameters of 4.5 cm or more (6).

TEE is generally less useful for characterizing aneurysms of the descending aorta, particularly those below the diaphragm. Thoracic endovascular aortic repair (TEVAR) is frequently utilized in these situations. Although there are a variety of manufacturers and models, the basic structure of an endograft is a polyester tube with either an endo- or exoskeleton of metal wires. The metallic structure can create reverberation artifacts, making TEE imaging of the actual endograft challenging (Figure 17.11). While intravascular ultrasound (IVUS) and fluoroscopy are the main imaging modalities for TEVAR placement, TEE can be used to detect leaks post-deployment with a sensitivity of more than 80% and specificity of approximately 70% (Figure 17.12) (15). In the case of type B dissections, successful deployment will cover the entry site, reducing flow into the false lumen and eventually causing it to thrombose (Video 17.7). Following TEVAR deployment, TEE can also be used to rule out a retrograde TAD.

Thoracoabdominal aneurysms are often done as staged repairs, with the ascending portion replaced first. In this situation, an "elephant trunk" is frequently placed for easy proximal connection or as a landing zone for stent deployment during the second stage of repair. The elephant trunk can be visualized floating in the descending aorta (Video 17.8). Color flow Doppler should be utilized to verify flow within it.

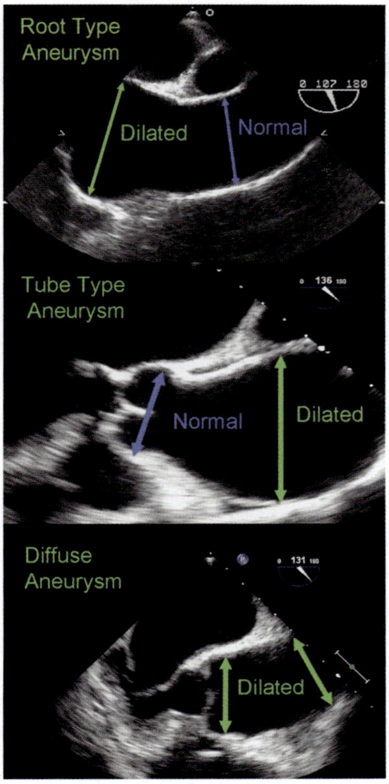

FIGURE 17.10 Types of ascending aortic aneurysms. Root-type aneurysms (top) are commonly found in patients with connective tissue disorders (eg, Marfan syndrome). The sinotubular junction is typically visible in both root and supracoronary (middle) types but is effaced and indistinguishable on TEE in cases of tubular (bottom) ascending aneurysms. TEE, transesophageal echocardiography.

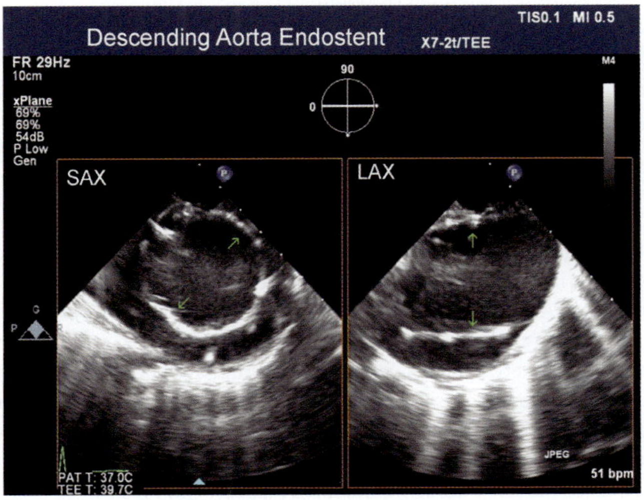

FIGURE 17.11 Descending aorta endostent. An endostent seen in the short-axis (SAX) and long-axis (LAX) views of the descending aorta. Green arrows denote the edges of the inner lumen of the stent.

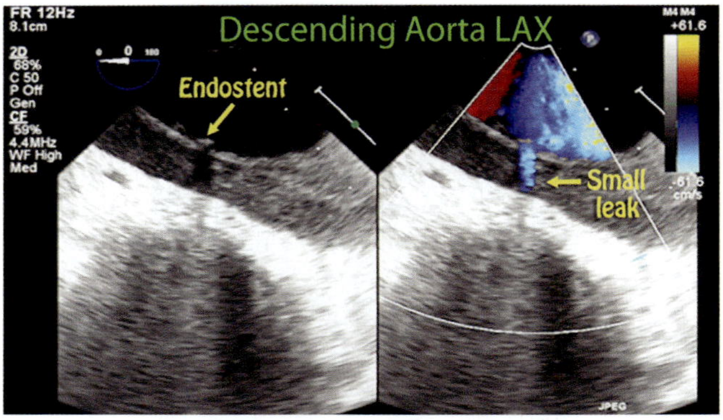

FIGURE 17.12 Small endoleak. Descending aorta long-axis (LAX) view with color flow Doppler compare demonstrating a small leak with flow into the false lumen of a type B aortic dissection.

AORTIC ATHEROMA

Cardiac surgery patients often have atherosclerotic disease, so the intraoperative echocardiographer will frequently encounter aortic plaques during TEE examination. From a surgical perspective, it is useful to know the location of severe plaques to avoid manipulation of those areas and potentially reduce the chance of embolic events. Plaques in the descending aorta are usually well visualized and may impact the decision to place an IABP or other mechanical support. However, as mentioned earlier, TEE can only visualize about 60% of the ascending aorta, missing the segments most frequently utilized for cannulation and cross-clamping.

Because of TEE's blind spots on the ascending aorta, epiaortic scanning can be employed to determine the location of atherosclerotic plaques in these areas. Guidelines for an intraoperative epiaortic examination have been published, which recommend using a high-frequency probe (≥7 MHz) in a sterile sheath that can be used in the surgical field (16). Linear array transducers provide the advantage of being able to be placed directly on the aorta but may not be wide enough to include all walls in a single image. A phased-array transducer, such as a pediatric transthoracic probe, can typically visualize all walls at once but must be held about 1 cm above the aortic wall to prevent near-field clutter. In either case, SAX views of the proximal, mid, and distal segments of the ascending aorta should be obtained (Figure 17.13).

The normal intimal layer of the aorta is less than 2 mm thick, and atherosclerosis first leads to an increase in this thickness. With disease progression, the atheroma becomes more complex in shape and protrudes into the lumen of the aorta (Figure 17.14). While several grading systems have been used to describe the severity of aortic atherosclerosis, the recommended approach is presented in Table 17.2 (17-19). Plaques with a mobile component have the greatest potential to embolize and represent the most severe grade in all classification systems (Video 17.9).

Intraaortic Balloon Pump Placement

TEE plays an important role in positioning IABPs in the operating room, particularly when they are placed under urgent circumstances. Aortic regurgitation of moderate or greater severity represents an absolute contraindication and should be ruled out prior to insertion. Other potential contraindications include aneurysms, dissections, and severe atherosclerosis. Placement of the IABP begins with inserting a guidewire into the descending aorta, which can be confirmed using TEE. Using the Seldinger technique, the balloon is then inserted into the aorta over the wire (Video 17.10). For positioning, the tip of the IABP should sit about 2 cm below the takeoff of the LSCA (Figure 17.15).

Estimating the distance of the IABP tip from the LSCA takeoff can be done by first obtaining a descending long-axis view of the aorta and putting the end of the tip in the center of the screen. This position can be marked by the echocardiographer pinching the shaft of the probe with the thumb and forefinger at the patient's mouth. The TEE probe is then withdrawn, keeping the thumb and forefinger on the same

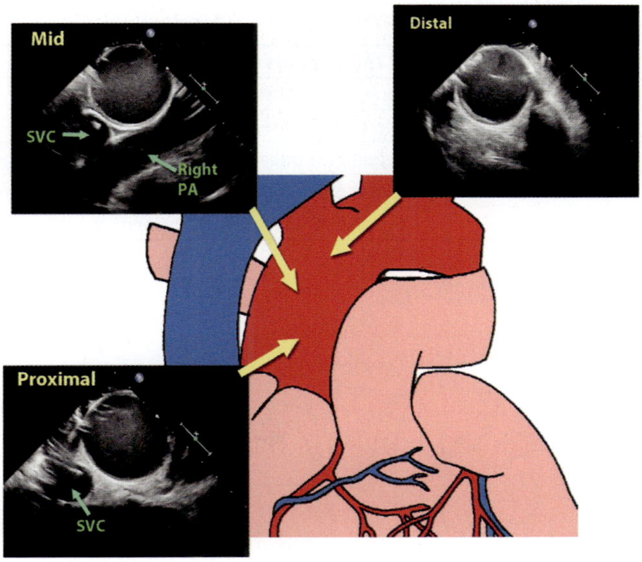

FIGURE 17.13 Epiaortic imaging of the ascending aorta. Aortic plaques in the blind spots of TEE can effectively be imaged using epiaortic ultrasound. The proximal ascending aorta begins just above the sinotubular junction. The superior vena cava (SVC) is seen on the right. The probe is then moved distally up the ascending aorta until the right pulmonary artery (PA) is seen posterior to the aorta. This marks the midportion of the ascending. As the epiaortic probe is moved even more distally, the right PA disappears from view. TEE, transesophageal echocardiography.

part of the probe, and turned slightly to the right to see the LSCA. The distance from the patient's mouth to the echocardiographer's thumb/forefinger represents the distance of the IABP tip to the LSCA takeoff (Videos 17.11 and 17.12) (20).

The acoustic impedance mismatch between blood and the gas-filled balloon is large, causing strong specular reflections and multiple shadowing and reverberation artifacts. Direct imaging of the actual balloon is only possible during systole when it is deflated. A correctly functioning IABP will have a characteristic

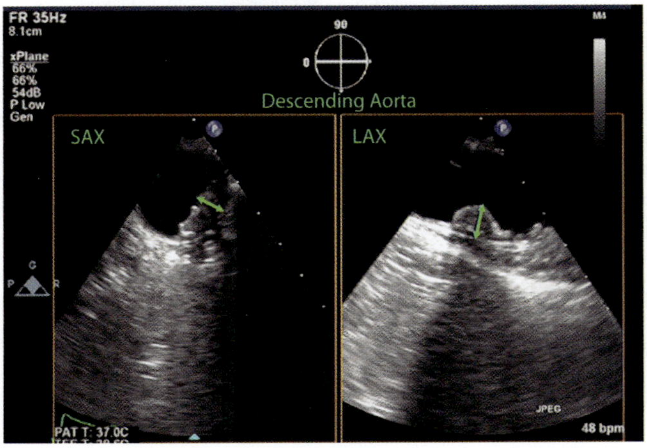

FIGURE 17.14 Measurement of an aortic plaque. The plaque is seen protruding into the lumen of the aorta in both short axis (SAX) and long axis (LAX). The maximal plaque height/intimal thickness (denoted by green arrows) is used to determine the grade of the lesion (see Table 17.2).

TABLE 17.2 Grading System for Aortic Atheroma Used in Cardiac Surgical Patients

Grade	TEE Findings
I	Normal intimal thickness (<2 mm)
II	Mild intimal thickening (2-3 mm)
III	Plaque protrudes >3-5 mm into the aortic lumen
IV	Plaque protrudes >5 mm into the aortic lumen
V	Any plaque with a mobile component

TEE, transesophageal echocardiography.

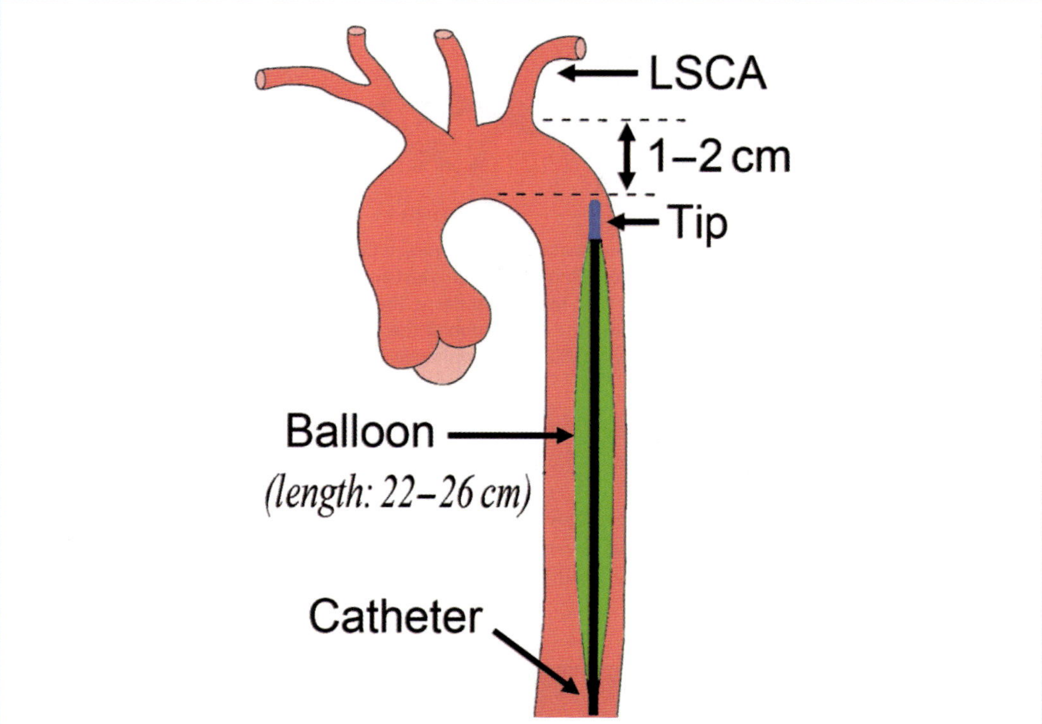

FIGURE 17.15 Correct placement of an intraaortic balloon pump (IABP). The tip of the balloon pump should generally rest 1 to 2 cm distal to the takeoff of the left subclavian artery (LSCA). Typical balloon lengths are 22 to 26 cm. (Reprinted with permission from Klopman MA, Chen EP, Sniecinski RM. Positioning an intraaortic balloon pump using intraoperative transesophageal echocardiogram guidance. *Anesth Analg*. 2011;113(1):40-43.)

pattern of inflation and deflation as seen in Video 17.13. Failure to see this pattern, particularly in the presence of gas bubbles in the descending aorta, should raise the possibility of balloon rupture, and the IABP should be removed from the patient.

CONCLUSION

The intraoperative echocardiographer needs to pay particular attention to the thoracic aorta. It is the site for both acute (dissections, IMHs) and progressive (aneurysms, atherosclerosis) diseases. Although not all segments can be evaluated using TEE, a systematic evaluation can help confirm diagnoses and guide surgical therapy.

REFERENCES

1. Goldstein S, Evangelista A, Abbara S, et al. Multimodality imaging of diseases of the thoracic aorta in adults: from the American Society of Echocardiography and the European Association of Cardiovascular Imaging. *J Am Soc Echocardiogr.* 2015;28:119-182.
2. Royse C, Royse A, Blake D, Grigg L. Assessment of thoracic aortic atheroma by echocardiography: a new classification and estimation of risk of dislodging atheroma during three surgical techniques. *Ann Thorac Cardiovasc Surg.* 1998;4(2):72-77.
3. Czerny M, Schmidli J, Adler S, et al. Current options and recommendations for the treatment of thoracic aortic pathologies involving the aortic arch: an expert consensus document of the European Association for Cardio-Thoracic Surgery (EACTS) and the European Society for Vascular Surgery (ESVS). *Eur J Cardiothorac Surg.* 2019;55:133-162.
4. Evangelista A, Isselbacher EM, Bossone E, et al. Insights from the international registry of acute aortic dissection: a 20-year experience of collaborative clinical research. *Circulation.* 2018;137:1846-1860.
5. Wolfe SB, Sundt TM, Isselbacher EM, et al. Survival after operative repair of acute type A aortic dissection varies according to the presence and type of preoperative malperfusion. *J Thorac Cardiovasc Surg.* 2022;22:1-13.
6. Isselbacher EM, Preventza O, Black JH, et al. 2022 ACC/AHA guideline for the diagnosis and management of aortic disease: a report of the American Heart Association/American College of Cardiology Joint Committee on Clinical Practice Guidelines. *Circulation.* 2022;146:e334-e482.
7. Hamid A, Gupta M, Rajiah PS, et al. The current and future role of imaging of thoracic aortic disease: a North American society for cardiovascular imaging commentary on the 2022 AHA/ACC guidelines for the diagnosis and management of aortic disease. *Int J Cardiovasc Imag.* 2024;40:5-14.
8. Meredith EL, Masani ND. Echocardiography in the emergency assessment of acute aortic syndromes. *Eur J Echocardiogr.* 2009;10(1):i31-i39.
9. Nauta FJH, Tolenaar JL, Patel HJ, et al. Impact of retrograde arch extension in acute type B aortic dissection on management and outcomes. *Ann Thorac Surg.* 2016;102:2036-2043.
10. Appelbe AF, Walker PG, Yeoh JK, et al. Clinical significance and origin of artifacts in transesophageal echocardiography of the thoracic aorta. *J Am Coll Cardiol.* 1993;21(3):754-760.
11. Maslow A, Atalay MK, Sodha M. Intramural Hematoma. *J Cardiothorac Vasc Anesth.* 2018;32:1341-1362.
12. Harris KM, Braverman AC, Eagle KA, et al. Acute aortic intramural hematoma: an analysis from the International Registry of Acute Aortic Dissection. *Circulation.* 2012;126:S91-S96.
13. Nathan DP, Boonn W, Lai E, et al. Presentation, complications, and natural history of penetrating atherosclerotic ulcer disease. *J Vasc Surg.* 2012;55(1):10-15.
14. Elefteriades JA, Mukherjee SK, and Mojibian H. Discrepancies in measurement of the thoracic aorta: JACC review topic of the week. *J Am Coll Cardiol.* 2020;76:201-217.
15. Nana PN, Brotis AG, Tsolaki V, et al. Transesophageal echocardiography during endovascular procedures for thoracic aorta diseases: sensitivity and specificity analysis. *J Cardiovasc Surg (Torino).* 2021;62(1):79-86.
16. Glas KE, Swaminathan M, Reeves ST, et al. Guidelines for the performance of a comprehensive intraoperative epiaortic ultrasonographic examination: recommendations of the American Society of Echocardiography and the Society of Cardiovascular Anesthesiologists; endorsed by the Society of Thoracic Surgeons. *J Am Soc Echocardiogr.* 2007;20(11):1227-1235.
17. Katz ES, Tunick PA, Rusinek H, et al. Protruding aortic atheromas predict stroke in elderly patients undergoing cardiopulmonary bypass: experience with intraoperative transesophageal echocardiography. *J Am Coll Cardiol.* 1992;20(1):70-77.
18. Trehan N, Mishra M, Kasliwal RR, Mishra A. Reduced neurological injury during CABG in patients with mobile aortic atheromas: a five-year follow-up study. *Ann Thorac Surg.* 2000;70:1558-1564.
19. Nohara H, Shida T, Mukohara N, Obo H, Higami T. Ultrasonic plaque density of aortic atheroma and stroke in patients undergoing on-pump coronary bypass surgery. *Ann Thorac Cardiovasc Surg.* 2004;10:235-240.
20. Klopman MA, Chen EP, Sniecinski RM. Positioning an intraaortic balloon pump using intraoperative transesophageal echocardiogram guidance. *Anesth Analg.* 2011;113(1):40-43.

QUESTIONS

1. **What is indicated by the yellow arrow (QFigure 17.1)?**

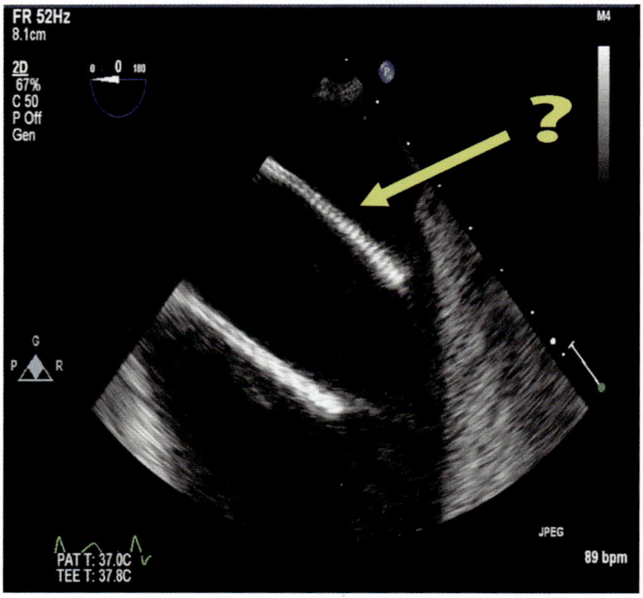

A. A dissection flap in the aortic arch
B. A graft dehiscence in the ascending aorta
C. The tip of an IABP
D. The distal end of a prosthetic graft

2. **Within which part of the aortic lumen is the letter "X" located (QFigure 17.2)?**

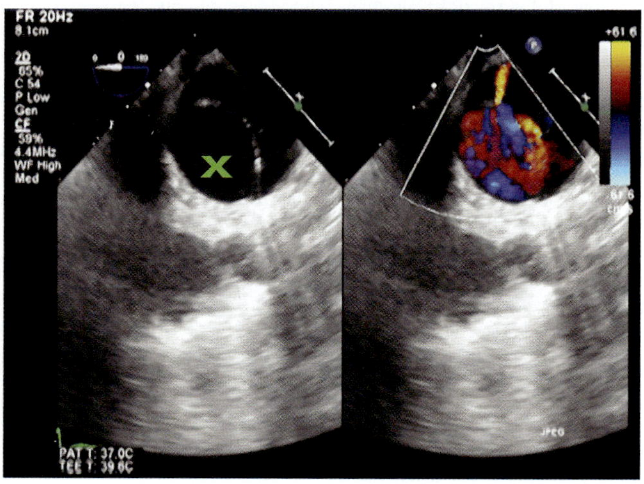

A. True lumen of a descending aortic dissection
B. The aortic root
C. False lumen of a descending aortic dissection
D. The aortic arch

3. In terms of "landing zones," where is the takeoff of the innominate artery located?
A. Zone 0
B. Zone 1
C. Zone 2
D. Zone 3

4. What pathology is demonstrated in QFigure 17.3?

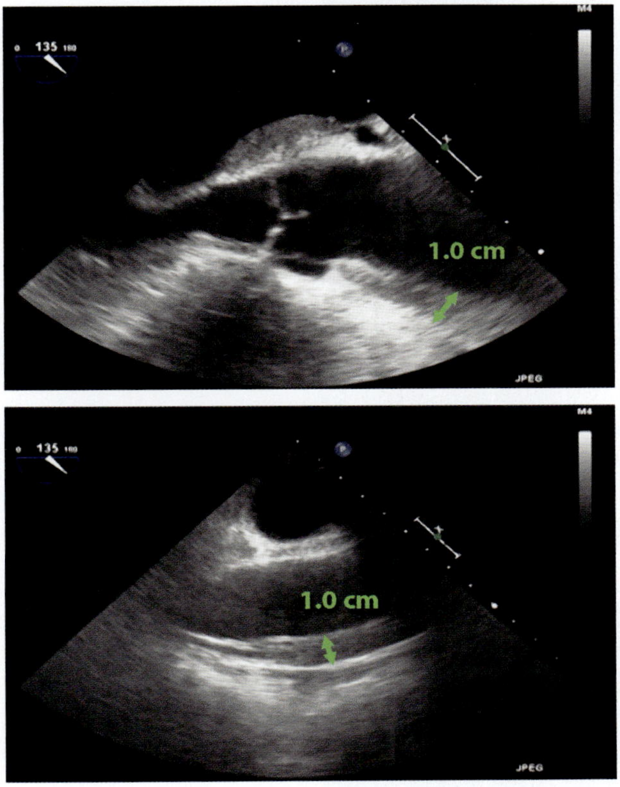

A. Supracoronary aneurysm
B. Thoracic aortic dissection
C. Intramural hematoma
D. Penetrating atherosclerotic ulcer

5. An otherwise healthy 57-year-old woman with a BiAV and normal ejection fraction is undergoing aortic valve replacement for severe aortic regurgitation. Which of the following baseline findings on intraoperative TEE would MOST likely change the planned operation?
A. An anomalous right pulmonary vein
B. A root diameter of 4.7 cm
C. A peak velocity of 3 m/s through the aortic valve
D. Smooth atheroma in the descending aorta extending 2 mm into the aortic lumen

6. Surgical intervention is appropriate in all of the following patients with aortic aneurysms listed below *except*:
A. A patient with a BiAV with an aneurysm measuring 4.8 cm
B. A patient undergoing coronary bypass grafting with an aneurysm that measures 4.1 cm
C. A patient with Marfan syndrome with an aneurysm that measures 4.4 cm
D. An asymptomatic patient with an aneurysm that measures 5.2 cm

7. **What grade of atheromatous disease of the descending aorta is shown in the following TEE image according to the Katz grading system (QFigure 17.4)?**

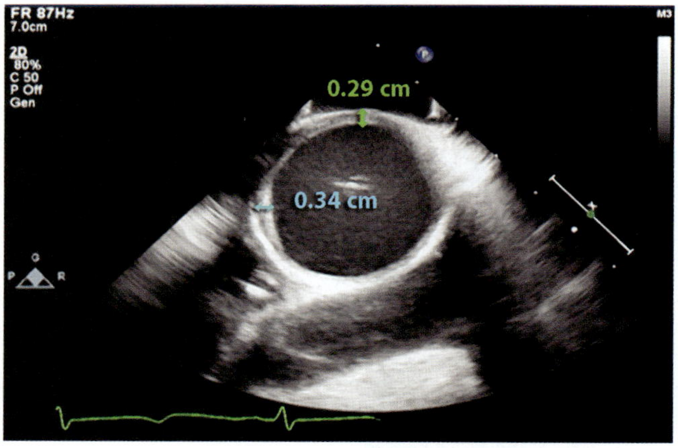

A. Grade II
B. Grade III
C. Grade IV
D. Grade V

8. **What aortic pathology is demonstrated?**
A. Mild aortic regurgitation
B. Acute aortic dissection
C. Intramural hematoma
D. None - this is reverberation artifact

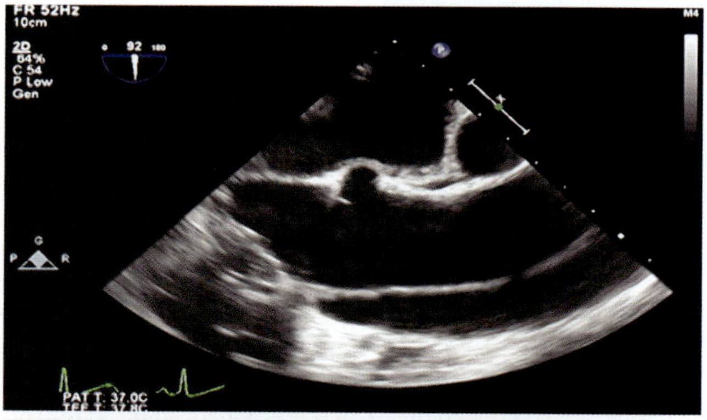

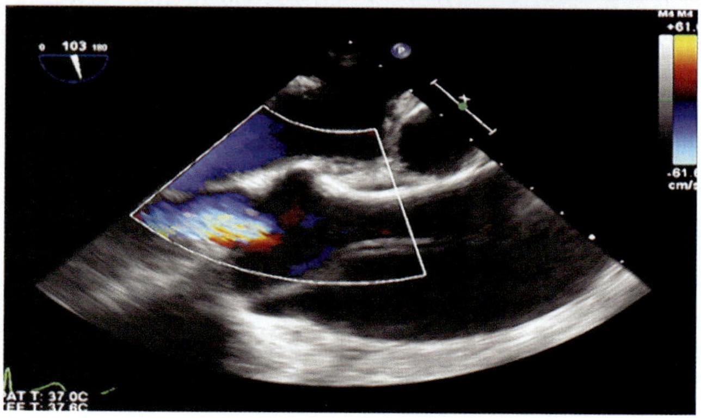

9. All of the following probes can be used to perform an epiaortic examination except:

A. Curvilinear probe
B. Linear array transducer
C. Phase array transducer
D. High-frequency transducer

10. What pathology is demonstrated in QFigure 17.6?

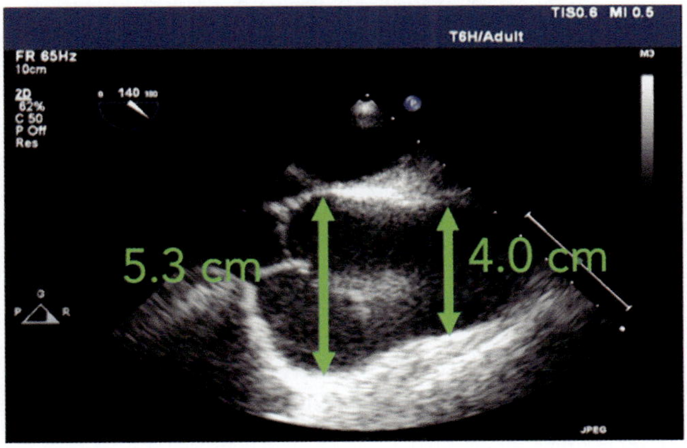

A. Aortic dissection
B. Intramural hematoma
C. Penetrating atherosclerotic ulcer
D. Grade IV atherosclerotic disease

ANSWERS

1. Correct Answer: D.
Rationale: The yellow arrow is pointing to the distal end of a prosthetic graft. This is an example of an "elephant trunk" that is commonly placed for staged repair of thoracoabdominal aneurysms. Note the striated appearance of the material. Although these can be mobile, they have a much different appearance from an aortic dissection flap or the tip of an IABP. Dehiscence of an aortic graft would likely be seen as a more irregularly shaped object. Additionally, the ascending aorta is not seen in long axis at an omniplane angle of 0°.

2. Correct Answer: A.
Rationale: The aorta is seen as a circle at an omniplane angle of 0°, indicating this is the descending aorta. The "X" is most likely located in the true lumen since it is the smaller of the two lumens and flow can be seen going out of it into the larger (false) lumen in the color flow Doppler frame.

3. Correct Answer: A.
Rationale: The European Association for Cardio-Thoracic Surgery (EACTS) and the European Society for Vascular Surgery (ESVS) divided the aorta into 12 "landing zones" (also called Ishimaru zones) for purposes of endovascular repair (2). Zone 0 is defined as extending from the STJ to the distal end of the takeoff of the innominate artery. Zone 1 lies under the common carotid artery takeoff and zone 2 under the LSCA takeoff. Zone 3 extends 2 cm below the distal end of the LSCA takeoff. Zone 4 extends from this area to the T6 level. Zone 5 extends below the diaphragm to the celiac trunk and generally represents the limit of reliable imaging by TEE. Zones 6 to 8 include the celiac trunk and renal artery takeoff, which can be seen in a small subset of patients. Zones 9, 10, and 11 include the abdominal aorta, femoral bifurcation, and iliac bifurcations respectively.

4. Correct Answer: C.
Rationale: This is a long-axis view of the ascending aorta at the level of the PA (circular vessel above the aorta). There is a thickening of approximately 1 cm below the level of the aortic intima (demonstrated by green arrows). Since this is greater than 5 mm, the pathology is most

correctly classified as an IMH. Based upon this measurement, as well as the markers on the right side of the image plane, no aneurysm is present. A TAD would show a mobile flap within the lumen of the aorta. A PAU would have an irregular protrusion into the lumen of the aorta.

5. **Correct Answer: B.**
Rationale: Patients with BiAV are at increased risk for aortic dissection, particularly when the aortic root is involved. Guidelines suggest that it is reasonable to undergo repair at an experienced center when the root or ascending diameter is 4.5 cm or more (12). Patients with BiAV may also have pulmonary vein anomalies, although they are usually clinically irrelevant. A peak velocity of 3 m/s is consistent with severe regurgitation and would support the planned operation. While grading systems differ, a nonmobile atheroma of less than 3 mm in the descending aorta is not likely to change any kind of management, including placement of any type of mechanical support.

6. **Correct Answer: B.**
Rationale: Current guidelines recommend repair of the aorta in asymptomatic patients without genetic risk factors when the maximal diameter is 5.0 cm or more. This threshold is lowered for patients with known connective tissue disorders such as Marfan syndrome, Loeys-Dietz syndrome, or certain genetic defects; surgical intervention can be considered at measurements as low as 4.0 cm in some of these patient populations. In patients undergoing cardiac surgery for some other reason, particularly those with a BiAV, it is reasonable to surgically address ascending aortic aneurysms with diameters 4.5 cm or more.

7. **Correct Answer: B.**
Rationale: The image shows a SAX-view of the descending aorta with an atheroma that measures 3.4 mm. According to the Katz grading system, Grade I disease is classified as normal intimal thickening and Grade II as intimal thickening without protrusion into the lumen. Plaques that protrude into the aortic lumen and measure less than 5 mm are Grade III, while protruding plaques of greater than 5 mm are classified as Grade IV. All mobile plaques are considered Grade V disease.

8. **Correct Answer: B.**
Rationale: Both images of the aorta are the mid-esophageal long axis, with the bottom image including color flow Doppler. While aortic regurgitation is present, it takes up almost the entire width of the left ventricular outflow tract and is certainly not mild in severity. A dissection flap is seen with 2 different omniplane angles, making an artifact unlikely. Flaps are not typical of isolated intramural hematomas.

9. **Correct Answer: A.**
Rationale: Guidelines for an intraoperative epiaortic examination have been published, which recommend using a high-frequency probe ($\geq$7 MHz) in a sterile sheath that can be used in the surgical field. Linear array transducers provide the advantage of being able to be placed directly on the aorta but may not be wide enough to include all walls in a single image. A phased-array transducer, such as a pediatric transthoracic probe, can typically visualize all walls at once but must be held about 1 cm above the aortic wall to prevent near-field clutter.

10. **Correct Answer: B.**
Rationale: This is a short view of the descending aorta. No flap is visible, so an aortic dissection is unlikely. This is an intramural hematoma, which is a thickening of the media and clearly has a diameter of greater than 5 mm. Atherosclerosis, either an ulcer or severe disease, would generally protrude into the lumen of the aorta. Additionally, this intramural hematoma has a smooth surface, rather than a jagged one expected of atherosclerosis.

18 Critical Care Echocardiography

Karel Huard, Etienne J. Couture, Marc-Antoine Lepage, and André Y. Denault

Critical care ultrasound (CCUS) comprises ultrasound evaluation of the heart, lungs, pleural space, intra-abdominal organs, and the nervous and vascular systems. CCUS is designed to be a series of simplified, focused examinations that can quickly rule in or out a diagnosis, or guide the practitioner to perform additional testing, imaging, or procedures. In this chapter, we focus on two of the most common issues encountered in the intensive care unit (ICU): hemodynamic instability and hypoxemia. We do not cover the use of central nervous system, renal, or vascular ultrasound to assess altered neurologic status, oligoanuria, or for vascular access. Interested reader can refer to several references regarding these applications (1-6).

A PROPOSED APPROACH TO HEMODYNAMIC INSTABILITY

The approach to a patient with hemodynamic instability should incorporate all relevant parameters, including history, physical examination, waveform analysis, electrocardiographic changes, and laboratory values. This assessment must include simultaneous conventional resuscitation management (Figure 18.1). There have been several proposed approaches for the use of CCUS in patients with hemodynamic instability. These include the **Fo**cused **C**ardiac **U**ltrasound or FOCUS (7), the **F**ocused **A**ssessed **T**ransthoracic **E**cho or FATE (8), the **F**ocused **A**ssessment with **S**onography in **T**rauma or FAST (9), the **R**apid **U**ltrasound for **Sh**ock and Hypotension or RUSH (10), and the **H**emodynamic **E**chocardiography **A**ssessment in **R**eal **T**ime or HEART (11) scan protocols. All of these emphasize the following three points: (1) The examination can be rapidly performed at the bedside by the treating physician; (2) the dynamic images are correlated with the clinical picture; (3) the examination should be repeated as often as needed to monitor disease progression or the effect of therapeutic interventions. While both transthoracic echocardiography (TTE) and transesophageal echocardiography (TEE) can be performed at the bedside, **this chapter focuses more on TTE**, as it is more commonly available to anesthesiologists and critical care physicians.

Most of the previously mentioned approaches are based on obtaining a sequence of images limited to specific organs in order to rule out specific conditions. So far, there is no evidence that one approach is superior to the other. At our institution, we prefer a pathophysiologic approach that integrates multiple pieces of information to distinguish among three categories of shock based on the concept of venous return (VR) (12-15).

In simple terms, shock can be approached using the concept of VR popularized by Guyton et al (16). In a steady state, VR is equal to cardiac output and is determined by a pressure gradient corresponding to the difference between the mean systemic venous pressure (P_{ms}) and the right atrial pressure (P_{ra}). VR is inversely proportional to the resistance to venous return (R_{vr}), as described by this equation:

$$\mathrm{VR} = \frac{P_{\mathrm{ms}} - P_{\mathrm{ra}}}{R_{\mathrm{vr}}}$$

This concept allows hemodynamic instability to be characterized from a VR perspective according to one of the following three fundamental mechanisms: (1) reduction in mean systemic venous pressure, (2) increase in right atrial (RA) pressure, and (3) increase in resistance to VR (Table 18.1). This approach will guide the application of bedside ultrasound in managing patients with hemodynamic instability. Initially, CCUS will be employed to assess the underlying mechanism of shock, followed by identifying the specific pathology.

Step 1. Ultrasound Imaging of the Inferior Vena Cava and Abdominal Venous Flow

Examination of the size and respiratory variation of the inferior vena cava (IVC) provides a starting point to rapidly identify possible mechanisms of hemodynamic instability. We recommend beginning with the assessment of the IVC for several reasons. First, ultrasound interrogation of the IVC from the

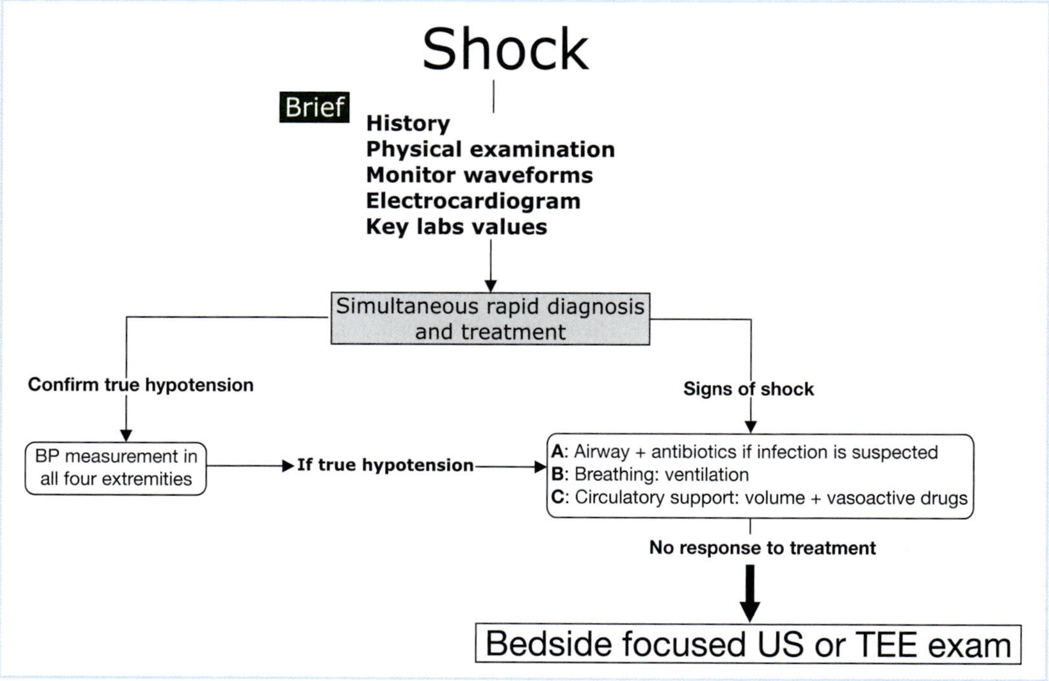

FIGURE 18.1 General approach to shock. In the presence of shock, a brief focused history and examination of the patient and the monitors is performed. In addition, key laboratory values and an electrocardiogram are obtained. Once hypotension is confirmed and the signs of shock are present, an ABC approach is proposed. If these initial steps do not correct the hemodynamic instability, bedside ultrasound (US) examination should be considered. BP, blood pressure; TEE; transesophageal echocardiography. (Reproduced by permission of Taylor and Francis Group, LLC, a division of Informa plc from Denault A, Vegas A, Lamarche Y, Tardif J, Couture P. *Basic Transesophageal and Critical Care Ultrasound*. Taylor and Francis, CRC Press; 2018.)

subcostal window has a high success rate in ICU patients. In patients where chest tubes or dressings obstruct access to this window, the IVC can be imaged through the liver from any right lower intercostal position, though the values of IVC diameter and collapsibility vary by location as the vessel is not consistently round (Figure 18.2) (15,17,18).

Second, IVC imaging offers important insights into the mechanism of shock. For example, if the IVC appears small and collapsible, reduced mean systemic venous pressure is more likely and cardiogenic shock less likely. Finally, the same acoustic window allows for the assessment of hepatic and portal vein flows, further elucidating the mechanism of shock (Figure 18.3) (19,20).

However, using the IVC to estimate mean systemic venous pressure in the ICU has its limitations, particularly in patients who are mechanically ventilated (Table 18.2) (21). Notably, the IVC provides a more accurate estimation of central venous pressure when assessed in both transverse and longitudinal views (22). This approach can also help avoid "mistaken identity" errors where either the aorta or the hepatic veins are erroneously identified as the IVC.

In summary, in an unstable patient with a small collapsible IVC, reduced mean systemic venous pressure should be suspected. Two potential mechanisms are vasodilation, as seen in septic shock, or reduced blood volume, as in hemorrhagic shock. In these patients, hepatic and portal venous flow will appear normal, prompting CCUS to shift focus toward identifying the underlying cause by assessing the thoracic cavity and abdomen.

When the IVC is large and noncollapsible, increased RA pressure from cardiogenic or obstructive shock should be considered. Concomitant findings of abnormal hepatic and portal venous flows are hallmarks of right heart dysfunction (3,19). The CCUS examination will subsequently focus on determining the etiology through the cardiac examination.

TABLE 18.1 Classification of Hemodynamic Instability Using the Concept of Venous Return

Reduced Mean Systemic Venous Pressure	Increased Right Atrial Pressure	Increased Resistance to Venous Return
Hemorrhagic/hypovolemic shock	**Myocardial**	**Supradiaphragmatic**
External bleeding	Systolic dysfunction	Cardiac tamponade
Internal bleeding	Diastolic dysfunction	Pneumothorax
• Thorax		Mediastinal tamponade
• Abdominal	**Valvular**	Dynamic hyperinflation (auto-PEEP)
• Pelvis	Acute valvular regurgitation	
• Long bones		**Infradiaphragmatic**
	Mechanical obstruction	Abdominal compartment syndrome
Distributive shock	Outflow tract obstruction	IVC obstruction
Septic	Pulmonary embolism	• IVC anastomosis
Nonseptic	Ventilatory	• Compressive tumors
• Anaphylactic	Hypoxemia	• Restrictive devices
• Endocrine: ↓ adrenal or thyroid function	Hypercapnia	
• Liver failure		
• Neurogenic		
• Neuroaxial blockade		
• Pharmacologic and toxic		
• Post CPR and CPB (postreperfusion)		
• Inflammatory		
– Burns		
– Pancreatitis		
– Multiple trauma		
– SIRS		

CPB, cardiopulmonary bypass; CPR, cardiopulmonary resuscitation; IVC, inferior vena cava; PEEP, positive end-expiratory pressure; SIRS, systemic inflammatory response syndrome. Reproduced with permission of Taylor and Francis Group, LLC, a division of Informa plc from Denault A, Vegas A, Lamarche Y, Tardif J, Couture P. *Basic Transesophageal and Critical Care Ultrasound*. Taylor and Francis, CRC Press; 2018.

Finally, increased resistance to VR arises when, despite a low RA pressure (normal cardiac function), and a high mean systemic venous pressure (adequate blood volume), blood is unable to reach the heart. Resistance may be at or above the level of the diaphragm, as seen in tension pneumothorax or tamponade, with a distended IVC. It may occur from extrinsic compression from an abdominal compartment syndrome where the IVC will be collapsed. In such situation, hepatic and portal venous flow are abnormal or absent (15,19).

Step 2. Critical Care Ultrasound in Patients With Reduced Mean Systemic Venous Pressure

In spontaneously breathing patients, reduced mean systemic venous pressure is typically associated with a small IVC that varies in dimensions with respiration. Another useful way to evaluate mean systemic venous pressure is to interrogate the hepatic venous flow (HVF) using pulsed-wave Doppler. Normal HVF generates a triphasic Doppler waveform that corresponds to the RA waveform (Figure 18.3). Reduced mean systemic venous pressure is typically associated with normal HVF. In certain cases of reduced mean systemic venous pressure, the HVF velocity can be increased because the hepatic vein is smaller in size and, consequently, blood flow velocity is higher. With positive pressure, regardless of the mode of ventilation, RA pressure will increase, affecting IVC diameter and respiratory variations. In this context, a small collapsible IVC can rule in low mean systemic venous pressure. A large or poorly varying IVC cannot effectively rule out low mean systemic venous pressure or rule in increased RA pressure.

Once reduced mean systemic venous pressure is identified in the context of hemodynamic instability, the next step is to determine its etiology. The two most likely causes are vasodilatation, as in septic shock, and reduced circulating blood volume, as in hemorrhagic shock. There are several ways to distinguish one from the other: Patients with hemorrhagic shock are typically cold and clammy as opposed to those with septic shock who are warm. Point-of-care or noninvasive measurement of hematocrit may differentiate between the two. However, in cases of acute hemorrhage, hematocrit values may initially remain normal, as the reduction in red blood cells is accompanied by a corresponding loss of plasma volume. Other clinical tools that can

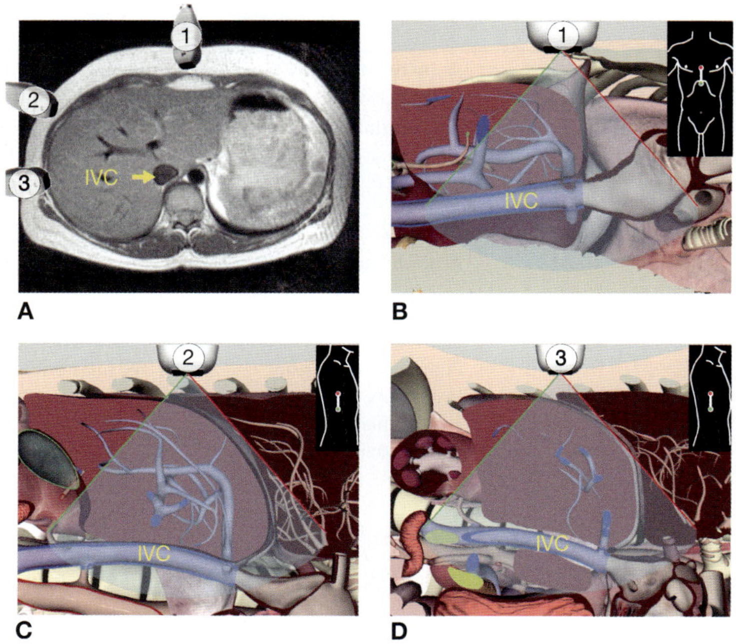

FIGURE 18.2 Inferior vena cava (IVC). A: Axial T1-weighted magnetic resonance image of the liver showing different positions of the ultrasound (US) probe that can be used to obtain a longitudinal view of the IVC. B-D: The subcostal (1), anterior axillary line (2), and posterior axillary line (3) positions using the Vimedix simulator are shown. The subcostal view is obtained in the supine patient by positioning the probe in the subcostal region with the probe marker placed toward the head at 12 o'clock. The US plane is directed toward the liver to show a longitudinal view of the IVC. The IVC can be distinguished from the pulsatile aorta by identifying the following criteria: (1) the IVC drains into the right atrium; (2) liver surrounds the IVC; (3) lack of pulsatility of the IVC (unless the presence of severe tricuspid regurgitation); and (4) hepatic veins draining into the IVC. (Reproduced with permission of Taylor and Francis Group, LLC, a division of Informa plc from Denault A, Vegas A, Lamarche Y, Tardif J, Couture P. *Basic Transesophageal and Critical Care Ultrasound*. Taylor and Francis, CRC Press; 2018.)

be used are invasive or noninvasive oximetry, which will typically be reduced in hemorrhagic shock but remain normal, or even increase, in vasodilatory shock (23,24).

Blood loss can be external or internal, including bleeding into the thoracic (Figure 18.4A; Video 18.1), peritoneal (Figure 18.5; Videos 18.2 and 18.3), or retroperitoneal space; pelvis; long bones; or gastrointestinal tract. Hemothorax and free fluid in the abdomen can easily be identified with CCUS. If blood loss is not the cause of the reduced mean systemic venous pressure, history, physical examination, and other ancillary testing can help determine if an alternate etiology of severe hypovolemia is present (hyperosmolar hyperglycemia state, burns, pancreatitis, cytokine release syndrome, etc). Otherwise, a distributive shock is to be considered. A septic process should be ruled out through appropriate investigations, including clinical and laboratory assessments. TTE views of the heart may reveal a vegetation secondary to infective endocarditis. Complex pulmonary effusion (Figure 18.4B) or lung consolidation associated with pneumonia (Figure 18.4C,D) can also be visualized with CCUS. However, diagnosing conditions such as liver abscess, cholecystitis, or pyelonephritis requires skills typically beyond CCUS. In addition, CCUS is of limited utility in some conditions associated with distributive shock, such as anaphylactic shock, neurogenic shock (with the exception of brain-heart axis involvement), pharmacologic central blockade, and adrenal crisis.

Step 3. Critical Care Ultrasound in Patients With Increased Right Atrial Pressure

In patients with elevated RA pressure and shock, a goal-directed bedside ultrasound examination must include views to assess the heart. TTE views are named first based on probe position (or "window"), namely, the parasternal, apical, and subcostal, and second by the axis (eg, long and short) or chambers visualized

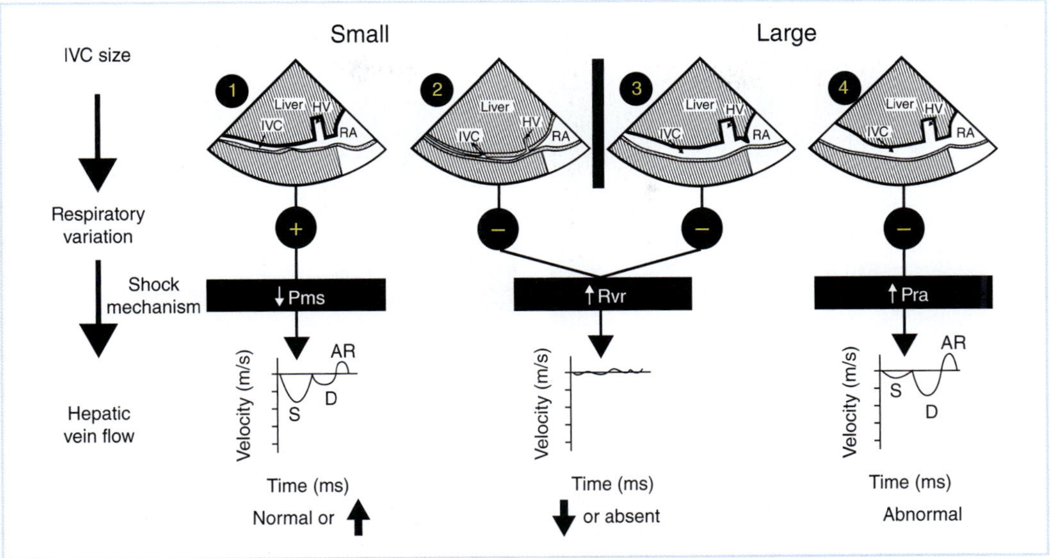

FIGURE 18.3 Shock mechanism. Algorithm to determine shock mechanism using inferior vena cava (IVC) size, respiratory variation during spontaneous ventilation, and hepatic venous flow. (1) In patients with reduced mean systemic venous pressure (P_{ms}), the IVC is small (<21 mm) with respiratory variation (>50%), and the hepatic venous flow typically displays a normal pattern. (2) In patients with increased resistance to venous return (R_{vr}), the IVC can be collapsed from an abdominal compartment syndrome or (3) distended from a mechanical obstruction at the junction of the IVC and right atrium (RA). The hepatic venous flow signal can be significantly reduced, monophasic, or absent in both situations. (4) In a situation where the right atrial pressure (P_{ra}) is increased, the IVC is dilated (>21 mm) without respiratory variation (<50%), and the HV Doppler will typically display a reduced systolic (S) to diastolic (D) velocity ratio. The cutoffs for IVC assessment presented here apply to nonmechanically ventilated patients. AR, atrial reversal hepatic venous flow velocity; D, diastolic hepatic venous flow velocity; HV, hepatic vein; S, systolic hepatic venous flow velocity. (Adapted from Via LL, Astuto M, Dezio V, et al. Agreement between subcostal and transhepatic longitudinal imaging of the inferior vena cava for the evaluation of fluid responsiveness: a systematic review. *J Crit Care*. 2022;71:154108; and reproduced by permission of Taylor and Francis Group, LLC, a division of Informa plc from Denault A, Vegas A, Lamarche Y, Tardif J, Couture P. *Basic Transesophageal and Critical Care Ultrasound*. Taylor and Francis, CRC Press; 2018.)

(eg, four-chamber, two-chamber) (Figure 18.6; Videos 18.4-18.7). A detailed approach to all the cardiac views is beyond the scope of this chapter (25). The most important ones and their critical role in CCUS are be discussed.

Parasternal Long- and Short-Axis Views

The parasternal window is found immediately adjacent to the sternum, typically in the third or fourth intercostal space. Images obtained in this window are greatly improved by left lateral decubitus positioning, which moves the heart closer to the chest wall. The parasternal long-axis view (Figure 18.6A,B) provides images of

TABLE 18.2 Limitations to Using the IVC to Estimate Mean Systemic Venous Pressure

Mechanical obstruction **Prominent Eustachian valve, web, tissue, tumor, thrombus, abdominal aortic aneurysm, foreign body such as IVC filters, narrowing of the IVC-right atrial junction**
Others Athletic training, low BMI, large body surface area, mechanical ventilation

BMI, body mass index; IVC, inferior vena cava.
Adapted from Beigel R, Cercek B, Luo H, Siegel RJ. Noninvasive evaluation of right atrial pressure. *J Am Soc Echocardiogr*. 2013;26(9):1033-1042.

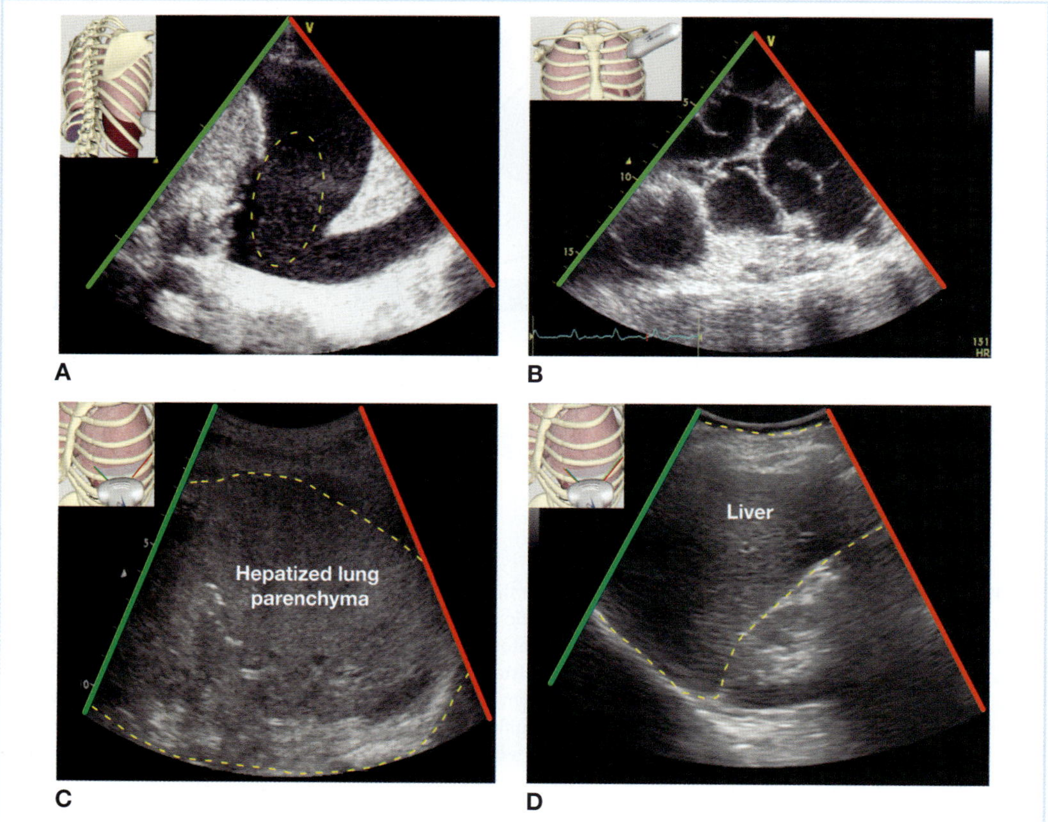

FIGURE 18.4 Reduced systemic venous pressure from a pulmonary etiology. A: Imaging of complex pleural effusion (hemothorax) in zone 4 using phased-array probe for lung ultrasound (Video 18.1). B: Imaging of heterogeneous pleural effusion with multiple septations suggesting an empyema in zone 5 using phased-array probe for lung ultrasound. C: Imaging of hepatized lung parenchyma in zone 8 using convex probe for lung ultrasound. D: Normal hepatic parenchyma. (Reproduced by permission of Taylor and Francis Group, LLC, a division of Informa plc from Denault A, Vegas A, Lamarche Y, Tardif J, Couture P. *Basic Transesophageal and Critical Care Ultrasound*. Taylor and Francis, CRC Press; 2018.)

the ascending and descending aorta, the aortic and mitral valves, the left atrium (LA) and left ventricle (LV), a small portion of the right ventricular outflow tract (RVOT), the left pleural space and, finally, the pericardial space. The anteroseptal and inferolateral walls of the LV are seen in this view (Video 18.1). By rotating the probe 90° clockwise, the parasternal short axis is imaged (Figure 18.4C,D). A view at the level of the papillary muscles allows for evaluation of interventricular septum curvature and wall motion abnormalities at the midventricular level. Cephalic tilting of the probe allows progressive visualization of the basal segments and mitral valve. Further cephalad tilting will demonstrate the aortic, tricuspid, and pulmonary valves and the RA and LA, RV, and pulmonary arteries. Caudal tilting from the midventricular level allows visualization of the apical segments and the apical cap. The parasternal short-axis view is one of the most useful to evaluate global and regional LV systolic function by looking at the thickening of the different segments at the basal, midpapillary, and apical levels. It can provide a rapid assessment of LV systolic function, which is helpful when considering, for instance, the addition of inotropic support.

Apical Four-Chamber and Two-Chamber Views

The apical four-chamber view is obtained by placing the probe at the ventricular apex, identified as the point of maximal impulse, near the anterior axillary line (Figure 18.6E,F). The apical four-chamber view provides a global picture of all four chambers. Chamber size and ventricular interdependence can be evaluated (Video 18.5).

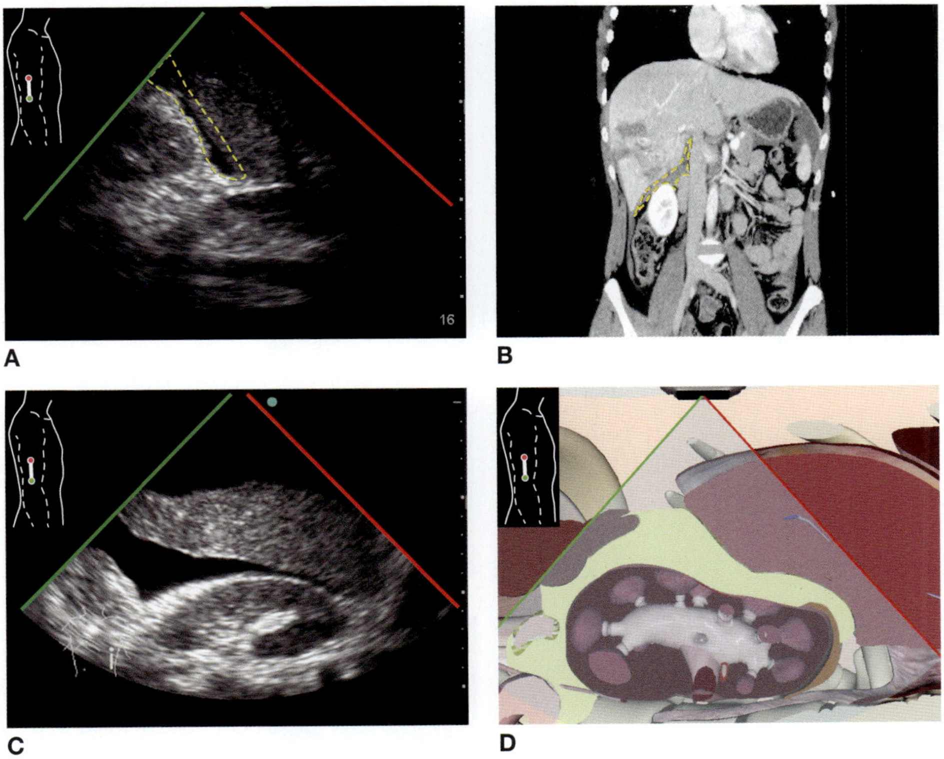

FIGURE 18.5 Reduced mean systemic venous pressure from abdominal etiology. Free intra-abdominal fluid is shown on the right middle axillary coronal abdominal ultrasound image of a 48-year-old patient with a liver laceration after a car accident. A: Free fluid (yellow dotted line) is seen in the hepatorenal space (Video 18.2) with (B) corresponding coronal computed tomography scan. C: Free fluid in a patient with ascites (Video 18.3) and (D) the corresponding Vimedix simulator image. (Reproduced by permission of Taylor and Francis Group, LLC, a division of Informa plc from Denault A, Vegas A, Lamarche Y, Tardif J, Couture P. *Basic Transesophageal and Critical Care Ultrasound*. Taylor and Francis, CRC Press; 2018.)

The inferoseptal and anterolateral walls can be assessed in the apical four-chamber view. Tricuspid and mitral valve Doppler interrogations to rule out regurgitation or stenosis can be done in this view. With a slight anterior tilt and/or slight clockwise rotation, the left ventricular outflow tract (LVOT) appears, and pulsed-wave Doppler can be applied to evaluate cardiac output. The apical two-chamber view is obtained by rotating the transducer 90° counterclockwise from this position. The apical two-chamber view allows visualization of the LV anterior and inferior walls.

Subcostal Four-Chamber and Inferior Vena Cava Views

A simple way to obtain a subcostal four-chamber view from the subcostal-IVC view is to rotate the ultrasound probe clockwise approximately 90° and tilt away from the spine (Figure 18.6G,H). This image can be difficult to obtain in patients with midline abdominal incisions or mediastinal chest tubes. During chest compressions, this view allows quick evaluation of tamponade, chamber size quantification, and cardiac activity (Video 18.7).

As previously noted, cases of cardiogenic shock and elevated venous pressures typically present with a distended IVC without respiratory variation and a reduced systolic-to-diastolic ratio in the HVF profile. Detailed evaluation of ventricular function has been reviewed in previous chapters. It is important to point out that myocardial depression is not always a consequence of ischemia. For example, a catecholamine-induced cardiomyopathy can be found in up to 60% of patients when an echocardiographic examination is performed within 3 days after admission for septic shock (26). In addition, regional wall motion abnormalities

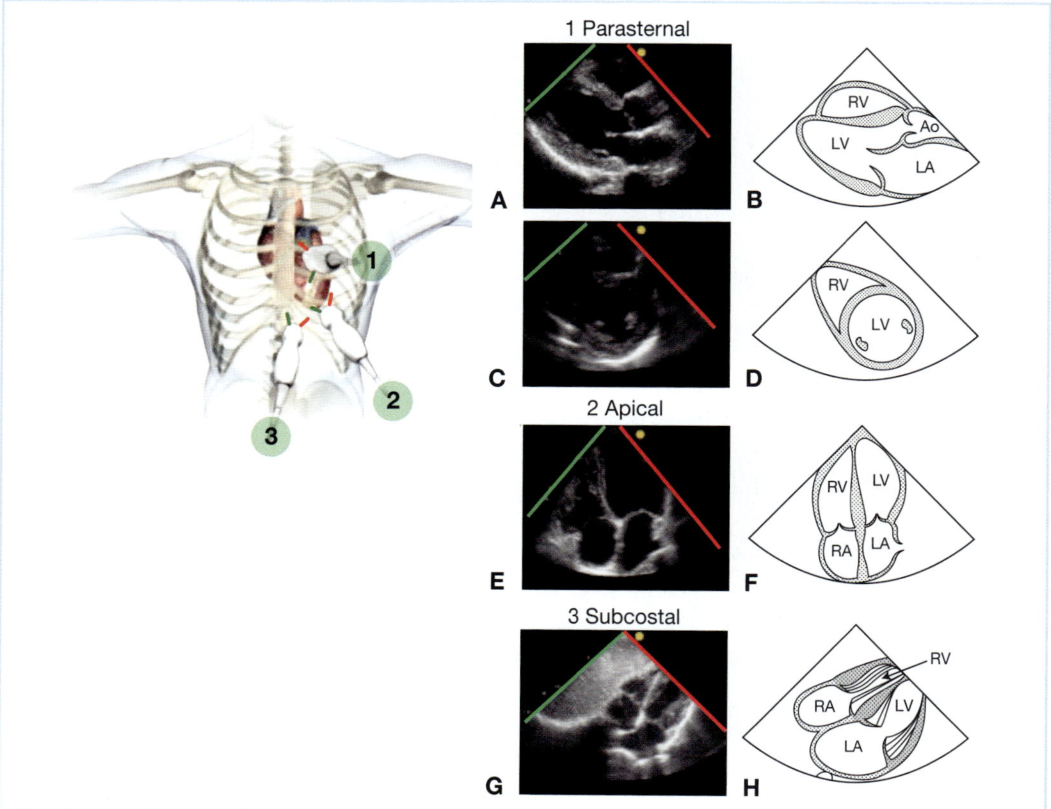

FIGURE 18.6 Focused cardiac ultrasound study (FOCUS) examination. The FOCUS examination includes these important transthoracic echocardiographic views. Scanning should be performed in a systematic, clockwise manner, from these main areas: (1) parasternal long-axis (LAX) (A,B) (Video 18.4) or short-axis (SAX) (C,D) (Video 18.5), (2) apical (E,F) (Video 18.6), and (3) subcostal (G,H) (Video 18.7) views. Ao, aorta; LA, left atrium; LV, left ventricle; RA, right atrium; RV, right ventricle. (Reproduced by permission of Taylor and Francis Group, LLC, a division of Informa plc from Denault A, Vegas A, Lamarche Y, Tardif J, Couture P. *Basic Transesophageal and Critical Care Ultrasound*. Taylor and Francis, CRC Press; 2018.)

can represent ischemic or nonischemic pathologies. Conditions such as Takotsubo syndrome or stress-induced cardiomyopathy will present in 50% to 80% of patients with dyskinetic ballooning of the entire LV apex with compensatory hyperkinesis of the basal segments (Figure 18.7; Videos 18.8 and 18.9) (27). It must be distinguished, with a coronary angiogram, from myocardial ischemia due to a left anterior descending artery occlusion, which can present with apical akinesia, anteroseptal, anterior, anterolateral walls hypokinesia in their mid and basal segments with preserved inferoseptal, inferior, and inferolateral motion.

Acute RV failure can occur from various conditions, including ischemia, pulmonary embolism, septic shock, or iatrogenic volume overload from massive resuscitation. This can occur on a background of chronic pulmonary hypertension (28,29). CCUS is useful to assess the consequences of acute increases in pulmonary artery pressure, such as RV dilatation with reduced tricuspid annular plane systolic excursion, the presence of the McConnell sign (akinesis of the RV free wall with normal wall motion of the apex), and small-sized and hyperdynamic LA and LV from less blood transiting to the left-sided chambers. CCUS performs better than the Wells score (30) but has limited ability to directly confirm pulmonary embolism unless concomitant clear visualization of the thrombus-in-transit associated with hemodynamic instability is present. A computed tomography pulmonary angiography remains the gold standard for the diagnosis of pulmonary embolism.

Both LVOT and RVOT obstruction (RVOTO) can increase LA and/or RA pressure (Figures 18.8 and 18.9; Videos 18.10-18.15) (31).

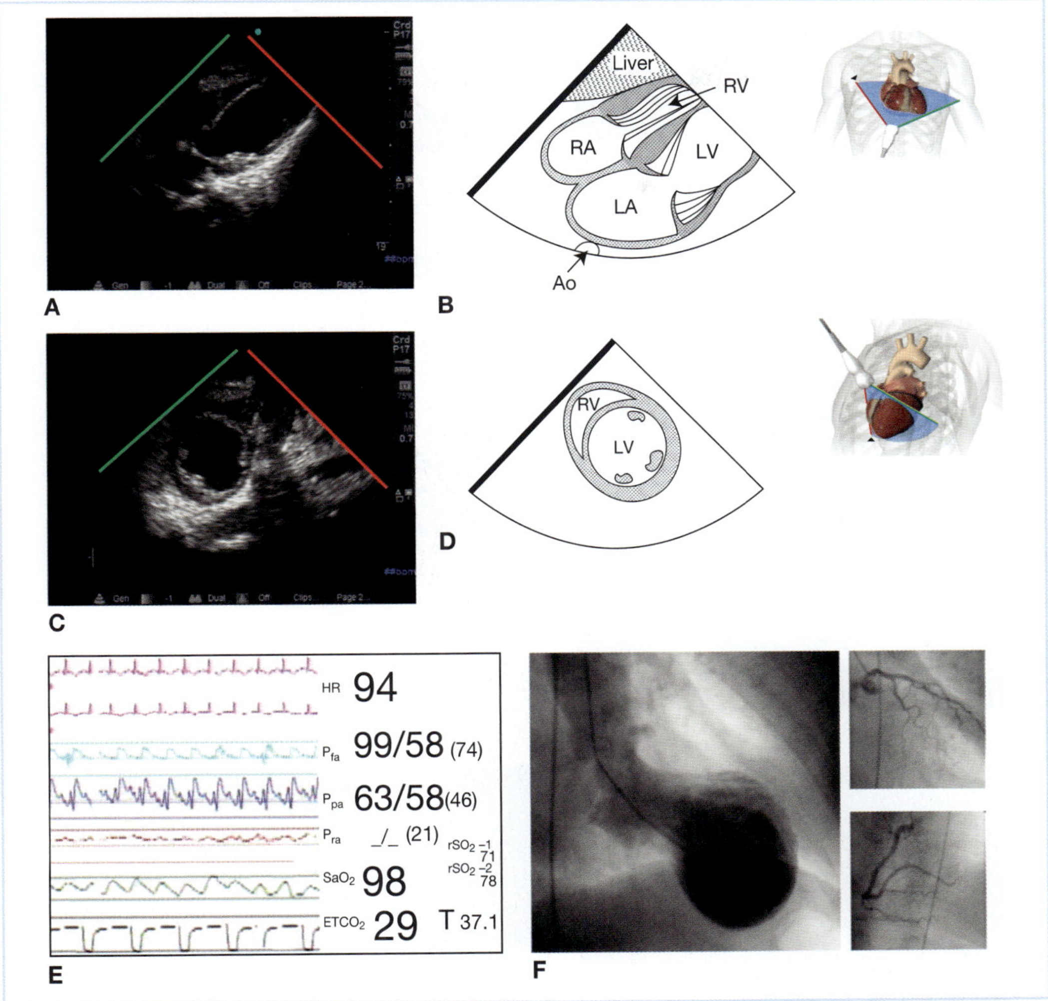

FIGURE 18.7 Takotsubo syndrome. Acute hemodynamic instability in a 73-year-old female after duodenal perforation. A,B: A subcostal view revealed the presence of severe left ventricular dysfunction with basal sparing (Video 18.8). C,D: Parasternal short-axis view confirms left ventricular dysfunction (Video 18.9). E: Left ventriculography shows apical dilatation with normal coronaries on angiography. Ao, aorta; $ETCo_2$, end-tidal carbon dioxide; HR, heart rate; LA, left atrium; LV, left ventricle; P_{fa}, femoral arterial pressure; P_{pa}, pulmonary artery pressure; P_{ra}, right atrial pressure; RA, right atrium; RV, right ventricle; Sao_2, oxygen saturation. (Reproduced by permission of Taylor and Francis Group, LLC, a division of Informa plc from Denault A, Vegas A, Lamarche Y, Tardif J, Couture P. *Basic Transesophageal and Critical Care Ultrasound*. Taylor and Francis, CRC Press; 2018.)

These conditions occur in patients with anatomic predispositions including ventricular hypertrophy or reduced ventricular dimensions, and in those receiving inotropic agents that can induce tachycardia and subsequently reduce ventricular filling time. Administration of fluid to increase preload, reduction of inotropic agents, and even initiation of short-acting beta-blockers to reduce both chronotropy and inotropy will often correct this condition. Mechanical compression of the RVOT can occur with an anterior left pneumothorax, in which case obstruction will initially be seen only in diastole (Figure 18.10; Video 18.16). It has also been described in the prone position (32) or with anterior mediastinal hematomas or tumors close to the RVOT (33).

A common cause of increased RA pressure is LV diastolic dysfunction (34). Dilated atria are typically present in this condition. Diastolic failure can be associated with either (1) a small LV and normal ejection fraction or (2) a dilated LV and reduced ejection fraction (35).

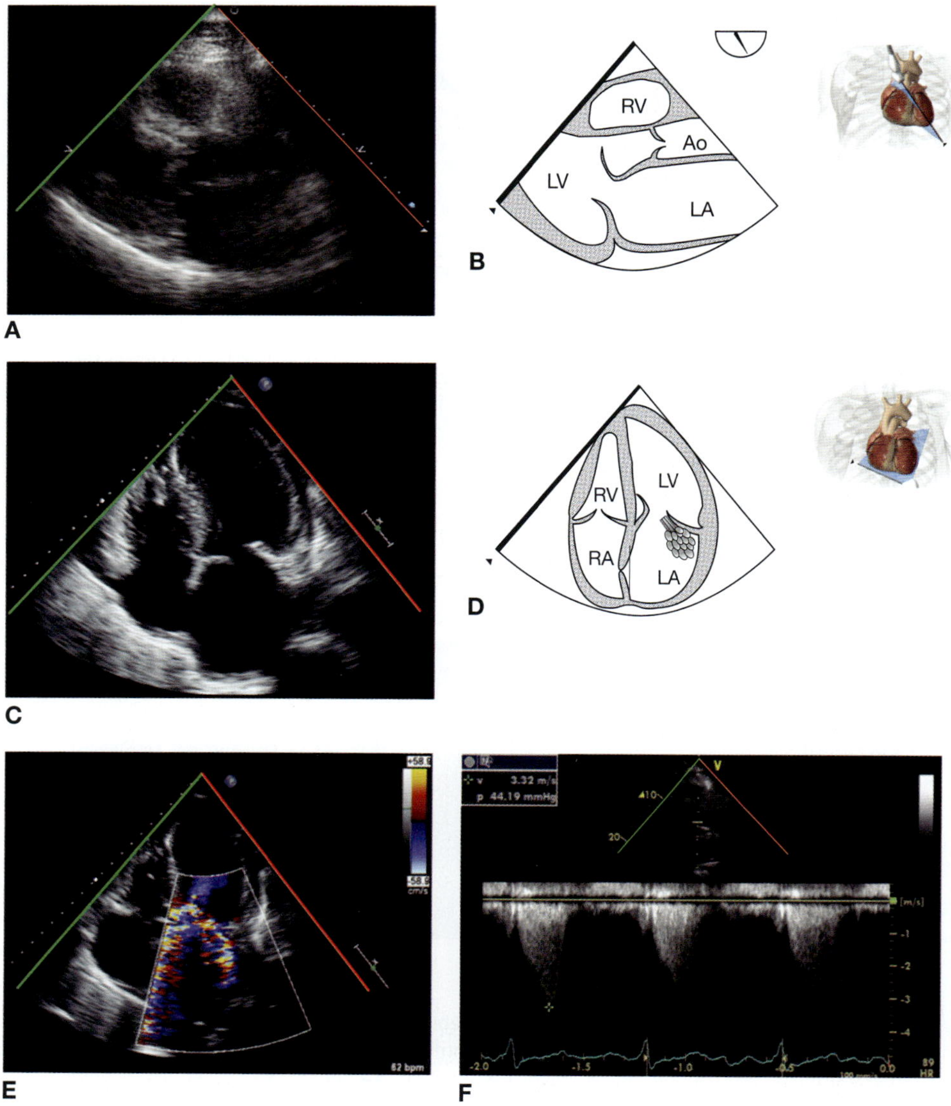

FIGURE 18.8 Left ventricular outflow tract (LVOT) obstruction. A,B: Parasternal long-axis view of a patient shows dynamic LVOT obstruction from systolic anterior motion of the anterior mitral valve leaflet (Video 18.10). C,D: Apical four-chamber view has a displacement of the anterior mitral valve leaflet against the interventricular septum (Video 18.11). E: This was associated with eccentric mitral regurgitation (Video 18.12). F: Dagger-shaped acceleration through the LVOT with 44-mm Hg pressure gradient using continuous-wave Doppler. Ao, aorta; LA, left atrium; LV, left ventricle; RA, right atrium; RV, right ventricle. (Reproduced by permission of Taylor and Francis Group, LLC, a division of Informa plc from Denault A, Vegas A, Lamarche Y, Tardif J, Couture P. *Basic Transesophageal and Critical Care Ultrasound*. Taylor and Francis, CRC Press; 2018.)

Lastly, both hypoxemia and hypercapnia can lead to RV failure secondary to acute increases in pulmonary artery and RA pressures. Combining both cardiac and lung ultrasound will be useful in such patients. Lung ultrasound can help to differentiate the etiology of hypoxemia, such as a pneumothorax, pleural effusion, lung consolidation, atelectasis, and lung congestion. B-lines, or comet tail artifacts, when distributed bilaterally and symmetrically, are typically associated with left heart failure (Figure 18.11; Videos 18.17-18.19) (36). In cases of unexplained hypoxemia with normal pulmonary compliance and ventilatory resistance, an intracardiac right-to-left shunt should be considered.

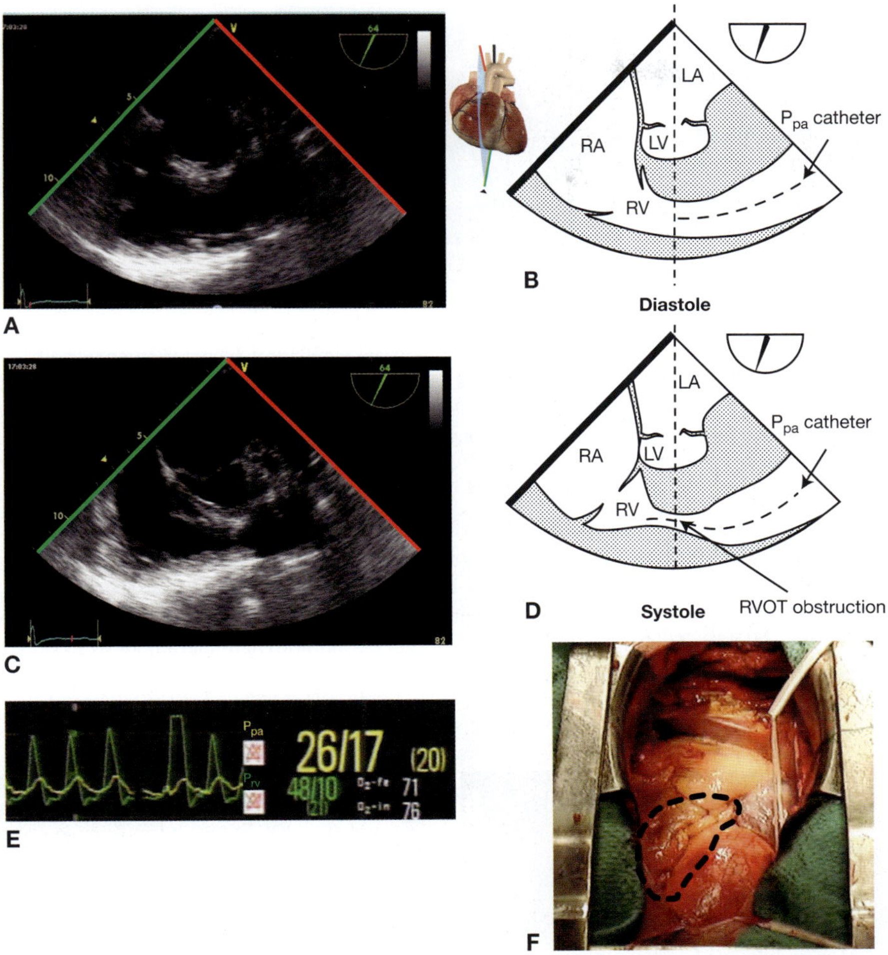

FIGURE 18.9 Right ventricular outflow tract (RVOT) obstruction. Midesophageal inflow-outflow views in (A,B) diastole and (C,D) systole show significant collapse of the RVOT during systole (Video 18.13). E: A 22-mm Hg pressure gradient is present using combined right ventricular pressure (P_{rv}) and pulmonary artery pressure (P_{pa}) waveforms (Video 18.14). F: Intraoperative aspect (Video 18.15). LA, left atrium; LV, left ventricle; RA, right atrium; RV, right ventricle. (Reproduced by permission of Taylor and Francis Group, LLC, a division of Informa plc from Denault A, Vegas A, Lamarche Y, Tardif J, Couture P. *Basic Transesophageal and Critical Care Ultrasound*. Taylor and Francis, CRC Press; 2018.)

Step 4: Critical Care Ultrasound in Increased Resistance to Venous Return

Hemodynamic instability from increased resistance to VR is less common and can be insidious. Failure to diagnose this condition, however, can have catastrophic consequences. A compressed IVC suggests an infradiaphragmatic etiology. For example, the IVC will typically be small or completely compressed and often barely visible in patients with abdominal compartment syndrome. The HVF Doppler will show a monophasic or absent waveform because the lower pressure gradient between the mean systemic venous pressure and the RA pressure reduces the antegrade HVF (Figure 18.3) (15,19).

Conversely, a dilated IVC suggests supradiaphragmatic pathology such as cardiac tamponade (Figure 18.12; Video 18.20), tension pneumothorax (Figure 18.13; Video 18.21), mediastinal tamponade, or dynamic lung hyperinflation due to intrinsic positive end-expiratory pressure (PEEP).

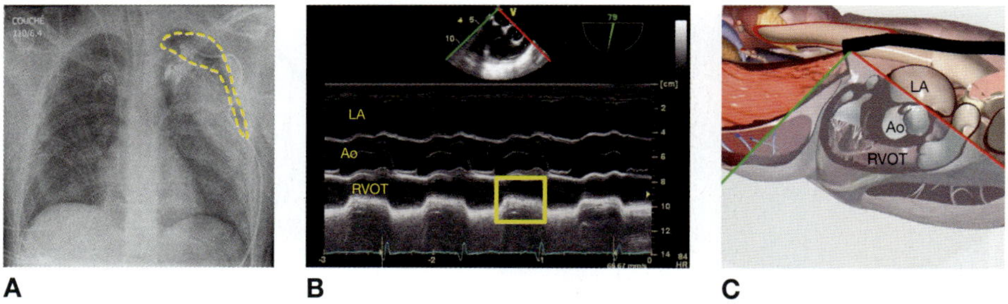

FIGURE 18.10 Right ventricular outflow tract (RVOT) obstruction from the left-sided pneumothorax. A: Chest radiograph shows a left pneumothorax (dotted area). B: Using transesophageal echocardiography, an M-mode from midesophageal four-chamber view shows diastolic obstruction of the RVOT from compression by the anterior portion of the left pneumothorax (Video 18.16). Ao, aorta; LA, left atrium. (Reproduced by permission of Taylor and Francis Group, LLC, a division of Informa plc from Denault A, Vegas A, Lamarche Y, Tardif J, Couture P. *Basic Transesophageal and Critical Care Ultrasound*. Taylor and Francis, CRC Press; 2018.)

In patients with iatrogenic IVC occlusion or intrinsic obstruction, the intrahepatic IVC will also be distended (Figure 18.14; Video 18.22). This condition can occur after liver and cardiac transplantation due to tight IVC anastomosis or from complications of IVC cannulation for cardiopulmonary bypass. The key echocardiographic features in such cases are narrowing of the IVC lumen and flow acceleration seen by color Doppler at the site of the IVC stenosis (19). Confirmation of the hemodynamic gradient by IVC catheterization can be performed when IVC stenting is considered. Figure 18.3 summarizes the type of shock according to the mechanism, the IVC dimension, and the HVF pattern (5).

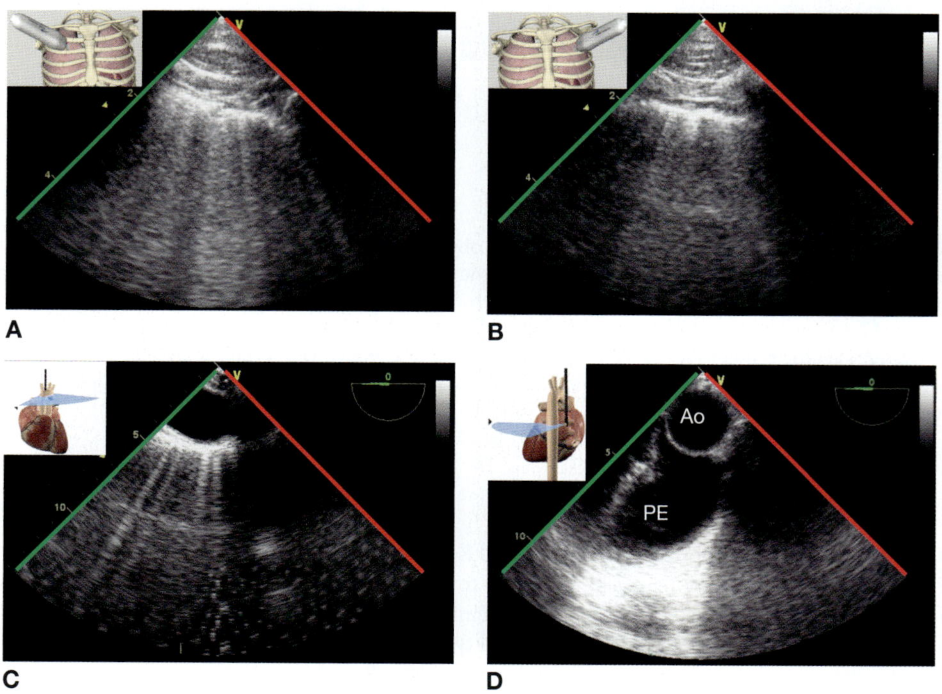

FIGURE 18.11 Congestive heart failure signs using lung ultrasound. A,B: Diffuse B-lines in zones 1 and 5 using critical care ultrasound (Videos 18.17 and 18.18). C: B-lines present below aortic arch using transesophageal lung ultrasound (Video 18.19). D: Left pleural effusion. Ao, aorta; PE, pleural effusion. (Reproduced by permission of Taylor and Francis Group, LLC, a division of Informa plc from Denault A, Vegas A, Lamarche Y, Tardif J, Couture P. *Basic Transesophageal and Critical Care Ultrasound*. Taylor and Francis, CRC Press; 2018.)

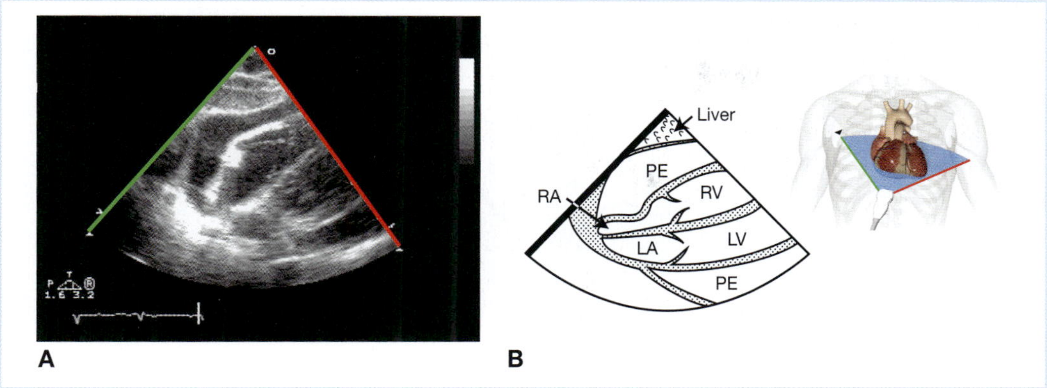

FIGURE 18.12 Cardiac tamponade. A,B: Transthoracic subcostal view shows late diastolic right atrial collapse and early diastolic right ventricle (RV) collapse (Video 18.20). C: Dilated inferior vena cava measured within 1.5 cm of the right atrial-inferior vena cava junction just before the hepatic vein (HV) junction. LA, left atrium; LV, left ventricle; PE, pericardial effusion; RA, right atrium. (Reproduced by permission of Taylor and Francis Group, LLC, a division of Informa plc from Denault A, Vegas A, Lamarche Y, Tardif J, Couture P. *Basic Transesophageal and Critical Care Ultrasound*. Taylor and Francis, CRC Press; 2018.)

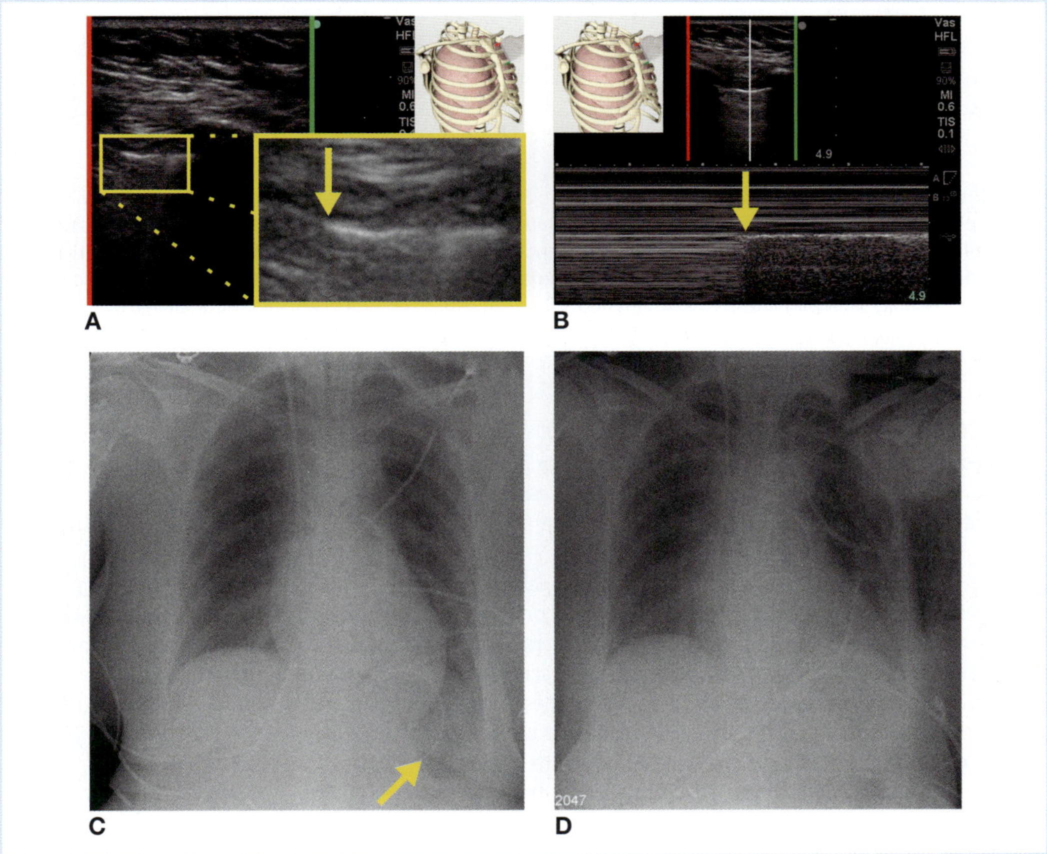

FIGURE 18.13 Pneumothorax. Lung ultrasound examination of zone 5 of the upper left lung shows a lung point using (A) two-dimensional (Video 18.21) and (B) M-mode imaging. The lung point is the transition point between a normal pleural interface and the separation of the viscera and parietal pleura by air (pneumothorax). It can be identified when the normal pleural interface and underlying B-lines seem to disappear. Supine chest radiographs show (C) a deep sulcus sign (arrow), which (D) disappears after chest tube insertion. (Reproduced by permission of Taylor and Francis Group, LLC, a division of Informa plc from Denault A, Vegas A, Lamarche Y, Tardif J, Couture P. *Basic Transesophageal and Critical Care Ultrasound*. Taylor and Francis, CRC Press; 2018.)

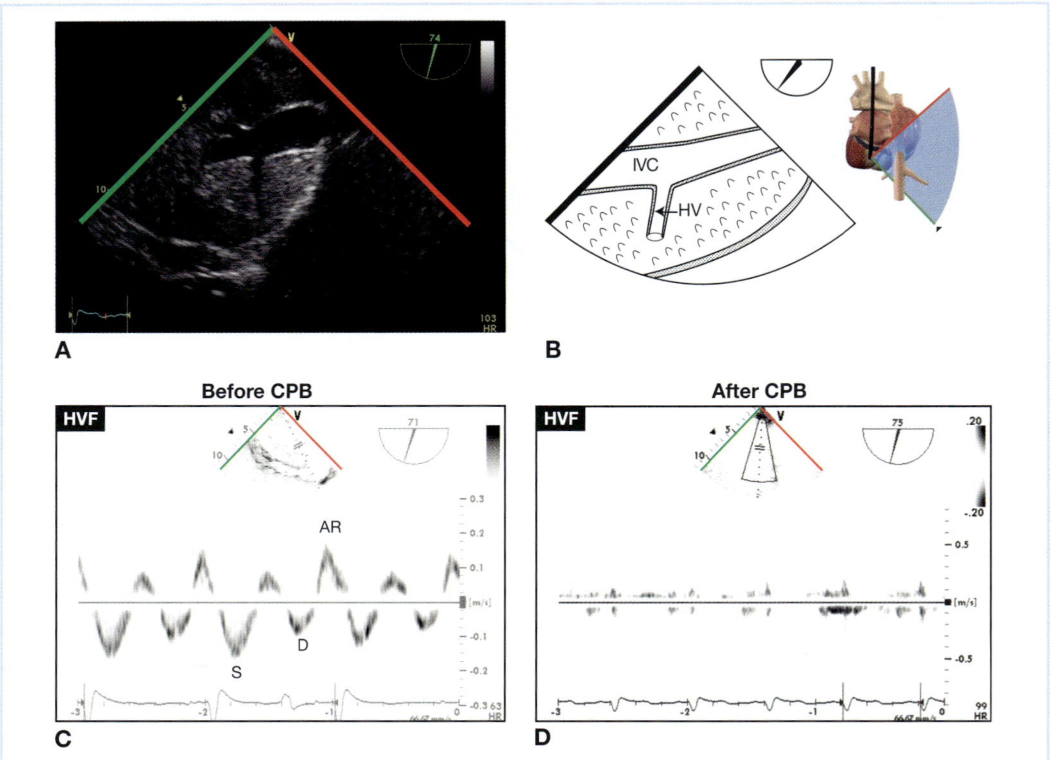

FIGURE 18.14 Inferior vena cava (IVC) occlusion during Fontan procedure. A,B: Transgastric IVC long-axis view from transesophageal echocardiography imaging shows a dilated IVC due to partial occlusion at the caval anastomosis following a Fontan procedure (Video 18.22). C,D: Hepatic venous flow (HVF) is present (C) before cardiopulmonary bypass (CPB) and is almost absent (D) after the procedure. AR, atrial reversal hepatic venous flow velocity; D, diastolic hepatic venous flow velocity; HR, heart rate; HV, hepatic vein; S, systolic hepatic venous flow velocity. (Reproduced by permission of Taylor and Francis Group, LLC, a division of Informa plc from Denault A, Vegas A, Lamarche Y, Tardif J, Couture P. *Basic Transesophageal and Critical Care Ultrasound*. Taylor and Francis, CRC Press; 2018.)

HYPOXEMIA AND LUNG ULTRASOUND

Most causes of hypoxemia are related to pulmonary pathology, which can often be rapidly diagnosed with ultrasound examination of the lungs and pleurae. Less commonly, cardiac conditions such as a right-to-left intracardiac shunt or pulmonary embolism may be the underlying cause. In these cases, lung ultrasound findings will generally be normal.

Lung ultrasound provides a real-time, fast, and easily repeatable bedside evaluation (37), particularly in circumstances where chest radiography (CXR) or computed tomography scan is not rapidly available. The lung ultrasound examination can be performed with the patient in a sitting or supine position, but since most critical care patients are supine, this approach is described here. For a patient examined in the supine position, the anterior thorax is subdivided into eight zones (Figure 18.15). All zones must be scanned to obtain a complete lung examination. To do so, the transducer is placed perpendicular to the long axis of the ribs, with the image showing two ribs cut in a transverse manner (Figure 18.16).

The hyperechoic linear structure between two ribs is the pleural interface. The visceral pleura moves in a synchronous manner with respiration to produce an artifactual movement called lung sliding. The lung parenchyma located under the pleural interface is wherein artifacts are observed. Both abdominal lateral upper quadrants must also be examined for pleural effusions. When using TEE, pleural effusion, atelectasis, or pneumonia might be easier to observe than lung sliding due to the latter being in the near-field clutter. Tables 18.3 and 18.4 depict the principal findings in lung and pleural ultrasound.

Many pleural effusion quantification methods have been published (38-40). Using TTE, estimation of pleural effusion can be done with a patient supine with head elevated (15°) by measuring the maximal distance between parietal and visceral pleura at the posterior axillary line with the probe oriented to obtain a transverse section perpendicular to the body axis with pleural separation visible as an anechoic or hypoechoic

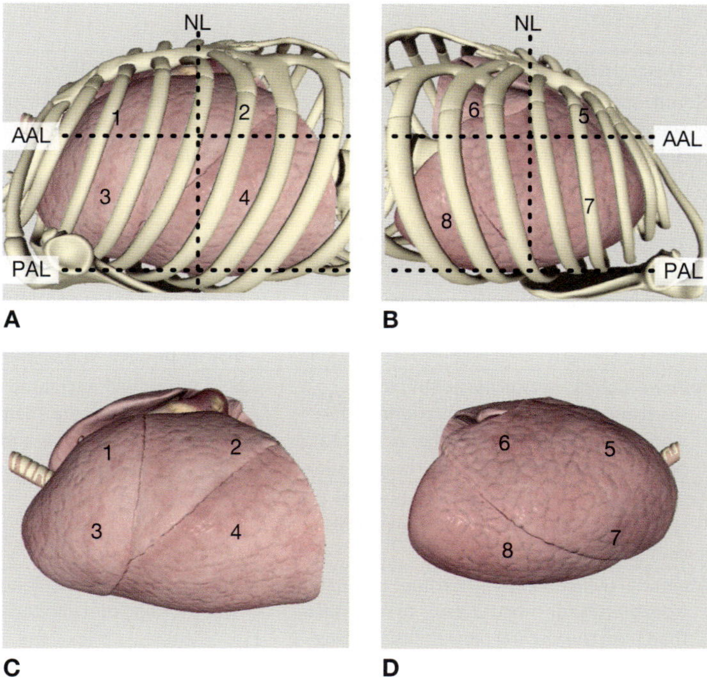

FIGURE 18.15 Lung ultrasound anatomic correlation. The correlation between the surface anatomy of the Volpicelli zones and the lung lobe is shown using the Vimedix simulator. A,C: Right anterior axillary line (AAL) corresponds to the anterior part of the right upper lobe and the middle lobe, whereas the right posterior axillary line (PAL) corresponds to the posterior part of the right upper lobe and the right inferior lobe. B,D: Left AAL corresponds to the anterior part of the left upper lobe, whereas left PAL corresponds to the posterior part of the left upper lobe and the left inferior lobe. NL, nipple line. (Reproduced by permission of Taylor and Francis Group, LLC, a division of Informa plc from Denault A, Vegas A, Lamarche Y, Tardif J, Couture P. *Basic Transesophageal and Critical Care Ultrasound*. Taylor and Francis, CRC Press; 2018.)

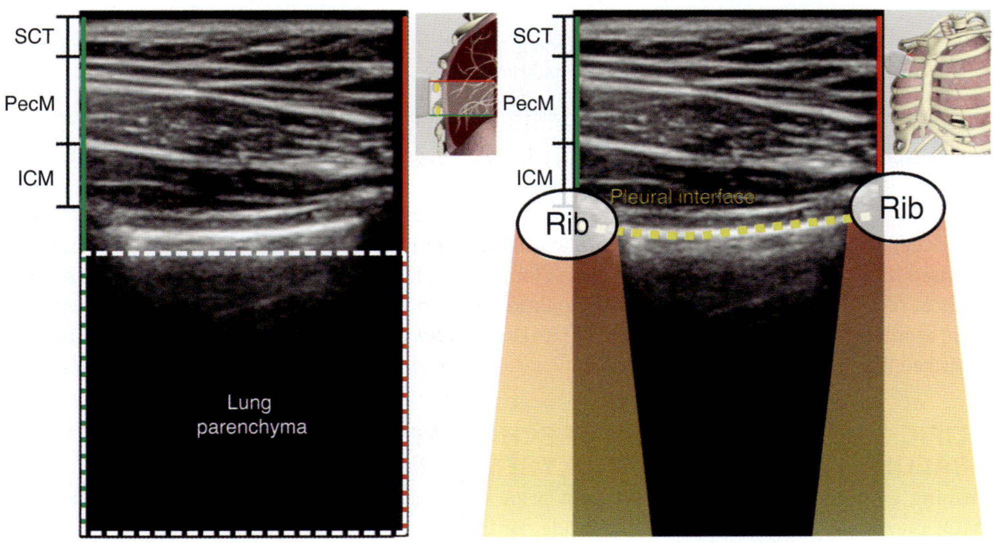

FIGURE 18.16 Landmarks using linear probe for two-dimensional lung ultrasound imaging. ICM, intercostal muscle; PecM, pectoralis muscle; SCT, subcutaneous tissue. (Adapted from Piette E, Daoust R, Denault A. Basic concepts in the use of thoracic and lung ultrasound. *Curr Opin Anaesthesiol*. 2013;26[1]:20-30; and reproduced by permission of Taylor and Francis Group, LLC, a division of Informa plc from Denault A, Vegas A, Lamarche Y, Tardif J, Couture P. *Basic Transesophageal and Critical Care Ultrasound*. Taylor and Francis, CRC Press; 2018.)

TABLE 18.3 Findings in Lung Ultrasound

Finding	Description	Diagnostic Utility
Lung sliding	Normal sliding motion of the visceral pleura against the parietal pleura with inflation and deflation of the lung	Absence associated with: pneumothorax, selective intubation, breath-hold, pleurodesis or other pleural fibrosing pathology, pneumonectomy or lobectomy, large parenchymal tumor, atelectasis
Lung pulse	Normal rhythmic movement of the pleural line caused by transmission of heart beats	Absence associated with pneumothorax
A-line	Normal horizontal repetitions of the pleural line generated by reverberation	Absent with lung consolidation Erased by B-line May be present with pneumothorax
B-line	Abnormal shiny vertical line arising from the pleura, moving along throughout the respiratory cycle. It erases other artifacts and does not fade. Also caused by reverberation.	May appear with increased lung parenchyma density; pulmonary edema, alveolo-interstitial syndrome, and atelectasis
Z-line	Normal hyperechoic vertical lines, but they do not erase other artifacts and fade gradually over a short distance.	No clinical utility
E-Line	Abnormal hyperechoic vertical lines originating from the skin or subcutaneous tissue rather than from the visceral pleura erasing other artifacts and reaching the end of the display	May appear with subcutaneous emphysema or a foreign metallic body
Lung point	Transition point between the presence and absence of lung sliding that corresponds to the beginning of the separation between parietal and visceral pleura	Presence is associated with pneumothorax. Accurately delineates the margin of the pneumothorax False positive at the junction between pleura and peritoneum and between pleura and pericardium
Seashore sign	In M-mode, normal lung sliding and parenchyma create a linear pattern in the tissue superficial to the pleural line with a granular appearance deep to the pleural line.	Normal finding
Barcode sign	The fixed subcutaneous tissue linear pattern is reverberated in the pneumothorax, giving the appearance of fixed horizontal lines extending into the far field.	Presence is associated with pneumothorax. See above for false positives. Lung pulse can be seen in M-mode too.

Reproduced by permission of Taylor and Francis Group, LLC, a division of Informa plc from Denault A, Vegas A, Lamarche Y, Tardif J, Couture P. *Basic Transesophageal and Critical Care Ultrasound*. Taylor and Francis, CRC Press; 2018.

layer between two pleural layers. This distance in millimeters or separation (Sep), multiplied by a factor of 20, can be used to estimate the amount of fluid in milliliters of a pleural effusion. (V [mL] = 20 × Sep [mm]) (38). Estimation of pleural fluid and detection of pulmonary and pleural pathologies in patients with limited acoustic windows can also be done using TEE (41). The approach to hypoxemia using lung ultrasound is summarized in Figure 18.17.

SPECIFIC CONSIDERATION: USE OF ECHOCARDIOGRAPHY FOR EXTRACORPOREAL MEMBRANE OXYGENATION

Performing a comprehensive echocardiogram prior to initiating extracorporeal membrane oxygenation (ECMO) may assist in patient selection, exclude contraindications, and guide the choice of configuration (42-44). Patients with severe acute respiratory distress syndrome (ARDS) may have limited TTE views. TEE provides better visualization of cardiac chambers, guidewires, and cannulas during ECMO cannulation without interfering with the sterile fields. It allows optimal positioning of cannula and reveals complications (45). During cannulation, TEE can confirm the guidewire position within the vena cava and RA for venovenous

TABLE 18.4 Lung Ultrasound Findings in Thoracic Pathology

Pathology	Lung Ultrasound Findings
Alveolo-interstitial	• Multiple B-lines • White lung
Cardiogenic pulmonary edema	• Homogeneously distributed and sized bilateral B-lines increasing in number in a gravity-dependent gradient • Absence of skip areas
ARDS	• Patchy areas of B-lines • Irregular pleural line • Small consolidations • Reduced lung sliding
Pulmonary fibrosis	• Bilateral B-lines • Irregular pleural thickening • Reduced lung sliding
Consolidation	• Lung hepatization
Atelectasis	• Lung hepatization • Mechanism for atelectasis (eg, pleural effusion) • Static air bronchograms • reduced lung sliding
Pneumonia	• Darker tissue • Static and dynamic bronchograms
Pulmonary embolism	• Often normal lung ultrasound • Small triangular or rounded well-demarcated consolidations without any blood flow on color Doppler
Pneumothorax	• Absence of lung sliding and lung pulse • Presence of lung point • Presence of barcode sign • Absence of seashore sign
Pleural fluid	• Homogeneously black if simple • Particles, echotexture and/or swirling, loculations if complex
Diaphragmatic paralysis	• Reduced or absent thickening and excursion during spontaneous inspiration

ARDS, acute respiratory distress syndrome.
Reproduced by permission of Taylor and Francis Group, LLC, a division of Informa plc from Denault A, Vegas A, Lamarche Y, Tardif J, Couture P. *Basic Transesophageal and Critical Care Ultrasound*. Taylor and Francis, CRC Press; 2018.

(VV) ECMO and vena cava and aorta for venoarterial (VA) ECMO. TEE views used to guide cannulation are beyond the scope of this chapter. Readers interested in this topic can refer to additional references for more details (43,45).

Echocardiography plays an essential role in the management of patients on VV and VA ECMO, beyond its role in guiding safe and adequate cannulation. Counterintuitively, echogenicity may improve with a lung rest strategy once on ECMO, and TTE may be sufficient to assess cardiac function and cannula position (46). Monitoring with TEE is otherwise essential to assess ventricular function, cannula position in case of suboptimal unloading while on VA ECMO, recirculation on VV ECMO, and aortic valve opening during VA ECMO support. Echocardiography can detect other significant ECMO complications such as cannula misplacement, especially with changes in intrathoracic pressures and lung volumes in patients on VV ECMO, vascular complication, thrombosis of cannula, pericardial tamponade, or pleural effusion (47). Importantly, ECMO changes the features of tamponade, and the effects of increased pericardial pressures may only appear late when ECMO flows are dropping or when reducing flows during a weaning trial on VA ECMO (48). Echocardiography is also central in the weaning process from VA ECMO to quantify cardiac function and recovery (49).

LIMITATIONS AND CAVEATS OF CRITICAL CARE ULTRASOUND

Hemodynamic instability during shock can be caused by a variety of mechanisms. Therefore, more than one intervention may be necessary to correct the shock condition. The most important aspect of hemodynamic instability management is to address the etiology of the shock condition. For instance, severe hemorrhagic

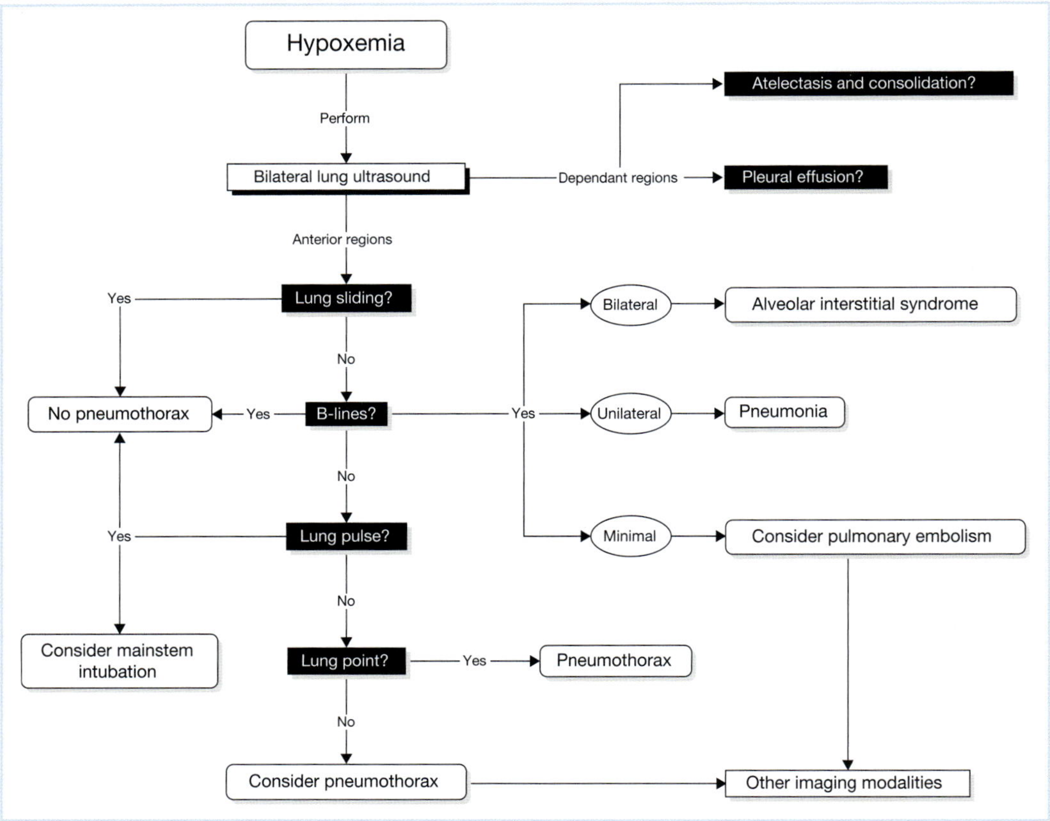

FIGURE 18.17 Lung ultrasound algorithm for hypoxemia. (Adapted from Piette E, Daoust R, Denault A. Basic concepts in the use of thoracic and lung ultrasound. *Curr Opin Anaesthesiol.* 2013;26[1]:20-30; and reproduced by permission of Taylor and Francis Group, LLC, a division of Informa plc from Denault A, Vegas A, Lamarche Y, Tardif J, Couture P. *Basic Transesophageal and Critical Care Ultrasound.* Taylor and Francis, CRC Press; 2018.)

shock can lead to outflow tract obstruction if the patient is under-resuscitated. Acute RV failure can be precipitated if excessive fluid resuscitation is undertaken, which, in turn, may lead to LV diastolic dysfunction through interventricular dependence. LV diastolic dysfunction can further lead to pulmonary edema and hypoxemia, which will then worsen RV failure.

In addition, although bedside ultrasound can estimate cardiac output, this does not describe the adequacy of oxygen transport, and additional tests such as arterial and venous blood gas for mixed venous oxygen tension, VA carbon dioxide difference, lactate levels, and noninvasive cerebral or somatic oxygen spectroscopy should be used as appropriate (50). Nevertheless, these latter techniques do not inform the clinician of the mechanism of reduced oxygen transport. Therefore, both oxygen transport variables and bedside CCUS are complementary tests when dealing with a patient in shock.

When adequate acoustic windows for TTE are unavailable, TEE examination can be a useful alternative. When used in this setting, TEE should not be limited to imaging the cardiac structures, and its use should be further extended to examine the lung (41,51) and the abdomen (52) to identify extracardiac pathologies.

CONCLUSION

In summary, CCUS is becoming an essential tool in the care of critically ill patients. This is reflected by the fact that in 2019, the first Critical Care Echocardiography examination under the National Board of Echocardiography was held in the United States (https://www.echoboards.org). Interestingly, this is 20 years after the first perioperative TEE examination was introduced. This highlights the fact that the use of CCUS is invaluable in the diagnosis and management of common critical situations, such as hemodynamic instability and hypoxemia.

REFERENCES

1. Troianos CA, Hartman GS, Glas KE, et al; Councils on Intraoperative Echocardiography and Vascular Ultrasound of the American Society of Echocardiography. Guidelines for performing ultrasound guided vascular cannulation: recommendations of the American Society of Echocardiography and the Society of Cardiovascular Anesthesiologists. *J Am Soc Echocardiogr.* 2011;24(12):1291-1318.
2. Harrer JU, Eyding J, Ritter M, et al. The potential of neurosonography in neurological emergency and intensive care medicine: monitoring of increased intracranial pressure, brain death diagnostics, and cerebral autoregulation—part 2. *Ultraschall Med.* 2012;33(4):320-331; quiz 332-336.
3. Tang WH, Kitai T. Intrarenal venous flow: a window into the congestive kidney failure phenotype of heart failure? *JACC Heart Fail.* 2016;4(8):683-686.
4. Grande D, Terlizzese P, Iacoviello M. Role of imaging in the evaluation of renal dysfunction in heart failure patients. *World J Nephrol.* 2017;6(3):123-131.
5. Denault A, Vegas A, Lamarche Y, Tardif J, Couture P. *Basic Transesophageal and Critical Care Ultrasound.* Taylor and Francis, CRC Press; 2018.
6. Robba C, Cardim D, Sekhon M, Budohoski K, Czosnyka M. Transcranial Doppler: a stethoscope for the brain-neurocritical care use. *J Neurosci Res.* 2018;96(4):720-730.
7. Kirkpatrick JN, Panebianco N, Díaz-Gómez JL, et al. Recommendations for cardiac point-of-care ultrasound nomenclature. *J Am Soc Echocardiogr.* 2024;37:809-819.
8. Holm JH, Frederiksen CA, Juhl-Olsen P, Sloth E. Perioperative use of focus assessed transthoracic echocardiography (FATE). *Anesth Analg.* 2012;115(5):1029-1032.
9. Scalea TM, Rodriguez A, Chiu WC, et al. Focused Assessment with Sonography for Trauma (FAST): results from an international consensus conference. *J Trauma.* 1999;46(3):466-472.
10. Perera P, Mailhot T, Riley D, Mandavia D. The RUSH exam: Rapid Ultrasound in SHock in the evaluation of the critically ill. *Emerg Med Clin North Am.* 2010;28(1):29-56, vii.
11. Faris JG, Veltman MG, Royse CF. Limited transthoracic echocardiography assessment in anaesthesia and critical care. *Best Pract Res Clin Anaesthesiol.* 2009;23(3):285-298.
12. Gelman S. Venous function and central venous pressure: a physiologic story. *Anesthesiology.* 2008;108(4):735-748.
13. Funk DJ, Jacobsohn E, Kumar A. The role of venous return in critical illness and shock-part I: physiology. *Crit Care Med.* 2013;41(1):255-262.
14. Denault A, Vegas A, Royse C. Bedside clinical and ultrasound-based approaches to the management of hemodynamic instability—part I: focus on the clinical approach: continuing professional development. *Can J Anesth.* 2014;61(9): 843-864.
15. Vegas A, Denault A, Royse C. A bedside clinical and ultrasound-based approach to hemodynamic instability—part II: bedside ultrasound in hemodynamic shock: continuing professional development. *Can J Anesth.* 2014;61(11):1008-1027.
16. Guyton AC, Lindsey AW, Abernathy B, Richardson T. Venous return at various right atrial pressures and the normal venous return curve. *Am J Physiol.* 1957;189(3):609-615.
17. Denault AY, Azzam MA, Beaubien-Souligny W. Imaging portal venous flow to aid assessment of right ventricular dysfunction. *Can J Anesth.* 2018;65(11):1260-1261.
18. Via LL, Astuto M, Dezio V, et al. Agreement between subcostal and transhepatic longitudinal imaging of the inferior vena cava for the evaluation of fluid responsiveness: a systematic review. *J Crit Care.* 2022;71:154108.
19. Hulin J, Aslanian P, Desjardins G, Belaidi M, Denault A. The critical importance of hepatic venous blood flow Doppler assessment for patients in shock. *A A Case Rep.* 2016;6(5):114-120.
20. Denault AY, Beaubien-Souligny W, Elmi-Sarabi M, et al. Clinical significance of portal hypertension diagnosed with bedside ultrasound after cardiac surgery. *Anesth Analg.* 2017;124(4):1109-1115.
21. Beigel R, Cercek B, Luo H, Siegel RJ. Noninvasive evaluation of right atrial pressure. *J Am Soc Echocardiogr.* 2013;26(9): 1033-1042.
22. Seo Y, Iida N, Yamamoto M, Machino-Ohtsuka T, Ishizu T, Aonuma K. Estimation of central venous pressure using the ratio of short to long diameter from cross-sectional images of the inferior vena cava. *J Am Soc Echocardiogr.* 2017;30(5):461-467.
23. Lecluyse V, Couture EJ, Denault AY. A proposed approach to cerebral and somatic desaturation in the intensive care unit: preliminary experience and review. *J Cardiothorac Vasc Anesth.* 2017;31(5):1805-1809.
24. Hu T, Collin Y, Lapointe R, et al. Preliminary experience in combined somatic and cerebral oximetry monitoring in liver transplantation. *J Cardiothorac Vasc Anesth.* 2018;32(1):73-84.
25. Denault AY, Langevin S, Lessard MR, Courval JF, Desjardins G. Transthoracic echocardiographic evaluation of the heart and great vessels. *Can J Anesth.* 2018;65(4):449-472.
26. Vieillard-Baron A, Caille V, Charron C, Belliard G, Page B, Jardin F. Actual incidence of global left ventricular hypokinesia in adult septic shock. *Crit Care Med.* 2008;36(6):1701-1706.
27. Hessel EA 2nd. Takotsubo cardiomyopathy and its relevance to anesthesiology: a narrative review. *Can J Anesth.* 2016; 63(9):1059-1074.

28. Parker MM, McCarthy KE, Ognibene FP, Parrillo JE. Right ventricular dysfunction and dilatation, similar to left ventricular changes, characterize the cardiac depression of septic shock in humans. *Chest*. 1990;97(1):126-131.
29. Romero-Bermejo FJ, Ruiz-Bailen M, Gil-Cebrian J, Huertos-Ranchal MJ. Sepsis-induced cardiomyopathy. *Curr Cardiol Rev*. 2011;7(3):163-183.
30. Nazerian P, Volpicelli G, Gigli C, et al; Ultrasound Wells Study Group. Diagnostic performance of wells score combined with point-of-care lung and venous ultrasound in suspected pulmonary embolism. *Acad Emerg Med*. 2017;24(3):270-280.
31. Zeng YH, Calderone A, Rousseau-Saine N, et al. Right ventricular outflow tract obstruction in adults: a systematic review and meta-analysis. *CJC Open*. 2021;3(9):1153-1168.
32. Neira VM, Gardin L, Ryan G, Jarvis J, Roy D, Splinter W. A transesophageal echocardiography examination clarifies the cause of cardiovascular collapse during scoliosis surgery in a child. *Can J Anesth*. 2011;58(5):451-455.
33. Young AM, Danter MR, Lewis JS Jr, Barton BR. Right ventricular hemangioma in the outflow tract: a rare cause of obstruction. *Ann Thorac Surg*. 2017;103(3):e245-e246.
34. Nagueh SF, Smiseth OA, Appleton CP, et al. Recommendations for the evaluation of left ventricular diastolic function by echocardiography: an update from the American Society of Echocardiography and the European Association of Cardiovascular Imaging. *Eur Heart J Cardiovasc Imaging*. 2016;17(12):1321-1360.
35. Aurigemma GP, Zile MR, Gaasch WH. Contractile behavior of the left ventricle in diastolic heart failure: with emphasis on regional systolic function. *Circulation*. 2006;113(2):296-304.
36. Miglioranza MH, Gargani L, Sant'Anna RT, et al. Lung ultrasound for the evaluation of pulmonary congestion in outpatients: a comparison with clinical assessment, natriuretic peptides, and echocardiography. *JACC Cardiovasc Imaging*. 2013;6(11):1141-1151.
37. Zanobetti M, Scorpiniti M, Gigli C, et al. Point-of-care ultrasonography for evaluation of acute dyspnea in the ED. *Chest*. 2017;151(6):1295-1301.
38. Balik M, Plasil P, Waldauf P, et al. Ultrasound estimation of volume of pleural fluid in mechanically ventilated patients. *Intensive Care Med*. 2006;32(2):318.
39. Usta E, Mustafi M, Ziemer G. Ultrasound estimation of volume of postoperative pleural effusion in cardiac surgery patients. *Interact Cardiovasc Thorac Surg*. 2010;10(2):204-207.
40. Remerand F, Dellamonica J, Mao Z, et al. Multiplane ultrasound approach to quantify pleural effusion at the bedside. *Intensive Care Med*. 2010;36(4):656-664.
41. Cavayas YA, Girard M, Desjardins G, Denault AY. Transesophageal lung ultrasonography: a novel technique for investigating hypoxemia. *Can J Anesth*. 2016;63(11):1266-1276.
42. Donker DW, Meuwese CL, Braithwaite SA, et al. Echocardiography in extracorporeal life support: a key player in procedural guidance, tailoring and monitoring. *Perfusion*. 2018;33(1_suppl):31-41.
43. Douflé G, Roscoe A, Billia F, Fan E. Echocardiography for adult patients supported with extracorporeal membrane oxygenation. *Crit Care*. 2015;19:326.
44. Platts DG, Sedgwick JF, Burstow DJ, Mullany DV, Fraser JF. The role of echocardiography in the management of patients supported by extracorporeal membrane oxygenation. *J Am Soc Echocardiogr*. 2012;25(2):131-141.
45. Morales Castro D, Abdelnour-Berchtold E, et al. Transesophageal echocardiography-guided extracorporeal membrane oxygenation cannulation in COVID-19 patients. *J Cardiothorac Vasc Anesth*. 2022;36(12):4296-4304.
46. Viau-Lapointe J, Douflé G. Transthoracic view of extracorporeal membrane oxygenation cannulae. *Am J Respir Crit Care Med*. 2019;199(10):e39-e40.
47. Cheng R, Hachamovitch R, Kittleson M, et al. Complications of extracorporeal membrane oxygenation for treatment of cardiogenic shock and cardiac arrest: a meta-analysis of 1,866 adult patients. *Ann Thorac Surg*. 2014;97(2):610-616.
48. Dragoi L, Teijeiro-Paradis R, Douflé G. When is tamponade not an echocardiographic diagnosis... or is it ever? *Echocardiography*. 2022;39(7):880-885.
49. Aissaoui N, El-Banayosy A, Combes A. How to wean a patient from veno-arterial extracorporeal membrane oxygenation. *Intensive Care Med*. 2015;41(5):902-905.
50. Denault A, Guimond JG. Does measuring veno-arterial carbon dioxide difference compare to predicting a hockey game's final score? *Can J Anesth*. 2021;68(4):445-453.
51. Piette E, Daoust R, Denault A. Basic concepts in the use of thoracic and lung ultrasound. *Curr Opin Anaesthesiol*. 2013;26(1):20-30.
52. Denault AY, Roberts M, Cios T, et al. Transgastric abdominal ultrasonography in anesthesia and critical care: review and proposed approach. *Anesth Analg*. 2021;133(3):630-647.
53. Denault AY, Chaput M, Couture P, Hebert Y, Haddad F, Tardif JC. Dynamic right ventricular outflow tract obstruction in cardiac surgery. *J Thorac Cardiovasc Surg*. 2006;132(1):43-49.
54. Maslow A, Stearns G, Bert A, et al. Monitoring end-tidal carbon dioxide during weaning from cardiopulmonary bypass in patients without significant lung disease. *Anesth Analg*. 2001;92(2):306-313.

QUESTIONS

1. **A 68-year-old female, diagnosed with anterolateral myocardial infarction (MI) in the emergency department, has multivessel disease on coronary angiography. The patient is transferred to the ICU while the operating room is prepared for urgent coronary revascularization. Just after arrival in the ICU, the patient suddenly deteriorates (blood pressure 80/40 mm Hg, heart rate 120/min, respiratory distress with an oxygen saturation [Sp_{O_2}] of 88% with a fraction of inspired oxygen [F_{IO_2}] of 100%).**

A focused ultrasound examination is performed showing the following findings:
- The IVC diameter is 20 mm with respiratory variations less than 50%.
- HVF shows a blunted S (S < D).
- Normal LV systolic function with tachycardia, left ventricular internal dimension (LVID) at end diastole of 5.5 cm and LVID at end systole of 4 cm
- Eccentric mitral valve regurgitation jet (vena contracta 0.7 cm)
- Lung ultrasound: diffuse bilateral B-lines in positions 1 and 5

According to the findings in the CCUS examination, what is your primary diagnosis?
A. Hypovolemia due to acute hemorrhage
B. Tamponade
C. Mitral valve pathology
D. Severe LV dysfunction

2. **Which of the following interventions is the *least appropriate* next step in managing hemodynamic instability in this patient?**
A. Fluid challenge with crystalloids
B. Dobutamine infusion
C. Insertion of an intra-aortic balloon pump (IABP)
D. Diuretics

3. **While the circulation is supported with inotropes and the insertion of an IABP is being performed, what would be the next best step in this patient?**
A. Call the surgeon and transfer the patient to the operating room for emergency surgery.
B. Call the surgeon and ask to perform thoracotomy on the ICU.
C. Call for/perform a comprehensive echocardiogram.
D. Call the cardiologist and have percutaneous angioplasty performed.

4. **The abovementioned patient underwent emergency surgery for mitral valve repair and coronary revascularization. A pulmonary artery catheter was inserted. Inotropic support with dobutamine 5 μg/kg/min was provided. Just after arrival in the ICU the patient suddenly deteriorates (blood pressure 90/60 mm Hg, heart rate 100/min, central venous pressure 5 mm Hg, cardiac index 1.8 L/min/m^2). A CCUS examination is performed showing the following findings:**
- IVC diameter 20 mm, respiratory variation greater than 50%, HVF showing a predominant systolic (S) velocity (S > D)
- LV being hyperdynamic, LVID at end diastole of 3.5 cm and LVID at end systole of 1 cm, LV septal thickness at end diastole 1.8 cm
- Eccentric mitral valve regurgitation jet (vena contracta 0.7 cm)

Which of the following is the most appropriate next step?
A. Fluid challenge with crystalloids
B. Norepinephrine infusion
C. Vasopressin infusion
D. Dobutamine infusion

5. **A similar patient underwent emergency surgery for mitral valve repair and coronary revascularization. A pulmonary artery catheter was inserted. Inotropic support with dobutamine 5 μg/kg was provided. Just after arrival in the ICU, the patient suddenly deteriorated (blood pressure 90/60 mm Hg, heart rate 100/min, central venous pressure 15 mm Hg, systolic pulmonary artery pressure 35 mm Hg, systolic RV pressure 55 mm Hg, cardiac index 1.8 L/min/m^2).**

A focused examination is performed showing the following findings:
- IVC diameter 25 mm, respiratory variation less than 50%, HVF showing a blunted S (S < D)
- LV being hyperdynamic, LVID at end diastole of 3.5 cm and LVID at end systole of 1 cm, LV septal thickness at end diastole 1.8 cm
- Trace mitral valve regurgitation with a central jet

Which of the following views is the most useful to further evaluate the underlying etiology of hemodynamic instability:

A. Subcostal four-chamber view
B. Parasternal short-axis view at aortic valve level
C. Parasternal short-axis view at midpapillary level
D. Apical four-chamber view

6. Despite your efforts to stabilize the patient, the patient further deteriorates and goes into cardiac arrest. When performing a focused transthoracic echo examination during advanced cardiac life support or cardiopulmonary resuscitation, which of the following is the preferred single view?

A. Subcostal four-chamber view
B. Parasternal long-axis view
C. Parasternal short-axis view
D. Apical two-chamber view

7. An ultrasound examination can be performed to discover potentially treatable causes of cardiac arrest. What is the best time to obtain a transthoracic echo image during advance cardiac life support?

A. Before cardiopulmonary resuscitation starts
B. As soon as the echo machine arrives
C. During immediate pulse check
D. During the pulse check but not before 5 cardiopulmonary resuscitation cycles (2 minutes)

8. An 81-year-old woman diagnosed with anterolateral MI was diagnosed with multivessel disease from a coronary angiogram. The patient is transferred to the ICU after coronary angiogram while the operating room is prepped for urgent revascularization surgery. Just after arrival in ICU, the patient suddenly deteriorates (blood pressure 80/40 mm Hg, heart rate 120/min, respiratory rate of 16/min with oxygen saturation of 96% on room air). A focused examination is performed showing the following findings:

- IVC: IVC diameter 6 mm, respiratory variation greater than 50%
- HVF: normal hepatic vein flow (S > D)
- TTE: hyperdynamic LV with an LVID at end diastole of 2.5 cm and LVID at end systole of 0.5 cm with "kissing papillary muscles" in the parasternal short-axis view. Hyperdynamic RV. RV/LV ratio less than 0.6. Normal valves, no effusions

Which of the following interventions is the most appropriate next step?

A. Fluid challenge with crystalloids
B. Dobutamine infusion
C. Norepinephrine infusion
D. Heparin infusion

9. After your initial evaluation and stabilization of the patient, you decide to proceed with the following examinations/procedures, *except*:

A. Perform lung and abdominal ultrasound to look for hemothorax/free fluid.
B. Perform computed tomographic angiography (CTA).
C. Call the surgeon and transfer the patient immediately to the operating room.
D. Check hemoglobin and order blood products.

10. The patient underwent emergency surgery for retroperitoneal hemorrhage after failed angiographic interventional treatment. During surgery, the patient received 10 L of fluids (blood products and crystalloids). The patient arrives in the ICU from the operating room intubated and mechanically ventilated. Blood pressure is 90/50 mm Hg, heart rate is 100/min, central venous pressure 21 mm Hg, Sa_{O_2} 92% with F_{IO_2} 60%, PEEP 5 cm H_2O, plateau pressure 30 cm H_2O. Somatic near-infrared spectroscopy (NIRS) monitoring of the lower extremities decreased, while values remained stable on the upper extremities. The patient remains oliguric after surgery.

Focused ultrasound examination shows:

- IVC: not visible
- HVF: very low velocity profile
- TTE: LV and RV function: normal to hyperdynamic; size: LVID end diastole of 4.0 cm and LVID at end systole of 2.2 cm, RV/LV ratio less than 0.6

Which of the following interventions is *least* appropriate at this point?

A. Fluid challenge with albumin 5%
B. Ultrasound examination of the bladder and kidneys
C. Ultrasound of the lower limb vasculature
D. Measure intra-abdominal pressure

11. **Despite deep sedation, paracentesis, and evacuation of intraluminal fluids, the patient remains hypotensive and acute renal failure persists. Meanwhile, pulmonary function deteriorates: Sa_{O_2} 88%, F_{IO_2} 80%, PEEP 5 cm H_2O, plateau pressure 30 cm H_2O**
    - TTE: LV and RV function: normal to hyperdynamic; size: LVID end diastole of 4.0 cm and LVID at end systole of 2.2 cm, RV/LV ratio less than 0.6
    - Lung ultrasound: hypoechoic layer between pleural layers: 2 cm right side, 1.5 cm left side. Right and left lower lobe atelectasis, only few B-lines

    Which of the following interventions is the most appropriate next step?

    A. Increase PEEP to 10 cm H_2O
    B. Increase F_{IO_2} to 100%
    C. Drain the right-sided pleural effusion
    D. Prone positioning

12. **With the measures taken above, pulmonary function slightly improves. Since the patient remains anuric, consistent with an abdominal compartment syndrome, the patient is again taken to the operating room for decompressive laparotomy. After readmission to the ICU, blood pressure is 110/55 mm Hg, heart rate is 90/min, central venous pressure 12 mm Hg, Sa_{O_2} 97% with F_{IO_2} 45%, and urine output 40 mL/h. After 10 hours, blood pressure is 95/45 mm Hg, heart rate 105/min, Sa_{O_2} drops to 89% despite an F_{IO_2} of 80%, and a PEEP of 15 cm H_2O. The patient is still deeply sedated and under neuromuscular blockade. Bedside echo shows:**
    - IVC 2.5 cm, no respiratory variation; HVF: S < D
    - Echo: moderate tricuspid regurgitation (TR), no effusions, and RV/LV ratio greater than 1 in the four-chamber view, tricuspid annular plane systolic excursion (TAPSE) 15 mm
    - Lung ultrasound: patchy areas of B-lines on the anterior chest bilaterally, irregular pleural line, reduced lung sliding

    Which of the following interventions is the most appropriate next step?

    A. Abdominal ultrasound
    B. CXR
    C. Magnetic resonance tomography of the chest
    D. Prone positioning

13. **With the measures taken above, pulmonary function slightly improves. Since the patient remains anuric, consistent with an acute compartment syndrome, the patient is again taken to the operating room for decompressive laparotomy. After readmission to the ICU, blood pressure is 110/55 mm Hg, heart rate is 90/min, central venous pressure 12 mm Hg, Sa_{O_2} 97% with F_{IO_2} 45%, and urine output 40 mL/h. After 10 hours, blood pressure is 95/45 mm Hg, heart rate 105/min, Sa_{O_2} drops to 89% despite an F_{IO_2} of 80%, and a PEEP of 15 cm H_2O. The patient is still deeply sedated and relaxed. Bedside CCUS shows:**
    - IVC 1.8 cm, respiratory variation greater than 50%; HVF: S > D
    - Echo: normal LV/RV function, RV/LV ratio less than 0.6, no significant valvular abnormality, no effusion. TAPSE 20 mm
    - Lung ultrasound: right and left lower lobes with areas of darker tissue and dynamic bronchograms

Which of the following interventions is the most appropriate next step?
A. Fluid challenge with crystalloids (2 L)
B. Dobutamine infusion
C. Norepinephrine infusion and broad-spectrum antibiotics
D. Prone positioning

14. Which of the following echo findings is most consistent with acute right heart failure following a massive pulmonary embolism?
A. Severe pulmonic insufficiency
B. RV free wall thickness greater than 1 cm
C. LV end-diastolic diameter of 8 cm
D. RV area greater than LV area

15. A 56-year-old patient with Ebstein anomaly is in the ICU and intubated and mechanically ventilated for decompensated RV failure. Shortly after intubation, Sa_{O_2} drops to 88% on an F_{IO_2} of 70%. CXR is unremarkable, and lung ultrasound is normal. Which of the following TEE views would be most helpful in determining the cause of this patient hypoxia?
A. Midesophageal four-chamber view
B. RV outflow
C. Transgastric short-axis view
D. Bicaval

16. A 56-year-old patient with Ebstein anomaly is in the ICU and intubated and mechanically ventilated for decompensated RV failure. Shortly after intubation, Sa_{O_2} drops to 88% on an F_{IO_2} of 70% and a PEEP of 5 cm H_2O. CXR is unremarkable.
- TEE: small LV, normal function, small RV with decreased RV function. Severely dilated RA (atrialization of the RV) due to Ebstein pathology. Moderate TR. Bulging of the interatrial septum and interventricular septum toward the left-sided chambers during systole and diastole. Color flow detects right-to-left shunt via a patent foramen ovale.

Which of the following interventions is the *least* appropriate next step?
A. Increase F_{IO_2} to 85%.
B. Increase PEEP to 10 cm H_2O.
C. Start intravenous diuretics.
D. Avoid hypercapnia.

17. When performing a focused TTE during advanced cardiac life support, which of the following is the preferred single view in order to rule out MI?
A. Subcostal four-chamber view
B. Parasternal long-axis view
C. Parasternal short-axis view
D. Apical four-chamber view

18. Which element on lung ultrasound is not useful to *exclude* a pneumothorax?
A. Sliding lung
B. B-lines
C. Lung pulse
D. Lung point

19. What is the likely mechanism of shock in a patient with a small IVC but significantly reduced flow velocity in the hepatic vein?
A. Hemorrhagic shock
B. Abdominal compartment syndrome
C. Septic shock
D. Cardiogenic shock

20. A 75-year-old woman arrives in the ICU from the emergency department with the diagnosis of urosepsis. The patient is intubated and mechanically ventilated. Blood pressure is 105/55 mm Hg, heart rate is 90/min, and the mixed venous oxygen saturation is 75%. Bedside CCUS shows moderate TR, no effusions, and RV area > LV area in the four-chamber view. Which of the following interventions is the most appropriate next step?

A. One liter of normal saline bolus
B. Dobutamine infusion
C. Norepinephrine infusion
D. Chest computed tomography and heparin infusion if positive

ANSWERS

1. Correct Answer: C.

Rationale: The mechanical complications of acute MI include papillary muscle rupture, LV free wall rupture, and rupture of the interventricular septum. According to the classification of hemodynamic instability using the concept of VR, acute mitral regurgitation (MR), as found in this patient, may lead to LV systolic dysfunction with pulmonary edema, pulmonary hypertension, and finally increased RA pressure. In this patient, a posteriorly directed regurgitant jet indicative of a flail anterior mitral valve leaflet from anterolateral papillary muscle rupture was diagnosed. Rupture of the anterolateral muscle is less common than posteromedial, since it has a dual blood supply (from the circumflex and left anterior descending arteries) and is associated with anterolateral MI as found in this patient. The posteromedial muscle is only supplied from the posterior descending artery, which makes it more susceptible to rupture.
Since mechanical complications of MI are associated with a high mortality if not rapidly treated, immediate recognition is crucial. Mechanical complications of acute MI can be identified with CCUS.

2. Correct Answer: A.

Rationale: Papillary muscle rupture leads to sudden hemodynamic deterioration, dyspnea, pulmonary edema, and cardiogenic shock. Immediate treatment to bridge to emergency surgery consists of afterload reduction to reduce volume overload and pulmonary congestion. Inotropes, vasodilators, diuretics, and IABP may be indicated to stabilize the patient.

3. Correct Answer: C.

Rationale: A comprehensive echo is required to confirm the diagnosis and to understand the underlying mechanism to proceed with surgery. Angioplasty could relieve the underlying coronary vessel disease but would be associated with the intake of oral platelet inhibitors and, therefore, increase the bleeding risk of this patient. In addition, mitral valve pathology would not be resolved. In this patient, a TEE was performed after intubation, confirming the suspected mechanism of anterolateral papillary muscle rupture due to anterolateral MI, leading to flail of the anterior mitral valve leaflet with severe eccentric (posteriorly directed) regurgitation. CCUS helps to rapidly understand the pathophysiology of shock. However, it should act as a trigger for further diagnostics/comprehensive echocardiography if its findings require more detailed examinations. The surgeon can be called after confirming the diagnosis.

4. Correct Answer: A.

Rationale: The patient most likely has severe MR due to systolic anterior motion (SAM) of the anterior mitral valve leaflet. Small ventricles with septal hypertrophy and post–mitral valve repair state may predispose to this condition. This process is worsened by hypovolemia and increased contractility. The first step would be to optimize LV volume and decrease inotropic support. If SAM persists, a comprehensive TEE should be performed to detect the need for revision of mitral valve repair.

5. Correct Answer: B.

Rationale: In this patient, RVOTO can occur in association with the use of inotropes. Small and hypertrophic ventricles are predisposed to develop RVOTO, which can be exaggerated by the use of inotropes. The best view to diagnose this pathology is the RVOT, either in the parasternal short axis with TTE or at the midesophageal level at about 45° to 60° with the TEE probe. RVOTO will equally lead to an increase in RA pressure. Continuous pressure waveform monitoring of the RV and pulmonary artery using the RV port of a pulmonary artery catheter is the easiest way of detecting this inotropic-related complication (53).

6. **Correct Answer: A.**
Rationale: In supine patients undergoing cardiopulmonary resuscitation, this is often the easiest and fastest four-chamber view to obtain. However, when available, TEE is the best monitoring modality because it allows continuous cardiac massage without interruption. In addition, it can be used to diagnose not only cardiac but also extracardiac conditions, such as hemothorax and abdominal bleeding.

7. **Correct Answer: D.**
Rationale: Ultrasound should be performed for nonshockable rhythm and minimize interruptions of cardiopulmonary resuscitation. A focused examination should not reduce or delay the time of chest compressions, should only be done during the pulse check, and should be an abbreviated examination.

8. **Correct Answer: A.**
Rationale: This patient shows a small IVC with respiratory variation and a normal HVF. Therefore, a cardiac origin for hemodynamic instability is unlikely. This is confirmed by the focused cardiac examination, showing the ventricles with hyperdynamic systolic function and a decrease in both LV end-diastolic and end-systolic size. According to the classification of hemodynamic instability using the concept of VR, a reduced mean systemic venous pressure due to hemorrhagic or hypovolemic shock is the most probable. This implies fluid responsiveness, and a bolus should be administered as a first step in order to stabilize the patient. In some patients, retroperitoneal hemorrhage can be seen using bedside ultrasound. It can occur after coronary angiography following the use of the femoral artery. The best diagnostic modality for retroperitoneal hemorrhage, however, is CTA of the abdomen.

9. **Correct Answer: C.**
Rationale: In this patient, hemorrhagic or hypovolemic shock is suspected. With ultrasound examination, a hemothorax or intra-abdominal bleeding can easily be excluded. However, this patient underwent coronary angiography via a femoral artery access. Besides coronary dissection and tamponade, hemorrhage from the puncture side with retroperitoneal bleeding is another procedural complication, which may lead to hemorrhagic shock. Besides initial volume resuscitation, vasopressor support may be needed in order to stabilize blood pressure. Compression of the puncture side may help control bleeding. Laboratory values including hemoglobin, hematocrit, lactate, and coagulation factors are needed to confirm or refute the diagnosis of hemorrhagic shock. If the patient is stabilized, one should proceed with further diagnostic and/or therapeutic tools such as CTA to identify the retroperitoneal bleeding. In case of hemodynamic instability and failure to stabilize the patient, immediate transfer to the operating room for emergency vascular surgery is indicated.

10. **Correct Answer: C**
Rationale: This patient is prone to suffer from an abdominal compartment syndrome, which equates to an increase in infradiaphragmatic resistance to VR. In patients who are oliguric, it is always crucial to exclude other causes of acute renal failure such as postrenal obstruction like an obstructed urinary catheter, which is easily done at the bedside with ultrasound. Abdominal imaging is also important to exclude higher amounts of intra-abdominal fluid/blood, which may contribute to abdominal compartment syndrome. Diagnosis of intra-abdominal hypertension is made by measuring the intra-abdominal pressure via the installation of 25-mL sterile saline into the bladder in supine, sedated, under neuromuscular blockade, and mechanically ventilated patient. Values are taken at end expiration. Abdominal compartment syndrome is confirmed if the intra-abdominal pressure is above 20 cm H_2O and organ dysfunction persists. Reduced leg somatic oximetry signals compared to cerebral and upper extremity is typical of abdominal compartment syndrome because the lower extremity venous congestion will result in increased near-infrared absorption signal (23,24).

11. **Correct Answer: A.**
Rationale: Increasing PEEP to 10 cm H_2O is the appropriate next step. In the presence of increased intra-abdominal pressure, it is important to optimize ventilation and alveolar recruitment using transmural airway

pressures: $P_{plateau}$ (transmural) = $P_{plateau}$ − intra-abdominal pressure. Therefore, protective lung ventilation is still guaranteed with a PEEP of 10 cm H_2O and will be the first option. Drainage of pleural effusion is another option, but in this patient, pleural effusions are small (estimates of the left side: 300 mL, right side: 400 mL), with no sign of atelectasis. We use lung ultrasound to personalize PEEP: We would give PEEP until the atelectasis disappears and stops if there is reduction in cardiac output estimated using end-tidal carbon dioxide (54).

12. **Correct Answer: B.**
Rationale: ARDS with secondary RV failure. According to the Berlin definition for the diagnosis of ARDS, a CXR or computed tomography is indicated to show bilateral opacities. In ARDS, B-lines can be present; however, they are not specific for pulmonary edema and could be associated with increased lung permeability.

13. **Correct Answer: C.**
Rationale: Distributive/septic shock with ventilator-associated pneumonia is the most common finding in this situation. The most important intervention if a distributive shock is suspected is the rapid use of broad-spectrum antibiotics. A small fluid challenge could be considered; however, in the presence of hypoxemia, vasopressors might be more appropriate.

14. **Correct Answer: D.**
Rationale: CCUS is limited in the diagnosis of pulmonary embolism because chronic conditions such as chronic obstructive pulmonary disease can be associated with pulmonary hypertension. In those patients, typically, RV hypertrophy is present. In any doubt, computed tomography of the chest should be considered.

15. **Correct Answer: D.**
Rationale: With a normal CXR, a right-to-left shunt needs to be ruled out. The bicaval view is the best view to rule out an atrial septal defect or patent foramen ovale. Ebstein anomaly can be associated with atrial septal defects. Most desaturation is associated with abnormal lung ultrasound. If the lung ultrasound is normal, a cardiogenic cause should be considered.

16. **Correct Answer: B.**
Rationale: Increasing PEEP will further increase intrathoracic pressure and, therefore, RV afterload. The right-to-left shunt will worsen with increased afterload. In such situations, increasing left-sided pressure with vasoactive agents may reverse the right-to-left shunt to a left-to-right shunt.

17. **Correct Answer: C.**
Rationale: In supine patients undergoing cardiopulmonary resuscitation, this is often the easiest and fastest four-chamber view to obtain. However, in order to rule out an MI, the short-axis view at the midpapillary level will allow interrogation of all the coronary artery territory. This will not be possible using a subcostal view.

18. **Correct Answer: D.**
Rationale: A lung point is a transition point between a normal sliding lung and the absence of sliding lung resulting most commonly from a pneumothorax. In the absence of all the other signs, the lung point should be searched carefully to diagnose a pneumothorax. All the other elements can be used to exclude a pneumothorax.

19. **Correct Answer: B.**
Rationale: In a situation where the VR will be compromised resulting in resistance to VR, the flow in the hepatic vein can be almost absent. In abdominal compartment syndrome, typically, the flow from the lower extremity and the abdominal organs will be significantly reduced. This explains the fact that typically the HVF is significantly reduced compared to the pulmonary venous flow (19). In those patients, the use of regional NIRS will show a significant reduction in the lower extremity values compared to the upper extremity, confirming the diagnosis (23,24).

20. **Correct Answer: D.**
Rationale: The patient has a dilated RV and TR suggestive of an acute pulmonary embolism. However, one cannot exclude a chronic underlying pulmonary problem. In addition, septic shock can cause RV dysfunction. Therefore, it is more prudent to exclude pulmonary embolism using computed tomography while maintaining blood pressure with vasoactive support once fluid responsiveness is ruled out and broad-spectrum antibiotics administered.

19 Transesophageal Echocardiography for Congenital Heart Disease in the Adult

Pablo Motta, Carolyn Taylor, and Wanda C. Miller-Hance

The spectrum of congenital heart disease (CHD) seen in adults varies widely, ranging from mild anomalies with no clinical repercussions to extremely complex malformations. Advances in medical and surgical care over the past several decades have dramatically extended life expectancy and increased survival rates in patients with CHD (1). This is the case even for those afflicted by the most severe congenital defects (2). The improvements in clinical care have led to an increasing and aging population of affected individuals (3,4). It is well recognized that at the current time, adults living with CHD outnumber affected children. As such, CHD is no longer to be considered a disease exclusive to childhood but a condition of relevance to all who provide perioperative care to this population, regardless of patient age.

Echocardiography represents the primary noninvasive imaging modality in the assessment of CHD and has significantly contributed to improvements in patient care. Other imaging techniques such as cardiac magnetic resonance and chest tomography are usually considered complementary to echocardiography. As technology evolved, the transesophageal imaging approach extended the applications of echocardiography to CHD as has been well documented in the literature (5). By allowing the acquisition of structural and functional information that is often not obtainable by transthoracic imaging, this modality has been invaluable to patient care. Transesophageal echocardiography (TEE) has been of particular benefit to those individuals with suboptimal transthoracic windows, as it significantly enhances the detailed characterization of congenital defects and the evaluation of hemodynamics. In the intraoperative setting, significant contributions of TEE in CHD include the assessment of the surgical intervention, detection of residual pathology, and surgical guidance if an immediate revision is warranted. TEE also plays a vital role in the cardiac catheterization and electrophysiology laboratories as an adjunct to therapeutic interventions and in the critical care setting.

This chapter reviews relevant aspects of CHD with emphasis on the application of TEE in the affected adult. Although many of the congenital cardiovascular malformations can be examined using the standard TEE views outlined in the comprehensive guidelines by the Society of Cardiovascular Anesthesiologists (SCA) and American Society of Echocardiography (ASE) (6), in some cases, the detailed examination of these lesions and associated hemodynamic perturbations requires alternative or modified planes of interrogation. This issue, along with the fact that these recommendations were primarily aimed for adults with structurally normal hearts, subsequently led to the development of guidelines for the comprehensive TEE evaluation in this unique congenital patient population (refer to the corresponding section later in the text) (7). These modified cross sections/sweeps are described as relevant to the pathology being discussed. For this discussion and specifically regarding suggested TEE imaging planes, we assume the more common anatomic arrangement of situs solitus and levocardia for each of the defects.

INCIDENCE AND PREVALENCE OF CONGENITAL HEART DISEASE IN THE ADULT POPULATION

CHD represents the most common major congenital malformation, occurring in approximately 1% of live births worldwide. This figure does not include the bicuspid aortic valve (Bic AV), occurring in 2% to 3% of the general population. At birth, the most common lesion is that of a ventricular septal defect (VSD). Other relatively common congenital pathologies include atrial septal defects (ASDs), pulmonary (pulmonic) stenosis (PS), and persistent patent ductus arteriosus (PDA). Beyond these defects, other less prevalent pathologies include tetralogy of Fallot (TOF), aortic stenosis (AS), coarctation of the aorta (CoA), atrioventricular septal defect (AVSD), and transposition of the great arteries (TGA) (refer to Table 19.1). Not surprisingly, the highest childhood survival rate in CHD occurs among those with simple lesions or milder forms of disease. However, overall outcomes in those with complex pathologies have improved significantly over the past several decades, representing a challenge to adult health care providers who look after these patients. Progress in CHD care is attributed to factors such as prenatal diagnosis, enhancements in diagnostic techniques including echocardiography, advances in medical and surgical strategies, definitive surgical repair at an earlier age, and overall improvements in intraoperative/postoperative management.

TABLE 19.1 Congenital Heart Disease in the Adult: Physiology, Epidemiology, Associated Pathology, Treatment, and Prognosis

Cardiac Pathology	Physiology	Epidemiology/Prevalence	Associated Lesions	Treatment/Prognosis
Aortic stenosis (AS)	• Obstruction to systemic blood flow • Increased LV afterload • LVH and decreased LV diastolic compliance • Myocardial supply-demand mismatch (possible ischemia)	• Bicuspid AV: most common congenital anomaly (2% of the population) and most common cause of AS in age < 65 y	• VSD • PDA • Ascending aortopathy	• For severe disease, transcatheter and surgical approaches available • Valvuloplasty associated with high incidence of reintervention (>25% in adult) • AV and ascending aortic surgery among the most common ACHD procedures
Atrial septal defect (ASD)	• Left-to-right shunt • Right-sided volume overload • Late symptoms (CHF, atrial arrhythmias, and rare PHTN)	• 30% of ACHD • PFO is present in ~25% of adults.	• Secundum: MV prolapse and/or regurgitation • Primum: cleft MV, ± regurgitation • Sinus venosus: anomalous pulmonary venous return	• Secundum defect may be amenable to transcatheter device closure. • Surgical closure if defect not suitable for percutaneous intervention • Treated 10-y survival 95%
Coarctation of the aorta	• Obstruction to systemic blood flow • Proximal hypertension • Increased LV afterload • LVH and decreased diastolic compliance • Collateral circulation	• 5%-8% of ACHD	• Bicuspid AV • VSD • MV anomalies • Left-sided obstructive lesions	• Balloon dilation ± stent placement vs surgery • If untreated, mortality 80% at 50 y
Congenital coronary artery anomalies	• Potential coronary ischemia • CHF if large fistula	• <1%	• Isolated lesion or seen in CHD (D-TGA, TOF, and other complex pathologies)	• Not always requires intervention • Coronary reimplantation and/or unroofing most common surgery • If occlusion of fistula indicated, transcatheter and/or surgical intervention • No long-term follow-up reported

(*continued*)

TABLE 19.1 Congenital Heart Disease in the Adult: Physiology, Epidemiology, Associated Pathology, Treatment, and Prognosis (*continued*)

Cardiac Pathology	Physiology	Epidemiology/Prevalence	Associated Lesions	Treatment/Prognosis
Congenitally corrected transposition	• Asymptomatic or symptoms related to intracardiac shunting and/or outflow obstruction • Presence or absence of cyanosis dependent on associated pathology • Adult symptoms: TR, RV failure, and CHB	• Rare lesion in the adult patient (accounts for ~0.5% of all CHD)	• VSD • Pulmonary outflow obstruction • TV anomalies (Ebstein like) • Atrioventricular block	• May require interventions such as closure of intracardiac communication(s), relief of outflow obstruction, TV repair or replacement, pacemaker insertion • Cardiac transplantation (if severe RV—systemic ventricular failure) • 15-y survival ~60%
D-Transposition	• Parallel circulation requiring intercirculatory mixing • Cyanotic lesion	• Most common form of CHD presenting in the neonatal period • High mortality if untreated early in life • Most adults have undergone a surgical intervention in childhood.	• VSD (20%) • LVOT obstruction • Coronary artery anomalies	• Post–atrial baffle procedure (Mustard or Senning) may require interventions for baffle leak/obstruction, TR, atrial arrhythmias, or RV (systemic) failure. • Post ASO infrequent need for reintervention • 20-y survival after ASO ~70%
Ebstein anomaly	• Wide disease spectrum • TR (variable severity) • Can be asymptomatic • Right heart failure • Atrial arrhythmias • If associated PFO/ASD can develop cyanosis • RV dysfunction	• Occurs in 0.5% of all patients with CHD	• PFO • ASD • Accessory atrioventricular connections	• TV repair/replacement • ASD closure • May require antiarrhythmic therapy and/or electrophysiologic evaluation and treatment • 10-y survival ~84%
Patent ductus arteriosus (PDA)	• Left-to-right shunt • Left-sided volume overload • Symptoms and PHTN depend on the size of the PDA	• 8% of ACHD	• Isolated or within the context of complex CHD • Bicuspid AV	• Transcatheter closure • Surgical (open vs VATS) • Treated 10-y survival ~95%
Pulmonary (pulmonic) stenosis	• Obstruction to pulmonary blood flow • Increased RV afterload • RVH with decreased diastolic compliance • Acyanosis unless severe and associated ASD/VSD • If severe, may result in CHF	• 10% of ACHD	• PFO • ASD (20%) • VSD • Obstructive subpulmonary hypertrophy	• Valvuloplasty/surgical valvotomy is highly effective. • Treated 25-y survival ~95%

Single ventricle	• "Passive" pulmonary circulation • Single systemic ventricle (left or right morphology) • Acyanosis after Fontan palliation in most cases except if fenestration present	• Group includes different pathologies.	• Depends on the anatomy	• Survival into adulthood requires palliative intervention(s) in childhood in most cases and eventual Fontan procedure. • "Older" Fontan modifications may require revision (in-hospital mortality ~11%). • Maze procedure for arrhythmias/pacemaker for atrioventricular synchrony and antiarrhythmic therapy • Potential long-term problems: protein-loosing enteropathy, plastic bronchitis, liver disease • Cardiac transplantation
Tetralogy of Fallot (TOF)	• Obstruction to RV outflow • Intracardiac shunting (left-to-right, right-to-left, or bidirectional) • Cyanosis usually present in childhood • Increased RV afterload • RVH, decreased RV diastolic compliance • Cyanotic spells associated with infundibular spasm in children	• Most common form of cyanotic CHD • Several variants (eg, pulmonary atresia with multiple aortopulmonary collaterals, absent pulmonary valve syndrome)	• Right aortic arch (25%) • PFO or ASD (Pentalogy of Fallot) • Persistent L-SVC to coronary sinus • Discontinuous PAs • Coronary artery anomalies	• Most surviving adults have undergone prior palliative or corrective procedures. • Long-term issues: pulmonary regurgitation, pulmonary valve/RVOT problems, residual shunts, RV dilation and dysfunction, LV dysfunction • Interventions in the adult frequently required (eg, pulmonary valve replacement, RV-PA conduit changes) • Treated 30-y survival ~86%-90%
Ventricular septal defect	• Left-to-right shunt • Left-sided volume overload • Early congestive symptoms and PHTN if defect large and long-standing	• Most common form of CHD in children • High incidence of spontaneous closure in childhood • Isolated VSD rare in the adult (10%-15% of ACHD) • Untreated defects in adults almost always small in size • Muscular defect may be secondary to septal infarct.	• Bicuspid AV • Coarctation of Ao • Occasionally RVOT obstruction (double-chambered RV) or subaortic membrane	• Surgical closure • Some defects (usually muscular VSDs and some perimembranous) may be amenable to device closure. • Residual defects associated with complex CHD • Treated 10-y survival, no PHTN—96%

ACHD, adult congenital heart disease; Ao, aorta; ASO, arterial switch operation; AV, aortic valve; CHB, complete heart block; CHD, congenital heart disease; CHF, congestive heart failure; D-TGA, d-transposition of the great arteries; L-SVC, left superior vena cava; LV, left ventricle; LVH, left ventricular hypertrophy; LVOT, left ventricular outflow tract; MV, mitral valve; PA, pulmonary artery; PFO, patent foramen ovale; PHTN, pulmonary hypertension; RV, right ventricle; RVH, right ventricular hypertrophy; RVOT, right ventricular outflow tract; TR, tricuspid regurgitation; TV, tricuspid valve; VATS, video-assisted thoracoscopic surgery; VSD, ventricular septal defect.

The prevalence of CHD is estimated at approximately 4 per 1,000 living adults, of which 30% is of moderate severity and nearly 10% represents complex disease. In the United States, this accounts for approximately 2 million adults (8). It is anticipated that the number of adults with congenital cardiovascular malformations will continue to increase worldwide, as well as the complexity of this patient group (9). This group of patients is known as the "adult with CHD (ACHD)," also referred to as the "grown-up with CHD" (GUCH) population.

CLASSIFICATION OF CONGENITAL HEART DISEASE

Given the broad spectrum of pathologies in CHD, several classification schemes have been proposed to facilitate our understanding of the defects and their associated physiologic impact. Malformations can be characterized, for example, according to the disease severity, presence or absence of cyanosis, or primary physiologic alteration.

Based on Severity of Disease

Defects have been stratified according to their severity or level of complexity into simple, moderate severity, and complex defects. This classification scheme has been utilized for recommendations regarding patient care, estimation of long-term problems, and expectation of potential outcomes. Intracardiac communications in their isolated forms typically represent simple defects. Mild PS and small PDAs are also considered simple forms of CHD. Moderate defects include, for example, CoA, TOF, and Ebstein anomaly. Complex pathology comprises all forms of cyanotic CHD, lesions associated with multiple concomitant defects, and single ventricles or univentricular hearts.

Based on the Presence or Absence of Cyanosis

In this scheme, congenital cardiac malformations are classified into acyanotic or cyanotic lesions based on whether the native physiology results in cyanosis. Conditions associated with cyanosis are usually characterized by restrictive pulmonary blood flow (in the presence of intracardiac shunting) or complete arterial and venous admixture. Cyanosis is less likely to occur in individuals with pulmonary overcirculation secondary to isolated intracardiac communications.

Based on the Physiology of the Defect

This classification algorithm based on the physiologic spectrum of CHD comprises four major categories: shunts, obstructions to either pulmonary or systemic blood flow, regurgitant pathologies, and mixed lesions. Shunt lesions can occur at the intracardiac or extracardiac levels. The direction and magnitude of shunting depend on the size of the communication and the relative resistances of the pulmonary and systemic vascular beds. Obstructive lesions can affect the inflow or outflow of blood and vary widely in severity. Regurgitant disease is rarely found in isolation and is frequently secondary to the primary pathology. In mixed lesions, which account for a significant number of cyanotic heart defects, there is mixing of the systemic and pulmonary venous returns.

GUIDELINES FOR TRANSESOPHAGEAL ECHOCARDIOGRAPHY IN CONGENITAL HEART DISEASE

The ASE document addressing guidelines for comprehensive TEE imaging in CHD describes techniques, protocols, and three-dimensional (3D)-TEE methods in this population (7). The reader is referred to this publication as an essential reference on the subject.

Key points to be emphasized from the comprehensive TEE imaging document in CHD include the following:

- The suggested imaging protocol includes 28 two-dimensional (2D) tomographic views. Many of these represent cross sections previously described in the TEE guidelines document by the SCA/ASE published in 2013, with modifications and additions given the congenital focus of the publication.
- TEE views outlined are to be regarded as a foundation, given the fact that numerous variants and a wide spectrum of abnormalities in CHD frequently necessitate modification of these key views and/or additional nonstandard views.
- TEE imaging in CHD relies on examining structures rather than previously defined views.

- There is a need not only for single-beat recordings in congenital TEE assessment but also for multiple-beat loops and sweeps that display the anatomic and spatial relationships among structures.
- Recommendations note the use of a combination of modalities that include 2D imaging and Doppler interrogation (spectral and color flow) in multiple views and the use of 3D imaging, as indicated, in evaluating any abnormalities.
- Consideration for the use of TEE, particularly during (1) transcatheter closure of septal defects for procedural guidance, measurement of defects, and visualization of hardware; (2) assessment of atrioventricular valves; and (3) evaluation of the left ventricular (LV) outflow/aortic valve (AV).

The ASE document on TEE screening for structural heart interventions also provides an outstanding guideline for acquiring essential information before interventional procedures, including those relevant to CHD (10). It should also serve as an excellent reference on the topic.

INDICATIONS FOR TRANSESOPHAGEAL ECHOCARDIOGRAPHY IN THE ADULT WITH CONGENITAL HEART DISEASE

The indications for TEE in patients with CHD fall within the major categories of (1) diagnostic use, (2) perioperative assessment, (3) procedural guidance in the cardiac catheterization/electrophysiology laboratories, and (4) critical care unit assessment. Regardless of the indication for the study, when performing TEE, it is essential to review in advance the details of the medical history, particularly as it pertains to the initial anatomy and prior interventions as many adult patients have complex pathology and have undergone multiple prior interventions. A review of transthoracic studies and any prior TEE images, as well as any other imaging examinations (eg, chest radiography, angiography, chest tomography, and cardiac magnetic resonance), is imperative as this facilitates an understanding of the anatomy and assists the echocardiographer regarding what to anticipate.

Transesophageal Echocardiography for Diagnostic Applications

Transthoracic echocardiography (TTE) can be suboptimal in adult patients due to poor windows related to obesity, muscle mass, or prior cardiothoracic interventions. This contrasts with young children, where TTE is diagnostic in most cases and only in rare instances is TEE used for this purpose. Particularly in the adult congenital population, TEE plays an important diagnostic role. The transesophageal imaging approach may also be superior in the evaluation of specific pathologies such as endocarditis and aortic root abscess, for exclusion of intracardiac thrombus prior to cardioversion or to identify an embolic source, for assessment of small intracardiac communications, anomalous pulmonary venous connections, aortic root/ascending aorta (Asc Ao) pathology, after complex interventions such as intracardiac baffles and Fontan procedures, conduits, and in the evaluation of prosthetic heart valves.

Transesophageal Echocardiography During Cardiothoracic Surgery

Imaging during cardiac surgery represents the most common indication for TEE in CHD. Extensive experience has demonstrated the ability of intraoperative imaging to improve the quality of the surgical interventions in these patients. As such, TEE has become the standard of care in centers that specialize in CHD, consistent with the indications outlined by various clinical practice guidelines.

Intraoperative imaging provides detailed anatomic and hemodynamic information prior to the planned surgical procedure and assists in the assessment of the quality of the repair. A major impact of TEE in CHD is seen when new prebypass information alters the planned surgical intervention or when the postbypass examination prompts immediate revision of hemodynamically significant defects. Intraoperative echocardiography in the congenital population, whether via the epicardial, transesophageal, or combined approaches, can alter the surgical plan in approximately 1% to 13% of cases and prompt a return-to-cardiopulmonary bypass (CPB) rate of 2% to 7%. Major impact of TEE is more likely to occur in younger patients with CHD, during reoperations, and in those undergoing valve repairs and complex outflow tract reconstructions. Failure to address significant residual pathology has been associated with high morbidity in the CHD population and, in some cases, accounts for perioperative mortality. Additional benefits of intraoperative TEE in patients with CHD include the recognition of complications associated with cannulation during CPB, detection of intracardiac air and facilitating cardiac de-airing, assessment of ventricular loading conditions and myocardial performance, detection of myocardial ischemia, and identification of problems associated with weaning from bypass.

Over the past several years, the applications of 3D-TEE have been extended to various congenital pathologies, including septal defects, valvar lesions, outflow tracts, and complex abnormalities of cardiac connections (11). The additional diagnostic information provided by the 3D technology has been shown to enhance 2D data in intraoperative clinical decision-making.

Transesophageal Echocardiography in the Cardiac Catheterization and Electrophysiology Laboratory

The most common indications for catheter-based interventions in the ACHD are valvular disease, closure of communications (intracardiac/vascular), and relief of vascular obstruction. Benefits include the acquisition of detailed anatomic and hemodynamic data before and during interventions, guidance by real-time evaluation of catheter placement across valves and vessels, immediate assessment of the procedural results, and monitoring for catheter-related complications (12). Transesophageal imaging can also facilitate transseptal puncture, catheter manipulation, and guide interventions in the electrophysiology laboratory. As the applications of 3D-TEE continue to evolve, this technology is likely to provide further benefits to the care of patients with CHD undergoing catheter-based interventions by enhancing the characterization of anatomic defects and providing guidance and monitoring during these procedures (13).

Transesophageal Echocardiography in the Critical Care Unit

In the critical care setting, TEE has been shown to be useful during evaluation of the hemodynamically unstable adult patient, particularly in those with limited TEE windows. Settings where TEE can be of particular benefit include in the assessment of pericardial fluid, endocarditis, cardiac tamponade physiology, and valve dysfunction. It can also provide additional information during the management of patients undergoing circulatory support strategies such as extracorporeal membrane oxygenation and in those with ventricular assist devices (VADs). TEE benefits in the critical care environment also include the assessment of volume status and ventricular function.

SELECTED CONGENITAL HEART DEFECTS

The section that follows provides an overview of selected congenital heart defects. A brief discussion of anatomy, pathophysiology, and management is presented as a background, followed by the general TEE evaluation of each anomaly. This information is summarized in Tables 19.1 and 19.2.

ATRIAL SEPTAL DEFECT

Anatomy

Defects that result in atrial level shunting are termed *atrial septal defects*. This may not necessarily imply a deficiency of the atrial septum itself. An overview of the embryologic processes involved in atrial septation, as depicted in Figure 19.1, facilitates our understanding of atrial septal anatomy and atrial communications that persist after atrial septation. Four main types of ASDs include ostium secundum, ostium primum, sinus venosus, and coronary sinus defects (Figure 19.2A). ASDs account for approximately 30% of all cases of CHD detected in adults and, in general, are more common in females.

Ostium secundum defects are typically located in the central portion of the interatrial septum in the region of the fossa ovalis and account for 70% of all atrial communications. Associated abnormalities include mitral valve prolapse and mitral regurgitation.

Ostium primum defects (also known as partial AVSDs) are located in the inferior aspect of the interatrial septum. They account for approximately 20% of ASDs and are associated with a cleft in the anterior mitral leaflet and consequent mitral regurgitation. This defect is considered within the spectrum of AVSDs and can be seen in patients with Down syndrome.

Sinus venosus defects occur posteriorly, adjacent to the entrance of the superior vena cava (SVC) or inferior vena cava (IVC) into the right atrium (RA). The superior defect is the most common type. They account for 5% to 10% of ASDs. In this lesion, straddling of the caval vein over the interatrial septum is commonly seen. These defects are often associated with partial anomalous pulmonary venous drainage from the right

TABLE 19.2 TEE Imaging Views and Postsurgical Assessment in Congenital Heart Disease

Lesion	TEE Planes and Information Provided	Postsurgical TEE Assessment
Aortic stenosis	ME AV SAX: AV morphology, valve motion ME AV LAX, ME 5-Ch, and DTG 5-Ch: valve morphology and motion, valvar regurgitation, Ao root size, subaortic and supra-aortic anatomy ME 5-Ch, TG LAX, and DTG 5-Ch: peak gradient across obstruction ME 4-Ch, ME 2-Ch, and TG Mid Pap SAX: LV hypertrophy and function	Residual/recurrent obstruction, Ao regurgitation, bioprosthetic/mechanical valve function, perivalvar leak (if prosthetic valve), ventricular function After Ross procedure: neoAV valve obstruction/regurgitation, function of right ventricular homograft, ventricular function (global and segmental)
Atrial septal defect (ASD)	ME 4-Ch: secundum and primum defects, mitral valve anatomy (prolapse)/competence ME bicaval: secundum and sinus venosus defect TG basal SAX: mitral valve cleft ME Rt pulm veins and Lt pulm veins: pulmonary venous return	Residual shunts Mitral stenosis/regurgitation Obstruction of pulmonary venous flows (sinus venosus ASD) Ventricular function
Coarctation of the aorta	UE Ao Arch SAX and LAX views of descending thoracic aorta and Ao Arch (if visible): posterior shelf, aliased color-flow Doppler (suboptimal angle of interrogation for spectral Doppler) ME 4-Ch, ME 2-Ch, ME AV LAX, and TG Mid Pap SAX: LV wall thickness and function, mitral valve morphology and function, AV, subvalvular and supravalvular Ao obstruction	Residual gradient, recoarctation, Ao aneurysm formation
Congenital coronary artery anomalies	ME AV SAX and ME LAX views in diastole	Assess repair (identify new coronary origin, unroofing, pathway from Ao to coronary arteries) Document flow in the coronary vessels by color Doppler Ventricular function (global and segmental)
Congenitally corrected transposition	ME 4-Ch, ME 2-Ch, ME 5-Ch, and TG Mid Pap SAX: ventricular morphology and function, TV function and associated lesions ME LAX, ME RV I-O, DTG RVOT, and DTG 5-Ch: pulmonary obstruction	Following double switch operation: Atrial baffle portion: baffle leaks, obstruction of venous pathways, AVV competence, function of systemic ventricle Arterial switch portion: outflow obstruction Residual intracardiac shunts
D-Transposition	ME 4-Ch: AVV regurgitation, associated intracardiac shunts, ventricular function ME 4-Ch and ME bicaval: systemic and pulmonary venous baffles TG Mid Pap SAX: ventricular function (global and segmental) ME 5-Ch, ME LAX, TG LAX, DTG RVOT, and DTG 5-Ch: ventriculoarterial connections and great artery anastomoses after arterial switch operation UE PA and modified views allowing visualization of pulmonary arteries	After Senning/Mustard procedure: baffle leaks, obstruction of venous pathways, function of systemic RV, AVV competence After arterial switch operation: supravalvar (Ao/pulmonary) stenosis or regurgitation, LV function Residual shunts Associated lesions
Ebstein anomaly	ME 4-Ch, ME Mod bicaval TV, and ME RV I-O: evaluation of TV (apical displacement and leaflet anatomy/mobility) 3D-TEE extremely useful ME 4-Ch and TG Mid Pap SAX: ventricular function	Residual TV insufficiency, TV stenosis RV size and function LV function

(continued)

TABLE 19.2 TEE Imaging Views and Postsurgical Assessment in Congenital Heart Disease (*continued*)

Lesion	TEE Planes and Information Provided	Postsurgical TEE Assessment
Patent ductus arteriosus	May be difficult to visualize by TEE, ductal flow might be detected in the UE PA, ME Asc Ao SAX, and ME RV I-O views by the presence of abnormal continuous flow into the PA by Doppler	Residual shunt, biventricular function
Pulmonary (pulmonic) stenosis	UE PA and ME Asc Ao SAX: evaluation of pulmonary valve, main PA and proximal branches, gradient assessment ME RV I-O and DTG RVOT: evaluation of outflow tract and gradient estimation	Residual pulmonary outflow tract obstruction, pulmonary regurgitation, RV size and function
Single ventricle	ME 4-Ch, ME 2-Ch, ME LAX, ME bicaval, TG Mid Pap SAX, TG RV I-O, DTG 5-Ch, DTG RVOT, and modified planes: atrioventricular and ventriculoarterial connections, outflow tracts ME 4-Ch: AVV competence Modified views as needed depending on the anatomy	Post-Fontan: cavopulmonary connection, Fontan baffle (patency/leak), Ao regurgitation, systemic outflow tract obstruction, AVV competence, ventricular function, adequacy of ASD Evaluation of thrombi (atrial or within Fontan pathway)
Tetralogy of Fallot	ME RV I-O, UE PA, and DTG RVOT: evaluation of RVOT, pulmonary valve, and estimation of outflow gradient ME AV LAX and DTG LAX: VSD and Ao override ME SAX, ME 4-Ch, and TG SAX: location and extension of VSD and additional VSDs ME AV SAX and ME AV LAX with color Doppler: evaluation of coronary arteries	Residual RVOT obstruction, pulmonary valve or conduit stenosis, residual shunts, ventricular function (RV and LV), Ao regurgitation
Ventricular septal defect (VSD)	ME 4-Ch, ME AV SAX, ME LAX, ME RV I-O and TG SAX (basal, Mid Pap and apical): perimembranous defect, presence of ventricular septal aneurysm, inlet and muscular VSDs, chamber sizes ME AV LAX and DTG LAX: evaluation of AV for regurgitation and prolapse/herniation	Residual shunts, AVV and semilunar valve competence, ventricular function

Ao, aortic; Asc Ao, ascending aorta; AV, aortic valve; AVV, atrioventricular valve; Ch, chamber; DTG, deep transgastric; I-O, inflow-outflow; LAX, long-axis; Lf, left; LV, left ventricle; ME, midesophageal; Mid Pap, mid papillary; PA, pulmonary artery; Pulm, pulmonary; Rt, right; RV, right ventricle; RVOT, right ventricular outflow tract; SAX, short-axis; SWMA, segmental wall motion abnormalities; TEE, transesophageal echocardiography; TG, transgastric; TV, tricuspid valve; UE, upper esophageal.

lung due to a deficiency of the wall that normally separates the pulmonary veins and the left atrium (LA), leading to pulmonary vein unroofing.

Coronary sinus defects (also called "unroofed coronary sinus") result from a communication between the coronary sinus (coronary sinus septum) and the LA. These defects are relatively rare (<2% of ASDs) and frequently occur in association with other malformations. They are typically seen within the context of a persistent left superior vena cava (L-SVC) draining to an unroofed coronary sinus. In this setting, the orifice of the coronary sinus is usually significantly dilated.

Pathophysiology

The physiologic consequence of an ASD is determined by the degree of shunting (predominant direction is usually left-to-right; Figure 19.2B). The size of the defect, ventricular compliances, and pulmonary artery (PA) pressures determine the magnitude of the shunt. A large defect leading to pulmonary overcirculation results in right-sided diastolic volume overload manifested as RA, right ventricular (RV), and PA dilation. Over time, atrial arrhythmias and heart failure can develop. Mild-to-moderate elevations of PA pressure can

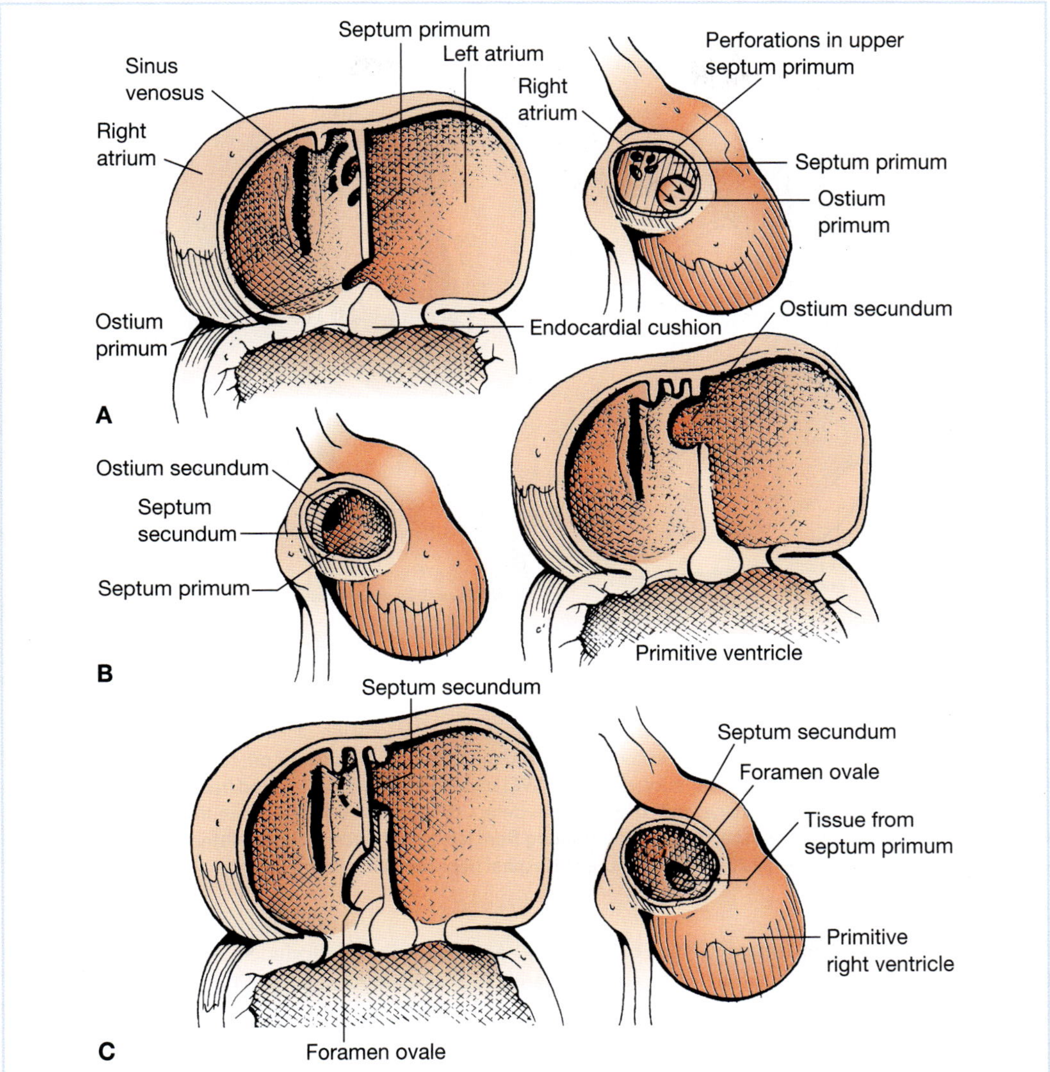

FIGURE 19.1 Stages of atrial septation. A: Atrial septation begins as early as the fifth week of gestation. As the septum primum grows inferiorly toward the endocardial cushions, the ostium secundum (labeled as perforations in the upper septum primum) forms in the posterior portion of the septum primum. Once the ostium secundum is formed, it ensures blood flow across the atrial septum in the fetus. After that, the septum primum completes its growth and becomes continuous with the developing endocardial cushions of the atrioventricular junction (arrows). B: The septum secundum develops parallel and to the right of the septum primum. It forms an incomplete partition. C: The remaining opening in the septum secundum is known as the *foramen ovale*. It is covered by a flap valve formed from septum primum tissue. Usually, this flap valve closes after birth when pressure in the left atrium increases, exceeding right atrial pressure.

be seen in older patients; however, severe pulmonary hypertension rarely occurs. Adults can remain asymptomatic, and an ASD may represent an incidental finding on echocardiography.

Management

Published guidelines by various professional organizations have outlined recommendations for closure of ASDs (14,15). Most patients with large defects undergo surgery. Selected ostium secundum defects may be amenable to percutaneous device closure in the cardiac catheterization laboratory. Several occluder devices

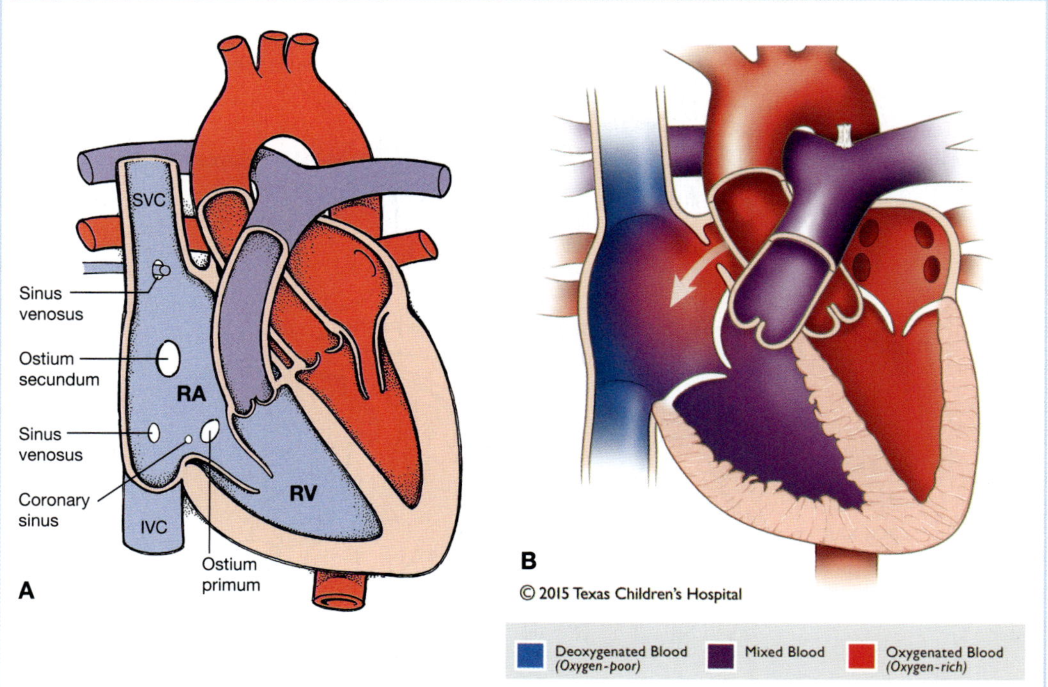

FIGURE 19.2 Atrial septal defects. A: The illustration depicts the typical location of the various interatrial communication as follows: centrally located ostium secundum defect, inferiorly located ostium primum defect, sinus venosus defect, near the entrance of either the superior vena cava (SVC) or inferior vena cava (IVC) and frequently associated with anomalous pulmonary venous drainage, and coronary sinus defect. B: The graphic displays a secundum-type atrial septal defect, and the arrow shows the usual direction of shunting from left-to-right across the interatrial communication. RA, right atrium; RV, right ventricle. (© 2015 Texas Children's Hospital [reprinted with permission].)

are currently available for different types of ASDs (eg, Amplatzer Septal Occluder, Gore Cardioform ASD Occluder) (16,17). A combination of fluoroscopy and TEE guidance usually guides placement of these devices. However, using 3D-TEE guidance may limit or even preclude the need for fluoroscopy. Intracardiac echocardiography offers an alternative to TEE imaging in some patients, usually those of the adolescent or adult age range. Suitability for transcatheter device occlusion of secundum ASDs includes the size of the defect and the presence of adequate rims of surrounding atrial septal tissue. Transcatheter device closure may also be considered in the patient with a patent foramen ovale (PFO) and a history of a cerebrovascular event, aiming to alter the risk of potential paradoxical emboli. Device closure of other types of interatrial communications is usually not favored due to the presence of critical structures surrounding the defect that could be compromised by the septal occluder.

Transesophageal Echocardiographic Evaluation

The TEE evaluation of the interatrial septum and atrial septal communications should follow established guidelines specifically developed for this assessment. Suggested cross sections for a focused examination of a *secundum ASD* include midesophageal (ME) four-chamber (4-Ch) (Figure 19.3; Video 19.1), ME bicaval, ME AV short-axis (SAX), ME RV inflow-outflow (I-O), and deep transgastric (DTG) atrial septal views (equivalent to ME bicaval view, obtained at ~90°). The region of the fossa ovalis and the flap of a PFO can be optimally imaged from the ME bicaval view. Additional cross sections may be useful in the assessment of other atrial level communications and their frequently associated pathology. In the case of a *primum ASD*, the ME 4-Ch view is diagnostic (Figure 19.4; Video 19.2), other useful views include the ME two-chamber (2-Ch), ME long-axis (LAX), and TG basal SAX views (for cleft mitral valve); for a *sinus venosus defect*, the ME bicaval view is notably helpful (Figure 19.5; Video 19.3) and cross sections that allow for imaging of

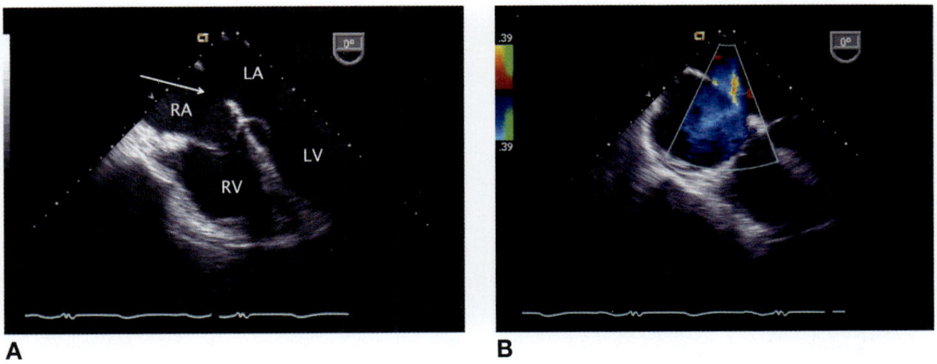

FIGURE 19.3 Secundum atrial septal defect. A: Midesophageal four-chamber view showing a moderate-size central defect in the atrial septum (arrow), typical of a secundum atrial septal defect. B: Corresponding color-flow Doppler image depicting left-to-right atrial level shunting (blue flow). LA, left atrium; LV, left ventricle; RA, right atrium; RV, right ventricle.

the pulmonary veins (ME right pulmonary veins and ME left pulmonary veins); for a *coronary sinus defect*, views that examine the coronary sinus (ME 4-Ch with retroflexion; Figure 19.6A; Video 19.4), ME 2-Ch, and those that allow for imaging of an associated L-SVC (sweep obtained by rotating probe leftward in the upper esophageal aortic arch [UE Ao Arch] SAX view).

Goals of the Two-Dimensional Examination

- Definition of defect type, location, size, shape, and number of orifices. Detection of a PFO or small interatrial communication may require the intravenous injection of agitated saline or other material that allows for contrast and a Valsalva maneuver (or equivalent) to increase RA pressure over LA pressure and identify right-to-left shunting.
- Evaluation of the entire atrial septum. Determination of defect size(s) and rims to assess suitability for transcatheter closure
  - Anterosuperior (aortic rim): ME AV SAX view, the distance between the aortic ring and the defect (note: lack of rim does *not* necessarily preclude device deployment)
  - Posterior: ME 4-Ch view, the gap between the coronary sinus and defect
  - Inferoanterior (atrioventricular rim, also referred to as mitral rim): ME 4-Ch, the space between the defect and atrioventricular valves

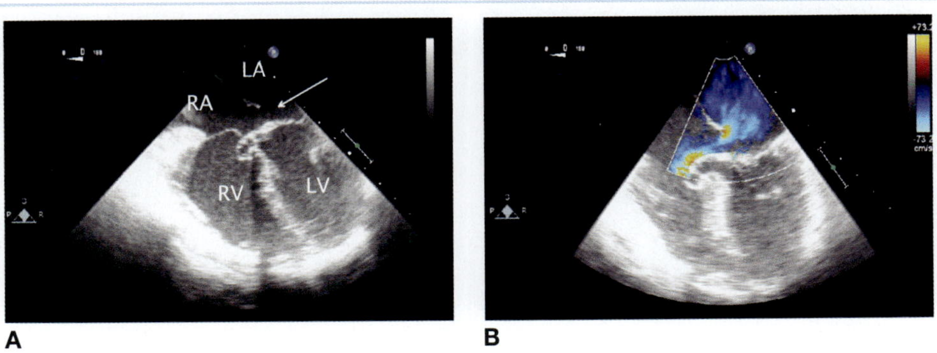

FIGURE 19.4 Primum atrial septal defect. A: Midesophageal four-chamber view depicting a relatively small defect in the inferior aspect of the atrial septum (arrow), a location characteristic of a primum atrial septal defect. B: Corresponding color-flow Doppler demonstrating left-to-right atrial level shunting across the defect. A tricuspid pouch (aneurysmal tissue) is seen billowing into the right ventricle (RV), representing remnants of endocardial cushion tissue. LA, left atrium; LV, left ventricle; RA, right atrium.

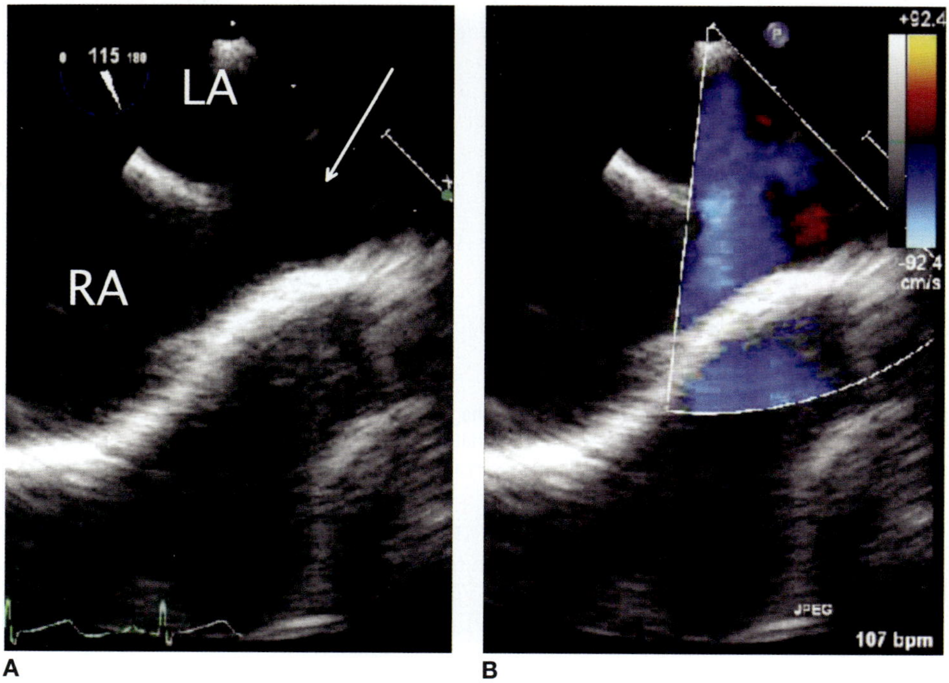

FIGURE 19.5 Sinus venosus atrial septal defect. A: Midesophageal bicaval view illustrating a communication in the interatrial septum (arrow) near the entrance of the superior vena cava. The findings are typical of a superior vena cava–type sinus venosus atrial septal defect. B: Corresponding color-flow mapping demonstrating left-to-right atrial level shunting across the communication. The superior vena cava frequently overrides this defect, which is usually associated with anomalous pulmonary venous drainage. LA, left atrium; RA, right atrium.

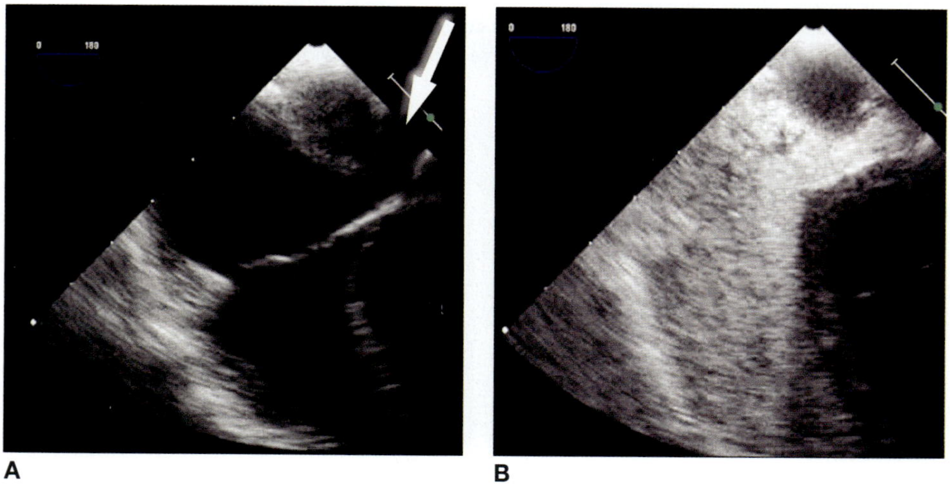

FIGURE 19.6 Dilated coronary sinus associated with a persistent left superior vena cava. A: Midesophageal four-chamber view with transesophageal echocardiography probe retroflexion showing a dilated coronary sinus (white arrow). B: The same view was obtained after injection of agitated saline into a left arm vein, displaying contrast in the coronary sinus and right atrium and confirming the presence of a persistent left superior vena cava connection draining into the coronary sinus.

    - Superior-posterior (SVC Rim): ME bicaval view, the distance between the SVC and the defect
    - Inferoposterior (IVC Rim): ME bicaval view, the gap between the IVC and the defect (deficient rim is unfavorable for percutaneous device closure)
- Assessment of mitral valve anatomy (evaluate for prolapse/cleft: prolapse may occur in association with secundum ASDs; a cleft in the anterior leaflet is commonly seen in partial AVSD)
- Evaluation of pulmonary venous drainage (all cases, particularly sinus venosus ASD)
- Examination of right-sided structures for dilation and motion of the interventricular septum (flattened or paradoxical motion related to volume load)
- Contrast echocardiography may help identify the presence of a persistent L-SVC in a coronary sinus communication (Figure 19.6B; Video 19.4) and confirm or exclude unroofing of the coronary sinus in a coronary sinus ASD.
- Evaluation of RV wall thickness, suggestive of pulmonary hypertension
- Assessment of ventricular function

Goals of the Doppler Examination

- Assessment of flow across defect: nature, direction, and mean velocity
- Detection of atrioventricular/semilunar valve regurgitation
- Measurement of tricuspid regurgitant jet velocity (V_{TR}) for estimation of PA systolic pressure (PASP) as follows: RV systolic pressure = $4\,(V_{TR})^2$ + RA pressure
  In the absence of RV outflow obstruction: PASP = RV systolic pressure
- Interrogation of pulmonary venous flows to determine drainage
- Estimation of shunt magnitude (pulmonary and systemic blood flows, Qp:Qs) in the absence of significant atrioventricular valve regurgitation

Goals of the Examination After Surgery

- Detection of residual interatrial shunting (color Doppler and contrast echocardiography) (Figure 19.7; Video 19.5)
- Evaluation of atrioventricular valve competence
- Examination of systemic and pulmonary venous pathways (depending on the defect and nature of intervention)
- Assessment of ventricular function

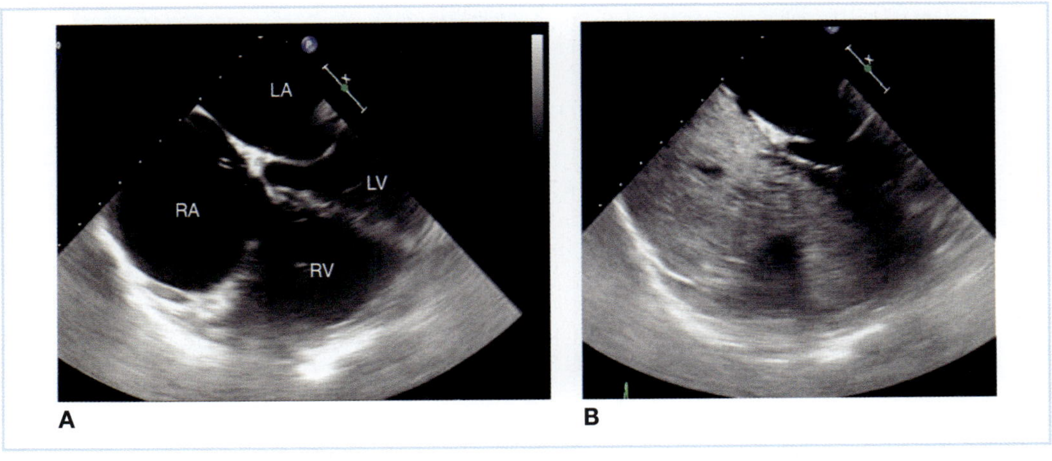

FIGURE 19.7 Postoperative patch closure of secundum atrial septal defect. A: Midesophageal four-chamber view depicting an autologous pericardial patch in the interatrial septum. B: Corresponding contrast injection into an arm vein using an agitated mixture of saline and blood, showing enhancement of right-sided structures and no contrast in the left heart excluding residual shunting. LA, left atrium; LV, left ventricle; RA, right atrium; RV, right ventricle.

Goals of the Examination During Transcatheter Intervention

- Determination of defect size and tissue margins or rims around the defect to facilitate device selection
- Assessment of the relation of defect/device to surrounding anatomic structures (Ao, pulmonary veins, venae cavae, atrioventricular valves, coronary sinus) and potential effects of the device on these structures
- Measurement of maximal defect diameter (balloon stretch sizing)
- Sizing for selection of occluder device and detection of leaks around the occluding balloon, if the "stop-flow technique" is used
- Live monitoring and guidance during device positioning, deployment, and determination of device stability
- Assessment of residual shunting (Figure 19.8; Video 19.6)
- Evaluation of proper positioning of device (documentation of unobstructed flow in systemic and adjacent pulmonary veins and lack of impingement in nearby structures prior to and following device deployment)
- Exclusion of complications related to the intervention (for device: embolization, erosion, pericardial effusion)

Applications of Three-Dimensional Imaging

- Enhances visualization of the anatomy of the interatrial septum and spatial details of the defect (size, location, number of defects, rims, shape, relationships between defect/device and adjacent anatomic structures). Various acquisition modes can be used (eg, 3D narrow-sector, zoomed, wide-angled gated).
- Allows for *en face* views and appreciation of changes in the configuration of the defect throughout the cardiac cycle (Figure 19.9A; Video 19.7)
- Facilitates continuous visualization of hardware and the 3D relations while monitoring device deployment (Figure 19.9B; Video 19.7); X-plane imaging provides simultaneous display of the defect and surrounding structures in orthogonal views.
- Evaluates for appropriate device position and entrapment of septal rims around the occluder
- Provides detailed assessment of residual shunts during device placement (Doppler flow analysis with live 3D color)
- Allows for characterization of associated anomalies such as mitral valve cleft in an ostium primum ASD (Figure 19.10; Video 19.8)
- Allows for assessment of ventricular volumes and ejection fraction
- Provides guidance during procedures requiring transseptal puncture

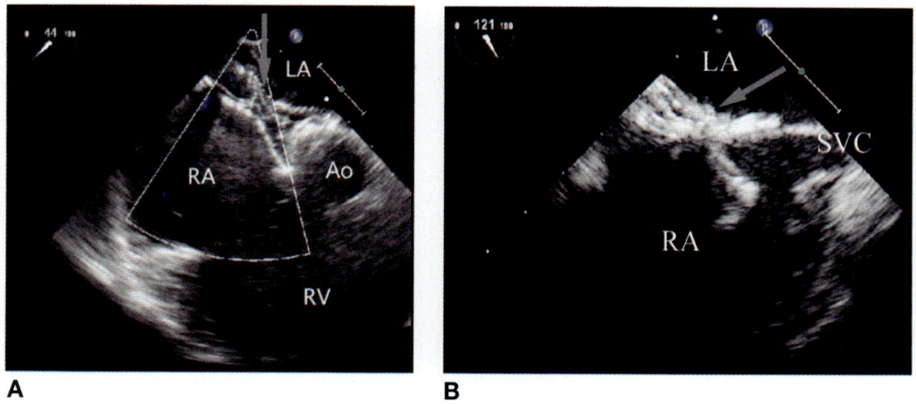

FIGURE 19.8 Atrial septal defect, occluder device. A: Midesophageal aortic valve short-axis view with rightward transducer rotation demonstrating an atrial septal defect closure device (gray arrow) straddling the interatrial septum. B: Midesophageal bicaval view (orthogonal cross-sectional view relative to panel A) depicting the device (gray arrow) appropriately placed across the atrial septal defect before deployment. Ao, aorta; LA, left atrium; RA, right atrium; RV, right ventricle; SVC, superior vena cava.

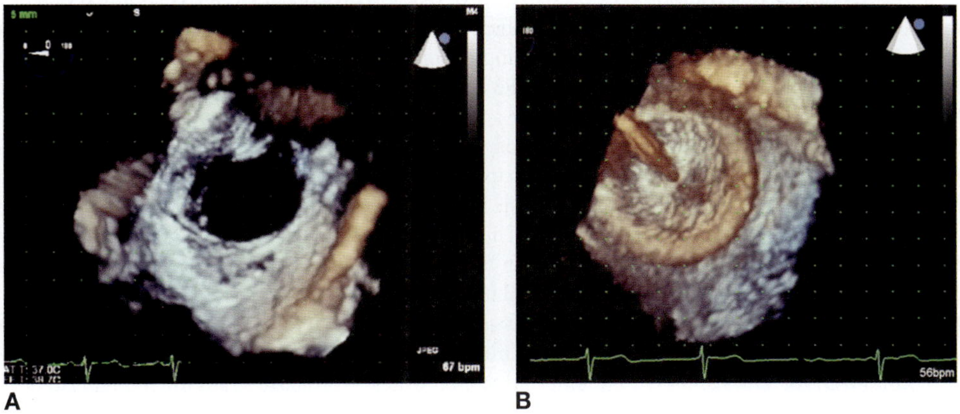

FIGURE 19.9 Atrial septal defect, transcatheter closure. A: Three-dimensional transesophageal echocardiography image of a secundum atrial septal defect viewed from the right atrial aspect with visible rims in all quadrants; B: The same view displaying the right atrial disc of the occluder device and the delivery cable before release.

VENTRICULAR SEPTAL DEFECT

Anatomy

The categorization of VSDs has been the subject of controversy and ongoing debate. However, for simplicity, these defects have been classified according to their location within the ventricular septum into four major types: perimembranous, muscular, doubly committed outlet, and inlet defects (Figure 19.11A). They can occur either in isolation or as part of complex malformations. An isolated VSD is the most common congenital cardiac pathology diagnosed in infancy. Because 60% of smaller defects close spontaneously and larger defects are usually repaired in childhood, VSDs account for only 10% to 15% of defects observed in adults with CHD.

Perimembranous defects account for approximately 70% of VSDs, involve most or all of the membranous septum, and can extend into the muscular region. Associated findings may include an aneurysm of the

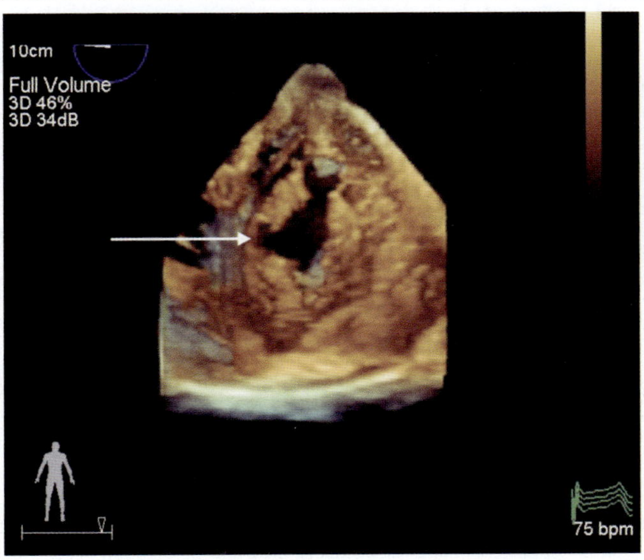

FIGURE 19.10 Cleft mitral valve associated with primum atrial septal defect. Transgastric short-axis view displays a cleft in the anterior mitral leaflet (arrow) by three-dimensional imaging.

membranous septum that is composed of tricuspid valve tissue. This appears as a tissue pouch on echocardiography and often limits shunting across the defect. Potential associated pathologies include a subaortic membrane or AV cusp herniation/prolapse (resulting in aortic regurgitation). A perimembranous VSD can also be seen when there is obstruction within the RV cavity related to muscular band hypertrophy, dividing it into two chambers (double chamber RV).

Muscular defects are defined by their location in the muscular portion of the ventricular septum. They account for 20% of VSDs, can be isolated or multiple ("Swiss cheese" type), and are often located in the central or apical portion of the trabecular septum. Post–myocardial infarction ventricular septal rupture can also result in a VSD as a rare complication. These may develop within a few days after a transmural myocardial infarction involving the septum and can be hemodynamically significant. Thus, not all muscular defects encountered in adult patients are congenital in nature.

Doubly committed outlet defects (also known as supracristal, subarterial, subpulmonary, infundibular, or conal VSDs) are located in the infundibular septum immediately below the pulmonary (pulmonic) valve (PV). They account for 5% of VSDs and are frequently associated with AV prolapse, resulting in regurgitation.

Inlet defects account for approximately 5% of VSDs and are located in close proximity to the atrioventricular valves in the posterior or inlet portion of the ventricular septum. These defects predominate in patients with Down syndrome. An associated primum ASD within the context of a common atrioventricular valve annulus is part of the defect known as a complete AVSD (canal defect or endocardial cushion defect).

Pathophysiology

The physiologic consequences of a VSD are determined by the size of the defect and the pulmonary vascular resistance. Moderate-to-large defects are associated with significant left-to-right shunting (Figure 19.11B), left heart dilation, and symptoms of heart failure. Pulmonary vascular changes can occur, leading to pulmonary

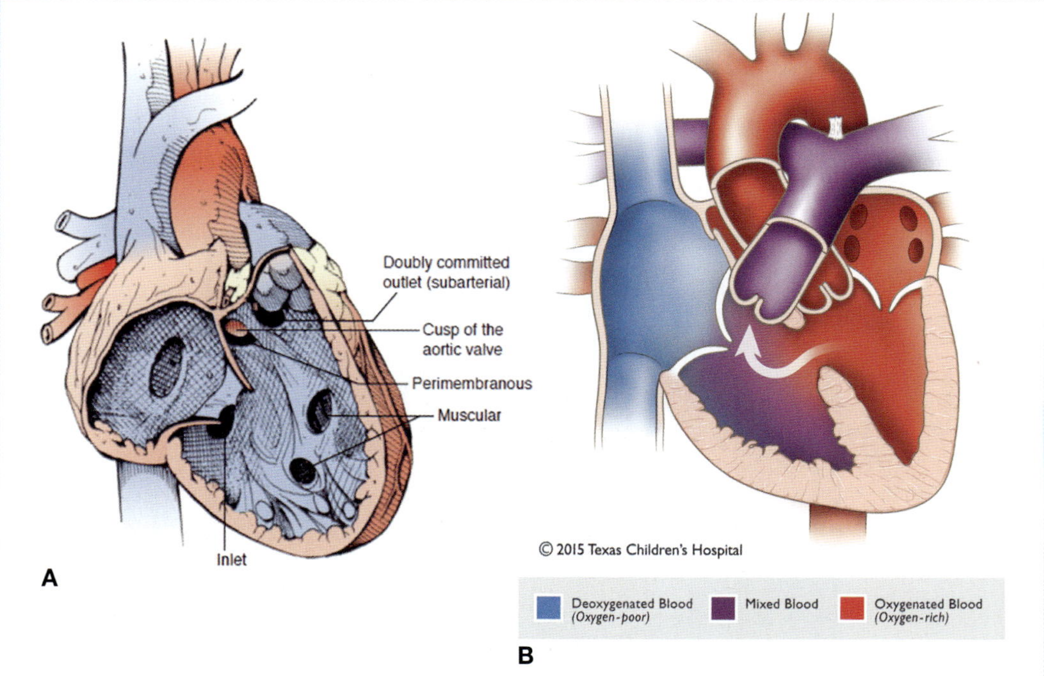

FIGURE 19.11 Ventricular septal defects. A: Graphic rendering of the interventricular septum as seen from the right ventricular aspect. Ventricular septal defects are classified by location into four major groups: perimembranous, muscular, doubly committed outlet (subarterial), and inlet defects. Muscular defects can occur anywhere in the trabecular interventricular septum. In this figure, a cusp of the aortic valve can be visualized through the perimembranous defect. B: Illustration showing left-to-right ventricular level shunting (arrow) across a ventricular septal defect. (© 2015 Texas Children's Hospital [reprinted with permission].)

hypertension in the patient with a large, long-standing VSD and substantial pulmonary overcirculation. This, in turn, can lead to a reversal in the direction of the shunt through the defect (right-to-left shunting) and resultant cyanosis. Increased pulmonary vascular resistance secondary to irreversible vascular changes leads to a condition known as Eisenmenger physiology, rarely seen today in developed countries. The affected adult has early mortality and is not considered a candidate for defect closure.

Management

Most symptomatic patients with a VSD require intervention. Surgical closure of an isolated defect is most frequently accomplished through a transatrial or transpulmonary approach. Thus, the location of the communication has important implications for surgical access to the defect and should be evaluated carefully by the perioperative echocardiographer. In selected cases, transcatheter device occlusion can also be an option (16). This has been more commonly applied to muscular communications due to the distant anatomic relationship of this type of defect to the atrioventricular valves/outflow tracts. In addition, these types of defects (particularly if multiple) can present significant challenges for surgical closure. In some cases, perimembranous defects may be amenable to device closure. A catheter-based intervention can be accomplished either percutaneously in the cardiac catheterization laboratory, as noted earlier being the most common setting, or in the operating room using a hybrid approach. The latter strategy uses a combination of surgical and interventional techniques. During a typical procedure, following a sternotomy, the free wall of the RV is punctured with a needle, a wire is inserted through the needle, and a sheath is placed across the wire. TEE guides device placement across the defect. Surgery for associated pathology, if necessary, can then be performed using conventional techniques.

Transesophageal Echocardiographic Evaluation

The systematic interrogation of the entire IVS requires multiple TEE views. The use of 2D imaging can identify each type of VSD. Suggested cross sections for a focused examination, depending on the type of defect include ME 4-Ch (Figures 19.12-19.14; Videos 19.9-19.11), ME five-chamber (5-Ch), ME AV SAX, ME LAX (Figure 19.15; Video 19.12), ME RV I-O, TG, and DTG views (Video 19.10).

Goals of the Two-Dimensional Examination

- Assessment of defect(s) location, size, number, and extension (Figures 19.12-19.15; Videos 19.9-19.12)
- Interrogation of associated abnormalities, including ventricular septal aneurysm (Figure 19.12; Video 19.9)
- Evaluation of AV for deformity (herniation or prolapse; Figure 19.15; Video 19.12)

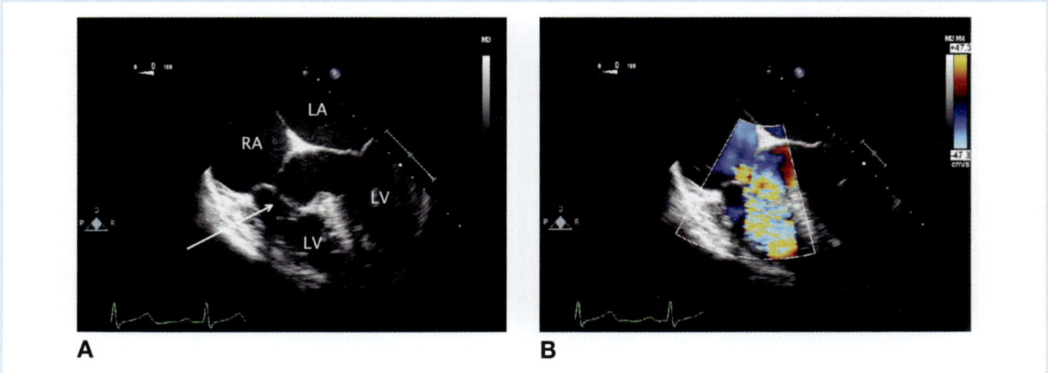

FIGURE 19.12 Perimembranous ventricular septal defect. A: Midesophageal four-chamber view depicting a large defect in the membranous region of the ventricular septum partially covered by aneurysmal tissue (arrow). B: Corresponding color-flow Doppler demonstrating significant left-to-right shunting across the defect. LA, left atrium; LV, left ventricle; RA, right atrium; RV, right ventricle.

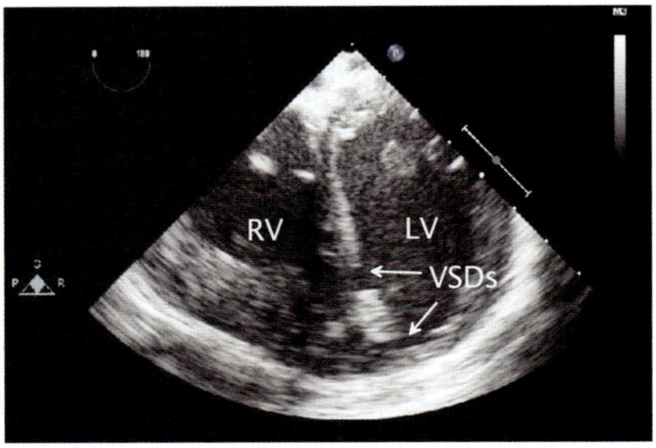

FIGURE 19.13 Muscular ventricular septal defects. The image displays two muscular ventricular septal defects (VSDs, arrows) as demonstrated in a transgastric left ventricular short-axis cross section. The larger defect is located in the mid-muscular region, and a second smaller one is seen at the apex. LV, left ventricle; RV, right ventricle.

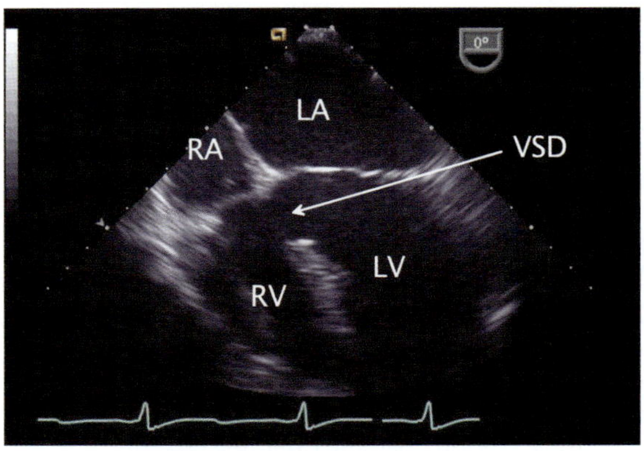

FIGURE 19.14 Inlet ventricular septal defect. Midesophageal four-chamber view depicting a large ventricular septal defect (VSD) in the inlet portion of the ventricular septum (arrow). Note that both atrioventricular valves appear to be at the same level in this defect, in contrast to the offset in the normal heart, where the tricuspid valve has a more apical insertion into the ventricular septum than the mitral valve. LA, left atrium; LV, left ventricle; RA, right atrium; RV, right ventricle.

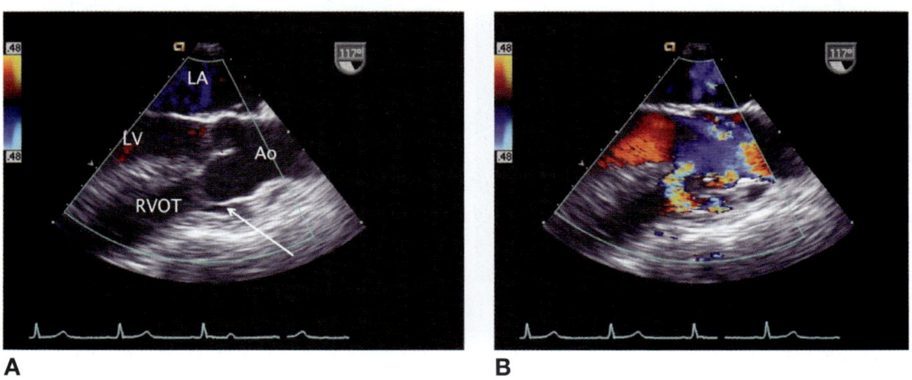

FIGURE 19.15 Supracristal (conal, subarterial) ventricular septal defect. A: Midesophageal aortic valve long-axis view demonstrating prolapse of the aortic valve (right coronary cusp; arrow) through a subarterial ventricular septal defect into the right ventricle. B: Systolic frame demonstrating color Doppler flow across the ventricular communication. Ao, aorta; LA, left atrium; LV, left ventricle; RVOT, right ventricular outflow tract.

- Examination of PAs and left-sided cardiac structures for dilation
- Inspection for findings suggestive of pulmonary hypertension (RV wall thickness and configuration of interventricular septum during systole)

Goals of the Doppler Examination

- Confirmation of the presence of the defect and evaluation for additional defects
- Determination of the nature, magnitude, and direction of shunt flow
- Detection of tricuspid, mitral, and aortic regurgitation (color Doppler)
- Estimation of PASP by:
  - Tricuspid regurgitant jet peak velocity (V_{TR})
  - VSD jet peak velocity (V_{VSD}):

$$\text{RV systolic pressure} = \text{Systolic arterial blood pressure} - 4\,(V_{VSD})^2$$

  In the absence of RV outflow obstruction:

$$\text{RV systolic pressure} = \text{PASP}$$

  In the absence of LV outflow obstruction:

$$\text{Systemic systolic blood pressure} = \text{LV systolic pressure}$$

- Determination of flow restriction across VSD (high-velocity VSD jet suggests restriction vs low-velocity flow of a nonrestrictive defect)
- Estimation of the magnitude of the shunt (pulmonary-to-systemic blood flow ratio) in the absence of significant atrioventricular valve regurgitation

Goals of the Examination After Surgery

- Detection of residual shunts and evaluation of hemodynamic significance
- Determination of potential changes in valvar regurgitation
- Assessment of ventricular function

Goals of the Examination During Transcatheter Intervention

- Determination of VSD anatomy, size, and relationship to ventricular inflows and outflows
- Evaluation of valvar competence
- Detection of leaks around the balloon, if balloon sizing is performed
- Guidance and monitoring during device positioning and deployment
- Evaluation of occluder device position in the ventricular septum relative to surrounding structures (Figure 19.16; Video 19.13)
- Assessment of leaks across the occluder device
- Early detection of complications related to device positioning

Applications of Three-Dimensional Imaging

- Improves visualization of defect (location, size, number, shape)
- Enhances characterization of structures surrounding defect(s) during transcatheter closure
- Allows for *en face* views of defects from RV and LV aspects of the ventricular septum
- Provides for assessment of the result of the intervention

PATENT DUCTUS ARTERIOSUS

Anatomy

During fetal life, the ductus arteriosus connects the PA to the proximal descending (Desc) Ao distal to the level of the origin left subclavian artery (Figure 19.17A). This muscular communication allows for RV output into the Desc Ao, bypassing the lungs under normal fetal conditions of increased pulmonary vascular resistance. Failure of closure of this communication in the neonatal period results in persistent ductal patency.

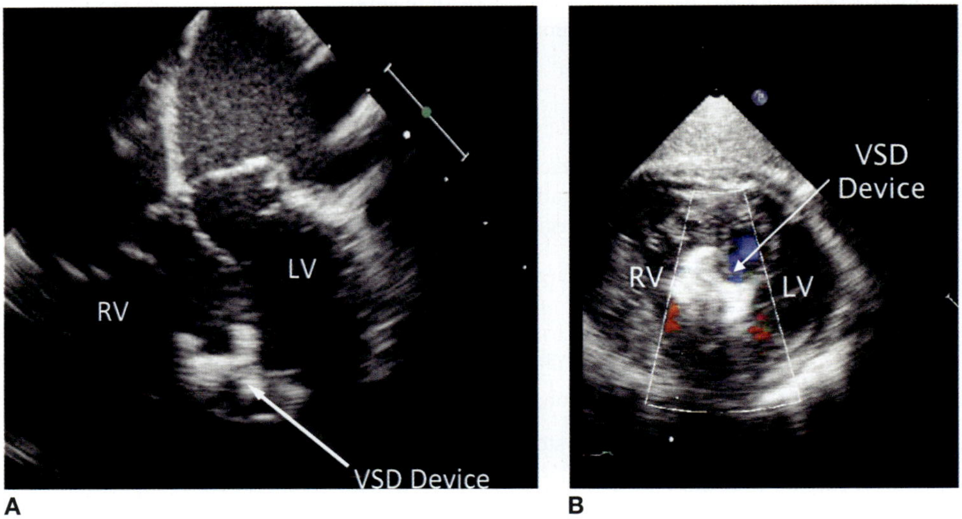

FIGURE 19.16 Muscular ventricular septal defect, transcatheter occlusion. A: Midesophageal four-chamber view showing a ventricular septal defect (VSD) occluder device (arrow) between the mid and apical muscular portion of the ventricular septum. B: Transgastric short-axis view with color-flow imaging displaying the VSD occluder device (arrow). LV, left ventricle; RV, right ventricle.

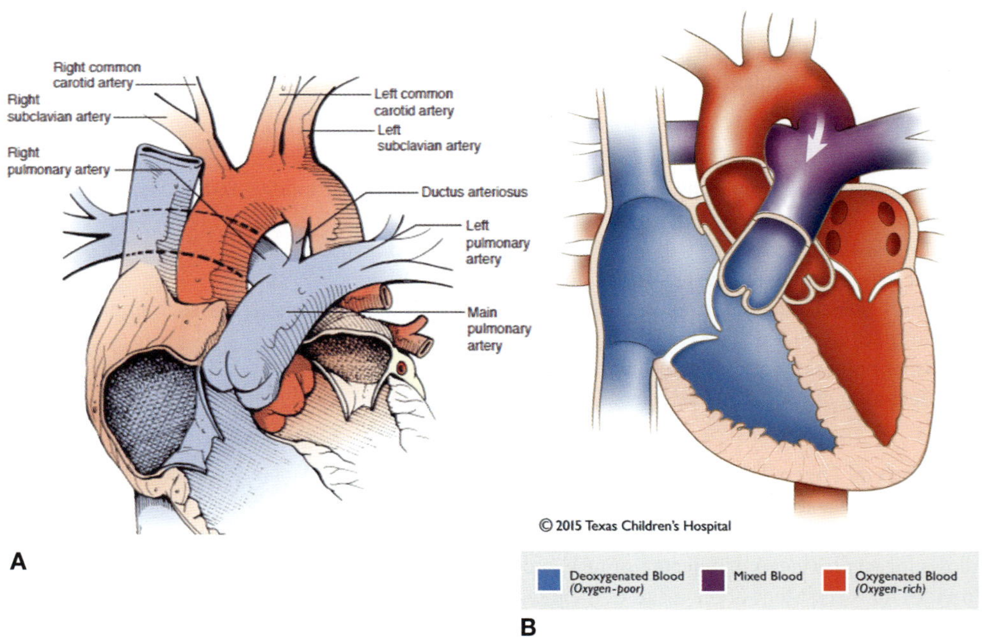

FIGURE 19.17 Patent ductus arteriosus. A: Diagram illustrating the ductus arteriosus as it connects the main pulmonary artery to the descending aorta. B: Sketch showing the usual direction of left-to-right shunting (arrow) across a patent ductus arteriosus. (© 2015 Texas Children's Hospital [reprinted with permission].)

This lesion accounts for approximately 8% of cases of CHD. As in many other defects, a PDA can be found either in isolation or in association with additional cardiac defects.

Pathophysiology

The physiologic consequences of a PDA are determined by the size of the communication and the relative systemic and pulmonary vascular resistances. Although a small PDA can have little or no physiologic consequences, hemodynamically significant left-to-right shunting (Figure 19.17B) in larger communications leads to pulmonary overcirculation and congestive symptoms and, if chronic, may increase pulmonary vascular resistance. Most individuals with a large shunt become symptomatic and require medical attention. A PDA in the adult patient, albeit rarely, can be associated with complications such as endarteritis, aneurysm formation, dissection, and rupture. Occasionally, in the older patients, left-to-right shunting and LV volume load are limited by an increased pulmonary vascular resistance, a finding associated with the development of Eisenmenger syndrome.

Management

Small- to moderate-sized communications may be suitable for percutaneous device occlusion. Surgical ligation of a PDA in the adult may be complicated by calcification of ductal tissue, increasing the risks of the procedure and potential need for cardiopulmonary or ventricular bypass. Interventions to obliterate the communication are contraindicated in the setting of pulmonary vascular obstructive disease.

Transesophageal Echocardiographic Evaluation

The use of TEE is not routine during transcatheter closure, nor surgical interventions for a PDA; however, it can be helpful in some cases. When utilized, the TEE examination is enhanced by color Doppler information superimposed on the 2D image. This assessment may require nonstandard views that allow for visualization of the site of ductal insertion into the main PA (MPA) or for detection of blood flow into the PA (Figure 19.18; Video 19.14).

Suggested cross sections for focused examination include UE PA, ME Asc Ao SAX, UE Ao Arch SAX, ME RV I-O, and ME Desc Ao LAX views.

Goals of the Two-Dimensional Examination

- Identification of the communication
- Evaluation of associated cardiac malformations

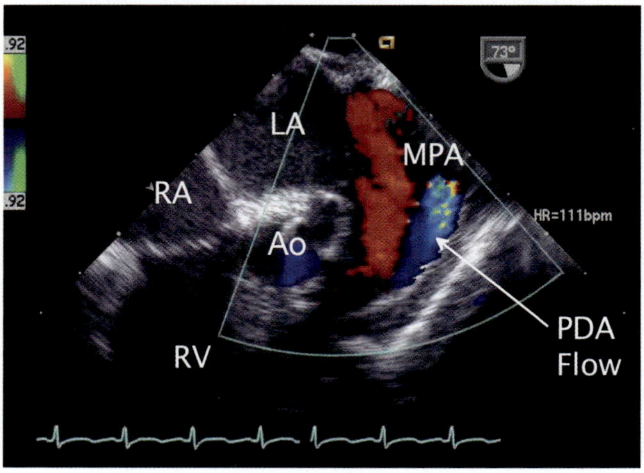

FIGURE 19.18 Patent ductus arteriosus. Midesophageal right ventricular inflow-outflow view depicting blue flow away from the transducer and into the main pulmonary artery (MPA) from a patent ductus arteriosus (PDA, arrow). Ao, aorta; LA, left atrium; RA, right atrium; RV, right ventricle.

- Examination of the size of the PAs/left-sided cardiac chambers (to assess the magnitude of the volume overload)
- Evaluation of RV wall thickness and septal configuration (as an indicator of the extent of RV and PA pressure elevation)
- Assessment of biventricular function

Goals of the Doppler Examination

- Detection of the presence and magnitude of ductal shunting
- Characterization of flow direction and velocity (flow typically continuous in nature into the PAs)
- Detection of retrograde flow in the thoracic Ao from ductal runoff
- Examination of valvar regurgitation
- Estimation of systolic PA pressure by tricuspid regurgitant jet and PDA jet

4 (Peak systolic left-to-right flow velocity of PDA jet)^2 = systolic pressure gradient between the Ao and PA

Goals of the Examination After Intervention

- Detection of residual ductal shunting
- Verification of unobstructed flow in adjacent structures

COARCTATION OF THE AORTA

Anatomy

Coarctation in adolescent and adult patients is usually characterized by narrowing of the thoracic Ao immediately opposite to the insertion site of the ligamentum arteriosum (juxtaductal) (Figure 19.19A). Typically, this results from a discrete obstructing shelf that projects into the aortic lumen. In some cases, diffuse Ao Arch and isthmic hypoplasia may be seen complicating the primary pathology, which is the most common manifestation of a CoA during infancy. Associated defects include a Bic AV in up to 50% of cases, PDA, VSD, and subaortic membrane. CoA accounts for approximately 6% of all CHD and is more common in males, and 20% of cases are diagnosed in adolescents or adults.

Pathophysiology

The primary physiologic consequence of CoA is increased LV afterload due to obstruction to blood flow. The systolic arterial blood pressure is increased proximal to the narrowing and decreased distally. This pressure gradient, whether minimal or significant, is exacerbated by exercise. Systemic hypertension occurs frequently and may result in hypertensive heart disease. The development of collateral vessels may be seen, accounting for the finding of rib notching on chest radiography. Most adults with CoA are asymptomatic, although recurrent epistaxis, headache, claudication, dizziness, and palpitations may occur. Significant complications include aortic dissection, rupture, endarteritis of the Ao, infective endocarditis, and LV failure. An association with cerebral aneurysms has been well described in affected individuals.

Management

The severity of the obstruction dictates the need for intervention. Options include surgical management (Figure 19.19B-D) or catheter-based interventions such as balloon dilation with or without stent placement.

Transesophageal Echocardiographic Evaluation

The surgical approach in uncomplicated CoA is via a thoracotomy incision. In this setting, TEE has a limited role. The indications for TEE in most patients with CoA involve the evaluation of associated defects that require CPB. The anterior position of the air-filled trachea relative to the esophagus limits the TEE examination of the distal Asc Ao and proximal Ao Arch, thereby making this a challenging lesion to examine by TEE comprehensively. This pathology is most reliably assessed by other imaging modalities, such as TTE, magnetic resonance imaging, and computed tomography. Suggested cross sections for focused TEE examination include UE Ao Arch SAX and LAX, and ME Desc Ao SAX and LAX (▶ Video 19.15).

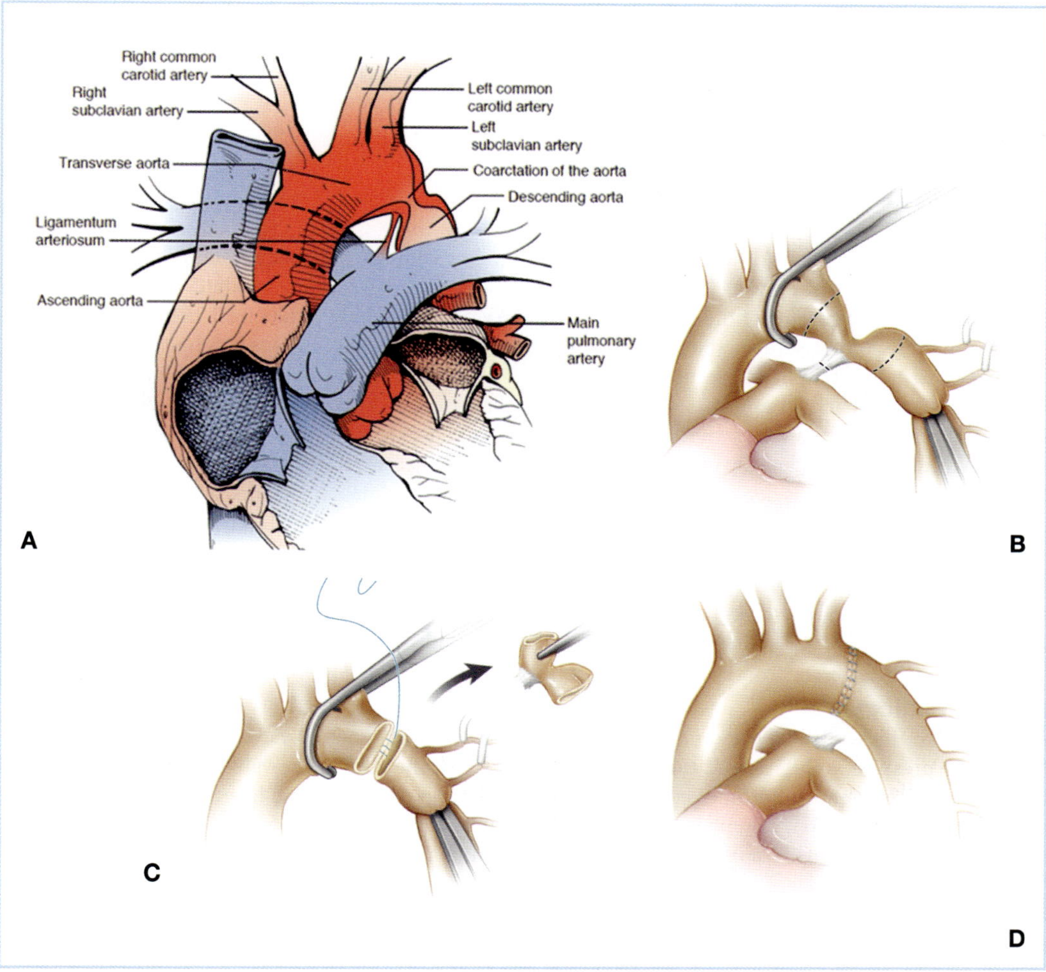

FIGURE 19.19 Coarctation of the aorta. A: Graphic representation depicting the aortic narrowing in coarctation. **B:** Illustration of one of the surgical approaches to coarctation repair involving aortic cross-clamping. C: Resection of the stenotic segment. D: End-to-end anastomosis. (Images in panels B, C, and D © 2015 Texas Children's Hospital [reprinted with permission].)

Goals of the Two-Dimensional Examination

- Limited evaluation of the Ao Arch/Ao for narrowing of Desc Ao distal to the left subclavian artery
- Evaluation of associated defects
- Determination of LV function and wall thickness
- Monitoring of LV function during aortic-clamp application

Goals of the Doppler Examination

- Detection of turbulent, eccentric jets or flow acceleration in the Desc Ao
- Determination of flow pattern (increased systolic velocity at the region of obstruction and continuous diastolic forward flow) and velocities across the area of narrowing and distally (this is complicated by the limited ability to align the Doppler beam to the direction of blood flow)
- Characterization of aortic pulsations distal to the obstruction (blunted pattern with decreased systolic upstroke in the presence of obstruction)
- Identification of flow in collateral vessels (color Doppler)
- As required for the assessment of associated pathology

Goals of the Examination After Surgery

- Detection of residual obstruction (challenging to assess due to suboptimal Doppler alignment with the direction of blood flow)
- Identification of complications related to the intervention
- Evaluation of coexisting defects

AORTIC STENOSIS

Anatomy

AS can occur at the subvalvar, valvar, and supravalvar levels. Although the isolated Bic AV usually does not require treatment in infancy or childhood, it is a well-known cause of morbidity in adult. This represents the most common malformation of the normally tricuspid AV and frequently results from commissural fusion. A "raphe" or false commissure may be present, and the resultant two leaflets or cusps may be equal or markedly different in size, resulting in an eccentric line of closure. A Bic AV can be associated with valvular stenosis and/or regurgitation and, in some cases, an aortopathy characterized by aortic root dilation. AS accounts for 6% of all CHD. In patients with symptomatic AS who are younger than 65 years of age, a Bic AV is the most common finding. The mechanism of the valve obstruction is frequently related to leaflet calcification. In most cases, aortic regurgitation is due to cusp prolapse or redundancy. Weakness in the media of the Asc/transverse Ao may predispose to aneurysm formation. Other associated defects include VSD, PDA, and CoA. Subaortic stenosis can occur due to a discrete membrane or muscular, more diffuse, tunnel-type obstruction. Pathologies such as hypertrophic cardiomyopathy can also be associated with LV outflow tract obstruction. Congenital supravalvar AS primarily involves the sinotubular junction but, in some cases, can affect the Asc Ao and arch vessels as an arteriopathy. This can be a feature of Williams syndrome.

Pathophysiology

A Bic AV can thicken, calcify, and display decreased mobility over time. As valve stenosis progresses, the LV systolic pressure increases, and the wall hypertrophies. As the area of the valve orifice becomes more restrictive and the stenosis becomes critical, LV systolic function decreases, and heart failure occurs. Aortic regurgitation may lead to a volume load on the LV, resulting in chamber dilation. Subvalvar and supravalvar stenoses also account for LV outflow obstruction and can impact AV function. Supravalvar AS can involve the coronary arteries and lead to myocardial ischemia. Patients affected by Williams syndrome can have other anatomic abnormalities (ie, peripheral PA stenosis), resulting in biventricular outflow tract obstruction, implying potentially significant anesthetic risks.

Management

Several strategies have been applied to patients with AV stenosis. Therapies, when necessary, include surgery and percutaneous interventions. Surgical valvotomy/valvuloplasty or valve replacements with a bioprosthesis, mechanical valve, or pulmonary autograft (Ross procedure) represent options. Aortic root replacement may also be needed. Transcatheter procedures may include balloon valvuloplasty and transcatheter aortic valve replacement (TAVR) in patients with severe AS (the latter is discussed in depth elsewhere in this textbook). Subvalvar and supravalvar aortic pathology associated with significant obstruction or impacting AV function usually requires surgical therapy.

Transesophageal Echocardiographic Evaluation

Methods to determine AV area and the severity of obstruction are addressed in other chapters. It should be mentioned that the use of planimetry by 2D imaging to estimate AV area is unreliable in patients with a Bic AV. 3D-TEE may provide an advantage in this regard. Suggested cross sections for focused TEE examination in subvalvar, valvar, and supravalvar AS include ME AV SAX and LAX, ME LAX, ME 5-Ch, TG LAX, and DTG 5-Ch. For evaluation of the Asc Ao: ME Asc Ao SAX and LAX, and UE Ao Arch LAX. Additional cross sections may be necessary when TEE is used for procedural guidance during TAVR.

Goals of the Two-Dimensional Evaluation

- Determination of AV morphology (cusps, commissures, fish-mouth appearance of a Bic AV) and systolic motion (doming) (Figure 19.20A; Video 19.16)

- Define site (valvar, subvalvar, supravalvar) and type of obstruction (Figures 19.20 and 19.21; Videos 19.16 and 19.17)
- Measurement of semilunar valve annular sizes (important in valve replacement and the Ross procedure where near matching of annular sizes is optimal) and assistance in TAVR valve sizing
- Identification of dilation of the Asc Ao (poststenotic or otherwise) (Figure 19.20B; Video 19.18)
- Detection of LV hypertrophy or dilation
- Assessment of global (ejection fraction) and segmental LV function
- Evaluation of the aortic root and Asc Ao
- Identification of associated pathology

Goals of the Doppler Examination

- Quantification of AV stenosis and aortic regurgitation
- Estimation of the gradient across the AV (TG LAX and DTG 5-Ch views are optimal for spectral Doppler interrogation; mean gradients correlate better with catheter-derived gradients than peak gradients; Figure 19.20C)

Goals of the Examination After Surgery

- Examination of results depending on the type of intervention (residual obstruction, aortic regurgitation, autograft, and pulmonary homograft function in Ross procedure, iatrogenic VSD)
- Evaluation of prosthetic valve function and exclusion of paravalvular leak(s) following valve replacement/implantation
- Assessment of ventricular function.

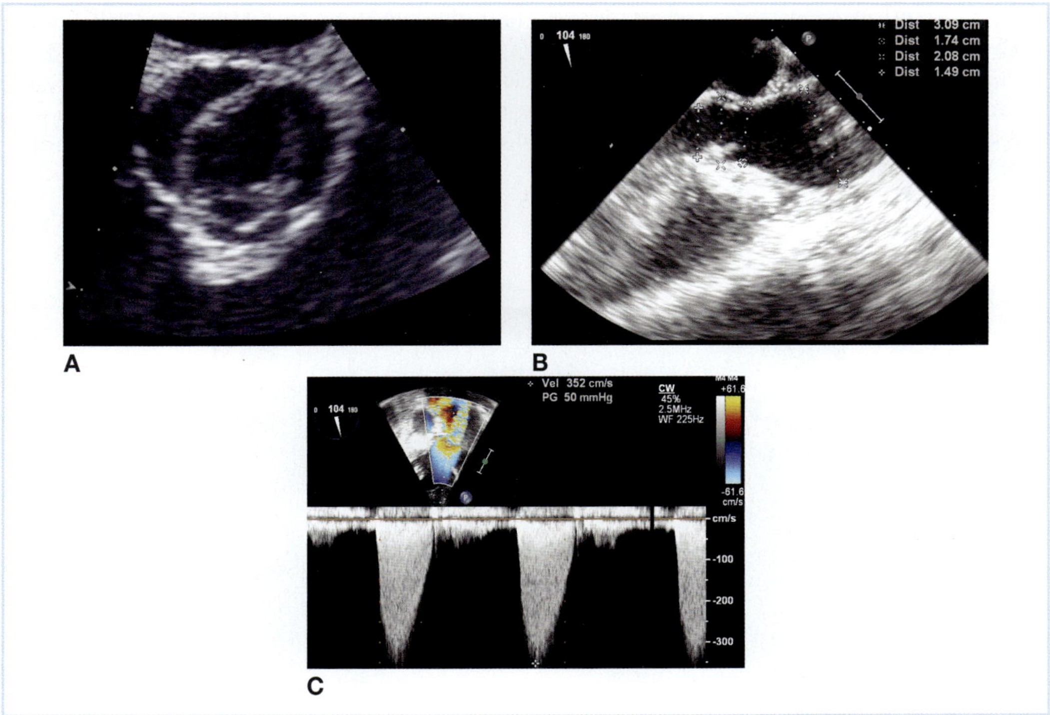

FIGURE 19.20 Bicuspid aortic valve. A: Midesophageal short-axis view of a bicuspid aortic valve demonstrating the "fish-mouth" appearance of the restrictive valvar opening during systole. Note that the valve leaflets are fused at the intercoronary commissure. B: Midesophageal long-axis view of a patient with a stenotic bicuspid aortic valve showing poststenotic ascending aortic dilation. C: Deep transgastric view showing flow acceleration across stenotic aortic valve with a peak velocity of 3.5 m/s (peak gradient of 50 mm Hg) consistent with moderate stenosis.

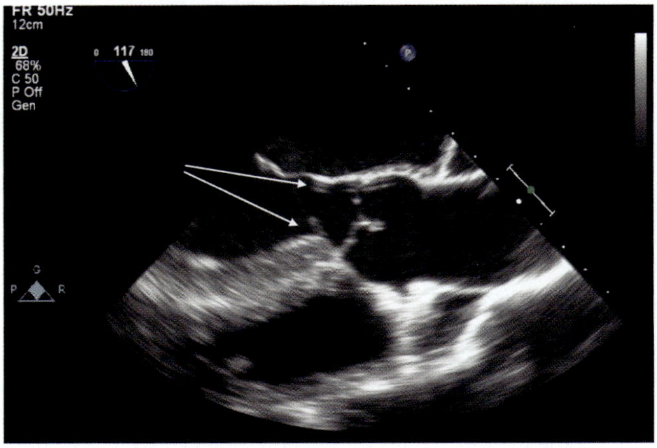

FIGURE 19.21 Subaortic stenosis. Midesophageal long-axis view displaying a discrete circumferential subaortic fibromuscular membrane (arrows).

Goals of the Examination During Transcatheter Intervention

- Assessment of results during interventions, such as balloon valvuloplasty
- Guidance during TAVR procedure and monitoring of complications

Applications of Three-Dimensional Imaging

- Enhances the characterization of AV anatomy (leaflet morphology) and pathology (Figure 19.22; Videos 19.17 and 19.19)
- Provides accurate measurements of the aortic annulus
- Facilitates the evaluation of regurgitant jets and the mechanism of regurgitation
- Assists with guidance during procedures associated with AV and root interventions (eg, closure of sinus of Valsalva aneurysm)

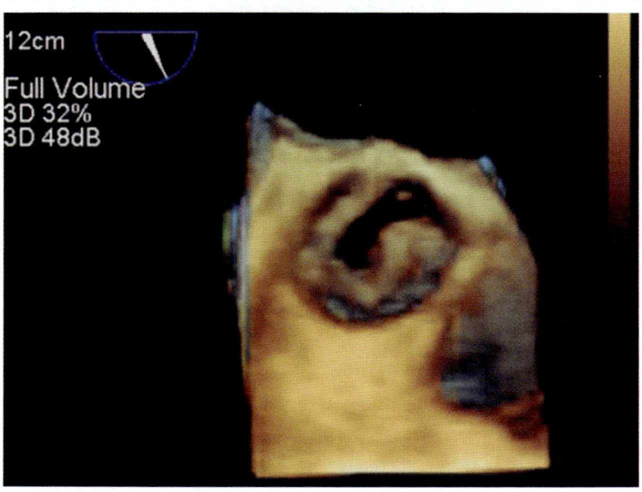

FIGURE 19.22 Bicuspid aortic valve. Zoomed three-dimensional transesophageal echocardiography short-axis image of a bicuspid aortic valve affected by endocarditis from a perspective above the level of the valve (*en face* view).

PULMONARY VALVE (PULMONIC) STENOSIS

Anatomy

A doming PV without clear leaflet separation is the most common pathology that causes congenital valvar PS. The orifice of the valve early in life ranges from a pinhole to several millimeters in diameter (Figure 19.23). Less commonly (10% of patients), valvar dysplasia and thickening are present with redundant leaflets that display reduced systolic excursion. PS can occur as an isolated lesion and accounts for approximately 10% of CHD in adults. Associated defects include ASD, VSD, and obstructive subpulmonary hypertrophy. Isolated stenosis of the supravalvar and subvalvar regions is less common than valvar stenosis.

Pathophysiology

The physiologic consequence of valvar PS is an elevation of RV systolic pressure and subsequent RV hypertrophy, proportional to the degree of obstruction. Most severity grading systems rely on Doppler-derived peak instantaneous transvalvar gradients (mild <36 mm Hg; moderate 36-64 mm Hg; severe >64 mm Hg). Mild valvar obstruction is usually not associated with symptoms. Moderate stenosis can result in dyspnea and fatigue during exertion. Patients with severe PS can manifest RV dilation and failure, although up to 25% may be symptom free. Typically, decisions for intervention are based on a combination of symptoms and valvar gradient. Patients with valvar dysplasia are more likely to develop symptoms. Occasionally, exertional chest pain and syncope are seen.

Management

Most symptomatic patients are treated with transcatheter balloon valvuloplasty. Pulmonary regurgitation can occur after the procedure, but overall, the long-term results are excellent. Those with a dysplastic PV may require surgery and, in some cases, valve replacement. Obstructive subpulmonic hypertrophy, if present, can regress after either intervention.

Transesophageal Echocardiographic Evaluation

Essential aspects of the examination include evaluation of not only the PV itself but also the immediate subvalvar and supravalvar regions. Suggested cross sections for focused TEE examination include ME Asc

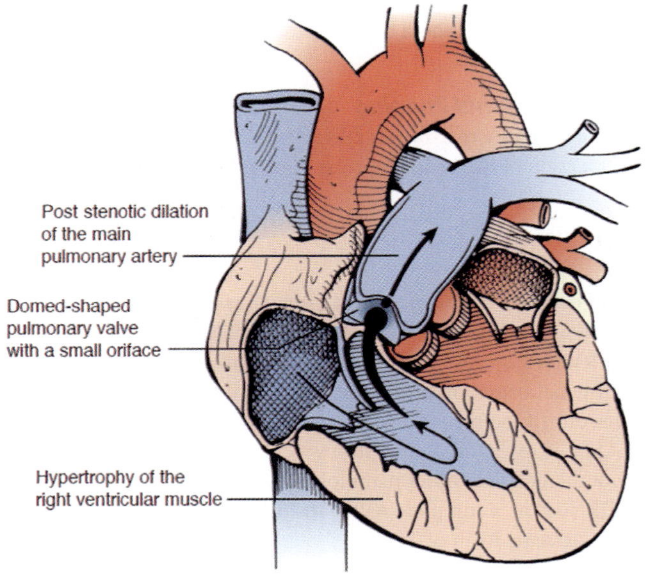

FIGURE 19.23 Pulmonary (pulmonic) stenosis. Graphic representation of pulmonary stenosis. In this pathology, the valve is usually domed shaped with a small orifice. There is hypertrophy of the right ventricle and poststenotic dilation of the main pulmonary artery. The arrows note the direction of blood flow across the right-sided cardiac structures.

Ao SAX, ME RV I-O, TG RV I-O, UE PA, and UE Ao Arch SAX. Additional views of the RV outflow tract (RVOT) can be obtained from the DTG window after rotating the imaging plane to approximately between 50° to 90° from the DTG 5-Ch view to obtain the DTG RVOT view. This modified view provides complementary anatomic information and facilitates gradient measurements.

Goals of the Two-Dimensional Evaluation

- Determination of PV morphology (thickening) and motion (tethering, doming). Planimetry is not feasible as the valve is not usually seen *en face*
- Measurement of annular size
- Evaluation of the subvalvar region, PA, and proximal branches. To image the right PA from the UE PA view, the transducer is rotated rightward; to display the left PA from the UE Ao Arch view, the transducer is slightly advanced and rotated leftward (examination of left PA may be limited by the interposed left bronchus). The UE PA view is also helpful in the left PA evaluation.
- Identification of poststenotic dilation of the PA
- Assessment of the RV, including systolic function, wall hypertrophy, and dilation. The position of the interventricular septum provides a crude estimation of RV systolic pressure.
- Identification of associated pathology (eg, atrial communication)

Goals of the Doppler Examination

- Identification of turbulent flow across the PV and/or pulmonary regurgitation
- Estimation of transpulmonary pressure gradient (peak and mean) using spectral Doppler in views that allow for optimal alignment with the direction of blood flow
- Evaluation of subvalvar and supravalvar regions to assess for associated obstruction
- Identification of tricuspid regurgitation and peak regurgitant velocity assessment for RV pressure estimation

Goals of the Examination After Surgery

- Examination/quantitation of residual pathology depending on the intervention (residual obstruction, pulmonary regurgitation)
- If valve replacement or an RV-to-PA conduit is placed, depending on the intervention, patency, valvar regurgitation, and paravalvular leak should be evaluated as appropriate.

Applications of Three-Dimensional Imaging

- Although diagnostic image quality may be feasible using 2D-TEE imaging, due to the far-field location of the PV relative to the location of the imaging probe during TEE, the role of 3D imaging is often limited.

TETRALOGY OF FALLOT

Anatomy

The classic constellation of defects in TOF includes a large nonrestrictive VSD, RV obstruction, an overriding Ao, and RV wall hypertrophy (Figure 19.24A). The obstruction can occur at any or at a combination of multiple levels across the RV outflow and PAs. It is well recognized that this anomaly encompasses a broad morphologic spectrum. The malformation represents the most common cyanotic cardiac defect (accounting for 10% of all CHD) and is one of the most prevalent lesions of moderate severity seen in adults. Associated defects include a PFO/ASD, PDA, additional VSDs, vascular anomalies (Ao Arch, coronary arteries, and systemic veins), aortic root dilation, and other pathologies. Variants of tetralogy display other defects besides the typical features of TOF, such as a complete AVSD in "tet-canal" patients. Pulmonary atresia with VSD is considered to represent an extreme form of TOF.

Pathophysiology

The clinical manifestations in patients with TOF relate primarily to the severity of RV outflow obstruction. This, along with the magnitude of ventricular level right-to-left shunting, accounts for the degree of cyanosis

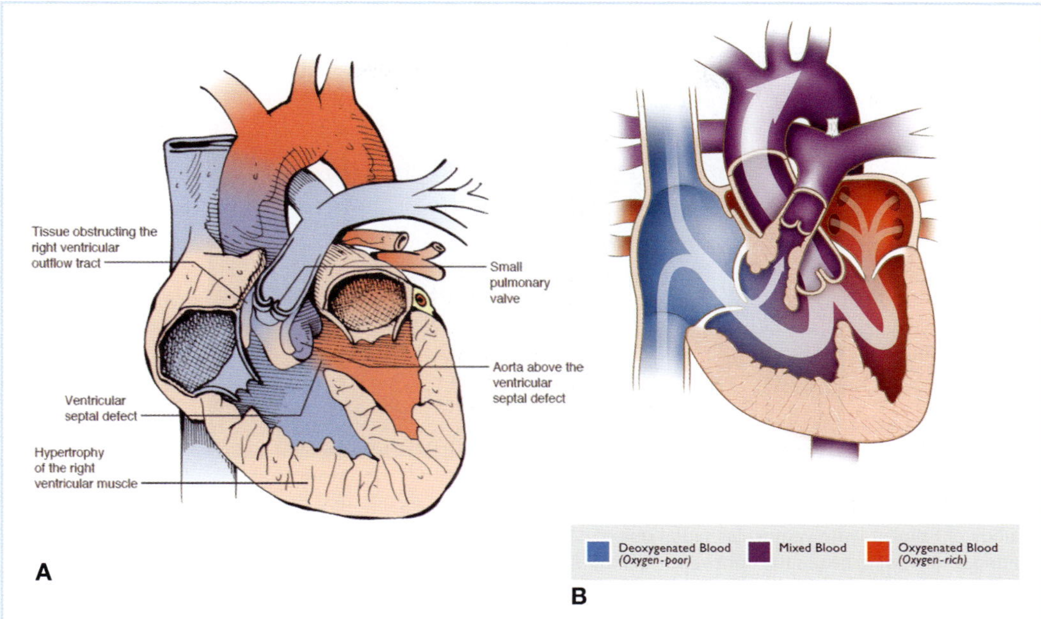

FIGURE 19.24 Tetralogy of Fallot. A: Classic features of this lesion include a ventricular septal defect, right ventricular outflow tract (RVOT) obstruction, right ventricular hypertrophy, and aortic override. The obstruction across the RVOT usually occurs at multiple levels. B: Illustration of tetralogy of Fallot depicting restricted flow across the RVOT (small arrow) and output into the aorta from both ventricles (large arrow). (© 2015 Texas Children's Hospital [reprinted with permission].)

(Figure 19.24B). The unrestrictive VSD and RV pressure at systemic levels results in RV hypertrophy. Although the diagnosis of TOF in most cases is made in infancy or childhood, this pathology may occasionally present in adulthood when the RV outflow obstruction is of minimal to mild severity.

Management

Most patients undergo palliative or "corrective" procedures early in life. Definitive surgery in TOF consists of relief of the RV outflow obstruction and closure of the VSD. When the size of the pulmonary annulus is restrictive, the repair requires the placement of a patch across this region (transannular patch). This disrupts PV integrity and results in some degree of pulmonary regurgitation that increases over time. Occasionally, placement of an RV-to-PA extracardiac conduit is necessary to establish RVOT continuity. Reintervention, either surgical or in the catheterization laboratory, may be required to address pulmonary regurgitation, residual or recurrent RV outflow obstruction, or a residual VSD. In some cases, indications for reoperation include endocarditis, severe aneurysmal dilation of the RV outflow/false aneurysm, or significant aortic regurgitation and progressive root dilation.

Transcatheter or percutaneous pulmonary valve (PPV) implantation is feasible in selected patients. PPV was initially primarily used in patients with RV-to-PA conduits; however, the introduction of larger self-expanding valves has extended its application to native and "patched" RVOTs. In general, these procedures are primarily facilitated by fluoroscopy and angiography but, in many cases, are also assisted by TEE. With the growing use of PPV implantation, both early and late complications have been observed. Early complications include valve migration or embolization, conduit rupture, and coronary artery compression. In contrast, late complications such as stent rupture and endocarditis have emerged as serious concerns. Factors such as younger age at implantation and an immediate postimplant valve peak gradient of 15 mm Hg or higher have been associated with an increased risk of endocarditis. Echocardiography is known to play an important role in diagnosing valve migration and PPV-related endocarditis.

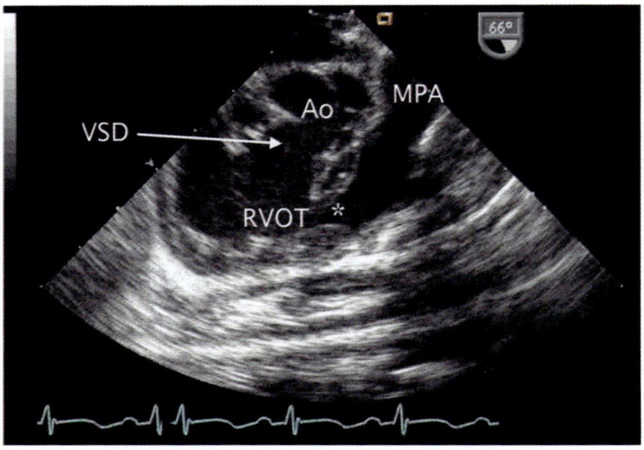

FIGURE 19.25 Tetralogy of Fallot. Midesophageal right ventricular inflow-outflow view displaying classic features of tetralogy of Fallot: a large ventricular septal defect (VSD, arrow) and anterior deviation of the conal septum (asterisk) resulting in narrowing across the right ventricular outflow tract (RVOT). Ao, aorta; MPA, main pulmonary artery.

Transesophageal Echocardiographic Evaluation

The characteristic echocardiographic finding in TOF is that of anterior, superior, and leftward deviation of the conal (infundibular or outlet) septum. This is optimally seen in the ME LAX, ME RV I-O (Figure 19.25; Video 19.20), TG RV I-O, and DTG RVOT views. The ventricular communication usually consists of a large subaortic defect (conoventricular defect) best demonstrated in the ME AV SAX and LAX, and ME 5-Ch views. Additional communications at the atrial and ventricular levels should be explored. Aortic override is best appreciated in the ME LAX (Figure 19.26; Video 19.21), ME AV LAX, ME 5-Ch, TG LAX, and DTG 5-Ch views. Evaluation of the RV outflow and PAs requires a combination of scanning planes that define the

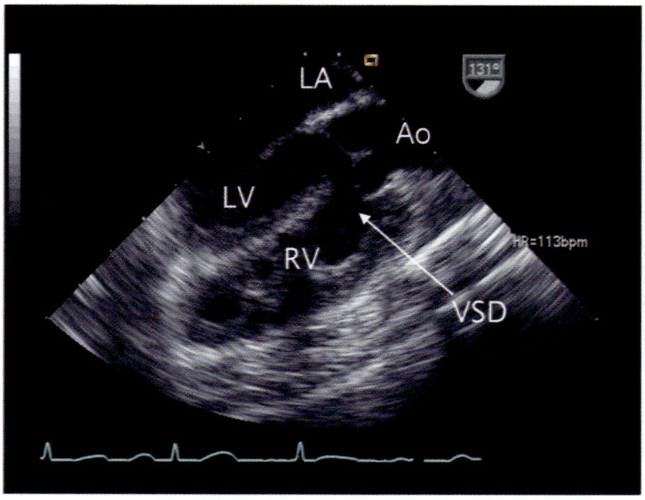

FIGURE 19.26 Tetralogy of Fallot, aortic override. Midesophageal long-axis view displays aortic override over the ventricular septal defect (VSD, arrow) in tetralogy. Ao, aorta; LA, left atrium; LV, left ventricle; RV, right ventricle.

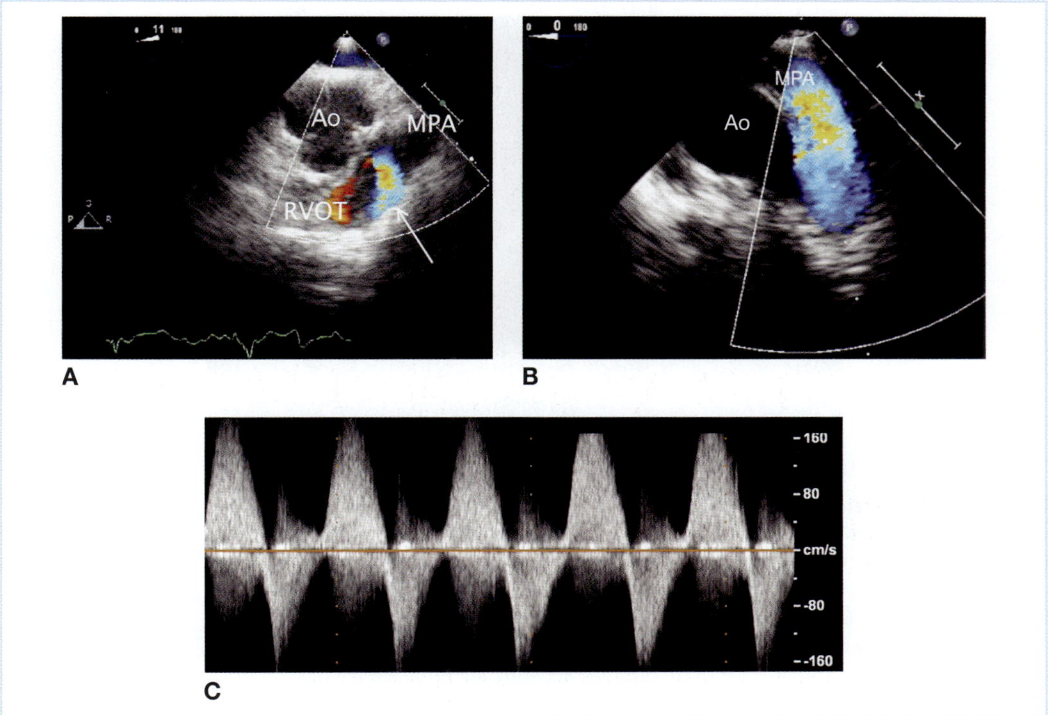

FIGURE 19.27 Tetralogy of Fallot, pulmonary regurgitation. A: Midesophageal aortic valve short-axis view depicts a diastolic color Doppler jet of pulmonary regurgitation (blue signal noted by arrow) in a patient after tetralogy repair. B: Color-flow mapping at the upper esophageal pulmonary artery view displaying the main pulmonary artery (MPA) in the long axis and demonstrating significant flow reversal (blue signal), typical of severe pulmonary regurgitation. C: Continuous-wave Doppler obtained in same view as panel B showing mild flow acceleration across the MPA (flow above the spectral baseline) and pulmonary regurgitant flow away from the transducer (depicted below the baseline) with a short deceleration time, supporting the diagnosis of free pulmonary regurgitation. Ao, aorta; RVOT, right ventricular outflow tract.

subvalvar, valvar, and supravalvar regions. The UE PA view is particularly helpful to visualize the branched PAs in TOF. TEE interrogation of the distal pulmonary bed and aortopulmonary collaterals, if suspected or present, is suboptimal at best because of the limited views of these structures. Suggested cross sections for focused TEE examination include ME 4-Ch, ME 5-Ch, ME LAX, ME AV SAX and LAX, ME RV I-O, ME Asc Ao SAX, TG LAX, TG RV I-O, and DTG views.

Reoperation in the patient with TOF is frequently related to pulmonary regurgitation (Figure 19.27; Video 19.22), resulting in RV dilation (Figure 19.28; Video 19.23) and, in some cases, RV dysfunction (Video 19.24) (18). This may also impair LV myocardial performance due to ventricular interdependence. Residual or recurrent obstruction at the level of the RVOT (Figure 19.29; Video 19.25), MPA/branches, or a residual intracardiac shunt may require reintervention. The same TEE views previously suggested for the initial repair can also be applied to this assessment.

As previously indicated, endocarditis and implanted device migration are significant complications post-PPV placement, both of which can be evaluated using TEE. Without any other anatomic explanation, a single or multiple echodensities along the valve (Figure 19.30; Video 19.26), particularly if an oscillating intracardiac mass is seen on the implanted PV or its supporting structures, should strongly raise the concern of endocarditis. Device misplacement or migration is also easily identified by TEE as, in these cases, the PPV appears positioned either above or below the annulus, potentially resulting in abnormal valve function (Figures 19.30 and 19.31; Video 19.26).

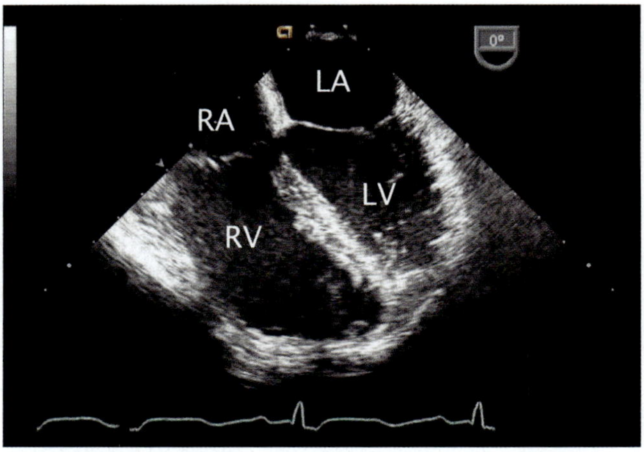

FIGURE 19.28 Tetralogy of Fallot, right ventricular dilation. Midesophageal four-chamber view demonstrating a volume-loaded, dilated right ventricle (RV) in a patient after tetralogy repair undergoing pulmonary valve replacement for severe regurgitation. LA, left atrium; LV, left ventricle; RA, right atrium.

Goals of the Two-Dimensional Examination

- Characterization of RVOT obstruction (distinguish tetralogy from double chamber RV, where there is also a VSD; however, anomalous muscle bundles account for midcavitary obstruction and, unlike tetralogy, no infundibular obstruction is usually present)
- Evaluation of PV annular dimensions, MPA, and branch PA sizes
- Definition of VSD (size, type, and location)
- Evaluation of the degree of aortic override and ventriculoarterial connection (distinguish from double outlet RV, where mitral-aortic fibrous continuity is lacking)
- Determination of aortic root dimension
- Exclusion/evaluation of associated pathology
- Confirmation of coronary artery anatomy
- Assessment of RV hypertrophy, biventricular function

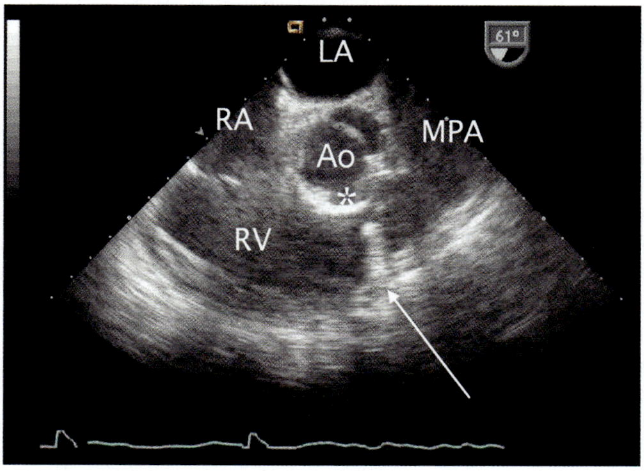

FIGURE 19.29 Tetralogy of Fallot, right ventricular outflow tract obstruction. Midesophageal right ventricular inflow-outflow view displaying recurrent muscular right ventricular outflow tract obstruction (arrow) in a patient with a history of tetralogy repair. The echogenic area noted with an asterisk indicates the ventricular septal defect patch. Ao, aorta; LA, left atrium; MPA, main pulmonary artery; RA, right atrium; RV, right ventricle.

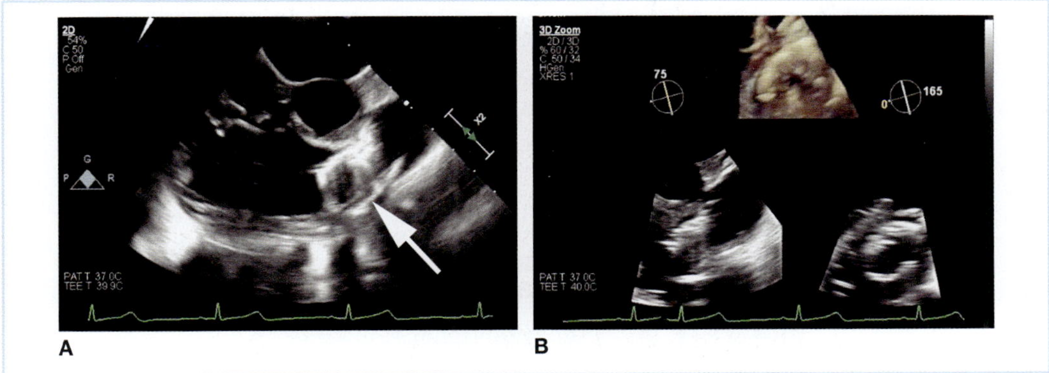

FIGURE 19.30 Tetralogy of Fallot, Melody valve endocarditis. A: Midesophageal right ventricular inflow-outflow view displaying a percutaneously implanted Melody (Medtronic) pulmonary valve located in the infundibular region. This suggests either valve misplacement or migration. B: X-plane imaging of the right ventricular outflow tract (75° and 165°) and three-dimensional reconstruction showing echo densities in the pulmonary aspect of the valve concerning for vegetations versus thrombi.

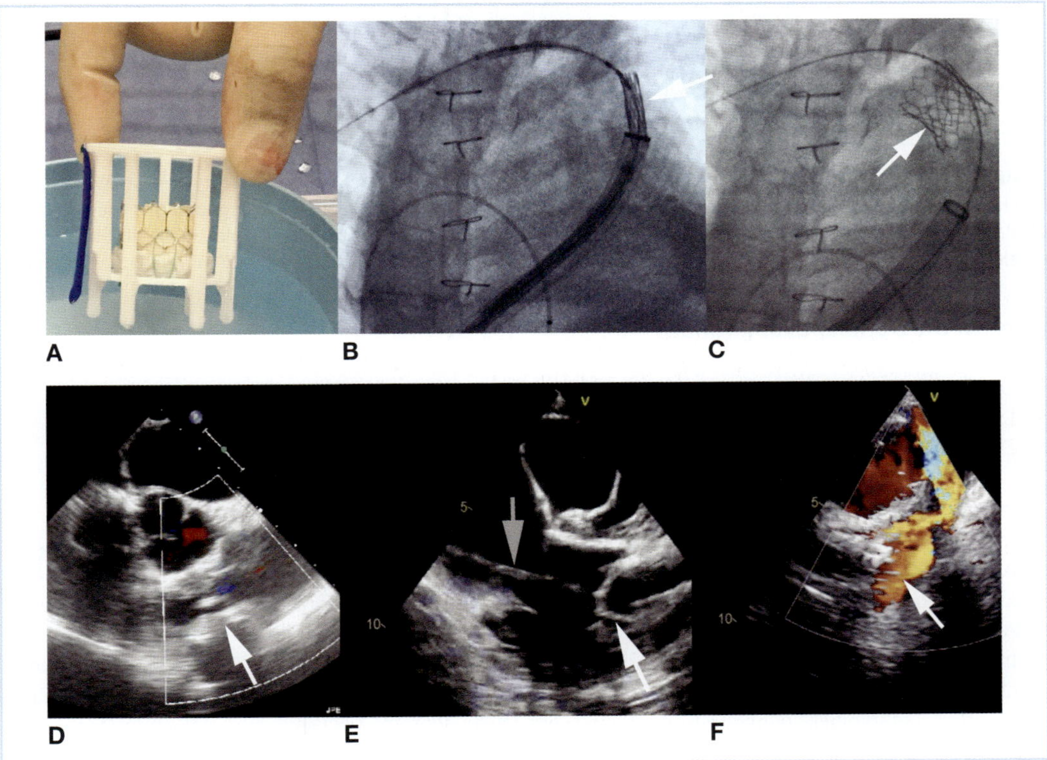

FIGURE 19.31 Tetralogy of Fallot, percutaneous pulmonary valve implantation and migration. A: SAPEIN 3 valve (Edwards Lifesciences) prior to implantation in pulmonary position (size 26 mm). B: Anteroposterior fluoroscopic view depicting the valve and delivery sheath prior to percutaneous deployment (white arrow). C: Same fluoroscopic view showing the deployed valve in the right ventricular outflow tract (white arrow). D: Post-deployment midesophageal right ventricular inflow-outflow image showing the implanted valve in subpulmonary position (white arrow) with a trivial jet of regurgitation. The image raised the question of valve malposition and because of concerns related to device instability, the patient was immediately taken to the operating room. E: Same transesophageal echocardiography view obtained in the operating room showing further valve prolapse into the right ventricle (white arrow). The deployment sheath that was left in place for stabilization is seen across the tricuspid valve (gray arrow). F: Color-flow Doppler across the prolapsed pulmonary valve with associated flow disturbance (white arrow). (Reprinted with permission from Andropoulos DB, Mossad EM, Gottlieb EA, eds. *Anesthesia for Congenital Heart Disease*. 4th ed. Wiley-Blackwell; 2023.)

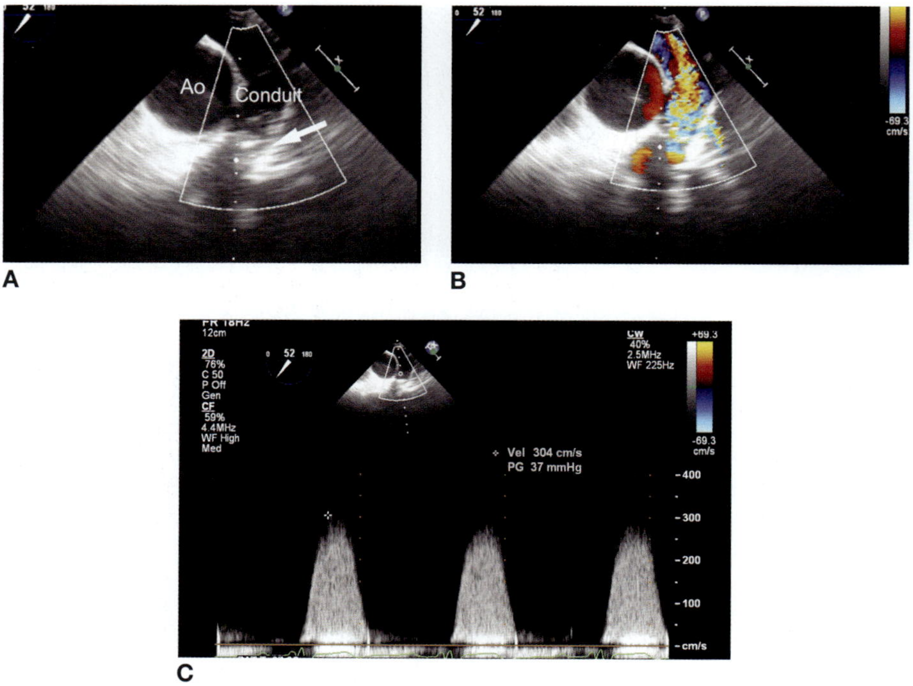

FIGURE 19.32 Tetralogy of Fallot, conduit obstruction. A: Upper esophageal pulmonary artery view showing a calcified right ventricular to main pulmonary artery conduit (white arrow). B: Color-flow Doppler imaging at the same level displaying turbulent flow across the conduit as manifested by flow aliasing. C: Spectral Doppler tracing illustrating flow acceleration across the conduit with a peak velocity of 3 m/s and a derived peak gradient of 37 mm Hg. Ao, aorta.

Goals of the Doppler Examination

- Characterization of flow across VSD (direction and velocity) and other intracardiac communications
- Definition of the level/severity of the RV outflow obstruction
- Evaluation of AV competence
- Detection of tricuspid regurgitation and peak regurgitant velocity for RV systolic pressure estimate

Goals of the Examination After Surgery

- Evaluation for residual pathology, such as RV outflow or conduit obstruction and intracardiac shunts
- Assessment of tricuspid, pulmonary, and AV competence
- Evaluation of tricuspid regurgitation and peak regurgitant velocity for estimation of RV systolic pressure
- Assessment of biventricular function
- In the patient undergoing reintervention following TOF repair: evaluation for pulmonary/conduit obstruction (Figure 19.32; Video 19.27) and/or regurgitation, presence of residual intracardiac shunts or other pathologies, configuration of interventricular septum, tricuspid and AV competence, and biventricular size and systolic function
- Interrogation of PV function after replacement (Video 19.28)

Goals of the Examination During Transcatheter Intervention

- TEE may be used during PV implantation for monitoring and to facilitate the procedure

Applications of Three-Dimensional Imaging

Also applicable to conotruncal defects discussed as follows:

- Evaluation of anatomy, particularly septal defects and outflows
- Simultaneous *en face* view of all three PV leaflets, allowing for a more detailed assessment of each leaflet and their coaptation

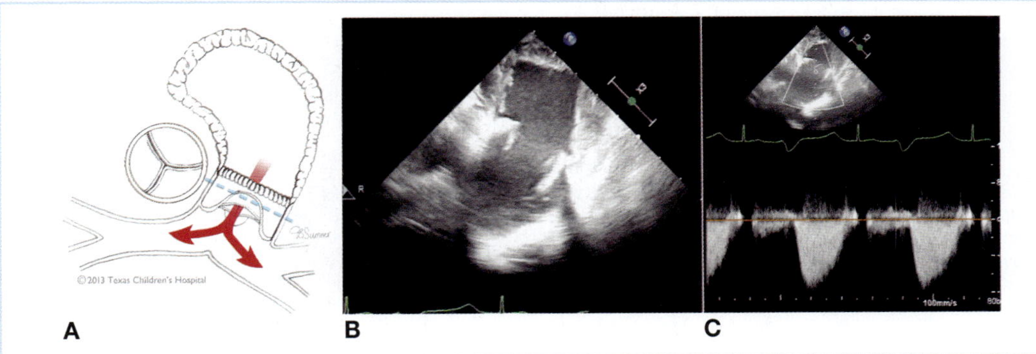

FIGURE 19.33 Tetralogy of Fallot, surgical pulmonary valve replacement (epicardial echocardiography). A: Diagrammatic representation of the right ventricular outflow view (RVOT) as obtained by epicardial imaging (transthoracic parasternal short-axis echocardiographic view equivalent) after pulmonary valve replacement. (© 2013 Texas Children's Hospital [reprinted with permission].) B: Epicardial echo image of the RVOT displaying a 27 mm Epic porcine bioprosthetic heart valve in pulmonary position (Abbott Laboratories). C: Pulsed-wave Doppler imaging in the same view, showing low-velocity forward flow across the valve.

- Visualization of the subvalvar apparatus and its spatial relationship to the PV and surrounding structures
- Determination of repair suitability
- Assessment of the surgical procedures and their complications
- Evaluation of ventricular volumes and ejection fraction

Epicardial Echocardiographic Evaluation

TEE has limitations when evaluating the PV and RVOT due to the anterior position of these structures relative to the esophagus, which can result in suboptimal image quality, particularly in the adult population. Epicardial echocardiography (EE) offers an alternative or complementary imaging modality to TEE in the interrogation of these structures and other settings (eg, poor TEE windows, arch reconstruction, inability to use TEE) (19-21). During surgery, EE is performed by the surgeon while placing an ultrasound probe covered by a sterile sheath directly onto the surface of the heart, providing the acquisition of real-time, high-resolution images. The epicardial RVOT view is favored for imaging of the RVOT and the PV (22). In this view, the probe is positioned over the RV scanning toward the RV outflow and PV, allowing for optimal 2D image resolution of these structures, color-flow Doppler assessment, and ideal Doppler alignment to assess any residual gradient and/or severity of pulmonary regurgitation (Figure 19.33; Video 19.28). In addition, the MPA bifurcation and proximal/mid right and left PA branches can be easily visualized. A limitation of this technique is the need for surgical expertise regarding probe positioning.

TRANSPOSITION OF THE GREAT ARTERIES

Anatomy

Dextro-transposition of the great vessels (D-TGA), also referred to as complete transposition, is characterized by concordance of the atrioventricular connection and discordance of the ventriculoarterial connection. In this malformation, a morphologic RA is connected to a morphologic RV; however, the RV ejects into the Ao. A morphologic LA drains into a morphologic LV, giving rise to the PA (Figure 19.34A). The abnormal origin of the great arteries typically results in a parallel relation of these structures rather than the normal crossover between the two. D-TGA accounts for 4% of all cases of CHD. Associated pathology may include PDA, ASD, VSD, obstruction to pulmonary blood flow, AV abnormalities, variation in the origin and course of the coronary arteries, and Ao Arch anomalies.

Pathophysiology

In D-TGA, the systemic and pulmonary circulations function in parallel rather than in series, leading to cyanosis in the neonatal period (Figure 19.34B). Mixing of the circulations is essential for survival.

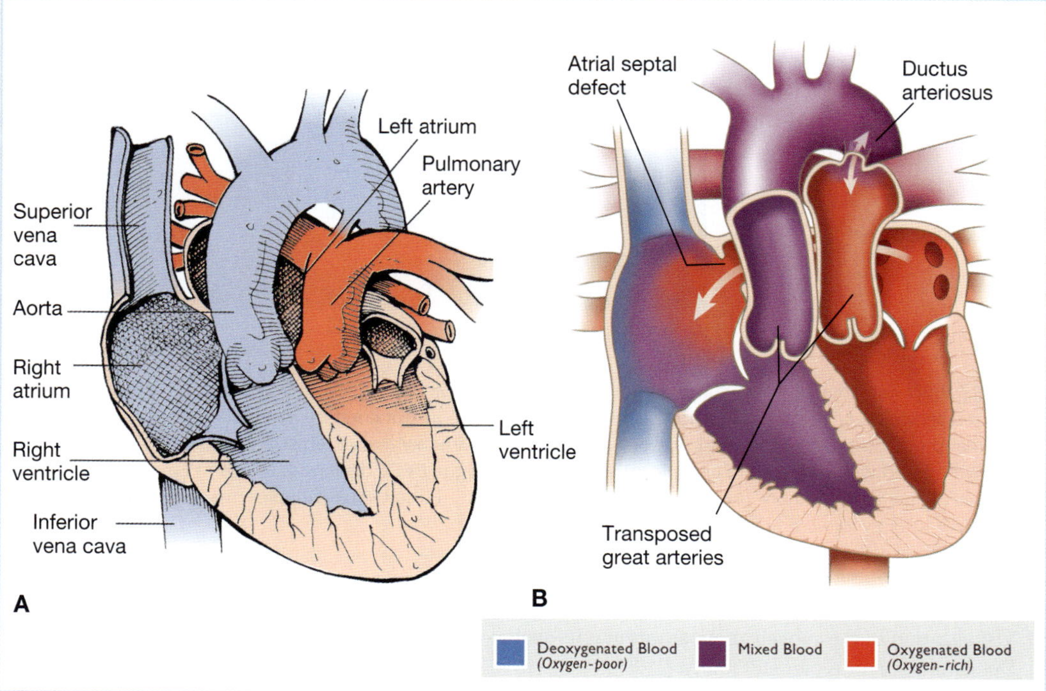

FIGURE 19.34 Transposition of the great arteries. A: Graphic depicting the anatomic features in D-transposition of the great arteries. In this lesion, the right atrium is connected to the right ventricle, giving rise to the aorta. The left atrium is connected to the left ventricle, which gives rise to the pulmonary artery. This abnormal relationship is referred to as atrioventricular concordance and ventriculoarterial discordance. B: Illustration displaying the parallel systemic and pulmonary circulations in transposition and the associated cyanosis. Mixing of the circulations is essential for survival and occurs at the ductal and atrial levels.

Management

The surgical management of this lesion has evolved dramatically over the years. In the past, most patients underwent either palliation or an atrial baffle procedure (Mustard or Senning operation; Figure 19.35). This is also referred to as an "atrial switch procedure." This intervention consists of redirecting the systemic venous blood through the mitral valve, LV, and PA, while the pulmonary venous return is diverted across the tricuspid valve, RV, and Ao. This allows for the separation of pulmonary and systemic circulations and physiologic correction but maintains the RV as the systemic pump. Most older adult patients are likely to have undergone this type of repair. Long-term issues following atrial switch procedures include dysfunction of the systemic RV, tricuspid (systemic) valve incompetence, obstruction of venous pathways/baffle leaks, arrhythmias, sudden cardiac death, and the late development of pulmonary vascular disease. Currently, the favored approach for infants with D-TGA is anatomic correction or the arterial switch operation (Jatene procedure; Figure 19.36). This involves transection of the great arteries above the valve sinuses and anastomoses to their appropriate respective ventricular outflows, in addition to translocation of the coronary arteries to the systemic outflow tract. At the time of this intervention, additional defects are also addressed. Problems after the arterial switch procedure are primarily related to supravalvar or branch PA stenosis, neoaortic root dilation/regurgitation, and coronary artery issues. Catheter-based interventions and/or reoperation may be required for progression of the primary pathology, recurrent disease, residua, or sequelae associated with prior surgical procedures. In cases of transposition where there are additional defects, interventions other than the arterial switch procedure might be indicated. For patients with transposition, VSD, and LV outflow tract obstruction, a Rastelli or Nikaidoh procedure might be performed. In the Rastelli operation, an intracardiac baffle is created that allows for LV output into the anterior Ao, and the RVOT is reconstructed. In the Nikaidoh procedure, the conal septum is divided, the Ao is posteriorly translocated to

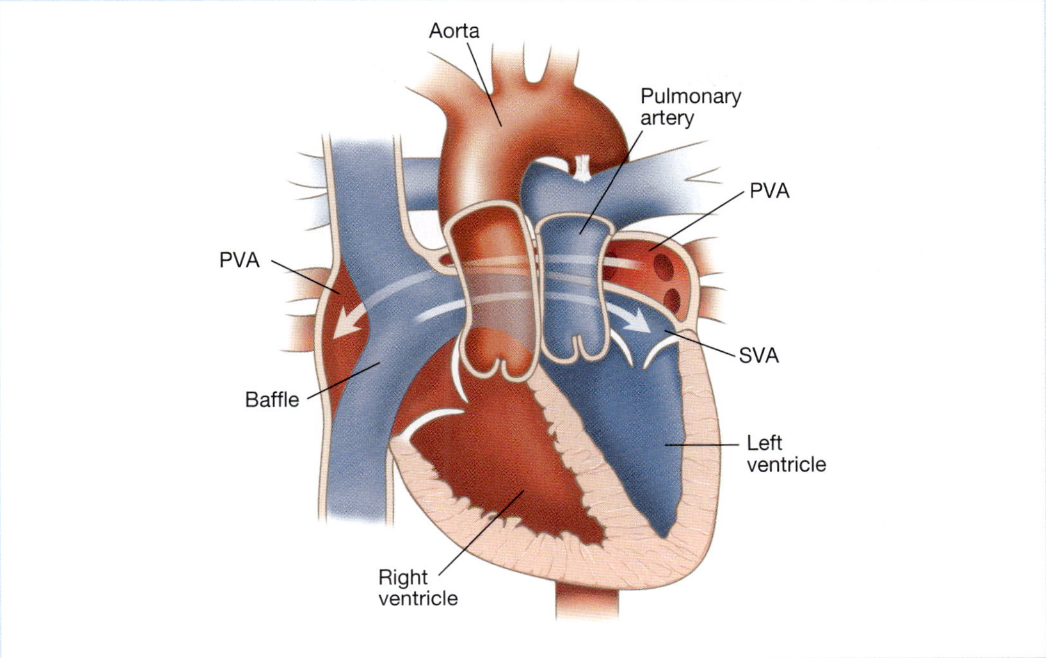

FIGURE 19.35 Transposition of the great arteries, atrial baffle procedure. The graphic depicts the direction of blood flow following an atrial redirection procedure. PVA, pulmonary venous atrium; SVA, systemic venous atrium.

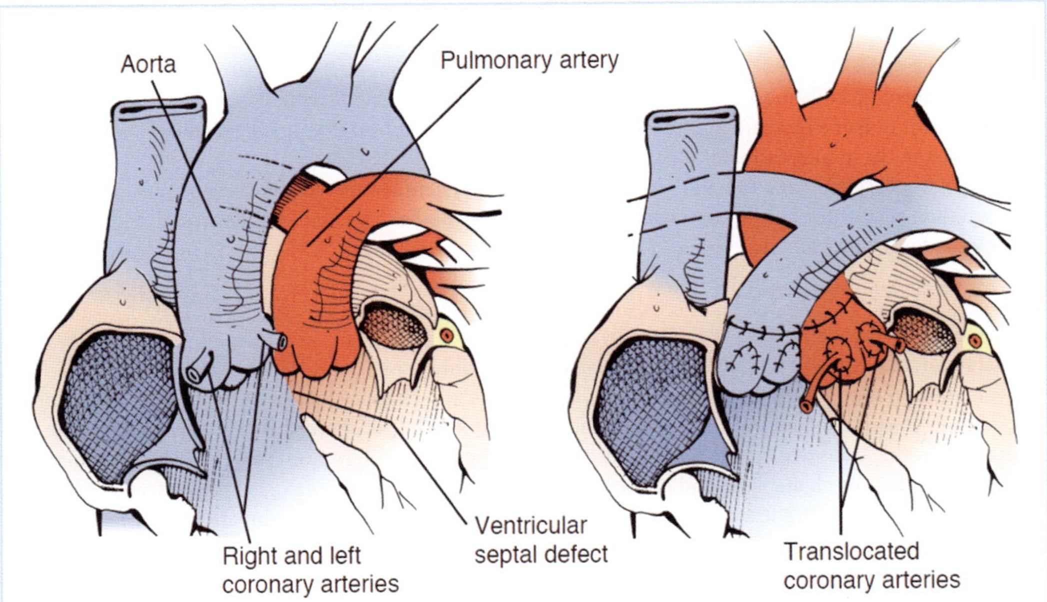

FIGURE 19.36 Transposition of the great arteries, arterial switch procedure. The aorta and main pulmonary artery are transected and anastomosed to their appropriate ventricular outflows in this surgical procedure. The coronary arteries are translocated to the systemic outflow tract. This diagrammatic representation depicts a ventricular septal defect, which is patch closed when the arterial switch operation is undertaken.

receive LV output, and the RVOT is reconstructed. These complex operations are each potentially associated with late complications that include residual VSD, subaortic obstruction (following Rastelli), conduit failure, and coronary problems (following Nikaidoh).

Transesophageal Echocardiographic Evaluation

The echocardiographic evaluation in D-TGA should include 2D imaging, spectral Doppler examination, color-flow mapping, and possibly contrast echocardiography (23). In addition, 3D imaging could be extremely helpful in some cases. Suggested cross sections for focused TEE examination include ME 4-Ch, ME 5-Ch, ME 2-Ch, ME commissural, ME LAX, ME AV SAX and LAX, ME bicaval, ME modified bicaval, ME RV I-O, TG basal and midpapillary (Mid Pap) SAX, and DTG views of both outflow tracts.

Goals of the Two-Dimensional Examination

- Assessment of atrioventricular and ventriculoarterial connections
- Evaluation of associated pathology, such as intracardiac communications and outflow tract obstruction
- Definition or confirmation of coronary anatomy in some cases
- Estimation of ventricular sizes and systolic function
- Abnormal chordal attachments across the VSD in patients with TGA/VSD that can alter intraoperative management and surgical approach; therefore, crossing chords should be carefully evaluated

Goals of the Doppler Examination

- Characterization of flow across intracardiac communications
- Assessment of outflow tract gradients
- Evaluation of valvar competence
- Estimation of PA pressure

Goals of the Examination After Surgery

For atrial baffle (atrial switch procedures):

- Visualization of systemic and pulmonary venous pathways (Figure 19.37; Video 19.29) to assess for obstruction; contrast administration through an arm or jugular vein facilitates this assessment (in the absence of obstruction, contrast rapidly courses from the SVC into the systemic venous atria and no contrast is seen from the IVC aspect of the baffle; if severe obstruction of superior limb, contrast is diverted through collaterals to the lower aspect of the systemic venous baffle)
- Assessment of baffle leaks (administration of agitated saline solution through a peripheral or central vein can assist in the identification of baffle leaks)
- Evaluation of systemic RV function and tricuspid valve (systemic atrioventricular valve) for regurgitation
- Estimation of LV pressure (pulmonary ventricle) using the peak velocity of the mitral regurgitant jet, allowing for PA pressure assessment

For arterial switch procedures:

- Evaluation of valvular regurgitation
- Evaluation of outflow tract for obstruction/arterial root dimensions
- Evaluation of the PAs (most of these operations involve a LeCompte maneuver where the MPA and its branches are brought forward in front of the Ao; it should be recognized that in this setting, the PAs drape over the Ao as this can be potentially confusing during imaging). Comprehensive assessment of PA branches might be challenging and may benefit from epicardial imaging.
- Examination of flow in the translocated coronary arteries (may benefit a combination of TEE and EE)
- Assessment of residual shunts (atrial and ventricular)
- Assessment of global and segmental ventricular function

For the Rastelli or Nikaidoh procedures:

- Evaluation for residual intracardiac shunts
- Evaluation of outflow tracts for obstruction
- Assessment of global and segmental ventricular function

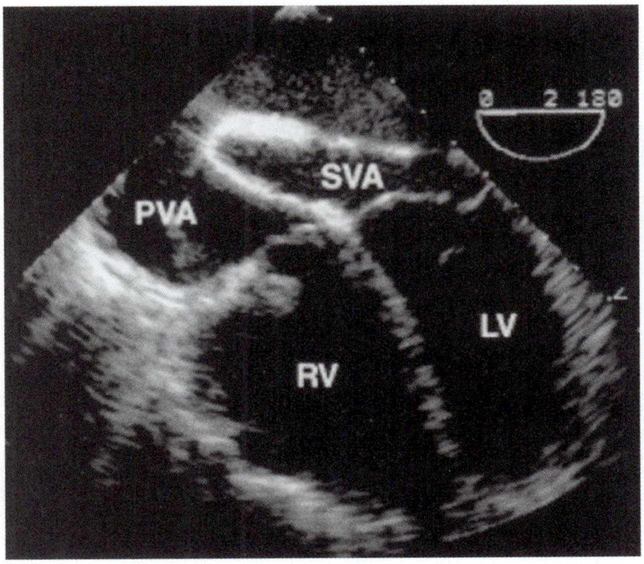

FIGURE 19.37 Transposition of the great arteries, atrial baffle procedure. Midesophageal four-chamber view illustrating the features of an atrial redirection procedure. In this procedure, venous returns from the systemic and pulmonary circulations are redirected using a baffle. This results in drainage of deoxygenated blood from the superior and inferior venae cavae into the systemic venous atrium (SVA), then through the mitral valve into the left ventricle (LV), being ejected into the pulmonary artery. Oxygenated blood from the pulmonary veins drains into the pulmonary venous atrium (PVA) and, through the tricuspid valve into the right ventricle (RV) being ejected into the aorta. The RV remains the systemic ventricle.

Goals of the Examination During Transcatheter Interventions

- Monitoring during transcatheter balloon dilation and possible stenting of venous pathway obstruction in atrial baffles
- Monitoring during transcatheter occlusion of intracardiac shunts (baffle leaks and residual ventricular communications)

CONGENITALLY CORRECTED TRANSPOSITION OF THE GREAT ARTERIES

Anatomy

Congenitally corrected transposition of the great arteries (CCTGA), also known as physiologically corrected transposition, is characterized by discordance between the atrioventricular and ventriculoarterial connections (double discordance). The RA connects to a morphologic LV that ejects into the PA, while the LA connects to a morphologic RV that ejects into the Ao (Figure 19.38A). This defect is relatively rare, accounting for less than 0.5% of all forms of CHD. Corrected transposition may also be referred to as levo-TGA (L-TGA) due to the abnormal looping pattern of the heart tube during development (L-loop) in most patients with this lesion. In this case, the Ao is oriented to the left (levo) rather than to the right (D-loop) as is normally the case. This defect in most cases is associated with cardiac anomalies, such as VSD, obstruction to pulmonary blood flow, and left atrioventricular (tricuspid) valve abnormalities (eg, Ebstein-like malformation or dysplasia).

Pathophysiology

In this lesion, the systemic venous return enters the PA being ejected by the LV; the pulmonary venous blood exits into the Ao as ejected by the RV. The serial arrangement of the systemic and pulmonary circulations results in normal physiology—hence the term "corrected." Patients with CCTGA require medical attention in most cases because of associated lesions, such as VSD (Figure 19.38B), PS, and/or regurgitation related to Ebstein-like (Ebsteinoid) malformation of the systemic tricuspid valve. In the absence of concomitant

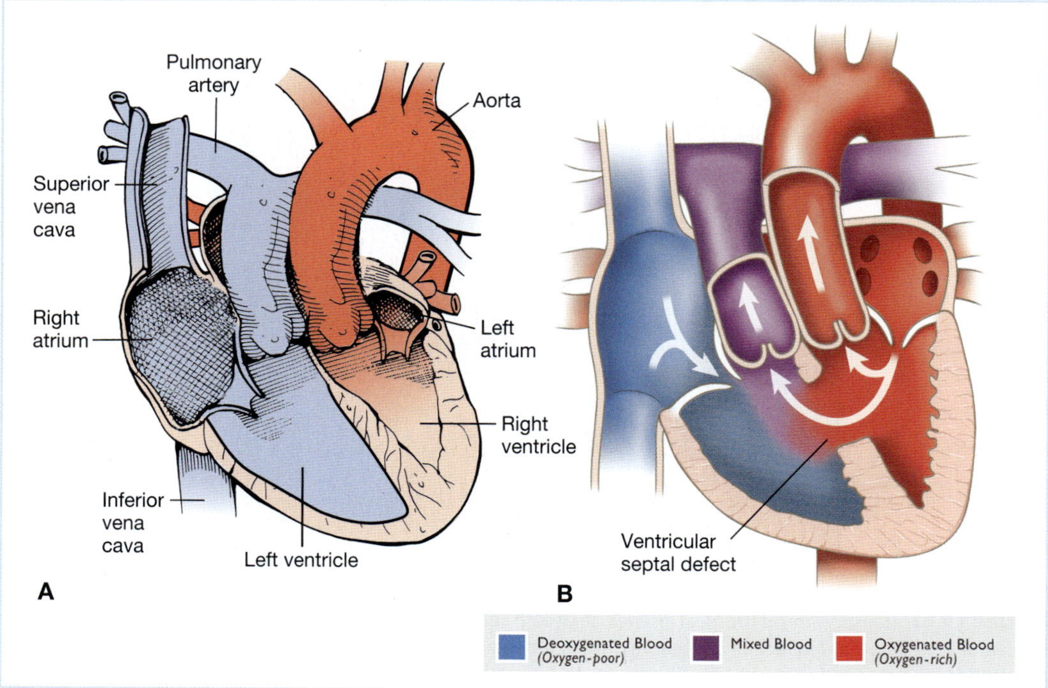

FIGURE 19.38 Congenitally corrected transposition. A: The graphic depicts the abnormal connections of the cardiac segments of this lesion. Note the "double discordant" atrioventricular and ventriculoarterial connections. B: The illustration displays the physiology of congenitally corrected transposition associated with a ventricular septal defect.

pathology, a small number of individuals can have relatively normal lives and even survive into the seventh and eighth decades. Unfortunately, in the majority, progressive systolic impairment of the systemic RV ensues, frequently associated with concomitant systemic (tricuspid) atrioventricular valve regurgitation, overt heart failure, and/or conduction defects prompting medical care.

Management

Most patients require surgery to address associated defects. Interventions include closure of intracardiac communications, relief of pulmonary outflow tract obstruction, and tricuspid valve repair/replacement (the so-called "classic repairs"). In view of late problems such as progressive dysfunction and failure of the RV in the systemic circulation and tricuspid regurgitation, in addition to the high incidence of reoperation, alternate strategies have been utilized. In some cases, more complex interventions such as "double switch procedures" (atrial redirection and arterial switch operation) or modifications thereof may be advised in infants, children, and adolescents. Under circumstances where the LV pressure is subsystemic and this chamber may not be able to assume the role of a systemic pump following this type of intervention (absent or restrictive VSD, or no pulmonary outflow obstruction), preliminary PA banding may be performed to train the LV over time. This approach may not be successful past adolescence. In patients with systemic RV dysfunction, palliative options include PA banding, tricuspid valve repair/replacement, cardiac resynchronization therapy, and mechanical circulatory support. Cardiac transplantation may be the only long-term option in adults with this defect and severe RV failure. A high incidence of atrioventricular block is seen in this lesion, and therefore, the frequent need for pacemaker placement/replacement is seen in this patient group.

Transesophageal Echocardiographic Evaluation

Definition of atrioventricular connections by echocardiography requires identification of the characteristic features that establish cardiac chamber morphology. The atrioventricular valves are associated with their

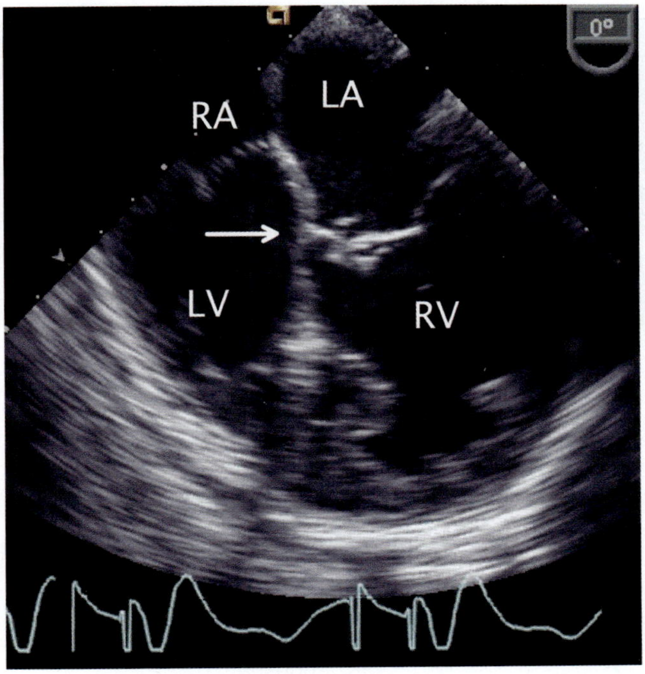

FIGURE 19.39 Congenitally corrected transposition. Midesophageal four-chamber view displays this lesion's abnormal (discordant) atrioventricular connection. The right atrium (RA) empties into the morphologic left ventricle (LV) through the mitral valve, and the left atrium (LA) empties into the morphologic right ventricle (RV) through the tricuspid valve. Note the apical displacement of the left-sided tricuspid valve (arrow), a frequently associated anomaly in this lesion.

corresponding ventricles; thus, the morphologic tricuspid valve will identify the RV and the morphologic mitral valve the LV. In the ME 4-Ch view, the morphologic RV is characterized by inferior insertion of the septal leaflet of the tricuspid valve to the ventricular septum (relative to the mitral valve; Figure 19.39; Video 19.30) and by the presence of the moderator band. The tricuspid valve characteristically displays attachments to the ventricular septum (septophilic), in contrast to the mitral valve (septophobic). The LV is identified by two distinct papillary muscles in the TG Mid Pap SAX view. Typically, in CCTGA, the Ao is anterior and to the left relative to the PA. Suggested cross sections for focused TEE examination include ME 4-Ch, ME 5-Ch, ME 2-Ch, ME LAX, TG Mid Pap SAX, TG LAX, TG RV I-O, and DTG views.

Goals of the Two-Dimensional Examination

- Determination of atrial arrangement, ventricular, and great artery morphologies
- Assessment of atrioventricular and ventriculoarterial connections
- Evaluation of associated defects (Figure 19.40; Videos 19.31-19.33). As with D-TGA/VSD, in CCTGA/VSD, abnormal chordal attachments crossing the VSD should be carefully assessed.
- Estimation of ventricular sizes and systolic function

Goals of the Doppler Examination

- Characterization of flow across intracardiac communications
- Assessment of outflow tracts for the presence and severity of obstruction
- Evaluation of atrioventricular valve regurgitation
- Estimation of LV pressure (pulmonary ventricle) using the peak velocity of the mitral regurgitant jet

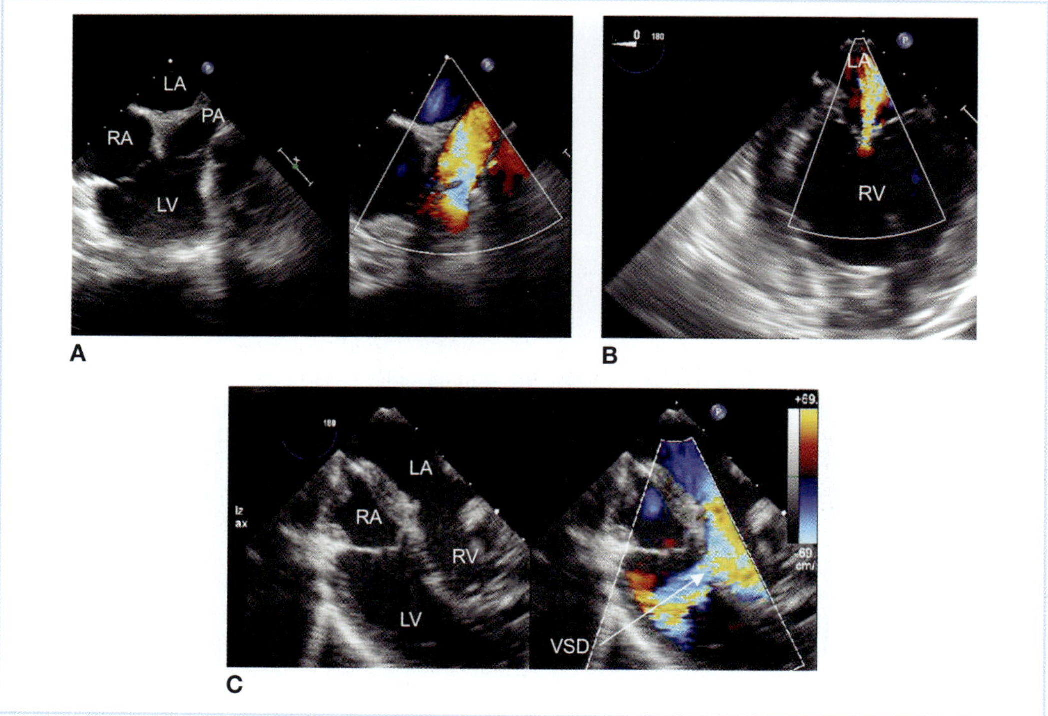

FIGURE 19.40 Congenitally corrected transposition, associated lesions. A: Modified midesophageal transesophageal echocardiography view showing a narrowed pulmonary outflow tract with color Doppler evidence of turbulent flow across this region in congenitally corrected transposition. B: Midesophageal four-chamber view with color-flow Doppler (focusing on the left-sided cardiac structures) in a patient with the same cardiac anomaly demonstrating severe systemic right ventricular (RV) dilation (left-sided ventricle) and associated tricuspid regurgitation. C: Midesophageal four-chamber two-dimensional and color Doppler imaging showing a muscular ventricular septal defect (VSD; arrow) with shunting from the systemic (left-sided) RV to the subpulmonary (right-sided) left ventricle (LV). LA, left atrium; PA, pulmonary artery; RA, right atrium.

Goals of the Examination After Surgery

- Evaluation of residual shunts, outflow obstruction, and systemic atrioventricular valve regurgitation
- Assessment of systolic function of the morphologic RV in the systemic circulation. The evaluation of LV global and segmental function is important following the double switch operation, given the coronary translocation.
- Interrogation of the atrial baffle in double switch procedures
- Determination of adequacy of PA banding if training or palliative strategy undertaken (band gradient, septal configuration, ventricular wall thickness)

EBSTEIN ANOMALY

Anatomy

The hallmark of Ebstein anomaly is apical displacement of the septal and, often, posterior tricuspid valve leaflets (Figure 19.41A). Classic findings include abnormal tricuspid leaflet morphology/dysplasia, a redundant sail-like anterior leaflet associated with varying degrees of regurgitation, and an atrialized inlet portion of the RV resulting in a reduction in the functional components of this chamber. This lesion is the most common form of congenital tricuspid valve disease and accounts for less than 1% of CHD. Frequent associated defects are atrial communications and RVOT anomalies.

Pathophysiology

The wide morphologic spectrum in this lesion, together with the concomitant presence of associated defects, accounts for the variable hemodynamic abnormalities and clinical manifestations. The severity of tricuspid

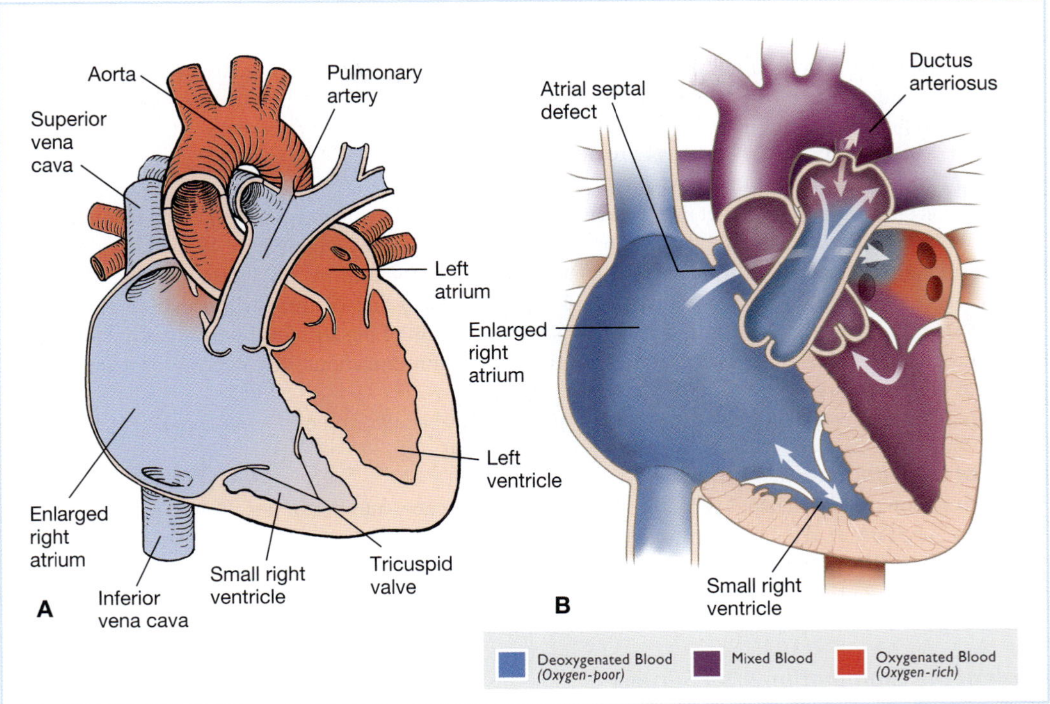

FIGURE 19.41 Ebstein anomaly. A: Graphic depicting the tricuspid valve displacement in Ebstein anomaly. B: The physiologic features of this lesion are characterized by tricuspid regurgitation, right atrial dilation, and a frequently associated atrial communication that may allow for right-to-left shunting in some cases.

regurgitation due to abnormal leaflet coaptation plays a major role, resulting in RA dilation and the development of arrhythmias, enlargement of an atrial communication, concomitant shunting, and heart failure symptoms (Figure 19.41B). Associated atrial level right-to-left shunting and/or pulmonary outflow tract obstruction account for the presence of cyanosis in some cases. Various degrees of RV hypoplasia and systolic functional impairment may be seen. Enlargement of the right cardiac chambers can lead to a leftward shift of the interventricular septum, also compromising the geometry and function of the LV.

Management

The adult with Ebstein anomaly may only require medical surveillance. Supraventricular arrhythmias, severe tricuspid regurgitation, and/or the presence of an atrial communication represent the most common indications for intervention in this patient group. Tricuspid valve repair or replacement may be necessary with closure of an existing interatrial communication. Atrial plication and/or a Maze procedure may also be indicated. In some cases, a concomitant bidirectional cavopulmonary connection is also performed to decrease the volume load to the RV and optimize LV preload, particularly within the context of a small or severely dilated RV chamber with decreased systolic function. This is referred to as a "one-and-a-half" ventricle approach.

Transesophageal Echocardiographic Evaluation

The tricuspid valve pathology and degree of valvar regurgitation are best assessed in the ME 4-Ch, ME modified bicaval, ME RV I-O, TG RV inflow, and TG RV I-O views. Important aspects to be examined include septal leaflet displacement, leaflet motion, adherence or tethering of septal and posterior leaflets to underlying myocardium, and chordal support apparatus. These may impact the feasibility of a successful repair. Cross sections that allow for RV functional assessment, such as the TG RV basal view and TG RV I-O views, are of benefit. In patients with Ebstein anomaly, the use of 3D-TEE is key for comprehensive assessment of the abnormal tricuspid valve.

Severity scoring systems have been proposed for Ebstein anomaly as predictors of prognosis. Among echocardiographic parameters, the Celermajer index has been utilized most widely primarily in the pediatric age group but also applied to adults. This index is measured as the ratio between area of the anatomic RA plus atrialized RV and combined areas of the remaining chambers as obtained by planimetry. The application of this index in clinical assessment and prognostic value in the adult continues to be debated.

Goals of the Two-Dimensional Examination

- Definition of tricuspid valve leaflet morphology, mobility, chordal attachments, and coaptation point (favorable factors for repair are a large mobile anterior leaflet with a free leading edge; Figure 19.42; Video 19.34)
- Determination of apical tricuspid septal leaflet displacement (>8 mm/m^2 distance compared to the level of attachment of the anterior mitral leaflet and indexed to body surface area is abnormal) (Figure 19.43)
- Assessment of RA, tricuspid annulus, and RV sizes; evaluation of the atrialized portion of the RV
- Evaluation of associated defects, such as intracardiac communications, RV outflow obstruction, and mitral valve prolapse
- Assessment of biventricular function (for RV: atrialized, trabecular, and outlet portions)

Goals of the Doppler Examination

- Interrogation of the tricuspid valve for regurgitation (presence, number of jets, origin, pattern, severity, peak regurgitant jet velocity); in most cases, the regurgitant jet originates below the level of the annulus
- Inspection of RVOT for obstruction and, if present, determination of gradient (severe leaflet displacement can lead to RV outflow obstruction)
- Interrogation of the atrial septum (presence of communication, size, direction of shunting)

Goals of the Examination After Surgery

- Evaluation of the tricuspid valve for stenosis and regurgitation
- Examination of prosthetic valve function as indicated
- Assessment of biventricular function
- Exclusion of residual intracardiac shunting (color Doppler and contrast study with agitated saline as needed)

Goals of the Examination During Transcatheter Intervention

- Monitoring and guidance during valve implantation or other percutaneous procedures addressing associated defects (eg, ASD device closure)
- Guidance during electrophysiologic procedures (eg, catheter ablations, transseptal puncture)

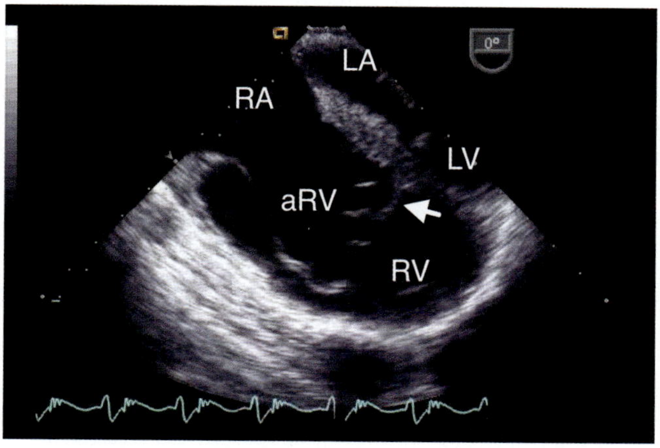

FIGURE 19.42 Ebstein anomaly. Midesophageal four-chamber view with rightward transducer rotation in a patient with Ebstein anomaly. Note the severe apical displacement of the tricuspid valve septal leaflet (arrow) from the valve annulus and the redundant anterior leaflet. The leaflet displacement results in an atrialized portion of the right ventricle (aRV). LA, left atrium; LV, left ventricle; RA, right atrium; RV, right ventricle.

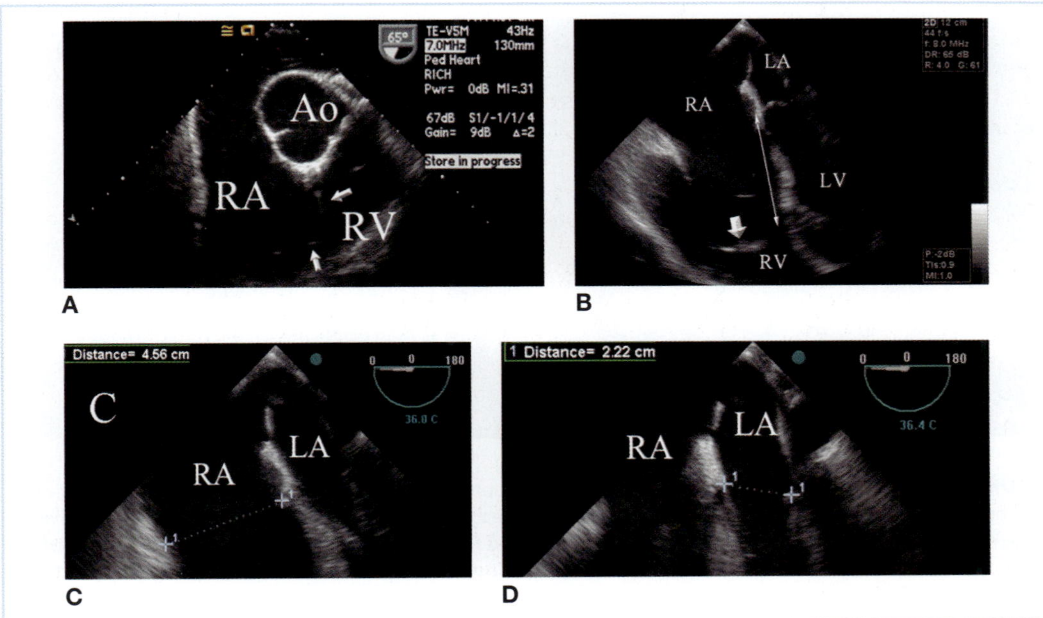

FIGURE 19.43 Ebstein anomaly. A: Midesophageal right ventricular inflow-outflow view showing apical displacement of the tricuspid valve leaflets (arrows). B: Midesophageal four-chamber view depicting the apically displaced leaflets (short arrow). The distance corresponding to the apical tricuspid septal leaflet displacement relative to the septal insertion of the anterior mitral leaflet is noted (long arrow). C,D: Same images as in panel B showing measurement of the "true" tricuspid valve annulus, which appears dilated (45 mm) in panel C and a corresponding normal mitral valve annulus of 22 mm in panel D. Ao, aorta; LA, left atrium; LV, left ventricle; RA, right atrium; RV, right ventricle.

Applications of Three-Dimensional Imaging

- Visualization of tricuspid valve leaflet morphology and coaptation (shown to correlate with intraoperative findings) (Figure 19.44; Video 19.35)
- Examination of the tricuspid valve apparatus in different planes
- Calculation of tricuspid valve area
- Assessment of chordal support apparatus
- Enhanced definition of regurgitant jets, analysis of jets in terms of origin, mechanism, and severity
- Visualization of the orifice of the tricuspid valve cone (*en face* view planimetry) following the da Silva cone reconstruction

SINGLE-VENTRICLE LESIONS OR UNIVENTRICULAR HEART

Anatomy

The spectrum of single ventricle or univentricular heart encompasses a wide variety of anatomic arrangements. In most cases, there is ventricular hypoplasia; thus, a single functional ventricular chamber is present. However, in some patients with a two-ventricle heart, a biventricular repair is not feasible, and a single-ventricle management strategy is undertaken. The latter group is functionally considered within the univentricular heart category. The major anatomic variants of single ventricle include tricuspid atresia, hypoplastic left heart syndrome, and double-inlet LV.

Pathophysiology

A common feature among these lesions is complete admixture of systemic and pulmonary venous blood at the atrial or ventricular level. Another frequent finding is systemic or pulmonary outflow tract obstruction.

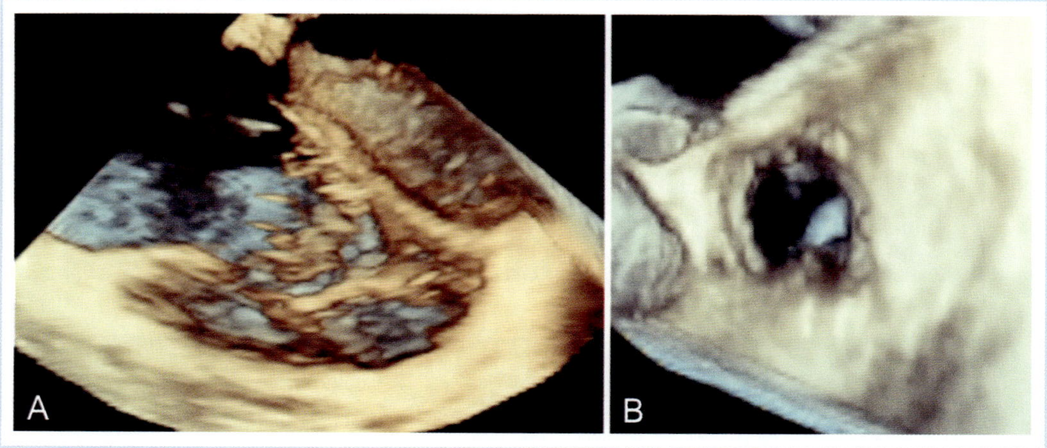

FIGURE 19.44 Ebstein anomaly. A: Three-dimensional midesophageal four-chamber view depicting in anatomic detail the abnormal dysplastic tricuspid valve (TV) in this defect. Note the dilated valvar annulus and the significant valve displacement into the right ventricle (RV), resulting in an atrialized RV. B: Following valve cone reconstruction, an *en face* three-dimensional image from an atrial perspective displays the reduced size of the TV annulus. (Images by courtesy of Dr. David W. Liddle, University of Pittsburg Medical Center).

Management

Surgical procedures attempt initially to protect the integrity of the pulmonary vascular bed and myocardium. Specific goals are to prevent pulmonary overcirculation, which may lead to elevation of PA pressure/pulmonary vascular resistance, ventricular overload, and myocardial dysfunction. The development of any of these may complicate the management of subsequent palliative strategies

Ductal-dependent systemic blood flow: In infants with LV hypoplasia (hypoplastic left heart syndrome) or other types of single ventricle with ductal-dependent systemic blood flow, the initial surgical intervention is a Norwood procedure. This consists of reconstruction of the hypoplastic Ao/arch, creation of a systemic-to-PA connection to provide a reliable source of pulmonary blood flow, and an atrial septectomy to ensure unrestricted egress of pulmonary venous blood into the systemic RV. Either a Sano connection (extracardiac graft from the single ventricle to the PA; Figure 19.45A) or a modified Blalock-Thomas-Taussig (BTT) shunt (Figure 19.45B) is placed (see later).

Ductal-dependent pulmonary blood flow: In patients with anatomic substrates associated with restricted or ductal-dependent pulmonary blood flow, a systemic-to-pulmonary connection is created to provide pulmonary blood flow. This typically consists of a Gore-Tex graft between an innominate or subclavian artery and a branch PA. An alternate potential source of pulmonary blood flow can include an RV-to-PA conduit. Ductal stent placement may be considered instead of a surgically created shunt in some cases.

PA band: In patients with excessive pulmonary blood flow, mechanical limitation of pulmonary overcirculation is accomplished by placement of band across the MPA (less frequently across the PA branches). This aims to protect the pulmonary vascular bed from high flow/pressure, preventing the development of pulmonary hypertension/vascular changes. The adequacy of the intervention can be assessed by estimation of the peak systolic pressure gradient across the PA band. This requires spectral Doppler interrogation and application of the simplified Bernoulli equation (pressure gradient = $4V^2$; where V = PA band peak velocity). Ideally, the band reduces the PASP to around one-third of the systemic systolic arterial blood pressure. Measurements of the internal vessel wall restricted by the band may also be used.

Glenn and Fontan procedures: The eventual goal of surgical palliation in the patient with single-ventricle physiology is the separation of the pulmonary and systemic circulations. At present, the favored approach is sequential diversion of the systemic venous blood directly into the pulmonary vascular bed. This consists of an initial Glenn anastomosis and a subsequent Fontan procedure. In the Glenn operation, a cavopulmonary connection is created, allowing for blood flow from the SVC into both PAs (bidirectional). This is a modification of the older classic Glenn operation, where the PAs were divided and flow was only into a single branch PA. The eventual separation of the pulmonary and systemic circulations in patients with single

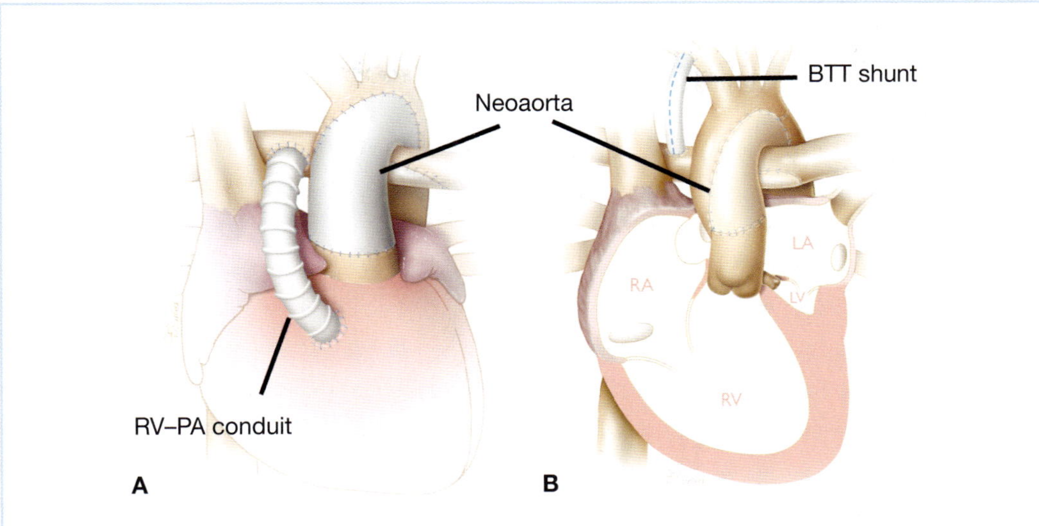

FIGURE 19.45 Hypoplastic left heart syndrome. A: Norwood procedure with Brawn's Sano modification. The graphic depicts the reconstructed aorta (neoaorta) and a ring conduit placed between the right ventricle (RV) and the pulmonary artery (PA), allowing for pulmonary blood flow. There is a complete mixing of the systemic and pulmonary venous returns at this palliative stage, resulting in cyanosis (single-ventricle physiology). B: Norwood procedure with modified Blalock-Thomas-Taussig (BTT) shunt (Gore-Tex graft) as the source of pulmonary blood flow. LA, left atrium; LV, left ventricle; RA, right atrium; RV, right ventricle. (Images in panels A and B © 2014 Texas Children's Hospital [reprinted with permission].)

ventricle requires a Fontan procedure to direct blood from the IVC into the PAs. This completes the total cavopulmonary connection.

The Fontan operation has been significantly modified over the years. It is likely that many adult patients have undergone procedures in the past that are no longer favored (eg, atriopulmonary Fontan connection). These interventions over time have been found to be associated with significant long-term morbidity, such as atrial arrhythmias, liver dysfunction, congestive heart failure, progressive ventricular dysfunction, protein-losing enteropathy, and stroke. These patients may need reoperation(s) to improve their physiologic condition including revision of the cavopulmonary connection to what is now considered a more hemodynamically favorable modification (ie, lateral tunnel or extracardiac Fontan [Figure 19.46]), optimization of cardiac rhythm, fenestration along the systemic venous pathway, mechanical circulatory support, and ultimately, if necessary, cardiac transplantation.

Transesophageal Echocardiographic Evaluation

Diagnostic assessment of the functional single ventricle requires a combination of imaging planes, including nonstandard views depending on the anatomy and the information of interest. In addition, sweeps are critically important, allowing for sequential cross sections to be obtained. In most cases, the examination addresses the nature of the interatrial communication, atrioventricular valve competence, outflow tract patency, and ventricular function. The ME 4-Ch view is particularly helpful in characterizing the atrioventricular connections (Figure 19.47; Video 19.36). Additional views contribute to the segmental analysis of the anatomy by defining the ventriculoarterial connections, ventricular morphology, and location of hypoplastic or rudimentary chambers. Color-flow and spectral Doppler interrogation are essential to determine valve competence and inflow/outflow tract obstruction. Suggested cross sections for focused TEE examination include ME 4-Ch, ME 5-Ch, ME 2-Ch, ME LAX, ME bicaval, and ME RV in-out (I-O) views. The TG and DTG views complement the anatomic details obtained in other windows. The dilated RA in the atriopulmonary connection is imaged in the ME 4-Ch (Figure 19.48; Video 19.37), ME Asc Ao SAX views, and modified views. The lateral tunnel and extracardiac Fontan connections can be seen in the ME 4-Ch, ME bicaval views, DTG views, and modified views.

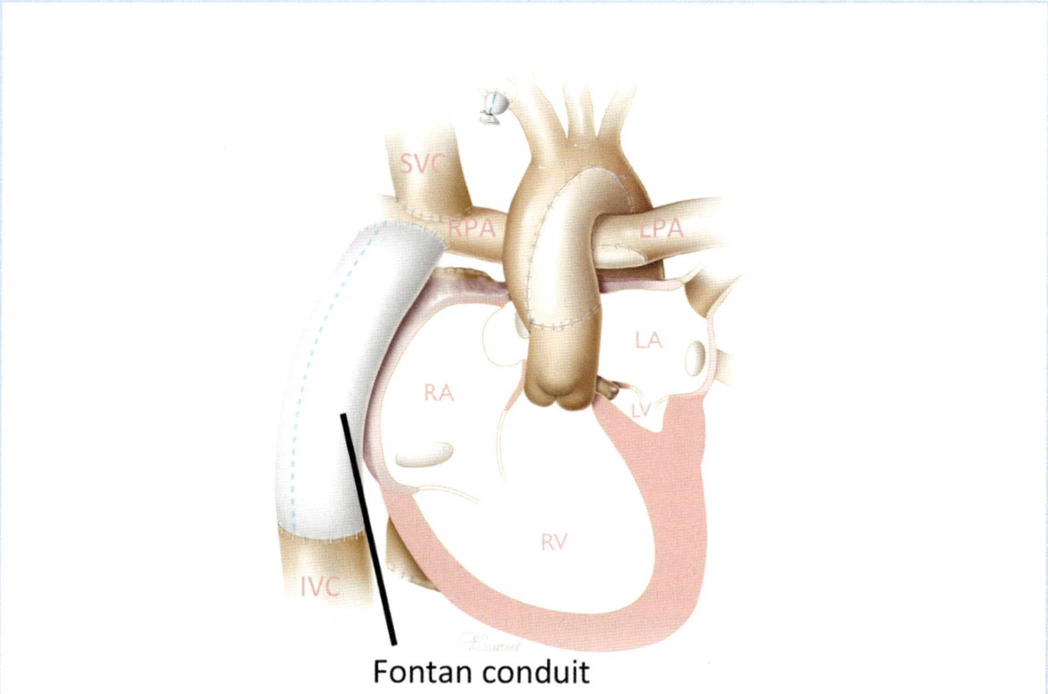

FIGURE 19.46 Extracardiac Fontan. Illustration showing extracardiac Fontan connection created by graft placement between the inferior vena cava (IVC) and the right pulmonary artery (RPA). The Glenn anastomosis between the superior vena cava (SVC) and RPA is seen. The procedures allow for a total cavopulmonary connection. Note the reconstructed aorta in hypoplastic left heart syndrome. LA, left atrium; LPA, left pulmonary artery; LV, left ventricle; RA, right atrium; RV, right ventricle. (© 2014 Texas Children's Hospital [reprinted with permission].)

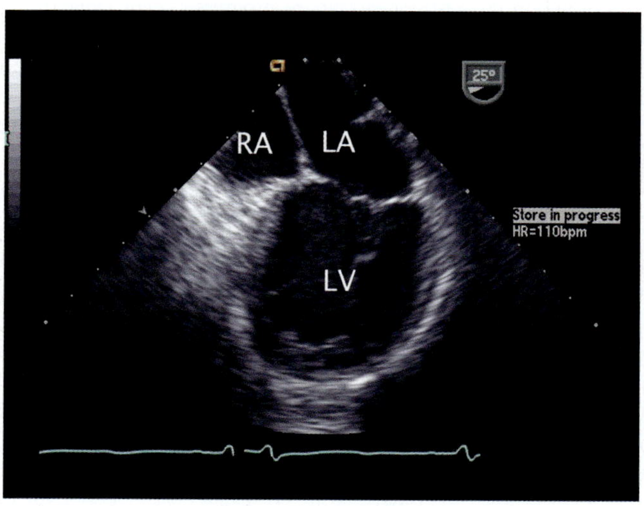

FIGURE 19.47 Single-ventricle, tricuspid atresia. Midesophageal four-chamber view demonstrating the echocardiographic findings in tricuspid atresia. The absent right atrioventricular connection and the severely hypoplastic right ventricle are seen. LA, left atrium; LV, left ventricle; RA, right atrium.

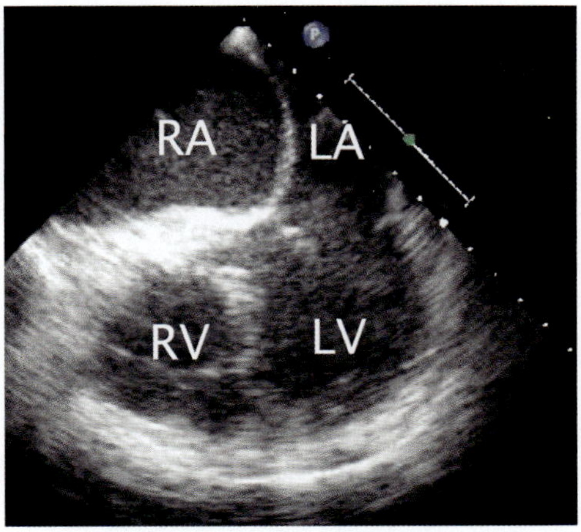

FIGURE 19.48 Atriopulmonary Fontan. Midesophageal four-chamber view in a patient with tricuspid atresia, following atriopulmonary Fontan connection. As is frequently the case, this Fontan modification in the long term resulted in severe right atrial (RA) dilation. LA, left atrium; LV, left ventricle; RV, right ventricle.

Goals of the Two-Dimensional Examination

- Assessment of atrioventricular and ventriculoarterial connections
- Evaluation of adequacy of the interatrial communication and systemic outflow tract patency
- Characterization of associated defects
- Estimation of ventricular chamber size(s) and function

Goals of the Doppler Examination

- Assessment of atrioventricular and semilunar valves for obstruction/regurgitation
- Estimation of gradient if outflow tract obstruction is present
- Evaluation of PA band gradient when intervention is undertaken (Figure 19.49)

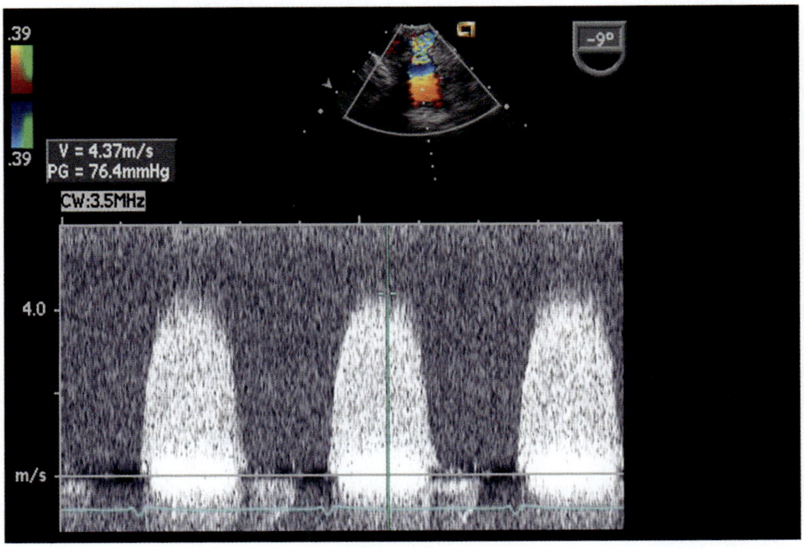

FIGURE 19.49 Pulmonary artery band. Spectral Doppler image obtained from interrogation across a pulmonary artery band. Using the simplified Bernoulli equation, the peak velocity obtained by continuous-wave Doppler across the band can be applied to estimate the right ventricular outflow tract systolic gradient.

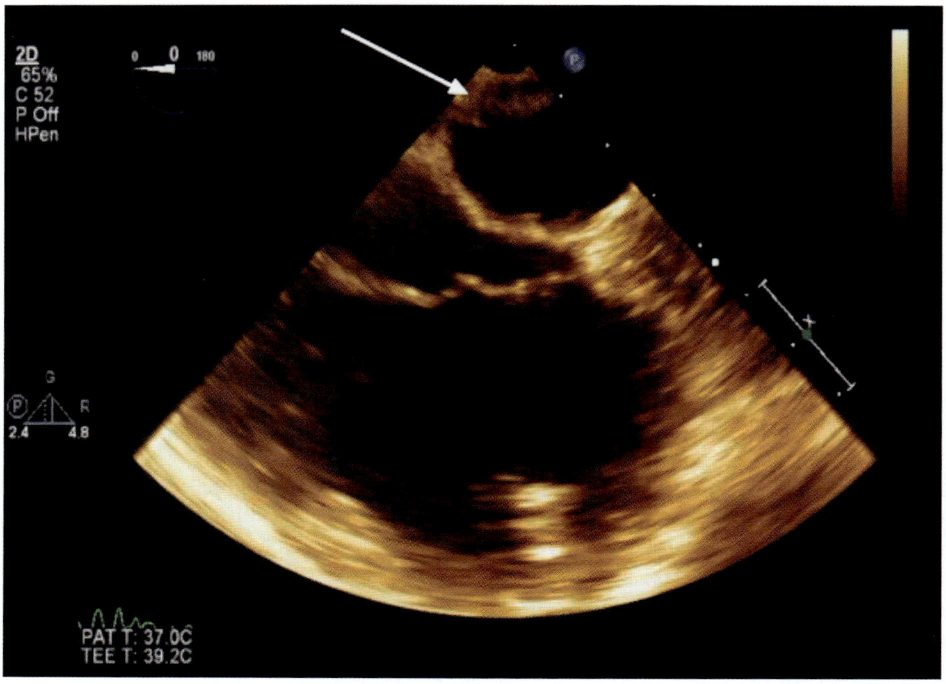

FIGURE 19.50 Lateral tunnel Fontan, thrombus. Image in a patient with dextrocardia and visceroatrial heterotaxy displaying a mass in the stented portion of the lateral tunnel Fontan connection highly suggestive of a thrombus (arrow).

Goals of the Examination After Surgery

- Evaluation of the adequacy of the intervention (imaging of a modified BTT shunt or Glenn connection is not always possible by TEE because of limited imaging planes)
- Determination of flow through the Sano (RV-to-PA) connection, if performed as part of the Norwood procedure
- Exclusion of obstruction to blood flow at the atrial level
- Assessment of patency across the Fontan connection, characterization of flow across the IVC pathway to PA
- Evaluation of Fontan fenestration (if present) in terms of size and gradient
- Assessment for thrombus in the Fontan circuit should be performed in all post-Fontan patients during TEE (Figure 19.50; Video 19.38). In the post-Fontan patient with a history of an arrhythmia, TEE may be indicated prior to cardioversion to exclude atrial thrombi, at which time the Fontan circuit should also be examined.
- Evaluation of valvar competence and ventricular function

Goals of the Examination During Transcatheter Intervention

- Monitoring during catheter interventions that may either create or obliterate a Fontan fenestration (a fenestration represents a "pop-off" allowing for right-to-left shunting and the maintenance of cardiac output under some circumstances)
- Guidance during procedures that require catheter-based interventions (eg, dilation, stenting, coiling)

CONGENITAL CORONARY ARTERY ANOMALIES

Anatomy

Anomalies of the coronary arteries of a congenital nature represent a diverse group of malformations. These are rare collectively. The most common are anomalies of origination and course (eg, anomalous origin of the coronary artery from the PA and anomalous origin from the inappropriate sinus potentially associated with an abnormal intramural or intra-arterial course or compromised orifice [Figure 19.51]), anomalies of

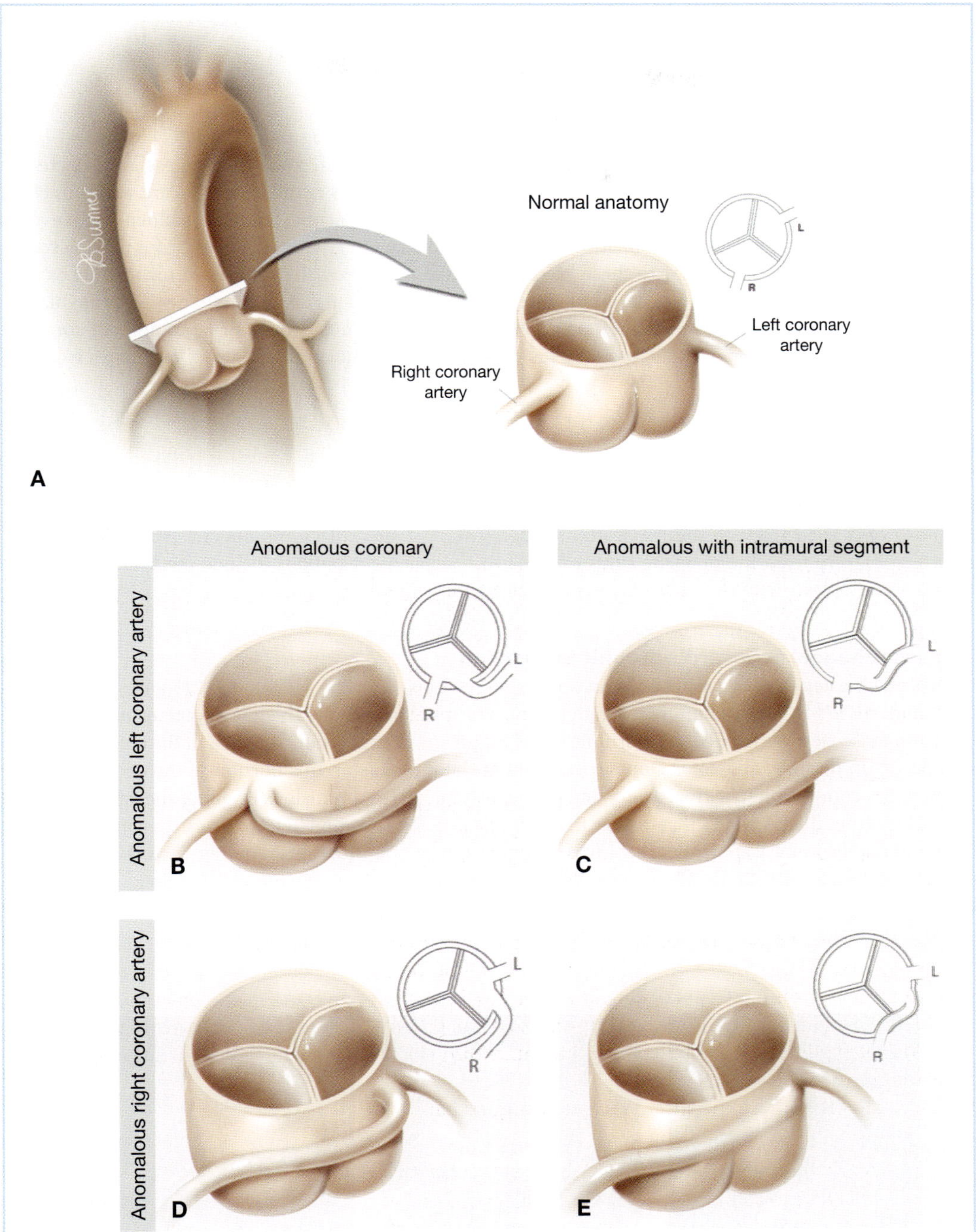

FIGURE 19.51 Anomalies of coronary artery origin and proximal course. A: Normal coronary anatomy. B: Anomalous left coronary artery origin from right aortic sinus of Valsalva. C: Anomalous left coronary artery origin from right aortic sinus of Valsalva with intramural course. D: Anomalous right coronary artery from left aortic sinus. E: Anomalous right coronary artery from left aortic sinus with intramural course. (Images in panels A-E © 2014 Texas Children's Hospital [reprinted with permission].)

intrinsic vessel anatomy (eg, ostial atresia and coronary aneurysm), and anomalies of coronary termination (eg, coronary fistula draining into a cardiac chamber/vascular structure).

Pathophysiology

The physiology and clinical manifestations of this congenital pathology are extremely variable. These anomalies may present as an incidental finding on echocardiography. In some cases, these are detected in the evaluation of a heart murmur or congestive symptoms (coronary fistula), or myocardial dysfunction (anomalous origin from PA). Chest pain, ventricular arrhythmias, syncope, and near-sudden death events are the main presentations of an anomalous origin of a coronary artery from the aortic root in adolescents and adults. Ischemia in patients with these lesions is considered the result of impaired myocardial oxygen delivery either at rest or during conditions of increased demand. This may be due to either acute angulation of a coronary artery origin, extrinsic compression along an anomalous course, or alterations in coronary blood flow related to a low diastolic pressure (as is the case when the coronary artery originates from the pulmonary root).

Management

The presentation of anomalies involving origination/course and intrinsic vessel anatomy in the adult patient is usually related to myocardial ischemia during exercise. Therefore, this entity is part of the differential diagnosis of cardiac arrest or sudden death in athletes. For patients with symptoms related to the origin of a coronary artery from the opposite sinus of Valsalva, management options include medical surveillance, coronary angioplasty with stent placement, or surgical intervention.

Transesophageal Echocardiographic Evaluation

The coronary arteries are visualized in multiple cross sections, with the ME AV SAX (Figure 19.52A), ME LAX, and ME RV I-O views representing, in most cases, a starting point. The imaging plane is to be modified from these views as needed to determine vessel origin and proximal course. Most of the coronary perfusion occurs in diastole, and color Doppler assessment should focus on this portion of the cardiac cycle to examine the connection to a great artery and characterize flow. For anomalous origin of the left main coronary artery from the PA, views that display the MPA (eg, ME RV I-O and UE PA) are also essential. The TEE examination of coronary anomalies that involve origin from an opposite sinus requires views that display the aortic root (Figure 19.52B,C; Videos 19.39 and 19.40). For the evaluation of fistulous connections, the examination should focus on cross sections that allow for the coronary blood flow to be followed into the site(s) of drainage.

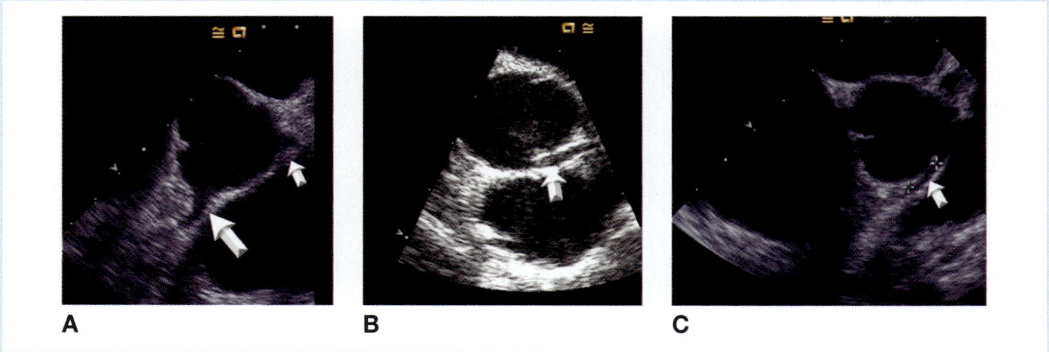

FIGURE 19.52 Coronary arteries. A: Midesophageal aortic short-axis view depicting normal origin of the coronary arteries from the aortic root as shown by the two arrows. B: Anomalous origin of left coronary artery from the right aortic sinus (arrow). C: Anomalous origin of right coronary artery from the left aortic sinus (arrow) with intramural segment (noted by crosshairs).

Goals of the Two-Dimensional Examination

- Evaluation of the origin of the coronary arteries
- Assessment of vessel course (evaluation for intra-arterial/intramural path)
- Determination of ventricular size and systolic function (global and segmental)

Goals of the Doppler Examination

- Interrogation with pulsed and color-flow Doppler to visualize the origin and course of the coronary arteries as well as the direction of blood flow (this may require adjustment in the echocardiographic settings to detect low-velocity flow signals)

Goals of the Examination After Surgery/Intervention

- Assessment of the results of the procedure (eg, evaluation of coronary origin, unroofing of intramural segment, successful occlusion of coronary fistula)
- Documentation of flow in the coronary vessels by spectral and color Doppler
- Evaluation of ventricular function (global and segmental)

END-STAGE HEART DISEASE IN ADULT WITH CONGENITAL HEART DISEASE

End-stage heart disease (ESHD) may be seen in patients with complex congenital conditions, such as functionally single ventricles or univentricular circulation (eg, post-Fontan palliation), systemic RV (eg, D-TGA after Mustard/Senning operation), severe PA hypertension/pulmonary vascular disease (eg, Eisenmenger syndrome), and severe valvular disease (eg, after complete AVSD repair). In fact, heart failure represents the leading cause of death in the population of ACHD. Orthotopic cardiac transplantation in this patient group is considered the primary treatment. However, it is well recognized that patients with ACHD may face longer waiting list times due to antibody sensitization related to prior blood product exposure and the need for specific grafts due, in many cases, to underlying pulmonary and systemic venous anomalies as well as unusual cardiac positions or situs abnormalities, among other issues. Although rare, the use of mechanical circulatory support in the form of VAD implantation has been applied in some cases, with reports documenting that early use may favorably impact survival partly related to improving physical condition and end-organ function (24).

In general, patients with ACHD represent a growing minority of adult cardiac transplants. Of note is that ailing Fontan patients often require multiorgan transplantation due to associated significant liver and kidney disease. In the transplanted patient with ACHD, the frequent need for reconstruction of the PAs along with longer ischemic times, the higher likelihood of future reinterventions, and a prior univentricular versus biventricular circulation may influence immediate- and long-term outcomes.

Transesophageal Echocardiographic Evaluation

Depending on the nature of the intervention in ESHD (cardiac transplantation, mechanical circulatory device support implantation, or other surgical strategies), the main goals of the TEE examination may differ (25). General objectives of the examination in these patients are listed below.

Goals of the Two-Dimensional Examination

- Assessment of cardiovascular anatomy (Video 19.41)
- Evaluation of ventricular function (Video 19.41)
- Exclusion of intracardiac thrombus

Goals of the Doppler Examination

- Detection of intracardiac shunts (eg, PFO) that could impact outcomes after VAD implantation
- Evaluation of any underlying significant valvular lesions that must be addressed during VAD placement (eg, aortic regurgitation)

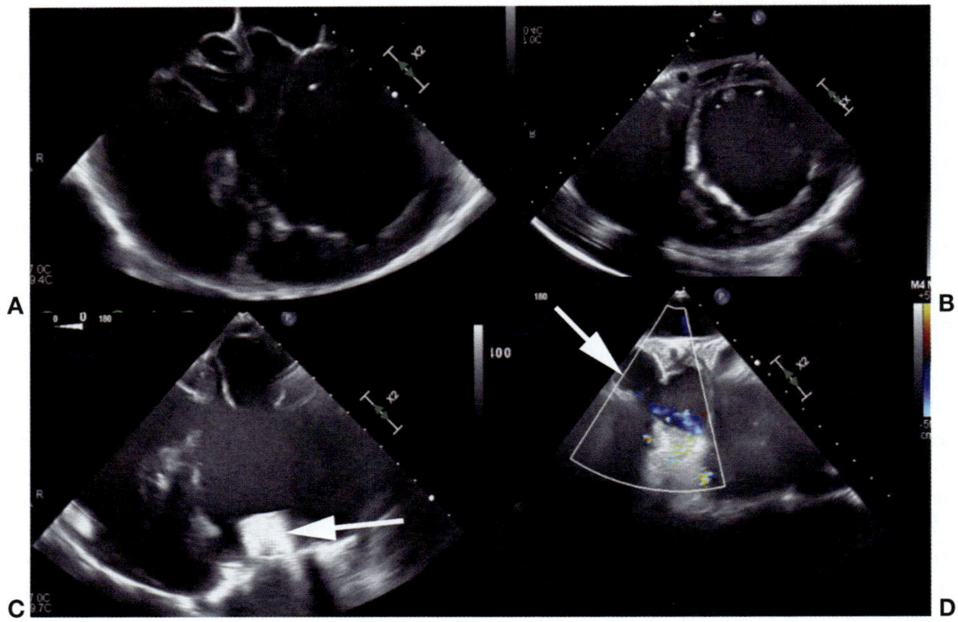

FIGURE 19.53 Post-Fontan procedure, end-stage heart disease. A: Midesophageal four-chamber view depicting the abnormal anatomy in an adult with heart failure and end-stage heart disease late after Fontan palliation for congenitally corrected transposition, hypoplastic left ventricle, and a straddling mitral valve. Note the smooth wall of the right-sided left ventricle and the trabeculated, left-sided right ventricle (RV). B: Transgastric view showing the biventricular dilation. C: Midesophageal four-chamber view post HeartMate 3 ventricular assist device (VAD) implantation (Abbott Laboratories) showing the inflow cannula in the RV apex (arrow). D: Midesophageal four-chamber view rotated to the right showing the fenestrated Fontan conduit (arrow). Although the fenestration was not closed as is usually the case during VAD placement to avoid cyanosis related to right-to-left intracardiac shunting, its size was significantly reduced.

Goals of the Examination After Surgery/Intervention

- Accurate device positioning after VAD implantation and patency of inflow and outflow, particularly in patients with a systemic RV, where trabeculations can complicate VAD inflow cannula placement (Figure 19.53; Video 19.42)
- Optimization of VAD settings
- Assessment of patency of anastomotic connections and graft function after cardiac transplantation, especially after extensive reconstructive surgeries
- After most procedures, evaluation of valve and ventricular function

TRANSESOPHAGEAL ECHOCARDIOGRAPHY FOR NONCARDIAC SURGERY IN ADULTS WITH CONGENITAL HEART DISEASE

The use of TEE during noncardiac surgery in the ACHD patient has not been explored to the same extent as in atherosclerotic, valvular heart disease, or other potentially high-risk adult settings. However, TEE in this patient group can be applied similarly in evaluating ventricular volume, function, and myocardial ischemia to optimize clinical care during noncardiac surgery. Patients with intracardiac shunts may benefit from TEE, given the potential for paradoxical emboli associated with specific interventions. In those with CHD and associated elevations in PA pressure and/or vascular resistance, TEE may also be considered to assist patient management. Intraoperative TEE can also be helpful in those with ACHD and limited cardiac reserve, poor exercise tolerance, or anyone with significant potential risk of perioperative morbidity during noncardiac procedures. It should be emphasized that adults with CHD can have concurrent acquired cardiovascular disease, increasing their risks for hemodynamic disturbances during noncardiac surgery and thus the potential benefits of intraoperative TEE.

LIMITATIONS OF TRANSESOPHAGEAL ECHOCARDIOGRAPHY IN CONGENITAL HEART DISEASE

Despite the significant contributions of TEE to CHD, some limitations should be acknowledged. Optimal interrogation of far-field structures, such as the RVOT and PA, can be challenging. Other anatomic structures of interest may not be amenable to imaging through the transesophageal approach (eg, left PA, distal branch PAs, Ao Arch). In this regard, epicardial imaging may complement the assessment (19).

With respect to the perioperative setting, it is recognized that a variety of factors (level of inotropic support, catecholamine state immediately after bypass, loading conditions, myocardial functional state) can impact the echocardiographic findings. These variables can underestimate or overestimate the hemodynamic severity of the condition in question. Therefore, decisions regarding return to bypass to address residual pathology should consider TEE findings along with many other parameters and the overall risk-benefit of reintervention.

SUMMARY

TEE has been shown to provide anatomic and hemodynamic information beyond that acquired with conventional transthoracic imaging. This is particularly relevant to characterizing cardiovascular anomalies and pathologies of a congenital nature. In the operating room, TEE allows for confirmation of preoperative diagnoses and modification of the surgical plan if necessary. This technology facilitates perioperative care by assisting in formulating anesthetic plans, guiding fluid management, and selecting inotropes/vasoactive drugs. Other known benefits of TEE, also applicable to the congenital patient, include continuous monitoring of myocardial function, detecting intracavitary/intravascular air, and assessing for myocardial ischemia. Evaluation of the repair in CHD and assessment of residual pathology to improve overall patient outcome represents one of the main attributes of this imaging modality. TEE is also extremely valuable in evaluating factors that can lead to difficulties during weaning from CPB and in guiding the surgical revision when indicated. The contributions of TEE have also been documented in the cardiac catheterization and electrophysiology laboratories during the monitoring of interventions, increasing the safety of these procedures while reducing exposure to ionizing radiation and contrast agents, and allowing for the immediate evaluation of complications. The number of adults with CHD continues to increase, and with that, the overall complexity of this population. It is anticipated that further advancements in ultrasound technology, including that of 3D/4D-TEE and associated techniques (eg photorealistic rendering of cardiac structures, blood speckle imaging) as well as artificial intelligence as applied to echocardiography, will continue to play a major role in the care of these patients.

REFERENCES

1. Abdurrahman L. Adult congenital heart disease update. *Curr Probl Pediatr Adolesc Health Care*. 2023;53:101399.
2. Warnes CA. Adult congenital heart disease: the challenges of a lifetime. *Eur Heart J*. 2017;38:2041-2047.
3. Thakkar AN, Chinnadurai P, Lin CH. Adult congenital heart disease: magnitude of the problem. *Curr Opin Cardiol*. 2017;32:467-474.
4. Dellborg M. Adult congenital heart disease. *Circulation*. 2024;149:1397-1399.
5. Wong PC, Miller-Hance WC. *Transesophageal Echocardiography for Pediatric and Congenital Heart Disease*. 2nd ed. Springer; 2021:810 p.
6. Hahn RT, Abraham T, Adams MS, et al. Guidelines for performing a comprehensive transesophageal echocardiographic examination: recommendations from the American Society of Echocardiography and the Society of Cardiovascular Anesthesiologists. *J Am Soc Echocardiogr*. 2013;26:921-964.
7. Puchalski MD, Lui GK, Miller-Hance WC, et al. Guidelines for performing a comprehensive transesophageal echocardiographic examination in children and all patients with congenital heart disease: recommendations from the American Society of Echocardiography. *J Am Soc Echocardiogr*. 2019;32:173-215.
8. Marelli AJ, Mackie AS, Ionescu-Ittu R, Rahme E, Pilote L. Congenital heart disease in the general population: changing prevalence and age distribution. *Circulation*. 2007;115:163-172.
9. Brida M, Gatzoulis MA. Adult congenital heart disease: past, present and future. *Acta Paediatr*. 2019;108:1757-1764.
10. Hahn RT, Saric M, Faletra FF, et al. Recommended standards for the performance of transesophageal echocardiographic screening for structural heart intervention: from the American Society of Echocardiography. *J Am Soc Echocardiogr*. 2022;35:1-76.
11. Simpson J, Lopez L, Acar P, et al. Three-dimensional echocardiography in congenital heart disease: an expert consensus document from the European Association of Cardiovascular Imaging and the American Society of Echocardiography. *J Am Soc Echocardiogr*. 2017;30:1-27.

12. Avesani M, Kang SL, Jalal Z, Thambo JB, Iriart X. Renaissance of cardiac imaging to assist percutaneous interventions in congenital heart diseases: the role of three-dimensional echocardiography and multimodality imaging. *Front Pediatr.* 2022;10:894472.
13. Jone PN. Applications of three-dimensional transesophageal echocardiography in congenital heart disease. *Echocardiography.* 2020;37:1665-1672.
14. Stout KK, Daniels CJ, Aboulhosn JA, et al. 2018 AHA/ACC Guideline for the management of adults with congenital heart disease: a report of the American College of Cardiology/American Heart Association Task Force on Clinical Practice Guidelines. *J Am Coll Cardiol.* 2019;73:e81-e192.
15. Baumgartner H, De Backer J. The ESC clinical practice guidelines for the management of adult congenital heart disease 2020. *Eur Heart J.* 2020;41:4153-4154.
16. Turner ME, Bouhout I, Petit CJ, Kalfa D. Transcatheter closure of atrial and ventricular septal defects: JACC focus seminar. *J Am Coll Cardiol.* 2022;79:2247-2258.
17. Li A, Aboulhosn JA. Update on transcatheter interventions in adults with congenital heart disease. *J Clin Med.* 2024; 13:3685.
18. Valente AM, Cook S, Festa P, et al. Multimodality imaging guidelines for patients with repaired tetralogy of fallot: a report from the American Society of Echocardiography: developed in collaboration with the Society for Cardiovascular Magnetic Resonance and the Society for Pediatric Radiology. *J Am Soc Echocardiogr.* 2014;27:111-141.
19. Ozturk E, Cansaran Tanidir I, Ayyildiz P, et al. The role of intraoperative epicardial echocardiography in pediatric cardiac surgery. *Echocardiography.* 2018;35:999-1004.
20. Stern KWD, Emani SM, Peek GJ, Geva T, Kutty S. Epicardial echocardiography in pediatric and congenital heart surgery. *World J Pediatr Congenit Heart Surg.* 2019;10:343-350.
21. Stauffer KJ, Brabender J, Reddy CD, et al. Intraoperative epicardial echocardiography or transoesophageal echocardiography in CHD: how much does it matter. *Cardiol Young.* 2023;33(5):718-725.
22. Reeves ST, Glas KE, Eltzschig H, et al. Guidelines for performing a comprehensive epicardial echocardiography examination: recommendations of the American Society of Echocardiography and the Society of Cardiovascular Anesthesiologists. *J Am Soc Echocardiogr.* 2007;20:427-437.
23. Cohen MS, Eidem BW, Cetta F, et al. Multimodality imaging guidelines of patients with transposition of the great arteries: a report from the American Society of Echocardiography developed in collaboration with the Society for Cardiovascular Magnetic Resonance and the Society of Cardiovascular Computed Tomography. *J Am Soc Echocardiogr.* 2016;29:571-621.
24. Schweiger M, Lorts A, Conway J. Mechanical circulatory support challenges in pediatric and (adult) congenital heart disease. *Curr Opin Organ Transplant.* 2018;23:301-307.
25. Nicoara A, Skubas N, Ad N, et al. Guidelines for the use of transesophageal echocardiography to assist with surgical decision-making in the operating room: a surgery-based approach: from the American Society of Echocardiography in collaboration with the Society of Cardiovascular Anesthesiologists and the Society of Thoracic Surgeons. *J Am Soc Echocardiogr.* 2020;33:692-734.

QUESTIONS

1. **The following TEE findings are characteristic of most patients with uncomplicated ASDs EXCEPT for:**
   A. RV dilation
   B. Left-to-right atrial level shunting
   C. A high tricuspid regurgitant jet Doppler velocity
   D. Spectral Doppler evidence of normal mitral inflow velocity

2. **Primum ASDs are commonly associated with which of the following congenital anomaly?**
   A. Mitral atresia
   B. Mitral valve cleft
   C. TGA
   D. Ebstein anomaly

3. **An enlarged coronary sinus is usually seen within the context of which of the following?**
   A. Sinus venosus ASD
   B. Persistent L-SVC
   C. Dilated LA
   D. TGA

4. **The ventricular communication in a complete AVSD is referred to as a(n):**
   A. Primum defect
   B. Malaligned defect
   C. Inlet defect
   D. Supracristal defect

5. **TEE in an adult patient followed for a perimembranous VSD displays a peak Doppler velocity of 5 m/s across the communication with optimal Doppler alignment and without evidence of RV outflow obstruction. At the time of the study, the noninvasive blood pressure measures 125/65 mm Hg. Based on this information, the estimated PASP is:**
   A. Suprasystemic level
   B. Half of the systemic blood pressure
   C. 36 mm Hg
   D. 25 mm Hg

6. **Which associated pathology in the patient with tetralogy of Fallot is BEST characterized in the ME AV SAX TEE view?**
   A. Coronary artery anomaly
   B. Right Ao Arch with aberrant left subclavian artery
   C. AVSD
   D. Distal left PA stenosis

7. **In the adult patient with a history of tetralogy of Fallot repaired in early childhood, the MOST common indication for reintervention later in life is due to:**
   A. Aortic root dilation and progressive aortic regurgitation
   B. Recurrence of RVOT obstruction
   C. Free pulmonary regurgitation with associated RV dilation
   D. Residual ventricular level shunting resulting in potential paradoxical embolism

8. **Which of the following long-term complications is MOST likely in the adult with D-TGA following an arterial switch operation during infancy?**
   A. Myocardial ischemia due to the coronary translocation
   B. Supravalvar PS related to the arterial anastomosis
   C. Systemic RV systolic dysfunction
   D. Atrial baffle leak

9. **Which of the following identifies the surgical intervention in the patient with a functional single ventricle that completes the total cavopulmonary connection?**
   A. Mechanical assist device that supports flow from the IVC into the MPA
   B. Glenn cavopulmonary connection
   C. Extracardiac Fontan operation
   D. Cardiac transplantation

10. **The following statement BEST describes the use of TEE in the catheterization laboratory in the ACHD undergoing an intervention:**
    A. Is more useful than in the perioperative setting.
    B. It is likely to be associated with probe-related complications.
    C. It completely avoids radiation exposure.
    D. Potentially limits procedural time and complications.

▶ANSWERS

1. **Correct Answer: C.**
   Rationale: ASDs are characterized by atrial level shunting, usually in the left-to-right direction. The RV volume overload resulting from the shunt is manifested as RV dilation. Although pulmonary hypertension is a potential complication of a long-standing atrial level shunt, this represents a relatively rare occurrence. When it occurs, if tricuspid regurgitation is present, the jet peak velocity would be expected to be high, reflecting the elevated RV and PA pressures, unlike a low regurgitant velocity in most cases. The mitral inflow velocity would be expected to be normal in most patients with ASDs, unlike when a ventricular level shunt is present ("flow-related" increased velocity).

2. **Correct Answer: B.**
   Rationale: A cleft in the anterior leaflet of the mitral valve is a frequent association in primum ASDs. The cleft is best demonstrated

in the TG basal view (*en face* view of the mitral valve). Color Doppler interrogation of the mitral valve in this view assists in the characterization of the regurgitant jet when present. There is not a recognized know association between primum ASDs and mitral atresia. In TGA, intercirculatory mixing is essential for survival, and this usually occurs at the atrial level in the form of a central defect that if not present or adequate can be created or enlarged by balloon atrial septostomy early in the neonatal period. Ebstein anomaly is frequently associated with a secundum type of ASD. This may contribute to volume loading of the right heart in the presence of significant tricuspid regurgitation.

3. **Correct Answer: B.**
   Rationale: A persistent L-SVC is usually associated with an enlarged coronary sinus. In some cases, this represents an anatomic variant and may be of no consequence, but it can have implications for venous cannulation during CPB, the administration of cardioplegia, and other surgical procedures in CHD. The systemic venous connection can be confirmed upon injection of agitated saline into a left arm or left neck vein as contrast would be seen draining across the coronary sinus into the RA.

4. **Correct Answer: C.**
   Rationale: AVSDs, also known as to as endocardial cushion or AV canal defects, are characterized by a common atrioventricular junction or region of the heart where the atrial and ventricular myocardium becomes contiguous, variable deficiencies in atrial and ventricular septation, and an abnormal structure of the atrioventricular valves. In the complete form of the defect, a large common atrioventricular valve is present. The communication in the inferior portion of the atrial septum is referred to as a primum ASD, and at the ventricular level, the typical defect is located in close proximity to the atrioventricular valves in the posterior or inlet portion of ventricular septum, thus the term "inlet defect." Although additional septal defects can be present in this lesion, these are more likely to involve the trabecular muscle (muscular type).

5. **Correct Answer: D.**
   Rationale: In the scenario presented, the data provided can be utilized to estimate the PASP. By applying the *simplified* Bernoulli equation to the peak velocity across the VSD as obtained by Doppler echocardiography, the pressure difference across the defect can be calculated (pressure gradient = 4 × velocity squared). By subtracting this calculated pressure gradient from the systemic systolic blood pressure, the RV systolic pressure or PASP can be derived as follows in the absence of obstruction across the RV outflow as indicated in this case:

$$\text{PASP (mm Hg)} = 125 - 4\,(5)^2$$

$$\text{PASP} = 125 - 100$$

$$\text{PASP} = 25 \text{ mm Hg}$$

6. **Correct Answer: A.**
   Rationale: Various associated lesions have been described in tetralogy of Fallot that include, among others, AVSD, abnormal Ao Arch sidedness and branching patterns, and anomalies in the origin and course of the coronary arteries that can impact surgical management. The ME AV SAX view facilitates the assessment of the origin of the coronary arteries and can identify anomalous origin and proximal course in tetralogy and other congenital defects. Although all congenital lesions/variants listed are known to be associated with tetralogy, these are best assessed in other TEE views or by alternate imaging modalities.

7. **Correct Answer: C.**
   Rationale: In patients with tetralogy of Fallot, several potential long-term issues require ongoing medical surveillance. Patching across the PV, also referred to as transannular patching, leads to pulmonary regurgitation, which usually increases in severity over time. This represents the most common indication for either surgical or catheter-based intervention later in life in tetralogy patients. Related to this problem, frequently performed surgical procedures in this population include PV placement/replacement or RV-to-PA conduit change/placement. Other less common causes of surgical reintervention include significant residual intracardiac shunts, RVOT obstruction, aneurysmal RVOT dilation, and increasing aortic regurgitation.

8. **Correct Answer: B.**
   Rationale: In the arterial switch operation, D-TGA are transected and anastomosed to their appropriate respective ventricles, the coronary arteries are translocated to the

"neoaorta," and any additional defects are repaired. The most common indication for reintervention after this type of surgery is related to obstruction at the level of the PA anastomosis (supravalvar PS). Improvements in surgical techniques over time have made this a less likely occurrence. Compromised myocardial blood flow has been described after an arterial switch operation, but in the long-term setting, it represents a less likely complication. The atrial switch procedure (Mustard or Senning operation), no longer favored for this lesion, can be associated with atrial baffle obstruction/leaks and eventual systemic RV failure.

9. Correct Answer: C.
Rationale: The Fontan procedure represents the final surgical palliative strategy that completes a total cavopulmonary in the patient with a functional single ventricle. By directing blood from the IVC into the PA without intervening pumping chamber, this achieves separation of the pulmonary and systemic circulations. The bidirectional Glenn operation is considered an intermediate step in the single-ventricle palliation pathway. Various configurations of VAD support have been proposed and even applied in the Fontan circulation to assist the systemic or pulmonary circulation, but these have not been used with the goal of creating a total cavopulmonary connection. In the setting of the failed Fontan circulation or single ventricle, cardiac transplantation, at times combined with liver or kidney transplantation, may represent the ultimate treatment option aiming to restore the normal biventricular circulation.

10. Correct Answer: D.
Rationale: The applications of TEE in the cardiac catheterization laboratory include the acquisition of detailed anatomic and hemodynamic data before and during the planned procedures, real-time evaluation of catheter placement across valves and vessels, and immediate assessment of the results of interventions(s). The modality is also known to limit procedural time and related complications. The role of TEE in the cardiac catheterization, although potentially different than that in the intraoperative setting, should not be considered more nor less useful. TEE is known to limit radiation exposure by complementing the information obtained by fluoroscopy and angiography; however, in most cases, it does not completely obviate the need for the use of radiation. The incidence of complications related to TEE probe insertion or manipulation has not been examined specifically in those in the cardiac catheterization environment but may not differ significantly from that reported in other settings where TEE is applied.

20 Cardiac Masses and Embolic Sources

Farid Jadbabaie

Transesophageal echocardiography (TEE) is an extremely useful imaging modality for the assessment of cardiac masses and sources of emboli (1,2). The enhanced resolution of TEE and proximity of the transducer to posterior cardiac structures enable visualization of small masses or thrombi in the atria, atrial appendages, or those attached to cardiac valves or devices that would otherwise be missed on transthoracic echocardiography. Moreover, additional techniques such as contrast echocardiography and three-dimensional (3D) imaging can provide further information on the vascularity of the mass and its spatial relationship to neighboring cardiac structures. In the evaluation of cardiac masses, it is essential to recognize the variants of normal cardiac anatomy as well as artifacts that can be mistaken for cardiac masses or thrombus (3,4). Normal structures such as pectinate muscle in the left atrial appendage (LAA) or the tissue fold between LAA and left upper pulmonary vein ("Coumadin ridge") can be mistaken for a thrombus or a small tumor (Figure 20.1). Similarly, a prominent Chiari network in the right atrium can be mistaken for a right atrial mass.

CARDIAC TUMORS

Primary cardiac tumors are very rare and account for 25% of all cardiac neoplasms in pathologic studies (5,6). Majority of primary cardiac tumors are benign without local invasion or metastatic spread. In contrast, malignant tumors often appear as large masses with invasion into the surrounding cardiac structures.

Myxoma

Myxoma is the most common primary cardiac tumor in adults and accounts for 30% of all primary cardiac neoplasms. Cardiac myxomas commonly arise from the left atrium but can also originate from the right atrium or the ventricles. These tumors are usually pedunculated and have a smooth surface. The most common attachment site is the fossa ovalis on the left side of the interatrial septum. Myxomas are slow-growing tumors and can remain asymptomatic for a long period of time. If undetected, myxomas can grow in size and occupy a significant portion of the left atrium, causing obstruction to flow across the mitral valve (Figure 20.2; ▶ Videos 20.1 and 20.2). Cardiac myxomas are friable and can often result in systemic embolization.

Lipoma

Lipomas are the second most common cardiac tumors in adults and account for 10% of all benign cardiac neoplasms (5). These tumors usually originate from ventricular myocardium and less commonly from atrial myocardium. These tumors often appear as a sessile mass with smooth surface and increased echogenicity. Lipomas are slow-growing tumors that can become large and cause obstruction to blood flow (Figure 20.3; ▶ Video 20.3). Cardiac lipomas should be distinguished from lipomatous hypertrophy of the interatrial septum, which is caused by the infiltration of mature fat cells and a characteristic appearance of the dumbbell-shaped thickening of the atrial septum with the sparing of fossa ovalis (7) (Figure 20.4; ▶ Video 20.4). Lipomatous hypertrophy is more commonly seen in older adults, especially older women, and usually has a benign clinical course.

Papillary Fibroelastoma

Papillary fibroelastoma (PFE) is the third most common primary cardiac tumor in adults. Fibroelastomas are small mobile tumors that commonly originate from the valvular leaflets but can arise from other endocardial surfaces. The aortic valve is the most common site of origin, followed by the mitral valve. These tumors often appear as a small (0.5-2 cm) pedunculated echo density, with multiple mobile fibrillar projections, which are attached to the valve leaflets (8-10) (Figure 20.5; ▶ Videos 20.5-20.7).

Fibroblastomas have a high potential for embolization, which is thought to be from either the embolization of tumor fragments or associated thrombi. The risk of embolization is higher as the tumor grows larger.

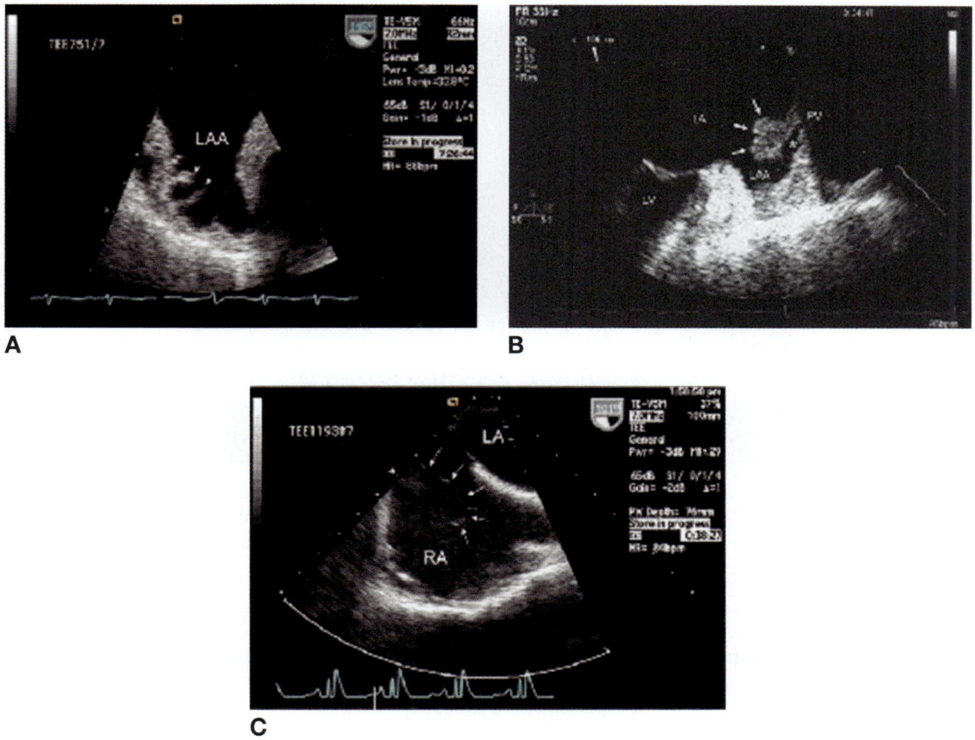

FIGURE 20.1 Normal cardiac structures can often be mistaken for cardiac masses or thrombus. Panel A shows a prominent pectinate muscle in the left atrial appendage mimicking a thrombus. An example of a prominent Coumadin ridge is shown in panel B, and an example of a prominent Chiari network is shown in panel C. LA, left atrium; LAA, left atrial appendage; LV, left ventricle; PV, pulmonary vein; RA, right atrium; asterisk, shows the posterior horn of LAA.

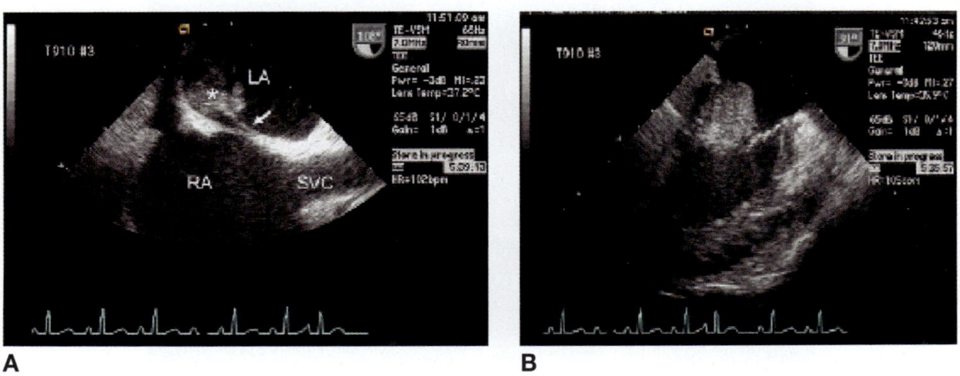

FIGURE 20.2 Example of a large myxoma in the left atrium (asterisk) with a stalk (arrow) attached to the atrial septum (panel A). Tumor prolapses into the left ventricle during diastole (panel B). LA, left atrium; RA, right atrium; SVC, superior vena cava.

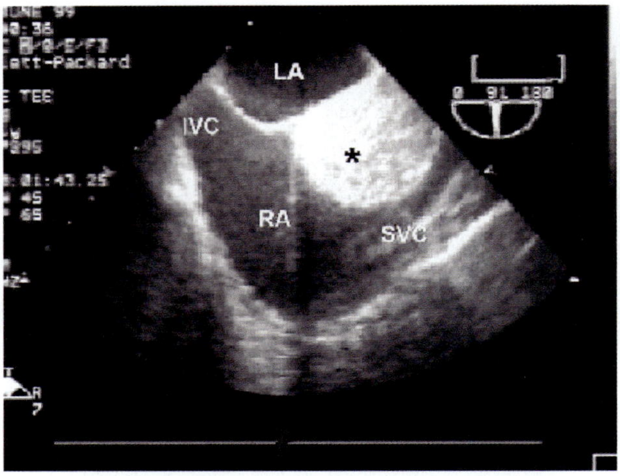

FIGURE 20.3 Example of a large lipoma (asterisk) involving the interatrial septum. Note the echogenicity of the tumor and acoustic shadowing. IVC, inferior vena cava; LA, left atrium; RA, right atrium; SVC, superior vena cava.

Valvular fibroelastomas are frequently confused with vegetations, given the size, location, and potential for embolization. In contrast to vegetations, fibroelastomas mostly arise from the aortic side of the aortic valve leaflets (8-10) and are not associated with significant valvular regurgitation (10). Prominent valvular (Lambl) excrescences are other conditions that can be confused with fibroelastomas (8). Valvular excrescences are commonly seen on commissural edges of the valve leaflets and comprise a small fibrous core covered by endothelial cells. These densities are commonly seen on TEE in all age groups and are not associated with embolic events (11). An example of a prominent Lambl excrescence on the aortic valve is shown in Figure 20.6 and Video 20.8.

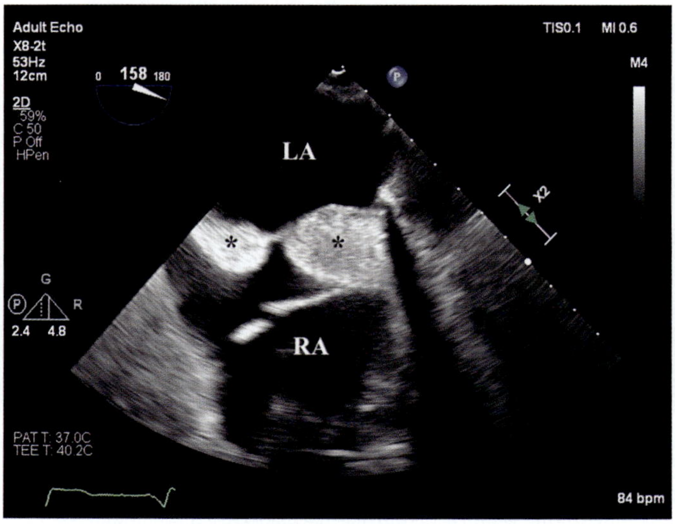

FIGURE 20.4 Example of lipomatous hypertrophy of interatrial septum (asterisks) is depicted. Note the characteristic "dumbbell-shape" appearance and sparing of fossa ovalis. LA, left atrium; RA, right atrium; SVC, superior vena cava.

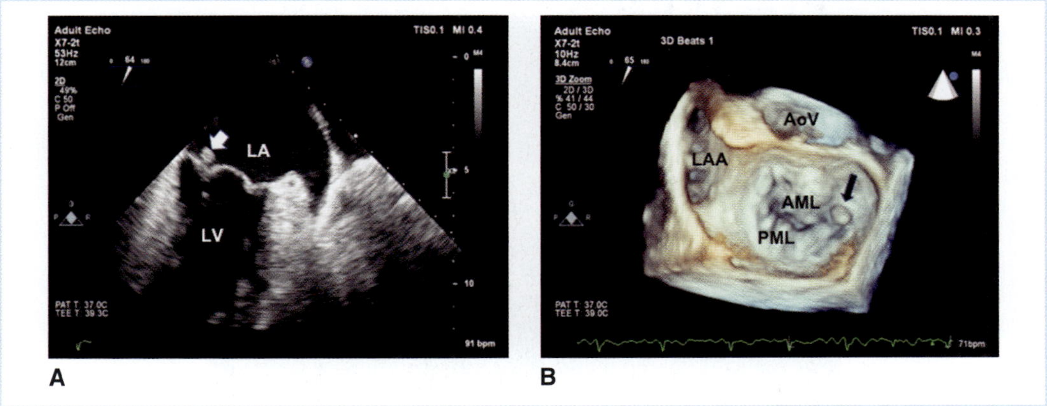

FIGURE 20.5 A: Example of a papillary fibroelastoma on mitral valve (arrow). B: Surgeon's view 3D image of same tumor (arrow). AML, anterior mitral leaflet; AoV, aortic valve; LA, left atrium; LAA, left atrial appendage; LV, left ventricle; PML, posterior mitral leaflet.

Rhabdomyoma

Rhabdomyomas are the most common primary cardiac tumor in children (4,5). Rhabdomyomas are almost always associated with tuberous sclerosis. They often appear as multiple tumors originating from the left or right ventricular myocardium. These tumors can become large and cause valvular or outflow tract obstruction. Asymptomatic rhabdomyomas are usually followed over time, as some of these tumors can spontaneously resolve.

Fibroma

Fibromas are the second most common benign cardiac tumors in children (4,5). Fibromas usually originate from the ventricles or the atrioventricular groove. A characteristic feature of fibroma is the presence of central calcification. Fibromas usually appear as a large, single intramural mass with multiple central densities. Singularity and presence of central calcification are key factors in differentiating fibromas from rhabdomyomas (Figure 20.7).

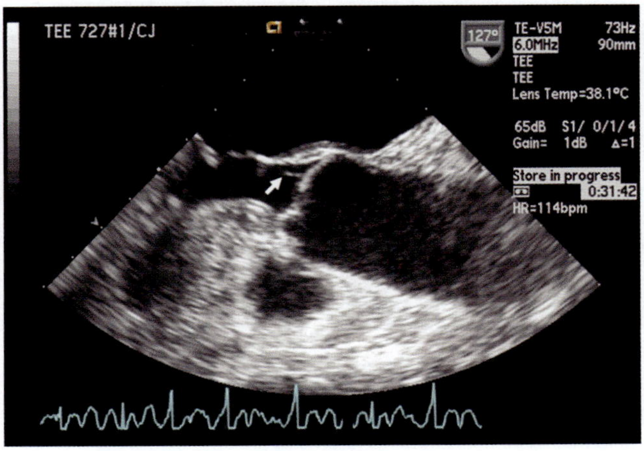

FIGURE 20.6 Example of a Lambl excrescence on the aortic valve leaflets (arrow).

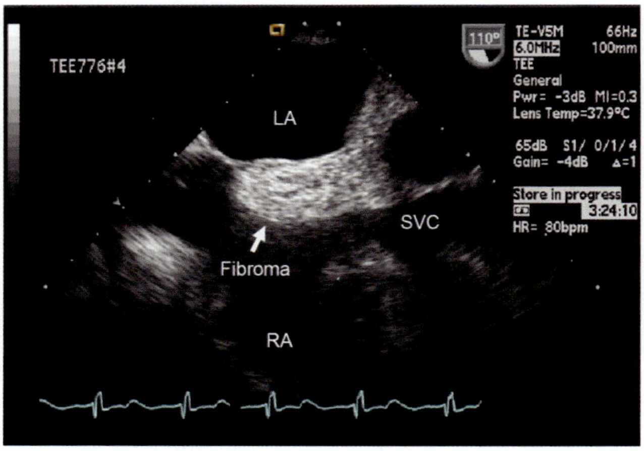

FIGURE 20.7 Example of a fibroma involving the medial left atrial wall and the atrial septum (arrow). LA, left atrium; RA, right atrium; SVC, superior vena cava.

Cardiac Sarcomas

Malignant tumors such as sarcomas are rare causes of cardiac neoplasms and usually originate from the ventricular myocardium. These tumors can become large and invade any cavity and surrounding structures with protruding mobile components and attached thrombi (Figure 20.8). One of the distinguishing features of malignant cardiac tumors is enhancement with ultrasound contrast, given their extensive vascularity.

Metastatic Tumors

Metastatic tumors involve the heart or the pericardium through local invasion (such as breast or lung cancer) or hematogenous spread (melanoma). Tumors that invade the heart locally can at times be seen on TEE as an external mass compressing or invading the cardiac chambers (Figure 20.9; Video 20.9).

Embolization

Most cardiac tumors have the potential for embolization. Emboli can be from tumor fragments or dissociation of attached thrombi. Certain tumors, such as fibroelastoma and myxoma, are associated with higher

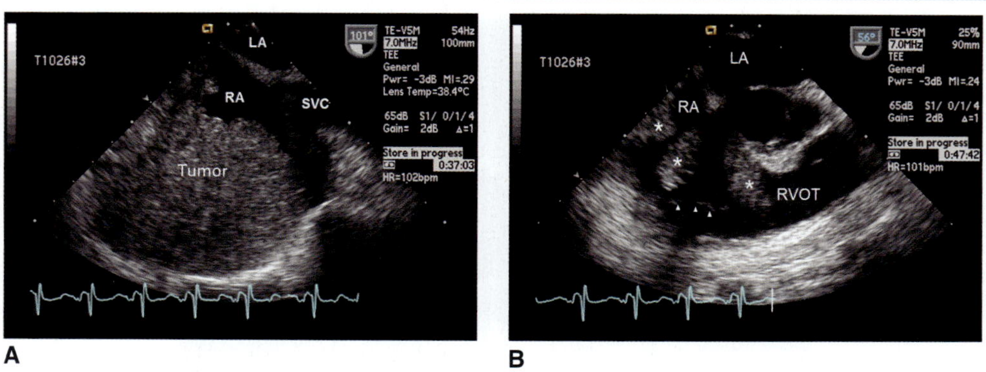

FIGURE 20.8 Midesophageal bicaval view of an angiosarcoma of the right atrium. In this image, a large mass is occupying the entire right atrium (panel A). Tumor fragments (asterisks) prolapse across the tricuspid valve (arrowheads) into the right ventricle and right ventricular outflow tract (panel B). LA, left atrium; RA, right atrium; RVOT, right ventricular outflow tract; SVC, superior vena cava.

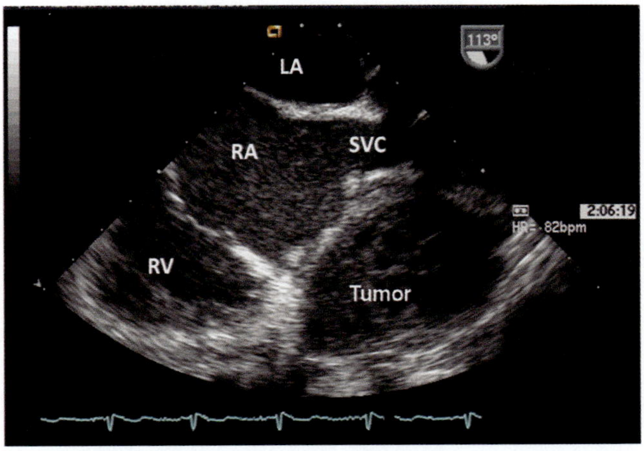

FIGURE 20.9 Example of a large extracardiac tumor manifesting as a heterogeneous mass anterior to the superior vena cava. LA, left atrium; RA, right atrium; RV, right ventricle; SVC, superior vena cava.

rates of embolization. In one study, 30% of patients with an incidental finding of fibroelastoma had symptoms consistent with systemic embolization on clinical follow-up (8). In rare instances, large tumor fragments from distant sites can be seen in transit through the inferior vena cava (IVC) and the right heart. Renal cell carcinoma is commonly associated with embolization and transit of tumor fragments through the right heart (Figure 20.10; Video 20.10).

INTRACARDIAC THROMBUS

Thrombi can be formed within any cardiac chamber and are often associated with an underlying abnormality leading to stasis of blood such as atrial fibrillation or in low-flow states associated with regional wall motion abnormalities. The most common site for intracardiac thrombus is the LAA in patients with atrial fibrillation or rheumatic mitral stenosis (Figure 20.11; Videos 20.11 and 20.12). Thrombus can also form on intracardiac devices such as pacemaker wires, septal closure devices, or indwelling catheters in the right heart (Figure 20.12; Video 20.13).

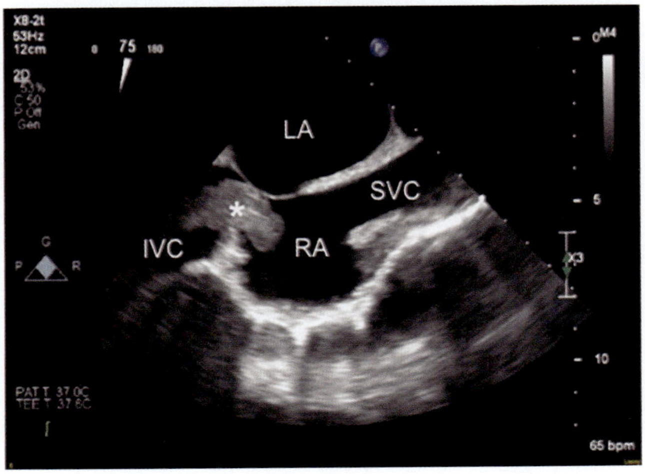

FIGURE 20.10 Example of a tumor fragment emboli in transit through IVC in the RA in a patient with renal cell carcinoma (asterisk). IVC, inferior vena cava; LA, left atrium; RA, right atrium; SVC, superior vena cava.

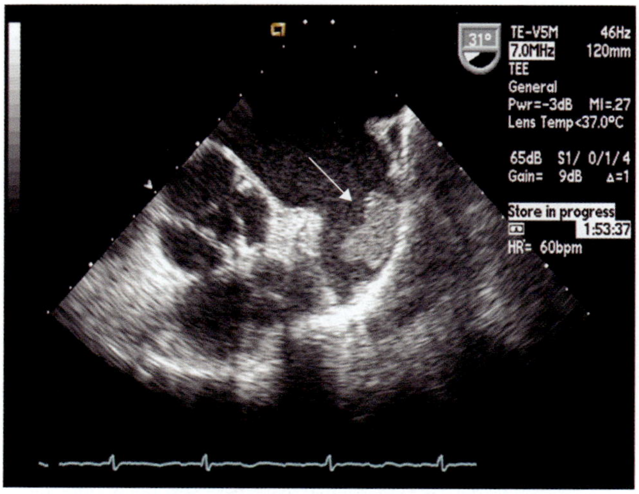

FIGURE 20.11 Midesophageal image of the left atrial appendage (LAA) at 30° is depicted. A large thrombus (arrow) is seen in the LAA.

Thrombus in the ventricles is almost always associated with an underlying wall motion abnormality. Fresh thrombi tend to be round and mobile, whereas chronic thrombi appear flat and laminated and are less mobile. Size and mobility are important predictors of systemic embolization (Figure 20.13; Video 20.14).

Practical Considerations in the Evaluation of Cardiac Masses

Current echocardiographic techniques are limited in the assessment of histology of cardiac masses. As one of our editors (JZ) is fond of saying "Ultrasound cannot make tissue diagnoses." As a result, it's important to obtain images at multiple planes (perpendicular views using transducer angle rotations or 3D imaging) to further characterize the size, shape, mobility, and anatomic location of any suspected mass. Anatomic features as well as associated clinical history and response to therapy may offer clues to the origin and type of the mass. For example, intracavitary masses associated with stagnation, regional wall motion abnormalities,

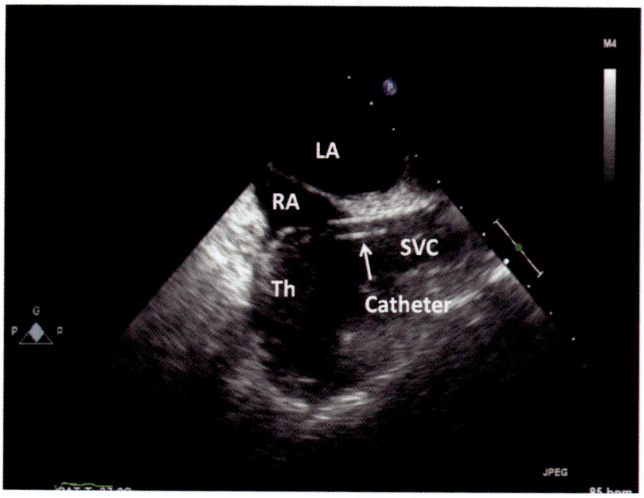

FIGURE 20.12 Example of a large thrombus (Th) in the right atrium (RA) is shown in a patient with indwelling hemodialysis catheter (arrow). LA, left atrium; SVC, superior vena cava.

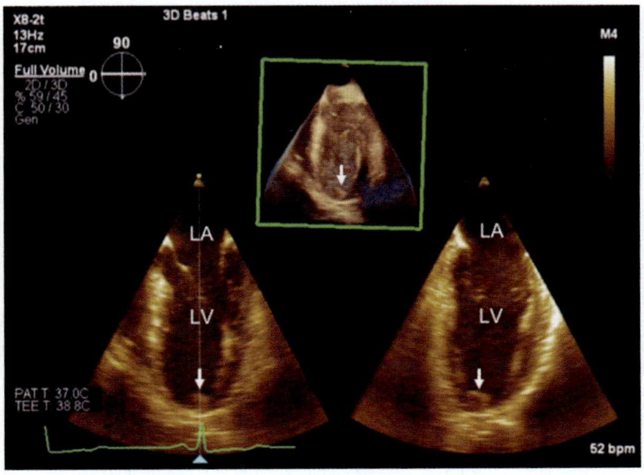

FIGURE 20.13 Midesophageal biplane view of the left ventricle in diastole showing a large apical thrombus (arrow) in a patient with apical hypokinesis. LA, left atrium; LV, left ventricle.

or intracardiac devices are likely thrombi. Furthermore, resolution of a mass on repeat imaging after a few weeks of anticoagulation is suggestive of thrombus (Figure 20.14).

Administration of ultrasound-enhancing agents (UEAs) can provide important information on the vascularity of the suspected mass (12). Malignant tumors are usually highly vascular and may take up UEA, whereas benign stromal tumors with low vascularity or organized thrombus will show low enhancement; fresh clots will appear as filling defects (Figure 20.15; Video 20.15).

When using UEA, it is essential to adjust the settings on echocardiography platforms (low mechanical index and harmonic imaging) to obtain good-quality contrast images. Echocardiographic characteristics of different cardiac masses are summarized in Table 20.1.

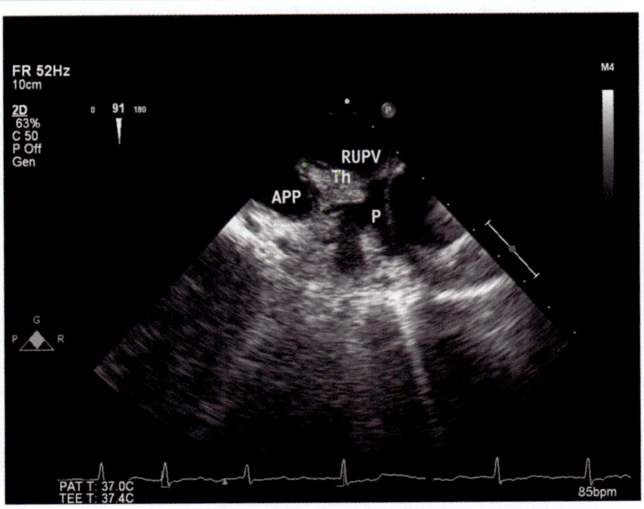

FIGURE 20.14 Example of a small thrombus (Th) in the oblique pericardial sinus (P) adjacent to the right upper pulmonary vein (RUPV) in a patient with a recent pulmonary vein ablation procedure for atrial fibrillation. Thrombus was resolved on repeat TEE after 4 weeks of anticoagulation. Small amount of fluid is seen in the pericardial space (P). App, left atrial appendage; TEE, transesophageal echocardiography.

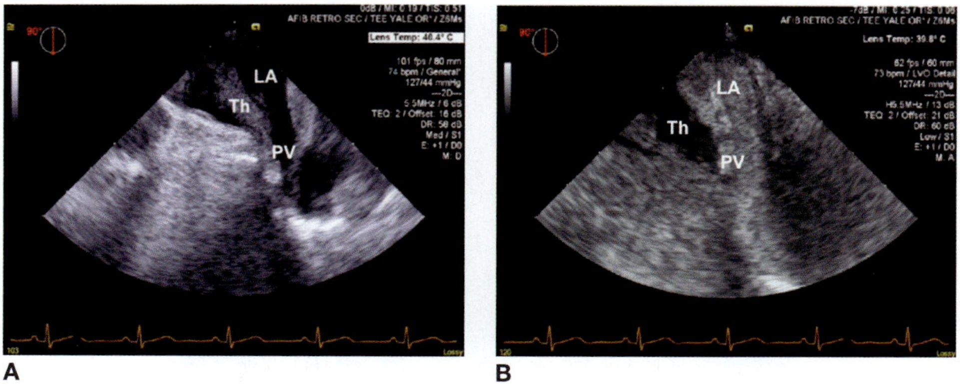

FIGURE 20.15 Panel A: Example of a large mass likely thrombus (Th) originating from the pulmonary vein (PV) and protruding into the left atrium (LA) as a highly mobile mass (see Video 20.15) in a patient with lung cancer. Panel B: After administration of intravenous echo contrast, the thrombus appears as a nonenhancing filling defect.

Transesophageal Echocardiography in the Assessment of Cardiac Sources of Emboli

Emboli originating from the heart or great vessels are common etiologic factors in stroke and peripheral arterial occlusions. More than 20% of all cases of ischemic stroke are embolic in origin. In as many as 40% of patients with stroke, despite intense clinical workup, the etiology is not identified. These patients with cryptogenic stroke are younger, with less evidence of generalized atherosclerosis (13,14). It has been shown that the incidence of a patent foramen ovale (PFO) is higher in this population, suggesting a potential role of paradoxical embolism as the etiologic factor. Atherosclerotic disease of the ascending aorta and aortic arch are other potential sources of emboli in older patients.

Cardiac sources of emboli can be further divided into probable (high embolic potential) and possible (low embolic potential) sources based on the strength of association and potential for embolization (1).

Probable Sources of Emboli With High Embolic Potential

Left Atrial Appendage Thrombus

Thrombus in the left atrium or LAA is a common source of systemic embolization, especially in patients with atrial fibrillation (Figures 20.11 and 20.16; Videos 20.11 and 20.12).

Left atrial clot is usually an extension of existing thrombus in the LAA. The LAA is an extension of the left atrial cavity and originates from the superior aspect of the left atrium anterior to the insertion site of the left upper pulmonary vein. The LAA usually comprises two or more lobes and is lined with pectinate muscle. The LAA is best visualized in the midesophageal position with the transducer at 30° to 60° rotation. With a gradual increase in the transducer rotation up to 150°, detailed views of the wall structure and number and location of lobes can be obtained. It is essential to image the appendage in multiple transducer angles and

TABLE 20.1 Echocardiographic Characteristics of Common Cardiac Masses

Mass Type	Appearance	Size and Location	Other
Myxoma	Large, smooth surface, mobile and pedunculated	Left atrium, right atrium	Minimal enhancement with echo contrast
Papillary fibroelastoma	Mobile pedunculated, multiple fibrillar projections	Small (<1 cm), attached to valvular structures/cords	No significant valvular regurgitation
Lipoma	Smooth surface, large, increased echogenicity	Ventricular and atrial myocardium	Minimal enhancement with ultrasound contrast
Thrombus	Stagnation, prior instrumentation, often mobile	Any size, commonly in low-flow areas such as atrial appendage or apex with wall motion abnormalities	No enhancement with contrast. Resolution after anticoagulation

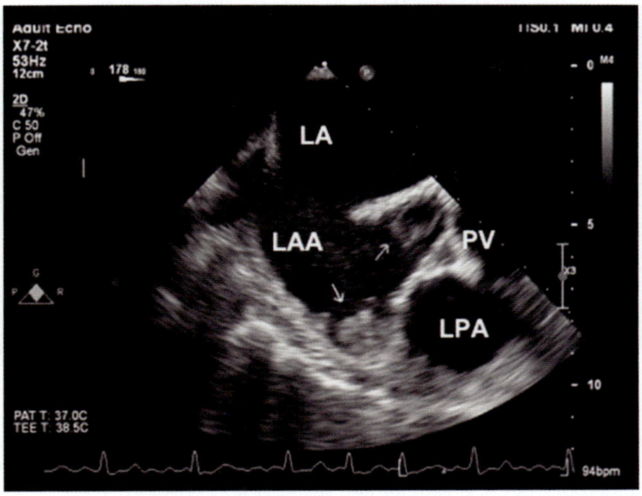

FIGURE 20.16 Example of thrombi in both the main lobe and posterior lobes on the left atrial appendage (LAA) (arrows) in a patient with chronic atrial fibrillation. The thrombus in the main lobe was easily detected; however, visualization of thrombus in the posterior lobe required higher transducer angle rotation and posterior tilting of the TEE probe. This serves as an important reminder to look in every lobe of the appendage (and there are often several) rather than just in the "tip." LA, left atrium; LAA, left atrial appendage; LPA, left pulmonary artery; PV, pulmonary vein.

in orthogonal views to be able to view all the lobes of the LAA and distinguish the pectinate muscle from a potential thrombus (Figures 20.16 and 20.17). Intravenous administration of UEA can be useful to distinguish pectinate muscle from other luminal densities such as thrombus, spontaneous echo contrast (SEC), or sludge (Figure 20.18, Panels A and B). In addition to two-dimensional (2D) images, a detailed examination of the atrial appendage should include an assessment of blood flow velocity by pulse wave Doppler. Decreased blood flow velocity (<40 cm/s) in the LAA has been shown to be associated with an increased risk of thromboembolic events.

Left Ventricular Thrombus

Thrombus in the left ventricle (LV) is usually associated with regional wall motion abnormalities. The majority of thrombi in the LV are located in the apex (Figure 20.13; Video 20.14). TEE is often limited in visualizing the apex, given its anterior location and relative distance from the transducer. The LV apex is

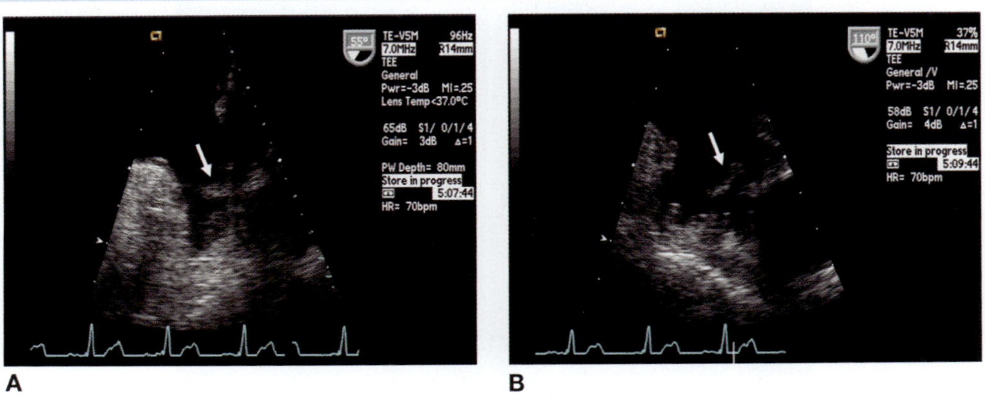

FIGURE 20.17 Example of a prominent pectinate muscle in the left atrial appendage (LAA) mimicking a thrombus (arrow) is depicted (panel A). Images obtained at an orthogonal plane from the same patient demonstrate that the density is a septation between lobes of the LAA (panel B) (arrow).

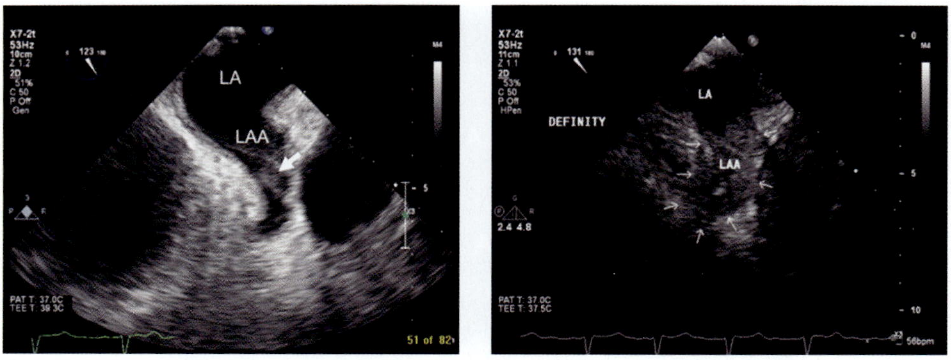

A B

FIGURE 20.18 Panel A: Example of dense spontaneous echo contrast in the left atrial appendage (LAA) (thick arrow) mimicking a thrombus. Panel B: Complete opacification of LAA without filling defects confirms the absence of thrombus. Small arrows mark the borders of LAA. LA, left atrium; LAA, left atrial appendage.

best seen in the ME LAX view with slight retroflexion of the probe. Administration of UEAs can further assist in identifying apical thrombi, which appear as filling defects in the ventricular apex. In contrast to TEE, transthoracic echocardiography is a better technique to assess the LV apex.

Complex Aortic Atheromas

Complex atherosclerotic plaques, defined as size >4 mm or with the presence of mobile components or ulcers, in the ascending aorta or aortic arch are another important source of stroke and embolization (15-17) (Figure 20.19; Videos 20.16 and 20.17).

These plaques are often associated with thrombi superimposed on ulcerated plaques. Thromboembolization, whether spontaneous or associated with surgical or endovascular interventional procedures, is the underlying mechanism for embolic events. In a study of 331 older patients (age >60) with stroke who underwent a diagnostic TEE, presence of large arch atheroma (>4 mm) was associated with an 11.9% per year incidence of repeat stroke in the 24-month follow-up period, which was 4 times higher than repeat stroke rate in patients with small plaques (<1 mm) (16). Large atheromas in the descending aorta are also associated with systemic emboli syndromes. In a case-control study of 250 patients with stroke who had TEE, the large atheroma of

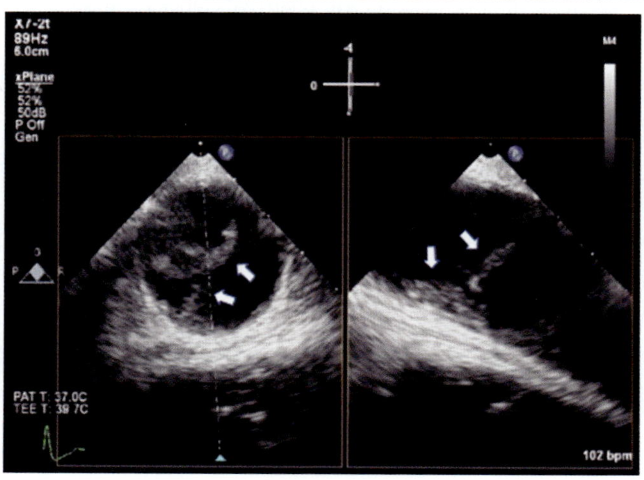

FIGURE 20.19 Biplane image of a large complex atheroma in the descending aorta with a highly mobile component (arrows) (see Video 20.16) in a patient presenting with emboli to the femoral artery.

the descending aorta was associated with an odds ratio of 1.5 for recurrent stroke as compared to matched controls (17). The causative role of smaller aortic atheroma in stroke and systemic embolic syndromes is less clear and may reflect the presence of diffuse atherosclerosis.

Endocarditis

Vegetation on any cardiac valve can also be a source of embolic events. Vegetation size (size >10 mm) and mobility on TEE are independent risk factors for embolic events (18).

Possible Sources of Emboli With Low Embolic Potential

Spontaneous Echo Contrast (Smoke)

SEC or smoke is an echogenic swirling pattern of blood flow in the left atrium associated with stagnation (Figure 20.20; Video 20.18). The exact mechanism of SEC is not well understood, but it is thought to be due to aggregation of red blood cells. The presence of SEC in the left atrium or LAA is associated with an increased risk of thromboembolism (19,20). It should be noted that gain settings on the echocardiography equipment should be optimized before any diagnosis of SEC is made since an increased gain setting can mimic SEC.

Paradoxical Embolus Through a Patent Foramen Ovale

Transit of a venous embolus through a PFO can lead to systemic embolization. This theory is further supported by a higher incidence of PFO in young patients with cryptogenic stroke and anecdotal reports of paradoxical embolus caught in transit across the septum (13,21) (Figure 20.21; Video 20.19).

Although the direct causative role of PFO in cryptogenic stroke is not established, recent clinical trial evidence of beneficial effect of PFO closure in reducing the risk of recurrent stroke in patients with cryptogenic stroke and PFO further supports the important association of PFO and cryptogenic stroke (22-24). Therefore, TEE for evaluation of the source of embolus should include a detailed evaluation of the atrial septum with color flow Doppler (CFD) and agitated saline bubble study to assess for the presence of PFO and right-to-left shunt. The atrial septum is best seen in the midesophagus with a transducer angle of 100° to 120° (ME bicaval view). A PFO can be seen by CFD demonstrating the flow across the foramen ovale or by an early appearance of agitated saline bubbles in the left atrium after intravenous injection of agitated saline contrast (Figure 20.22; Videos 20.20 and 20.21). PFOs can be easily closed via a percutaneous approach using an Amplatzer occluder device. TEE is often performed to guide device implantation. It is important to recognize the correct

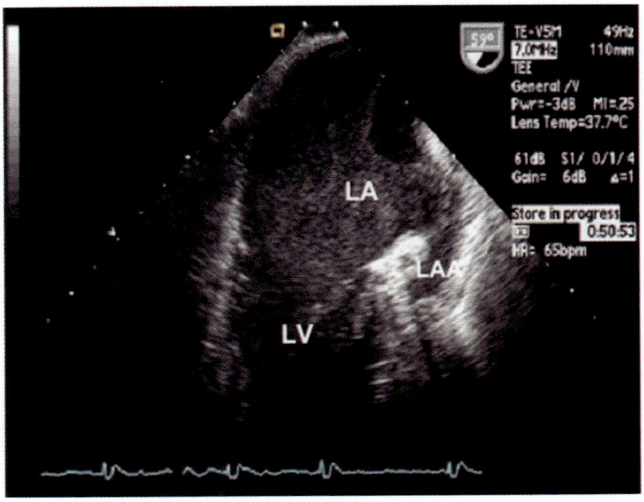

FIGURE 20.20 Midesophageal image of the left atrium demonstrating increased left atrial size and spontaneous echo contrast. LA, left atrium; LAA, left atrial appendage; LV, left ventricle.

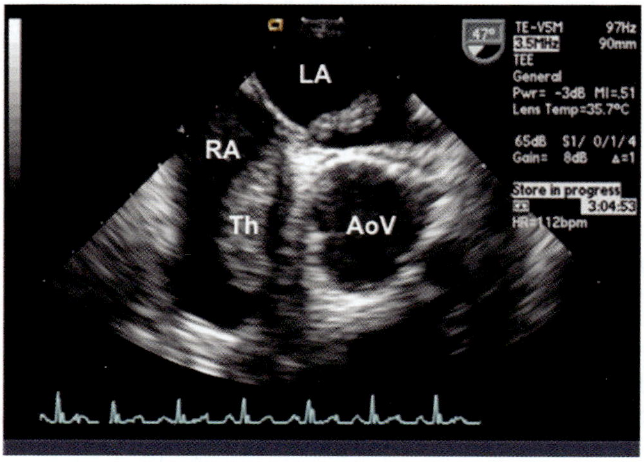

FIGURE 20.21 Midesophageal view of a large thrombus in transit (Th) across a patent foramen ovale in a patient who presented with pulmonary emboli and renal infarcts. AoV, aortic valve; LA, left atrium; RA, right atrium.

implantation position, as improper implantation can lead to device migration and embolization requiring surgical intervention.

Transesophageal Echocardiography During Percutaneous Procedures to Reduce the Risk of Emboli

Patients with atrial fibrillation and an increased risk of stroke are treated with systemic anticoagulation to reduce the risk of thromboemboli originating from LAA (1). Occlusion of the LAA is a viable alternative to anticoagulation in patients who cannot tolerate anticoagulation due to an increased risk of bleeding. The Watchman percutaneous left atrial occlusion device is recently approved as an alternative to anticoagulation in patients with an increased risk of bleeding. This device is delivered through venous access and a transseptal approach under echocardiographic guidance. TEE is an essential tool to assist in procedure planning and guide delivery of the device during the procedure (25) (Figure 20.23).

During the planning stage, morphology and dimensions of the LAA are evaluated by TEE to guide appropriate device size selection. During the procedure, with live TEE guidance using 3D-derived multiplane

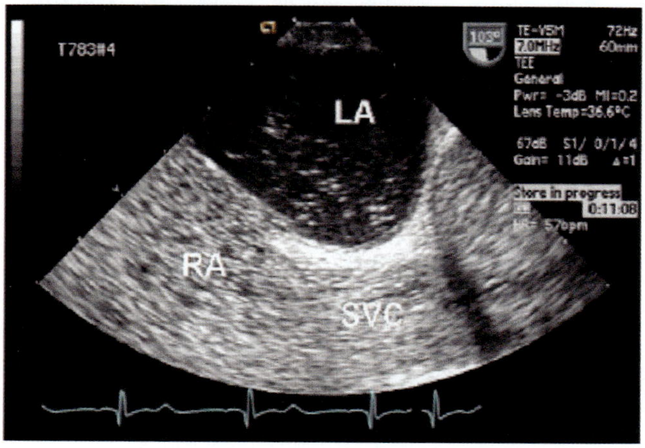

FIGURE 20.22 Midesophageal bicaval view after intravenous injection of agitated saline demonstrating the passage of saline bubbles across a patent foramen ovale into the left atrium. LA, left atrium; RA, right atrium; SVC, superior vena cava.

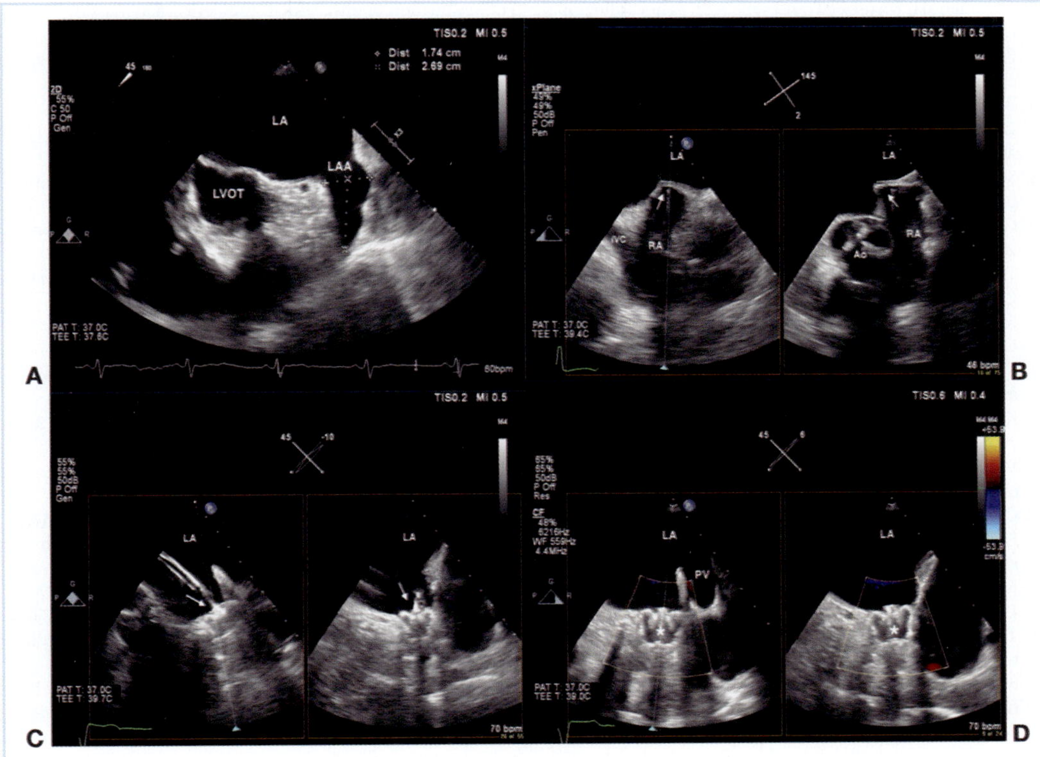

FIGURE 20.23 TEE-guided closure of left atrial appendage with Watchman device. A: Appropriate device size is selected based on TEE-derived measurements of LAA orifice size, depth, and shape. B: Optimal positioning of transseptal catheter is guided and confirmed on biplane TEE. Arrows show tenting of intra-atrial septum caused by transseptal puncture needle. C: Delivery and positioning of the device into LAA is guided on biplane TEE images. Arrows point to the device attached to the delivery system. D: Well-positioned device (Asterix) after release from the delivery system; color Doppler imaging is used to evaluate for the presence of peri-device leak. A peri-device leak with a jet width greater than 5 mm on color Doppler is considered significant and may require device repositioning before the device is released. A0, aortic valve; LA, left atrium; LAA, left atrial appendage; LVOT, left ventricular outflow tract; PV, pulmonary vein; RA, right atrium; TEE, transesophageal echocardiography.

imaging, the transseptal puncture is performed and the device is positioned and deployed in LAA. Prior to release of device from delivery system, a detailed TEE examination of the LAA, closure device, and surrounding cardiac structures is performed for assessment of appropriate positioning, device stability, and detection of peri-device leak. Device stability is assured with an assessment of appropriate device compression post insertion as well as direct observation of device after a tugging maneuver. Peri-device regurgitation is assessed with color Doppler imaging after adjustment of Nyquist limit to allow for detection of low-velocity flows. Any color Doppler width greater than 5 mm is considered unacceptable and may require device repositioning. Lastly, after the release of the device, repeat TEE imaging is obtained to assess for potential complications (26) such as perforation and pericardial effusion.

REFERENCES

1. Saric M, Armour AC, Arnaout MS, et al. Guidelines for the use of echocardiography in the evaluation of a cardiac source of embolism. *J Am Soc Echocardiogr*. 2016;29:1-42.
2. Cohen A, Donal E, Delgado V, et al. EACVI recommendations on cardiovascular imaging for the detection of embolic sources: endorsed by the Canadian Society of Echocardiography. *Eur Heart J Cardiovasc Imaging*. 2021;22:e24-e57.
3. Peters PJ, Reinhardint S. The echocardiographic evaluation of intracardiac masses: a review. *J Am Soc Echocardiogr*. 2006;19(2):230-240.

4. Goldman JH, Foster E. Transesophageal echocardiographic (TEE) evaluation of intracardiac and pericardial masses. *Cardiol Clin*. 2000;18(4):849-860.
5. Pino PG, Moreo A, Lestuzzi C. Differential diagnosis of cardiac tumors: general consideration and echocardiographic approach. *J Clin Ultrasound*. 2022;50(8):1177-1193.
6. Basso C, Rizzo S, Valente M, et al. Cardiac masses and tumors. *Heart*. 2016;102(15):1230-1245.
7. O'Connor S, Recavarren R, Nichols LC, et al. Lipomatous hypertrophy of the interatrial septum: an overview. *Arch Pathol Lab Med*. 2006;130(3):397-399.
8. Sun JP, Asher CR, Yang XS, et al. Clinical and echocardiographic characteristics of papillary fibroelastomas: a retrospective and prospective study in 162 patients. *Circulation*. 2001;103(22):2687-2693.
9. Gowda RM, Khan IA, Nair CK, et al. Cardiac papillary fibroelastoma: a comprehensive analysis of 725 cases. *Am Heart J*. 2003;146(3):404-410.
10. Tamin SS, Maleszewski JJ, Scott CG, et al. Prognostic and bioepidemiologic implications of papillary fibroelastomas. *J Am Coll Cardiol*. 2015;65(22):2420-2429.
11. Roldan CA, Shively BK, Crawford MH. Valve excrescences: prevalence, evolution and risk for cardioembolism. *J Am Coll Cardiol*. 1997;30(5):1308-1314.
12. Kirkpatrick JN, Wong T, Bednarz JE, et al. Differential diagnosis of cardiac masses using contrast echocardiographic perfusion imaging. *J Am Coll Cardiol*. 2004;43(8):1412-1419.
13. Kizer JR, Devereux RB. Clinical practice: patent foramen ovale in young adults with unexplained stroke. *N Engl J Med*. 2005;353(22):2361-2372.
14. Wu LA, Malouf JF, Dearani JA, et al. Patent foramen ovale in cryptogenic stroke: current understanding and management options. *Arch Intern Med*. 2004;164(9):950-956.
15. Cui X, Li Y, Liu J, et al. Aortic arch atheroma and the risk of stroke: a meta-analysis. *J Evid Based Med*. 2014;7(3):185-191.
16. French Study of Aortic Plaques in Stroke Group, Amarenco P, Cohen A, et al. Atherosclerotic disease of the aortic arch as a risk factor for recurrent ischemic stroke. *N Engl J Med*. 1996;334(19):1216-1221.
17. Amarenco P, Cohen A, Tzourio C, et al. Atherosclerotic disease of the aortic arch and the risk of ischemic stroke. *N Engl J Med*. 1994;331(22):1474-1479.
18. Thuny F, Di Salvo G, Belliard O, et al. Risk of embolism and death in infective endocarditis: prognostic value of echocardiography: a prospective multicenter study. *Circulation*. 2005;112(1):69-75.
19. Bernhardt P, Schmidt H, Hammerstingl C, et al. Patients with atrial fibrillation and dense spontaneous echo contrast at high risk: a prospective and serial follow-up over 12 months with transesophageal echocardiography and cerebral magnetic resonance imaging. *J Am Coll Cardiol*. 2005;45(11):1807-1812.
20. Zhao Y, Ji L, Liu J, et al. Intensity of left atrial spontaneous echo contrast as a correlate for stroke risk stratification in patients with nonvalvular atrial fibrillation. *Sci Rep*. 2016;6:27650.
21. Cramer SC. Patent foramen ovale and its relationship to stroke. *Cardiol Clin*. 2005;23(1):7-11.
22. Søndergaard L, Kasner SE, Rhodes JF, et al. Patent foramen ovale closure or antiplatelet therapy for cryptogenic stroke. *N Engl J Med*. 2017;377(11):1033-1042.
23. Mas JL, Derumeaux G, Guillon B, et al. Patent foramen ovale closure or anticoagulation vs. antiplatelets after stroke. *N Engl J Med*. 2017;377:1011-1021.
24. Saver JL, Carroll JD, Thaler DE, et al. Long-term outcomes of patent foramen ovale closure or medical therapy after stroke. *N Engl J Med*. 2017;377(11):1022-1032.
25. Vainrib AF, Harb SC, Jaber W et al. Left atrial appendage occlusion/exclusion: procedural image guidance with transesophageal echocardiography. *J Am Soc Echocardiogr*. 2018;31(4):454-474.
26. Thakker R, Faluk MA, Modi S, Ahmad M. Echocardiography in percutaneous left atrial appendage occlusion and related complications. *Echocardiography*. 2023;40(12):1325-1335.

▶QUESTIONS

1. Which one of the following statements is *true:*

A. The Coumadin ridge is the tissue fold between LAA and left upper pulmonary vein that can often be mistaken for a thrombus or a small tumor.

B. The Chiari network is a remnant of fetal circulation that appears as a mobile density in the left atrium and can be confused with a left atrial mass.

C. Lipomatous hypertrophy of the intra-atrial septum is commonly seen in women and is associated with a benign course.

D. All of the above

2. All of the following statements are true *except:*

A. Primary cardiac tumors are very rare and comprise a minority of all cardiac neoplasms.

B. Metastatic tumors involve the heart or pericardium through local invasion or hematogenous spread.

C. Echocardiography is an effective technique in identifying the tissue origin of cardiac masses.

D. Lack of enhancement of cardiac mass with UEA suggests slow-growing benign tumors.

3. **All of the following statements are true *except:***
   A. A myxoma is the most common primary cardiac tumor in adults.
   B. Cardiac myxomas are pedunculated masses that commonly arise from the atrioventricular valves.
   C. A myxoma is a slow-growing tumor and can remain asymptomatic for a long period of time.
   D. A myxoma can grow in size and occupy a significant portion of the cardiac chambers.

4. **All of the following statements are true *except:***
   A. Fibroelastomas are mobile tumors that appear as a small (0.5-2 cm) pedunculated echo density on valvular structures.
   B. Fibroelastomas are often associated with valvular calcifications.
   C. Fibroblastomas have high potential for embolization.
   D. In contrast to vegetations, fibroelastomas are not associated with significant valvular regurgitations.

5. **Which one of the following statements is *true:***
   A. Rhabdomyomas are the uncommon primary cardiac tumors in children.
   B. Rhabdomyomas are almost always associated with tuberous sclerosis.
   C. Asymptomatic rhabdomyomas are usually followed over time, as some of these tumors can spontaneously resolve.
   D. B and C

6. **Which of the following malignancies is associated with tumor fragment embolization through IVC?**
   A. Lymphoma
   B. Melanoma
   C. Renal cell carcinoma
   D. Non-small-cell lung carcinoma

7. **All of the following statements are true *except:***
   A. Intracardiac thrombi are associated with stasis of blood.
   B. Thrombus can be formed on intracardiac devices such as pacemaker wires.
   C. Thrombus in the ventricles is almost always associated with underlying wall motion abnormality.
   D. Thrombus size and mobility are not predictors of systemic embolization.

8. **Which of the following statements are *true:***
   A. SEC or smoke is an echogenic swirling pattern of blood flow in the left atrium and is a marker of stagnation.
   B. The presence of SEC in the left atrium or LAA is associated with increased risk of thromboembolism.
   C. SEC is commonly seen in atrial fibrillation.
   D. All of the above

9. **All of the following statements are true *except:***
   A. Lambl excrescences are commonly seen on commissural edges of the aortic valve leaflets.
   B. Larger Lambl excrescences are often confused with valvular vegetations.
   C. Similar to vegetations, Lambl excrescences are associated with valvular regurgitations.
   D. Lambl excrescences are not associated with embolic events.

10. **A 45-year-old patient with stroke underwent a TEE procedure to evaluate the source of emboli. Which one of the following has a high probability of being the source of emboli?**
   A. Small PFO with left-to-right shunt
   B. Thrombus in LAA
   C. 2-mm Nonmobile plaque in descending aorta
   D. Small Lambl excrescence on the aortic valve

ANSWERS

1. **Correct Answer: D.**
   Rationale: Several normal cardiac structures can be mistaken for cardiac masses including the tissue ridge between posterior wall of LAA and anterior wall of left upper pulmonary vein (the coumadin ridge) or remnants of the Chiari

network, which is lacy mobile remnant of fetal circulation in the right atrium. Lipomatous hypertrophy of the atrial septum is commonly seen in older women and is due to fat infiltration in the atrial septal tissue. This entity is distinct from lipomas since lipomas have a well-defined capsule.

2. **Correct Answer: C.**
Rationale: Echocardiography is a poor technique in the determination of tissue histology and identification of the origin of tumors. Administration of UEAs will help distinguish malignant tumors with high vascularity from slow-growing benign tumors such as cardiac myxoma. Primary cardiac tumors comprise a minority of cardiac tumors; the most common cardiac tumors are metastatic from remote sites.

3. **Correct Answer: A.**
Rationale: Cardiac myxomas are slow-growing benign cardiac neoplasms with low vascularity that are often pedunculated and attached to interatrial septum in the left atrium but can occur in other cardiac chambers. These slow-growing tumors can remain undetected and present as large mobile intracavity masses interfering with blood flow across the mitral valve.

4. **Correct Answer: B.**
Rationale: PFEs are common, small benign cardiac tumors often attached to valvular structures (aortic and mitral valves) and are hallmarked by frondlike projections. Larger fibroelastomas are associated with an increased risk of stroke from embolization of tumor fragments or associated thrombi. In contrast to valvular vegetations, fibroelastomas are not associated with infection and inflammation and are not associated with valvular dysfunction and regurgitation.

5. **Correct Answer: D.**
Rationale: Rhabdomyomas are the most common primary cardiac tumors in children and are almost always associated with tuberous sclerosis. Rhabdomyomas can present as multiple masses affecting the ventricular myocardium. Rhabdomyomas are usually followed over time, as some of these tumors can spontaneously resolve.

6. **Correct Answer: C.**
Rationale: Renal cell carcinoma is associated with embolization of tumor fragments through IVC. Both lymphoma and renal cell carcinoma can affect the heart through local extension to pericardial space. Melanoma is associated with a high incidence of hematogenous metastasis to the myocardium.

7. **Correct Answer: D.**
Rationale: Stagnation, hypercoagulability, and foreign material (Virchow triad) are three factors that contribute to thrombosis. Intracardiac thrombi form in areas with blood flow stasis, such as LAA or in the ventricular cavity adjacent to regions with severe wall motion abnormality. Pacemaker/implantable cardioverter-defibrillator (ICD) leads are often niduses for small thrombi in the right atrium. Risk of embolization is higher with larger thrombi with increased mobility.

8. **Correct Answer: D.**
Rationale: SEC is a smoke-like echogenic swirling pattern of blood flow seen in cardiac chambers in the setting of blood flow stagnation and is thought to be due to rouleaux formation of red blood cells in low-flow states. SEC is often seen in the left atrium in the setting of atrial fibrillation and is associated with a higher risk of thromboembolization.

9. **Correct Answer: C.**
Rationale: Lambl or valvular excrescences are small (1-2 mm) growths attached to commissural surface of the valves (most commonly aortic valve). These growths are composed of an avascular fibroelastic core covered with a single endothelial layer. Larger Lambl excrescences can be mistaken for vegetations; however, Lambl excrescences are not associated with valvular dysfunction and regurgitation. There is no clear association between Lambl excrescences and the risk of stroke.

10. **Correct Answer: B.**
Rationale: Although choices A and C are associated with an increased risk of emboli, they have low embolic potential. Risk of paradoxical emboli is low in patients with small PFO and left-to-right shunt. Although large (>4 mm) and mobile aortic atheromas are associated with an increased risk of emboli, this risk is lower with small nonmobile atheromas. Risk and potential for embolization are higher in the presence of thrombus in the LAA. There is no clear association between valvular excrescences and embolic stroke.

21 3D Transesophageal Echocardiography Imaging

Marcus Salvatori and Annette Vegas

Rapid technological advances have made three-dimensional transesophageal echocardiography (3DTEE) commonplace in the perioperative setting as a standard and affordable feature of modern ultrasound (US) systems. Over the past 20 years, the early complexity of offline 3DTEE imaging has quickly progressed with streamlined workflows into single-button acquisition, real-time (RT) imaging, multiplanar reconstruction (MPR), and US machine–integrated software analysis. An optimized 3DTEE dataset yields more information about a structure than a two-dimensional (2D) transesophageal echocardiography (TEE) interrogation at multiple transducer angles. Understanding a 3D structure from several 2D images is time-consuming, inefficient, and, more importantly, variable and subjective.

Despite its prevalence, 3DTEE technology remains underutilized owing to perceived barriers, including (a) the steep learning curve for image acquisition and optimization, (b) prohibitive time requirement, (c) poor temporal resolution, and (d) difficulties in image interpretation. There is the perception that 3DTEE is a "supplemental" or "accessory" component of a focused TEE examination. Even echocardiographers experienced in 3DTEE underutilize this powerful imaging tool at a fraction of its true potential, despite growing evidence demonstrating its superiority.

Despite these obstacles, proficiency in 3DTEE has become an essential skill in the perioperative setting. 3DTEE shows entire structures from any perspective, in contrast to 2D imaging that relies on a mental reconstruction of serial images. The opportunity to view an entire moving structure in a single display is an invaluable visual aid to the echocardiographer and surgeon to better establish and communicate individual patient anatomy.

This chapter is a practical guide for echocardiographers seeking to incorporate and optimize 3DTEE as an integral part of their perioperative practice. Part 1 summarizes the physics and US principles underlying 3DTEE. Familiarity with these concepts is essential to understanding 3D imaging, limitations, and artifacts. Part 2 reviews the practical aspects and clinical applications of 3DTEE for each major cardiac structure. Finally, Part 3 discusses the future directions in 3DTEE technology.

THE SCIENCE OF 3D ULTRASOUND

There are fundamental differences between 2D and 3D echocardiographic imaging related to image acquisition, display, and interpretation. 2D imaging uses sector-based scanning, in which piezoelectric crystals arranged in a single row acquire a thin sector of information and display one 2D image (slice) at a time. Conversely, 3D imaging uses volume-based scanning, in which piezoelectric crystals arranged as a matrix acquire pyramidal 3D datasets containing a volume of information.

Creation of a US 3D image involves four basic steps: (1) data acquisition, (2) data storage, (3) data processing, and (4) image display (Figure 21.1). This requires using special US probes to obtain raw US data and integrated US machine software to process this into 3D datasets for displaying a 3D image.

Transesophageal Echocardiography Probes

The modern adult 2DTEE multiplane transducer comprises a linear phased array of 64 to 128 piezoelectric crystals arranged in a circular transducer face. Sequential activation of the crystals generates a 2D, sector-shaped, flat US plane. Mechanical or electronic rotation of the US plane in 1° increments through 180° generates a conical-shaped scan (Figure 21.2). A standard 2D multiplane TEE probe can create 3D images, but this is time-consuming and requires offline reconstruction.

3DTEE and 2DTEE probes are similar in size and have an operating frequency of 3 to 8 MHz. However, 3DTEE probes contain a single piezoelectric crystal partitioned into thousands of elements arranged in a matrix of rows and columns. Whereas the composition of conventional piezoelectric crystals is PZT (lead zirconate titanate), these probes use an alternative type of piezoelectric crystal. Proprietary TEE probes

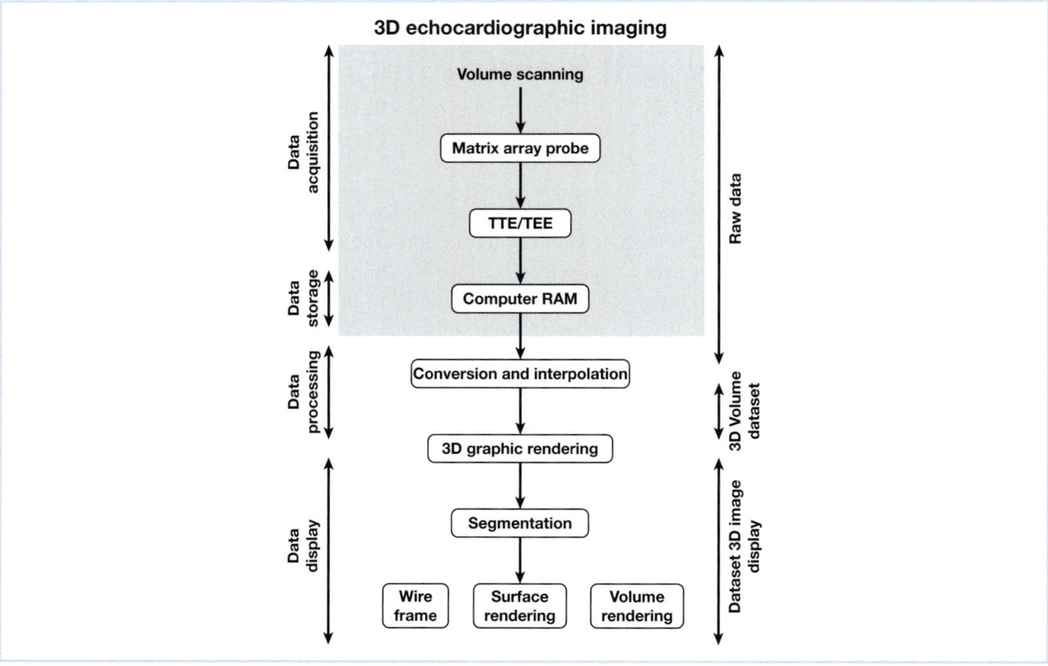

FIGURE 21.1 3D imaging. 3D echocardiographic imaging includes four stages: data acquisition, data storage, data processing, and data display. RAM, random access memory; TEE, transesophageal echocardiography; TTE, transthoracic echocardiography.

(Philips Healthcare and General Electric [GE] HealthCare) have a matrix array arrangement of 2,500 piezoelectric elements in 50 rows by 50 columns to cover a square transducer face (Table 21.1). Each element can be activated independently (fully sampled), focused, and steered. This generates a steerable US beam in the azimuthal (*x-y*) and the elevational (*x-z*) planes that create a scanned pyramidal 3D volume (Figure 21.2). The Siemens (Siemens Medical Solutions) Z6Ms 4DTEE probe uses a 48 × 48 matrix array of 2,304 elements. This probe also contains an application-specific integrated circuit (ASIC) that enables instantaneous acquisition of large 3D volumes of the entire heart at high volume rates without electrocardiogram (ECG) gating.

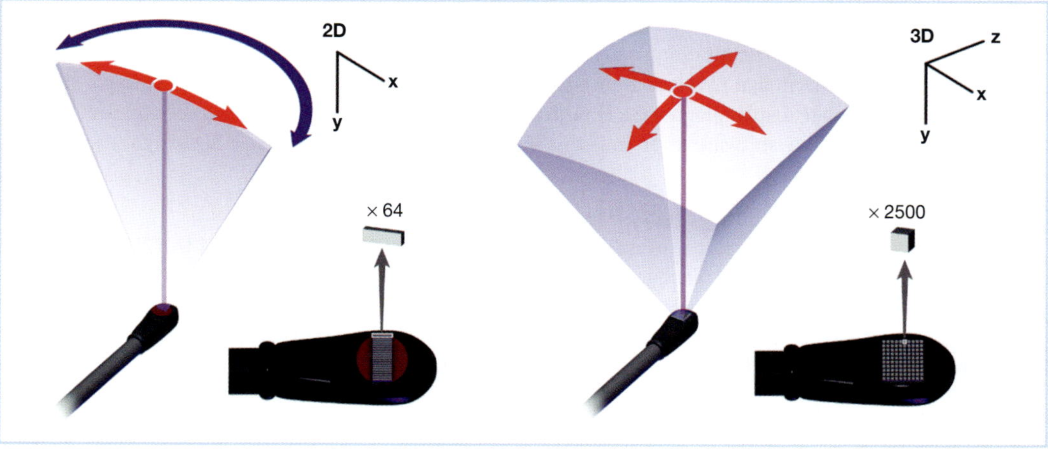

FIGURE 21.2 Transesophageal echocardiography transducers. This shows a comparison between a 64-crystal linear array in a 2DTEE probe and 2,500 crystals in a matrix array 3DTEE probe. TEE, transesophageal echocardiography. (Images courtesy of Michael Corrin.)

TABLE 21.1 Vendors and Equipment for 3DTEE

Vendor	Philips Healthcare	General Electric Healthcare	Siemens Medical Solutions
	Andover, MA, USA	Wauwatosa, WI, USA	Mountain View, CA, USA
Probe	X7-2t, X8-2t, X11-4t	6VT, 9VT-D	Z6Ms, V5Ms
Transducer Frequency	5-7 MHz	3-8 MHz	3-7 MHz
3D Modes	Live Zoom Full volume Color	Bird's view 4D zoom Medium, large Color	Icon
Biplane	xPlane (2 planes)	Multi D (3 planes)	Icon
Analytic Software	QLAB QLAB Advanced MVQ TomTec	TomTec	4D Volume Analysis e-Sie Valves

MVQ, mitral valve quantification. TEE, transesophageal echocardiography.

In addition, all 3DTEE probes can simultaneously display two or more independent 2D scanning planes (biplane or multiplane) and perform all the standard 2D functions, including M-mode and Doppler modes (spectral, color, and tissue).

Data Acquisition

Initial 3D data acquisition obtains US characteristics of many single points within a volume of tissue. Beamforming is a technique that manipulates US signals to be directionally/spatially sent or received from a crystal. In the modern 3DTEE systems, beamforming occurs both in the probe as fine (micro) beamforming and on the US machine computer system as coarse beamforming. This approach ensures a small probe and thin cable with less power consumption. There is a complex proprietary algorithm for each vendor that processes the emitting and returning US signals.

Spatial Versus Temporal Resolution

Temporal resolution for 3D echo is the volume rate in **volumes per second** (VPS), although the frame rate (FR) often appears on the display. Obtaining a 3D volume requires more scanning time than for a 2D slice, resulting in a lower volume rate. The ideal 3D dataset has a sufficient spatial resolution to discern fine anatomic detail, combined with the temporal resolution to capture the movement of large structures with high fidelity. These are competing goals, as higher spatial resolution requires more scan lines per volume, adding to the time required for acquisition and processing. Partial mitigation of this trade-off may involve reducing the volume size and imaging depth. The following equation best illustrates the complex interdependence of temporal resolution, sector size, volume depth, and spatial resolution:

$$\text{Volume rate} = \frac{1{,}540 \times \text{no. of parallel received beams}}{2 \times \left(\text{volume width} / \text{lateral resolution}\right)^2 \times \text{volume depth}}.$$

Modern US systems have features designed to increase the volume rate, such as parallel beamforming (1), frame reordering (2), multiline transmission (3), high pulse repetition (4), interpolation/high-volume rate imaging mode, and virtual array. See relevant references for an advanced discussion of each.

Real-Time Versus Multibeat Acquisition

3D data acquisition occurs as either single-beat or ECG-triggered multibeat imaging (MBI) acquisition. Older technology using MBI did not display the image immediately, and the displayed image did not change with probe movement. Modern systems enable RT display of 3D datasets in all imaging modes. The term RT refers to any 3D dataset that changes on the display synchronously with probe movement.

RT, single-beat acquisitions are convenient, acquired rapidly, and resistant to rhythm disturbances, movement, and cautery artifacts, but at the cost of low temporal and spatial resolution. Single-beat acquisitions can effectively image smaller structures, such as the aortic valve (AV), with adequate spatial and temporal resolution if the sector size is sufficiently narrow.

However, 3D images of larger structures, such as the left ventricle (LV), are best acquired using gated MBI to improve temporal resolution. Merging subvolumes from consecutive heartbeats creates a single loop of gated images. The same portion of the ECG wave (usually the R-wave) triggers the recording of each subvolume with rapid data reconstruction synchronous with the ECG. MBI is exquisitely sensitive to artifacts, especially for higher beats (3+). Arrhythmias, electrocautery artifacts, and probe movement will affect the ability to stitch together seamlessly the subvolumes. A demarcation line, termed a stitch artifact, appears between the subvolumes, distorting the anatomic structures and potentially affecting analysis (see "Artifacts" section for more detail).

Data Acquisition Modes

There are five acquisition modes for 3D imaging: (1) simultaneous 2D multiplane, (2) 3D narrow volume, (3) 3D zoom, (4) 3D wide angled (full volume), and (5) 3D color flow Doppler (CFD). Current technology allows the acquisition of 3D datasets of variable user-adjusted sizes for display in RT for all the 3D modes (Figure 21.3A; Video 21.1). As with 2D imaging, larger 3D volumes and adding CFD reduce the temporal resolution. 3D images can appear as static or moving objects. The term 4D refers to a moving (dynamic) 3D object, with time considered as the fourth dimension.

Multiplane (ie, xPlane by Philips or Triplane by GE) uses a single-button activation to show cardiac structures from different transducer angles simultaneously in a split-screen display (Figure 21.4A,B). As these are 2D images, this mode often goes unrecognized as a feature of 3D imaging functionality. Simultaneous multiplane imaging is invaluable for aligning planes through cardiac structures, distinguishing potential artifacts, and guiding percutaneous interventions (Figure 21.4C; Video 21.2). Superimposing CFD on the multiplane display can help identify the origin of regurgitant jets.

3D narrow volume uses a single-button activation to display a small 3D volume of the 2D image by including some elevational width (*x-z* plane). The operator can manually expand the 3D dataset in lateral and elevational size, albeit reducing the FR. This is a useful mode to check for general 3D image quality and image small structures (Figure 21.3B).

3D zoom uses a multistep single-button activation to display a user-defined subsection of 3D pyramidal volume centered on a specific region of interest (eg, mitral valve [MV]). The acquisition involves positioning an adjustable box on two orthogonal 2D images to encompass the desired 3D volume, followed by a rotation of the 3D volume to display the structure of interest (Figure 21.3C).

3D full volume uses a single-button activation to obtain a large 3D volume as a single beat or, more often, as an MBI acquisition to improve temporal resolution (Figure 21.3D). The user defines the 3D volume size by adjusting the lateral and elevational size or position using simultaneously displayed 2D images.

3D color flow Doppler (3D CFD) obtains a large amount of information (3D volume and 3D CFD), resulting in low temporal resolution (FR <20 Hz). The acquisition of a 3D CFD dataset is by either (1) first optimizing a 3D volume, then activating the CFD button or (2) applying CFD to a 2D image, then activating the 3D live mode button. Current technology requires the MBI acquisition of small 3D pyramidal volumes in any 3D mode to improve FR and show the entire color jet in 3D (Figure 21.3E). The Siemens US system, equipped with the Z6Ms true volume TEE probe, uses proprietary technology to display large-volume 3D datasets with superimposed 3D CFD at high volume rates (40 VPS) and without ECG gating. This technology better visualizes blood flow in RT.

Optimizing 3D Data Acquisition

High-quality 3D imaging relies on the acquisition of US data optimized for gain, compression, transducer frequency, line density, depth, and sector size (Figure 21.5). Generally, 2D image quality predicts the quality of the associated 3D dataset. Undergain leads to echo dropout and a loss of information that is irrecoverable in postprocessing (Figure 21.6). Overgain is similarly deleterious, with an associated drop in resolution, loss of depth perception, and a compromised 3D image. The 2012 American Society of Echocardiography (ASE)

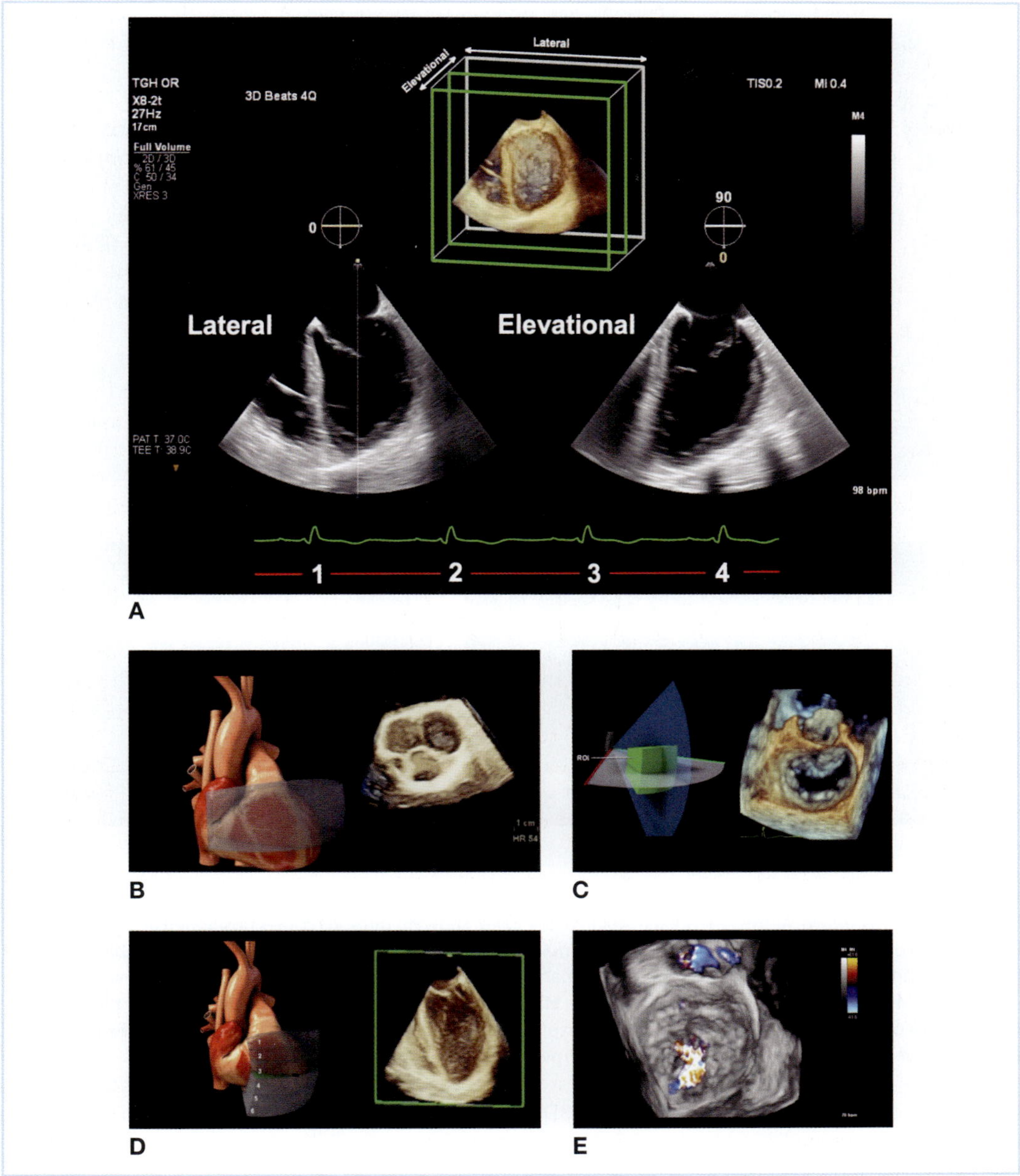

FIGURE 21.3 3D imaging modes. A: In all imaging modes, the user can define the 3D volume size by adjusting the elevational (*x-z*) and lateral (*x-y*) widths. The larger the 3D volume, the lower the temporal resolution. Multibeat acquisition improves temporal resolution with timing to the R-wave of consecutive heartbeats and merging of each subvolume to create a large 3D volume. B: 3D *Live* of an en face view of the aortic valve with the right coronary cusp at the 6 o'clock position. C: 3D *Zoom* of an enface view of the mitral valve from the left atrium in the surgeon's perspective. D: 3D *Full-volume* multibeat acquisition of a midesophageal four-chamber view shown with 50% cropping of the 3D dataset. E: Color flow Doppler imposed over the mitral and aortic valves showing mitral regurgitation but with low spatial and temporal resolution. (B and C, courtesy of Annette Vegas and the website https://pie.med.utoronto.ca/; see also Video 21.1.)

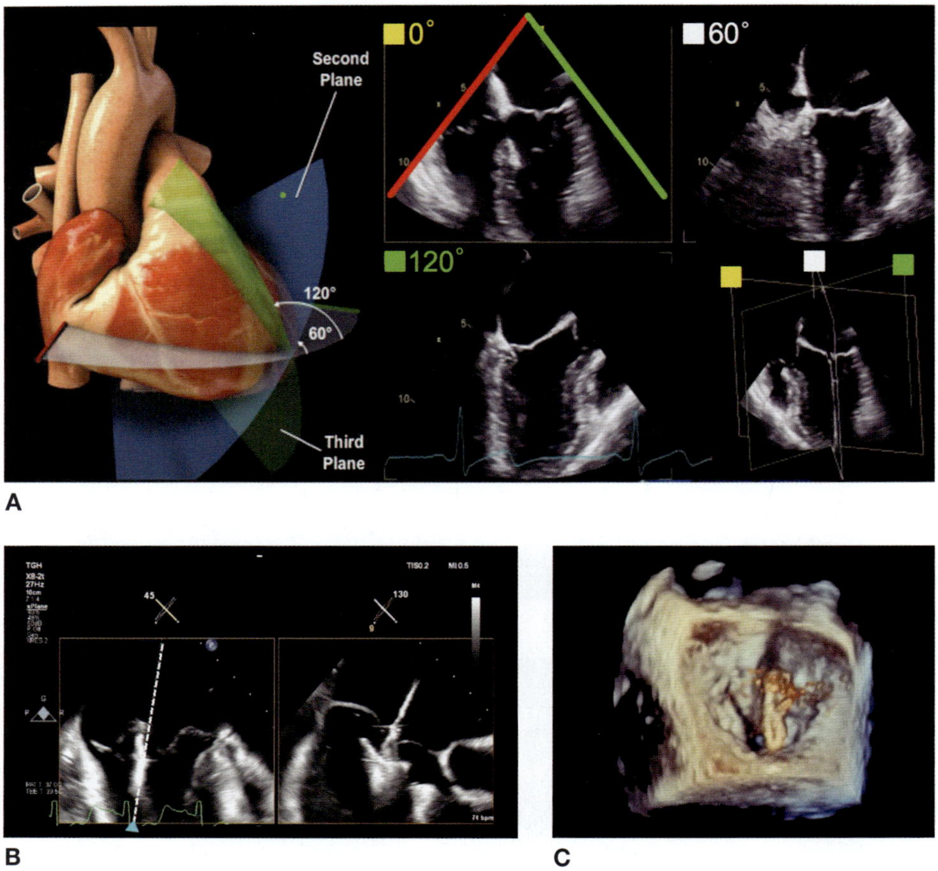

FIGURE 21.4 Multiplane imaging. A 3D matrix array probe can simultaneously display multiple real-time images from different angles, as shown. A: This is a triplane image of the heart, showing three 2D planes positioned at 0°, 60°, and 120° in a single display. B: Biplane imaging shows two 2D images in a single display. The left image is the fixed base view. The user can obtain the other view by adjusting the blue triangular marker in the base view. This is a biplane view of the mitral valve (MV) at 45° and 130° during the positioning of a MitraClip across the valve. C: The 3D enface view of the MV shows the MitraClip positioned perpendicular above the coaptation line between the A2 and P2 segments of the MV leaflets. (A, courtesy of Annette Vegas and the website https://pie.med.utoronto.ca/; see also Video 21.2.)

guidelines recommend that optimal settings for 3DTEE include midrange gain and compression, with higher time gain compensation (TGC) to allow for maximal postprocessing flexibility. It is important to tailor depth and sector size to the area of interest while still capturing the anatomic features essential to landmark and orientate the 3D image.

Data Storage and Processing

The acquired US raw data undergoes near-instantaneous transmission, storage, and processing in the random access memory (RAM) of the US system. RAM is a temporary data store that enables rapid processing of large datasets without time-intensive transmission to and from the unit's hard drive. Modern US systems have sufficient RAM that processing time is negligible, even when performing complex functions on large-volume datasets.

Data processing comprises three integrated steps: conversion, interpolation, and segmentation that transform the scanned raw data into a 3D dataset necessary to create a 3D object (Figure 21.1). Conversion positions and assigns *x-y-z* coordinates (Cartesian volume) to each of the scanned raw data points, identifying their echogenic characteristics with a known position in space. Interpolation fills the gaps between all the known points in space to generate a 3D dataset comprising voxels or volume elements (Figure 21.7). A voxel

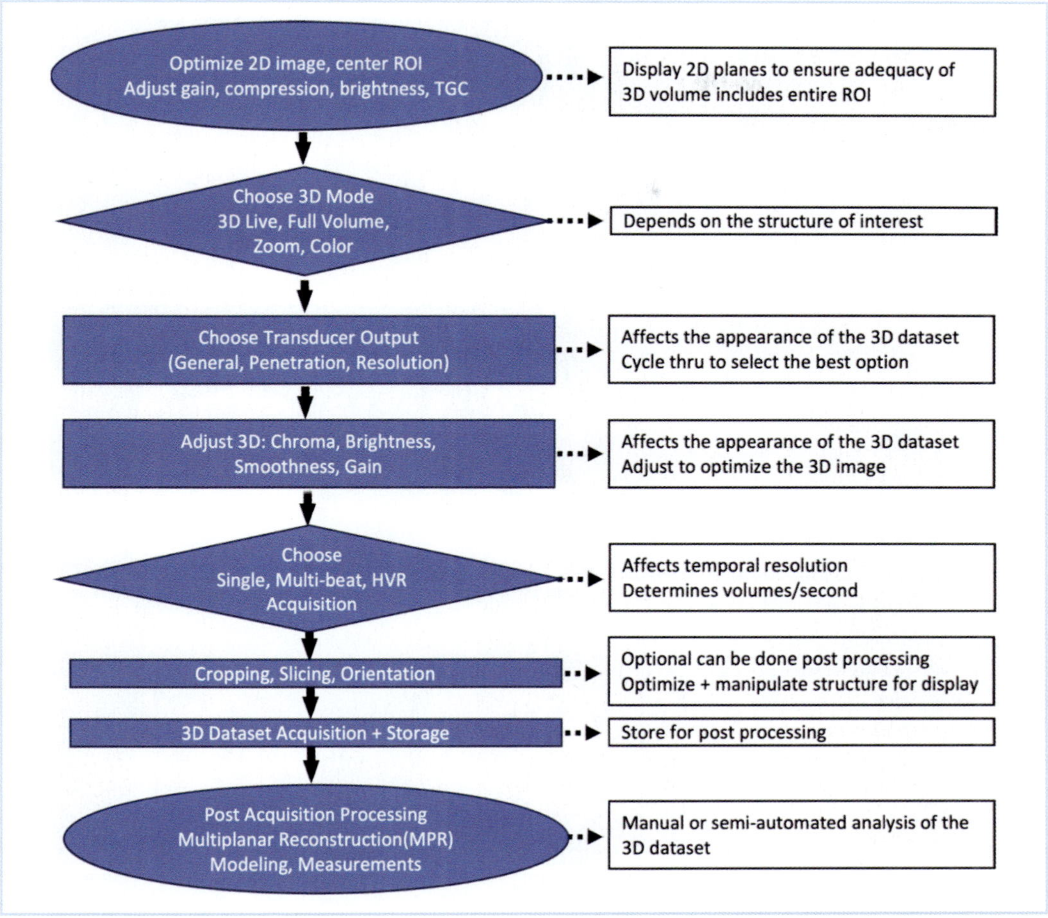

FIGURE 21.5 3D image acquisition and optimization. The algorithm describes how to acquire and optimize 3D images across all 3D imaging modes. HVR, high volume rate; ROI, region of interest; TGC, time gain compression.

is a (vo)lume of pi(xel)s that encrypts the physical characteristics and location of the smallest cube in a dataset, which is used for 3D display. The voxel size is inversely proportional to the 3D image resolution. Larger voxels resulting in poorer resolution occur when raw data are available for fewer points in the scanned volume and interpolation fills wider gaps. Segmentation is the first step in graphic rendering, during which there is an identification of the object to be rendered and separation from surrounding structures in the 3D dataset. Software filters enable separation by differentiating cardiac tissue from blood, pericardial fluid, and are based on their dissimilar ability to reflect US.

3D Image Display

Rendering is a graphics term for generating an image from a dataset (2D or 3D) of multiple spatial elements. Following segmentation, the 3D dataset undergoes one of three increasingly complex graphic rendering techniques: wireframe, surface, or volume rendering, to display the 3D object (Figure 21.8; Video 21.3).

Wireframe rendering is the simplest and fastest way to create a visible 3D object. A series of equidistant points on the surface of a 3D object are defined and connected with lines (wires) to form a mesh of small polygonal tiles. Smoothing algorithms can refine the narrow angles and make the object appear more real. This technique is relevant for structures with flat surfaces, such as the LV and the atrial cavities.

Surface rendering extends the wireframe technique by defining more points on the surface of a 3D object, making the lines joining them invisible. It generates 3D objects with detailed solid surfaces but an empty

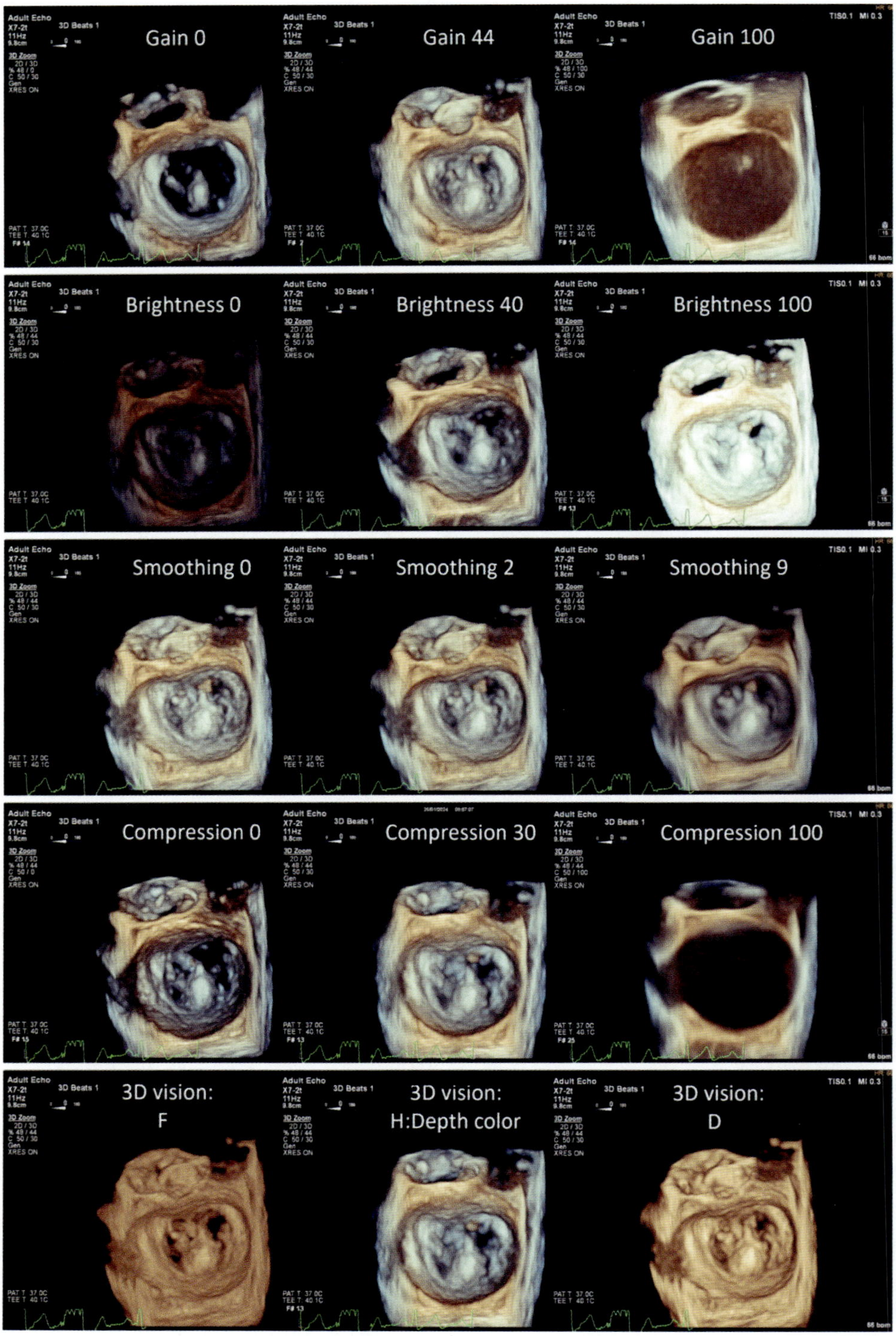

FIGURE 21.6 3D image optimization. Adjustments of 3D settings include gain, brightness, smoothing, compression, and vision map, all of which alter the display of the 3D image in real-time or stored images.

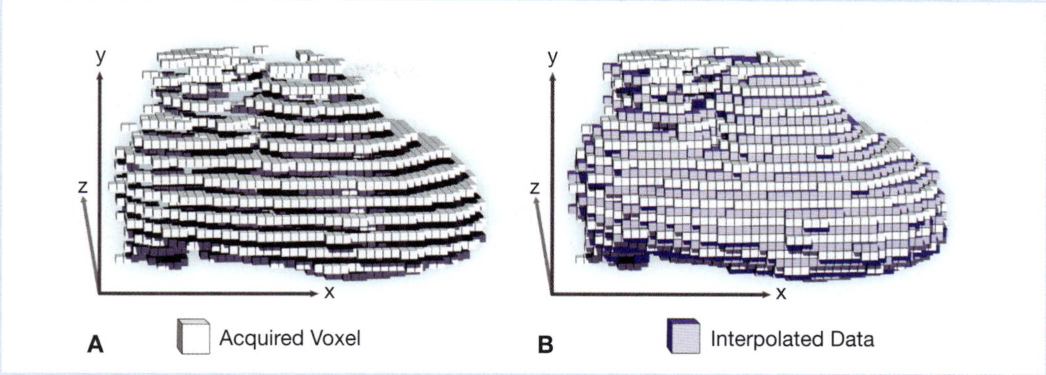

FIGURE 21.7 Interpolation. Data processing of the raw data creates a 3D dataset that comprises voxels through (A) conversion (white) and (B) interpolation (purple). Conversion positions each ultrasound data point in space. Interpolation fills in the gaps to create the 3D dataset. The more interpolation, the worse the spatial resolution.

hollow inner core. This makes possible the morphologic assessment of the corresponding anatomic structure (eg, cardiac valves) and determination of cavity volume (eg, LV volume).

Volume rendering retains all the 3D data and displays a 3D object with full details of the surface and inner structure. This display of each voxel of the 3D dataset permits a "virtual dissection" of the 3D object.

Despite being composed of voxels, 3D objects appear on the screen as pixels of a 2D image. Perspective, light casting, depth color coding, and newer options described below offer a visual sense of depth and reality. Any rendered 3D object can freely rotate on the display and appear in any orientation and from any perspective.

Postprocessing Optimization

Ideally, the optimization of 3D datasets should be prior to acquisition (see "Optimizing 3D Data Acquisition" section). Cropping techniques remove extraneous parts of the image to better focus on areas of interest, anatomic structures, and pathologies. Manipulation of the 3D image is essential for positioning structures in a standard anatomic orientation, facilitating interpretation and comparison across studies. Contemporary US systems offer fully or semiautomated software packages for advanced interrogation and data extraction from the 3D dataset. Offline third-party software may provide more detailed analysis for future intervention planning. Postprocessing is crucial to unlocking the information available for clinical applications, allowing for comprehensive evaluation and effective communication among medical professionals.

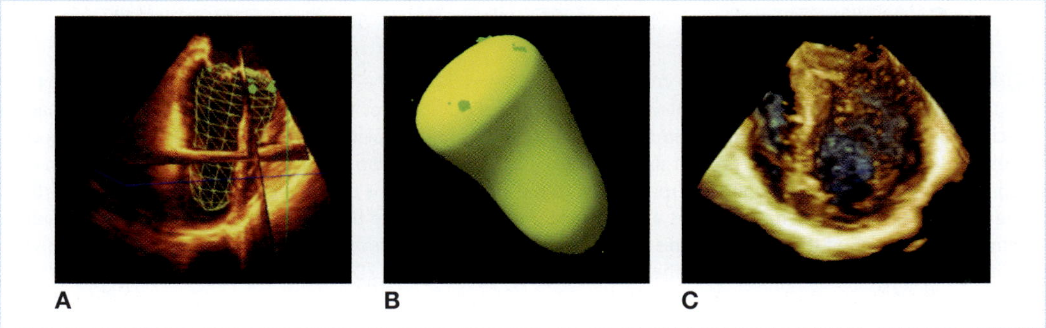

FIGURE 21.8 Graphic rendering. The display of 3D data can be as (A) wireframe, (B) surface, or (C) volume rendered, as shown for the left ventricle (see also Video 21.3).

Cropping and Orientation

A powerful advantage of 3DTEE is the ability to crop, rotate, and orientate a 3D volume to appear from any perspective on the display. The operator can crop images using a crop box with six standard orthogonal planes, an arbitrary cropping plane freely oriented in space, and a fixed plane aligned to the structure of interest or autocrop, which removes 50% of the 3D dataset (Figure 21.9).

Notably, cropping can occur after data acquisition but before storage or on stored images, with different implications. Cropping prior to data storage effectively decreases the volume size, thus increasing temporal and spatial resolution. However, the image cannot be subsequently uncropped, as the data are excluded from

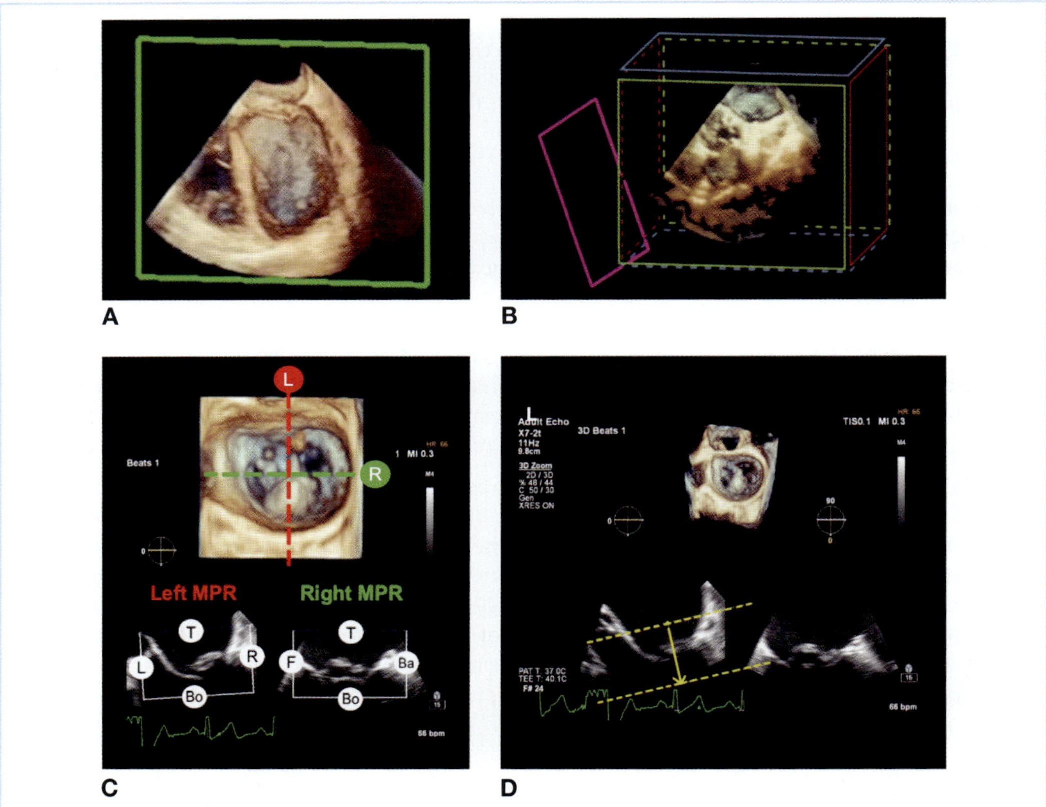

FIGURE 21.9 Cropping options. A: Auto crop. This tool removes 50% of the 3D image by cropping the front portion from the original 2D plane. This is a display of a full-volume acquisition for the left ventricle in the midesophageal four-chamber view/plane with the green square representing the cropped plane. B: Box crop/plane crop. The box crop tool uses a cube with six sides to represent six orthogonal planes that can crop the 3D image. The fixed planes can crop independently but not simultaneously, perpendicular to the 3D image. This is useful to crop crudely the outer portions of the 3D image. The plane crop tool uses a crop plane (in purple) that the user can move freely to align and adjust to remove any portion of the 3D image. This permits refinement of the 3D image. C: iCrop (Phillips machines). This is a simplified cropping box tool that displays the 3D image and two orthogonal 2D planes, right and left multiplanar reconstruction (MPR). Aligning the cropping box over the region of interest in either the right or left 2D image allows adjustment of the top (T), bottom (Bo), front (F), back (Ba), right (R), and left sides of the box. The results of cropping appear in the 3D image. D: Parallel Crop/2-click crop (GE machines)/Quick view (Phillips machines). This is a simple and quick tool to crop structures from a larger 3D image. This is like the iCrop tool and displays the 3D image and two 2D planes. The operator can position a plane to a region of interest represented by a dashed line and arrow. Clicking and dragging the dotted line toward the arrow crops the 3D image, which appears from this perspective. This example shows the mitral valve from the left atrial perspective with much of the left atrium removed.

storage and processing. Cropping on stored datasets is reversible and amenable to serial adjustments but does not improve spatial or temporal resolution.

Before cropping, it is helpful to orient the structure on the display using adjacent structures in the dataset because it is possible to lose spatial orientation after cropping the surrounding structures. Newer software includes presets that automatically orientate the 3D image to show the MV, AV, and left atrial appendage (LAA) from midesophageal (ME) two-chamber or four-chamber captures.

Gain, Compression, Brightness, and Smoothing

Postprocessing adjustment of gain, compression (contrast ratio), brightness (increasing whiteness), and smoothing (reducing image coarseness) can improve 3D image quality but cannot fully correct gross imbalances during data acquisition (Figure 21.6).

Vendor-Specific Image Enhancement

Each vendor offers proprietary software packages designed to refine images and enhance details to improve 3D perception. These enhancement packages can better delineate cardiac structures such as MV morphology and improve diagnostics in adult congenital heart disease (ACHD).

For example, Philips enhancement features include Vision, Chroma Mapping, and TruVue (Figure 21.10). Vision applies preset combinations of contrast, transparency, lighting, and compositing algorithms (labeled A-H) onto 3D images to affect the spatial filtering and depth of colorization. Chroma Mapping (settings 1-8) alters the intensity and combination of the colors used in the display to enhance variations in depth (Figure 21.10A). TrueVue provides 3D photorealistic rendering that simulates the texture of cardiac tissue. TrueVue Light adds a virtual light source that can be repositioned to enhance contrast and shadows from different angles independent of the viewing perspective (Figure 21.10B). TrueVue Glass makes the tissue transparent, enhancing the spatial relationships between heart structures (Figure 21.10C; Video 21.4).

Image enhancement software from GE includes high definition (HD) Color, Flexilight, Ultra Definition (UD) Clarity, and UD Speckle Reduce. HD Color allows semitransparent visualization of the source of high-velocity jets to better delineate spatial relationships. Flexilight renders photorealistic light source–based illumination of cardiac structures. The UD Clarity and UD Speckle Reduce options can reduce signal noise to enhance the definition of significant boundaries.

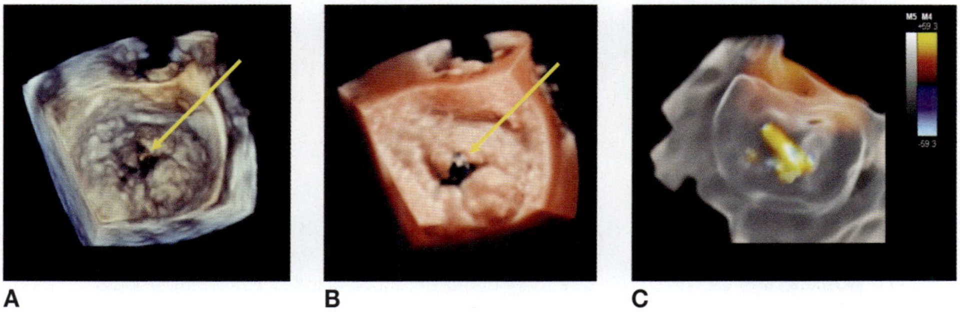

FIGURE 21.10 3D display options. 3DTEE en face views of the mitral valve (MV) from the left atrial perspective in the surgeons orientation show a midsystolic frame of a pathologic MV with Barlow disease. The valve pathology includes bileaflet prolapse, a coaptation gap, a flail of the A2 segment of the anterior mitral valve leaflet (AMVL), and a ruptured chorda tendineae flicking in and out of the LA. Different display options can better highlight the pathology. A: A conventional 3D render where brown shading is closer and blue shading is further from the viewer. B: Tissue rendering using transillumination adds a virtual light source to create a photorealistic image with shadows that highlight structures and enhance depth perception. This example better shows the leaflet prolapse and ruptured chordae (arrow). C: Transillumination imaging with transparency renders the tissue translucent, highlighting the interface between tissue and blood. Superimposing color flow Doppler on the transparent tissue can aid in identifying the origin of a mitral regurgitation jet (see also Video 21.4). TEE, transesophageal echocardiography.

Quantification Analysis Models

Multiplanar Reconstruction and Measurements

A drawback of 3DTEE is the inability to perform measurements directly on 3D images in RT. This limitation results from parallax error, defined as the difference in the apparent position of an object depending on the line of sight. 3D acquisition captures objects from multiple angles simultaneously, each with unique viewing perspectives, causing discrepancies in the perceived position of anatomic structures.

Measurements in the 3D dataset therefore require using US machine software for MPR of the structure of interest. MPR displays regions of the dataset based on three 2D planes (coronal, sagittal, and transverse), which the operator can move independently and align through structures (Figure 21.11). Although time-consuming, MPR permits slice-by-slice (tomographic) control of data points from a stored 3D dataset.

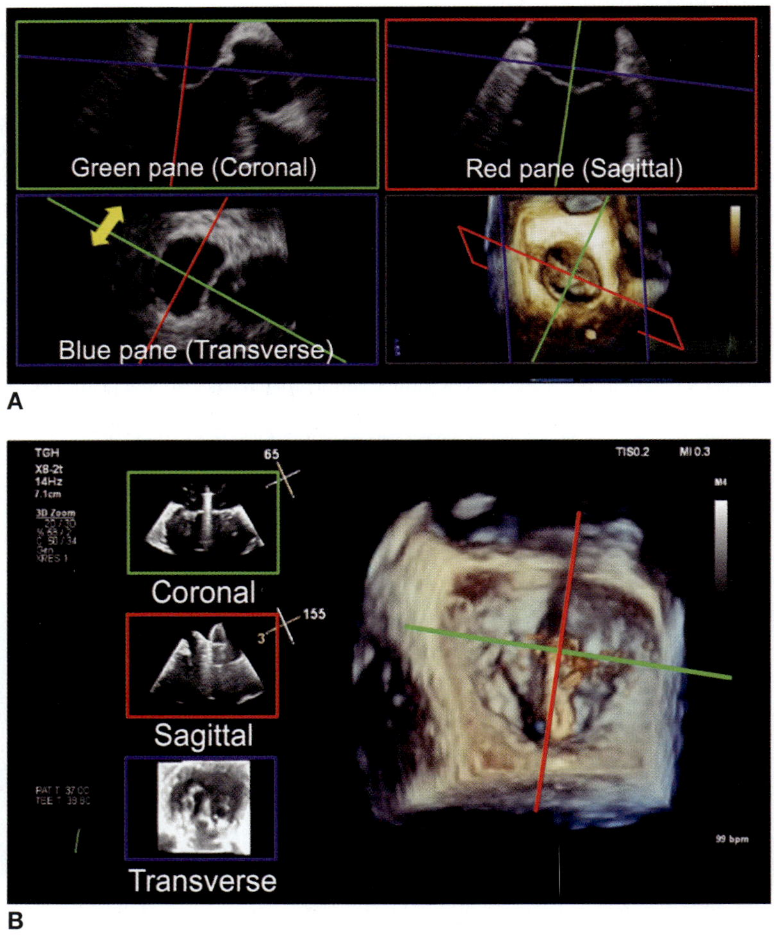

FIGURE 21.11 Multiplanar reconstruction (MPR). The MPR technique slices a (A) stored or (B) live 3D dataset to create multiple 2D images. Locking the planes to be perpendicular allows the user to align planes through the major (coronal and sagittal) and minor (transverse) axes. Each pane allows the user to adjust two planes. The green pane is the coronal plane while adjusting the red and blue planes. The red pane is a sagittal plane while adjusting the blue and green planes. The blue pane is a transverse plane generated from the 3D dataset and allows adjustment of the red and green planes. In this example of a mitral valve (MV), the user aligns the blue plane through the annulus in the red and green panes, giving a transverse (short-axis) image of the MV annulus in the blue pane. The red plane is perpendicular to the coaptation line and the green plane is through the commissure. Scrolling the green plane in the blue pane shows the coaptation of segments of the anterior and posterior leaflets in the green pane.

MPR software allows precise measurements of cardiac structures such as valve leaflet length, defect size, valve annulus dimensions, valve orifice area, regurgitant orifice area, and vena contracta (VC) area. 3D imaging has proven reliable and comparable to other imaging techniques, such as CT and cardiac magnetic resonance (CMR) imaging for measuring annular dimensions, valve area, chamber volume, and components of a regurgitant CFD jet. However, unlike 2D imaging, there are currently few validated 3DTEE-specific values to distinguish abnormalities or grade the severity of valvular pathologies.

Live 3D MPR simultaneously displays multiple imaging planes (typically two long-axis views and one short-axis [SAX] view) and a 3D view, without or with color Doppler. This option is valuable during percutaneous catheter procedures as it (1) avoids the errors of parallax, (2) obtains 2D views that are physically impossible with conventional 2D imaging, and (3) limits the need to change views and probe positions.

Postprocessing Analysis Software

Proprietary software programs (Table 21.1) available on the US machines and at workstations allow the analysis of stored 3D datasets: QLAB (Philips Healthcare), TomTec (TomTec), and eSie Valves (Siemens Medical Solutions). TomTec and eSie Valves can read transthoracic echocardiography (TTE) and TEE 3D datasets generated by different vendors, while QLAB is vendor specific. All use a semiautomated method to create dynamic or static models of cardiac structures, which will be discussed in the "Clinical Applications" section.

Artifacts

3DTEE is susceptible to the same artifacts as 2D imaging, although imaging enhancements and lack of familiarity can cause many artifacts to appear larger and more realistic (Figure 21.12; Video 21.5). Furthermore, 3D imaging is uniquely susceptible to artifacts that arise from postprocessing. Case reports describe diagnostic errors resulting from the misinterpretation of 3D artifacts.

Stitching artifacts are unique to ECG-gated MBI, in which narrow sectors combine to capture large-volume 3D datasets over consecutive cardiac cycles. Any coarse movements of the probe or region of interest between beats cause misalignment of the individual sectors during subsequent reconstruction, creating a fractured image. Minimize stitching artifact by ensuring conditions are optimal for MBI, including normal sinus rhythm, stationary probe position, static surgical field, and patient breath-hold to minimize respiratory variation.

Shadowing artifacts arise from the inability of US to pass through a strong reflector. Imaging of a catheter results in a lack of tissue of a similar shape below the catheter, which resembles a tear in tissue.

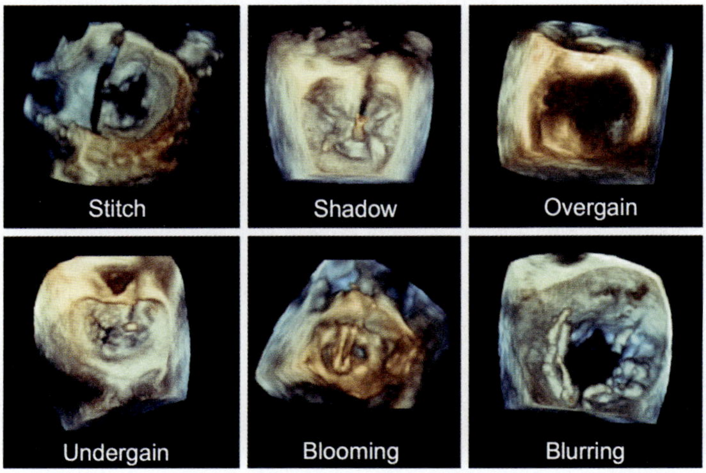

FIGURE 21.12 Artifacts. The artifacts in 3D images include stitch, shadowing, overgain, undergain, blooming, and blurring as described in more detail in the text (see also Video 21.5).

Overgain appears as brown speckles, which may obscure structures or mimic clinical findings (foreign bodies, vegetations, etc). Reducing the 2D gain and optimizing the TGC improves the visualization of structures.

Dropout artifacts occur in both 2D and 3D imaging, although the mechanism and implications for image interpretation differ. In 2D imaging, dropout occurs from undergain or dense structures impeding the path of the US beam, resulting in poor visibility of far-field structures. In 3D imaging, undergain, parallel beam alignment, or inadequate signal strength result in tissue loss for structures furthest away from the probe, which can give the false appearance of holes or defects. This is problematic when visualizing the interatrial septum (IAS), in which an intact fossa ovalis may appear as a patent foramen ovale (PFO). Dropout can also create false fenestrations in valve leaflets. The borders of these 3D dropout artifacts are often coarse and blurred, in contrast to the well-defined borders characterizing true defects. Optimization of gain settings and probe position may eliminate this artifact, although definitive testing with a formal bubble study for a septal defect is sometimes necessary.

A blurring artifact can make thin structures appear coarse, thick, and ill-defined. Blurring is a function of "nonisotropic voxels" that arise from differing resolutions of the axial, lateral, and elevational orientations of a 3D dataset. Thin structures such as sutures and chordae are most susceptible. Optimization of gain settings and probe position may eliminate this artifact.

Blooming artifact affects visualization around metallic or echo-dense structures such as mechanical valves, valve clips, and mechanical circulatory support cannulae. Metals refract US beams, resulting in thick, indistinct borders that make objects appear falsely large. Comparing multiple 2D and 3D images can help to delineate the true dimensions.

Limitations

As with any emergent technology, one must weigh the utility of 3DTEE against perceived and actual limitations, such as artifacts, resolution, skill acquisition, and societal recommendations.

The ideal conditions for 3D imaging include normal sinus rhythm, stationary probe position, static surgical field, and optimized 2D images. These requirements may not be possible during critical periods of the operation when 3D imaging would be most valuable. Similarly, stillness and prolonged breath holds are challenging in awake patients under conscious sedation.

Spatial and temporal resolution compete with 3D imaging. Poor spatial resolution prevents accurate endocardial border tracking for automated volume quantification. Poor temporal resolution with large-volume datasets and CFD may require MBI, which is limited by stitching artifacts. Low temporal resolution reduces the number of images available for assessment, which is significant when quantifying blood flow or performing chamber quantification. The expectation is that spatial and temporal resolution will improve with advances in hardware, processing power, and software enhancements.

The steep learning curve to proficiency in 3DTEE is a powerful deterrent for echocardiographers confident that their 2D skill set answers all pertinent questions. Even modern training and certifications do not ensure or assess competence in 3D imaging as a necessary requirement. Although 3D imaging can approximate surgical views, many surgeons still prefer to communicate through the lens of 2DTEE, with which they are most accustomed. Continuing medical education initiatives have inconsistent benefits, as the acquisition of 3D images returns to baseline within 6 months of a one-day workshop.

Recent ASE guidelines for both surgical decision-making in the operating room and intervention for structural heart disease expect all perioperative echocardiographers to be proficient in 3DTEE. However, there have been no revisions to the seminal 2012 European Association of Echocardiography (EAE)/ASE 3DTEE guidelines despite continual advancements in both software and hardware, culminating in new, powerful imaging modes. The 2013 ASE Guidelines for Performing a Comprehensive TEE Examination incorporate seven recommended 3D views but without the rigor or specifics of the 2D views recommendations. Furthermore, although quantitative assessment of cardiac structures is now possible through semi-automated parametric models, there are few published values to identify abnormalities or grade the severity of valvular pathologies.

CLINICAL APPLICATIONS

TEE imaging uses standardized protocols, which for 3DTEE represent a structure-based approach in contrast to 2D imaging, which uses a view-based approach. The opportunity to assess a structure from a single display obviates the need to reconstruct the structure from multiple 2D images. Guidelines exist for 3D echocardiographic image acquisition and standardized display orientation (Figure 21.13).

3DTEE complements 2DTEE by better visualizing individual patient anatomy and pathology and is superior to 2DTEE in assessing valvular pathology, ventricular function, cardiac masses, and congenital heart lesions (Table 21.2). It is indispensable for RT guidance during percutaneous interventions for structural heart disease.

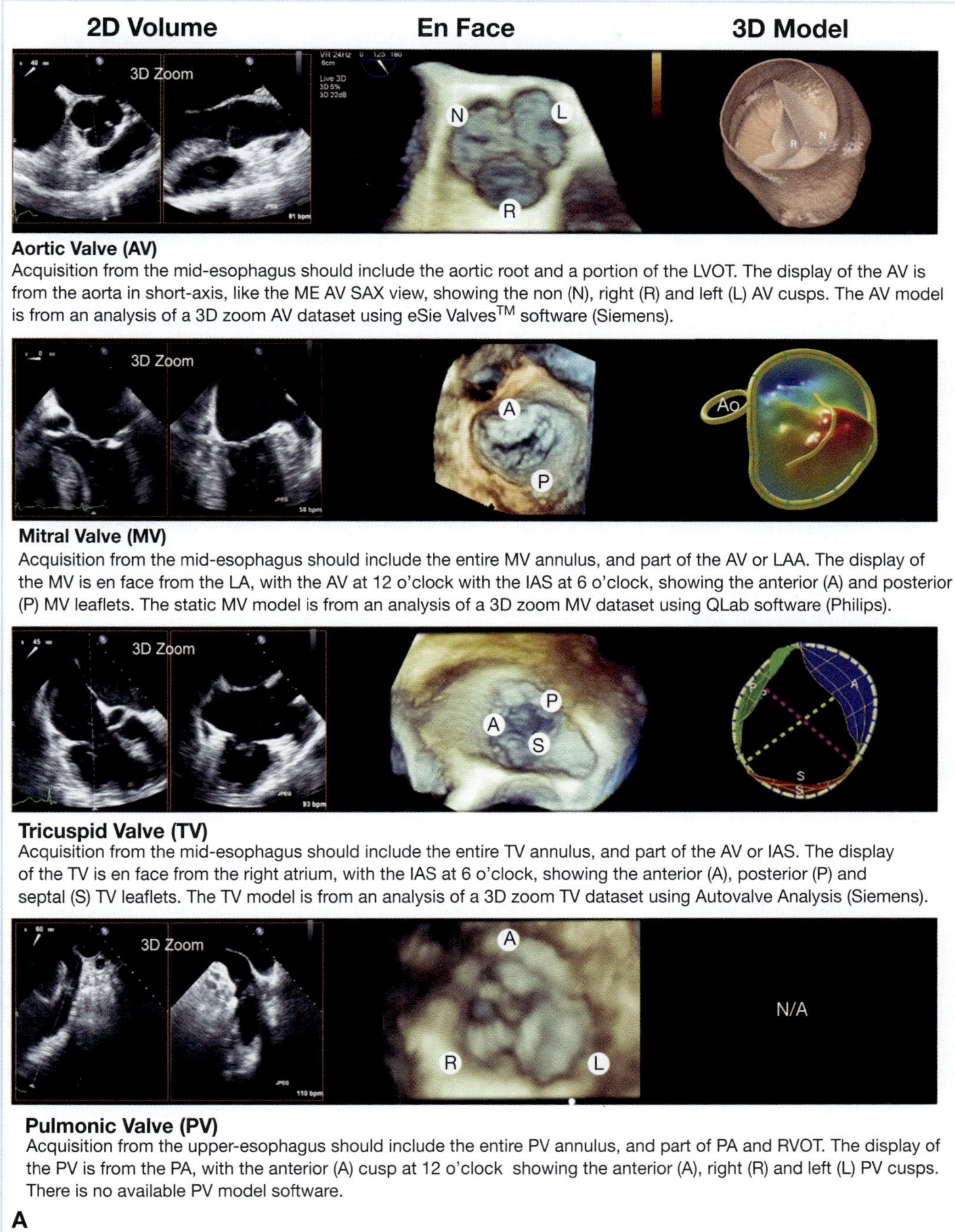

FIGURE 21.13 Cardiac structures in 3D. This figure shows the acquisition, display, and models of different heart components. A: shows the cardiac valves; B: shows the ventricles and interatrial septum. AV, aortic valve; IAS, interatrial septum; IVC, inferior vena cava; LA, left atrium; LAA, left atrial appendage; LVOT, left ventricular outflow tract; ME, midesophageal; PA, pulmonary artery; RVOT, right ventricular outflow tract; SAX, short axis; SVC, superior vena cava.

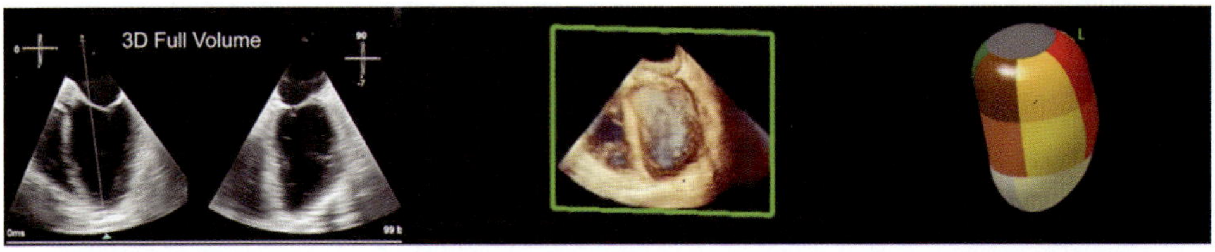

Left Ventricle (LV)
Acquisition from the mid-esophagus should include the entire LV, including the apex and endocardium.
The display of the LV is from the mid-esophagus with 50% crop showing the LV cavity.
The dynamic LV model is from an analysis of a Full Volume LV dataset using QLab software (Philips).

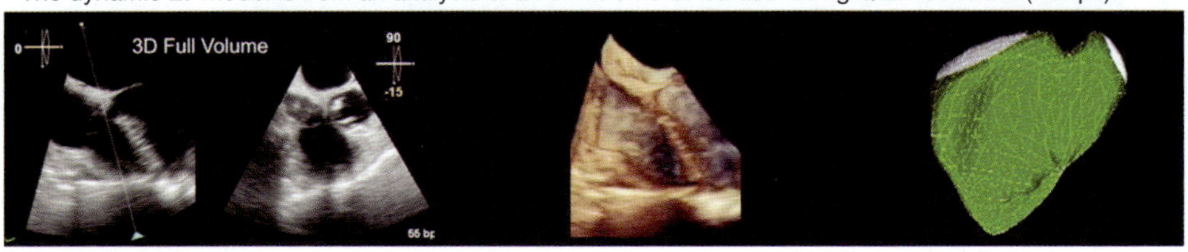

Right Ventricle (RV)
Acquisition from the mid-esophagus should include the entire RV, including the TV, apex and RVOT.
The display of the RV is from the mid-esophagus with 50% crop showing the RV cavity.
The dynamic RV model is from an analysis of a Full Volume RV dataset using TomTec software (Philips).

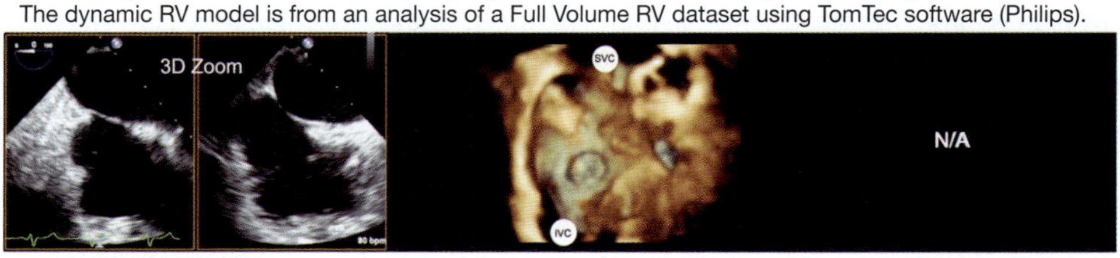

Inter-atrial Septum (IAS)
Acquisition from the mid-esophagus should include the entire IAS, including the SVC and IVC.
The display of the IAS is from the RA with the SVC at 11 o'clock.
There is no available IAS model software.

B

FIGURE 21.13 (*continued*)

TABLE 21.2 Clinical Utility 3DTEE

Structure	Clinical Utility
Mitral valve (MV)	Clefts, perforations, models
Mitral regurgitation	Mechanism, VCA, 3D PISA
Mitral stenosis	MVA (using MPR)
Aortic root	Anatomy, model
Aortic regurgitation	Mechanisms, root dimensions, cusp measurements, VCA
Aortic stenosis	LVOT area, AVA by planimetry
Tricuspid valve (TV)	Identify specific leaflets, annulus size
Left ventricle	Volumes, EF, strain, RWMA
Right ventricle	Volumes, EF
Cardiac masses	Location, attachment size
Congenital heart disease	Complex anatomy, 3D printing
3D model printing	Complex anatomy, educational tools
Percutaneous procedures	Transseptal puncture, device closure (PFO, ASD, VSD, paravalvular), valves (MV, TV, TAVI, valve in valve), LAA occluder

ASD, atrial septal defect; AVA, aortic valve area; EF, ejection fraction; LAA, left atrial appendage; LVOT, left ventricular outflow tract; MPR, multiplanar reconstruction; MVA, mitral valve area; PFO, patent foramen ovale; PISA, proximal isovelocity surface area; RWMA, regional wall motion abnormality; TAVI, transcatheter aortic valve implantation; VCA, vena contracta area; VSD, ventricular septal defect.

Left Ventricle

Quantification of Left Ventricular Volumes and Systolic Function

The primary advantage of 3D analysis in chamber quantification is the ability to refine the position of orthogonal planes to identify accurately the true apex, thus minimizing the foreshortening, malrotation, and angulation that underestimate chamber volume by 2D imaging. Quantification starts with the acquisition of an LV full-volume (FV) 3D dataset guided by a split-screen display of orthogonal views (Figure 21.14A; Video 21.6). The FV dataset is the only 3D imaging modality that can capture the entire LV volume at a sufficient FR of at least 25 VPS for dynamic assessment by software analysis. Volume rendering is useful for identifying structural abnormalities such as intracavitary thrombi and masses, but surface rendering by analytical software is the ideal image display for chamber quantification and global and regional functional measurements.

The operator can use US machine software (3DQ QLAB by Philips and 4D Cardio-View by TomTec) to measure LV volumes from FV 3D datasets by two methods: 3D-guided biplanes or direct volumetric analysis. The 3D-guided biplane method allows the user to position two perpendicular 2D planes to intersect the LV long axis at the true apex. This simultaneous display of ideal ME four-chamber and two-chamber 2D views permits the user to apply manually the modified Simpson biplane method of disks to the end-systolic and end-diastolic frames to measure the LV volume, ejection fraction (EF), and mass. This method minimizes LV foreshortening using TEE but still relies on geometric assumptions.

Direct volumetric analysis using special US machine software (3DQ Advanced, QLAB by Philips and 4D LV analysis by TomTec) semiautomatically creates a surface-rendered cast of the LV cavity (Figure 21.14B). This analysis measures LV volume throughout the entire cardiac cycle to determine end-diastolic volume (EDV) and end-systolic volume (ESV), with calculations of the stroke volume and EF. This method accurately

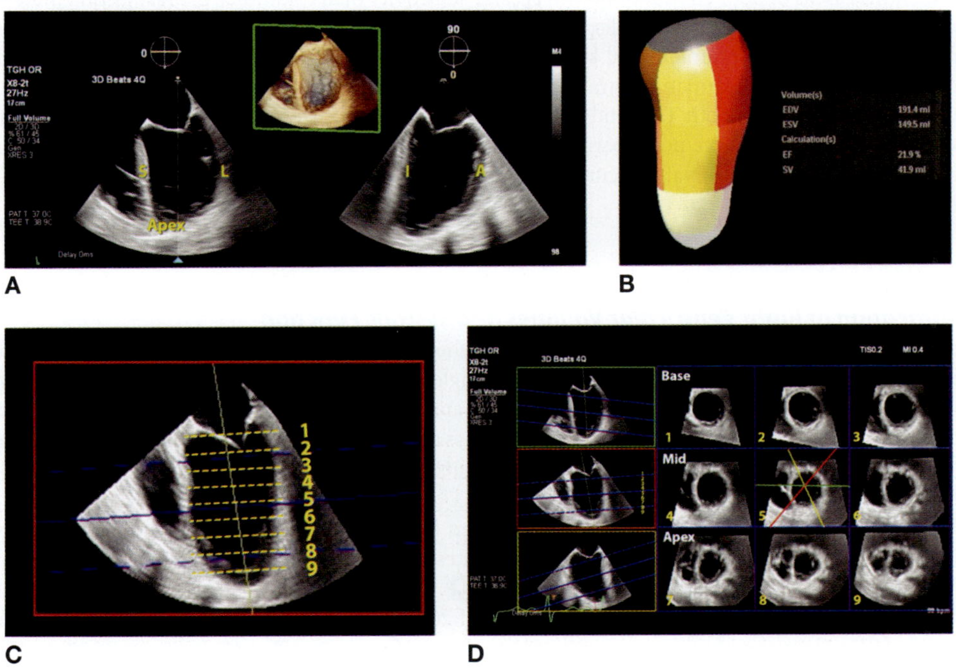

FIGURE 21.14 3D imaging and assessment of the left ventricle (LV). A: A 3D full-volume acquisition of the LV over four beats gives a frame rate of 27 Hz. B: Semiautomated analysis of this 3D dataset using specialized software creates a dynamic 3D volumetric model of the LV by tracking the endocardial border across the cardiac cycle. Color coding of the myocardial segments is according to a 17-segment model. Measures of LV volumes and ejection fraction occur without geometric assumptions. C, D: Analysis using multiplanar reconstruction of the 3D dataset can slice and display the LV across multiple short-axis planes, allowing the identification of regional wall motion abnormalities. A, anterior; EDV, end-diastolic volume; EF, ejection fraction; ESV, end-systolic volume; I, inferior; L, lateral; S, septal; SV, stroke volume (see also Video 21.6).

quantifies LV volumes, particularly in patients with an abnormal ventricular shape or regional wall motion abnormalities (RWMAs). There is better alignment through the cardiac apex, the inclusion of more endocardial surface during analysis, and the lack of geometric shape assumption. Limitations of this 3D method include lack of reproducibility, poor spatial and temporal resolution, and the inaccuracy of endocardial surface tracking.

A meta-analysis of 3D echocardiographic studies evaluating LV volumes and EF showed larger volumes than 2DTTE, CMR, and CT techniques, but with less variability than 2D measurements. 3DTEE better correlated with CMR measurements than 2D (5). In the perioperative setting, 3DTEE yielded larger volumes than 2DTEE for ESV and EDV, although EF was comparable (6). Notably, 3D imaging had equivalent acquisition times, but longer analysis times compared to 2D (6).

Regional and Segmental Dyssynchrony

The LV analysis software can perform 17-segment analysis of LV function and assess LV synchronicity. Evaluation of regional LV wall motion by 3DTEE is based on a change in LV chamber subvolume over time from altered segmental myocardial contractility. Unlike standard 2DTEE, there is no direct measurement of myocardial thickening or displacement of individual segments. Another option uses a multislice tool in MPR to display on the screen the LV at multiple levels in simultaneous SAX slices like a CT scan, enabling qualitative assessment for RWMAs (Figure 21.14C).

Deformation imaging, also known as myocardial strain analysis, assesses myocardial function by measuring the change in myocardial length throughout the cardiac cycle. Strain and strain rate (strain/time) measurements quantify deformation using speckle tracking software. "Speckle tracking" identifies and tracks the movement of a unique US pattern, speckles, generated by a myocardial area through the cardiac cycle. Strain identifies areas of poor contractility with greater sensitivity than traditional global ejection indices and displays each segment on a "Bullseye" display. Traditional 2D strain parameters include global longitudinal strain, radial strain, and circumferential strain. Offline analyses of 3D datasets using specialized software allow new and enhanced deformation parameters, including area strain and principal strain. These advanced software packages apply to both TTE and TEE datasets and enhance the ability to assess myocardial function comprehensively. However, poor spatiotemporal resolution and significant intervendor variability affect the standardization of normal values, currently impeding the incorporation of strain measurements into guidelines.

Right Ventricle

Quantification of Right Ventricular Volumes and Systolic Function

The crescent geometry of the right ventricle (RV) with the inlet, apical, and outlet portions lying in different tomographic planes makes it difficult to capture in a single 2D view. Similarly, 2D measures of systolic function such as RV fractional area change (FAC), tricuspid annular plane systolic excursion (TAPSE), and tissue Doppler-derived lateral annular systolic velocity (S') assess a single tomographic plane, and may overrepresent the longitudinal excursion. These 2D measures of RV function have low interobserver concordance and poor correlation with CMR measurements.

Right ventricular ejection fraction (RVEF) measured by 3D echocardiography is the only index of RV systolic function suggested by guidelines that incorporates all RV regions with their relative contributions to both longitudinal and radial shortening (Figure 21.15; ▶ Video 21.7). An adequate RV 3D dataset is an FV acquisition that encompasses the entire RV at an FR of 20 to 25 VPS. Guidelines recommend offline measurement of RV volume and function using special analytic software (TomTec 4D RV Function) from RV 3D datasets when feasible.

3DTTE assessment of RV function via disc summation method shows reduced interobserver variability compared to 2D assessments of RV function (7). Unlike 2D assessments that rely on geometric assumptions and limited views, 3DTEE captures the entire RV, allowing for more accurate and reproducible measurements. In a comparison of several imaging modalities (2D echo, 3D echo, radionuclide ventriculography, cardiac CT, gated single-photon emission CT, and invasive cardiac cine ventriculography), 3DTEE and CT-derived RVEF measurements best correlated with CMR (8). Meta-analyses have shown a general trend toward underestimation of 3DTEE RV volumes compared to CMR, although RVEF is comparable (9).

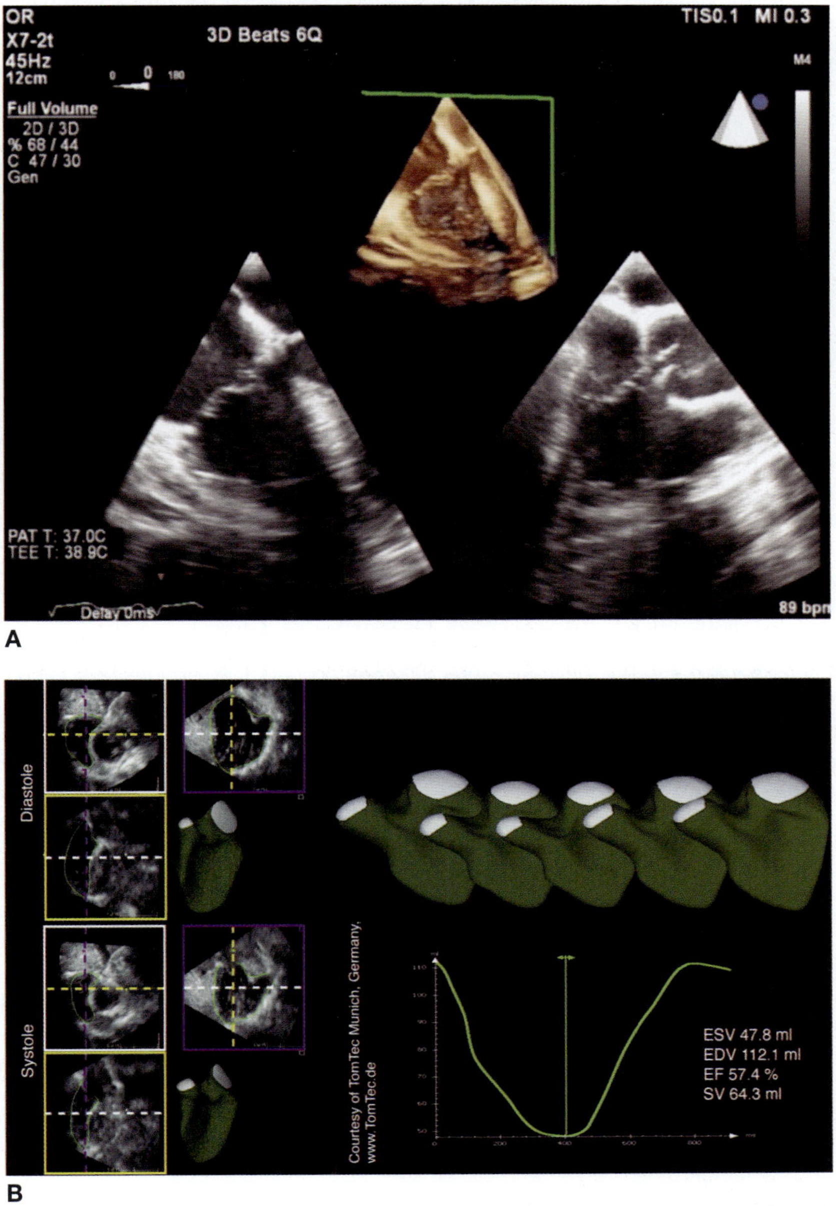

FIGURE 21.15 3D imaging and assessment of the right ventricle. A: An adequate 3D dataset of the right ventricle (RV) should include the inflow and outflow portions, as shown in the midesophageal 4C and inflow-outflow views. The size of the dataset should include the entire tricuspid valve annulus and a portion of the intra-atrial septum or aortic valve to aid in the orientation of the 2D image. B: Offline analysis of the RV full-volume 3D dataset by specialized software (TomTec) creates a dynamic model of the RV endocardial border and measures RV volumes and ejection fraction (see also Video 21.7). (TomTec®, Munich Germany.)

Mitral Valve

Mitral Valve Anatomy

All 3D imaging modes can examine the MV with excellent spatial resolution. Zoom or FV MBI 3D dataset acquisitions also provide good temporal resolution but may generate stitch artifacts, which can complicate image interpretation.

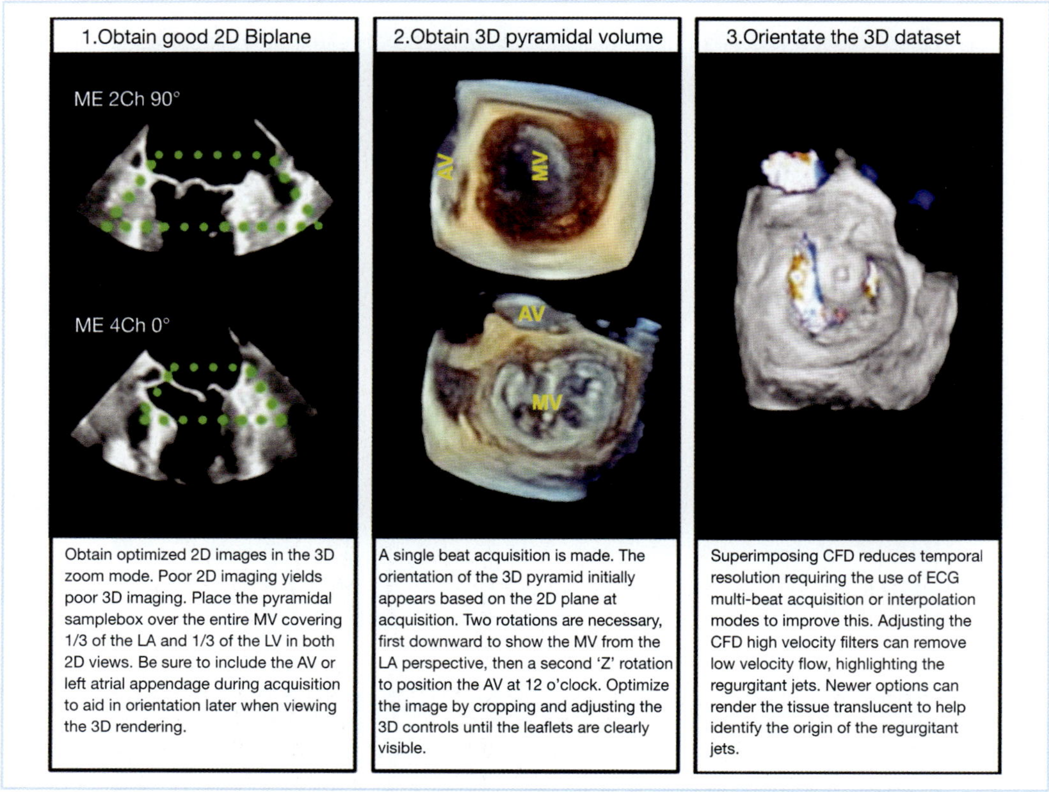

FIGURE 21.16 3D imaging of the mitral valve. This summarizes the directions to obtain the surgical en face view of the MV. Specific steps vary between different vendor platforms but are broadly similar. AV, aortic valve; CFD, color flow Doppler; LA, left atrium; LV, left ventricle; ME, midesophageal; MV, mitral valve (see also Video 21.8).

The en face perspective of the MV in the surgeon's orientation as viewed from the LA with the AV at the top of the image (12 o'clock) and the LAA on the left is widely used to display the MV in 3DTEE (Figure 21.16; Video 21.8). This image shows details of MV anatomy, including the individual scallops of the posterior leaflet and commissures. Manipulation of the 3D image can better define clefts, perforations, and complex degenerative MV pathology involving both leaflets and commissures. Examination of the subvalvular structures uses the LV perspective.

Mitral Valve Assessment

There are different options for using a 3D dataset to evaluate the MV, including (1) cropping, (2) angled views, (3) MPR, and (4) MV models. An intraoperative assessment of the MV is evolving from a qualitative to a more precise quantitative approach for evaluating anatomic structure and function.

The en face MV view can foreshorten the extent of mitral leaflet motion and may underestimate MV prolapse. Rotating the en face view through 360° provides additional perspectives from "angled views" (Figure 21.17A; Video 21.9), anterolateral commissure, posterior scallops, and posteromedial commissure views. Systematic use of these views is less time-consuming than additional processing by software, enabling accurate identification in RT of prolapsed segments involving both commissures and each leaflet.

The echocardiographer can use the 3D narrow volume mode to examine the MV in the ME four-chamber view by adjusting the elevational width to show the entire MV. Examination of opposing MV segments by cropping through the valve can identify coaptation pathology without using specialized software (Figure 21.17B).

An alternative method to analyze leaflet motion in relation to the annulus applies specialized MPR software to a Zoom or FV 3D dataset of the MV. This enables the precise evaluation of specific leaflet lengths,

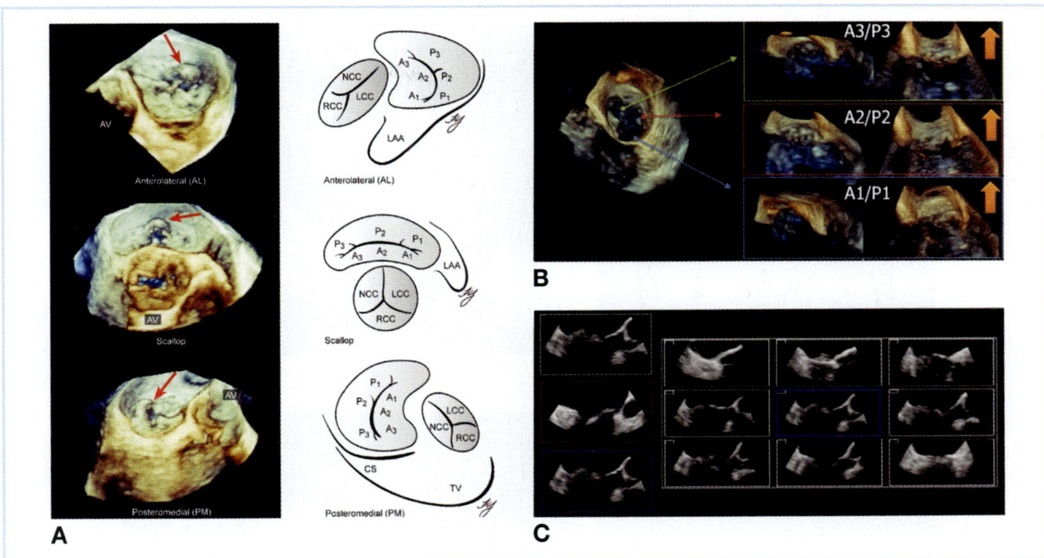

FIGURE 21.17 Mitral valve assessment. Currently, 3DTEE can assess the mitral valve (MV) using real-time and offline analytic techniques. A: Besides the en face view, angled views obtained from manipulating an MV 3D dataset can improve the visualization of pathology. The anterolateral, scallop, and posteromedial orientations for the MV show a flail P2 segment (red arrow) with multiple torn chordae. B: The MV Live 3D dataset can examine the MV by changing the elevational width to scroll through coapting segments. Tilting the dataset up (orange arrow) helps to identify MV leaflet pathology. C: Analysis using QLAB (3DQ, Philips Healthcare) multiplanar views can precisely identify the prolapse of individual MV segments. LCC, left coronary cusp; NCC, noncoronary cusp; RCC, right coronary cusp. (Illustrations in A are with permission from Frances Yeung and images from Vegas A, Meineri M, Jerath A. *Real-Time Three-Dimensional Transesophageal Echocardiography. A Step-by-Step Guide*. Springer; 2012 used with kind permission from Springer Science+Business Media.) (see also Video 21.9.)

coaptation length, and the region of billowing or prolapse. In addition, all vendors provide the ability to multislice the MV from commissure to commissure using MPR in a 2D image from the 3D dataset. This method uses MPR to examine MV coaptation through precut sagittal cuts, providing detailed insights into the valve's function and potential pathologies (Figure 21.17C).

Construction of dynamic or static 3D MV models using proprietary software (Philips QLAB MVQ, TomTec 4D MV Assessment, and Siemens eSie Valves) can yield detailed quantitative information about the MV (Figure 21.18). Most software is semiautomated with some user input to generate the model. The novel parameters derived from these 3D models have afforded greater insight into MV dynamics and pathology. The perioperative use of 3DTEE may provide surgeons with additional information about MV pathology to guide individual patient management.

Mitral Regurgitation

CFD identifies mitral regurgitation (MR) jets from defective leaflet coaptation, perforations, or paravalvular leaks. 3DTEE is more accurate than 2DTEE in identifying the mechanism of MR. The origin, direction, and components of flow convergence, VC, and jet area for the regurgitant jet can characterize regurgitation severity.

Identifying the origin and direction of eccentric and multiple jets from different MV pathologies can be difficult using 2D CFD, but easier using 3D CFD. Rendering the tissue or the CFD in the 3D dataset translucent (Figure 21.10C) may help to identify the origin of a regurgitant jet, jet direction, and the variability of jet geometry.

Qualitative, semiquantitative, and quantitative methods can assess MR jets, each with limitations. 3DTEE improves accuracy compared to 2DTEE, specifically for measuring the vena contracta area (VCA) and the

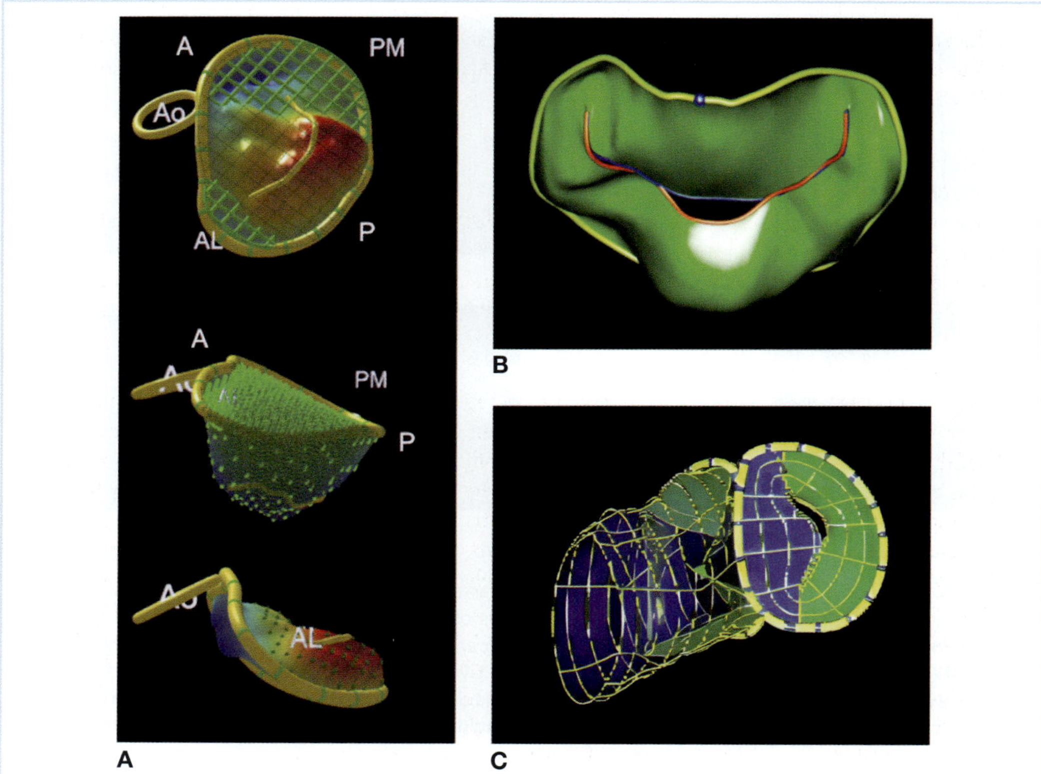

FIGURE 21.18 Mitral valve analysis software. Commercial software is available to analyze 3D valve datasets. A: QLAB Mitral Valve Quantification (MVQ, Philips Healthcare) creates a static 3D model for the mitral valve (MV) with multiple measurements depending on the pathology. B: TomTec 4D MV Assessment (Munich, Germany) provides a dynamic diastolic MV model by analyzing MV 3D datasets from any vendor. C: eSie Valves (Siemens Medical Solutions) also analyzes 3D datasets from any vendor to display a unique dynamic model of both the mitral and aortic valves. A, anterior; AL, antero-lateral; Ao, aorta; P, posterior; PM, postero-medial. ([A] MVQ, Philips Healthcare, Andover, MA; [B] Munich, Germany; [C] Courtesy of Siemens Medical Solutions USA, Inc.)

flow convergence proximal iso velocity area (PISA) by using MPR to align planes through the components of the MR jet. Both 3D TTE and 3DTEE (10) have a better correlation with gold-standard CMR than 2D imaging, particularly for eccentric, multiple, and late-systolic regurgitant jets (11). A single study suggests that the 3DTTE measure of VCA greater than 0.4 cm^2 correlates with severe MR (12). However, to date, no guidelines incorporate parameters measured from 3DTEE datasets in assessing MR severity (11). The 2021 European Society of Cardiology (ESC)/European Association for Cardio-Thoracic Surgery (EACTS) valvular heart disease guidelines now suggest CMR as a valid alternative for quantifying MR in patients with inconsistent or discordant echocardiographic parameters.

Mitral Stenosis

Conventional echocardiographic assessment of mitral stenosis (MS) relies heavily on transmitral pressure gradients, which may be inaccurate in interatrial shunting, irregular rhythms, LV dysfunction, severe diastolic dysfunction, or aortic regurgitation (AR). Supportive indices such as PISA, pressure half-time (PHT), and the continuity equation are sensitive to misalignment and cannot always be easily or quickly attained. Although the 2DTEE transgastric basal SAX view can allow planimetry of the open orifice, overestimation is common, as any single orthogonal plane may not capture the smallest orifice area.

MV area (MVA) from planimetry of a 3D dataset overcomes the limitations of planimetry by 2DTEE by identifying the narrowest orifice using either a direct or MPR approach. The MPR approach involves the simultaneous display of three orthogonal views through the MV to improve identification of the narrowest orifice. The direct planimetry approach crops the 3D dataset to identify the smallest orifice, which is traced directly. Severely calcified valves are susceptible to blooming artifacts, underestimating the orifice area due to falsely thickened edges. A comparative study using 3DTEE showed that direct planimetry correlated with the 3D MPR approach at MVA values less than 1.5 cm^2. In MVA above 1.5 cm^2, direct planimetry underestimates the MVA compared to the 3D MPR approach (13).

Aortic Valve

Aortic Root Anatomy

All 3D modes can image the AV, but the normal thin, pliable cusps and a heavily calcified valve are more difficult to image, though 3D AV modeling may overcome this. The 3D dataset should display the AV en face from the aorta or left ventricular outflow tract (LVOT) in an orientation with the right coronary cusp (RCC) position inferior at 6 o'clock (Figure 21.19). An FR of 25 VPS is necessary for dynamic assessment.

Aortic Valve Assessment

2D measurements of the aortic annulus diameter are susceptible to underestimation if the imaging plane is not in the center of the aortic root, with alignment between the left and noncoronary commissures and the middle of the RCC. Simultaneous biplane images can confirm this central alignment. Small refinements of orthogonal plane alignment reveal that the AV annulus often has an asymmetric shape, contrary to the circular assumption made by 2DTEE. 3D echocardiography more accurately determines the AV area (AVA) via direct measurement independent of geometric assumptions (see the "Aortic Stenosis" section that follows).

MPR from an AV 3D dataset can determine accurately the dimensions of the LVOT, aortic annulus, AV orifice, aortic root, and proximal ascending aorta. In situations of aortic root distortion from dilation or aneurysmal pathology, using MPR, the operator can manipulate a plane through each sinus, assessing its size, asymmetry, and suitability for repair. During transcatheter aortic valve implantation (TAVI), 3DTEE can estimate the AV annulus size with good correlation but with slight underestimation of CT measurements. Notably, relying on CT measurements alone may lead to prosthesis oversizing. There is less risk of post-TAVI paravalvular regurgitation when 3DTEE and CT measurements agree (14).

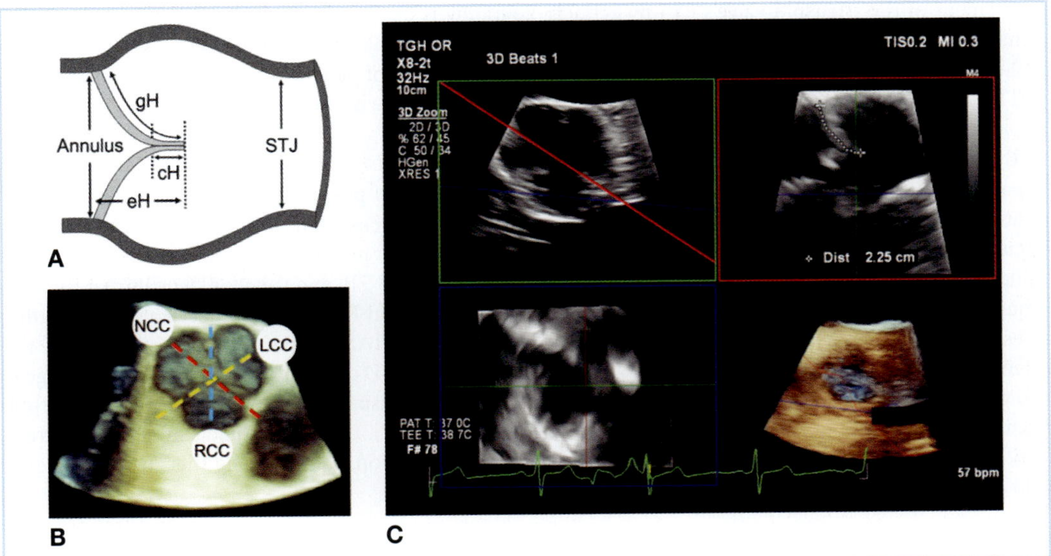

FIGURE 21.19 3D imaging of the aortic valve. A: This diagram of the aortic root in the long axis shows the geometric height (gH), coaptation height (cH), and effective height (eH), which are all important measurements made during aortic valve (AV) sparing surgery. B: Three dotted lines on this 3D AV dataset in the short axis show planes through the commissures, leaflet tips, and the coaptation base in diastole. These planes guide the measurements mentioned previously. C: This shows the measurement of the geometric height of the NCC using multiplanar reconstruction (MPR). The AV appears in a short axis in the green box, with the red plane aligned across the middle of the NCC body and the right and left commissure in diastole. The user can trace the geometric height of the NCC in the red box. LCC, left coronary cusp; NCC, noncoronary cusp; RCC, right coronary cusp; STJ, sinotubular junction.

The eSie Valves (Siemens Medical Solutions) software is available on the Acuson US machine for MV and AV analysis. It takes seconds to use this semiautomated software to construct patient-specific dynamic 3D MV, AV, and aortic root models with simultaneous display of the aortic-mitral complex (Figure 21.18C). A comprehensive biometric and kinematic measurement suite is available in a numeric or graphic output, as well as mapped to the model.

Aortic Regurgitation

Complex AR jets may be eccentric with a noncircular regurgitant orifice, making VC width measurements and estimates of the effective regurgitant orifice area (EROA) from the PISA radius less accurate by 2DTEE. EROA and VCA measurements by 3DTEE have a better correlation with CMR measurements (11). 3DTEE is especially valuable during assessments for AV repair or valve-sparing root procedures. MPR planes derived from an aortic root 3D dataset provide precise measurements that 2DTEE cannot achieve, such as the measure of geometric height, which is the curved distance along each individual cusp (Figure 21.19). It is easier using a 3D dataset to assess each cusp for partial or complete prolapse, which is difficult in 2D because of poor alignment between the noncoronary and left coronary cusps.

Aortic Stenosis

Guideline recommendations for the evaluation of aortic stenosis (AS) comprise both flow-dependent (velocity and pressure gradients) and flow-independent measures of AVA (planimetry, continuity equation) (15). Doppler assessments may be inaccurate in small aorta size, LV dysfunction, subaortic stenosis, or high LVOT gradients. The operator can evaluate AVA from a 3D dataset using MPR by either direct planimetry of the smallest valve orifice or by applying planimetry of the LVOT area to the continuity equation. However, in a comparison of 2D versus 3DTEE, AVA calculation by the continuity equation using conventional 2D best correlated with ex vivo scanning of the excised stenotic AV (16). Both planimetry (2DTEE) and MPR (3DTEE) significantly overestimated AVA (16).

Tricuspid Valve

Tricuspid Valve Anatomy

Assessment of the tricuspid valve (TV) by echocardiography is challenging because of the complex, nonplanar geometry of the annulus and asymmetric cusp anatomy. Visualization of the entire TV with all three leaflets in a single display is only attainable by 2DTTE in 5% to 10% of patients (17), and unobtainable from 2DTEE ME views. Thin leaflets and the distance of the valve from the probe further compromise the spatial resolution required for detailed assessment.

By comparison, 3D echocardiography can visualize all TV leaflets simultaneously by TTE in 85% to 90% of patients and from 3DTEE transgastric approach in 65% to 70% of patients (17). 3DTEE views from the right atrium (RA) or RV should orientate the TV with the septal cusp inferior at the 6 o'clock position (Figure 21.20A; Video 21.10). The RA perspective best evaluates primary tricuspid regurgitation (TR), while the RV perspective better assesses the commissures, functional TR, and valvular stenosis. An FV MBI acquisition should capture the essential landmarks while achieving an FR of 20 VPS necessary for dynamic assessment (17). Sector size must be wide enough to encompass the IAS and part of the AV to facilitate the orientation of the 3D image. It may be necessary to acquire multiple 3D datasets from ME, lower esophageal, and transgastric levels because of the US beam alignment. The TV cusps are best visualized closed in systole from the esophagus, but open during diastole from the stomach (17). Dropout artifacts are common from thin leaflets, valve distance from the probe, and an oblique orientation, so increasing the TGC and overall gain may minimize dropout (17).

Tricuspid Valve Assessment

Poor-quality 3D datasets often limit the assessment of TV leaflet pathology but can better evaluate annulus size than 2D images. There are currently no commercially available software packages designed for quantitative analysis of TV annulus or leaflet geometry. Therefore, the operator must rely on MPR to make leaflet and annulus measurements and for planimetry of the TV orifice (Figure 21.20B). The nonplanar geometry of the TV can prevent the alignment of a single plane through all the hinge points in a 3D dataset. Even with this limitation, measurements of TV annular diameter obtained from 3D datasets have a better correlation with CMR than 2D measurements, which consistently underestimate.

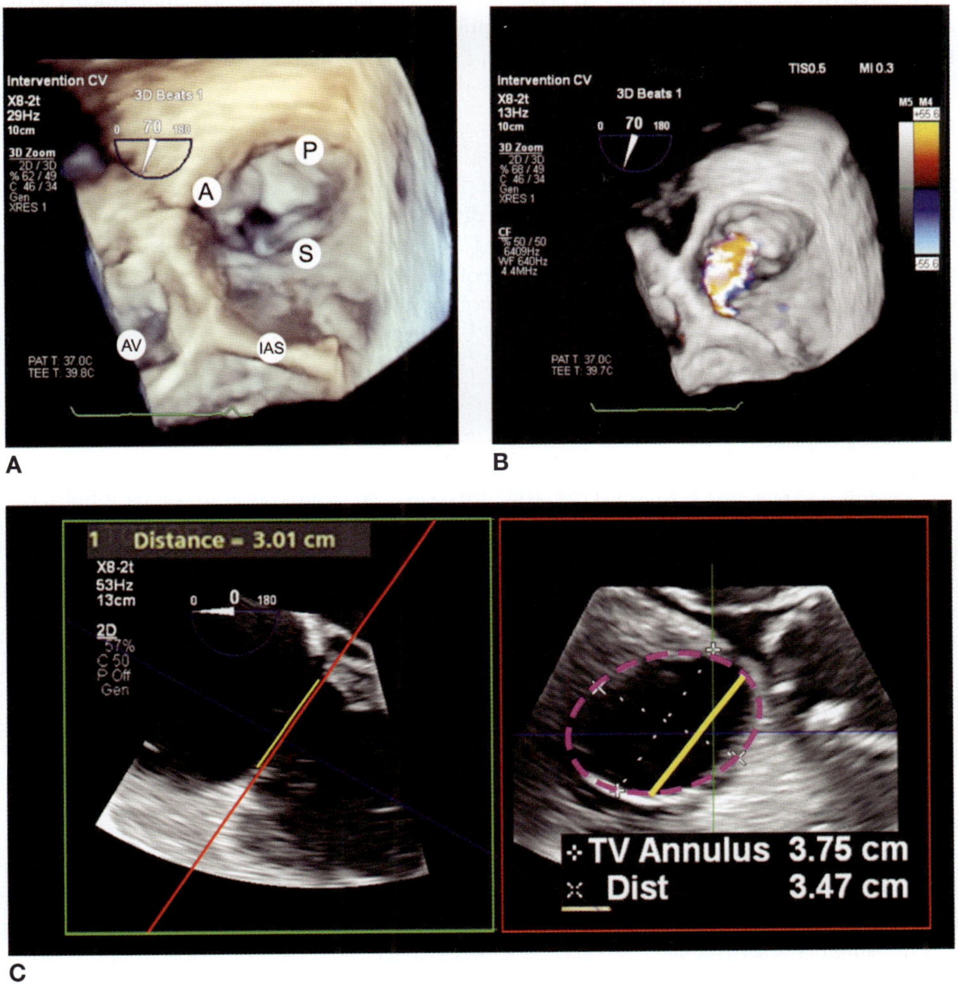

FIGURE 21.20 3D imaging of the tricuspid valve. A: This is a 3D image of the TV in short axis from the right atrial perspective as per guidelines. B: The same 3D dataset with color flow Doppler superimposed identifies the tricuspid regurgitant jet. C: This MPR of the TV annulus shows the green box of a standard midesophageal RV-focused view with the yellow line representing a TV annular measurement during diastole. A red MPR plane position in the green box is across the valve annulus, as shown in the red box. The tricuspid annulus has an oval shape. The maximum diameter is 3.75 cm, which differs from the 2D measurement of 3.01 cm obtained in the green box. A, anterior leaflet; AV, aortic valve; IAS, intra-atrial septum; MPR, multiplane reconstruction; P, posterior leaflet; S, septal leaflet; TV, tricuspid valve (see also Video 21.10).

Tricuspid Regurgitation

It is difficult to grade TR accurately using the 2D measures recommended by the ASE (11). Hemodynamic variables and jet eccentricity affect jet area, which is a semiquantitative measure of TR severity. Incorrect assumptions of a circular TR regurgitant orifice make 2D measures of TR VC width only moderately sensitive and specific, and TR PISA radius often underestimates TR severity. Volume status, atrioventricular dissociation, and RV compliance can impact corollary measures of TR severity, such as inferior vena cava diameter and hepatic vein flow reversal. Current data suggest that a 2D VCA greater than 0.4 cm^2 reflects severe TR (18).

Methods evaluating TR from 3D datasets include regurgitant orifice area planimetry, VC width, VC area, or PISA radius. The 3D VCA correlates strongly with the EROA, moderately with the VC width, and weakly with the jet area/right atrial area ratio (19). It is most effective for assessing primary TR in patients with sinus rhythm (11). These 3DTEE measures are less susceptible to the errors and geometric assumptions made during 2D assessment.

Tricuspid Stenosis

Tricuspid stenosis (TS) is a rare entity associated with congenital lesions, carcinoid, endocarditis, or rheumatic heart disease (15). Grading TS severity with 2DTEE relies entirely on flow parameters (mean gradient and PHT). This is because the tricuspid orifice is difficult to view en face with 2DTEE, which precludes planimetry. Planimetry of the narrowest orifice using MPR from a 3D dataset overcomes this limitation. However, the ASE guidelines note that quantification of the TV orifice area by 3D echocardiography is neither standardized nor sufficiently validated and thus not recommended (15).

Pulmonic Valve

Pulmonic Valve Anatomy

The pulmonic valve (PV) is the most difficult valve to visualize using 2DTEE, even for experienced echocardiographers. Although several windows can image the PV, this is inconsistent because of the thin leaflets, far-field position, and shadowing from nearby structures (20). 2DTEE images of the upper esophageal (UE) aortic arch SAX view are obtainable in only 72% of patients, with only 53% of patients having high-quality images (21). It is difficult with 2DTEE to show an en face view of the PV displaying all three leaflets.

En face views of all three leaflets are attainable using 3DTEE, allowing the detailed morphologic assessment of cusps, coaptation, PV annular diameter, and PV orifice area. The best 3D capture of the PV is from FV or zoom acquisitions in the UE aortic arch SAX view. Shown from the RV or pulmonary artery (PA) perspective, the PV orientation has the anterior cusp at the 12 o'clock position. However, the absence of nearby landmarks makes orientation very challenging. A wide-sector angle capturing the AV which may serve as a reference point at the 6 o'clock position. As with the TV, increasing the TGC and overall gain may minimize dropout in the 3D dataset.

Pulmonic Valve Assessment

A good 3D dataset of the PV may offer insights into PV pathology. There are currently no commercially available software packages designed for quantitative analysis of the PV annulus or leaflet geometry. Therefore, the operator uses MPR to make leaflet measurements and to planimeter the PV. A comparison of PV annular diameter measurements across imaging modalities shows that 3DTTE correlated best with surgical measurements, whereas 2DTTE and CT scans consistently provided underestimates (22). There are no published cross-modality comparisons of PV assessment involving 3DTEE.

Pulmonic Regurgitation

Trivial to mild pulmonic regurgitation (PR) is a common finding, detectable in 30% of patients (20). The relative lack of data regarding PR quantification has societal guidelines adopting AV methodologies and parameters for the PV with varying degrees of effectiveness (11). Primary PR without associated pulmonary hypertension can be difficult to visualize by CFD because of the low velocity, laminar flow, and brief duration of the PR jet. The evaluation of PR by 2D CFD echocardiography includes jet length, color jet area, proximal jet or VC width, and ratio of proximal PR jet width/pulmonary annulus, all of which can be difficult to capture routinely (11). 3DTEE with MPR of a 3D dataset may theoretically allow planimetry of the regurgitant orifice area, VCA, and PR jet width. However, data are sparse on the role of 3D echocardiography in assessing PR. The ASE guidelines state that the practical application of these techniques for PR quantification is not well established, and no studies have compared PR quantification across imaging modalities (11).

Pulmonic Stenosis

Pulmonic stenosis (PS) is almost entirely a congenital disease. Like the TV, the grading of PS depends on flow-derived measures. The continuity equation and PISA method are feasible but not validated measurements of the PV area. 2D planimetry is not feasible because of inadequate imaging planes. Planimetry using MPR on a 3D dataset is possible but not validated nor recommended at present.

SHUNTS

A 3D Zoom or FV acquisition of the IAS from ME views should encompass the entire IAS and include the superior vena cava (SVC) and inferior vena cava (IVC). Presentation of the IAS can be from the RA or LA perspective with the orientation of the IAS such that the SVC appears at 11 o'clock. This facilitates the diagnosis and treatment of common pathologies, such as a PFO or atrial septal defect (ASD) (Figure 21.21; Video 21.11).

3D imaging of the interventricular septum (IVS) requires FV acquisition to capture sufficient sector size and FR. The optimal acquisition angle depends on the type of defect, categorized as (1) supracristal, (2) perimembranous, (3) inlet, or (4) muscular. Although the IVS can appear from either the RV or LV perspective, the IVS components appear by convention from the RV. En face 3DTEE imaging and MPR permit detailed measurements of irregularly shaped ventricular septal defects (VSDs) and rims, allowing more precise device sizing. RT imaging during device closure ensures precise orientation with fewer adjustments than with 2D imaging (23).

Congenital Heart Disease

CHD poses challenges for expert echocardiographers because of abnormal structures, connections, communications, and prior surgical interventions. Recognizing these challenges, the 2019 ASE guidelines provide recommendations for performing a comprehensive TEE examination in children and adults with CHD. Owing to the innumerable anatomic variations of CHD, these guidelines emphasize structure-based over view-based algorithms, aligning well with the 3D workflow. Single tomographic views rarely capture complex anatomy, and the guidelines specifically recommend 3D structural and color Doppler imaging wherever appropriate. Thus, 3DTEE may be useful during Fontan or baffle thrombus analysis, imaging of atriopulmonary connections, and guidance of interventional fenestration closure or creation. The recent availability of mini 3DTEE probes (X11-4t from Philips and 9VT-D from GE) for use in pediatric patients weighing 5 kg or more will be invaluable for the diagnosis and perioperative assessment of CHD in pediatrics.

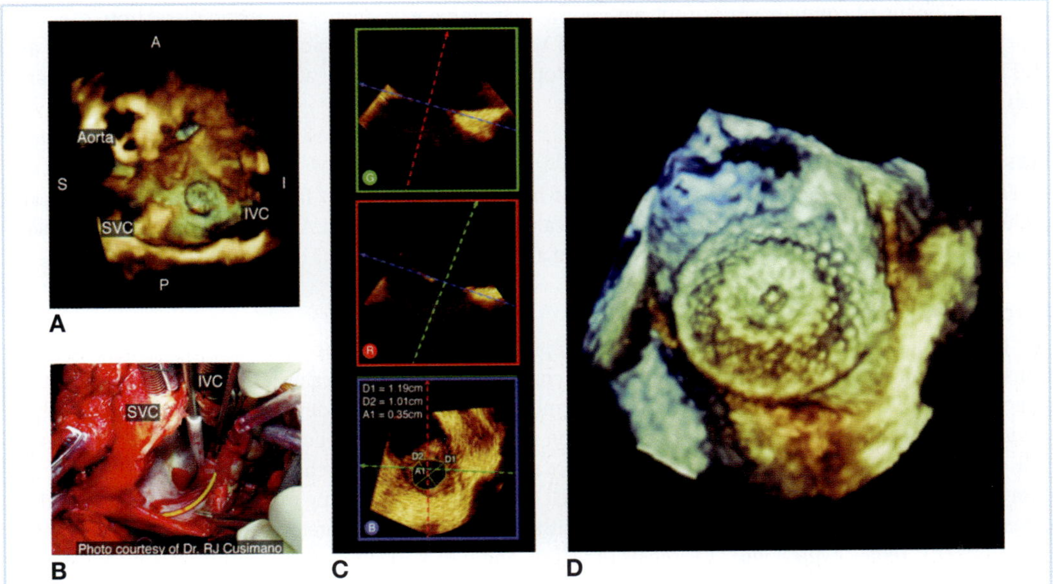

FIGURE 21.21 3D imaging of the interatrial septum. Patent foramen ovale (PFO) and atrial septal defect (ASD) closure. A: Interrogation of the interatrial septum can use a full-volume 3D dataset oriented to be viewed from the right atrium. B: Surgical view of the PFO. C: The size and location of this ASD secundum are assessed using QLAB (3DQ, Philips Healthcare) by positioning planes parallel (B, blue) and through the center of the defect (G, green and R, red). D: 3D Zoom from the left atrium of the deployed Amplatzer device used to close the ASD. A, anterior; I, inferior; IVC, inferior vena cava; P, posterior; S, superior; SVC, superior vena cava. (A: From Vegas A, Meineri M, Jerath A. *Real Time Three-Dimensional Transesophageal Echocardiography. A Step-by-Step Guide*. Springer; 2012 used with kind permission from Springer Science + Business Media; see also Video 21.11.)

TABLE 21.3 RT 3DTEE for Procedural Interventions

Procedure	Preprocedure	Intraprocedure	Postprocedure
ASD	Size, location, multiplicity Relation to structures	TSP ASD size	Device stability Residual flow
TAVI	AV morphology AV annulus size Aortic root dimensions Coronary height MR severity	Guidewires Valve position Residual AI	Valve stability Paravalvular leak LV dysfunction Pericardial effusion
Valve clips	Valve morphology Regurgitant severity	TSP Device position Clip location	Clip stability Residual regurgitation Orifice size Valve gradient
LAA occluder	LAA morphology LAA dimensions Thrombus	TSP Device size/type Device position	Device stability LAA flow MV relationship Pericardial effusion
Paravalvular leak	Defect size, location Regurgitant volume	Guidewires Device sizing Device location	Device stability Residual leak

AI, aortic insufficiency; ASD, atrial septal defect; LAA, left atrial appendage; LV, left ventricle; MV, mitral valve; TAVI, transcatheter aortic valve implantation; TSP, transseptal puncture.

Aorta

3DTEE can image the entire aorta, excluding the blind spot, to assess aortic pathology. The 3D images can reveal the details of complex aortic root pathology, including aortic aneurysm, aortic dissection, pseudoaneurysm of the intravalvular fibrosa, and sinus of Valsalva aneurysm. Epiaortic scanning, multiplane, and 3DTEE narrow volume mode can better show the topographic definition of atheromatous disease compared with 2DTEE.

Masses

3DTEE can show the location and attachment of intracardiac masses to facilitate surgical planning and evaluate for a source of embolism. The operator can examine the entire LAA for thrombus using biplane images or the 3D zoom mode. The measurement of any mass size can occur in 2D or 3D using MPR.

Percutaneous Interventions

The field of interventional echocardiography has rapidly matured out of the need to support more complex transcatheter procedures of an interventional structural heart program. Regardless of the type of structural intervention, TEE plays a critical role in (1) confirming the diagnosis, (2) device sizing, (3) intraprocedural guidance, and (4) postdevice evaluation of function and procedural complications (Table 21.3). The use of TEE to guide the placement of percutaneous device closure of holes in the heart, including ASD, VSD, and paravalvular leaks of prosthetic valves, has been well described. 3DTEE using multiplane, Live MPR, and 3D datasets enables RT guidance and assessment of catheter-based valvular interventions including transseptal puncture, MV repair (MitraClip), TV repair (TriClip), and TAVI. 3DTEE offers significant advantages over 2DTEE by providing more accurate spatial orientation, detailed anatomic visualization, and comprehensive assessment of device-tissue interactions, which enhances procedural guidance and outcomes.

FUTURE DIRECTIONS

The pervasiveness of 3D US in modern cardiology and cardiac surgery is remarkable for a technology widely available for less than 15 years. Continuous advancements in probe technology offer a promise to increase image resolution and FR with smaller transducers.

Progress in the computation power of graphic processing units has culminated in in vivo experiments with 3D ultrafast imaging. Instead of using focused beams that create one scan line at a time, ultrafast imaging uses multiplane waves at various angles that reconstruct one full image in one emission. The typical US systems have 2D imaging FRs of 50 to 200 Hz, while an ultrafast 2D system can achieve 20,000 Hz. By comparison to a standard 3D system which samples up to a few tens of volumes/s, an ultrafast system can sample 2,325 volumes/s at a depth of 12 cm. Higher FRs enhance temporal resolution for large 3D volumes, allowing for a more accurate evaluation of pathology, especially when using CFD. This enhanced temporal resolution is critical for capturing dynamic cardiac events and providing detailed flow information, which improves diagnostic accuracy and clinical decision-making.

Artificial intelligence (AI) promises to revolutionize 2D and 3D echocardiography. Current 2DTTE AI applications are facilitating fewer human-machine interactions during measurements by using automatic algorithms for functional (eg, strain/speckle tracking, EF, regional wall movement), linear, Doppler, and complex modeling. The expectation is for similar improvements in 3DTEE. Automated tools for chamber quantification and valve modeling are already available, replacing early computational methods that relied on mathematical rules for automation. Powerful proof-of-concept studies show that deep-learning neural networks can correctly identify 2DTEE views, valve leaflets, prosthetic valves, and Doppler traces. Machine learning algorithms can already quantify MR severity with 99% accuracy (24) and identify rheumatic valves with 72% accuracy (25). The FDA approval of an AI software that acquires diagnostic-quality 2D TTE images opens the door to integration with TEE.

Regardless of advances in 3D acquisition, there is a loss of valuable data when transferring these images to a 2D display. New technologies in development may allow echocardiographers, surgeons, and proceduralists to interact with data in 3D. 3D printing, holographic displays, stereo monitors, and virtual, augmented, and mixed reality allow the tangible manipulation and interrogation of complex datasets. 3D echocardiographic data used to create 3D visualizations in a virtual reality application led surgeons to modify their planned surgical approach in 60% of cases.

Fused imaging allows proceduralists to layer fluoroscopy or CT data over echo data to create augmented reality images to guide device delivery, determine balloon sizing, or assess device stability. Communication and integration across imaging platforms can enhance the strengths and capabilities of each modality synergistically.

Cardiac 5D echocardiography, pioneered by Samsung Medison (Seoul, South Korea), is a volumetric echocardiography concept that heavily relies on automatic software processing to deliver sharp, high-definition live images. Currently available for transabdominal fetal medicine clinical applications, it is expected to be integrated into TEE. The fifth dimension in this concept represents the full automation of data processing to produce higher-standard images than the current 3D technology.

SUMMARY

3DTEE has quickly integrated into perioperative workflows to enhance the diagnostic capabilities of modern US systems. Emerging guidelines and practice standards expect 3DTEE proficiency from all echocardiographers, which begins with understanding the technology, physics, limitations, and errors that characterize this powerful tool. Although still perceived as an accessory to 2D imaging, 3DTEE continues to demonstrate superiority in many aspects of routine examination, including structural measurements and identification of valvular pathology. As spatial and temporal resolutions improve, the use of 3DTEE will continue to expand to improve perioperative outcomes.

REFERENCES

1. Muraru D, Badano L. Physics and technical principles of three-dimensional echocardiography. In: Badano LP, Lang RM, Muraru D, eds. *Textbook of Three-Dimensional Echocardiography*. Switzerland Springer Nature; 2019.
2. Perrin DP, Vasilyev NV, Marx GR, et al. Temporal enhancement of 3D echocardiography by frame reordering. *JACC Cardiovasc Imaging*. 2012;5:300-304.
3. Denarie B, Bjastad T, Torp H. Multi-line transmission in 3-D with reduced crosstalk artifacts: a proof of concept study. *IEEE Trans Ultrason Ferroelectr Freq Control*. 2013;60:1708-1718.
4. Skaug TR, Amundsen BH, Hergum T, et al. Quantification of aortic regurgitation using high-pulse repetition frequency three-dimensional colour Doppler. *Eur Heart J Cardiovasc Imaging*. 2014;15:615-622.
5. Rong LQ. An update on intraoperative three-dimensional transesophageal echocardiography. *J Thorac Dis*. 2017;9:S271-S282.
6. Meris A, Santambrogio L, Casso G, et al. Intraoperative three-dimensional versus two-dimensional echocardiography for left ventricular assessment. *Anesth Analg*. 2014;118:711-720.
7. Chua S, Levine RA, Yosefy C, et al. Assessment of right ventricular function by real-time three-dimensional echocardiography improves accuracy and decreases interobserver variability compared with conventional two-dimensional views. *Eur J Echocardiogr*. 2009;10:619-624.

8. Pickett CA, Cheezum MK, Kassop D, et al. Accuracy of cardiac CT, radionucleotide and invasive ventriculography, two- and three-dimensional echocardiography, and SPECT for left and right ventricular ejection fraction compared with cardiac MRI: a meta-analysis. *Eur Heart J Cardiovasc Imaging.* 2015;16:848-852.
9. Shimada YJ, Shiota M, Siegel RJ, et al. Accuracy of right ventricular volumes and function determined by three-dimensional echocardiography in comparison with magnetic resonance imaging: a meta-analysis study. *J Am Soc Echocardiogr.* 2010;23:943-953.
10. Shanks M, Siebelink HM, Delgado V, et al. Quantitative assessment of mitral regurgitation: comparison between three-dimensional transesophageal echocardiography and magnetic resonance imaging. *Circ Cardiovasc Imaging.* 2010;3:694-700.
11. Zoghbi WA, Adams D, Bonow RO, et al. Recommendations for noninvasive evaluation of native valvular regurgitation: a report from the American Society of Echocardiography Developed in Collaboration with the Society for Cardiovascular Magnetic Resonance. *J Am Soc Echocardiogr.* 2017;30:303-371.
12. Zeng X, Levine RA, Hua L, et al. Diagnostic value of vena contracta area in the quantification of mitral regurgitation severity by color Doppler 3D echocardiography. *Circ Cardiovasc Imaging.* 2011;4:506-513.
13. Toufan Tabrizi M, Faraji Azad H, Khezerlouy-Aghdam N, Sakha H. Measurement of mitral valve area by direct three dimensional planimetry compared to multiplanar reconstruction in patients with rheumatic mitral stenosis. *Int J Cardiovasc Imaging.* 2022;38(6):1341-1349.
14. Willson AB, Webb JG, Freeman M, et al. Computed tomography-based sizing recommendations for transcatheter aortic valve replacement with balloon-expandable valves: comparison with transesophageal echocardiography and rationale for implementation in a prospective trial. *J Cardiovasc Comput Tomogr.* 2012;6:406-414.
15. Baumgartner H, Hung J, Bermejo J, et al. Echocardiographic assessment of valve stenosis: EAE/ASE recommendations for clinical practice. *J Am Soc Echocardiogr.* 2009;22:1-23; quiz 101-102.
16. Shirazi S, Golmohammadi F, Tavoosi A, et al. Quantification of aortic valve area: comparison of different methods of echocardiography with 3-D scan of the excised valve. *Int J Cardiovasc Imaging.* 2021;37:529-538.
17. Muraru D, Hahn RT, Soliman OI, et al. 3-Dimensional echocardiography in imaging the tricuspid valve. *JACC Cardiovasc Imaging.* 2019;12:500-515.
18. Tribouilloy CM, Enriquez-Sarano M, Capps MA, et al. Contrasting effect of similar effective regurgitant orifice area in mitral and tricuspid regurgitation: a quantitative Doppler echocardiographic study. *J Am Soc Echocardiogr.* 2002;15:958-965.
19. Chen TE, Kwon SH, Enriquez-Sarano M, et al. Three-dimensional color Doppler echocardiographic quantification of tricuspid regurgitation orifice area: comparison with conventional two-dimensional measures. *J Am Soc Echocardiogr.* 2013;26:1143-1152.
20. Taskesen T, Gill EA. Pulmonary valve assessment by three-dimensional echocardiography. *Echocardiography.* 2022;39:1001-1009.
21. Taskesen T, Prabhu SJ, Steinberg ZL, et al. Feasibility of pulmonary valve imaging using transesophageal echocardiography upper esophageal view. *Echocardiography.* 2019;36:930-937.
22. Hadeed K, Hascoet S, Amadieu R, et al. 3D transthoracic echocardiography to assess pulmonary valve morphology and annulus size in patients with Tetralogy of Fallot. *Arch Cardiovasc Dis.* 2016;109:87-95.
23. Mani A, Harikrishnan S, Sasidharan B, et al. Utility of 3D echocardiography for device sizing during transcatheter ASD closure: a comparative study. *J Cardiovasc Imaging.* 2023;31:180-187.
24. Moghaddasi H, Nourian S. Automatic assessment of mitral regurgitation severity based on extensive textural features on 2D echocardiography videos. *Comput Biol Med.* 2016;73:47-55.
25. Martins J, Nascimento ER, Nascimento BR, et al. Towards automatic diagnosis of rheumatic heart disease on echocardiographic exams through video-based deep learning. *J Am Med Inform Assoc.* 2021;28:1834-1842.

QUESTIONS

1. Which statement is true regarding the crystals in current 3DTEE probes?

A. The transducer crystal is composed of PZT.
B. The transducer contains 250 crystals.
C. The transducer crystals are arranged in a circle.
D. The elements are fully sampled.

2. Which 3D mode has the lowest temporal resolution for a single-beat acquisition?

A. 3D Live
B. 3D Full volume
C. 3D color Doppler
D. 3D Zoom

3. Which is not an artifact in 3D images?

A. Blooming
B. Stitch
C. Conversion
D. Blurring

4. **Postprocessing to optimize a 3D image includes adjusting all except:**
   A. Gain
   B. Line density
   C. Brightness
   D. Smoothing

5. **The inability to perform measurements directly on a 3D image is because of:**
   A. Poor spatial resolution
   B. Parallax error
   C. Poor temporal resolution
   D. Uncalibrated measuring tool

6. **Which is a disadvantage of using LV 3D models to estimate LV volumes?**
   A. Poor spatial resolution
   B. Lack of geometric model
   C. Assessment over the cardiac cycle
   D. Good cardiac apex alignment

7. **Which is the best option for assessing global right ventricular function by 3DTEE?**
   A. RV EF
   B. RV FAC
   C. RV tricuspid annulus systolic excursion
   D. RV 3D strain

8. **Which is the most reliable technique to measure the length of the leaflets of the MV?**
   A. From 2DTEE images
   B. Directly from a 3D MV image
   C. Using MPR
   D. Creating a 3D model

9. **In the en face view of the TV from the RA, what is the location of the IAS?**
   A. 6 o'clock
   B. 3 o'clock
   C. 9 o'clock
   D. 12 o'clock

10. **Experimental 3D ultrafast imaging can achieve VPS rates of:**
    A. 20
    B. 200
    C. 2,000
    D. 20,000

ANSWERS

1. **Correct Answer: D.**
   Rationale: 3DTEE probes contain a single piezoelectric crystal partitioned into thousands of elements arranged in a matrix of rows and columns. Whereas the composition of conventional piezoelectric crystals is PZT (lead zirconate titanate), 3DTEE probes use an alternative type of piezoelectric crystal. Each element can be activated independently (fully sampled), focused, and steered.

2. **Correct Answer: C.**
   Rationale: 3D color Doppler obtains a large amount of information (3D volume and 3D CFD), resulting in the lowest temporal resolution (FR <20 Hz) in a single-beat acquisitio

3. **Correct Answer: C.**
   Rationale: "Conversion" is one of the three integrated steps of data processing, together with interpolation and segmentation.

Conversion positions and assigns x-y-z coordinates (Cartesian volume) to each of the scanned raw data points, identifying their echogenic characteristics with a known position in space.

4. **Correct Answer: B.**
Rationale: Postprocessing adjustment of gain, compression (contrast ratio), brightness (increasing whiteness), and smoothing (reducing image coarseness) can improve 3D image quality but cannot fully correct gross imbalances during data acquisition. Time gain compensation and line density are fundamental properties of the acquisition and cannot be changed in postprocessing.

5. **Correct Answer: B.**
Rationale: The inability to perform measurements directly on 3D images in real time results from parallax error, defined as the difference in the apparent position of an object depending on the line of sight. 3D acquisition captures objects from multiple angles simultaneously, each with unique viewing perspectives, causing discrepancies in the perceived position of anatomic structures.

6. **Correct Answer: A.**
Rationale: 3D LV models accurately quantify LV volumes with better alignment through the cardiac apex, the inclusion of more endocardial surface during analysis, and the lack of geometric shape assumption. Limitations of this 3D method include lack of reproducibility, poor spatial and temporal resolution, and the inaccuracy of endocardial surface tracking software.

7. **Correct Answer: C.**
Rationale: RVEF measured by 3D echocardiography is the only index of RV systolic function that incorporates all RV regions with their relative contributions to both longitudinal and radial shortening. 2D measures of systolic function such as RV FAC, TAPSE, and tissue Doppler-derived lateral annular systolic velocity (*S′*) assess a single tomographic plane and may overrepresent the longitudinal excursion.

8. **Correct Answer: A.**
Rationale: Applying specialized MPR software to a Zoom or FV 3D data set of the MV enables precise evaluation of specific leaflet lengths, coaptation length, and the region of billowing or prolapse. Measurements directly from the 3D image are not possible due to parallax error.

9. **Correct Answer: A.**
Rationale: 3DTEE views from the RA or RV should orientate the TV with the septal cusp inferior at the 6 o'clock position (Figure 21.20A; Video 21.10).

10. **Correct Answer: C.**
Rationale: The typical US systems have 2D imaging frame rates of 50 to 200 Hz, while an ultrafast 2D system can achieve frame rates of 20,000 Hz. By comparison, to a standard 3D system that samples up to a few tens of volumes per second, an ultrafast system can sample 2,325 volumes/s at a depth of 12 cm.

22 Common Artifacts and Pitfalls of Clinical Echocardiography

Fabio Guarracino and Albert C. Perrino, Jr

Echocardiography provides noninvasive, real-time insights into cardiac structure and function. Although advancements in ultrasound technology have made echocardiography more accessible and reliable, it remains subject to various artifacts and pitfalls that can complicate interpretation. Artifacts—visual distortions caused by technical or physical factors—are common, and without careful analysis, they can lead to misdiagnosis or unnecessary intervention. Additionally, operator experience, patient anatomy, and equipment limitations introduce challenges that every clinician must be prepared to recognize.

Clinically important imaging artifacts result from the interplay of the ultrasound system, the patient, and the interpreting echocardiographer (1,2). Knowledge of the types of artifacts that occur during a standard transesophageal echocardiographic (TEE) examination is of paramount importance for the correct interpretation of the echo data. The most common artifacts seen in clinical practice are the result of (1) normal or variant anatomic structures that are misdiagnosed, (2) the physical limitations of ultrasound imaging, and (3) undesirable interactions of ultrasound with tissues or medical devices (3). In this chapter, we first explore the most frequently encountered artifacts in clinical echocardiography, offering insights into their origins and practical strategies for distinguishing artifacts from true pathology. Second, we review common interpretive pitfalls and discuss approaches to enhance accuracy, focusing on the importance of technical proficiency, anatomic knowledge, and a structured approach to image interpretation. Last, we discuss the various artifacts commonly encountered in 2D imaging, 3D imaging, and Doppler examinations.

NORMAL ANATOMIC VARIANTS IN TWO-DIMENSIONAL IMAGING

Both novice and experienced echocardiographers may call normal structures abnormal. These normal variants can affect the intraoperative diagnosis and lead to an inappropriate surgery. Careful evaluation and consideration of the common variants discussed in the subsequent text can help limit problems related to misdiagnosis.

Crista Terminalis

The crista terminalis has been misinterpreted as a right atrial tumor or thrombus. This prominent muscular ridge can be differentiated from an anomaly by its characteristic appearance and position. The crista terminalis originates at the junction of the right atrium and superior vena cava and runs longitudinally toward the inferior vena cava. The crista terminalis separates the trabeculated appendage of the atrium from the smooth tubular portion. The structure is best visualized in the midesophageal (ME) bicaval view (4) (Figure 22.1).

Eustachian Valve or Chiari Network

The eustachian valve is often misdiagnosed as an intra-atrial thrombus. The eustachian valve (called a *Chiari network* when fenestrated) is the remnant of the embryologic right venous valve, which is important in utero to direct inferior vena cava blood flow across the fossa ovalis. The filamentous structures can be differentiated from thrombus by their characteristic "insertion" into the atrial wall. They are best visualized in the ME bicaval view, in which they can be seen originating from the junction of the right atrium and inferior vena cava (Figure 22.1).

Lipomatous Hypertrophy of the Atrial Septum

Myxomas, the most common cardiac tumors, often originate from the interatrial septum and typically involve the fossa ovalis. Lipomatous hypertrophy of the atrial septum can mimic atrial masses such as myxomas. The characteristic "dumbbell" shape seen in the ME four-chamber or ME bicaval view differentiates lipomatous hypertrophy from other structures. The appearance is caused by fatty infiltration of the atrial septum with *sparing* of the fossa ovalis (Figure 22.2).

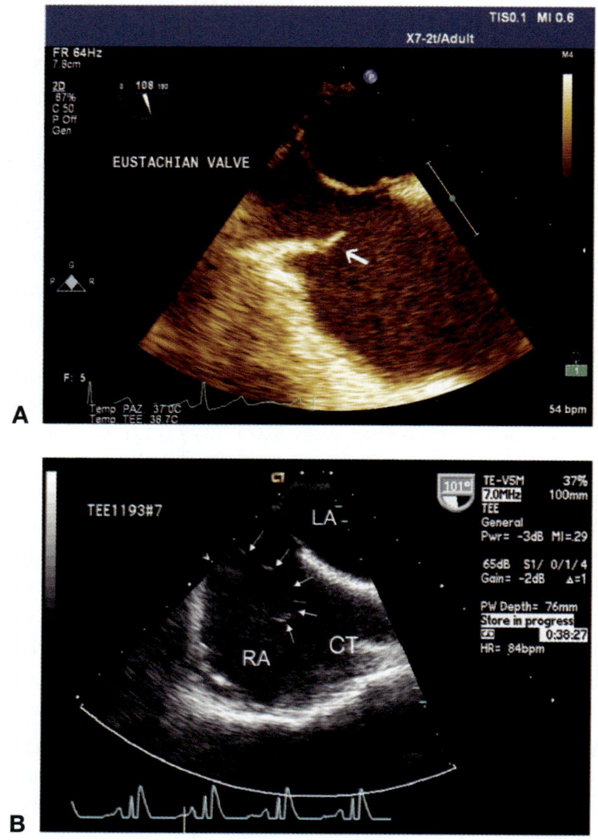

FIGURE 22.1 A: The eustachian valve is easily seen in this midesophageal bicaval view. B: A prominent Chiari network (arrows). CT, crista terminalis; LA, left atrium; RA, right atrium.

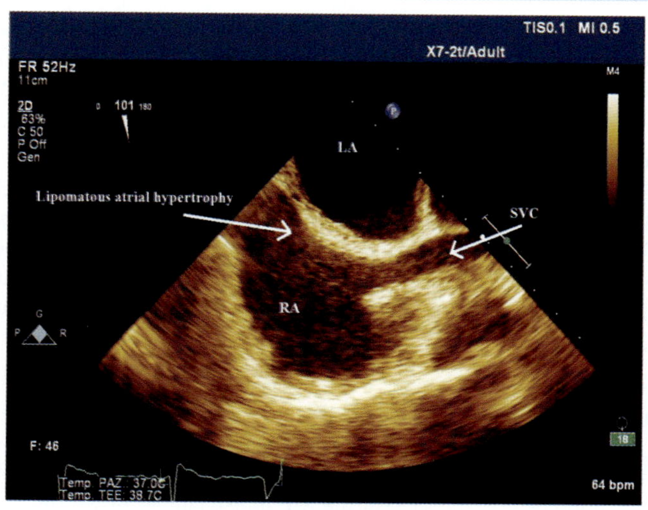

FIGURE 22.2 The characteristic dumbbell shape of a lipomatous atrial septum with sparing of the fossa ovalis is seen in this midesophageal bicaval view. LA, left atrium; RA, right atrium; SVC, superior vena cava.

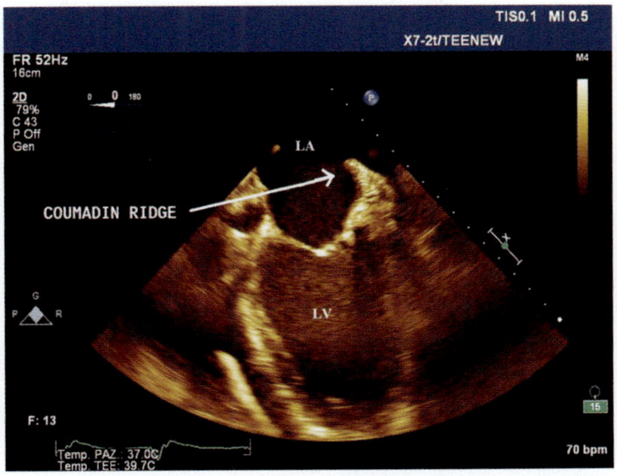

FIGURE 22.3 A Coumadin ridge is seen between the left atrial appendage and the left upper pulmonary vein (LUPV). LA, left atrium; LV, left ventricle.

Coumadin Ridge

A prominent muscle ridge is formed between the left atrial appendage and the atrial insertion of the left upper pulmonary vein. This prominence is often misdiagnosed as thrombus and is referred to as the *Coumadin ridge* or *"Q-tip" sign*. The lack of mobility and characteristic location, best seen in the ME two-chamber view, help distinguish it from an abnormal structure (Figure 22.3).

Pericardial Sinuses

Pericardial sinuses (or folds) between the atria and great vessels can give rise to echolucent spaces despite only minimal amounts of pericardial fluid. The transverse and oblique sinuses of the pericardium can easily mimic pericardial cysts or abscesses. Pericardial fat seen in these extracardiac structures can also mimic intracardiac thrombus (Figure 22.4).

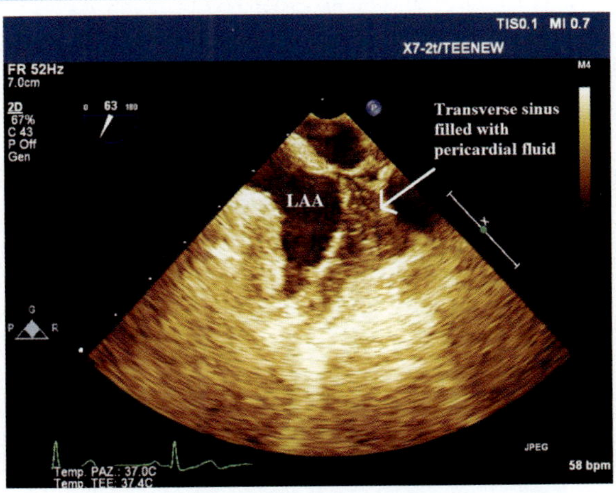

FIGURE 22.4 Transverse sinus filled with pericardial fluid can be seen in this midesophageal view at 60°. LAA, left atrial appendage.

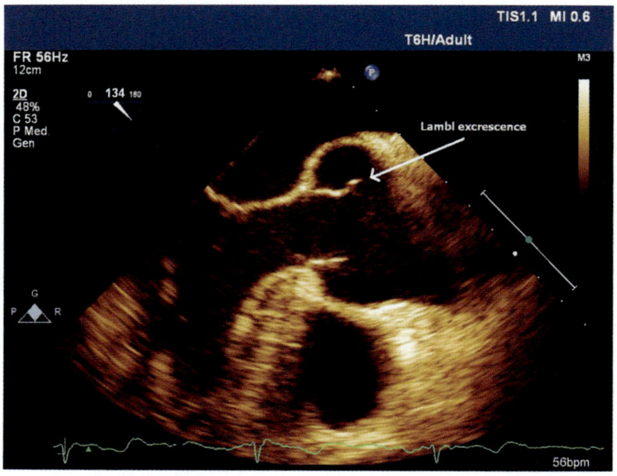

FIGURE 22.5 A Lambl excrescence is seen on the aortic valve (arrow).

Lambl Excrescences

Fine filamentous strands, Lambl excrescences, can be seen originating from the aortic valve of older adult patients. These structures can be differentiated from valvular vegetations by their characteristic "delicate" appearance in the absence of any clinical evidence of endocarditis (Figure 22.5).

Moderator Band and False Tendon

The moderator band of the right ventricle has been misinterpreted as an intracardiac mass (5). This specialized cardiac trabeculation runs from the right ventricular free wall to the interventricular septum. It is often best seen in the ME four-chamber view (Figure 22.6A). In contrast, a false tendon is an anatomic variant of the left ventricle consisting of fibromuscular string(s) coursing from the interventricular septum to the region about the papillary muscles (Figure 22.6B). They are best detected in ME longitudinal views and can be mistaken for subaortic membranes and pseudoaneurysms.

Pleural Effusion

Pleural effusions of the left side of the chest can mimic aortic dissection. In the descending aorta long-axis view, a pleural effusion will parallel the course of the aorta and have the appearance of a true lumen–false

A

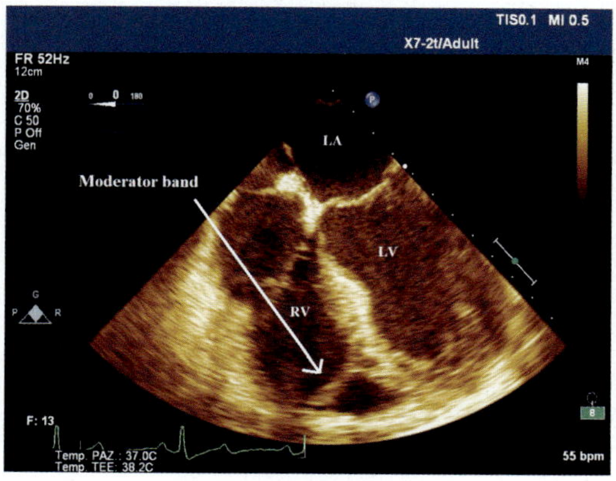

FIGURE 22.6 A: The moderator band of the right ventricle is seen in this midesophageal four-chamber view.

B
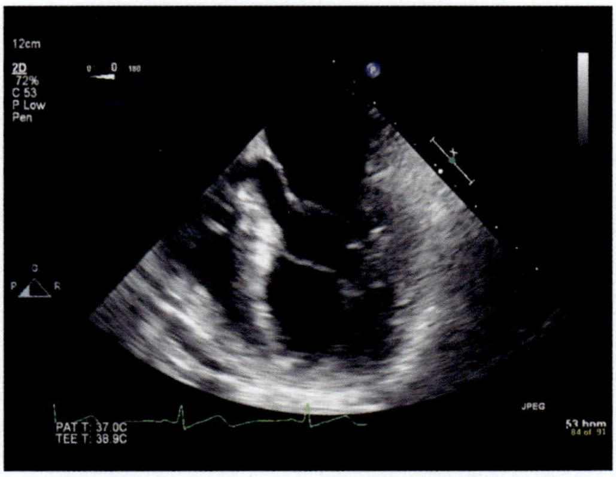

FIGURE 22.6 (*continued*) B: In contrast, a left ventricular false tendon. LA, left atrium; LV, left ventricle; RV, right ventricle.

lumen dissection. Changing to the descending aorta short-axis view and identifying the characteristic triangular shape of a left-sided pleural effusion easily confirm the diagnosis of effusion versus dissection (Figure 22.7). To inspect for a right-sided pleural effusion, the probe is turned progressively leftward from the descending aortic views to examine the right posterior chest.

TWO-DIMENSIONAL ECHOCARDIOGRAPHIC IMAGING ARTIFACTS

Suboptimal Image Quality

The inability to visualize cardiac structures because of suboptimal image quality remains a challenge in TEE diagnosis. Most commonly, improper settings of the ultrasound unit are to blame, but patient anatomy, acoustic interfaces (eg, air between the probe and the stomach or esophageal wall, hiatal hernia), and sonographer skill play definite roles. Adjustments in machine settings coupled with minor manipulations of the ultrasound probe can lead to substantial improvement of low-quality images. This topic is discussed further in Chapter 23: Techniques and Tricks for Optimizing Transesophageal Images.

Air between the transducer surface and tissue, more often encountered in transgastric (TG) views than in transesophageal views, causes severe image degradation to the point of complete inability to image. *Gastric suctioning before the TEE examination can rectify the poor acoustic transmission caused by an air-tissue interface.*

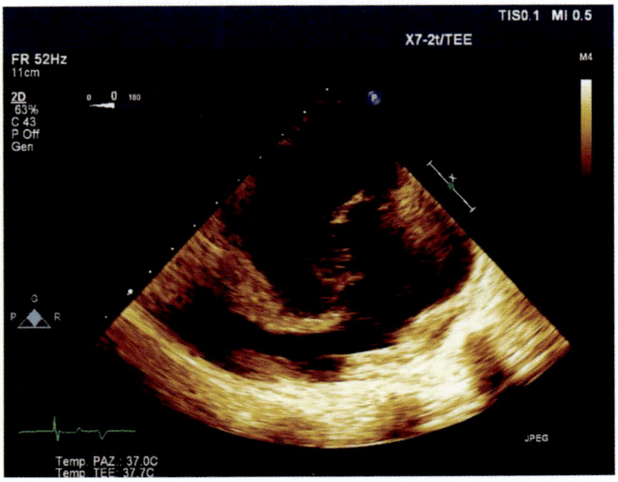

FIGURE 22.7 A pleural effusion is seen in a transverse plane.

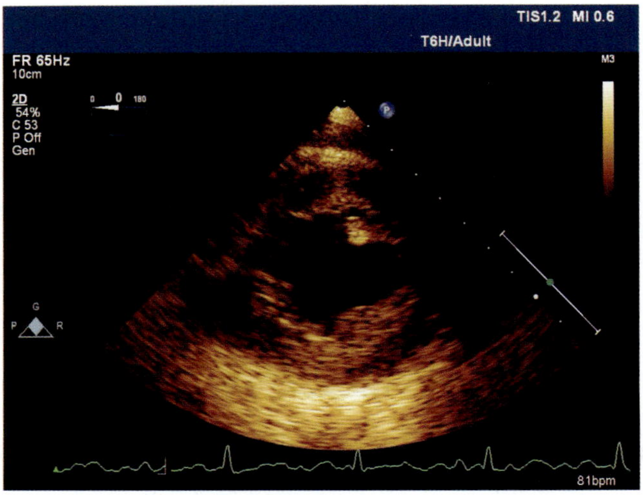

FIGURE 22.8 Transgastric mid short-axis view demonstrating septal and lateral wall dropout.

Imaging is also frequently suboptimal when the cardiac structure of interest lies parallel to the ultrasound beam. A common example of this artifact is "dropout" of the lateral and septal walls in the TG short-axis and ME four-chamber views (Figure 22.8). As specular reflections are maximized when tissue interfaces lie perpendicular to the ultrasound beam, this artifact is best overcome by repositioning the ultrasound probe to a more favorable vantage point. Another example of this phenomenon is the impaired ability to visualize thin linear structures, such as the chordae tendineae of the mitral valve, when they are parallel to the ultrasound beam (ME five-chamber view) (Figure 22.9A). However, when these structures are interrogated perpendicular to the beam (eg, TG two-chamber view), they are easily visualized (Figure 22.9B).

Acoustic Shadowing

Acoustic shadowing occurs when the ultrasound beam meets an interface of two structures with marked differences in acoustic impedance. Common examples include structures with a high level of acoustic impedance, such as calcific aortic or mitral valves (Figure 22.10A).

A

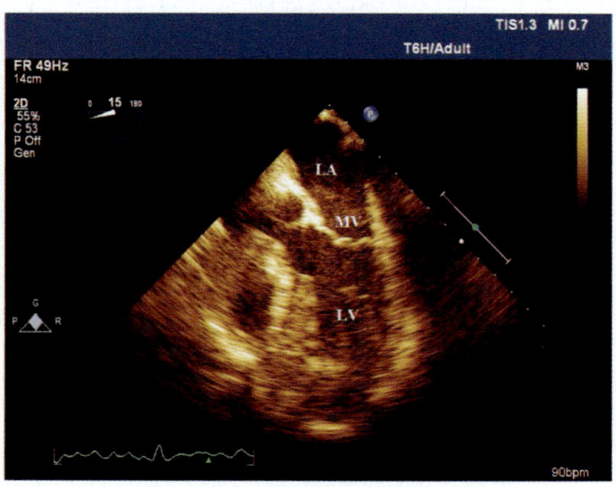

FIGURE 22.9 A: Mitral valve and apparatus imaged with chordae tendineae parallel to the ultrasound beam (midesophageal five-chamber view).

B
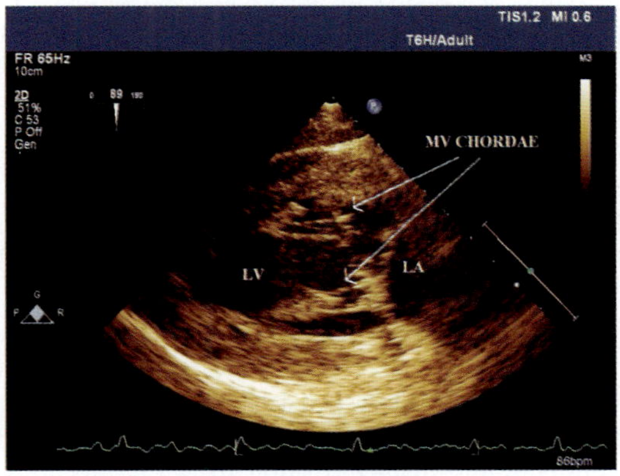

FIGURE 22.9 (*continued*) B: Markedly improved delineation of the chordae tendineae with the ultrasound beam perpendicular to the chordae tendineae (transgastric long-axis view). LA, left atrium; LV, left ventricle; MV, mitral valve.

A
B
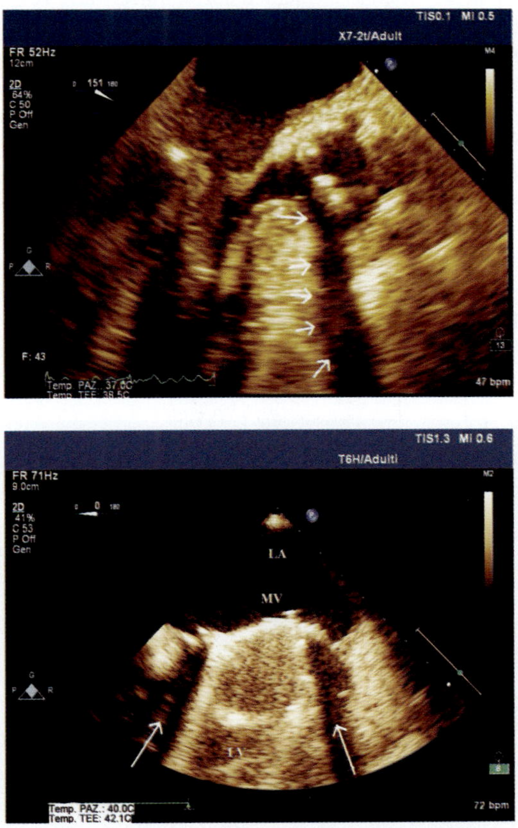

FIGURE 22.10 A: In this view a broad area of the distal scan is not visible due to shadowing from a calcific aortic valve (arrows). B: Acoustic shadowing caused by a prosthetic mitral valve ring imaged in the midesophageal four-chamber view. The arrows point to the long axial shadows. LA, left atrium; LV, left ventricle; MV, mitral valve.

Such structures strongly reflect and scatter the ultrasound signal, thereby limiting distal penetration of the sound waves. Similarly, mechanical prostheses and the struts of bioprosthetic valves produce shadowing. The resultant image reveals an echo-dense structure with a lack of signal in the sector beyond the structure (Figure 22.10B).

Lateral Resolution

The 2D image is created from a series of individual ultrasound beams or scan lines. Since structures lying between any two beams are not interrogated, the machine creates their display by averaging information received from the adjacent beams. This causes two problems. First, determinations of the size of a structure between beams (lateral resolution) are never as precise as measurements made along the beam's path (axial resolution). Consequently, most systems' axial resolution is at least twice the lateral resolution. Second, with sector scans, the ultrasound scan lines are closest to each other in the near field and the distance between them increases with increasing depth. Since this results in decreasing lateral resolution with increasing depth, while axial resolution remains constant, shape distortion artifact occurs. This typically appears as a lateral stretching of small, strongly echogenic objects, such as intracardiac catheters, bubbles, or wires. Round structures, such as intracardiac contrast agents or air, appear markedly elongated, as seen in Figure 22.11.

Side Lobe and Beam Width

Side lobes are weak beams emitted outside the path of the main ultrasound beam. Although weak, when they encounter an echo-dense structure such as a calcified aorta, mitral valve ring, or any prosthetic material or catheter (Figure 22.12A), the resulting reflection can be strong enough to be detected. When this occurs, the scanner misplaces these echoes in the image, incorrectly assuming they were generated by structures lying in the path of the main beam. The artifact is displayed at the appropriate distance from the transducer but at the wrong lateral position. Since the ultrasound beam sweeps the entire scan sector, side lobe artifacts often appear as narrow, curvilinear densities smeared over the entire scan sector.

Beam width artifacts differ from side lobe artifacts in that they are produced by the main ultrasound beam itself. They occur because each display pixel is generated from the data produced by a 3D, cone-shaped ultrasound wave. Thus, structures adjacent to the beam's center (in the lateral or elevational planes) that lie *within* the cone-shaped main beam are displayed. This creates artifacts that appear as structures or catheters in the wrong position, flaps in the aorta (Figure 22.12B), or elongated structures. Beam width artifacts also occur with spectral Doppler and are discussed later.

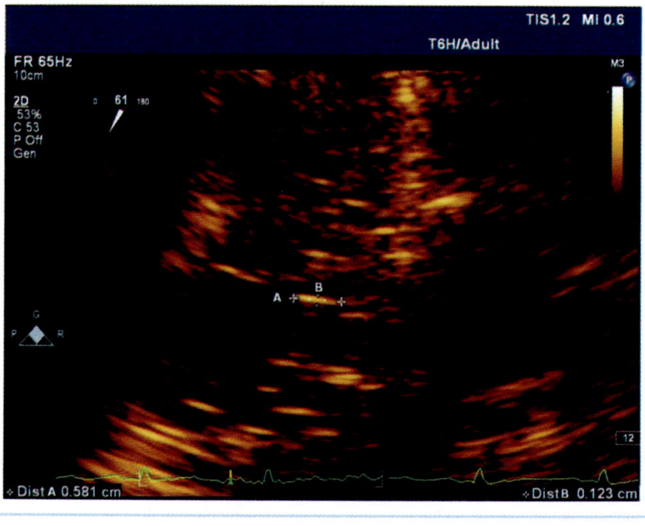

FIGURE 22.11 Discrepancy between axial and lateral sizes of microbubbles as a consequence of resolution artifact. Dist A and Dist B indicate lateral and axial dimensions, respectively.

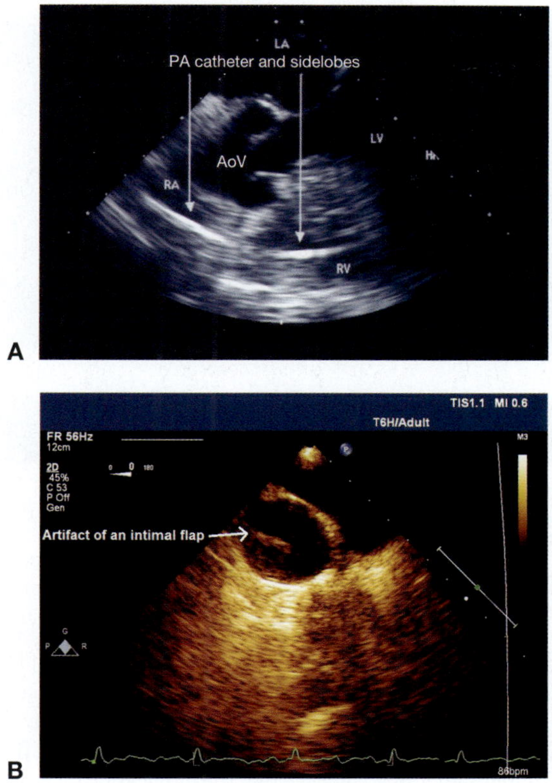

FIGURE 22.12 A: Side lobe artifact from a pulmonary artery catheter appearing as an echo-dense bright linear structure. B: A beam width artifact of aortic wall imaged in the ascending aorta. AoV, aortic valve; LA, left atrium; LV, left ventricle; RA, right atrium; RV, right ventricle.

Reverberation and Mirroring

Reverberations are caused by the repeated back-and-forth reflection of an ultrasound wave between two strong specular reflectors. This phenomenon leads to two types of imaging artifacts. In the first, multiple linear densities are produced in the area of the imaging sector distal to the reflecting structures (Figure 22.13). The second type of artifact occurs when the strong echoes are reflected from the transducer itself. The reflection

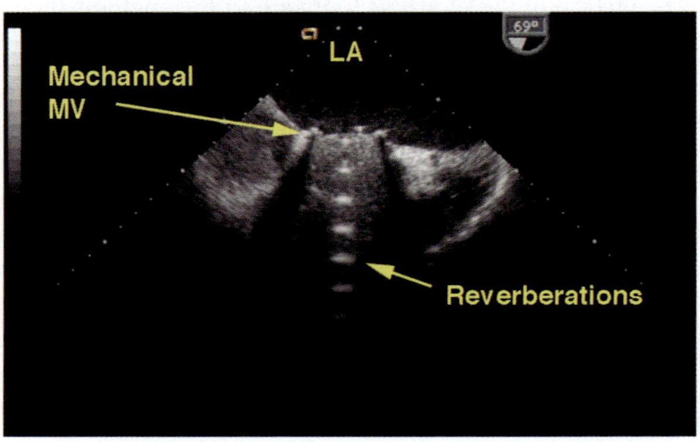

FIGURE 22.13 Reverberation artifact resulting from a mechanical mitral valve is easily seen distal to the valve. LA, left atrium; MV, mitral valve.

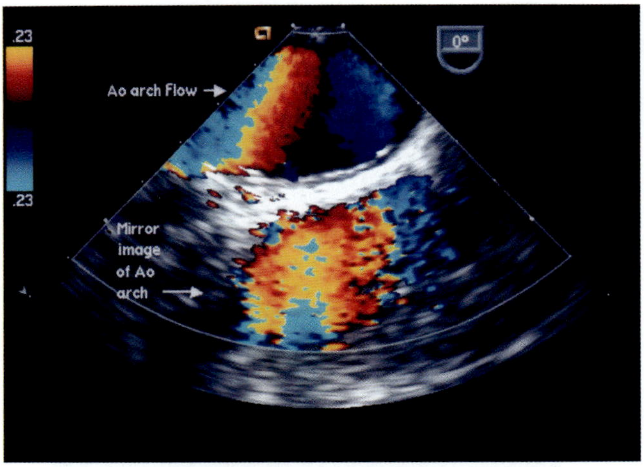

FIGURE 22.14 A mirror image of the true aortic arch is seen in the far field. Note that the false arch is the same size as the true structure. The color flow Doppler signals are also duplicated. Ao, aorta.

then travels back to the same target, where it is echoed a second time toward the detecting transducer. As a result, an artifact is produced that appears as a duplication or "mirror image" of the structure in the far field. Since this second trip doubles the travel time, the target structure is imaged once at the correct distance and a second time at twice the distance from the transducer. The descending thoracic aorta in both the transverse and longitudinal scans is a common source of this type of reverberation artifact. The vessel is imaged correctly in the near field and falsely duplicated immediately below. The duplicating reverberation artifact also extends in this case to color flow imaging (Figure 22.14).

Electronic Noise

Electronic noise, of which electrocautery is the major source, causes an imaging artifact that resembles a "snowed image" pattern. Viewing cardiac anatomy through this snowstorm is an annoying reality of echocardiographic imaging during surgery (Figure 22.15).

ARTIFACTS IN SPECTRAL AND COLOR FLOW DOPPLER

Spectral and color flow Doppler are susceptible to several of the mechanisms of artifact production that occur in 2D imaging; however, the appearance of the artifacts is quite different. In addition, the Doppler examinations are susceptible to a number of artifacts unique to this method such as aliasing and artifacts that result from incorrect alignment between the ultrasound beam and blood flow (6).

Aliasing

A shortcoming of pulsed-wave Doppler systems, which includes color flow Doppler, is that the maximal blood velocities that can be accurately quantified are limited by the pulse repetition frequency. Specifically, any Doppler frequency shift greater than one-half of the pulse repetition frequency, known as the *Nyquist limit*, results in a distorted spectral signal. The distortion in the Doppler signal, called ***aliasing***, causes several types of artifacts in the pulsed-wave spectral signal or color flow map. Common examples include "wraparound" of the spectral signal (see Figure 5.10) and red-blue stippling on the color flow map (see Figure 5.14).

Acoustic Shadowing in Color Flow

Strong specular reflectors result in acoustic shadowing not only with 2D imaging but also with Doppler modes. This artifact can be misinterpreted as a lack of blood flow in the shadowed region and is commonly seen during the interrogation of prosthetic or heavily calcified valves (Figure 22.16).

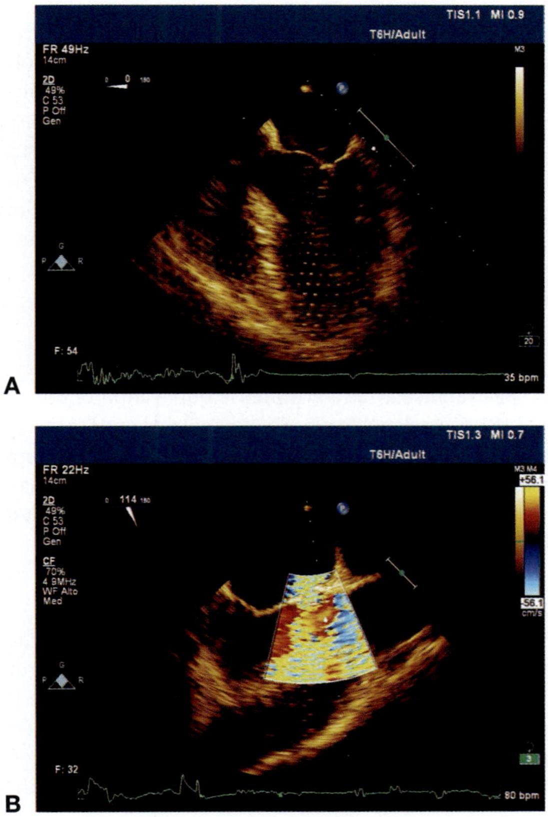

FIGURE 22.15 A: Electrocautery artifacts in the midesophageal five-chamber view. B: Electrocautery interference with color Doppler shown in a midesophageal long-axis view.

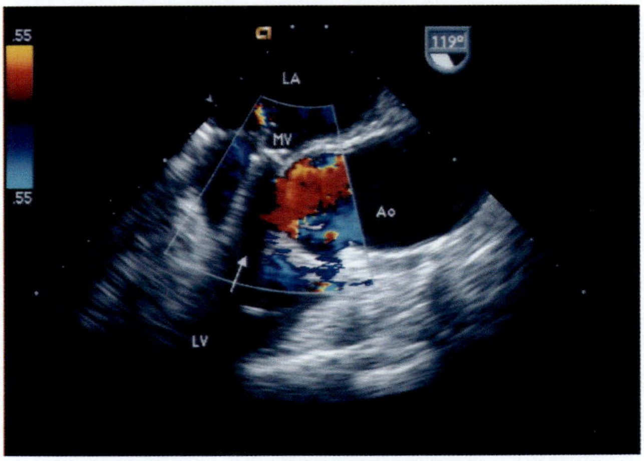

FIGURE 22.16 Acoustic shadowing in color flow Doppler caused by a prosthetic mitral valve ring in the midesophageal aortic valve long-axis view. The arrow points to the long axial shadow. Ao, aorta; LA, left atrium; LV, left ventricle; MV, mitral valve.

Nonparallel Beam Angle

Since the Doppler shift is proportional to the cosine of the angle between the path of the ultrasound beam and that of the blood flow, blood flow velocities are underestimated when the orientation of the ultrasound beam is not parallel to the blood flow. With color flow Doppler, this artifact typically occurs when the course of a vessel is oblique to the ultrasound beam. The blood flow perpendicular to the path of the Doppler beam is color-coded black (ie, no flow). Also, as the Doppler beam sweeps across the imaging sector, it intersects the blood path at varying angles, causing a peculiar artifact in the color flow map. For example, if the blood flow in an artery is directed from left-to-right across the ultrasound sector, the color mapper will characterize the flow in the left side of the sector red (ie, directed toward the transducer) and the blood flow in the right side of the sector blue (ie, moving away from the transducer). Therefore, an image is created in which it appears as if the blood were colliding in the middle portion of the vessel (Figure 22.17).

Mirroring

This artifact appears in the spectral display as a symmetric duplication of the actual flow signal, but in the opposite direction (Figure 22.18). It is related to a process known as *quadrature phase demodulation*, which allows the echo system to separate the Doppler-shifted signal from the complex returning signal. The demodulation procedure uses a second, weaker signal that is generated out of phase with the broadcast signal. However, excessive gain in the system causes the weak but incompletely canceled signal to be displayed as a mirror image of the actual flow signal.

Color Flow Reverberation and Gain-Related Anomalies

As discussed previously, reverberations are secondary reflections that occur when ultrasound is reflected a second time, typically from the transducer, highly reflective tissue, or intracardiac materials (eg, a pulmonary artery catheter). In the case of secondary reflections from the transducer face, a ghost of the primary image often appears at twice the distance of the actual target from the transducer, hence the term "mirror image." With Doppler reverberation, the reflected signal from a moving target is stronger than the original signal, so that the color intensity of the ghost is increased in comparison with that of the primary target (Figures 22.14 and 22.19).

Beam Width Flow Artifacts

The 2D image is actually constructed from 3D volumetric ultrasound signals. Just as beam width artifacts can occur in the 2D image, it also becomes possible to detect blood flow lying outside the displayed 2D image.

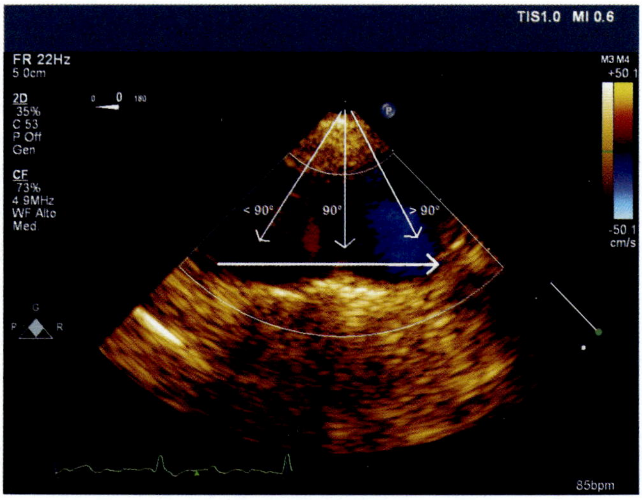

FIGURE 22.17 Nonparallel beam angle color flow Doppler artifact in the aortic arch. The direction of blood flow is indicated by the horizontal arrow. The angled arrows indicate the direction of the Doppler ultrasound interrogating beam.

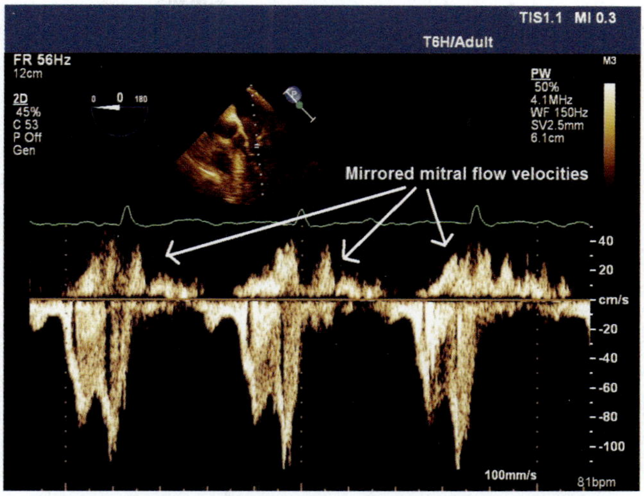

FIGURE 22.18 Pulsed-wave Doppler mirroring artifact. Transmitral flow and its weaker mirrored signal.

An example of this phenomenon is shown in Figure 22.20A, in which interrogation of the interventricular septum reveals high-velocity flow. This is not the result of a ventricular septal defect but an artifact caused by blood flow in the left ventricular outflow tract, which lies in a plane just anterior to the TG short-axis view seen in Figure 22.20B.

Range Ambiguity With Pulsed-Wave Doppler

One of the main advantages of pulsed-wave Doppler is the ability to range gate a sample volume. However, strongly reflected signals originating from blood flow at 2 or 3 times the depth of the pulsed-wave sample volume arrive at the transducer simultaneously with those produced from subsequent pulse signals reflected from the target. This artifact is particularly problematic when high-pulse–repetition frequency Doppler is employed. These signals are displayed and can be misinterpreted as blood flow within the target volume (Figure 22.21).

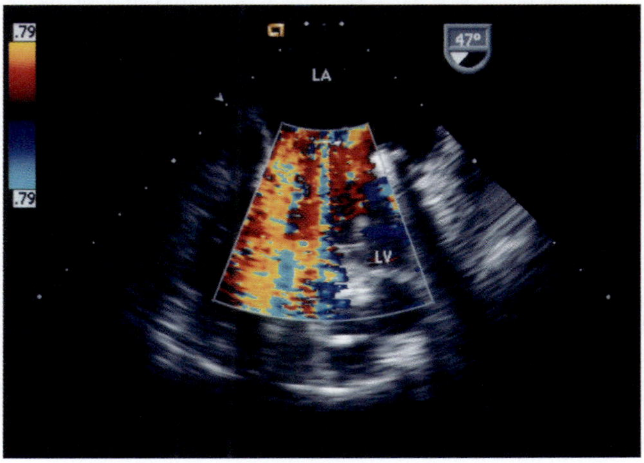

FIGURE 22.19 Color flow Doppler reverberations are seen distal to a mechanical mitral valve in this midesophageal commissural view. LA, left atrium; LV, left ventricle.

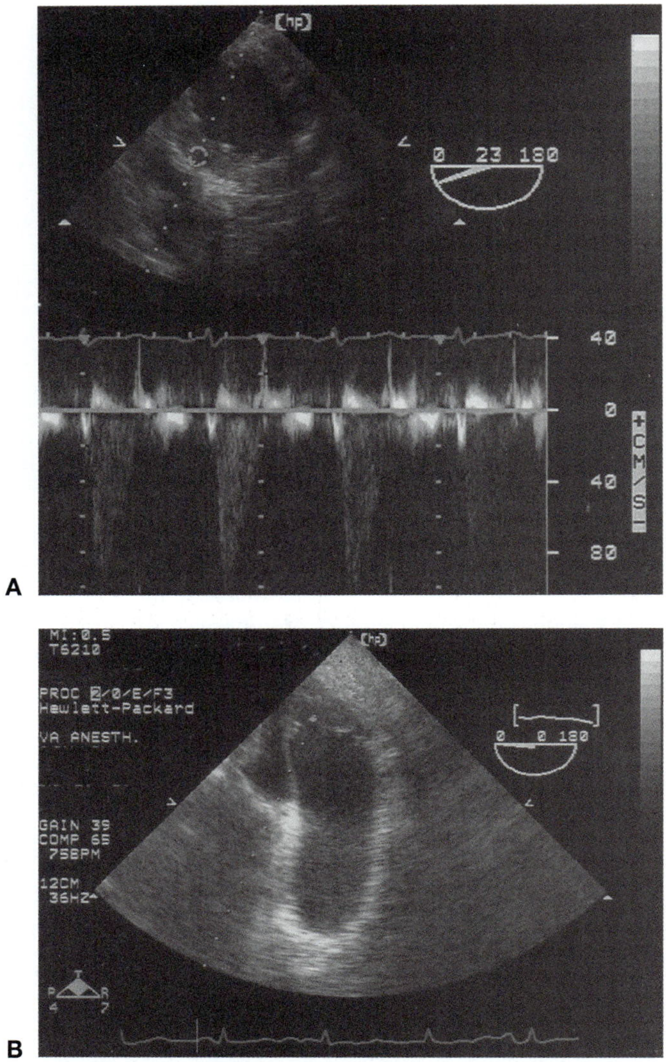

FIGURE 22.20 A: From the transgastric (TG) mid short-axis view, the pulsed-wave sample volume is shown placed on the interventricular septum. Spectral signals show high-velocity flow during systole. This is not caused by an interventricular septal defect; rather, it is an artifact of blood flow from the adjacent left ventricular outflow tract (LVOT), which lies just anterior to the imaged plane. B: With slight anteroflexion of the probe, the LVOT is visualized in the deep TG long-axis view.

THREE-DIMENSIONAL ECHOCARDIOGRAPHIC IMAGING ARTIFACTS

3D imaging strongly depends on 2D imaging optimization, and thus the same types of artifacts affect it as in 2D-TEE. So as with 2D-TEE, the inability to visualize cardiac structures with 3D-TEE because of suboptimal image quality remains a challenge and depends on the settings of the ultrasound unit and sonographer skills. Of course, patient anatomy and acoustic interfaces also play a role in 3D-TEE. Reverberations, shadowing, gain variation, and electronic noise, of which electrocautery is the major source, all cause imaging artifacts on 3D images, and the mechanisms are the same as in 2D.

3D image acquisition on TEE can occur either in real-time (live) mode or electrocardiogram (ECG) gated over multiple heartbeats (see Chapter 21: 3D Transesophageal Echocardiography Imaging). Several mechanisms affecting 3D image acquisition and postprocessing cause artifacts that are unique to 3D-TEE.

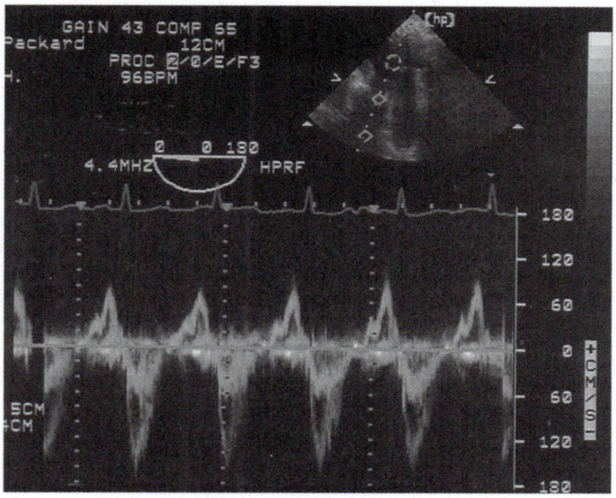

FIGURE 22.21 Top: In the deep transgastric long axis, the pulsed-wave Doppler sample volume is positioned at the tips of the mitral valve leaflets. Note that the left ventricular outflow tract and ascending aorta lie in the path of the beam in the far field. Bottom: The displayed pulsed-wave spectral signal shows not only the diastolic flow through the mitral valve but also the left ventricular outflow tract and aortic blood flow velocities during systole. These measurements of the far-field velocities are at exactly 2 and 3 times the distance to the primary measurement. HPRF, high-pulse–repetition frequency.

Artifacts Unique to Three-Dimensional TEE

The following artifacts are unique to 3D-TEE: reconstruction (stitching) artifacts, dropout artifacts, amplification (blurring) artifacts, and blooming artifacts (7) (Figure 21.4).

- *Stitching artifacts* are reconstruction artifacts typical of full-volume acquisition. A correct 3D image acquisition requires regular heart rhythm and no breathing/patient/probe movements to obtain the highest 3D spatial and temporal resolution. Therefore, arrhythmias, electrocautery, and patient (breathing activity or spontaneous movements) or probe movements will affect the ability to stitch together the subvolumes, leading to demarcation lines between the subvolumes (stitching artifacts), which distort the anatomic structures.
- *Dropout artifacts* typically appear as a lack of tissue on 3D images. The involved mechanism is a loss of ultrasound data due to poor echocardiographic signal strength. The dropout artifacts may be misinterpreted as anatomic abnormalities such as tissue defects or perforation. Interatrial septum and valve leaflets (more typically aortic valve leaflets) are vulnerable to dropout artifacts, leading to misdiagnosis of septal defect or valve perforation.
- *Amplification artifacts* result in anatomic structures appearing thicker than they actually are. This happens particularly with thin and elongated structures (ie, mitral valve chordae). These artifacts depend on the different orientations among axial, lateral, and elevation resolutions, which produce "nonisotropic voxels." Depending on which of the resolutions are used to generate the 3D image, an elongated and thin structure may appear increased in size.
- *Blooming artifact* refers to the appearance of fringes beyond the borders of metallic structures when they are met by ultrasound. More often this artifact may be seen in mechanical bileaflet valve prosthesis.

SUMMARY

Recognizing and understanding common artifacts and pitfalls in clinical echocardiography is fundamental to the accurate interpretation and effective use of this powerful diagnostic tool. As we have seen, artifacts can arise from a range of factors, including technical limitations, patient anatomy, and equipment settings. Differentiating between true pathologic findings and artifacts demands both technical expertise and a critical eye. By incorporating a structured approach to image acquisition, optimizing settings, and routinely verifying findings, clinicians can minimize errors and improve diagnostic accuracy. Ultimately, a solid grasp of these common artifacts and potential pitfalls is essential for delivering reliable, high-quality assessments, and for preventing clinical errors that can impact patient care.

REFERENCES

1. Otto CM, Pearlman AS. *Textbook of Clinical Echocardiography*. Elsevier; 2022.
2. Feigenbaum H. *Feigenbaum's Echocardiography*. 8th ed. Lippincott Williams & Wilkins; 2015.
3. Pepi M, Tamborini G. Echocardiography artifacts: recognizing and avoiding misinterpretation. *Heart*. 2016;102(3):148-151.
4. Akcay M, Bilen ES, Bilge M, et al. Prominent crista terminalis: as an anatomic structure leading to atrial arrhythmias and mimicking right atrial mass. *J Am Soc Echocardiogr. 2007*;20(2):197.e9-e10.
5. De Cara JM, Lang RM, Pellikka PA, et al. Pitfalls in the echocardiographic assessment of the right ventricle. *J Am Soc Echocardiogr*. 2008;21(6):675-683.
6. Rittgers SE. Signal processing of Doppler information. *Echocardiography*. 1987;4(1):7-14.
7. Faletra FF, Ramamurthi A, Dequarti MC, et al. Artifacts in three-dimensional transesophageal echocardiography. *J Am Soc Echocardiogr*. 2014;27(5):453-462.

QUESTIONS

1. **What is the most common type of imaging artifact?**
   A. Acoustic shadowing
   B. Reverberation
   C. Suboptimal image quality
   D. Mirroring

2. **Which of the following assumptions of the ultrasound (US) imaging system can be disrupted when artifacts occur?**
   A. The echoes travel in straight lines from the transducer.
   B. The echoes come back to the transducer after a single reflection.
   C. The time that the US wave employs to return to the transducer provides the distance between the transducer and the reflective structure.
   D. All of the above

3. **Acoustic shadowing can result from:**
   A. High attenuation
   B. Refraction
   C. Enhancement
   D. None of the above

4. **Acoustic shadowing will produce a dark area:**
   A. Proximal to the strong reflector
   B. Distal to the strong reflector
   C. Left of the strong reflector
   D. Right of the strong reflector

5. **Axial resolution artifacts occur when:**
   A. Two objects lying perpendicular to the main US beam are displayed as a single structure.
   B. Two objects lying parallel to the main US beam are displayed as a single structure.
   C. The US system employs shorter spatial pulse length.
   D. The US system employs shorter pulse duration.

6. **In most imaging systems, axial resolution is at least:**
   A. Equal to lateral resolution
   B. Twice the lateral resolution
   C. Ten times the lateral resolution
   D. Half of the lateral resolution

7. **The diameter of the US main beam impacts:**
   A. Temporal resolution
   B. The number of scan lines
   C. Axial resolution
   D. Lateral resolution

8. **The artifacts correlated to the lateral resolution are:**
   A. A double image of the object of interest
   B. A single image of two objects orientated perpendicular to the main beam
   C. Multiple equidistance bright signals
   D. None of the above

9. **Range ambiguity depends on the failure of which of the following fundamental assumptions?**
   A. The time that a single reflection employs to return back to the transducer only depends on the distance between the reflector and the transducer itself.
   B. The echoes detected by the system are those generated by the most recent pulse emitted by the transducer.
   C. A and B
   D. All the echoes are generated by the US main beam.

10. **Aliasing artifacts are typical of:**
    A. 2D US
    B. Color Doppler and pulsed Doppler
    C. Continuous-wave Doppler
    D. None of the above

11. **Which of the following factors are not related to aliasing in spectral Doppler imaging?**
    A. Pulse repetition frequency
    B. Nyquist limit
    C. "Wraparound"
    D. Lateral resolution

12. **The crista terminalis is located in the:**
    A. Right atrium
    B. Left atrium
    C. Right ventricle
    D. Left ventricle

13. **The moderator band is located in the:**
    A. Right atrium
    B. Left atrium
    C. Right ventricle
    D. Left ventricle

14. **The eustachian valve is located in the:**
    A. Right atrium
    B. Right ventricle
    C. Left atrium
    D. Left ventricle

15. **The Coumadin ridge is located in the:**
    A. Right atrium
    B. Right ventricle
    C. Left atrium
    D. Left ventricle

16. Which of the following statements is NOT true of a lipomatous atrial septum?
A. It has a dumbbell shape.
B. The fatty infiltration is echo dense.
C. The fossa ovalis is thickened.
D. The fossa ovalis is spared.

17. In an interrogation of flow with spectral Doppler, a nonparallel beam angle will:
A. Overestimate the true velocity.
B. Underestimate the true velocity.
C. Correctly measure the velocity.
D. Spectral Doppler does not measure velocities.

18. Side lobe artifacts:
A. Are true structures outside the path of the main beam
B. Are true structures in the path of the main beam
C. Are incorrectly displayed in the two-dimensional sector
D. A and C

19. Reverberation artifacts will not produce:
A. Multiple linear densities
B. Dual structures in an axial orientation
C. Dual structures in a left-right orientation
D. A duplication that is the same size as the original

20. The comet tails are atypical examples of:
A. Reverberation
B. Ringdown
C. Multipath
D. Mirroring

21. Dropout artifacts typically appear as:
A. A lack of tissue on 3D images
B. A lack of sound on Doppler signal
C. A drop of color pixels
D. None of the above

22. Blooming artifact more often occurs in:
A. In mechanical bileaflet valve prosthesis
B. Biologic calcified prosthesis
C. Guidewires
D. A+B

ANSWERS

1. Correct Answer: C.
Rationale: Ultrasound impacting interfaces with a high level of acoustic impedance often results in acoustic shadowing artifact.

2. Correct Answer: D.
Rationale: Refraction and reverberation disrupt assumptions A, B, and C.

3. Correct Answer: A.
Rationale: High attenuation results in low-energy US, resulting in acoustic shadowing distally.

4. Correct Answer: B.
Rationale: The shadow lies distal to the reflector as little US penetrates beyond it.

5. Correct Answer: B.
Rationale: Axial resolution affects imaging of objects parallel to the main US beam. Shorter pulse durations and short spatial pulse lengths improve axial resolution.

6. Correct Answer: B.
Rationale: Lateral resolution is related to the distance between scan lines, which is

greater than the pulse length, which defines axial resolution.

7. **Correct Answer: D.**
Rationale: Large diameter beams blur information across a greater lateral region, which decreases lateral resolution.

8. **Correct Answer: B.**
Rationale: Lateral resolution is related to objects lying perpendicular to the main beam in the axis of beam sweep (ie, between two scan lines) whereas axial resolution pertains to objects parallel to the beam.

9. **Correct Answer: C.**
Rationale: Returning echoes that derive from multiple reflections or are the result of strong reflections of prior pulses returning from greater depth can lead to range ambiguity.

10. **Correct Answer: B.**
Rationale: Aliasing artifacts relate to pulsed Doppler modalities (ie, pulsed Doppler and color Doppler) due to the Nyquist limit.

11. **Correct Answer: D.**
Rationale: Pulse repetition frequency and Nyquist limit determine the maximum velocity before aliasing of a signal. "Wraparound" is the classic spectral profile of an aliased signal.

12. **Correct Answer: A.**
Rationale: Crista terminalis is a muscular ridge in the right atrium.

13. **Correct Answer: C.**
Rationale: The moderator band is a trabeculation in the right ventricle.

14. **Correct Answer: A.**
Rationale: The Eustachian valve is an anatomic remnant found in the right atrium.

15. **Correct Answer: C.**
Rationale: The Coumadin ridge is located in the left atrium and can be misdiagnosed as thrombus.

16. **Correct Answer: C.**
Rationale: With lipomatous atrial septum, the fossa ovalis is typically normal giving it a dumbbell appearance.

17. **Correct Answer: B.**
Rationale: The Doppler equation calculates velocity as inversely proportional to the cosine of the beam angle of incidence with blood flow. As such, a nonparallel beam will lead to velocity underestimations unless the cosine factor is included.

18. **Correct Answer: D.**
Rationale: Side lobe artifacts are generated from interactions outside the path of the main beam, which are falsely displayed as if they were generated from structures along the main beam path.

19. **Correct Answer: C.**
Rationale: Reverberations are due to specular reflections along the beam path.

20. **Correct Answer: A.**
Rationale: Reverberations can lead to the characteristic multireflection comet tail appearance. Mirroring appears as a doubled image in the far field at twice the distance as the original.

21. **Correct Answer: A.**
Rationale: Dropout is an imaging artifact related to poor signal strength, resulting in images showing "holes" or volumes with lack of tissue.

22. **Correct Answer: A.**
Rationale: Strong reflections radiating from metallic valves result in 3D blooming artifacts. Calcified structures can result in acoustic shadowing artifacts.

23 Techniques and Tricks for Optimizing Transesophageal Images

Andrew Roscoe

When performing a transesophageal echocardiogram (TEE), image optimization is essential to give the sonographer the opportunity to clearly visualize pertinent structures in order to make an accurate assessment and the correct diagnosis. This chapter discusses the relevant machine "knobology" and settings to optimize image quality.

TWO-DIMENSIONAL IMAGING

Transducer Frequency

Modern echocardiography technology allows the sonographer to select from a range of TEE-transmitted frequencies. Higher-frequency ultrasound will give better axial resolution, but more attenuation will occur with reduced penetration to visualize structures further from the transducer. Conversely, lower-frequency ultrasound undergoes less attenuation, but provides poorer axial resolution. In addition, a higher-frequency transducer is associated with an increased focal depth and less divergence of the ultrasound beam, improving lateral resolution.

Depth

The depth control determines the maximal distance to be displayed on the image. Increasing the depth allows objects further from the transducer to be visualized, but decreases the size of the nearer structures and may reduce the frame rate, although this is less of a problem with newer systems with faster processing capabilities (Figure 23.1; Video 23.1A-D). To optimize the image, the depth should be limited to just beyond the structure of interest.

Sector Width

Using a maximal sector width of up to 90° displays a greater array of cardiac structures on the monitor for the sonographer to visualize and assess. However, the wider the sector, the slower the frame rate (Figure 23.2; Video 23.2A,B). When interrogating fast-moving structures, the sector width should be narrowed to maintain better temporal resolution.

Image Resolution

Axial resolution is the ability to distinguish two objects as separate entities parallel to the ultrasound beam. It is related to both spatial pulse length and transducer frequency. Axial resolution is improved by using a higher transmitted frequency.

Lateral resolution is the ability to distinguish two objects as separate entities perpendicular to the ultrasound beam. It is optimal when the ultrasound beam width is at its narrowest: the focal depth. A higher transmitted frequency causes less ultrasound beam divergence and improves lateral resolution. Some modern systems now offer "confocal" technology, which uses a "beamforming software algorithm" to optimize lateral resolution at all depths of the image.

Temporal resolution is the frame rate of the 2D image. In standard 2D imaging, the image is updated at 40 to 80 frames per second, which appears as "real time" to the human eye. When the frame rate decreases below 15 frames per second, the human eye can detect the image is not real time. Frame rate can be maximized by reducing the depth, sector width, line density, and the size of any color flow Doppler (CFD) window (Figure 23.3; Video 23.3A-D). Motion (M) mode provides the highest temporal resolution.

Focus

The focus (focal depth) is the point at which the ultrasound beam is at its narrowest, and thus lateral resolution is at its optimal. Structures proximal to the focal depth, in the near field (Fresnel zone), still appear

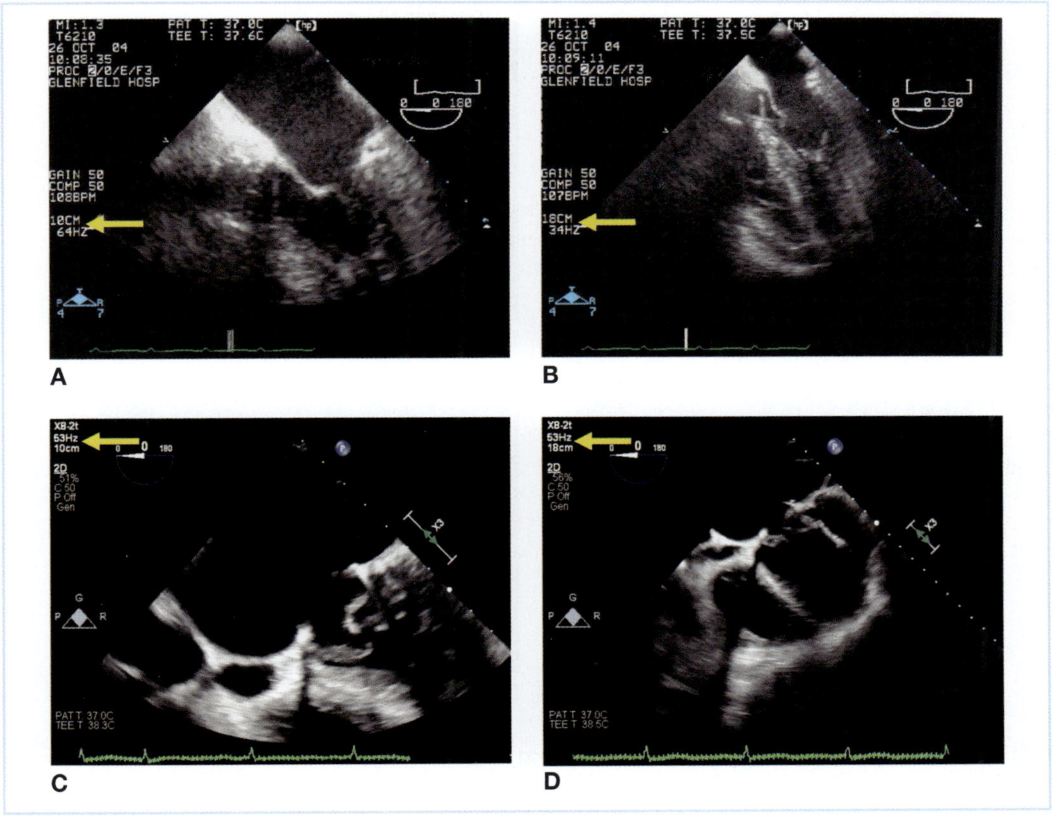

FIGURE 23.1 Midesophageal four-chamber view of the mitral valve, showing the effect of image depth on frame rate (arrow). A: Older system, 10 cm depth, frame rate 64 per second. B: Older system, 18 cm depth, frame rate 34 per second. C: Newer system, 10 cm depth, frame rate 53 per second. D: Newer system, 18 cm depth, frame rate 53 per second (see Video 23.1A-D).

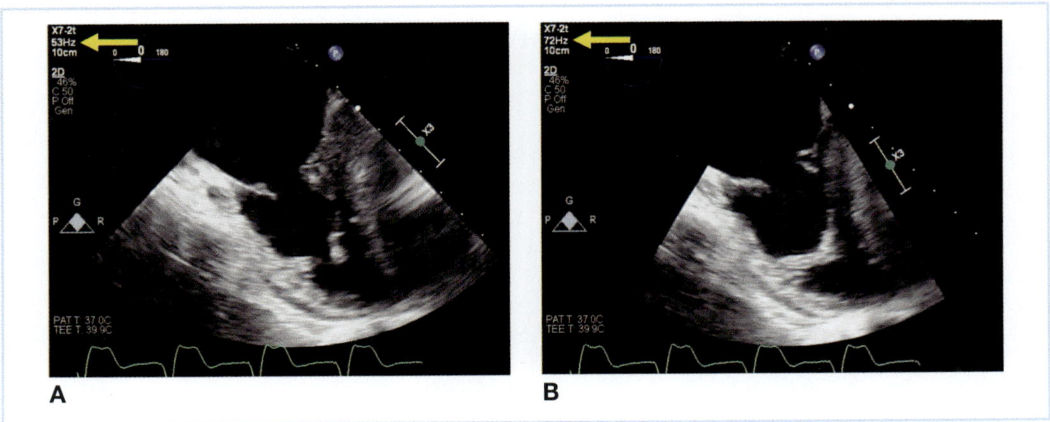

FIGURE 23.2 Midesophageal four-chamber modified view of the tricuspid valve showing the effect of sector width on frame rate frame rate (arrow). A: Full sector width, frame rate 53 per second. B: Narrowed sector width, frame rate 72 per second (see Video 23.2A,B).

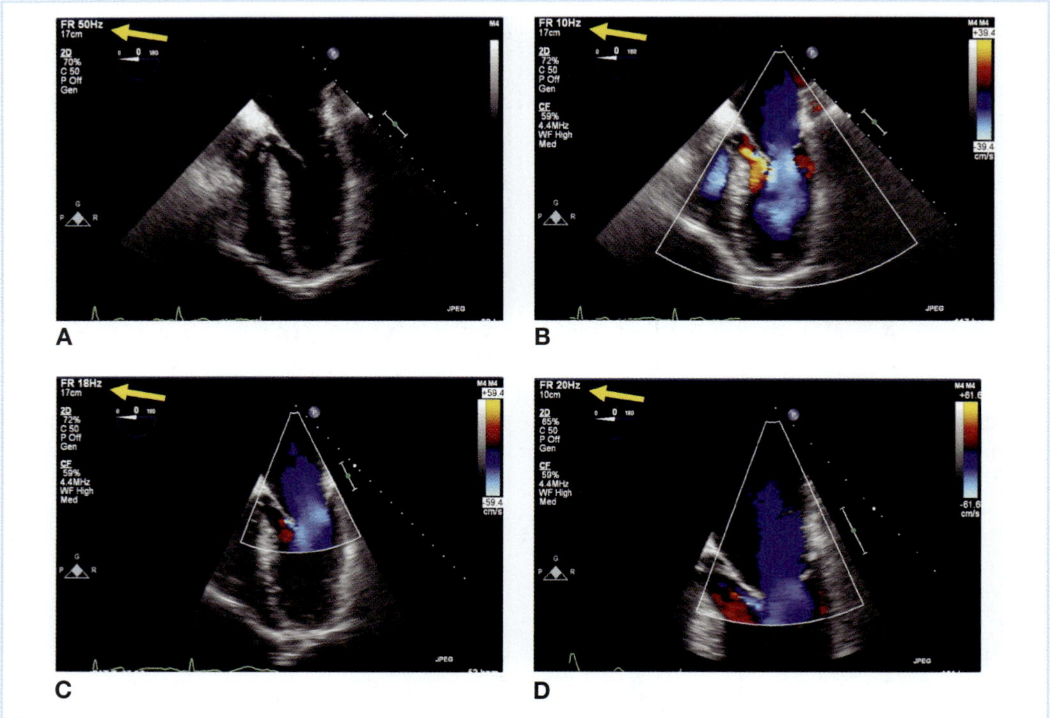

FIGURE 23.3 Midesophageal four-chamber view depicting factors affecting frame rate (arrow). A: 17-cm depth, frame rate 50 per second. B: 17-cm depth with large color flow Doppler box, frame rate 10 per second. C: 17-cm depth with reduced sector size and color flow Doppler box, frame rate 18 per second. D: 10-cm depth with reduced sector size and color flow Doppler box, frame rate 20 per second (see Video 23.3A-D).

clear, as the ultrasound beam remains relatively narrow. Structures beyond the focal depth, in the far field (Fraunhofer zone), typically appear less well defined, as the beam width diverges significantly and lateral resolution deteriorates. The focus should be positioned at the most appropriate depth to optimize the lateral resolution at the level of the structure being evaluated (Figure 23.4; Video 23.4A,B).

Zoom

The zoom feature allows the sonographer to magnify a specific region of the display monitor.

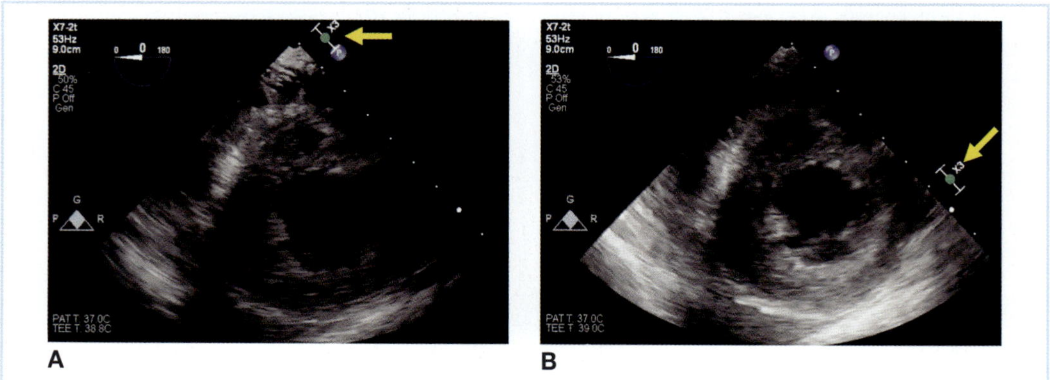

FIGURE 23.4 Transgastric short-axis mid-papillary view of the left ventricle showing the effect of *Focus* position (arrow) on image quality. A: *Focus* set in near field, resulting in reduced resolution in far field. B: *Focus* set in optimal position, resulting in improved resolution in far field (see Video 23.4A,B).

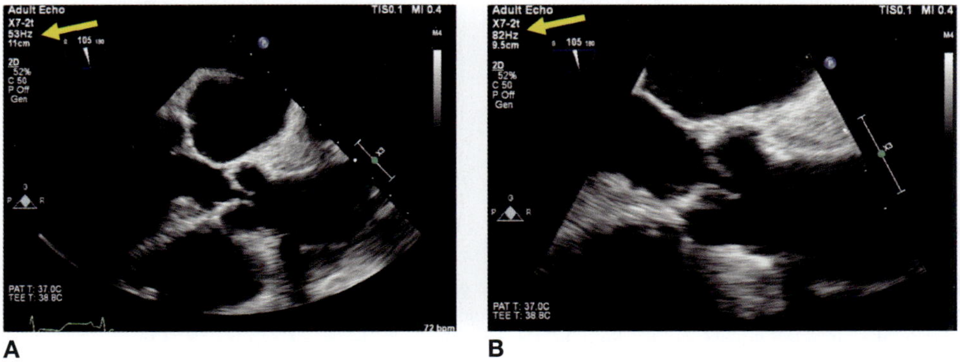

FIGURE 23.5 Midesophageal long-axis view of the aortic valve showing the effect of *Zoom* setting on frame rate (arrow). A: 11-cm depth, frame rate 53 per second. B: *Zoom* box over the aortic valve, frame rate 82 per second (see Video 23.5A,B).

In addition to aiding in the interrogation of the relevant cardiac structure, it will increase the frame rate (Figure 23.5; Video 23.5A,B).

Gain

The appropriate gain setting is important for the correct interpretation of the echocardiogram. Increasing the gain control will boost the amplitude of all ultrasound signals displayed on the monitor, including unwanted "noise" signals. In addition, both the duration and width of the displayed signals may be increased, impacting image resolution (1). The use of excessively high gain settings produces an overly bright image, linear structures may appear thickened, endocardial border definition is blurred, and spontaneous echocardiography contrast (SEC) may be erroneously diagnosed. Inadequately low gain settings result in returning signals of low amplitude not being displayed on the monitor, leading to nondetection of SEC and potential intracardiac thrombus (Figure 23.6; Video 23.6A-C). Typically, the gain control is set to the middle of the range, and minor adjustments are made according to the brightness of the display, the amplitude of the structures being interrogated, and the ambient light.

Time Gain Compensation

Time gain compensation (TGC) allows the sonographer to increase or decrease the amplitude of ultrasound signals returning from a specific depth in the display (Figure 23.7; Video 23.7A,B). Due to attenuation, signals returning from further away will naturally have a lower amplitude than those nearer to the transducer. Traditionally, the TGC controls were set to boost signals from the far field. However, more modern systems now account for this attenuation, and for most scanning, the controls can be set in a mid position. When there is a strong reflector close to the transducer, the TGC can be used to reduce the amplitude displayed in the near field.

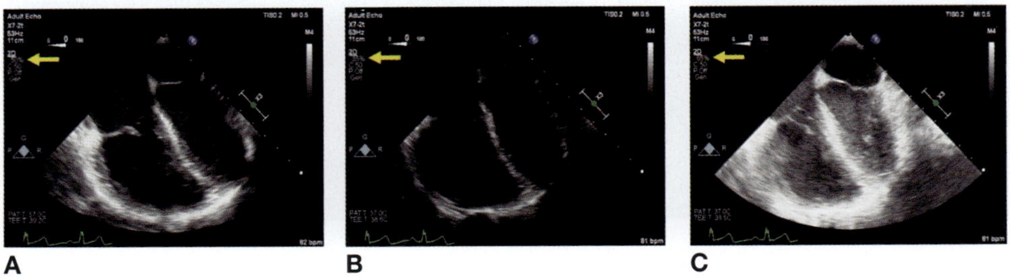

FIGURE 23.6 Midesophageal four-chamber view with different *gain* settings (arrow). A: Gain 50. B: Gain 35. C: Gain 65 (see Video 23.6A-C).

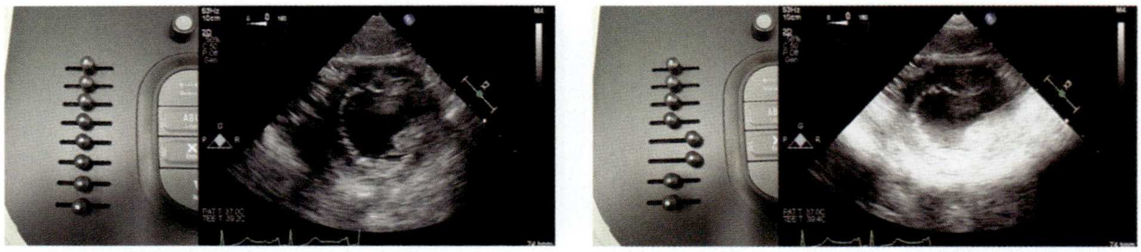

A B

FIGURE 23.7 Transgastric short-axis mid-papillary view of the left ventricle. A: *Time gain compensation* set to mid-position default setting. B: *Time gain compensation* sliding controls five and six shifted to the right, boosting the amplitude of the returning signal from the distal third quarter of the display (see Video 23.7A,B).

Lateral Gain Compensation

The lateral gain compensation (LGC) controls can be used to increase or decrease the amplitude of signals returning from different sectors on the display. It is occasionally used to boost weaker lateral signals to assist with endocardial border definition (Figure 23.8; Video 23.8A,B).

Compression

The compression control is a postprocessing setting that alters the range of gray scale on the display (1). Turning the dial clockwise increases the compression value on the monitor and increases the dynamic range: this results in more shades of gray, from black to white, being displayed on the monitor. Turning the dial anticlockwise will decrease the shades of gray shown, and the image will appear more "black and white" (Figure 23.9; Video 23.9A-C). Although the precise compression setting is a personal preference, extremes of compression should be avoided.

Harmonic Imaging

As an ultrasound wave passes through tissue, nonlinear propagation causes energy at the fundamental frequency (f_O) to be converted into its higher, harmonic frequencies ($2f_O$, $3f_O$, etc), particularly in the high-amplitude central part of the beam, but less so for the side lobes and artifacts. Harmonic imaging uses this phenomenon by displaying returning signals with the second harmonic energy ($2f_O$) and suppressing weaker artifactual echoes at the fundamental frequency (2). This effectively eliminates "noise" and produces a clearer image.

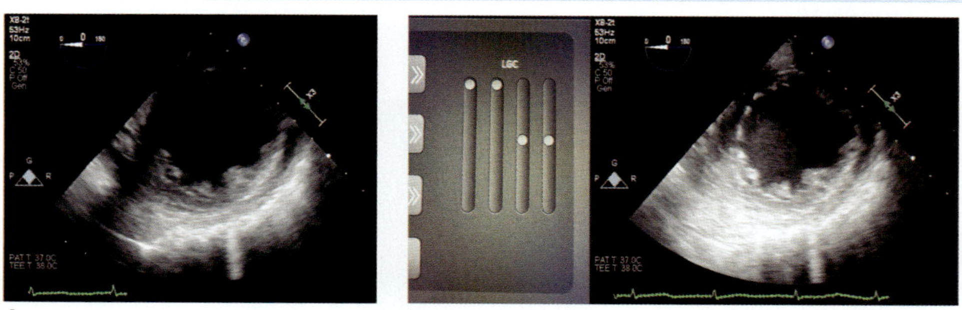

A B

FIGURE 23.8 Transgastric short-axis mid-papillary view of the left ventricle. A: *Lateral gain compensation* set to mid-position default setting. B: *Lateral gain compensation* boosting the signals returning from left sector, improving inferoseptal endocardial border visualization (see Video 23.8A,B).

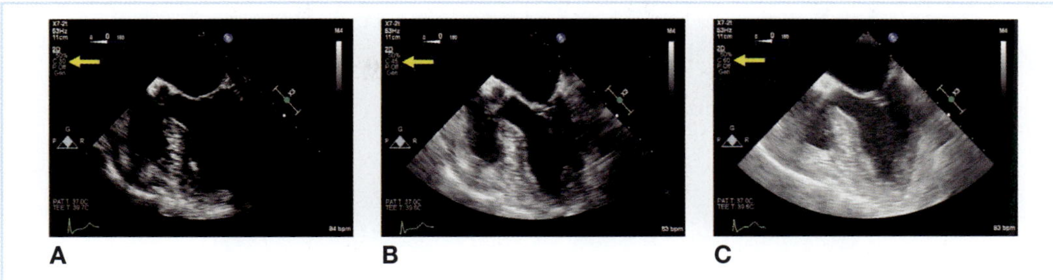

FIGURE 23.9 Midesophageal four-chamber view with different *compression* settings (arrow). A: Compression 30. B: Compression 45. C: Compression 60 (see Video 23.9A-C).

Contrast Imaging

Ultrasound-enhancing agents (UAEs) can be utilized to improve the contrast between different cardiac structures and evaluate real-time intracardiac blood flow. Applications include detection of patent foramen ovale, chamber opacification to identify intracardiac thrombus, and the enhancement of endocardial border definition. Signals reflected by the contrast microbubbles generate nonlinear, harmonic signals ($2f_O$), which increases the “contrast-to-tissue” signal ratio. Typically, a low mechanical index (MI) setting (<0.3) is selected to reduce contrast microbubble destruction (3).

DOPPLER IMAGING

Color Flow Doppler

When utilizing the CFD function, the *region of interest* CFD box should be limited to encompass only the relevant cardiac structures being interrogated. An oversized box will decrease the frame rate and significantly worsen temporal resolution.

The *color scale* displays the range of velocities encoded on the image. The highest and lowest velocities displayed represent the Nyquist limit. The color scale needs to be adjusted according to the structure being assessed: for evaluation of valvular heart disease, the Nyquist limit should be set at 50 to 70 cm/s (4); for interatrial septal defects, 35 to 40 cm/s (5); for other structures, it is important to appreciate the expected velocities of the blood flow to allow for optimal settings (Figure 23.10; Video 23.10A-C).

In specific situations, such as the calculation of proximal isovelocity surface area, the Nyquist limit is typically decreased (~30 cm/s) to produce aliasing, which creates an adequately sized flow convergence hemisphere (Figure 23.11; Video 23.11). Moving the CFD box further from the transducer into the far field may cause the Nyquist limit to decrease, as the pulse repetition frequency is reduced.

Increasing the *color gain*, like the 2D *gain* function, will amplify returning signals. To optimize the color gain, it is increased until color speckles appear in areas of tissue and then decreased slightly until these

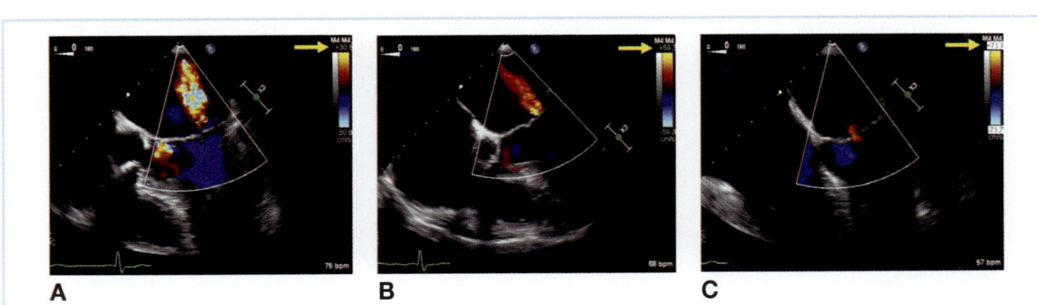

FIGURE 23.10 Midesophageal four-chamber view with color flow Doppler depicting the effect of Nyquist limit (arrow) on the size of the mitral valve regurgitation jet. A: Nyquist limit 30 cm/s. B: Nyquist limit 59 cm/s. C: Nyquist limit 71 cm/s (see Video 23.10A-C).

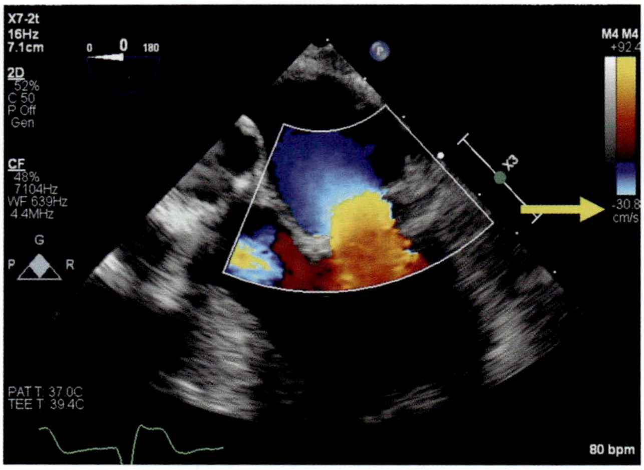

FIGURE 23.11 Midesophageal four-chamber view with color flow Doppler interrogation of the mitral valve. The color scale baseline has been shifted to decrease the Nyquist limit to 30 cm/s (arrow) in the direction of blood flow away from the transducer, to create aliasing of the flow convergence, and allow calculation of the proximal isovelocity surface area (see Video 23.11).

speckles disappear. When color gain is set too high, the size of regurgitant jets may be overestimated; when set too low, the jet size will be underestimated (Figure 23.12; Video 23.12A-C).

Variance color flow mapping shows the dispersion of velocities around the mean velocity by adding a green hue to the CFD image. It accentuates turbulent flow and may be used when attempting to identify small turbulent jets.

Spectral Doppler

A spectral Doppler display is obtained by implementing spectral analysis of the Doppler signal. As with any Doppler function, correct alignment of the ultrasound is paramount. Newer systems possess a feature that allows for correction of the angle of insonation if precise alignment is not feasible. *Pulse-wave Doppler* (PWD) is generally utilized for the lower velocity signals (<2 m/s) and will display blood flow at a specific location. The PWD sample volume envelope should be large enough to include the region of interest, but not so large that it will detect adjacent unwanted signals. *Continuous-wave Doppler* (CWD) can be used for very high-velocity signals, as it does not suffer from aliasing artifact. However, range ambiguity is a drawback.

The spectral Doppler *baseline* and *scale* settings should be adjusted to allow the whole of the returning signals to be displayed and maximized. As the returning backscatter signals from blood are generally lower than that of tissue, the spectral Doppler *gain* setting needs to be increased. However, increasing the gain will also amplify any background noise. In addition, when the *gain* is set too high, the system cannot accurately distinguish the direction of flow, generating a spectral mirroring artifact, where the true Doppler signal

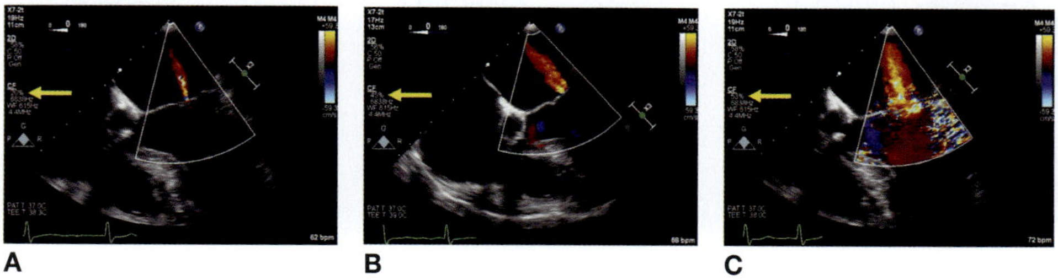

FIGURE 23.12 Midesophageal four-chamber view with color flow Doppler depicting the effect of *color gain* (arrow) on the size of the mitral valve regurgitation jet. A: color gain 20%. B: Color gain 45%. C: Color gain 53% (see Video 23.12A-C).

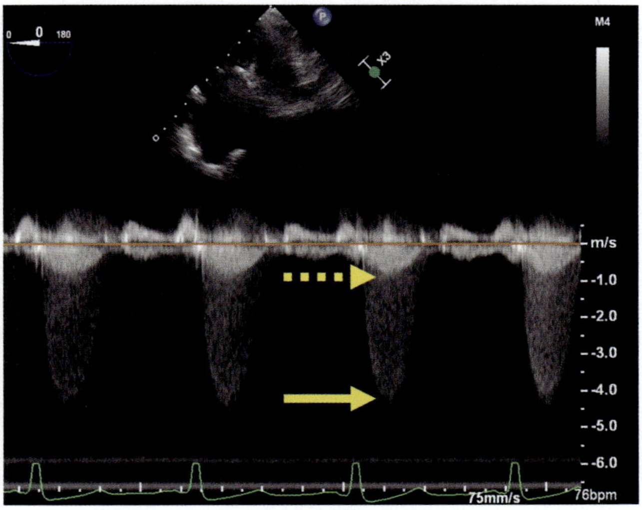

FIGURE 23.13 Spectral display of continuous-wave Doppler interrogation through the aortic valve in the deep transgastric view. *Gain* is reduced to show a double envelope: peak aortic valve velocity (arrow); peak left ventricular outflow tract velocity (dashed arrow).

appears in the reverse direction simultaneously (6). Decreasing the spectral gain setting can help to display the "double envelope" in CWD when evaluating left ventricular outflow and aortic valve Doppler velocities (Figure 23.13). The spectral gain must be adjusted for each individual spectral display.

THREE-DIMENSIONAL IMAGING

The first step in optimizing three-dimensional (3D) imaging is to obtain high-quality 2D images. Undergaining causes echo dropout, potentially eliminating important structures from the dataset. Overgaining reduces resolution and results in a loss of 3D perspective of the image. Ideally, the *gain* and *compression* settings should be set in the midrange, and the 2D image slightly overgained using the TGC settings, which allows for better postprocessing optimization (Figure 23.14; Video 23.13A-C).

3D volumes must encompass the whole of the structure being evaluated, but should be kept as small as feasible to maintain spatial resolution, without compromising temporal resolution.

For gated data sets, where sector slices are stitched together from consecutive beats, the electrocardiogram (ECG) is adjusted to ensure a prominent R wave is present, and a breath hold is recommended to reduce translational motion of cardiac structures, which may result in stitching artifacts on the 3D reconstruction (Figure 23.15; Video 23.14) (7).

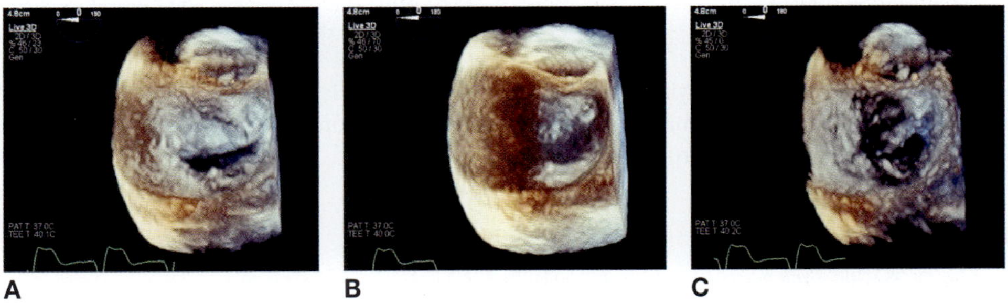

FIGURE 23.14 3D en face view of the mitral valve. A: Appropriate gain setting, allowing visualization of the mitral valve leaflets. B: High gain setting, causing mitral valve leaflets to be partly obscured. C: Low *gain* setting, causing dropout of anatomic structures (see Video 23.13A-C).

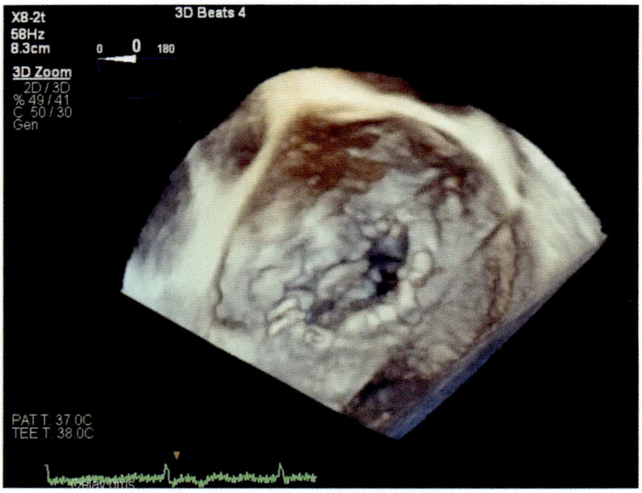

FIGURE 23.15 3D zoom en face view of the mitral valve, with four-beat acquisition, showing stitching artifact (see Video 23.14).

ARTIFICIAL INTELLIGENCE

Artificial intelligence (AI) is now being introduced into echocardiography with the goal of minimizing interobserver and intraobserver variability, facilitating the analysis of large data sets, and permitting imagers to perform and interpret exams with increased accuracy. Machine learning and more complex deep learning algorithms and convoluted neural networks can accurately perform pattern recognition and are being developed to assess contractility, diastolic function, and valvular diseases; to monitor disease progression; and to guide treatment options (Video 23.15).

The technology offers a means to minimize the variability between novice and expert readers and improve efficiency. Recently, after brief training, novices using AI software were able to successfully acquire sets of 10 cardiac images between 61% and 98% of the time. Although imaging success was less than that by trained sonographers, the authors concluded that AI software allowed qualitative analysis in 84% of images acquired by novices (8). Current AI technology, using automated border detection for calculating ejection fraction, is increasingly accurate for good to moderate images compared to manual tracing. Using a global longitudinal strain (GLS) model, the acquisition time is decreased from 5 to 10 minutes to 10 seconds as well as being able to detect more subtle changes in left ventricular ejection fraction. This has been used to assess patients undergoing chemotherapy as well as being fast and reproducible.

The application of AI is rapidly expanding within echocardiography. The ability of AI to guide image acquisition and analyze data holds great promise. As AI models are reliant on echocardiographers for image acquisition, current AI is used to assist manual acquisition, structure identification, and subsequent analysis (9).

SUMMARY

A good understanding of the underlying ultrasound and Doppler physics principles allows the echocardiographer to utilize the assortment of machine settings to appropriately optimize the image acquisition and to enhance the evaluation of cardiac structures.

REFERENCES

1. Weyman AE. *Principles and Practice of Echocardiography*. 2nd ed. Lea & Febiger; 1994:3-28.
2. Hoskins PR, Martin K, Thrush A, eds. *Diagnostic Ultrasound: Physics and Equipment*. 3rd ed. CRC Press; 2019:77-104.
3. Porter TR, Mulvagh SL, Abdelmoneim SS, et al. Clinical applications of ultrasonic enhancing agents in echocardiography: 2018 ASE guidelines update. *J Am Soc Echocardiogr*. 2018;31(3):241-274.
4. Zoghbi WA, Adams D, Bonow RO, et al. Recommendations for noninvasive evaluation of native valvular regurgitation. *J Am Soc Echocardiogr*. 2017;30(4):303-371.

5. Silvestry FE, Cohen MS, Armsby LB, et al. Guidelines for the echocardiographic assessment of atrial septal defect and patent foramen ovale. *J Am Soc Echocardiogr.* 2015;28(8):910-958.
6. Hoskins PR, Martin K, Thrush A, eds. *Diagnostic Ultrasound: Physics and Equipment.* 3rd ed. CRC Press; 2019:171-189.
7. Lang RM, Badano LP, Tsang W, et al. EAE/ASE recommendations for image acquisition and display using three-dimensional echocardiography. *J Am Soc Echocardiogr.* 2012;25(1):3-46.
8. Mor-Avi V, Khandheria B, Klempfner R, et al. Real-time artificial intelligence-based guidance of echocardiographic imaging by novices: image quality and suitability for diagnostic interpretation and quantitative analysis. *Circ Cardiovasc Imaging.* 2023;16(11):e015569.
9. Barry T, Farina JM, Chao CJ, et al. The role of artificial intelligence in echocardiography. *J Imaging.* 2023;9(2):50.

QUESTIONS

1. Compared to a higher-frequency transducer, a lower-frequency transducer will:
A. Provide better axial resolution
B. Provide better lateral resolution
C. Have an increased focal depth
D. Penetrate further into tissue with less attenuation

2. Axial resolution:
A. Improves with increased *gain*
B. Is the ability to distinguish two objects parallel to the ultrasound beam
C. Improves by decreasing transducer frequency
D. Improves with an increase in spatial pulse length

3. Temporal resolution is improved by:
A. Increasing sector width
B. Adding CFD box
C. Increasing line density
D. Reducing image depth

4. The following statements regarding the focal depth are all true except:
A. It is the point where the ultrasound beam is at its narrowest.
B. It is determined by transducer diameter.
C. It is not determined by transducer frequency.
D. It is the point where lateral resolution is optimal.

5. Increasing the gain setting:
A. May cause linear structures to appear thickened
B. Always improves image quality
C. Removed unwanted "noise" signals
D. Improved lateral resolution

6. The TGC control:
A. Can be used to decrease the brightness at a specific depth on the display
B. Can be used to boost the amplitude of a sector of the image
C. Improves lateral resolution distal to the focus
D. Affects the length of the Fresnel zone

7. Which of the following is true regarding the compression control:
A. Setting a high *compression* value creates a more "black and white" image on the display.
B. Can be used to reduce near-field clutter from a strong reflector
C. It is a postprocessing control.
D. Setting a low compression value can lead to misdiagnosis of spontaneous echo contrast.

8. Increasing the size of the CFD region of interest box:
A. Reduces temporal resolution
B. Increases the Nyquist limit
C. Decreases the *color gain*
D. Increases the *variance* on the color flow mapping

9. When using CFD to assess the interatrial septum for a patent foramen ovale defect, the recommended setting for the Nyquist velocity limit is:
A. 20 to 30 cm/s
B. 35 to 40 cm/s
C. 45 to 50 cm/s
D. 50 to 70 cm/s

10. Increasing the gain setting when using CWD:
A. Will result in overestimation of peak velocity
B. May cause spectral mirroring artifact
C. Will enhance double envelope evaluation of aortic valve stenosis
D. May increase the risk of aliasing artifact

ANSWERS

1. Correct Answer: D.
Rationale: A low-frequency transducer undergoes less attenuation and therefore penetrates further into tissue. However, it provides poorer axial resolution compared to a high-frequency transducer. Focal depth is determined by both transducer diameter and frequency:

Focal depth = $(\text{diameter})^2 \times (\text{frequency}/6)$.

Lateral resolution is determined by ultrasound beam width. A low-frequency transducer has a shorter focal depth and more beam divergence, leading to poorer lateral resolution.

2. Correct Answer: B.
Rationale: Axial resolution is the ability to distinguish two objects as separate entities parallel to the ultrasound beam. It is related to both transducer frequency and spatial pulse length. Axial resolution improves with higher-frequency ultrasound and shorter spatial pulse length.

3. Correct Answer: D.
Rationale: Temporal resolution can be maximized by reducing the depth, sector width, line density, and the size of any CFD window.

4. Correct Answer: C.
Rationale: The focus (focal depth) is the point at which the ultrasound beam is at its narrowest and thus lateral resolution is at its optimal. Focal depth is determined by both transducer diameter and frequency:

Focal depth = $(\text{diameter})^2 \times (\text{frequency}/6)$.

5. Correct Answer: A.
Rationale: The use of excessively high *gain* settings produces an overly bright image, linear structures may appear thickened, endocardial border definition is blurred, and SEC may be erroneously diagnosed. The *gain* setting has no effect on lateral resolution.

6. Correct Answer: A.
Rationale: The LGC controls can be used to increase or decrease the amplitude of signals returning from different sectors on the display. TGC allows the sonographer to increase or decrease the amplitude of ultrasound signals returning from a specific depth in the display. When there is a strong reflector close to the transducer, the TGC can be used to reduce the amplitude displayed in the near field. TGC has no effect on lateral resolution or focal depth.

7. Correct Answer: C.
Rationale: The *compression* control is a postprocessing setting that alters the range of gray scale on the display. Turning the dial clockwise increases the dynamic range and more shades of gray, from black to white, are displayed on the monitor. Turning the dial anticlockwise will decrease the shades of gray shown, and the image will appear more "black and white." Compression set very high, displaying many shades of gray, may lead to misdiagnosis of SEC in the cardiac chambers.

8. Correct Answer: A.
Rationale: When utilizing the CFD function, the *region of interest* CFD box should be limited to encompass only the relevant cardiac structures being interrogated. An oversized box will decrease the frame rate and significantly worsen temporal resolution. If increasing the size of the CFD box also moves the CFD box further from the transducer into the far field, then the Nyquist limit may

decrease, as the pulse repetition frequency is reduced.
The CFD box size has no effect on *color gain* or *variance* settings.

9. **Correct Answer: B.**
Rationale: The color scale needs to be adjusted according to the structure being assessed: for evaluation of interatrial septal defects, 35 to 40 cm/s: reference (5).

10. **Correct Answer: B.**
Rationale: Increasing spectral Doppler *gain* will amplify any background noise, and when the *gain* is set too high, the system cannot accurately distinguish the direction of flow, generating a spectral mirroring artifact, where the true Doppler signal appears in the reverse direction simultaneously. Decreasing the spectral gain setting can help to display the "double envelope" in CWD when evaluating left ventricular outflow and aortic valve Doppler velocities. CWD can be used for very high-velocity signals, as it does not suffer from aliasing artifact.

Appendices

A Cardiac Cross-Section Criteria

ME Asc aortic SAX	Probe adjustment: neutral	Sector depth: (~6 cm)
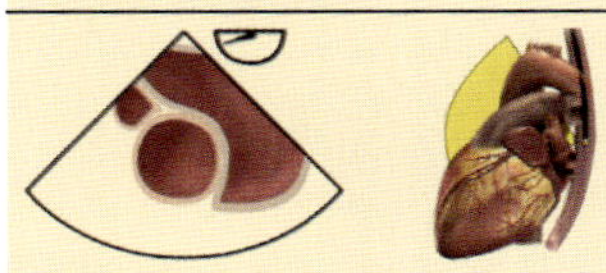	**Primary diagnostic issue(s)** Aortic atherosclerosis Aortic dissection Pulmonary artery pathology (emboli, dilation, etc)	**Required structures** Aorta in cross section in transverse plane (0°) Pulmonary artery (main and proximal right)
ME right pulmonary vein	Probe adjustment: neutral	Sector depth: (~6 cm)
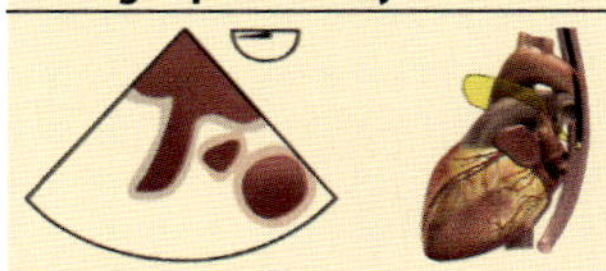	**Primary diagnostic issue(s)** Spectral PW Doppler interrogation of right upper pulmonary vein	**Required structures** Right atrium Right pulmonary veins Superior vena cava
ME Asc aortic LAX	Probe adjustment: neutral	Sector depth: (~6 cm)
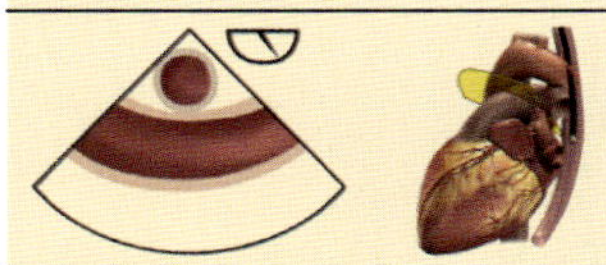	**Primary diagnostic issue(s)** Aortic atherosclerosis Aortic dissection	**Required structures** Ascending aorta in long axis Right pulmonary artery in cross section
ME AV SAX	Probe adjustment: neutral	Sector depth: (~10 cm)
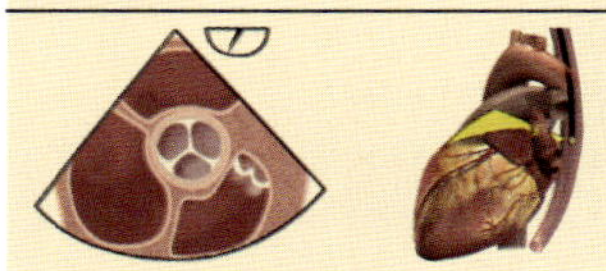	**Primary diagnostic issue** Aortic stenosis Valvular morphology	**Required structures** Aortic valve Superior intra-atrial septum Left and right atrium RV outflow tract
ME RV inflow-outflow	Probe adjustment: neutral	Sector depth: (~10 cm)
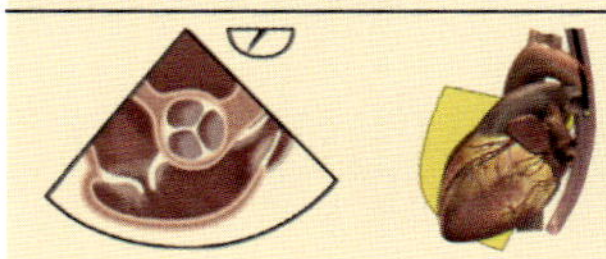	**Primary diagnostic issue(s)** Pulmonic valve disease Pulmonary artery pathology RVOT pathology	**Required structures** Pulmonic and tricuspid valve Superior intra-atrial septum Main pulmonary artery (at least 1 cm distal to the pulmonic valve) RVOT (at least 1 cm proximal to the pulmonic valve)
ME modified bicaval TV	Probe adjustment: neutral	Sector depth: (~12 cm)
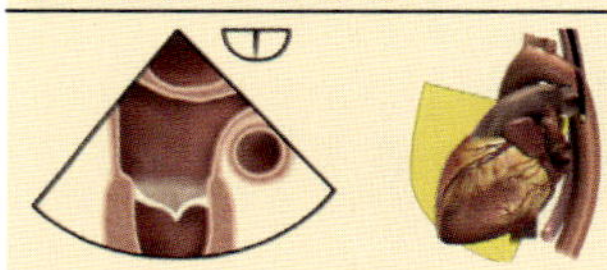	**Primary diagnostic issue(s)** Interrogation of spectral Doppler TV flow	**Required structures** Left and right atrium Mid intra-atrial septum Tricuspid valve Superior and inferior vena cava
ME AV LAX	Probe adjustment: neutral	Sector depth: (~10 cm)
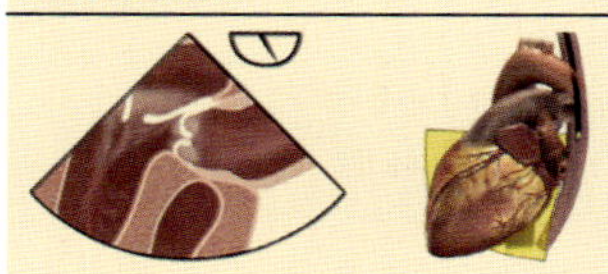	**Primary diagnostic issue(s)** Aortic valve pathology Aortic pathology (ascending and root) Left ventricular outflow tract pathology	**Required structures** LVOT (at least 1 cm proximal to the aortic valve) Aortic valve Ascending aorta Mitral valve (A2-P2 segments)

ME bicaval view	Probe adjustment: neutral	Sector depth: (~10 cm)
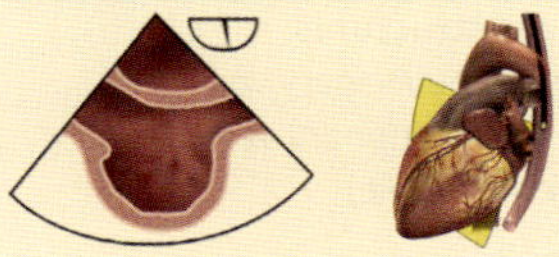	**Primary diagnostic issue(s)** Atrial septal defect Tumor	**Required structures** Right atrial free wall (or appendage) Superior vena cava (at least its entry into the right atrium) Interatrial septum Inferior vena cava
UE right pulmonary vein	Probe adjustment: neutral	Sector depth: (~10 cm)
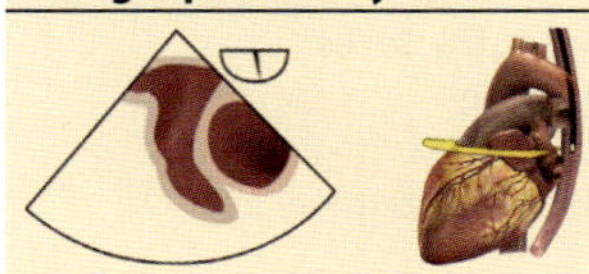	**Primary diagnostic issue(s)** Interrogation of pulmonary venous flow	**Required structures** Right upper pulmonary vein Right lower pulmonary vein (when possible) Left atrium Superior vena cava
UE left pulmonary vein	Probe adjustment: neutral	Sector depth: (~12 cm)
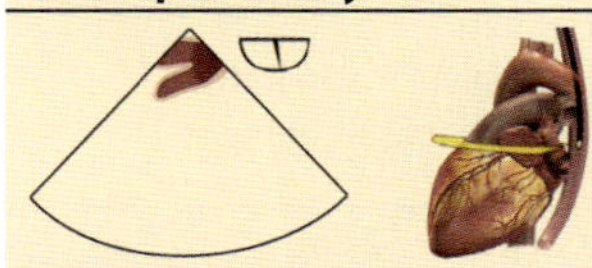	**Primary diagnostic issue(s)** Inspection and interrogation of pulmonary vein flow	**Required structures** Right and left pulmonary veins
ME five chamber	Probe adjustment: neutral-anteflexed	Sector depth: (~14 cm)
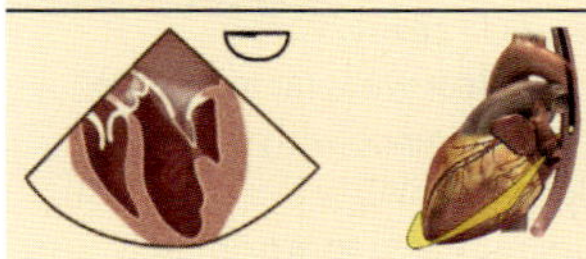	**Primary diagnostic issue(s)** Atrial septal defect Chamber enlargement/dysfunction Mitral disease Detection of intracardiac air	**Required structures** Left and right atrium Left and right ventricle Mitral valve Left ventricular outflow tract
ME four chamber	Probe adjustment: neutral-retroflex	Sector depth: (~14 cm)
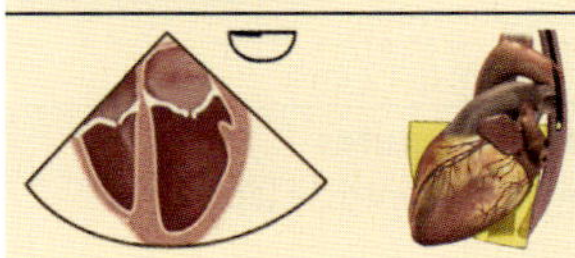	**Primary diagnostic issue(s)** Atrial septal defect Chamber enlargement/dysfunction Mitral disease Tricuspid disease Detection of intracardiac air	**Required structures** Left atrium Left ventricle Mitral valve Tricuspid valve (maximum annular dimension)
ME mitral commissural	Probe adjustment: neutral	Sector depth: (~12 cm)
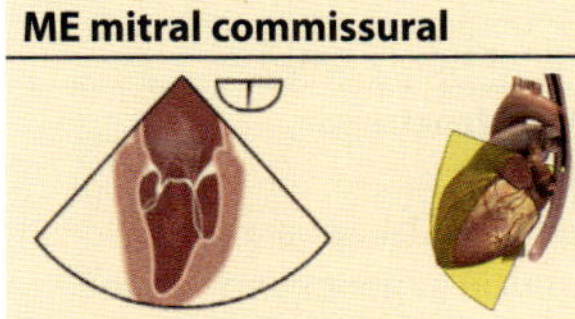	**Primary diagnostic issue(s)** Localization of mitral valve pathology	**Required structures** Mitral valve (P1, P3, and A2 scallops) Papillary muscles/chordae tendineae Left atrium Left ventricle
ME two chamber	Probe adjustment: neutral	Sector depth: (~14 cm)
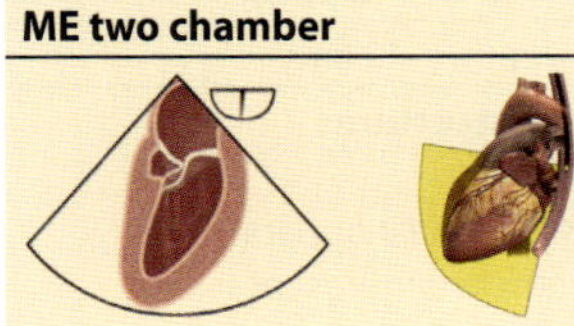	**Primary diagnostic issue(s)** Left atrial appendage mass/thrombus LV apex pathology LV systolic dysfunction (apical segments)	**Required structures** Left atrial appendage Coronary sinus (SAX) Mitral valve Left ventricular apex (ie, maximum LV length)
ME left atrial appendage view	Probe adjustment: neutral	Sector depth: (~10 cm)
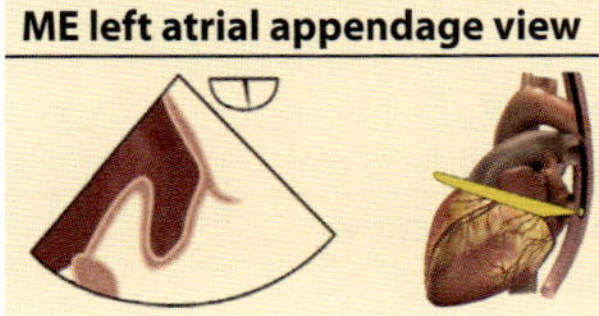	**Primary diagnostic issue(s)** Inspection and diagnosis of LAA thrombus	**Required structures** Left atrium Left atrial appendage Left upper pulmonary vein

(continued)

ME left pulmonary vein | Probe adjustment: neutral | Sector depth: (~10 cm)

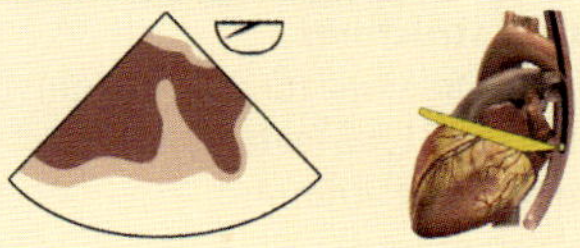

Primary diagnostic issue(s)
- Interrogation of pulmonary venous flow

Required structures
- Left upper pulmonary vein
- Left lower pulmonary vein (when possible)
- Left atrium
- Left atrial appendage

ME LAX | Probe adjustment: neutral | Sector depth: (~12 cm)

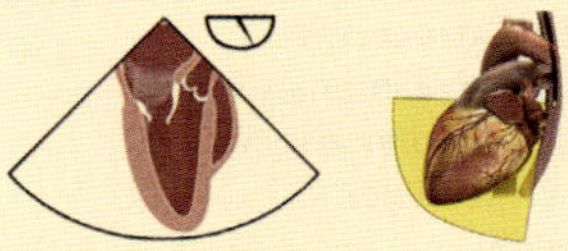

Primary diagnostic issue(s)
- Mitral valve pathology
- Left ventricular outflow tract pathology

Required structures
- Left ventricle
- Mitral valve
- Left ventricular outflow tract

TG Basal SAX | Probe adjustment: neutral | Sector depth: (~12 cm)

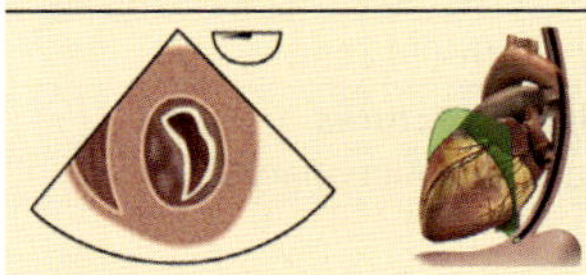

Primary diagnostic issue(s)
- LV systolic dysfunction (basal segments)
- Mitral valve pathology

Required structures
- Mitral leaflets
- Mitral subvalvular apparatus
- Left ventricle (basal segments)

TG mid SAX | Probe adjustment: neutral | Sector depth: (~12 cm)

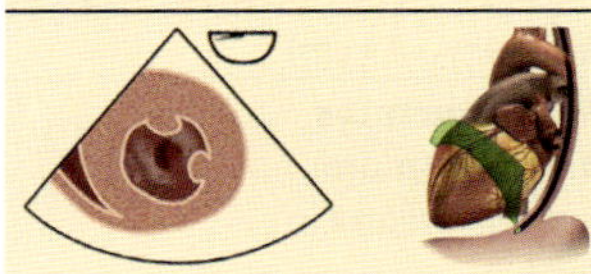

Primary diagnostic issue(s)
- Hemodynamic instability
- LV enlargement
- LV hypertrophy
- LV systolic dysfunction (global and regional)

Required structures
- Left ventricle cavity
- Left ventricular walls (at least 50% of circumference with visible endocardium)
- Papillary muscles (approximately equal in size and continuous with ventricular wall)

TG apical SAX | Probe adjustment: neutral-anteflex | Sector depth: (~12 cm)

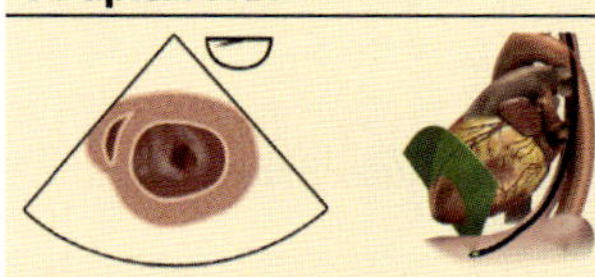

Primary diagnostic issue(s)
- LV systolic dysfunction (apical segments)

Required structures
- Left and right ventricle (apical segments)

TG two chamber | Probe adjustment: neutral | Sector depth: (~12 cm)

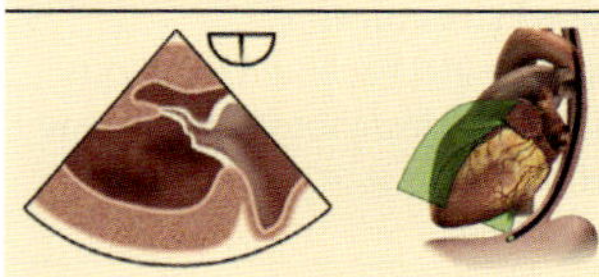

Primary diagnostic issue(s)
- LV systolic dysfunction (anterior and inferior: basal segments)

Required structures
- Mitral leaflets
- Mitral subvalvular apparatus
- Left ventricle (anterior and inferior: basal + mid segments)

TG LAX | Probe adjustment: neutral-leftward | Sector depth: (~12 cm)

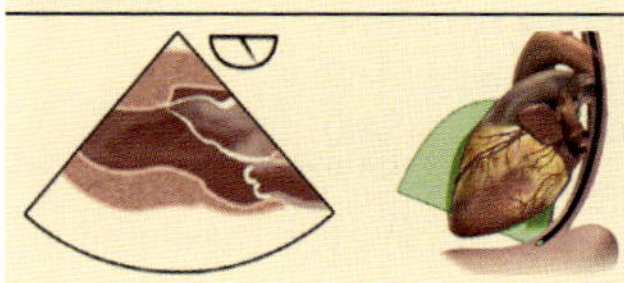

Primary diagnostic issue(s)
- LV systolic dysfunction (anteroseptal and posterior: basal segments)

Required structures
- Mitral leaflets
- Mitral subvalvular apparatus
- Left ventricle (anteroseptal and inferolateral: basal + mid segments)
- LVOT
- Aortic valve

TG RV inflow | Probe adjustment: neutral-rightward | Sector depth: (~12 cm)

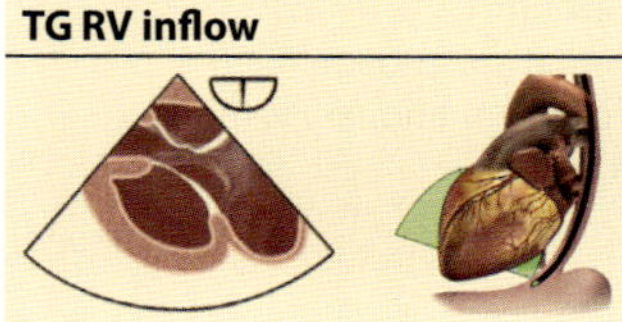

Primary diagnostic issue(s)
- RV systolic dysfunction
- Tricuspid valve pathology

Required structures
- Tricuspid leaflets
- Tricuspid subvalvular apparatus
- Right ventricle

Deep TG five chamber	Probe adjustment: neutral	Sector depth: (~16 cm)
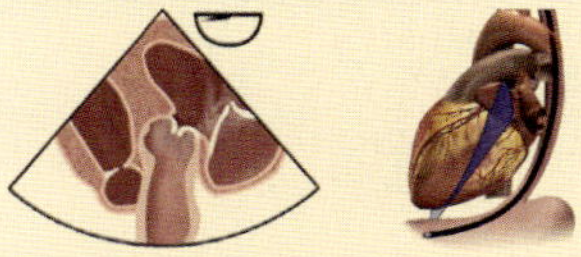	**Primary diagnostic issue(s)** Aortic valve pathology LVOT pathology	**Required structures** Left ventricle Left ventricular outflow tract Aortic valve Aorta
TG right ventricle basal	Probe adjustment: neutral	Sector depth: (~12 cm)
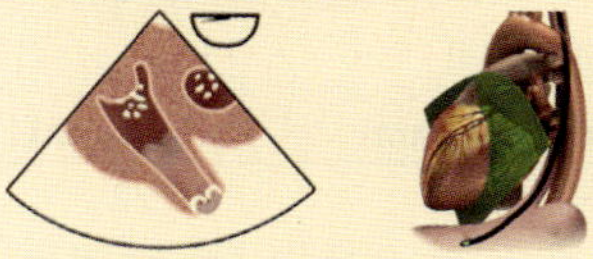	**Primary diagnostic issue(s)** RV systolic dysfunction (basal segments) Tricuspid valve pathology	**Required structures** Tricuspid valve leaflets (anterior, septal, and posterior) Right ventricle (basal segments)
TG RV inflow-outflow	Probe adjustment: neutral-rightward	Sector depth: (~14 cm)
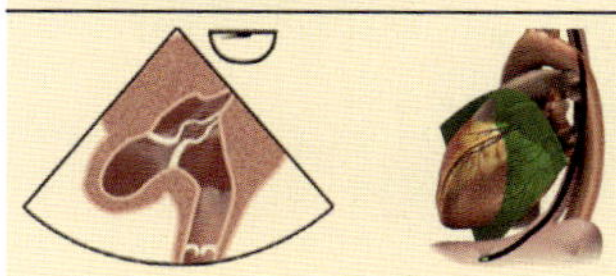	**Primary diagnostic issue(s)** RV systolic dysfunction RVOT pathology Pulmonary artery pathology	**Required structures** Right atrium Tricuspid valve Right ventricle Right ventricular outflow tract Main pulmonary artery
Desc aortic SAX	Probe adjustment: neutral	Sector depth: (~6 cm)
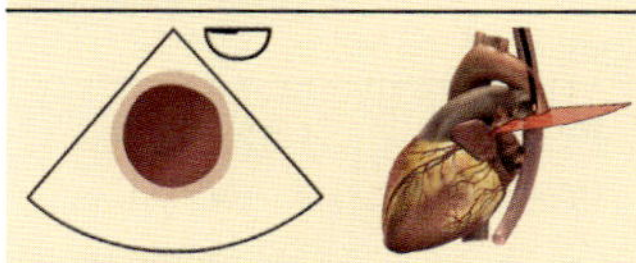	**Primary diagnostic issue** Aortic atherosclerosis Aortic dissection	**Required structures** Descending aorta in cross section in transverse plane (0°)
Desc aortic LAX	Probe adjustment: neutral	Sector depth: (~6 cm)
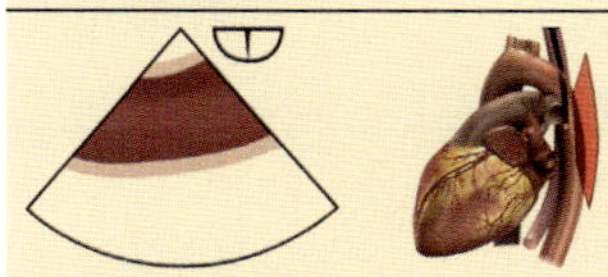	**Primary diagnostic issue(s)** Aortic atherosclerosis Aortic dissection	**Required structures** Descending aorta in long axis in longitudinal plane (90°)
UE aortic arch SAX	Probe adjustment: neutral	Sector depth: (~6 cm)
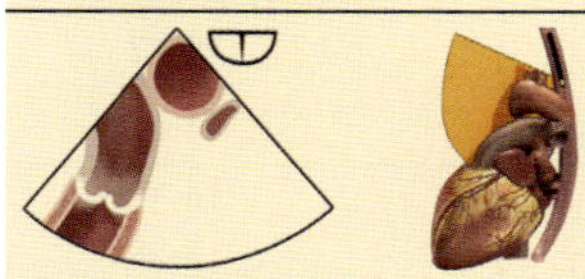	**Primary diagnostic issue(s)** Aortic atherosclerosis Aortic dissection	**Required structures** Aortic arch in cross section Main pulmonary artery (often not well seen)
UE aortic arch LAX	Probe adjustment: neutral	Sector depth: (~6 cm)
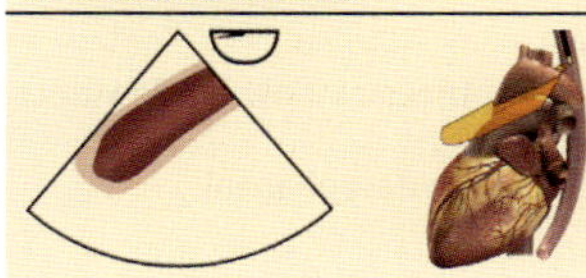	**Primary diagnostic issue(s)** Aortic atherosclerosis Aortic dissection Visualization of aortic cannulation site	**Required structures** Distal ascending aorta/aortic arch

Asc, ascending; Des, descending; LAA, left atrial appendage; LAX, long axis; LV, left ventricle; ME, midesophageal; ME AV SAX, midesophageal aortic valve short axis; PW, pulsed wave; RV, right ventricular; RVOT, right ventricular outflow tract; SAX, short axis; TG, transgastric; TV, tricuspid valve; UE, upper esophageal.

Based on Hahn RT, Abraham T, Adams MS, et al; American Society of Echocardiography; Society of Cardiovascular Anesthesiologists. Guidelines for performing a comprehensive transesophageal echocardiographic examination: recommendations from the American Society of Echocardiography and the Society of Cardiovascular Anesthesiologists. *Anesth Analg*. 2014;118(1):21-68.

B Cardiac Dimensions

TABLE B.1 Reference Values for Normal Adult TEE Measurements

Parameter		Mean ± SD (mm)	Range (mm)
	Right pulmonary artery diameter[a]	17 ± 3	12-22
	Left upper pulmonary vein diameter	11 ± 2	7-16
Left atrial appendage	Length	28 ± 5	15-43
	Diameter	16 ± 5	10-28
	Superior vena cava diameter	15 ± 3	8-20
	Right ventricular outflow tract diameter[b]	27 ± 4	16-36
Left atrium[c]	Anteroposterior diameter	38 ± 6	20-52
	Medial-lateral diameter	39 ± 7	24-52
Right atrium[c]	Anteroposterior diameter	38 ± 5	28-52
	Medial-lateral diameter	38 ± 6	29-53
	Tricuspid annular diameter[c]	28 ± 5	20-40
	Mitral annular diameter[c]	29 ± 4	20-38
	Coronary sinus diameter	6.6 ± 1.5	4-10
Left ventricle[d]	Anteroposterior diameter (diastole)	43 ± 7	33-55
	Medial-lateral diameter (diastole)	42 ± 7	23-54
	Anteroposterior diameter (systole)	28 ± 6	18-40
	Medial-lateral diameter (systole)	27 ± 6	18-42
	Aortic root diameter[b]	28 ± 3	21-34
Descending thoracic aorta diameter	Proximal	21 ± 4	14-30
	Distal	20 ± 4	13-28

SD, standard deviation; TEE, transesophageal echocardiography.
[a]Right pulmonary artery diameter measured in midesophageal ascending aorta short-axis view.
[b]Aortic root and right ventricular outflow tract diameters measured in the midesophageal right ventricular inflow-outflow tract view.
[c]Atrial (end systole) and both mitral and tricuspid annular (mid-diastole) diameters measured in the midesophageal four-chamber view.
[d]Left ventricular dimensions measured in transgastric mid short-axis view.
Adapted from Cohen G, White M, Sochowski R, et al. Reference values for normal transesophageal measurements. *J Am Soc Echocardiogr*. 1995;8:221-230.

C Hemodynamic Calculations

Pressure Estimated	Required Measurements	Formula	Normal Values
CVP	IVC size and respiratory collapse (quiet spontaneous ventilation)	<2.1 cm >20% collapse	<5 mm Hg
Right ventricular/pulmonary artery systolic pressure (RVSP/PASP)	Peak velocity TR CVP (estimated or measured) (assumes no PS)	$RVSP = 4(V_{TR})^2 + CVP$	≤34 mm Hg
Right ventricular/pulmonary artery systolic pressure (RVSP/PASP)	Systolic blood pressure (SBP) Peak velocity VSD (assumes no AS or LVOT obstruction)	$RVSP = SBP - 4(V_{VSD})^2$	≤34 mm Hg
Pulmonary artery diastolic pressure (PADP)	End-diastolic velocity PR CVP (estimated or measured)	$PADP = 4(V_{PR\ ED})^2 + CVP$	0-8 mm Hg
Pulmonary artery mean pressure (mPAP)	Early diastolic velocity PR CVP (estimated or measured)	$mPAP = 4(V_{early\ PI})^2 + CVP$	≤20 mm Hg
Pulmonary vascular resistance (PVR)	Peak velocity TR RVOT spectral Doppler envelope	$PVR = 10 \times (V_{TR}/V_{TI\ RVOT}) + 0.16$	<2.0 Wood units
Left atrial pressure (LAP)	Peak velocity MR SBP (assumes no AS or LVOT obstruction)	$LAP = SBP - 4(V_{MR})^2$	3-15 mm Hg
Left atrial pressure (LAP)	Peak velocity ASD CVP (estimated or measured)	$LAP = 4(V_{ASD})^2 + CVP$	3-15 mm Hg
LV end-diastolic pressure (LVEDP)	End-diastolic velocity AR Diastolic blood pressure (DBP)	$LVEDP = DBP - 4(V_{AR})^2$	3-15 mm Hg
LV dP/dT	MR spectral Doppler envelope TMR (3 m/s) − TMR (1 m/s)	$LV\ dP = 4V^2_{MR}\ (3\ m/s) - 4V^2_{MR}\ (1\ m/s)$ $LV\ dP/dT = dP/TMR\ (3\ m/s) - TMR\ (1\ m/s)$	>1,200 mm Hg/s

AR, aortic regurgitation; AS, aortic stenosis; ASD, atrial septal defect; CVP, central venous pressure; IVC, inferior vena cava; LVOT, left ventricular outflow tract; MR, mitral regurgitation; PR, pulmonic regurgitation; PR ED, pulmonic regurgitation end-diastolic; PS, pulmonic stenosis; RVOT, right ventricular outflow tract; TMR, trans-mitral regurgitation; TR, tricuspid regurgitation; VSD, ventricular septal defect.

D Valve Prostheses

Albert T. Cheung

TABLE D.1 Normal Doppler Echocardiographic Values of Aortic Valve Prosthesis

Valve	Size	Peak Gradient (mm Hg)	Mean Gradient (mm Hg)	Effective Orifice Area (cm^2)
Abbott *Epic*	21		19.1 ± 8.2	1.0 ± 0.3
	23		13.9 ± 6.0	1.4 ± 0.5
	25		12.1 ± 5.1	1.5 ± 0.5
	27		11.4 ± 4.1	1.6 ± 0.4
	29		7.5 ± 3.3	2.4 ± 1.1
Abbott *Trifecta*	19		10.7 ± 4.6	1.41 ± 0.24
	21		8.1 ± 3.5	1.63 ± 0.29
	23		7.2 ± 2.8	1.81 ± 0.30
	25		6.2 ± 2.7	2.02 ± 0.32
	27		4.8 ± 2.0	2.20 ± 0.20
	29		4.7 ± 1.6	2.35 ± 0.22
Arbor Surgical *Trilogy*	21	21 ± 8	11 ± 6	1.9 ± 0.2
	23	15 ± 7	8 ± 4	2.0 ± 0.3
ATS *Bileaflet*	19	47.0 ± 12.6	25.3 ± 8.0	1.1 ± 0.3
	21	23.7 ± 6.8	15.9 ± 5.0	1.4 ± 0.5
	23		14.4 ± 4.9	1.7 ± 0.5
	25		11.3 ± 3.7	2.1 ± 0.7
	27		8.4 ± 3.7	2.5 ± 0.1
	29		8.0 ± 3.0	3.1 ± 0.8
ATS AP *Bileaflet*	18		21.0 ± 1.8	1.2 ± 0.3
	20	21.4 ± 4.2	11.1 ± 3.5	1.3 ± 0.3
	22	18.7 ± 8.3	10.5 ± 4.5	1.7 ± 0.4
	24	15.1 ± 5.6	7.5 ± 3.1	2.0 ± 0.6
	26		6.0 ± 2.0	2.1 ± 0.4
ATS *3F Enable*	21	27.0 ± 8.4	15.0 ± 4.6	1.1 ± 0.4
	22	25.7 ± 10.8	14.5 ± 6.0	1.4 ± 0.4
	25	20.3 ± 7.4	11.4 ± 4.0	1.6 ± 0.5
	27	16.8 ± 6.3	9.4 ± 3.3	1.9 ± 0.5
	29	14.3 ± 6.7	7.8 ± 3.8	2.4 ± 0.8
Baxter Perimount *Stented bovine pericardial*	19	32.5 ± 8.5	19.5 ± 5.5	1.3 ± 0.2
	21	24.9 ± 7.7	13.8 ± 4.0	1.3 ± 0.3
	23	19.9 ± 7.4	11.5 ± 3.9	1.6 ± 0.3
	25	16.5 ± 7.8	10.7 ± 3.8	1.6 ± 0.4
	27	12.8 ± 5.4	4.8 ± 2.2	2.0 ± 0.4
Biocor *Stented porcine*	23	30.0 ± 0.7	20 ± 6.6	1.3 ± 0.3
	25	23.0 ± 7.9	16 ± 5.1	1.7 ± 0.4
	27	22.0 ± 6.5	15.0 ± 3.7	2.2 ± 0.4
Extended Biocor *Stentless*	19-21	17.5 ± 6.5	9.6 ± 3.6	1.4 ± 0.4
	23	14.7 ± 7.3	7.7 ± 3.8	1.7 ± 0.4
	25	14.0 ± 4.3	7.4 ± 2.5	1.8 ± 0.4
Bioflo *Stented bovine pericardial*	19	37.2 ± 8.8	26.4 ± 5.5	0.7 ± 0.1
	21	28.7 ± 6.2	18.7 ± 5.5	1.1 ± 0.1

TABLE D.1 Normal Doppler Echocardiographic Values of Aortic Valve Prosthesis (*continued*)

Valve	Size	Peak Gradient (mm Hg)	Mean Gradient (mm Hg)	Effective Orifice Area (cm^2)
Bjork-Shiley	21	38.9 ± 11.9	21.8 ± 3.4	1.1 ± 0.3
Single tilting disk	23	28.8 ± 11.2	15.7 ± 5.3	1.3 ± 0.3
	25	23.7 ± 8.2	13.0 ± 5.0	1.5 ± 0.4
	27		10.0 ± 2.0	1.6 ± 0.3
Carbomedics Reduced *Bileaflet*	19	43.4 ± 1.2	24.4 ± 1.2	1.2 ± 0.1
Carbomedics Standard	19	38.0 ± 12.8	18.9 ± 8.3	1.0 ± 0.3
Bileaflet	21	26.8 ± 10.1	12.9 ± 5.4	1.5 ± 0.4
	23	22.5 ± 7.4	11.0 ± 4.6	1.4 ± 0.3
	25	19.6 ± 7.8	9.1 ± 3.5	1.8 ± 0.4
	27	17.5 ± 7.1	7.9 ± 3.2	2.2 ± 0.2
	29	9.1 ± 4.7	5.6 ± 3.0	3.2 ± 1.6
Carbomedics TopHat	21	30.2 ± 10.9	14.9 ± 5.4	1.2 ± 0.3
Bileaflet	23	24.2 ± 7.6	12.5 ± 4.4	1.4 ± 0.4
	25		9.5 ± 2.9	1.6 ± 0.32
Carpentier-Edwards	19	32.1 ± 3.4	24.2 ± 8.6	1.2 ± 0.3
Pericardial	21	25.7 ± 9.9	20.3 ± 9.1	1.5 ± 0.4
Stented bovine pericardial	23	21.7 ± 8.6	13.0 ± 5.3	1.8 ± 0.3
	25	16.5 ± 5.4	9.0 ± 2.3	
Carpentier-Edwards	19	43.5 ± 12.7	25.6 ± 8.0	0.9 ± 0.2
Standard	21	27.7 ± 7.6	17.3 ± 6.2	1.5 ± 0.3
Stented porcine	23	28.9 ± 7.5	16.1 ± 6.2	1.7 ± 0.5
	25	24.0 ± 7.1	12.9 ± 4.6	1.9 ± 0.5
	27	22.1 ± 8.2	12.1 ± 5.5	2.3 ± 0.6
	29		9.9 ± 2.9	2.8 ± 0.5
Carpentier	19	34.1 ± 2.7		1.1 ± 0.1
Supra-Annular	21	28.0 ± 10.5	17.5 ± 3.8	1.4 ± 0.9
Stented porcine	23	25.3 ± 10.5	13.4 ± 4.5	1.6 ± 0.6
	25	24.4 ± 7.6	13.2 ± 4.8	1.8 ± 0.4
	27	16.7 ± 4.7	8.8 ± 2.8	1.9 ± 0.7
Cryolife	19		9.0 ± 2.0	1.5 ± 0.3
Stentless	21		6.6 ± 2.9	1.7 ± 0.4
	23		6.0 ± 2.3	2.3 ± 0.2
	25		6.1 ± 2.6	2.6 ± 0.2
	27		4.0 ± 2.4	2.8 ± 0.3
Edwards Duromedics	21	39.0 ± 13		
Bileaflet	23	32.0 ± 8.0		
	25	26.0 ± 10.0		
	27	24.0 ± 10.0		
Edwards	19		17.6 ± 7.8	1.1 ± 0.2
Inspiris Resilia	21		12.6 ± 4.7	1.3 ± 0.3
	23		10.1 ± 3.8	1.6 ± 0.4
	25		9.6 ± 6.2	1.8 ± 0.5
	27		8.2 ± 3.5	2.2 ± 0.6
Edwards	19		13.9 ± 3.9	1.1 ± 0.1
Intuity	21		11.6 ± 3.6	1.3 ± 0.1
	23		10.4 ± 3.5	1.7 ± 0.2
	25		9.1 ± 3.2	1.9 ± 0.2
	27		8.3 ± 3.7	2.2 ± 0.2
Edwards Mira	19		18.2 ± 5.3	1.2 ± 0.4
Bileaflet	21		13.3 ± 4.3	1.6 ± 0.4
	23		14.7 ± 2.8	1.6 ± 0.6
	25		13.1 ± 3.8	1.9

(*continued*)

TABLE D.1 Normal Doppler Echocardiographic Values of Aortic Valve Prosthesis (*continued*)

Valve	Size	Peak Gradient (mm Hg)	Mean Gradient (mm Hg)	Effective Orifice Area (cm^2)
Edwards *Mosaic*	21		13.3 ± 5.3	1.4 ± 0.4
	23		11.8 ± 4.9	1.6 ± 0.5
	25		10.6 ± 4.4	1.8 ± 0.5
	27		9.1 ± 4.0	2.0 ± 0.5
	29		8.6 ± 2.9	2.3 ± 0.6
Hancock *Stented porcine*	21	18.0 ± 6.0	12.0 ± 2.0	
	23	16.0 ± 2.0	11.0 ± 2.0	
	25	15.0 ± 3.0	10.0 ± 3.0	
Hancock II *Stented porcine*	21		14.8 ± 4.1	1.3 ± 0.4
	23	34.0 ± 13.0	16.6 ± 8.5	1.3 ± 0.4
	25	22.0 ± 5.3	10.8 ± 2.8	1.6 ± 0.4
	29	16.2 ± 1.5	8.2 ± 1.7	1.6 ± 0.2
Homograft *Homograft valves*	17-19		9.7 ± 4.2	4.2 ± 1.8
	19-21			5.4 ± 0.9
	20-21		7.9 ± 4.0	3.6 ± 2.0
	20-22		7.2 ± 3.0	3.5 ± 1.5
	22	1.7 ± 0.3		5.8 ± 3.2
	22-23		5.6 ± 3.1	2.6 ± 1.4
	22-24			5.6 ± 1.7
	24-27		6.2 ± 2.6	2.8 ± 1.1
	26	1.4 ± 0.6		6.8 ± 2.9
	25-28			6.2 ± 2.5
Intact *Stented porcine*	19	40.4 ± 15.4	24.5 ± 9.3	
	21	40.9 ± 15.6	19.6 ± 8.1	1.6 ± 0.4
	23	32.7 ± 9.6	19.0 ± 6.1	1.6 ± 0.4
	25	29.7 ± 15.0	17.7 ± 7.9	1.7 ± 0.3
	27	25.0 ± 7.6	15.0 ± 4.5	
Ionescu-Shiley *Stented bovine pericardial*	17	23.8 ± 3.4		0.9 ± 0.1
	19	19.7 ± 5.9	13.3 ± 3.9	1.1 ± 0.1
	21	26.6 ± 9.0		
	23		15.6 ± 4.4	
Labcor-Santiago *Stented bovine pericardial*	19	18.6 ± 5.0	11.8 ± 3.3	1.2 ± 0.1
	21	17.5 ± 6.6	8.2 ± 4.5	1.3 ± 0.1
	23	14.8 ± 5.2	7.8 ± 2.9	1.8 ± 0.2
	25	12.3 ± 3.4	6.8 ± 2.0	2.1 ± 0.3
Labcor Synergy *Stented porcine*	21	24.3 ± 8.1	13.3 ± 4.2	1.1 ± 0.3
	23	27.3 ± 13.7	15.3 ± 6.9	1.4 ± 0.4
	25	22.5 ± 11.9	13.2 ± 6.4	1.5 ± 0.4
	27	17.8 ± 7.0	10.6 ± 4.6	1.8 ± 0.5
MCRI On-X *Bileaflet*	19	21.3 ± 10.8	11.8 ± 3.4	1.5 ± 0.2
	21	16.4 ± 5.9	9.9 ± 3.6	1.7 ± 0.4
	23	15.9 ± 6.4	8.6 ± 3.4	1.9 ± 0.6
	25	16.5 ± 10.2	6.9 ± 4.3	2.4 ± 0.6
Medtronic Advantage *Bileaflet*	23		10.4 ± 3.1	2.2 ± 0.3
	25		9.0 ± 3.7	2.8 ± 0.6
	27		7.6 ± 3.6	3.3 ± 0.7
	29		6.1 ± 3.8	3.9 ± 0.7
Medtronic *Avalus*	19		17.1 ± 5.0	1.11 ± 0.25
	21		14.5 ± 4.3	1.25 ± 0.25
	23		12.1 ± 3.8	1.47 ± 0.32
	25		11.7 ± 4.0	1.57 ± 0.31
	27		10.3 ± 4.2	1.77 ± 0.41

TABLE D.1 Normal Doppler Echocardiographic Values of Aortic Valve Prosthesis (*continued*)

Valve	Size	Peak Gradient (mm Hg)	Mean Gradient (mm Hg)	Effective Orifice Area (cm²)
Medtronic Freestyle	19		13.0 ± 3.9	
Stentless	21		9.1 ± 5.1	1.4 ± 0.3
	23	11.0 ± 4.0	8.1 ± 4.6	1.7 ± 0.5
	25		5.3 ± 3.1	2.1 ± 0.5
	27		4.6 ± 3.1	2.5 ± 0.1
Medtronic-Hall	20	34.4 ± 13.1	17.1 ± 5.3	1.2 ± 0.5
Single tilting disk	21	26.9 ± 10.5	14.1 ± 5.9	1.1 ± 0.2
	23	26.9 ± 8.9	13.5 ± 4.8	1.4 ± 0.4
	25	17.1 ± 7.0	9.5 ± 4.3	1.5 ± 0.5
	27	18.9 ± 9.7	8.7 ± 5.6	1.9 ± 0.2
Medtronic Mosaic	21		14.2 ± 5.0	1.4 ± 0.4
Stented porcine	23	23.8 ± 11.0	13.7 ± 4.8	1.5 ± 0.4
	25	22.5 ± 10.0	11.7 ± 5.1	1.8 ± 0.5
	27		10.4 ± 4.3	1.9 ± 0.1
	29		11.1 ± 4.3	2.1 ± 0.2
Mitroflow *Stented bovine pericardial*	19	18.6 ± 5.3	13.1 ± 3.3	1.1 ± 0.2
Monostrut Bjork-Shiley	19		27.4 ± 8.8	
Single tilting disk	21	27.5 ± 3.1	20.5 ± 6.2	
	23	20.3 ± 0.7	17.4 ± 6.4	
	25		16.1 ± 4.9	
	27		11.4 ± 3.8	
Prima	21	28.8 ± 6.0	13.7 ± 1.9	1.4 ± 0.7
Stentless	23	21.5 ± 7.5	11.5 ± 4.9	1.5 ± 0.3
	25	22.1 ± 12.5	11.6 ± 7.2	1.8 ± 0.5
Omnicarbon	21	37.4 ± 12.8	20.4 ± 5.4	1.3 ± 0.5
Single tilting disk	23	28.8 ± 9.1	17.4 ± 4.9	1.5 ± 0.3
	25	23.7 ± 8.1	13.2 ± 4.6	1.9 ± 0.5
	27	20.1 ± 4.2	12.4 ± 2.9	2.1 ± 0.4
Omniscience	21	50.8 ± 2.8	28.2 ± 2.2	0.9 ± 0.1
Single tilting disk	23	39.8 ± 8.7	20.1 ± 5.1	1.0 ± 0.1
Starr-Edwards	23	32.6 ± 12.8	22.0 ± 9.0	1.1 ± 0.2
Caged ball	24	34.1 ± 10.3	22.1 ± 7.5	1.1 ± 0.3
	26	31.8 ± 9.0	19.7 ± 6.1	
	27	30.8 ± 6.3	18.5 ± 3.7	
	29	29.0 ± 9.3	16.3 ± 5.5	
Sorin Bicarbon	19	30.1 ± 4.5	16.7 ± 2.0	1.4 ± 0.1
Bileaflet	21	22.0 ± 7.1	10.0 ± 3.3	1.2 ± 0.4
	23	16.8 ± 6.1	7.7 ± 3.3	1.5 ± 0.2
	25	11.2 ± 3.1	5.6 ± 1.6	2.4 ± 0.3
Sorin Pericarbon	19	36.5 ± 9.0	28.9 ± 7.3	1.2 ± 0.5
Stentless	21	28.0 ± 13.3	23.8 ± 11.1	1.3 ± 0.6
	23	27.5 ± 11.5	23.2 ± 7.6	1.5 ± 0.5
Sorin Perceval	S (21)		10.1 ± 4.2	1.3 ± 0.3
Sutureless	M (23)		9.4 ± 5.5	1.5 ± 0.4
	L (25)		8.5 ± 4.6	1.5 ± 0.4
	XL (27)		9.7 ± 4.7	1.6 ± 0.4
St. Jude Medical	19	28.5 ± 10.7	17.0 ± 7.8	1.9 ± 0.1
Haem Plus	21	16.3 ± 17.0	10.6 ± 5.1	1.8 ± 0.5
Bileaflet	23	16.8 ± 7.3	12.1 ± 4.2	1.7 ± 0.5

(*continued*)

TABLE D.1 Normal Doppler Echocardiographic Values of Aortic Valve Prosthesis (*continued*)

Valve	Size	Peak Gradient (mm Hg)	Mean Gradient (mm Hg)	Effective Orifice Area (cm^2)
St Jude Medical Regent *Bileaflet*	19	20.6 ± 12	11.0 ± 4.9	1.6 ± 0.4
	21	15.6 ± 9.4	8.0 ± 4.8	2.0 ± 0.7
	23	12.8 ± 6.8	6.9 ± 3.5	2.3 ± 0.9
	25	11.7 ± 6.8	5.6 ± 3.2	2.5 ± 0.8
	27	7.9 ± 5.5	3.5 ± 1.7	3.6 ± 0.5
St Jude Medical Standard *Bileaflet*	19	42.0 ± 10.0	24.5 ± 5.8	1.5 ± 0.1
	21	25.7 ± 9.5	15.2 ± 5.0	1.4 ± 0.4
	23	21.8 ± 7.5	13.4 ± 5.6	1.6 ± 0.4
	25	18.9 ± 7.3	11.0 ± 5.3	1.9 ± 0.5
	27	13.7 ± 4.2	8.4 ± 3.4	2.5 ± 0.4
	29	13.5 ± 5.8	7.0 ± 1.7	2.8 ± 0.5
St Jude Medical *Stentless*	21	22.6 ± 14.5	10.7 ± 7.2	1.3 ± 0.6
	23	16.2 ± 9.0	8.2 ± 4.7	1.6 ± 0.6
	25	12.7 ± 8.2	6.3 ± 4.1	1.8 ± 0.5
	27	10.1 ± 5.8	5.0 ± 2.9	2.0 ± 0.3
	29	7.7 ± 4.4	4.1 ± 2.4	2.4 ± 0.6

Data are expressed as mean ± SD.
Adapted from: Zoghbi WA, Jone PN, Chamsi-Pasha MA, et al. Guidelines for the evaluation of prosthetic valve function with cardiovascular imaging. *J Am Soc Echocardiogr.* 2024;37(1):2-63.

TABLE D.2 Normal Doppler Echocardiographic Values for Mitral Valve Prosthesis

Valve	Size	Peak Gradient (mm Hg)	Mean Gradient (mm Hg)	Peak Velocity (m/s)	Pressure Half-Time (ms)	Effective Orifice Area (cm²)
Abbott	27		6.1 ± 2.9			1.4 ± 0.7
Epic	29		5.5 ± 1.7			1.5 ± 0.5
	31		4.8 ± 1.4			1.6 ± 0.3
	33		4.1 ± 1.6			1.5 ± 0.3
Biocor	27	13 ± 1				
Stentless bioprosthesis	29	14 ± 2.5				
	31	11.5 ± 0.5				
	33	12 ± 0.5				
Bioflo pericardial	25	10 ± 2	6.3 ± 1.5			2 ± 0.1
Stented bioprosthesis	27	9.5 ± 2.6	5.4 ± 1.2			2 ± 0.3
	29	5 ± 2.8	3.6 ± 1			2.4 ± 0.2
	31	4.0	2.0			2.3
Björk-Shiley	23			1.7	115	1.72 ± 0.6
Tilting disk	25	12 ± 4	6 ± 2	1.75 ± 0.38	99 ± 27	1.81 ± 0.54
	27	10 ± 4	5 ± 2	1.6 ± 0.49	89 ± 28	2.1 ± 0.43
	29	7.83 ± 2.93	2.83 ± 1.27	1.37 ± 0.25	79 ± 17	2.2 ± 0.3
	31	6 ± 3	2 ± 1.9	1.41 ± 0.26	70 ± 14	
Björk-Shiley monostrut	23		5.0	1.9		
Tilting disk	25	13 ± 2.5	5.57 ± 2.3	1.8 ± 0.3		
	27	12 ± 2.5	4.53 ± 2.2	1.7 ± 0.4		
	29	13 ± 3	4.26 ± 1.6	1.6 ± 0.3		
	31	14 ± 4.5	4.9 ± 1.6	1.7 ± 0.3		
Carbomedics	23			1.9 ± 0.1	126 ± 7	
Bileaflet	25	10.3 ± 2.3	3.6 ± 0.6	1.3 ± 0.1	93 ± 8	2.9 ± 0.8
	27	8.79 ± 3.46	3.46 ± 1.03	1.61 ± 0.3	89 ± 20	2.9 ± 0.75
	29	8.78 ± 2.9	3.39 ± 0.97	1.52 ± 0.3	88 ± 17	2.3 ± 0.4
	31	8.87 ± 2.34	3.32 ± 0.87	1.61 ± 0.29	92 ± 24	2.8 ± 1.14
	33	8.8 ± 2.2	4.8 ± 2.5	1.5 ± 0.2	93 ± 12	
Carpentier-Edwards	27		6 ± 2	1.7 ± 0.3	98 ± 28	
Stented bioprosthesis	29		4.7 ± 2	1.76 ± 0.27	92 ± 14	
	31		4.4 ± 2	1.54 ± 0.15	92 ± 19	
	33		6 ± 3		93 ± 12	

(continued)

TABLE D.2 Normal Doppler Echocardiographic Values for Mitral Valve Prosthesis (*continued*)

Valve	Size	Peak Gradient (mm Hg)	Mean Gradient (mm Hg)	Peak Velocity (m/s)	Pressure Half-Time (ms)	Effective Orifice Area (cm²)
Carpentier-Edwards	27		3.6	1.6	100	
pericardial	29		5.25 ± 2.36	1.67 ± 0.3	110 ± 15	
Stented bioprosthesis	31		4.05 ± 0.83	1.53 ± 0.1	90 ± 11	
	33		1.0	0.8	80	
Carpentier-Edwards	25		4.0 ± 1.0	1.7 ± 0.10	67 ± 21.5	1.75 ± 0.53
Perimount	27		6.3 ± 1.65	1.7 ± 0.27	74 ± 20.6	1.88 ± 0.52
Stented pericardial	29		6.0 ± 1.41	1.8 ± 0.19	76 ± 17.9	2.02 ± .57
	31		5.5 ± 1.06	1.8 ± 0.20	80 ± 21.8	2.09 ± 0.48
	33		6.1 ± 1.86	1.7 ± 0.23	77 ± 13.2	2.24 ± 0.97
Duromedics	27	13 ± 6	5 ± 3	1.61 ± 0.4	75 ± 12	
Bileaflet	29	10 ± 4	3 ± 1	1.40 ± 0.25	85 ± 22	
	31	10.5 ± 4.33	3.3 ± 1.36	1.38 ± 0.27	81 ± 12	
	33	11.2	2.5		85	
Edwards	25		4.9 ± 1.2			1.1 ± 0.4
Mitris	27		4.1 ± 1.4			1.2 ± 0.3
	29		4.1 ± 1.5			1.5 ± 0.6
	31		3.9 ± 2.0			1.4 ± 0.5
	33		3.3 ± 1.4			1.5 ± 0.7
Hancock I or not specified	27	10 ± 4	5 ± 2			1.3 ± 0.8
Stented bioprosthesis	29	7 ± 3	2.46 ± 0.79		115 ± 20	1.5 ± 0.2
	31	4 ± 0.86	4.86 ± 1.69		95 ± 17	1.6 ± 0.2
	33	3 ± 2	3.87 ± 2		90 ± 12	1.9 ± 0.2
Hancock II	25		8.3 ± 1.71	2.1 ± 0.28	76 ± 19.8	1.42 ± 0.29
Stented	27		6.1 ± 1.33	2 ± 0.28	81 ± 18.9	1.62 ± 0.47
bioprosthesis	29		6.7 ± 2.20	2.0 ± 0.31	77 ± 15.1	1.83 ± 0.68
	31		6.0 ± 1.58	2.0 ± 0.32	76 ± 12.1	1.70 ± 0.41
	33		5.5 ± 1.64	1.9 ± 0.50	65 ± 8.7	2.71 ± 0.77
Hancock pericardial	29		2.61 ± 1.39	1.42 ± 0.14	105 ± 36	
Stented bioprosthesis	31		3.57 ± 1.02	1.51 ± 0.27	81 ± 23	
Ionescu-Shiley	25		4.87 ± 1.08	1.43 ± 0.15	93 ± 11	
Stented bioprosthesis	27		3.21 ± 0.82	1.31 ± 0.24	100 ± 28	
	29		3.22 ± 0.57	1.38 ± 0.2	85 ± 8	
	31		3.63 ± 0.9	1.45 ± 0.06	100 ± 36	
Ionescu-Shiley low profile	29		3.31 ± 0.96	1.36 ± 0.25	80 ± 30	
Stented bioprosthesis	31		2.74 ± 0.37	1.33 ± 0.14	79 ± 15	

Labcor-Santiago pericardial	25	8.7	4.5		97	2.2
Stented bioprosthesis	27	5.6 ± 2.3	2.8 ± 1.5		85 ± 18	2.12 ± 0.48
	29	6.2 ± 2.1	3 ± 1.3		80 ± 34	2.11 ± 0.73
Lillehei-Kaster	18			1.7	140	
Tilting disk	20			1.7	67	
	22			1.56 ± 0.09	94 ± 22	
	25			1.38 ± 0.27	124 ± 46	
Medtronic-Hall	27			1.4	78	
Tilting disk	29			1.57 ± 0.1	69 ± 15	
	31			1.45 ± 0.12	77 ± 17	
Medtronic Intact Porcine	29		3.5 ± 0.51	1.6 ± 0.22		
Stented bioprosthesis	31		4.2 ± 1.44	1.6 ± 0.26		
	33		4 ± 1.3	1.4 ± 0.24		
	35		3.2 ± 1.77	1.3 ± 0.5		
Medtronic	25		8.3 ± 1.71	2.1 ± 0.28	76 ± 19.8	1.42 ± 0.29
Mosaic	27		6.1 ± 1.33	2 ± 0.28	81 ± 18.9	1.62 ± 0.47
	29		6.7 ± 2.20	2.0 ± 0.31	77 ± 15.1	1.83 ± 0.68
	31		6.0 ± 1.58	2.0 ± 0.32	76 ± 12.1	1.70 ± 0.41
	33		5.5 ± 1.64	1.9 ± 0.50	65 ± 8.7	2.71 ± 0.77
Mitroflow	25		6.9	2.0	90	
Stented bioprosthesis	27		3.07 ± 0.91	1.5	90 ± 20	
	29		3.5 ± 1.65	1.43 ± 0.29	102 ± 21	
	31		3.85 ± 0.81	1.32 ± 0.26	91 ± 22	
Omnicarbon	23		8.0			
Tilting disk	25		6.05 ± 1.81	1.77 ± 0.24	102 ± 16	
	27		4.89 ± 2.05	1.63 ± 0.36	105 ± 33	
	29		4.93 ± 2.16	1.56 ± 0.27	120 ± 40	
	31		4.18 ± 1.4	1.3 ± 0.23	134 ± 31	
	33		4 ± 2			
On-X	25	11.5 ± 3.2	5.3 ± 2.1			1.9 ± 1.1
Bileaflet	27-29	10.3 ± 4.5	4.5 ± 1.6			2.2 ± 0.5
	31-33	9.8 ± 3.8	4.8 ± 2.4			2.5 ± 1.1

(continued)

TABLE D.2 Normal Doppler Echocardiographic Values for Mitral Valve Prosthesis (*continued*)

Valve	Size	Peak Gradient (mm Hg)	Mean Gradient (mm Hg)	Peak Velocity (m/s)	Pressure Half-Time (ms)	Effective Orifice Area (cm^2)
Sorin Allcarbon	25	15 ± 3	5 ± 1	2 ± 0.2	105 ± 29	2.2 ± 0.6
Tilting disk	27	13 ± 2	4 ± 1	1.8 ± 0.1	89 ± 14	2.5 ± 0.5
	29	10 ± 2	4 ± 1	1.6 ± 0.2	85 ± 23	2.8 ± 0.7
	31	9 ± 1	4 ± 1	1.6 ± 0.1	88 ± 27	2.8 ± 0.9
Sorin Bicarbon	25	15 ± 0.25	4 ± 0.5	1.95 ± 0.02	70 ± 1	
Bileaflet	27	11 ± 2.75	4 ± 0.5	1.65 ± 0.21	82 ± 20	
	29	12 ± 3	4 ± 1.25	1.73 ± 0.22	80 ± 14	
	31	10 ± 1.5	4 ± 1	1.66 ± 0.11	83 ± 14	
St Jude Medical	23		4.0	1.5	160	1.0
Bileaflet	25		2.5 ± 1	1.34 ± 1.12	75 ± 4	1.35 ± 0.17
	27	11 ± 4	5 ± 1.82	1.61 ± 0.29	75 ± 10	1.67 ± 0.17
	29	10 ± 3	4.15 ± 1.8	1.57 ± 0.29	85 ± 10	1.75 ± 0.24
	31	12 ± 6	4.46 ± 2.22	1.59 ± 0.33	74 ± 13	2.03 ± 0.32
Starr-Edwards	26		10.0			1.4
Caged ball	28		7 ± 2.75	1.7 ± 0.3	125 ± 25	1.9 ± 0.57
	30	12.2 ± 4.6	6.99 ± 2.5	1.7 ± 0.3	110 ± 25	1.65 ± 0.4
	32	11.5 ± 4.2	5.08 ± 2.5			1.98 ± 0.4
	34		5.0			2.6
Stentless quadrileaflet	26		2.2 ± 1.7	1.6	103 ± 31	1.7
bovine pericardial	28			1.58 ± 0.25		1.7 ± 0.6
Stentless bioprosthesis	30			1.42 ± 0.32		2.3 ± 0.4
Wessex	29		3.69 ± 0.61	1.66 ± 0.17	83 ± 19	
Stented bioprosthesis	31		3.31 ± 0.83	1.41 ± 0.25	80 ± 21	

Data are expressed as mean ± SD.
Adapted from Zoghbi WA, Jone PN, Chamsi-Pasha MA, et al. Guidelines for the evaluation of prosthetic valve function with cardiovascular imaging. *J Am Soc Echocardiogr.* 2024;37(1):2-63.

TABLE D.3 Normal Doppler Echocardiographic Values of Tricuspid Valve Prosthesis

Valve	Size	Peak E-Velocity (m/s)	Mean Gradient (mm Hg)	Pressure Half-Time (ms)	Effective Orifice Area (EOA) (cm^2)
Carbomedics	31	1.4 ± 0.19	4.0 ± 1.63	78	2.01 ± 0.51
standard	33	1.2 ± 0.16	3.4 ± 1.19	98 ± 9.7	2.33 ± 0.43
Mechanical bileaflet					
Carpentier-	27	1.5 ± 0.26	5.2 ± 1.69	130 ± 45.4	1.34 ± 0.22
Edwards Duraflex	29	1.7 ± 0.27	6.0 ± 1.95	102 ± 26.5	1.54 ± 0.38
Bioprosthesis	31	1.5 ± 0.27	5.7 ± 1.67	115 ± 40.8	1.57 ± 0.39
	33	1.5 ± 0.26	5.6 ± 2.10	116 ± 39.7	1.69 ± 0.44
	35	1.5 ± 0.25	5.3 ± 1.61	83 ± 26.5	1.63 ± 0.38
Carpentier-Edwards	29	± 0.21	2.0 ± 1.41	94 ± 2.8	2.16 ± 0.43
Perimount	31	± 0.20	3.7 ± 1.53	74 ± 26.2	2.12 ± 0.53
pericardial	33	1.4 ± 0.21	3.9 ± 1.07	137 ± 53.0	1.93 ± 0.43
Bioprosthesis					
Medtronic Hancock II	31	1.6 ± 0.19	5.7 ± 1.37	-	1.40 ± 0.21
Bioprosthesis	33	1.4 ± 0.28	5.5 ± 3.54	-	1.40 ± 0.59
	35	1.3 ± 0.32	5.3 ± 0.58	-	2.11 ± 0.23
Medtronic Mosaic	25 (*n* = 1)	1.6	4.0	80	1.37
Bioprosthesis	27	1.6 ± 0.17	5.5 ± 0.58	-	1.53 ± 0.16
	29	1.5 ± 0.21	6.0 ± 2.00	115 ± 13.4	1.96 ± 0.39
	31	1.5 ± 0.21	5.2 ± 1.43	144 ± 28.6	1.74 ± 0.52
	33	1.4 ± 0.19	4.3 ± 1.30	139 ± 56.5	2.00 ± 0.53
Starr-Edwards	30 (*n* = 1)	1.5	5.0	132	2.07
Caged ball	32	1.5 ± 0.44	4.0 ± 1.00	N/A	1.87 ± 0.33
	34	1.8 ± 0.28	5.7 ± 1.63	118 ± 32.9	1.81 ± 0.48
St. Jude Medical	29 (*n* = 1)	1.6	6.0	-	2.84
Biocor	31	1.5 ± 0.34	5.1 ± 1.36	106 ± 48.5	1.67 ± 0.30
Bioprosthesis	33	1.3 ± 0.23	3.9 ± 1.20	125 ± 45.7	1.92 ± 050
St. Jude Medical	27	1.1 ± 0.32	2.4 ± 1.27	77 ± 14.6	2.54 ± 0.64
Standard	29	1.2 ± 0.21	2.6 ± 1.13	100 ± 35.2	2.20 ± 0.33
Mechanical bileaflet	31	1.4 ± 0.31	3.3 ± 1.21	81 ± 13.5	2.49 ± 0.45
	33	1.3 ± 0.22	3.2 ± 1.24	82 ± 18.8	2.46 ± 0.59

Data are expressed as mean ± SD.
Adapted from Blauwet LA, Burkhart HM, Dearani JA, et al. Comprehensive echocardiographic assessment of mechanical tricuspid valve prostheses based on early post-implantation echocardiographic studies. *J Am Soc Echocardiogr*. 2011;24(4): 414-424; and Blauwet LA, Danielson GK, Burkhart HM, et al. Comprehensive echocardiographic assessment of the hemodynamic parameters of 285 tricuspid valve bioprostheses early after implantation. *J Am Soc Echocardiogr*. 2010;23(10):1045-1059.

TABLE D.4

Tendyne Valve (Mitral Position)

Profile	Sizes	AP Range (mm)	IC Range (mm)	Perimeter (mm)
Standard (SP)	29S, 33S, 33M, 33L, 35M, 37S, 37L, 39M, 41S	32.5-40.5	43.5-52.5	130-156
Low (LP)	29S, 29L, 33S, 35M, 37M	29.0-36.5	42.5-49.5	119-150

Parameter	Target Value	Notes
Mean Gradient	≤6 mm Hg, ideally 3-5 mm Hg	Consistent across valve sizes
Peak LVOT Gradient	≤20-30 mm Hg	Assessed for LVOT obstruction

EVOQUE Valve (Tricuspid Position)

Valve Size (mm)	Systolic/Diastolic Diameters	Includes Derived Annular Diameter Range
44	Systole: 36.5-43 mm Diastole: 39.6-45.5 mm	Perimeter-derived
48	Systole: 40-47 mm Diastole: 43.2-49.5 mm	
52	Systole: 45-51 mm Diastole: 46.8-53.5 mm	
Valve Size Range	**Mean Gradient (Typical)**	**Gradient Target by Size?**
44-56 mm	~2-4 mm Hg	Not specified—Uniform across sizes

Trifecta Valve (Aortic Position)

Valve Size (mm)	Discharge Mean (mm Hg)	Discharge Peak (mm Hg)	1-Year Mean (mm Hg)
19	~9-13.5	~17-25	~10-11
21	~8.1-8.7	~16	~8-10
23	~6.9-10.5	~12.8-21	~7-11
25	~6.9	~12.6-25	~6.2-8.7
27	~4.8	~9.6-25.3	~4.7-7.4
29	—	—	~4.7

Latest Valves

Category	Valve	Geography/ Approval	Notable Features
Surgical (SAVR)	Avalus Ultra	Europe (October 2024)	Low profile, PEEK frame, valve-in-valve ready
Transcatheter (TAVR)	SAPIEN 3 Ultra RESILIA	Europe (CE: July 2025)	RESILIA tissue, dry-packaging, enhanced durability
Regional TAVR	Renatus	China NMPA (February 2025)	Balloon-expandable; elderly patients (≥70 years)

E Classification of the Severity of Valvular Disease

TABLE E.1 Echocardiographic Indices of Aortic Regurgitation Severity

Parameter	Mild	Moderate	Severe	Caveats
Structural Parameters				
Leaflets	Variable	Variable	Flail, wide coaptation defect	• Not reliable
LV size	Normal	Variable	Usually dilated	• Enlarged in other conditions • Normal in acute AR
Quantitative Doppler Parameters[a]				
Jet/LVOT height[b] (%) Jet/LVOT area[b] (%)	<25 <5	25-45, 46-64 5-20, 21-59	≥65 ≥60	• Variable in eccentric jets • Affected by direction and shape of jets
VC width[b] (cm)	<0.3	0.3-0.6	>0.6	• Problematic with multiple jets • May be less accurate in noncircular orifice
RVol (mL) RF (%) ERO area (cm^2)	<30 <30 <0.1	30-44, 45-59 30-39, 40-49 0.1-0.19 0.20-0.29	≥60 ≥50 ≥0.30	• Requires multiple measurements • Technically challenging • Time consuming
Qualitative Doppler Parameters				
Jet density	Faint	Dense	Dense	• Overlap between moderate and severe AR
Regurgitant slope (m/s^2) Pressure half-time (ms)	Slow >500	≥2 200-500	≥3 <200	• Effected by aortic and LV compliance • May be less accurate if beam is not oriented with jet
Diastolic flow reversal	Brief, early diastolic reversal	Intermediate	Prominent holodiastolic reversal	• Brief reversal is normal. • May be present in stiff aorta (in the absence of severe AR)

AR, aortic regurgitation; ERO, effective regurgitant orifice; LV, left ventricular; LVOT, left ventricular outflow tract; RF, regurgitant fraction; RVol, regurgitant volume; VC, vena contracta.
[a]Quantitative parameters allow for subclassification of moderate regurgitation into mild-to-moderate and moderate-to-severe AR.
[b]Performed at a Nyquist limit of 50-70 cm/s.

TABLE E.2 Grading Severity of Aortic Stenosis

	Aortic Sclerosis	Mild	Moderate	Severe
Peak velocity (m/s)	≤2.5	2.6-2.9	3.0-4.0	≥4.0
Mean gradient (mm Hg)		<20	20-40	≥40
AV area (cm^2)		>1.5	1.0-1.5	<1.0
AV area index (cm^2/m^2)		>0.85	0.60-0.85	<0.6
Velocity ratio		>0.50	0.25-0.50	<0.25

AV, aortic valve.
Adapted from Baumgartner H, Hung J, Bermejo J, et al. Recommendations on the echocardiographic assessment of aortic valve stenosis: a focused update from the European Association of Cardiovascular Imaging and the American Society of Echocardiography. *J Am Soc Echocardiogr*. 2017;30(4):372-392.

TABLE E.3 Summary of Assessment Methods to Grade Severity of Mitral Regurgitation

			Severity		
Modality	**Method**	**Type of Assessment**	**Mild**	**Moderate**	**Severe**
2D	Leaflet motion	Qualitative	Normal or abnormal		Flail or restricted
	Leaflet morphology	Qualitative	Normal or abnormal		Typically abnormal leaflets
	Coaptation defect	Qualitative	Absent		Presence of coaptation defect
	Mobile echodensity	Qualitative	Important but not associated directly with severity		
	LA size	Qualitative	Normal	Normal/enlarged	Enlarged
Color flow Doppler	Vena contracta width	Semiquantitative	<3 mm	3-6 mm	≥7 mm (or >8 for biplane)
	Flow convergence zone	Qualitative	None or small	Intermediate	Large
	Flow convergence radius	Quantitative (used for PISA)	(Adjust Nyquist in the direction of jet and measure parallel to the ultrasound beam)		
	Color flow jet size/shape	Qualitative	Small and central	Intermediate	Very large or eccentric with Coanda effect
Continuous-wave Doppler	MR jet density	Qualitative	Faint	Dense	
	MR jet profile	Qualitative	Parabolic		Triangular
	Peak velocity	Quantitative	(Measurement used for PISA calculation)		
Pulsed-wave Doppler	MV inflow pattern	Semiquantitative	E<A	E>A	E>>A
	MV inflow peak velocity	Semiquantitative	<1 m/s	Variable	≥1.2 m/s
	Pulmonary vein flow	Semiquantitative	Systolic dominant	Systolic blunting	Systolic flow reversal
	VTI_{mitral}/VTI_{LVOT}	Semiquantitative	<1	1-1.4	>1.4
3D	Annulus size	Semiquantitative	Annulus should have 4:3 ratio and is dilated when approaching 1:1 ratio.		
3D CFD	Vena contracta area	Quantitative	>0.2 cm^2	0.2-0.4 cm^2	≥0.4 cm^2
Multimodality	PISA PISA = $(2 \times \pi \times r^2 \times V_{alias})/V_{max}$	Quantitative	>0.2 cm^2	0.2-0.4 cm^2	≥0.4 cm^2
	Regurgitant volume[b]	Quantitative	<30 mL	30-44 mL[a] 44-59 mL[a]	≥60 mL
	Regurgitant fraction[b]	Quantitative	<30%	30-39 mL[a] 40-49 mL[a]	≥50%

CFD, color flow Doppler; CWD, continuous-wave Doppler; EROA, effective regurgitant orifice area; LA, left atrium; LVOT SV, left ventricular outflow tract stroke volume; MR, mitral regurgitation; MV, mitral valve; PISA, proximal isovelocity surface area; VTI, velocity-time integral.

[a]Guidelines subcategorize moderate MR into mild-to-moderate MR and moderate-to-severe MR based on the subgrouping indicated, respectively.

[b]This could be performed using 3D volumetric analysis to determine the total volume change and subtract forward flow via LVOT stroke volume to determine regurgitant volume and fraction. Or the EROA combined with MR VTI (CWD) can be used to determine MR flow and then compare to 3D volumes or LVOT SV calculation to determine regurgitant volume and fraction.

TABLE E.4 Mitral Stenosis Grading

	Progressive		
	Mild	**Moderate**	**Severe**
Valve area (cm^2)	>2.5	2.5-1.6	≤1.5
Pressure half-time (milliseconds)	<100	100-149	≥150
Mean gradient (mmHg)*	<5	5-9	≥10
Systolic pulmonary artery pressure (mmHg)	<30	30-49	≥50

*At a heart rate of 60-80 beats per minute.
Adapted from Pandian NG, Kim JK, Arias-Godinez JA, et al. Recommendations for the use of echocardiography in the evaluation of rheumatic heart disease: a report from the American Society of Echocardiography. *J Am Soc Echocardiogr*. 2023;36(1):3-28, with permission from Elsevier.

TABLE E.5 Grading the Severity of Chronic Tricuspid Regurgitation by Echocardiography

	Mild	**Moderate**	**Severe**		
■ **Structural**					
TV morphology	**Normal or mildly abnormal leaflets**	Moderately abnormal leaflets	**Severe valve lesions** (eg, flail leaflet, severe retraction, large perforation)		
RV and RA size	Normal	Normal/mild dilation	Usually dilated[a]		
IVC diameter	Normal, <2 cm	Normal to mildly dilated, 2.1-2.5 cm	Dilated, >2.5 cm		
■ **Qualitative Doppler**					
Color flow jet area[b]	**Small, narrow, central**	Moderate central	**Large central jet** or eccentric wall-impinging jet of variable size		
Flow convergence zone	**Not visible, transient or small**	Intermediate in size and duration	**Large throughout systole**		
CWD jet	**Faint/partial/** parabolic	Dense, parabolic, or triangular	Dense, often triangular		
■ **Semiquantitative**					
Color flow jet area (cm^2)[b]	Not defined	Not defined	>**10**		
VCW (cm)[b]	<0.3	0.3-0.69	Severe	Massive	Torrential
			0.7-1.3	1.4-2.0	≥2.1
PISA radius (cm)[c]	≤0.5	0.6-0.9	>**0.9**		
Hepatic vein flow[d]	Systolic dominance	Systolic blunting	**Systolic flow reversal**		
Tricuspid inflow[d]	**A-wave dominant**	Variable	E wave, >1.0 m/s		
■ **Quantitative**					
EROA (cm^2)	<0.20	0.20-0.39[e]	Severe	Massive	Torrential
			0.40-0.59	0.60-0.79	≥0.80
RVol (mL/beat)	<30	30-44[e]	≥45		
3D VCA or quantitative EROA[f] (cm^2)			Severe	Massive	Torrential
			0.75-0.94	0.95-1.14	≥1.15

Bolded signs are considered specific for their tricuspid regurgitation grade.
2D, two-dimensional; 3D, three-dimensional; CWD, continuous-wave Doppler; EROA, effective regurgitant orifice area; IVC, inferior vena cava; PISA, proximal isovelocity surface area; RA, right atrium; RV, right ventricle; RVol, regurgitant volume; TV, tricuspid valve; VCA, vena contracta area; VCW, vena contracta width.
[a]RV and RA size can be within normal range in patients with acute severe tricuspid regurgitation.
[b]With Nyquist limit of greater than 50 to 70 cm/s.
[c]With baseline Nyquist limit shift of 28 cm/s.
[d]Signs are nonspecific and are influenced by many other factors (RV diastolic function, atrial fibrillation, RA pressure).
[e]There are little data to support further separation of these values.
[f]3D VCA and quantitative Doppler EROA cutoffs may be larger than PISA EROA.
Adapted from Zoghbi WA, Adams D, Bonow RO, et al. Recommendations for noninvasive evaluation of native valvular regurgitation: a report from the American Society of echocardiography developed in collaboration with the society for cardiovascular magnetic resonance. *J Am Soc Echocardiogr*. 2017;30(4):303-371; Davidson LJ, Tang GHL, Ho EC, et al. The tricuspid valve: a review of pathology, imaging, and current treatment options: a scientific statement from the American Heart Association. *Circulation*. 2024;149(22):e1223-e1238.

TABLE E.6 Findings Indicative of Hemodynamically Significant Tricuspid Stenosis

■ **Specific findings**	
Mean pressure gradient	≥5 mm Hg
Inflow time–velocity integral	>60 cm
T½	≥190 ms
Valve area by continuity equation	≤1 cm^2
■ **Supportive findings**	
Enlarged right atrium ≥ moderate	
Dilated inferior vena cava	

Adapted from Baumgartner H, Hung J, Bermejo J, et al. Echocardiographic assessment of valve stenosis: EAE/ASE recommendations for clinical practice. *J Am Soc Echocardiogr*. 2009;22:1-23.

TABLE E.7 Grading the Severity of Pulmonic Regurgitation by Echocardiography

	Mild	**Moderate**	**Severe**
■ **Structural**			
PV morphology	Normal	Normal or abnormal	Abnormal
RV size	Normal[a]	Normal or dilated	Dilated[b]
Jet size, color Doppler[c]	Thin (usually <10 mm in length) with a narrow origin	Intermediate	Broad origin; variable depth of penetration
Ratio of PR jet width/ pulmonary annulus			>0.7 cm[d]
Jet density and contour (CWD)	Soft	Dense	Dense; early termination of diastolic flow
Deceleration time of the PR spectral Doppler signal			Short, <260 ms
Pressure half-time of PR jet			<100 ms[f]
PR index[e]		<0.77	<0.77
Diastolic flow reversal in the main or branch of PA (PWD)			Prominent
Pulmonic systolic flow (VTI) compared to systemic flow (LVOT VTI) by PWD[g]	Slightly increased	Intermediate	Greatly increased
RF[h]	<20%	20%-40%	>40%

CMR, cardiovascular magnetic resonance; CWD, continuous-wave Doppler; LVOT, left ventricular outflow tract; PA, pulmonary artery; PR, pulmonic regurgitation; PV, pulmonic valve; PWD, pulsed-wave Doppler; RF, regurgitation fraction; RV, right ventricle; RVol, regurgitant volume; VTI, velocity-time integral.

[a]Unless there are other reasons for RV enlargement.

[b]Exception: acute PR.

[c]At a Nyquist limit of 50-70 cm/s.

[d]Identifies a CMR-derived PR fraction ≥40%.

[e]Defined as the duration of the PR signal divided by the total duration of diastole, with this cutoff identifying a CMR-derived PR fraction >25%.

[f]Not reliable in the presence of high RV end-diastolic pressure.

[g]Cutoff values for RVol and fraction are not well validated.

[h]RF data primarily derived from CMR with limited application with echocardiography.

Adapted from Zoghbi WA, Adams D, Bonow RO, et al. Recommendations for noninvasive evaluation of native valvular regurgitation: a report from the American Society of Echocardiography developed in collaboration with the Society for Cardiovascular Magnetic Resonance. *J Am Soc Echocardiogr*. 2017;30(4):303-371.

TABLE E.8 Grading Severity of Pulmonary Stenosis

	Mild	Moderate	Severe
Peak velocity (m/s)	<3	3-4	>4
Peak gradient (mm Hg)	<36	36-64	>64

Adapted from Baumgartner H, Hung J, Bermejo J, et al. Echocardiographic assessment of valve stenosis: EAE/ASE recommendations for clinical practice. *J Am Soc Echocardiogr*. 2009;22:1-23.

Index

Note: Page numbers followed by *f* and *t* indicate figure and table respectively.

B

D

E

N

O

P

U

V

W

Z